Roach's Introductory Clinical Pharmacology

Roach's Introductory Clinical Pharmacology

SUSAN M. FORD, MN, RN, CNE
Adjunct Nursing Faculty
Bates Technical College
Tacoma, Washington

SALLY S. ROACH, MSN, RN, CNE
Associate Professor
University of Texas
Brownsville, Texas

EDITION 10

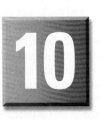

. Wolters Kluwer | Lippincott Williams & Wilkins
Health
Philadelphia · Baltimore · New York · London
Buenos Aires · Hong Kong · Sydney · Tokyo

Executive Editor: Christopher Richardson
Senior Product Manager: Amy Millholen
Developmental Editor: Robin Levin Richman
Production Product Manager: Marian Bellus
Design Coordinator: Stephen Druding
Senior Marketing Manager: Dean Karampelas
Compositor: Aptara, Inc.
Printer: C & C

10th Edition

Library of Congress Cataloging-in-Publication Data

Ford, Susan M.
    Roachs introductory clinical pharmacology / Susan M. Ford, Sally S. Roach.—10th ed.
        p. ; cm.
    Includes index.
    ISBN 978-1-4511-8671-0
    I. Roach, Sally S.   II. Title.   III. Title: Introductory clinical pharmacology.
    [DNLM: 1. Pharmacological Phenomena—Nurses' Instruction.   2. Drug Therapy—Nurses' Instruction.
3. Pharmaceutical Preparations—administration & dosage—Nurses' Instruction.   4. Pharmacology, Clinical—methods—Nurses' Instruction. QV 37]

    RM301.28
    615.5′8—dc23

                                                                                                2013016037

Care has been taken to confirm the accuracy of the information presented and to describe generally accepted practices. However, the authors, editors, and publisher are not responsible for errors or omissions or for any consequences from application of the information in this book and make no warranty, express or implied, with respect to the content of the publication. The authors, editors, and publisher have exerted every effort to ensure that drug selection and dosage set forth in this text are in accordance with the current recommendations and practice at the time of publication. However, in view of ongoing research, changes in government regulations, and the constant flow of information relating to drug therapy and drug reactions, the reader is urged to check the package insert for each drug for any change in indications and dosage and for added warnings and precautions. This is particularly important when the recommended agent is a new or infrequently employed drug. Some drugs and medical devices presented in this publication have Food and Drug Administration (FDA) clearance for limited use in restricted research settings. It is the responsibility of the health care provider to ascertain the FDA status of each drug or device planned for use in his or her clinical practice.

LWW.com

Reviewers

Preface

Why This Book?

Roach's Introductory Clinical Pharmacology is one in a series of textbooks designed for the Licensed Practical/Vocational Nurse (LPN/LVN). As a front-line provider you are often times the first person to interact with a patient in the health care system. This textbook is designed to provide learners with a clear, concise introduction to pharmacology. The ease in reading lets you gain practical information on how to approach the patient about the drugs being prescribed. The basic explanations presented in this text are *not* intended to suggest that pharmacology is an easy subject. As we know it, drug therapy is one of the most important and complicated treatment modalities in modern health care.

As a novice provider, this book gives you the introduction you need to begin gaining knowledge about drugs and medication management. The learner may find that certain drugs or drug dosages available when this textbook went to publication may no longer be available. Likewise, there may be new drugs on the market that were not approved by the U.S. Food and Drug Administration (FDA) at the time of publication. With the availability of computers, smart phones, and Internet resources, current information is always there for verification of any drug question and should be checked when you do have a question before administering a drug. Don't forget that your colleagues, clinical pharmacists, and primary health care providers are also resources for information concerning a specific drug, including dosage, adverse reactions, contraindications, precautions, interactions, or administration.

What's New in This Edition?

The tenth edition of *Roach's Introductory Clinical Pharmacology* reflects the ever-changing science of pharmacology and the nurse's responsibilities in administering pharmacologic agents. Content is arranged to help the learner connect concepts and information. **Key terms** and **drug class lists** are now easily accessible at the beginning of every chapter. A **new chapter (47)** adds to your understanding about the drugs used to deal with the changes of aging on the urinary and reproductive systems. Every chapter begins with a **case study** to help you connect people to the drugs they take.

Key Themes in the New Edition

Mathematics and Prevention of Medication Errors

Chapter improvements are designed to support your learning of pharmacologic concepts. **Chapter 3** provides you with ways to look at medication calculation using principles of safe practical information rather than mathematical formulas used in traditional math classes. You are guided through the chapter on the basics such as name, dose, and drug strength, then shown how to apply these elements in calculating medication doses from pill to liquid form. Learning focuses on reducing medication errors that result from mathematical mistakes rather than on the traditional arithmetic exercises. Up to seven dosage calculations for each chapter are provided when the textbook is used with the accompanying Study Guide. Should you wish to review math and less frequently used calculations, they are provided in Appendix F.

Communication Among Patients, Family, and Health Care Providers

Health literacy and communication are key components in **Chapter 5**. The patient–provider relationship has changed; patients are assuming a greater role and responsibility in their health care. Providers need to know the importance of good communication, health literacy, and cultural competence to practice patient-centered care. Your ability to use outcome strategies and communicate what you do to **support patient and family confidence** in learning self-management skills of medication administration is highlighted in patient teaching information.

Simple, Logical Drug Classification

Pharmacologic concepts are made easy and practical in the drug chapters, too. In Unit II, learning the different types of antibacterial drugs can be challenging. In this edition we have simplified the task by **grouping the drugs according to what they do to a bacterial cell**. This presentation helps in understanding how the different classes are similar and what to look for in terms of similar actions or adverse reactions. Unit III has a greater emphasis on teaching you **pain assessment strategies** as well as the drugs for pain relief. One of the main categories of drugs to treat **Alzheimer's disease**, the **cholinesterase inhibitors**, was moved to Unit IV and is now grouped with other drugs that affect the central nervous system. Lastly, diuretics work in the urinary system primarily to treat diseases like hypertension, so the chapter on **diuretics with cardiovascular system drugs** now appears in Unit VIII.

What Makes This Book Unique?

The unique feature of this book is **drug therapy from a nursing perspective**. Publishers give you many choices of textbooks offering information on drug action and activity. This text is written *by* nurses *for* nurses in easy-to-read language and is designed to teach you not only about the drugs but also how to relay this information to patients. The more you understand the drugs and their effects on the human body, the better you can help your patients understand and deal with the drugs they are taking. The **nursing process** uses a step-by-step method to show how medications are used in the care of patients. Elements of the nursing process—assessment, analysis, planning, intervention, and evaluation—show you basic and practical nursing skills to help people understand the treatment, to meet their health care needs, and to improve adherence to treatment, all designed for better patient outcomes.

This textbook is written by authors bringing well over 30 years of nursing experience each from working in mental health settings, acute care hospitals, operating rooms, ambulatory clinics, home health, and hospice settings, as well as holding nursing certification in areas such as oncology, holistic nursing, and medical surgical clinical nurse specialist. As certified nurse educators (CNEs) and from experiences of teaching at vocational, associate degree, and baccalaureate nursing programs, the authors understand how to design and communicate learning in a way that will maximize your knowledge of pharmacology.

User's Guide

Unit Structure and Organization

Learners are more successful when they know *how* to use the textbook as well as what is in the textbook. Here are some quick tips on how to use your textbook more effectively. Thirteen units offer 54 chapters providing information in learnable segments that are not overwhelming to the learner. Organization of the text in this manner allows you to move about the book easily when these areas are covered in your program curriculum.

The book starts with the basic fundamentals of drug therapy. Then units about infection and pain, followed by units about drugs related to different body systems. These units are written in a head-to-toe sequence, making the specific drugs easier to find.

Learning about drug therapy is easier when you can connect the information with life-like clinical experiences. In Chapter 5 you will be introduced to a group of clients in the clinic setting. Their stories establish for you a context in which to begin learning about the selected drugs and their real-world application.

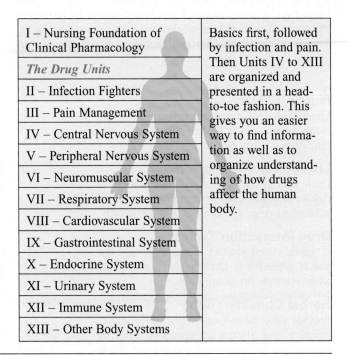

I – Nursing Foundation of Clinical Pharmacology	Basics first, followed by infection and pain. Then Units IV to XIII are organized and presented in a head-to-toe fashion. This gives you an easier way to find information as well as to organize understanding of how drugs affect the human body.
The Drug Units	
II – Infection Fighters	
III – Pain Management	
IV – Central Nervous System	
V – Peripheral Nervous System	
VI – Neuromuscular System	
VII – Respiratory System	
VIII – Cardiovascular System	
IX – Gastrointestinal System	
X – Endocrine System	
XI – Urinary System	
XII – Immune System	
XIII – Other Body Systems	

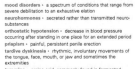

22

Antidepressant Drugs

LEARNING OBJECTIVES

On completion of this chapter, the student will:

1. Define depression and identify symptoms of a major depressive episode.
2. Name the different types of antidepressant drugs.
3. Discuss the uses, general drug actions, general adverse reactions, contraindications, precautions, and interactions of the antidepressant drugs.
4. Discuss important preadministration and ongoing assessment activities that the nurse should perform on the patient taking an antidepressant drug.
5. List nursing diagnoses particular to a patient taking an antidepressant drug.
6. Discuss ways to promote an optimal response to therapy, how to manage common adverse reactions, and important points to keep in mind when educating patients about the use of antidepressant drugs.

KEY TERMS

bipolar disorder • a mood disorder characterized by severe swings from extreme hyperactivity to depression
dysphoric • characterized by extreme or exaggerated sadness, anxiety, or unhappiness
endogenous • pertaining to something that normally occurs or is produced within the organism

mood disorders • a spectrum of conditions that range from severe debilitation to an exhaustive elation
neurohormones • secreted rather than transmitted neuro-substances
orthostatic hypotension • decrease in blood pressure occurring after standing in one place for an extended period
priapism • painful, persistent penile erection
tardive dyskinesia • rhythmic, involuntary movements of the tongue, face, mouth, or jaw and sometimes the extremities
tyramine • amino acid, commonly found in fermented foods such as cheese and red wine
unipolar depression • mental disorder of low mood, low self-esteem, and loss of interest/pleasure; also known as major mood disorder

DRUG CLASSES

Selective serotonin reuptake inhibitors (SSRIs)
Serotonin/norepinephrine or dopamine/norepinephrine

reuptake inhibitors (SNRIs or DNRIs)
Tricyclic antidepressants (TCAs)
Monoamine oxidase inhibitors (MAOIs)

PHARMACOLOGY IN PRACTICE

Mr. Phillip has been severely depressed for about 2 months, following the death of his wife in a car accident. One week ago, the primary care provider prescribed Zoloft 100 mg orally daily. His family is concerned because he is still depressed. Mr. Phillip's daughter is concerned because he feels drowsy and can't seem to get up until 11 a.m. or noon on most days. They are requesting that the dosage be increased. Read about the antidepressants and determine what should happen next.

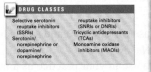

Beginning of the Chapter

The chapter opening page is designed to guide you, the learner, in organizing your study routine as you learn the essential elements of drug therapy in each chapter.

Learning Objectives

These define what you will learn in a specific chapter. Review the objectives first to help you understand what you need to learn after reading the chapter.

Key Terms

With accompanying definitions, the Key Terms help you build your vocabulary. Look for **bold type** in the text at first mention of the word in the chapter to remind you of the definition.

Drug Classes

This gives you a sense of how drugs are grouped according to like properties. Learning these groupings helps you identify potential errors and safety concerns.

Pharmacology in Practice

Each chapter features a case study about an individual dealing with an issue related to drugs featured in the chapter. Scenarios focus on assessment, administration, or teaching issues that have an impact on real-life patients. Their stories help you to focus your attention on the concepts important to patient care.

Drug Information

Consistent Framework

Each chapter presents the drugs in such a way that you learn to recognize and respond to patient questions quickly and accurately. Illustrated concepts guide you as each chapter features information about the drug class in a logical and sequential order as **Action, Uses, and Adverse Reactions**—the concepts you, the nurse, deal with on a consistent basis. This is followed by **Contraindications, Precautions, and**

Interactions—all items typically reviewed earlier and considered by other health providers, yet at the same time important for you to know to provide safe drug administration to your patients.

Special Features

Special features are sprinkled throughout the text to direct you to priority information about the drugs or individuals who will receive the drugs.

Nursing Alerts

Quickly identify urgent nursing actions in the management of the patient receiving a specific drug or drug category.

Lifespan Considerations

Draw your attention to specific populations at risk or needing specific administration considerations (e.g., gerontology and pediatric).

Drug Interaction Tables

A quick visual scan of these tables can tell you if a patient is likely to have a problem when multiple drugs are given.

Herbal Considerations

Provide information on herbs and complementary and alternative remedies used by patients under your care. Additional information is provided in Appendix D where examples of a number of natural products are provided.

> **! NURSING ALERT**
> After administering penicillin IM in the outpatient setting, ask the patient to wait in the area for at least 30 minutes. Anaphylactic reactions are most likely to occur within 30 minutes after injection.

> **LIFESPAN CONSIDERATIONS**
> **Gerontology**
> Older adults who are debilitated, chronically ill, or taking oral antibiotics for an extended period are more likely to develop a superinfection.

Interacting Drug	Common Use	Effect of Interaction
cimetidine	Decrease gastric secretions	Increased effectiveness of the 5-HT agonist
oral contraceptives	Birth control	Increased effectiveness of the 5-HT agonist

> **HERBAL CONSIDERATIONS**
> Ephedra (Ma Huang) and the many substances of the *Ephedra* genus have been used medicinally (e.g., *E. sinica* and *E. intermedia*). Ephedra (ephedrine) preparations

Nursing Process and Drug Therapy

Uniquely presented, nursing actions regarding drug information are provided in the context of a nurse's clinical practice. The nursing process is featured as a practical guide to connect patients and drug therapy.

ASSESSMENT	Here are the questions to ask for the information needed both before and during drug therapy.
ANALYSIS AND PLANNING	Offering suggestions on how people may respond to specific drugs or drug therapy.
IMPLEMENTATION	**Promoting an Optimal Response** Gives you specific information to use for effective and safe administration. **Monitoring and Managing Patient Needs** Gives you a number of strategies to use in your practice as a nurse to help patients deal with the drugs they are taking. **Educating the Patient and Family** LPN/LVNs are the first and often primary contacts in many clinics and offices. You will be the one to teach and provide information to patients and families about the drugs. Here are practical tools and methods to help you work with people to be sure they are taking medications correctly and watching for signs and symptoms.
EVALUATION	Bulleted lists highlight important measures and help you decide whether the strategies you use provide the best outcomes while building confidence in your patient's abilities to adhere to medication plans.

End of the Chapter

Here is where you determine what you have learned from reading each chapter. Information is summarized in an easy-to-read format, giving you the opportunity to demonstrate what you learned by applying information in the chapter case study. Once you review the chapter, use the review questions to demonstrate your skill as you would when you take the NCLEX-PN examination.

Pharmacology in Practice: Think Critically

Each chapter ends with a return to the case study patient. Realistic patient care situations help learners apply the material contained in the chapter by exploring options and making clinical judgments related to the administration of drugs. The case histories of seven patients are used, and different aspects of care are presented in different chapters like puzzle pieces, making connections for learners to appreciate the complex issues in providing care to both individuals and families.

Key Points

Key points are summarized and the important concepts of the chapter are listed to help you determine if you have mastered the learning objectives.

Summary Drug Tables

Conveniently placed, these tables provide a list of drugs from the classes discussed in each chapter. Names, uses, frequent adverse reactions, and general dosing information are given in an accessible format.

PHARMACOLOGY IN PRACTICE
THINK CRITICALLY

Lillian's first visit to the clinic was a year ago. Her blood pressure was 156/98 and lab work drawn that day was cholesterol = 320, LDL = 178, HDL = 20.

The following information from her medical record today shows that T = 98.6°F, P = 104, R = 18, and BP = 136/92. Lab work drawn had the following values: cholesterol = 256, LDL = 160, HDL = 36.

How can you use this information to help encourage Mrs. Chase to continue her medication? What information would you give the patient concerning her constipation?

KEY POINTS

- Atherosclerosis is a disorder in which lipid deposits accumulate on the lining of blood vessels. Cholesterol and triglycerides are two lipids in our blood; elevation of one or both is termed hyperlipidemia.
- Antihyperlipidemic drugs decrease cholesterol and triglycerides in the blood. When included with lifestyle changes such as diet modifications, physical activity, smoking cessation, and weight management, the risk of coronary heart disease is lessened.
- HMG-CoA reductase inhibitors are frequently called "statin" drugs. These drugs lower the blood level of LDL

cholesterol and triglycerides. Bile acid resins and fibric acid derivatives act in a similar manner to reduce cholesterol by binding with bile so the liver will use more, putting less in the system.

- Common adverse reactions include headache, dizziness, insomnia, and GI complaints such as increased flatulence and constipation. Patients taking bile acid resins need to be alert for bleeding tendencies. Those taking niacin have experienced a sensation of warmth, flushing, and itching; a reduction in dose diminishes the reactions.

Summary Drug Table ANTIHYPERLIPIDEMIC DRUGS

Generic Name	Trade Name	Uses	Adverse Reactions	Dosage Ranges
HMG-CoA Reductase Inhibitors (Statins)				
atorvastatin *ah-tor'-vah-stah'-tin*	Lipitor	Reduce risk of coronary heart disease (CHD) events, hyperlipidemia, familial hypercholesterolemia	Headache, diarrhea, sinusitis	10–80 mg/day orally
fluvastatin *floo-vah-stah'-tin*	Lescol	Atherosclerosis, hyperlipidemia, familial hypercholesterolemia	Headache, back pain, upper respiratory infection, flu-like syndrome	20–80 mg/day orally
lovastatin *loe-vah-stah'-tin*	Mevacor, Altoprev	Reduce risk of CHD events, atherosclerosis, hyperlipidemia, familial hypercholesterolemia	Headache, flatulence, infection	10–80 mg/day orally in single or divided doses Adolescents: 10–40 mg/day orally

(table continues on page 364)

Chapter Review

● Chapter Review
Know Your Drugs

Clients sometimes know a medication by the brand (or trade) name and not the generic name. To help you recognize both names, match the brand name with the generic name of the same medication.

Generic Name	Brand Name
1. carvedilol	A. Cardura
2. clonidine	B. Catapres
3. doxazosin	C. Coreg
4. nadolol	D. Corgard

Calculate Medication Dosages

1. A client in long-term care is ordered 50 mg of atenolol. The drug bubble pack card comes in 25-mg tablets per dose. How many tablets does the nurse remove from the bubble pack card?

2. The physician orders 0.4 mg of tamsulosin (Flomax) daily before breakfast. The drug is available in 0.4-mg capsules. The nurse instructs the client to take _____.

● Prepare for the NCLEX®
Build Your Knowledge

1. Antiadrenergic drugs block which of the following transmitters?
   1. serotonin
   2. norepinephrine
   3. dopamine
   4. acetylcholine

2. A client is to receive a β-adrenergic drug for hypertension. Before the drug is administered, the most important assessment the nurse performs is _____.
   1. weighing the client
   2. obtaining blood for laboratory tests
   3. taking a past medical history
   4. taking the blood pressure on both arms

3. When an adrenergic blocking drug is given for a life-threatening cardiac arrhythmia, which of the following activities would the nurse expect to be a part of client care?
   1. daily electrocardiograms
   2. fluid restriction to 1000 mL/day
   3. daily weights
   4. cardiac monitoring

4. To prevent complications when administering a β-adrenergic blocking drug to an elderly client, the nurse would be particularly alert for _____.
   1. vascular insufficiency (e.g., weak peripheral pulses and cold extremities)
   2. complaints of an occipital headache
   3. insomnia
   4. hypoglycemia

5. The client with glaucoma will likely receive a(n) _____.
   1. α/β-adrenergic blocking drug
   2. α-adrenergic blocking drug
   3. β-adrenergic blocking drug
   4. antiadrenergic drug

Apply Your Knowledge

6. When norepinephrine is blocked in the sympathetic nervous system, which of the following occurs?
   1. heart rate increase
   2. blood pressure lowers
   3. GI system slows
   4. bronchi constrict

7. Mr. Garcia was seen with a blood pressure of 210/120 and has taken one dose of metoprolol and returned for a blood pressure reading. Which of the following blood pressures should be reported to the primary health care provider immediately?
   1. 150/100
   2. 200/100
   3. 250/130
   4. 170/80

Alternate-Format Questions

8. The primary health care provider prescribes 60 mg propranolol to be given via the GI tube. The drug is available in an oral solution of 5 mg/mL. The nurse uses a total of 30 mL of warm water to flush before and after administering the drug. The total volume of fluid for this procedure was:
   1. 35 mL of water and drug solution
   2. 42 mL of water and drug solution
   3. 65 mL of water and drug solution
   4. 72 mL of water and drug solution

9. Select the terms that describe drugs that block the sympathetic branch of the ANS. **Select all that apply.**
   1. sympathomimetic
   2. sympatholytic
   3. antiadrenergic
   4. anticholinergic

10. A client has just had a dose increase to 12.5 mg of carvedilol. The client has a bottle with 3.125-mg tablets and insists on finishing the bottle before buying a different strength. The nurse tells the client to take_____.

To check your answers, see Appendix G.

thePoint *For more NCLEX-style questions, log on to http://thepoint.lww.com to access more than 1000 questions.*

Chapter Review

Know Your Drugs

Use the matching exercise to identify drug names and connect generic with brand names to help you recognize the potential for and prevention against using the wrong drug.

Calculate Medication Dosages

Practice the math skills to learn accurate drug dosing and recognize the potential for error, thus ensuring that you give the correct dose.

Prepare for the NCLEX®

Here questions allow you to test your knowledge of the material.

Build Your Knowledge – information and fact-based questions are presented to get you "warmed up" to apply what you've learned.

Apply **Your Knowledge** – keyed to the actual 2011 NCLEX-PN test plan (see examples in Appendix H), these application and analysis questions about concepts in the chapter help you apply what you've learned as well as prepare for the NCLEX-PN examination.

Alternate-Format Questions – provide you experience in applying what you've learned in a different manner.

Special Features

Questions are structured like the NCLEX examination. The design helps you become familiar with the language and format of NCLEX testing.

Patient or Client

In this section of each chapter, you see wording change from "patient" to "client." This is specifically designed because often you are taught using the terms *patient, resident, consumer,* or *client.* The ability to recognize the interchange of words helps you to adapt to testing format.

Numbered (1, 2, 3, 4) Distractors

The NCLEX provides a single question on a computer screen. The options you are given are listed as numbers. Distracter options in these questions are labeled 1, 2, 3, 4 instead of A, B, C, D—again, to simulate the NCLEX-PN examination.

Teaching/Learning Package

Resources for the Learner
Online Student Resources

Learning goes where you go! Free access to all your LWW resources at thePoint, at http://thepoint.lww.com/Ford10e Student resources on thePoint include eBook, NCLEX alternative-format tutorial, more than 1,000 NCLEX-style questions in an easy and accessible form, watch & learn videos, concepts in action animation 3-D depictions of pharmacology concepts, a Spanish-English audio glossary, and monographs of the 100 most commonly prescribed drugs.

Study Guide to Accompany Roach's Introductory Clinical Pharmacology, 10th Edition

Completely revised – offering exercises, puzzles, and the same seven patients as the textbook in real-life case studies connected to situations in the textbook.

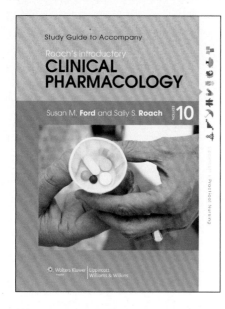

✓ PrepU

Practice makes perfect. And this is the perfect practice.
PrepU is an adaptive learning system designed to improve students' competency mastery and provide instructors with real-time analysis of their students' knowledge at both a class and individual student level.

PrepU demonstrates **formative assessment**—it determines what students know *as* they are learning and focuses them on what they are struggling with so they don't spend time on what they already know. Feedback is immediate and remediates students back to this specific text so they know where to go back to the text, read, and help understand a concept.

Adaptive and Personalized

No student has the same experience—PrepU recognizes when a student has reached "mastery" of a concept before moving the student on to higher levels of learning. This will be a different experience for each student based on the number of questions he or she answers and whether he or she answers them correctly. Each question is also "normed" by all students in PrepU around the country—how every student answers a specific question generates the difficulty level of each question in the system. This adaptive experience allows students to practice at their own pace and study much more effectively.

Personalized Reports

Students get individual feedback about their performance, and instructors can track class statistics to gauge the level of understanding. Both get a window into performance to help identify areas for remediation. Instructors can access the average mastery level of the class, students' strengths and weaknesses, and how often students use PrepU. Students can see their own progress charges and strengths and weaknesses—so they can continue quizzing in areas where they are weaker.

Mobile Optimized

Students can study anytime, anywhere with PrepU, as it is mobile optimized. More convenience equals more quizzing and more practice for students!

There is a PrepU resource available with this book! For more information, visit http://thepoint.lww.com/PrepU

Resources for the Instructor
thePoint

Classroom resources: PowerPoint presentations; Guided Lecture Notes; Discussion Topics; Assignments; Image Bank.

Even more NCLEX-style questions: this time presented within a test generator that allows you to create and edit your own exams.

Acknowledgments

Special thanks

To Sally S. Roach for trusting and believing in my efforts to continue the legacy of her book.

Dedication

To two very special women in my life, Sylvia Jones and Viola Oberholtzer. Sylvia is the first nurse I ever met, because she is my mother—and encouraged me to become a nurse, too. Aunt Vi (Viola O.), the person who told me to look at alternative routes to the Registered Nurse pathway, encouraging me to start at the community college and advance from there. Without the support of these two women in my life, I would not be authoring this book now.

Appreciation

To my extended family, friends, colleagues and students-turned-fellow nurses—thanks for being there with ideas and stories to share.

To my sister, Nancy Rauch, the high school math and science teacher—thanks for helping with application-based math.

To Bonnie, Pam, and Marion, the friends who kept my Beats Per Minute up as I worked on this project.

To my family–Jerry, Stephanie, Eric and Peter, you inspire me on a daily basis to be the best nurse possible.

Acknowledgments

To the team of people that make this book (and many others that you use) go from an idea to a bound copy. Amy Millholen–Senior Product Manager, a woman I feel privileged to have met in person; she kept me on task and motivated. Robin Levin Richman–Senior Developmental Editor, with her witty support and editorial assistance; she kept this book factual. Susan Caldwell–Medical Illustrator, made my case study patients come to life, along with her other drawings to improve this edition. Zack Shapiro–Editorial Assistant, he dealt with my e-mails, sent the resources I needed, and the first person I met face to face at LWW. Christopher Richardson–Executive Editor, for supporting the ideas I have that might not always make sense. To these people I offer a special word of thanks. My gratitude also goes to all those associated with Wolters Kluwer Health|Lippincott Williams & Wilkins who worked in any way on the design, production, and preparation of this book.

Contents

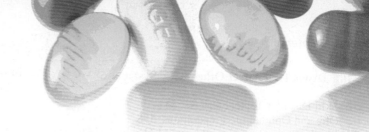

Nursing Foundation of Clinical Pharmacology

Unit I provides a foundation for understanding pharmacology in the context of nursing clinical practice. Three of the five chapters specifically discuss concepts focal to nursing: drug administration, nursing process, and patient teaching. The general principles of pharmacology and the mathematics involved in dosage calculation are concepts used by all providers involved with patients and medications and are included in their own chapters. This first unit of study is the foundation to build understanding of drug therapy in the subsequent units. Provided is a brief summary of the content in each chapter.

Basic principles are covered in Chapter 1, beginning with how drugs are derived from natural sources, such as plants, or made synthetically. Other concepts include how drug categories are based on the body system they influence or the way they are made chemically. Some drugs require a prescription (those given under the supervision of a licensed health care provider) or may be purchased as nonprescription (those obtained over the counter and designated as safe when taken as directed). When taken by a patient, drugs undergo a series of steps to be processed, utilized, and eliminated by the body—this is the basis for the study of pharmacology for health care providers.

Administration of a drug is primarily the responsibility of the nurse and is discussed in Chapter 2. Nurses have the duty to safely provide patient care by correctly administering the medication prescribed by the primary health care provider. This is achieved by learning and following the principles of drug administration, proper technique, and using medication systems correctly.

Your ability to correctly calculate mathematical problems is one of the most important steps in providing safe care to patients. Multiple steps in drug administration and delivery help to ensure accuracy in those math calculations. Chapter 3 provides both the opportunity to practice calculations and an overview of the tasks that you will undertake to be sure doses of drugs are correct before administration.

Most patients experience problems of anxiety or deficient knowledge regarding new medication routines. The nursing process is used to help members of the health care team provide effective patient care. This process is used to develop an individualized care and teaching plan for the patient. These concepts are covered in Chapter 4.

It is crucial that the patient understand the important information about the medication prescribed, including the dosage, how to take the medication, the expected

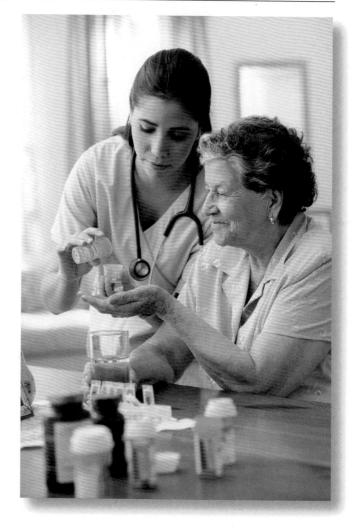

effect, and adverse reactions. In Chapter 5, components needed for successful patient teaching are described. Additionally, a group of individuals receiving nursing care in an ambulatory setting are introduced. Their stories are designed to help nurses understand how all this information is used in the nursing care of patients receiving drug therapy. You will learn how concepts are put into practice using case studies throughout the textbook.

By understanding the basic principles of pharmacology, you can build a sound knowledge base of the drugs used to help patients maintain their highest levels of wellness.

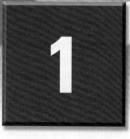

General Principles of Pharmacology

KEY TERMS

absorption • a drug is moved from site of administration to body fluids; first process during pharmacokinetics

adverse reaction • undesirable drug effect

allergic reaction • immediate hypersensitive reaction by the immune system; it presents as itching, hives, swelling, and difficulty breathing

anaphylactic shock • sudden, severe hypersensitivity reaction with symptoms that progress rapidly and may result in death if not treated; also called *anaphylactic reaction* or *anaphylactoid reaction*

angioedema • localized wheals or swellings in subcutaneous tissues or mucous membranes, which may be due to an allergic response; also called *angioneurotic edema*

controlled substances • drugs that have the potential for abuse and dependency, both physical and psychological

cumulative drug effect • when the body is unable to metabolize and excrete one dose of a drug before the next is given

distribution • drug moves from circulation to body tissue or a target site

drug idiosyncrasy • any unusual or abnormal response that differs from the response normally expected to a specific drug and dosage

drug tolerance • decreased response to a drug, requiring an increase in dosage to achieve the desired effect

excretion • elimination of a drug from the body

first-pass effect • action by which an oral drug is absorbed and carried directly to the liver, where it is inactivated by enzymes before it enters the general bloodstream

half-life • time required for the body to eliminate 50% of a drug

herbal medicine • type of complementary/alternative therapy that uses plants or herbs to treat various disorders; also called *herbalism*

hypersensitivity • undesirable reaction produced by a normal immune system

metabolism • drug is changed to a form that can be excreted

metabolite • inactive form of the original drug

nonprescription drugs • drugs that are designated by the U.S. Food and Drug Administration (FDA) to be safe (if taken as directed) and obtainable without a prescription; also called *over-the-counter* (OTC) drugs

pharmaceutic • pertaining to the phase during which a drug dissolves in the body

pharmacodynamics • study of the drug mechanisms that produce biochemical or physiologic changes in the body

pharmacokinetics • study of drug transit (or activity) after administration

physical dependency • habitual use of a drug, where negative physical withdrawal symptoms result from abrupt discontinuation

prescription drugs • drugs the federal government has designated as potentially harmful unless their use is supervised by a licensed health care provider, such as a nurse practitioner, physician, or dentist

psychological dependency • compulsion or craving to use a substance to obtain a pleasurable experience

receptor • *in pharmacology,* a reactive site on the surface of a cell; when a drug binds to and interacts with the receptor, a pharmacologic response occurs

teratogen • drug or substance that causes abnormal development of the fetus, leading to deformities

toxic • poisonous or harmful

Pharmacology is the study of drugs and their action on living organisms. A sound knowledge of basic pharmacologic principles is essential for nurses to administer medications safely and monitor patients who receive these medications. This chapter gives a basic overview of pharmacologic principles that you will need to understand when administering medications. The chapter also discusses drug development, federal legislation affecting the dispensing and use of drugs, and the use of **herbal medicines** as they relate to pharmacology.

Drugs have changed the way in which health care providers treat patients over the last century. In the early 1900s, individuals died of infections, from medical and surgical causes, due in part to lack of sanitary conditions and the fact that medicines to combat infection did not exist. The discovery of drug substances has changed an infection from being a death sentence into a deviation in health status. Additionally, patients lacking certain substances in their bodies, such as insulin, or diagnosed with cancerous tumors can now live long and productive lives due to drug therapy.

Medications are derived from natural sources, such as plants and minerals, or synthetically produced in a laboratory. Examples of natural sources include digitalis, which is an extract from the foxglove plant that acts as a potent heart medication. On the other hand, mipomersen is a chemically engineered drug being studied to target specific cell components in people with high cholesterol.

Drug Names

The first task in learning about drug therapy is to understand how drugs are named. Throughout the process of development, drugs may have several names assigned to them: a chemical name, a generic (nonproprietary, official) name, and a trade (or brand) name. These different names can be confusing. When you have a clear understanding of the different names used, you promote patient safety by reducing errors.

The chemical name is the scientific term that describes the molecular structure of a drug; it typically is the chemical components of the drug. The generic name is considered the official name of a drug and is the name given to a drug that can be made or marketed by any company; it is nonproprietary (meaning it is not owned by any specific agency). This name is typically written in smaller letters on a container. The generic name is the official name that is given a drug by the U.S. Food and Drug Administration (FDA). It also is the name found in the *National Formulary* or the *U.S. Pharmacopeia* for an approved drug.

When a drug name is followed by a trademark symbol ™ or a registered trademark symbol ®, this signifies that it is the trade or brand name. The trade name is selected by a specific company for marketing purposes. To avoid confusion, it is best to use the generic name. Table 1.1 identifies the various names and provides an explanation of each.

Drug Classes and Categories

A drug may be classified by the chemical type of the active ingredient or by the way it is used to treat a particular condition. Each drug can be classified into one or more drug classes. To help learn these classes a list will be included on each chapter's title page. For instance, in Unit II, drugs that retard or destroy pathogens are classified as anti-infectives. In each chapter, these drugs are further categorized by the way they work (such as antivirals) or their chemical structure (e.g., penicillins). Additionally, once a drug is approved for use, the FDA assigns it to one of the following categories: prescription, nonprescription, or controlled substance.

> **! NURSING ALERT**
>
> Study the patterns used in the naming of drugs. This may help you to identify names and prevent medication errors. Certain portions of the drug name may be similar in specific drug classes or categories. For example, beta (β)-adrenergic blocking drug names end with "lol." *Atenolol, metoprolol,* and *propranolol* are all antihypertensive drugs from the same category.

Table 1.1 Drug Names

Drug Name	Example	Explanation
Chemical name (scientific name)	Example: ethyl 4-(8-chloro-5, 6-dihydro-11*H*-benzo[5,6] cyclohepta[1,2-*b*]-pyridin-11-ylidene)-1-piperidinecarboxylate	Gives the exact chemical makeup of the drug and placing of the atoms or molecular structure; the chemical name is not capitalized.
Generic name (official or nonproprietary name)	Example: loratadine	Name given to a drug before it becomes official; may be used in all countries, by all manufacturers; the generic name is not capitalized.
Trade name (brand name)	Example: Claritin®	Name that is registered by the manufacturer and is followed by the trademark symbol; the name can be used only by the manufacturer; a drug may have several trade names, depending on the number of manufacturers; the first letter of the trade name is capitalized.

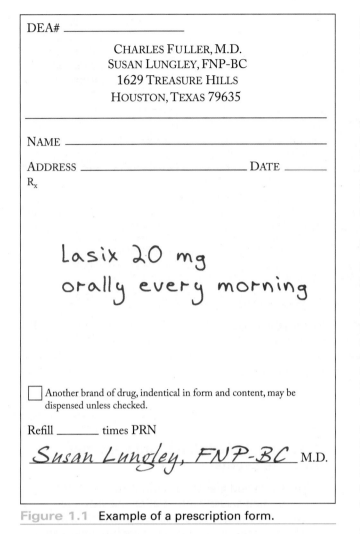

DEA# _____

CHARLES FULLER, M.D.
SUSAN LUNGLEY, FNP-BC
1629 TREASURE HILLS
HOUSTON, TEXAS 79635

NAME _____

ADDRESS _____ DATE _____

R$_x$

Lasix 20 mg
orally every morning

☐ Another brand of drug, indentical in form and content, may be dispensed unless checked.

Refill _____ times PRN

Susan Lungley, FNP-BC _____ M.D.

Figure 1.1 Example of a prescription form.

Prescription Drugs

Prescription drugs, also called *legend drugs,* are the largest category of drugs. Prescription drugs are prescribed by a licensed health care provider. The prescription (Fig. 1.1) contains the name of the drug, the dosage, the method and times of administration, and the signature of the licensed health care provider prescribing the drug.

Prescription drugs are designated by the federal government as potentially harmful unless their use is supervised by a licensed health care provider, such as a nurse practitioner, physician, or dentist. Supervision is important because, although these drugs have been tested for safety and therapeutic effect, prescription drugs may cause different reactions in some individuals.

In institutional settings, the nurse administers the drug and monitors the patient for therapeutic effect and **adverse reactions**. Some drugs have the potential to be **toxic** (harmful). You will play a critical role in evaluating the patient for toxic effects. When these drugs are prescribed to be taken at home, you will provide patient and family education about the drug.

Nonprescription Drugs

Nonprescription drugs are designated by the FDA as safe (when taken as directed) and can be obtained without a

prescription. These drugs are also referred to as over-the-counter (OTC) drugs and may be purchased in a variety of settings, such as a pharmacy, drugstore, or the local supermarket. Over-the-counter drugs include those given for symptoms of the common cold, minor aches and pains, constipation, diarrhea, and heartburn.

These drugs are not without risk and may produce adverse reactions. For example, acetylsalicylic acid, commonly known as aspirin, is potentially harmful and can cause gastrointestinal (GI) bleeding and salicylism (see Chapter 13). Labeling requirements give the consumer important information regarding the drug, dosage, contraindications, precautions, and adverse reactions. Consumers are urged to read the directions carefully before taking OTC drugs.

Controlled Substances

Controlled substances are the most carefully monitored of all drugs. These drugs have a high potential for abuse and may cause physical or psychological dependency. **Physical dependency** is the habitual use of a drug, in which negative physical withdrawal symptoms result from abrupt discontinuation; it is the body's dependence on repeated administration of a drug. **Psychological dependency** is a compulsion or craving to use a substance to obtain a pleasurable experience; it is the mind's desire for the repeated administration of a drug. One type of dependency may lead to the other.

The Controlled Substances Act of 1970 established a schedule, or classification system, for drugs with abuse potential. The act regulates the manufacture, distribution, and dispensing of these drugs. The Controlled Substances Act divides drugs into five schedules, based on their potential for abuse and physical and psychological dependence. Appendix A describes the five schedules.

Prescription practices of the primary health care provider for controlled substances are monitored by the Drug Enforcement Agency (DEA). Under federal law, limited quantities of certain schedule V drugs may be purchased without a prescription, with the purchase recorded by the dispensing pharmacist. In some cases, state laws are more restrictive than federal laws and impose additional requirements for the sale and distribution of controlled substances. In hospitals or other agencies that dispense controlled substances, the scheduled drugs are counted every 8 to 12 hours to account for each injectable, tablet, or other form of the drug. Any discrepancy in the number of drugs must be investigated and explained immediately.

Drug Development

Drug development is a long and arduous process that can take from 7 to 12 years, and sometimes longer. The FDA has the responsibility for approving new drugs and monitoring drugs currently in use for adverse or toxic reactions. The development of a new drug is divided into the pre-FDA phase and the FDA phase. During the pre-FDA phase, a manufacturer conducts in vitro testing (testing in an artificial environment, such as a test tube) using animal and human cells to discover new drugs. This testing is followed by studies in live animals. The manufacturer then makes application to the FDA for Investigational New Drug (IND) status.

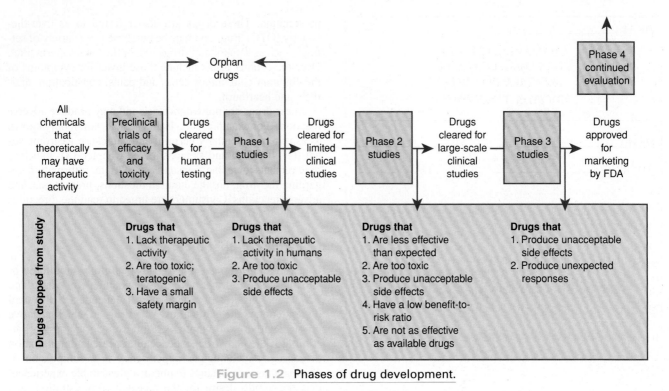

Figure 1.2 Phases of drug development.

Next, clinical (i.e., human) testing of the new drug begins. Clinical testing involves three phases, with each phase involving a larger number of people (Fig. 1.2). All effects, both pharmacologic and biologic, are noted. Phase 1 involves 20 to 100 individuals who are healthy volunteers. If Phase 1 studies are successful, the testing moves to Phase 2, in which tests are performed on people who have the disease or condition for which the drug is thought to be effective. If those results are positive, the testing progresses to Phase 3, in which the drug is given to large numbers of patients in medical research centers to provide information about adverse reactions. Phase 3 studies offer additional information on dosing and safety. Clinical trial studies can extend for many years.

A New Drug Application (NDA) is submitted after the investigation of the drug in Phases 1, 2, and 3 is complete and the drug is found to be safe and effective. With the NDA, the manufacturer submits all data collected concerning the drug during the clinical trials. A panel of experts, including pharmacologists, chemists, physicians, and other professionals, reviews the application and makes a recommendation to the FDA. The FDA then either approves or disapproves the drug for use.

After FDA approval, continued surveillance is done to ensure safety. Postmarketing surveillance (Phase 4) occurs after the manufacturer places the drug on the market. During this surveillance, an ongoing review of the drug occurs with particular attention given to adverse reactions. Health care providers are encouraged to help with this surveillance by reporting adverse effects of drugs to the FDA by using MedWatch (Display 1.1) or the Institute for Safe Medication Practices (ISMP) Medication Errors Reporting Program (MERP).

Display 1.1 MedWatch and Reporting Adverse Events

- The U.S. Food and Drug Administration (FDA) established a safety information and adverse event reporting program called MedWatch, by which nurses or other health care providers can learn about or report observations of serious adverse drug effects. Anyone can access the website (http://www.fda.gov/medwatch/index.html) to obtain safety alerts on drugs, devices, or dietary supplements.

- A drug must be used and studied for many years before all of the adverse reactions are identified. Nurses play an important role in monitoring for adverse reactions. The website provides a standardized form for reporting, which can be submitted electronically or downloaded, filled out, and mailed/faxed in to the program. It is important to submit reports, even if there is uncertainty about the cause–effect relationship. The FDA protects the identity of those who voluntarily report adverse reactions.

- The FDA considers serious adverse reactions those that may result in death, life-threatening illness, hospitalization, or disability or those that may require medical or surgical intervention. This form also is used to report an undesirable experience associated with the use of medical products (e.g., latex gloves, pacemakers, infusion pumps, anaphylaxis, blood, blood components).

Special Food and Drug Administration Programs

Although it takes considerable time for most drugs to get FDA approval, the FDA has special programs to meet different needs. Examples of these special programs include the orphan drug program and accelerated programs for urgent needs.

Orphan Drug Program

The Orphan Drug Act of 1983 was passed to encourage the development and marketing of products used to treat rare diseases. The act defines a rare disease as a condition affecting fewer than 200,000 individuals in the United States or a condition affecting more than 200,000 persons in the United States but for which the cost of producing and marketing a drug to treat the condition would not be recovered by sales of the drug. The National Organization of Rare Disorders reports that there are more than 6800 rare disorders that affect approximately 30 million individuals. Examples of rare disorders include multiple myeloma, cystic fibrosis, and phenylketonuria.

The act provides for incentives such as research grants, protocol assistance by the FDA, and special tax credits to encourage manufacturers to develop orphan drugs. If the drug is approved, the manufacturer has 7 years of exclusive marketing rights. More than 360 new drugs have received FDA approval since the law was passed. Examples of orphan drugs include Valortim for anthrax infection, TOL-101 for acute organ transplant rejection, and atiprimod for the treatment of multiple myeloma.

Accelerated Programs

Accelerated approval of drugs is offered by the FDA as a means to make promising products for life-threatening diseases available on the market, based on preliminary evidence and before formal demonstration of patient benefit. The approval that is granted is considered a "provisional approval," with a written commitment from the pharmaceutical company to complete clinical studies that formally demonstrate patient benefit. This program seeks to make lifesaving investigational drugs available before granting final approval to treat diseases that pose a significant health threat to the public. If the drug continues to prove beneficial, the process of approval is accelerated.

One example of a disease that qualified as posing a significant health threat is acquired immunodeficiency syndrome (AIDS). When first diagnosed, because AIDS was so devastating to the individuals affected and because of the danger the disease posed to public health, the FDA and pharmaceutical companies worked together to shorten the IND approval process for some drugs that show promise in treating AIDS. This accelerated process allowed primary health care providers to administer medications that indicated positive results in early Phase 1 and 2 clinical trials, rather than wait until final approval was granted.

Drug Activity within the Body

Once in the body, drugs act in certain ways or phases. Oral drugs go through three phases: the *pharmaceutic* phase, *pharmacokinetic* phase, and *pharmacodynamic* phase (Fig. 1.3).

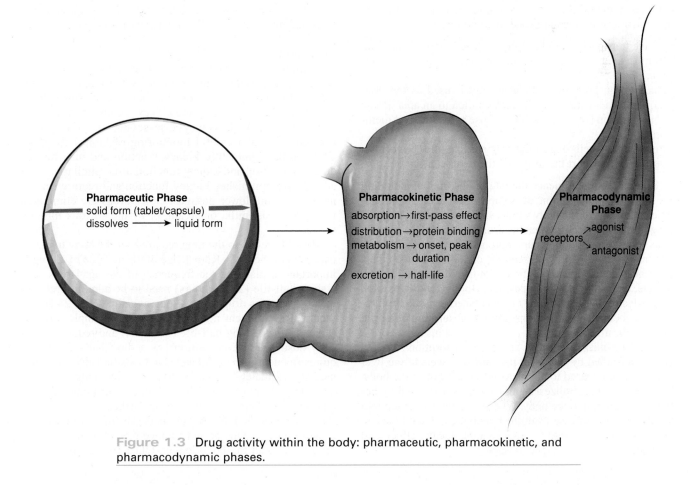

Figure 1.3 Drug activity within the body: pharmaceutic, pharmacokinetic, and pharmacodynamic phases.

Liquid and parenteral drugs (drugs given by injection) go through the latter two phases only.

Pharmaceutic Phase

In the **pharmaceutic** phase, the drug dissolves. Drugs must be a soluble liquid to be absorbed. Drugs that are liquid or drugs given by injection (parenteral drugs) are already dissolved and are absorbed quickly. A tablet or capsule (solid forms of a drug) goes through this phase as it disintegrates into small particles and dissolves into the body fluids in the GI tract. Tablets that have an enteric coating or time-release capsules do not disintegrate until they reach the alkaline environment of the small intestine.

Pharmacokinetic Phase

Pharmacokinetics refers to the transportation activity of drugs in the body after administration. These activities include absorption, distribution, metabolism, and excretion. Subcomponents of these pharmacokinetic activities include transport, first-pass effect during absorption, and half-life during excretion of the drug.

Absorption

Absorption involves moving the drug from the site of administration into the body fluids and is the process by which a drug is made available for use in the body. It occurs after dissolution of a solid form of the drug or after the administration of a liquid or parenteral drug. In this process, the drug particles in the GI tract are moved into the body fluids. This movement can be accomplished in several ways:

- Active transport—cellular energy is used to move the drug from an area of low concentration to one of high concentration.
- Passive transport—no cellular energy is used as the drug moves from an area of high concentration to an area of low concentration (small molecules diffuse across the cell membrane).
- Pinocytosis—cells engulf the drug particle (the cell forms a vesicle to transport the drug into the inner cell).

Several factors influence the rate of absorption, including the route of administration, the solubility of the drug, and specific conditions of the body's tissues. The most rapid route of drug absorption occurs when the drug is given by the intravenous route. Absorption occurs more slowly when the drug is administered orally, intramuscularly, or subcutaneously. This is because the complex membranes of the GI mucosal layers, muscle, and skin delay drug passage. Bodily conditions such as lipodystrophy (the atrophy of subcutaneous tissue from repeated subcutaneous injections) inhibits absorption of a drug given in the affected site.

The **first-pass effect** may also affect absorption. When a drug is absorbed by the small intestine, it travels to the liver before being released to circulate within the rest of the body. The liver may metabolize a significant amount of the drug before releasing it into the body. When the drug is released into the circulation from the liver, the remaining amount of active drug may not be enough to produce a therapeutic effect, and the patient will need a higher dosage.

Distribution

The systemic circulation transports and distributes drugs to various body tissues or target sites. **Distribution** of an absorbed drug in the body depends on protein binding, blood flow, and solubility.

When a drug travels through the blood, it comes into contact with proteins such as the plasma protein *albumin*. The drug can remain free in the circulation or bind to the protein. Only free drugs can produce a therapeutic effect. Drugs bound to protein are pharmacologically inactive. Only when the protein molecules release the drug can the drug diffuse into the tissues, interact with receptors, and produce a therapeutic effect. A drug is said to be highly protein bound when more than 80% of the circulating drug is bound to protein.

A drug is distributed quickly to areas with a large blood supply, such as the heart, liver, and kidneys. In other areas, such as the internal organs, skin, and muscle, distribution of the drug occurs more slowly.

Solubility, or the drug's ability to cross the cell membrane, affects its distribution. Lipid-soluble drugs easily cross the cell membrane, whereas water-soluble drugs do not.

Metabolism

Metabolism, also called *biotransformation*, is the process by which the body changes a drug to a more or less active form that can be excreted. Usually the resulting form is a **metabolite** (an inactive form of the original drug). In some drugs, one or more of the metabolites may have some drug activity. Metabolites may undergo further metabolism or may be excreted from the body unchanged. Most drugs are metabolized by the liver, although the kidneys, lungs, plasma, and intestinal mucosa also aid in the metabolism of drugs.

Excretion

The elimination of drugs from the body is called **excretion**. After the liver renders drugs inactive, the kidney excretes the inactive compounds from the body. Also, some drugs are excreted unchanged by the kidney without liver involvement. Patients with kidney disease may require a dosage reduction and careful monitoring of kidney function. Children have immature kidney function and may require dosage reduction and kidney function tests. Similarly, older adults have diminished kidney function and require careful monitoring and lower dosages. Other drugs are eliminated in sweat, breast milk, or breath, or by the GI tract through the feces.

Half-life refers to the time required for the body to eliminate 50% of the drug. Knowledge of the half-life of a drug is important in planning the frequency of dosing. Drugs with a short half-life (2 to 4 hours) need to be administered frequently, whereas drugs with a long half-life (21 to 24 hours) require less frequent administration. For example, digoxin (Lanoxin) has a long half-life (36 hours) and requires once-daily dosing. However, aspirin has a short half-life and requires frequent dosing. It takes five to six half-lives to eliminate approximately 98% of a drug from the body. Although half-life is fairly stable, patients with liver or kidney disease may have problems excreting a drug. Difficulty in excreting a drug increases the half-life and increases the risk of toxicity, because these organs do not remove the substances and the drug remains in the body longer. Older patients or patients with impaired kidney or liver function require frequent diagnostic tests measuring renal or hepatic function.

Onset, Peak, and Duration

The therapeutic effect of a drug determines the timing of drug administration. Three pharmacokinetic factors are important when considering how a drug acts in the body:

* *Onset of action*—time between administration of the drug and onset of its therapeutic effect
* *Peak concentration*—when absorption rate equals the elimination rate (not always the time of peak response)
* *Duration of action*—length of time the drug produces a therapeutic effect

These factors are taken into consideration when determining the dose schedule of a specific drug. This ensures that proper blood levels are maintained in the body for the drug to work properly.

Pharmacodynamic Phase

Pharmacodynamics is the study of the drug mechanisms that produce biochemical or physiologic changes in the body. Pharmacodynamics deals with the drug's action and effect in the body. After administration, most drugs enter the systemic circulation and expose almost all body tissues to possible effects of the drug. This exposure in all tissue causes the drug to produce more than one effect in the body. The primary effect of a drug is the desired or therapeutic effect. Secondary effects are all other effects, desirable or undesirable, produced by the drug.

Most drugs have an affinity for certain organs or tissues and exert their greatest action at the cellular level on those specific areas, which are called *target sites*. A drug exerts its action by one of two main mechanisms:

1. Alteration in cellular function
2. Alteration in cellular environment

Alteration in Cellular Function

Most drugs act on the body by altering cellular function. A drug cannot completely change the function of a cell, but it can alter its function. A drug that alters cellular function can increase or decrease certain physiologic functions, such as increasing heart rate, decreasing blood pressure, or increasing urine output.

Receptor-Mediated Drug Action

Many drugs act through drug–**receptor** interaction. The function of a cell is altered when a drug interacts with a receptor. This occurs when a drug molecule selectively joins with a reactive site—the receptor—on the surface of a cell. When a drug binds to and interacts with the receptor, a pharmacologic response occurs.

An *agonist* is a drug that binds with a receptor and stimulates the receptor to produce a therapeutic response. An *antagonist* is a drug that joins with receptors but does not stimulate the receptors. The therapeutic action in this case consists of blocking the receptor's function.

Receptor-Mediated Drug Effects

The number of available receptor sites influences the effects of a drug. When only a few receptor sites are occupied, although many sites are available, the response will be small. When the drug dose is increased, more receptor sites are used, and the response increases. When only a few receptor sites are available, the response does not increase when more of the drug is administered. However, not all receptors on a cell need to be occupied for a drug to be effective. Some extremely potent drugs are effective even when the drug occupies few receptor sites.

Alteration in Cellular Environment

Some drugs act on the body by changing the cellular environment, either physically or chemically. Physical changes in the cellular environment include changes in osmotic pressure, lubrication, absorption, or the conditions on the surface of the cell membrane.

An example of a drug that changes osmotic pressure is *mannitol,* which produces a change in the osmotic pressure in brain cells, causing a reduction in cerebral edema. A drug that acts by altering the cellular environment by lubrication is sunscreen. An example of a drug that acts by altering absorption is activated charcoal, which is administered orally to absorb a toxic chemical ingested into the GI tract. The stool softener *docusate* is an example of a drug that acts by altering the surface of the cellular membrane. Docusate has emulsifying and lubricating activity that lowers the surface tension in the cells of the bowel, permitting water and fats to enter the stool. This softens the fecal mass, allowing easier passage of the stool.

Chemical changes in the cellular environment include inactivation of cellular functions or alteration of the chemical components of body fluid, such as a change in the pH. For example, antacids neutralize gastric acidity in patients with peptic ulcers.

Other drugs, such as some anticancer drugs and some antibiotics, have as their main site of action the cell membrane and various cellular processes. They incorporate themselves into the normal metabolic processes of the cell and cause the formation of a defective final product, such as a weakened cell wall, which results in cell death, or reduce a needed energy substrate that leads to cell starvation and death.

Pharmacogenomics

Most pharmacodynamic mechanisms deal with principles that affect each cell in the same way, whereas *pharmacogenomics* is the study of how people's responses to medications are variable due to individual genetic variation. In other words, the genetic makeup of a person can affect the pharmacodynamics of a drug. This discovery was made during the Human Genome Project when many scientists were able to determine the different components of the human genetic code. *Pharmacogenetics* is the creation of individualized drug therapy that allows for the best choice and dose of drugs.

Drug Use, Pregnancy, and Lactation

The use of any medication (prescription or nonprescription) carries a risk of causing birth defects in the developing fetus. Drugs administered to pregnant women, particularly during the first trimester (3 months), may have teratogenic effects. A **teratogen** is any substance that causes abnormal development of the fetus, often leading to severe deformation. Some drugs are classified as teratogens.

To prevent teratogenic effects, the FDA has established five categories suggesting the potential of a drug for causing birth defects (Appendix A). Information regarding the pregnancy category of a specific drug is found in reliable drug literature, such as the inserts accompanying drugs and approved drug references. In general, most drugs are contraindicated during pregnancy and lactation unless the potential benefits of taking the drug outweigh the risks to the fetus or the infant.

During pregnancy, no woman should consider taking any drug, legal or illegal, prescription or nonprescription, unless the drug is prescribed or recommended by the primary health care provider. Smoking or drinking any type of alcoholic beverage also carries risks, such as low birth weight, premature birth, and fetal alcohol syndrome. Children born of mothers using addictive drugs, such as cocaine or heroin, often are born with an addiction to the drug abused by the mother. Women who are pregnant should also be very careful about the use of herbal supplements because these products can act like drugs. Women should not take an herbal supplement without discussing it first with her primary health care provider.

When a mother breastfeeds, her child has a risk of exposure to harmful medications. A number of drugs can be excreted in breast milk. Therefore, if a mother is lactating (breastfeeding), some of the drug she is taking may be ingested and absorbed by the infant or breastfeeding child. It is important for both mothers and nurses to know the potential of exposure to a breastfeeding child when the mother is taking a drug.

The National Library of Medicine provides a free online database with information on drugs and lactation called Lact-Med (http://toxnet.nlm.nih.gov/cgi-bin/sis/htmlgen?LACT). This website is geared to the health care practitioner and nursing mother and contains over 450 drug records. It includes information such as maternal levels in breast milk, infant levels in blood, and potential effects in breastfeeding infants. A pharmacist, Dr. Thomas Hale, from Texas Tech University has developed a system of lactation risk categories similar to that of the FDA pregnancy risk categories for drugs. Drugs are assigned an L1 to L5 risk according to the drug's transmission in breast milk and the effect it may have on the child. Hale's listing of certain drugs may differ from those published by organizations such as the American Academy of Pediatrics, yet it is a good starting point for discussion with mothers who are breastfeeding.

Drug Reactions

Drugs produce many reactions in the body. The following sections discuss adverse drug reactions, allergic drug reactions, **drug idiosyncrasy, drug tolerance, cumulative drug effect,** and toxic reactions.

Adverse Drug Reactions

Patients may experience one or more adverse reactions or side effects when they are given a drug. Adverse reactions are undesirable drug effects. Adverse reactions may be common or may occur infrequently. They may be mild, severe, or life-threatening. They may occur after the first dose, after a few doses, or after many doses. Often, an adverse reaction is unpredictable, although some drugs are known to cause certain adverse reactions in many patients. For example, drugs used in treating cancer are very toxic and are known to produce adverse reactions in many patients receiving them. Other drugs produce adverse reactions in fewer patients. Some adverse reactions are predictable, but many adverse drug reactions occur without warning.

Some texts use both the terms *side effects* and *adverse reactions,* using *side effects* to explain mild, common, and nontoxic reactions and *adverse reactions* to describe more severe and life-threatening reactions. For the purposes of this text, only the term *adverse reaction* is used, with the understanding that these reactions may be mild, severe, or life-threatening.

Allergic Drug Reactions

An **allergic reaction** is an immediate **hypersensitivity** reaction. Allergy to a drug usually begins to occur after more than one dose of the drug is given. On occasion, the nurse may observe an allergic reaction the first time a drug is given, because the patient has received or taken the drug in the past.

A drug allergy occurs because the individual's immune system responds to the drug as a foreign substance called an *antigen.* When the body responds to the drug as an antigen, a series of events occurs in an attempt to render the invader harmless. Lymphocytes respond by forming *antibodies* (protein substances that protect against antigens). Common allergic reactions occur when the individual's immune system responds aggressively to the antigen. Chemical mediators released during the allergic reaction produce symptoms ranging from mild to life-threatening.

Even a mild allergic reaction produces serious effects if it goes unnoticed and the drug is given again. Any indication of an allergic reaction is reported to the primary health care provider before the next dose of the drug is given. Serious allergic reactions require contacting the primary health care provider immediately, because emergency treatment may be necessary.

Some allergic reactions occur within minutes (even seconds) after the drug is given; others may be delayed for hours or days. Allergic reactions that occur immediately often are the most serious.

Allergic reactions are manifested by a variety of signs and symptoms observed by the nurse or reported by the patient. Examples of some allergic symptoms include itching, various types of skin rashes, and hives (urticaria). Other symptoms include difficulty breathing, wheezing, cyanosis, a sudden loss of consciousness, and swelling of the eyes, lips, or tongue.

Anaphylactic shock is an extremely serious allergic drug reaction that usually occurs shortly after the administration of a drug to which the individual is sensitive. This type of allergic reaction requires immediate medical attention. Symptoms of anaphylactic shock are listed in Table 1.2.

All or only some of these symptoms may be present. Anaphylactic shock can be fatal if the symptoms are not identified and treated immediately. Treatment is to raise the blood pressure, improve breathing, restore cardiac function, and treat other symptoms as they occur. Epinephrine (adrenalin) may be given by subcutaneous injection in the upper extremity or thigh and may be followed by a continuous intravenous infusion. Hypotension and shock may be treated with fluids and vasopressors. Bronchodilators are given to relax the smooth muscles of the bronchial tubes. Antihistamines

Body System	Symptoms
Respiratory	Bronchospasm Dyspnea (difficult breathing) Feeling of fullness in the throat Cough Wheezing
Cardiovascular	Extremely low blood pressure Tachycardia (heart rate >100 bpm) Palpitations Syncope (fainting) Cardiac arrest
Integumentary	Urticaria (hives) Angioedema Pruritus (itching) Sweating
Gastrointestinal	Nausea Vomiting Abdominal pain

Table 1.2 **Symptoms of Anaphylactic Shock**

and corticosteroids may also be given to treat urticaria and angioedema (swelling).

Angioedema (angioneurotic edema) is another type of allergic drug reaction. It is manifested by the collection of fluid in subcutaneous tissues. Areas that are most commonly affected are the eyelids, lips, mouth, and throat, although other areas also may be affected. Angioedema can be dangerous when the mouth is affected, because the swelling may block the airway and asphyxia may occur. Difficulty in breathing and swelling in any area of the body are reported immediately to the primary health care provider.

Drug Idiosyncrasy

Drug idiosyncrasy is a term used to describe any unusual or abnormal reaction to a drug. It is any reaction that is different from the one normally expected from a specific drug and dose. For example, a patient may be given a drug to help him or her sleep (e.g., a hypnotic). Instead of falling asleep, the patient remains wide awake and shows signs of nervousness or excitement. This response is idiosyncratic because it is different from what one expects from this type of drug. Another patient may receive the same drug and dose, fall asleep, and after 8 hours be difficult to awaken. This, too, is abnormal and describes an overresponse to the drug.

The cause of drug idiosyncrasy is not clear. Study in the science of genetics can give us insight into possible explanations. The inability to tolerate certain chemicals and drugs is believed to be due to a genetic deficiency. Pharmacogenetics, the study of ways that specific genes can enhance sensitivity or resistance to certain drugs, helps to explain some drug idiosyncrasies. A pharmacogenetic disorder is a genetically determined abnormal response to normal doses of a drug. This abnormal response occurs because of inherited traits that cause abnormal metabolism of drugs. For example, individuals with glucose-6-phosphate dehydrogenase (G6PD) deficiency have abnormal reactions to a number of drugs.

These patients exhibit varying degrees of hemolysis (destruction of red blood cells) when these drugs are administered. More than 100 million people are affected by this disorder. Examples of drugs that cause hemolysis in patients with a G6PD deficiency include aspirin, chloramphenicol, and the sulfonamides.

Drug Tolerance

Drug tolerance is a term used to describe a decreased response to a drug, requiring an increase in dosage to achieve the desired effect. Drug tolerance may develop when a patient takes certain drugs, such as opioids and tranquilizers, for a long time. The individual who takes these drugs at home increases the dose when the expected drug effect does not occur. The development of drug tolerance is a sign of physical drug dependence. Drug tolerance may also occur in the hospitalized patient. When the patient begins to ask for the drug at more frequent intervals, the nurse needs to assess whether the dose is not adequate based on the disease process or whether the patient is building a tolerance to the drug's effects.

Cumulative Drug Effect

A cumulative drug effect may be seen in those people with liver or kidney disease because these organs are the major sites for the breakdown and excretion of most drugs. This drug effect occurs when the body is unable to metabolize and excrete one (normal) dose of a drug before the next dose is given. Thus, if a second dose of the drug is given, some drug from the first dose remains in the body. A cumulative drug effect can be serious because too much of the drug can accumulate in the body and lead to toxicity.

Patients with liver or kidney disease are usually given drugs with caution because a cumulative effect may occur. When the patient is unable to excrete the drug at a normal rate, the drug accumulates in the body, causing a toxic reaction. Sometimes, the primary health care provider lowers the dose of the drug to prevent a toxic drug reaction.

Toxic Reactions

Most drugs can produce toxic or harmful reactions if administered in large dosages or when blood concentration levels exceed the therapeutic level. Toxic levels build up when a drug is administered in dosages that exceed the normal level or if the patient's kidneys are not functioning properly and cannot excrete the drug. Some toxic effects are immediately visible; others may not be seen for weeks or months. Some drugs, such as lithium or digoxin, have a narrow margin of safety, even when given in recommended dosages. It is important to monitor these drugs closely to detect and avoid toxicity.

Drug toxicity can be reversible or irreversible, depending on the organs involved. Damage to the liver may be reversible, because liver cells can regenerate. However, hearing loss from damage to the eighth cranial nerve caused by toxic reaction to the anti-infective drug streptomycin may be permanent. Sometimes drug toxicity can be reversed by administering another drug that acts as an antidote. For example, in serious instances of digitalis toxicity, the drug Digibind may be given to counteract the effect.

Carefully monitor the patient's blood level of drug to ensure that the level remains within the therapeutic range. Any deviation should be reported to the primary health care provider. Because some drugs can cause toxic reactions even in recommended doses, you should be aware of the signs and symptoms of toxicity of commonly prescribed drugs.

Minimizing Drug Reactions Through Pharmacogenomics

Drug developers are also researching ways to target cell structures and selected cells to minimize reactions in other body tissues, thereby reducing or eliminating adverse reactions. Genetic specialists search for genetic variations associated with drug efficiency. The goal of pharmacogenomics is the creation of drugs that can be tailor-made for individuals, target specific cells in the body, and adapt to each person's own individual genetic makeup.

Drug Interactions

It is important when administering medications to be aware of the various drug interactions that can occur, especially *drug–drug interactions* and *drug–food interactions.* This section gives a brief overview of drug interactions. Specific drug–drug and drug–food interactions are discussed in subsequent chapters.

Drug–Drug Interactions

A drug–drug interaction occurs when one drug interacts with or interferes with the action of another drug. For example, taking an antacid with oral tetracycline causes a decrease in the effectiveness of the tetracycline. The antacid chemically interacts with the tetracycline and impairs its absorption into the bloodstream, thus reducing the effectiveness of the tetracycline. Drug categories known to cause interactions with other drugs include oral anticoagulants, oral hypoglycemics, anti-infectives, antiarrhythmics, cardiac glycosides, and alcohol. Drug–drug interactions can produce effects that are additive, synergistic, or antagonistic.

Additive Drug Reaction

An *additive drug reaction* occurs when the combined effect of two drugs is equal to the sum of each drug given alone. The equation $1 + 1 = 2$ is sometimes used to illustrate the additive effect of drugs. For example, taking the drug heparin with alcohol will increase bleeding.

Synergistic Drug Reaction

Drug *synergism* occurs when drugs interact with each other and produce an effect that is greater than the sum of their separate actions. The equation $1 + 1 = 3$ may be used to illustrate synergism. Drug synergism is exemplified when a person takes both a hypnotic and alcohol. When alcohol is taken shortly before or after the hypnotic drug, the action of the hypnotic increases considerably. The individual experiences a drug effect that is greater than each drug taken alone. On occasion, the occurrence of a synergistic drug effect is serious and even fatal.

Antagonistic Drug Reaction

An *antagonistic* drug reaction occurs when one drug interferes with the action of another, causing neutralization or a decrease in the effect of one of the drugs. For example, protamine is a heparin antagonist. This means that the administration of protamine completely neutralizes the effects of heparin in the body and blood clotting will happen in the body.

Drug–Food Interactions

When a drug is given orally, food may impair or enhance its absorption. A drug taken on an empty stomach is absorbed into the bloodstream more quickly than when the drug is taken with food in the stomach. Some drugs (e.g., captopril) must be taken on an empty stomach to achieve an optimal effect. Drugs that should be taken on an empty stomach are administered 1 hour before or 2 hours after meals. Other drugs—especially drugs that irritate the stomach, result in nausea or vomiting, or cause epigastric distress—are best given with food or meals. This minimizes gastric irritation. The nonsteroidal anti-inflammatory drugs (NSAIDs) and salicylates are examples of drugs that are given with food to decrease epigastric distress. Still other drugs combine with a food, forming an insoluble food–drug mixture. For example, when tetracycline is administered with dairy products, a drug–food mixture is formed that is not absorbable by the body. When a drug cannot be absorbed by the body, no pharmacologic effect occurs.

Factors Influencing Drug Response

Certain factors may influence drug response and are considered when the primary health care provider prescribes and the nurse administers a drug. These factors include age, weight, sex, disease, and route of administration.

Age

The age of the patient may influence the effects of a drug. Infants and children usually require smaller doses of a drug than adults. Immature organ function, particularly of the liver and kidneys, can affect the ability of infants and young children to metabolize drugs. An infant's immature kidneys impair the elimination of drugs in the urine. Liver function is poorly developed in infants and young children. Drugs metabolized by the liver may produce more intense effects for longer periods. Parents must be taught the potential problems associated with administering drugs to their children. For example, a safe dose of a nonprescription drug for a 4-year-old child may be dangerous for a 6-month-old infant.

Elderly patients may also require smaller doses, although this may depend on the type of drug administered. For example, the elderly patient may be given the same dose of an antibiotic as a younger adult. However, the same older adult may require a smaller dose of a drug that depresses the central nervous system, such as an opioid. Changes that occur with aging affect the pharmacokinetics (absorption, distribution, metabolism, and excretion) of a drug. Any of these processes may be altered because of the physiologic changes that occur with aging. Table 1.3 summarizes the changes that occur with aging and their possible pharmacokinetic effects.

Table 1.3 Factors Altering Drug Response in Children and Older Adults

Body System Changes	Children/Infants	Older Adults
Gastric acidity	Higher pH—slower gastric emptying resulting in delayed absorption	Higher pH—slower gastric emptying resulting in delayed absorption
Skin changes	Less cutaneous fat and greater surface area—faster absorption of topical drugs	Decreased fat content—decreased absorption of transdermal drugs
Body water content	Increased body water content—greater dilution of drug in tissues	Decreased body water content—greater concentration of drug in tissues
Serum protein	Less protein—less protein binding creating more circulating drug	Less protein—less protein binding creating more circulating drug
Liver function	Immature function—increased half-life of drugs and less first-pass effect	Decreased blood flow to liver—delayed and decreased metabolism of drug
Kidney function	Immature kidney function—decreased elimination, potential for toxicity at lower drug levels	Decreased renal mass and glomerular filtration rate—increased serum levels of drugs

Polypharmacy is the taking of numerous drugs that can potentially react with one another. This is seen particularly in elderly patients who may have multiple chronic diseases; polypharmacy leads to an increase in the number of potential adverse reactions. Although multiple drug therapy is necessary to treat certain disease states, it always increases the possibility of adverse reactions. You need good assessment skills to detect any problems when monitoring the geriatric patient's response to drug therapy.

Weight

In general, dosages are based on a weight of approximately 170 lb, which is calculated to be the average weight of men and women. A drug dose may sometimes be increased or decreased because the patient's weight is significantly higher or lower than this average. With opioids, for example, higher- or lower-than-average dosages may be necessary, depending on the patient's weight, to produce relief of pain.

Sex

The sex of an individual may influence the action of some drugs. Women may require a smaller dose of some drugs than men. This is because many women are smaller and have a different body fat–to-water ratio than men.

Disease

The presence of disease may influence the action of some drugs. Sometimes disease is an indication for not prescribing a drug or for reducing the dose of a certain drug. Both hepatic (liver) and renal (kidney) disease can greatly affect drug response.

In liver disease, for example, the ability to metabolize or detoxify a specific type of drug may be impaired. If the average or normal dose of the drug is given, the liver may be unable to metabolize the drug at a normal rate. Consequently, the drug may be excreted from the body at a much slower rate than normal. The primary health care provider may then decide to prescribe a lower dose and lengthen the time between doses because liver function is abnormal.

Patients with kidney disease may exhibit drug toxicity and a longer duration of drug action. The dosage of drugs may be reduced to prevent the accumulation of toxic levels in the blood or further injury to the kidney.

Route of Administration

Intravenous administration of a drug produces the most rapid drug action. Next in order of time of action is the intramuscular route, followed by the subcutaneous route. Giving a drug orally usually produces the slowest drug action.

Some drugs can be given only by one route; for example, antacids are given only orally. Other drugs are available in oral and parenteral forms. The primary health care provider selects the route of administration based on many factors, including the desired rate of action. For example, the patient with a severe cardiac problem may require intravenous administration of a drug that affects the heart. Another patient with a mild cardiac problem may experience a good response to oral administration of the same drug.

Nursing Implications with Drug Actions

Many factors can influence drug action. Consult appropriate references or the clinical pharmacist if there is any question about the dosage of a drug, whether other drugs the patient is receiving will interfere with the drug being given, or whether the oral drug should or should not be given with food.

Drug reactions are potentially serious. Observe all patients for adverse drug reactions, drug idiosyncrasy, and evidence of drug tolerance (when applicable). It is important to report all drug reactions or any unusual drug effect to the primary health care provider.

Use good judgment when reporting adverse drug reactions to the primary health care provider. Accurate observation and evaluation of the circumstances are essential; record all observations in the patient's record. If there is any question regarding the events that are occurring, withhold the drug and immediately contact the primary health care provider.

Herbal Medicine and Health Care

Herbal medicine, herbalism, and herbal therapy are all names used for complementary/alternative therapy that uses plants or herbs to treat various disorders. Individuals worldwide use herbal therapy and dietary supplements extensively. According to the World Health Organization (WHO), 80% of the world's population relies on herbs for a substantial part of their health care. Herbs have been used by virtually every culture in the world throughout history. For example, Hippocrates prescribed St. John's wort, currently a popular herbal remedy for depression. Native Americans use plants such as coneflower, ginseng, and ginger for therapeutic purposes. Herbal therapy is part of the group of nontraditional therapies commonly known as complementary and alternative medicine (CAM).

Complementary and Alternative Medicine

The National Center for Complementary and Alternative Medicine (NCCAM) is one of the 27 institutes and centers that make up the National Institutes of Health (NIH). The NCCAM explores complementary and alternative healing practices through scientific research. It also trains CAM scientists and disseminates the information gleaned from the research it conducts. Among the various purposes of the NCCAM is to evaluate the safety and efficacy of widely used natural products, such as herbal remedies and dietary and food supplements. The NCCAM is dedicated to developing programs and encouraging scientists to investigate CAM treatments that show promise. The NCCAM budget has steadily grown, reflecting the public's interest and need for CAM information that is based on rigorous scientific research.

The NCCAM defines CAM as a "group of diverse medical and health care systems, practices, and products that are not presently considered to be part of conventional medicine." Examples of complementary therapies are relaxation techniques, massage, aromatherapy, and healing touch. Complementary therapies are often used with traditional health care to "complement" conventional medicine. Alternative therapies, on the other hand, are therapies used in place of or instead of conventional or Western medicine. The term *complementary/alternative therapy* often is used as an umbrella term for many therapies from all over the world.

Dietary Supplement Health and Education Act

Herbs are not sold and promoted in the United States as drugs. In addition to vitamins and minerals, herbs are classified as dietary or nutritional supplements. *Nutritional* or *dietary substances* are terms used by the federal government to identify substances that are not regulated by the FDA but purported to be effective for use to promote health. This means that they do not have to meet the same standards as drug and OTC medications for proof of safety and effectiveness and what the FDA calls "good manufacturing practices."

Because natural products cannot be patented in the United States, it is not profitable for drug manufacturers to spend the millions of dollars and the 7 to 12 years needed to study and develop these products as drugs. In 1994, the U.S. government passed the Dietary Supplement Health and Education Act (DSHEA). This act defines substances such as herbs, vitamins, minerals, amino acids, and other natural substances as "dietary supplements." The act permits general health claims such as "improves memory" or "promotes regularity" as long as the label also has a disclaimer stating that the supplements are not approved by the FDA and are not intended to diagnose, treat, cure, or prevent any disease. The claims must be truthful and not misleading and supported by scientific evidence. Some manufacturers have abused the law by making exaggerated claims, but the FDA has the power to enforce the law, which it has done, and these claims have decreased.

Educating Patients About Herbs and Dietary Supplements

The use of herbs and dietary supplements to treat various disorders is common. Herbs are used for various effects, such as boosting the immune system, treating depression, and promoting relaxation. Individuals are becoming more aware of the benefits of herbal therapies and dietary supplements. Advertisements, books, magazines, and Internet sites concerning these topics are prolific. People eager to cure or control various disorders take herbs, teas, megadoses of vitamins, and various other natural products. Although much information is available on dietary supplements and herbal therapy, obtaining the correct information can be difficult at times. Medicinal herbs and dietary substances are available at supermarkets, pharmacies, health food stores, and specialty herb stores and through the Internet. The potential for misinformation abounds. Because these substances are "natural products," many individuals incorrectly assume that they are without adverse effects. When any herbal remedy or dietary supplement is used, it should be reported to the nurse and the primary health care provider. Many of these natural substances have strong pharmacologic activity, and some may interact with prescription drugs or be toxic in the body. For example, *comfrey,* an herb that was once widely used to promote digestion, can cause liver damage. Although it may still be available in some areas, it is a dangerous herb and is not recommended for use as a supplement.

When obtaining the drug history, always question the patient about the use of herbs, teas, vitamins, or other dietary supplements. Many patients consider herbs as natural and therefore safe. Some also neglect to report the use of an herbal tea as part of the health care regimen because they do not think of it as such. Explain to the patient that just because an herbal supplement is labeled "natural," it does not mean the supplement is safe or without harmful effects. Herbal supplements can act the same way as drugs and can cause medical problems if not used correctly or if taken in large amounts. Display 1.2 identifies teaching points to consider when discussing the use of herbs and dietary supplements with patients.

Because herbal supplements are not regulated by the FDA, products lack standardization with regard to purity and potency. In addition, multiple ingredients in products and batch-to-batch variation make it difficult to determine if reactions occur as a result of the herb itself. To assist with the identification of herb–drug interactions, report any potential interactions to the FDA through its MedWatch program (see Display 1.1). It is especially important to take special care when patients are taking any drugs with a narrow therapeutic index (the difference between the minimum therapeutic and minimum toxic drug concentrations is small—such as warfarin, a blood thinner) and herbal supplements. Because the absorption, metabolism, distribution, and elimination characteristics of most herbal

Display 1.2 Teaching Points When Discussing Herbal Therapy

- *Herbal preparations are not necessarily safe because they are natural.* Unlike prescription and over-the-counter (OTC) medicines, herbal products and supplements do not have to be tested to prove they work well and are safe before they're sold. Also, they may not be pure. They might contain other ingredients, such as plant pollen, that could make you sick. Sometimes they contain drugs that are not listed on the label, such as steroids or estrogens.
- *If you have health problems, there may be an increased danger in taking herbal preparations.* These conditions include blood-clotting problems, cancer, diabetes, an enlarged prostate gland, epilepsy, glaucoma, heart disease, high blood pressure, immune system problems, psychiatric problems, Parkinson's disease, liver problems, stroke, and thyroid problems.
- *If you are going to have surgery, be sure to tell your doctor if you use herbal products.* Herbal products can cause problems with surgery, including bleeding and problems with anesthesia. Stop using herbal products at least 2 weeks before surgery, or sooner if your doctor recommends it.
- *Herbal products can change the way prescription and OTC drugs work.* Herbal health products or supplements can affect the way the body processes drugs. When this happens, your medicine may not work the way it should. This may mean the drugs aren't absorbed at high enough levels to help the conditions for which they are prescribed. This can cause serious problems. You should be especially cautious about using herbal health products or supplements if you take a drug in one of the following categories:
  - Drugs to treat depression, anxiety, or other psychiatric problems
  - Antiseizure drugs
  - Blood thinners
  - Blood pressure medicine
  - Heart medicine
  - Drugs to treat diabetes
  - Cancer drugs
  If you take any of these drugs, talk to your doctor before taking any type of herbal product or supplement.
- *Herbal products can cause other problems, too.* You should not take more than the recommended dose of any herbal health product or supplement. The problems that these products can cause are much more likely to occur if you take too much or take them for too long.

Adapted with permission from *Herbal products and supplements: What you should know.* Retrieved June 19, 2012, from the American Academy of Family Physicians FamilyDoctor.org website: http://familydoctor.org/familydoctor/en/drugs-procedures-devices/over-the-counter/herbal-products-and-supplements.html

products are poorly understood, much of the information on herb–drug interactions is speculative. Herb–drug interactions are sporadically reported and difficult to determine.

Although a complete discussion about the use of herbs is beyond the scope of this book, it is important to remember that the use of herbs and dietary supplements is commonplace in many areas of the country. To help you become more aware of herbal therapy and dietary supplements, Appendix D gives an overview of selected common herbs and dietary supplements. In addition, "alerts" related to herbs and dietary supplements appear throughout this text to alert the student to valuable information and precautions.

KEY POINTS

- Each drug has several names: a chemical name (chemical structure), a generic (nonproprietary, official—any company can use) name, and a trade (or brand) name.
- Drugs are classified by use (such as anti-infectives) and categorized by their potential to be harmful (prescription, nonprescription, and controlled substances).
- Controlled substances are restricted by a schedule system (C-I to V), and monitored by the DEA because they have higher abuse potential that can result in physical and/or psychological dependency.
- The FDA has strict controls for research, study, and production of drug substances; these processes can take many years between substance discovery and actual marketing of a drug. There are special programs to speed this process for rare diseases or life-threatening conditions.
- The three main phases of drug activity are pharmaceutic, pharmacokinetic, and pharmacodynamic.
- Principles involved in pharmacokinetics include the following: absorption involves moving the drug from the site of administration; the drug is then distributed to tissues via the body circulation; metabolism changes the drug for use; and the drug is finally eliminated by the kidneys or made inactive by the liver and eliminated via the GI system.
- Principles of pharmacodynamics involve the biochemical movement of drugs into a cell; by the receptors on cells; by altering the environment around the cell to gain entry.
- Drugs can cause problems to an unborn fetus and are classified as to their safety.
- Adverse reactions to drugs can range from minor GI distress to anaphylactic shock.
- Drugs interact with many foods or other drugs, resulting in reactions less than or greater than when given alone.
- Age, weight, sex, disease, and route of administration all influence a person's response to drug therapy.
- Herbal preparations are not considered drugs, yet they should be considered part of a medical routine.

● Chapter Review
● Prepare for the NCLEX-PN

Build Your Knowledge

1. The best definition of *pharmacology* would be:

   1. the study of plants and living organisms
   2. making of chemical compounds for illnesses
   3. the study of drugs and their action on living organisms
   4. monitoring and accounting for substances used to make people well

2. A client tells the nurse that he is taking Claritin. Which type of drug name is this?

   1. chemical
   2. official
   3. brand
   4. generic

3. A new drug will be given to healthy volunteers to see what happens. In what phase of clinical trial is the drug being currently tested?

   1. Preclinical
   2. Phase 1
   3. Phase 2
   4. Phase 3

4. A newly admitted client has a history of liver disease. In planning care, the nurse must consider that liver disease may result in a(n) _____.

   1. increase in the excretion rate of a drug
   2. impaired ability to metabolize or detoxify a drug
   3. need to increase the dosage of a drug
   4. decrease in the rate of drug absorption

5. A client asks the nurse to define a hypersensitivity reaction. The nurse begins by telling the client that a hypersensitivity reaction is also called a(n) _____.

   1. synergistic reaction
   2. antagonistic reaction
   3. drug idiosyncrasy
   4. allergic reaction

6. In monitoring drug therapy, the nurse is aware that a synergistic drug effect may be defined as _____.

   1. an effect greater than the sum of the separate actions of two or more drugs
   2. an increase in the action of one of the two drugs being given
   3. a neutralizing drug effect
   4. a comprehensive drug effect

Apply Your Knowledge

7. A client has a rash and pruritus. As the nurse, you suspect an allergic reaction and immediately assess him for other more serious symptoms. What question would be most important to ask the client?

   1. Are you having any difficulty breathing?
   2. Have you noticed any blood in your stool?
   3. Do you have a headache?
   4. Are you having difficulty with your vision?

8. Under the Controlled Substances Act, schedule II to V drugs are typically accounted for in the health care setting. Which of the following drugs would the nurse least expect to be counted during change-of-shift duties?

   1. opioids
   2. antidiarrheals with codeine
   3. anabolic steroids
   4. heroin

Alternate-Format Questions

9. Arrange the following steps of pharmacokinetics correctly:

   1. absorption
   2. distribution
   3. elimination
   4. metabolism

10. Identify the drug responses seen in children. **Select all that apply.**

   1. pH of gastric acid is higher
   2. decreased body water
   3. less protein, less binding of drug
   4. greater amount of circulating drug

To check your answers, see Appendix G.

the**Point** *For more NCLEX-style questions, log on to http://thepoint.lww.com to access more than 1000 questions.*

2

Administration of Drugs

Drug administration is a fundamental nursing responsibility. Understanding the basic concept of administering drugs is critical to perform this task safely and accurately. In addition to administering the drug, you will monitor the therapeutic response (desired response) and report adverse reactions. In the ambulatory setting, you are responsible for teaching the patient and family members the information needed to administer drugs safely in the home.

The (Five + 1) Rights of Drug Administration

The nurse who administers a drug assumes the responsibility for accuracy in preparation of the medication. Responsibility includes both preparing and administering the prescribed drug. Accuracy in preparation is provided by a procedure termed the five "rights" of drug administration:

1. Right patient
2. Right drug
3. Right dose
4. Right route
5. Right time

In recent years, the concern for increasing medication errors has produced a sixth right:

6. Right *documentation*

Right Patient

When administering a drug, you must be certain that the patient receiving the drug is the patient for whom the drug has been ordered. It is important to use two methods to identify the patient before administering the medication. Identifiers can include visual as well as verbal methods. A visual identifier may include checking the patient's name on his or her wristband (Fig. 2.1). If there is no written identification verifying the patient's name, you should obtain a wristband or other form of identification before administering the drug. You may also ask the patient to identify him- or herself and request another unique identifier such as date of birth. However, do not ask, "Are you Mr. Jones?" Some patients, particularly those who are confused or have difficulty hearing, may respond by answering "yes" even though that is not their name. Some long-term care or rehabilitation care facilities have pictures of the patient available, which allows

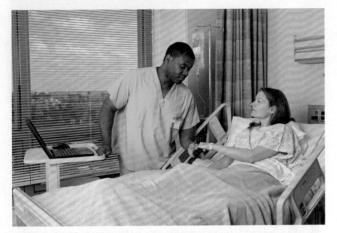

Figure 2.1 In following the "five + 1 rights" of medication administration, you always verify that the "right patient" is receiving the medication by using two identifiers, one of which is checking the patient's identification bracelet.

the nurse to verify the correct patient. If pictures are used to identify patients, it is critical that they are recent and bear a good likeness of the individual.

Right Drug

Drug names can be confused, especially when the names sound similar or the spellings are similar. Hurriedly preparing a drug for administration or failing to look up questionable drugs can put you at increased risk for administering the wrong drug. Appendix B identifies examples of drugs that can easily be confused. An error in drug name or amount can be found when you compare the medication administration record (MAR): (1) with the container label, (2) as the item is removed from the cart, and (3) before the actual administration of the drug (Fig. 2.2).

Right Dose, Right Route, and Right Time

Written orders are obtained from a primary health care provider for the administration of all drugs. The primary health care provider's order must include the patient's name, the drug name, the dosage form and route, the dosage to be administered, and the frequency of administration. The primary health care provider's signature must follow the drug order. In an emergency, you may administer a drug with a verbal order from the primary health care provider. However, the primary health care provider must write and sign the order as soon as the emergency is over.

If a verbal order is given over the telephone, write down the order, repeat back the information exactly as written, and then ask for a verbal confirmation that it is correct. Any order that is unclear should be questioned, particularly unclear directions for the administration of the drug, illegible handwriting on the primary health care provider's order sheet, or a drug dose that is higher or lower than the dosages given in approved references.

Right Documentation

After the administration of any drug, record the process immediately (Fig. 2.3). Immediate documentation is particularly important when drugs are given on an as-needed (PRN) basis. For example, most analgesics require 20 to 30 minutes before the drug begins to relieve pain. A patient may forget that he or she received a drug for pain, may not understand that the administered drug was for pain, or may not know that pain relief is not immediate, and may ask another nurse for the drug again. If the administration of the analgesic was not recorded, the patient might receive a second dose of the analgesic shortly after the first dose. This kind of situation can be extremely serious, especially when opioids or other central nervous system depressants are administered. Immediate documentation prevents accidental administration of a drug by another individual. Proper documentation is essential to the process of administering drugs correctly.

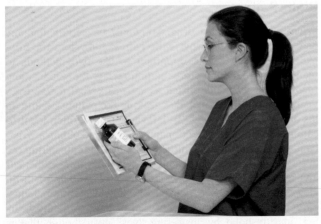

Figure 2.2 Before administering the medication, compare the medication, the container label, and the medication record to ensure that the patient receives the "right drug" and the "right dose."

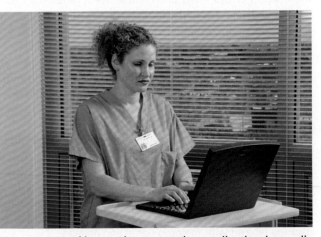

Figure 2.3 Always document the medication immediately after the drug is administered.

General Principles of Drug Administration

Considerations in Drug Administration

You must have factual knowledge of each drug, the reasons for use of the drug, the drug's general action, the more common adverse reactions associated with the drug, special precautions in administration (if any), and the normal dose ranges before you administer the drug to a patient.

When drugs are given frequently, you will become familiar with their pharmacologic information. Yet, when drugs are given less frequently or when a new drug is introduced, you should obtain information from reliable sources, such as the drug package insert, Internet sources, or the hospital department of pharmacy. It is important to check current and approved references for all drug information.

Take patient considerations, such as allergy history, previous adverse reactions, patient comments, and change in patient condition, into account before administering the drug. Before giving any drug for the first time, ask the patient about any known allergies and any family history of allergies. This includes allergies not only to drugs but also to food, pollen, animals, and so on. Patients with a personal or family history of allergies are more likely to experience additional allergies and must be monitored closely.

If the patient makes any statement about the drug or if there is any change in the patient, these situations are carefully considered before the drug is given. Examples of situations that require consideration before a drug is given include:

- Problems that may be associated with the drug, such as nausea, dizziness, ringing in the ears, and difficulty walking. Any comments made by the patient may indicate the occurrence of an adverse reaction. Withhold the drug until references are consulted and the primary caregiver contacted. The decision to withhold the drug must have a sound rationale and be based on knowledge of pharmacology.
- Patient or family comments stating that the drug looks different from the one previously received, that the drug was just given by another nurse, or that the patient thought the primary health care provider discontinued the drug therapy.
- A change in the patient's condition, a change in one or more vital signs, or the appearance of new symptoms. Depending on the drug being administered and the patient's diagnosis, these changes may indicate that the drug should be withheld and the primary health care provider contacted.

The Medication Order

Before a medication can be administered in a hospital or other agency, you must have a physician's order. Medications are ordered by the primary health care provider, such as a physician, dentist, or, in some cases, an advanced nurse practitioner. Common orders include the standing order, the single order, the PRN order, and the STAT (to be done immediately) order. See Display 2.1 for an explanation of each.

Display 2.1 Types of Medication Orders

Standing Order: This type of order is pre-established and approved for use by nurses and other health care providers under specific conditions in the absence of a health care provider. They may be drug orders for presurgical/procedure or postsurgical/procedure nursing care. *Example:* Cefotetan 1 gram IV 30 minutes preoperatively

Single order: An order to administer the drug one time only. *Example:* Valium 10 mg IM at 10:00 a.m.

PRN order: An order to administer the drug as needed. *Example:* Percocet 1–2 tablets orally q 4 hr PRN for pain

STAT order: A one-time order given as soon as possible. *Example:* Morphine 10 mg IV STAT for cardiac pain

---

Preparing a Drug for Administration

When preparing a drug for administration, observe the following guidelines:

- Always check the health care provider's written orders and verify any questions with the primary health care provider before preparing the medication.
- Be alert for drugs with similar names. Some drugs have names that sound alike but are very different (see Appendix B). To give one drug when another is ordered could have serious consequences.
- Perform hand hygiene immediately before preparing a drug for administration. Do not let your hands touch medication, especially topical preparations that you may absorb through the tissue of the hands.
- Always check and compare the label of the drug with the MAR three times: (1) when the drug is taken from its storage area, (2) immediately before removing the drug from the container, and (3) before administering the drug to the patient.
- Never remove a drug from an unlabeled container or from a package whose label is illegible. Do not remove the wrappings of the unit dose until the drug reaches the bedside of the patient who is to receive it. After administering the drug, document immediately on the MAR drug record.
- Never crush tablets or open capsules without first checking with the clinical pharmacist. Some tablets can be crushed or capsules can be opened and the contents added to water or a tube feeding when the patient cannot swallow a whole tablet or capsule. Some tablets have a special coating that delays the absorption of the drug. Crushing the tablet may destroy the drug's properties and result in problems such as improper absorption of the drug or gastric irritation. Capsules are gelatin and dissolve on contact with a liquid. The contents of some capsules do not mix well with water and therefore are best left in the capsule. If the patient cannot take an oral tablet or capsule, consult the primary health care provider because the drug may be available in liquid form.

• Never give a drug that someone else has prepared. The individual preparing the drug must administer the drug.
• Place drugs requiring special storage in the storage area immediately after they are prepared for administration. This rule applies mainly to drugs that need refrigeration, but may also apply to drugs that must be protected from exposure to light or heat.

Preventing Medication Errors

Medication errors include any event or activity that can cause a patient to receive the wrong dose, the wrong drug, an incorrect dosage of the drug, a drug by the wrong route, or a drug given at the incorrect time. Errors may occur in transcribing medication orders, when the drug is dispensed, or in administration of the drug. As a nurse and the medication administrator, you serve as the last defense against medication errors. When a medication error occurs, report it immediately so that any necessary steps to counteract the action of the drug or any observation can be made as soon as possible. In most institutions, if you made the error or discovered the error you must complete an unusual occurrence report and notify the primary care provider. It is important to report errors even when the patient suffers no harm.

Medication errors occur when one or more of the five + 1 rights have not been followed. Each time a drug is prepared and administered, the five + 1 rights must be a part of the procedure. In addition to consistently practicing the five + 1 rights, you should adhere to the following precautions to help prevent drug errors:

• Confirm any questionable orders.
• When calculations are necessary, verify them with another nurse.
• Listen to the patient when he or she questions a drug, the dosage, or the drug regimen.
• Never administer the drug until the patient's questions have been adequately researched.
• Avoid distractions and concentrate on only one task at a time.

A significant number of errors can be made during administration of a drug. Errors most commonly occur because of a failure to administer a drug that has been ordered, administration of the wrong dose or strength of a drug, or administration of a drug at the wrong time. Two drugs often associated with errors are insulin and heparin.

Innovative nurses are using various methods to study and reduce medication errors in cost-effective ways. Workplace distractions are one of the biggest issues being addressed by these nurses. Bright vests, mats on the floor, and "Do Not Disturb" signs are used to help lessen the number of people who interrupt the nurse as medications are being prepared and given to patients. An example is illustrated in Figure 2.4.

A number of agencies have instituted policies and practices to help in the reporting and reduction of errors. These practices (termed *Just Culture*) focus on finding the system problem, not punishing the person who made the error. Therefore, it is even more important for you and other nurses to report errors and omissions so problems can be discovered and changed.

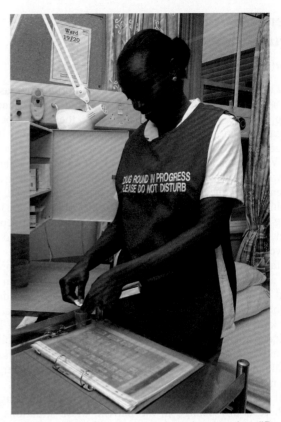

Figure 2.4 Reducing interruptions by wearing "Do Not Disturb" apparel is a cost-effective way to reduce drug errors.

National Patient Safety Goals

To evaluate the safety and quality of care provided by various accredited health care organizations, the Joint Commission establishes National Patient Safety Goals (NPSG) on a yearly basis. These goals are established to help accredited organizations address specific areas of concern with regard to patient safety. Several of these goals directly affect medication administration. For example, one of the first goals written that affects medication safety was the 2009 NPSG requiring improvement in the accuracy of patient identification. To meet this goal, institutions were required to use the two-identifier rule, where two methods must be used to identify the patient (other than the patient's room number) when administering medication or blood products. Another important standard that institutions desiring accreditation must follow is to compile a list of abbreviations, symbols, and acronyms *not* to be used throughout the institution. The Joint Commission has developed its own list of abbreviations that may no longer be used in any written medical documents (e.g., care plans, medical orders, nurses' notes). This list is referred to as the "minimum list." See Table 2.1 for the official "Do Not Use" list. Facilities accredited by the Joint Commission are required to be in compliance with the National Patient Safety Standards. Current information on these standards can be found at the Joint Commission website (http://www.jointcommission.org/standards_information/npsgs.aspx).

The list of error-prone abbreviations shown in Table 2.2 includes more abbreviations that are easily misinterpreted;

Table 2.1 Joint Commission Official "Do Not Use" List*

Abbreviation	Potential Problem	Use Instead
U (unit)	Mistaken as 0 (zero), 4 (four), or "cc"	Write "unit"
IU (international unit)	Mistaken as IV (intravenous) or 10 (ten)	Write "international unit"
Q.D., QD, q.d., qd (daily)	Mistaken for each other	Write "daily" and "every other day"
Q.O.D., QOD, q.o.d., qod (every other day)	The period after the "Q" can be mistaken for an "I" and the "O" can be mistaken for "I"	
Trailing zero (X.0 mg)†	Decimal point is missed	Write X mg
Lack of leading zero (.X mg)		Write 0.X mg
MS	Can mean morphine sulfate or magnesium sulfate	Write "morphine sulfate" or "magnesium sulfate"
MSO₄ and MgSO₄	Confused for one another	

*Applies to all orders and medication-related documentation that is handwritten (including free-test computer entry) or on preprinted forms.

†Exception: A "trailing zero" may be used only where required to demonstrate the level of precision of the value being reported, such as for laboratory results, imaging studies that report size of lesions, or catheter/tube sizes. It may not be used in medication orders or other medication-related documentation.

© The Joint Commission, 2012 Reprinted with permission.

therefore, providers are attempting to standardize terminology to reduce error.

The Institute for Safe Medication Practices

The Institute for Safe Medication Practices (ISMP) is a nonprofit organization devoted to the study of medication errors and their prevention. In addition to offering safety and educational information, it contains a section called the Medication Errors Reporting Program. This program is designed to identify the number and type of drug errors occurring around the country. It is a program similar to the MedWatch program of the U.S. Food and Drug Administration (FDA). The goal of this voluntary reporting system is to collect data and disseminate information that will prevent such errors in the future. A link to the report form may be found online at http://www.ismp.org/. You are urged to participate in this important program as a means of protecting the public by identifying ways to make drug administration safer.

Drug Distribution Systems

Primary or specialty providers order drugs for administration. Pharmacists dispense the medications, and nurses carry out the actual administration. Several drug distribution systems are available to be used to carry out the process. A brief description of three methods follows.

Unit Dose System

The **unit dose** system is a method in which drug orders are filled and medications dispensed to fill each patient's medication orders for a 24-hour period. The pharmacist dispenses each dose (unit) in a package that is typically labeled by the manufacturer and contains one tablet or capsule, a premeasured amount of a liquid drug, a prefilled syringe, or one suppository. Enough packaged drug for 1 day is placed in drawers in a special portable medication cart with a drawer for each patient. If the drug does not come individually packaged, a clinical pharmacist also may prepare unit doses. The pharmacy restocks the cart each day with the drugs needed for the next 24-hour period. If the cart is portable, you will take the drug cart to each patient's room. Once every 24 hours, it goes back to the pharmacy to be refilled and for new drug orders to be placed.

Table 2.2 Error-Prone Abbreviations

> (greater than) < (less than)	Misinterpreted as the number "7" or the letter "L"; confused with one another	Write "greater than" or "less than"
Abbreviations for drug names	Misinterpreted because of similar abbreviations for multiple drugs	Write drug names in full
Apothecary units	Unfamiliar to many practitioners; confused with metric units	Use metric units
@	Mistaken for the number "2" (two)	Write "at"
cc (cubic centimeter)	Mistaken for U (units) when poorly written	Write "mL" for milliliters
μg (microgram)	Mistaken for mg (milligrams), resulting in 1000-fold overdose	Write "mcg" or "micrograms"

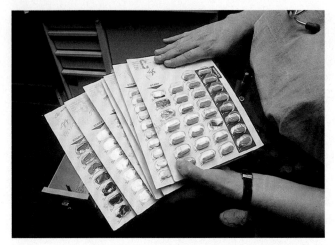

Figure 2.5 Multiunit dose packs, frequently used for medication administration in long-term care settings.

In facilities where patients may stay for a long time, such as long-term care, the drug may be packaged using a multiunit dose method. With this system, individual doses are "bubble" packed onto a card that may hold up to 60 individual doses (Fig. 2.5). Cards are labeled for individual patients and may hold 1 to 2 months' supply of a drug. These cards are then stored in slots for individual patients in a locked medication cart. When administering a drug, obtain the patient's card and pop the individual dose out of the card, returning the card with its remaining doses to the medication cart.

Automated Medication Management System

Automated or computerized management systems (Fig. 2.6) are used in most hospitals or agencies distributing drugs. Drug orders are managed in the pharmacy from physician

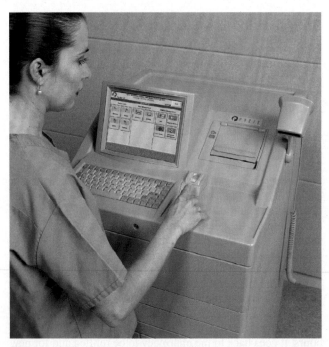

Figure 2.6 An automated medication system.

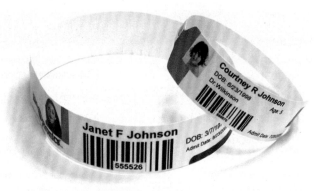

Figure 2.7 Bar-coded, point-of-care patient wrist bands used for medication administration.

orders that are sent from the individual floors or units. Each floor or unit has a medication station in which medications are placed in specific drawers. Medications are individually packaged as in the unit dose system. The difference is that there is more drug in the tray if a number of patients are prescribed the same medication. Once the order is entered into the system, you may enter the patient's name and the drug to be administered at the unit's automated medication station. The drawer with the specific drug opens for you to remove the drug, and then using a computer touch screen, the dose is automatically recorded into the computerized system. Print out this information for individual patients as their MAR if the facility uses paper charting.

Bar-Coded Point-of-Care Medication System

Some hospitals use a bar-code scanner in the administration of drugs. This system is the most effective way to reduce medication administration errors. To use this system, a bar code is placed on the patient's hospital identification band when the patient is admitted to the hospital (Fig. 2.7). The bar codes, along with bar codes on the drug unit dose packages, are used to identify the patient and to record and charge routine and PRN drugs. Additionally, provider identification badges are scanned during the procedure, thus identifying the nurse giving the medication. The scanner also keeps an ongoing inventory of controlled substances, which eliminates the need for controlled substance counts at the end of each shift.

Because of the serious consequences of administering the wrong drug, newer and more sophisticated automated systems to administer drugs are being constantly researched to provide the best safety to patients.

Administration of Drugs by the Oral Route

The oral route is the most frequent route of drug administration and rarely causes physical discomfort in patients. Oral drug forms include tablets, capsules, and liquids. Some capsules and tablets contain sustained-release drugs, which dissolve over an extended period. Administration of oral drugs is relatively easy for patients who are alert and can swallow.

Nursing Responsibilities

Observe the following points when giving an oral drug:

- Verify that the patient is able to swallow and is not nauseated or vomiting. Place the patient in an upright position. It is difficult, as well as dangerous, to swallow a solid or liquid when lying down.
- Assess the patient's need for assistance in holding the tablet or capsule or holding a glass of water. Some patients with physical disabilities cannot handle or hold these objects and may require assistance.
- Make sure that a full glass of water is readily available. Advise the patient to take a few sips of water before placing a tablet or capsule in the mouth.
- Instruct the patient to place the pill or capsule on the back of the tongue and tilt the head back to swallow a tablet or slightly forward to swallow a capsule. Encourage the patient first to take a few sips of water to move the drug down the esophagus and into the stomach, and then to finish the whole glass.
- Give the patient any special instructions, such as drinking extra fluids or remaining in bed, that are pertinent to the drug being administered.
- Never leave a drug at the patient's bedside to be taken later unless there is a specific order by the primary care provider to do so. Some units, such as postpartum, may offer self-administered medications. A few drugs (e.g., antacids or stool softeners) may be ordered to be left at the bedside.
- Patients with a nasogastric feeding tube or gastrostomy tube (also called the enteral route) may be given their oral drugs through the tube. Before administration, check the tube for placement. Dilute and flush liquid drugs through the tube. However, crush tablets and dissolve them in water before administering them through the tube. Flush the tube with water after the drugs are placed in the tube to clear the tubing completely.

- Instruct the patient to place buccal drugs in the mouth against the mucous membranes of the cheek in either the upper or lower jaw. They are absorbed slowly from the mucous membranes of the mouth. Examples of drugs given buccally are lozenges and troches.
- Certain drugs are also given by the sublingual (placed under the tongue) route. These drugs must not be swallowed or chewed and must be dissolved completely before the patient eats or drinks. Nitroglycerin is commonly given sublingually.

Infrequent Dosing of Drugs

Soon, many drugs will be available for once-a-week, or even once-a-year, administration. The doses are designed to replace daily doses of drugs. One of the first was alendronate (Fosamax), a drug used to treat osteoporosis (see Chapter 30). In 2001, the FDA approved two strengths for this drug to be given once a week. In clinical trials, once-a-week dosing showed no greater adverse reactions than the once-daily regimen. Since that time other drugs have been developed for dosing infrequently. A similar product, ibandronate (Boniva), is administered once a month for the treatment of osteoporosis. Infrequent dosing may prove beneficial for those experiencing mild adverse reactions in that the reactions would be experienced less frequently than every day.

Administration of Drugs by the Parenteral Route

Parenteral drug administration entails giving a drug by the **intradermal, subcutaneous, intramuscular (IM),** or **intravenous (IV)** route (Fig. 2.8). Other routes of parenteral administration that may be used by the primary health care provider are intradural (into the dural space of the spine), intra-arterial (into an artery), intracardiac (into the heart), and intra-articular (into a joint). In some instances, intra-arterial drugs are

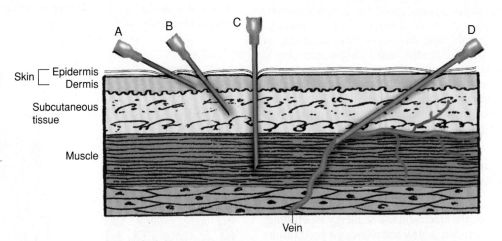

Figure 2.8 Needle insertion for parenteral drug. (**A**) Intradermal injection: a 26-gauge, 3/8-inch-long needle is inserted at a 10-degree angle. (**B**) Subcutaneous injection: a 25-gauge, 1/2-inch-long needle is inserted at an angle (45 to 90 degrees) that depends on the size of the patient. (**C**) Intramuscular injection: a 20- to 23-gauge, 1- to 3-inch-long needle is inserted into the relaxed muscle at a 90-degree angle with a quick (dart-throwing) type of hand movement. (**D**) Intravenous injection: the diameter (18 to 26 gauge) of the needle used depends on the substance to be injected and on the site of injection.

administered by a nurse. However, administration is not by direct arterial injection but by means of a catheter that has been placed in an artery.

Nursing Responsibilities

Observe the following points when giving a drug by the parenteral route:

- Wear gloves for protection from the potential of a blood spill when giving parenteral drugs. The risk of exposure to infected blood is increasing for all health care workers. The Centers for Disease Control and Prevention (CDC) recommends that gloves be worn when touching blood or body fluids, mucous membranes, or any broken skin area. This recommendation is referred to as **Standard Precautions**, which combine the Universal Precautions for Blood and Body Fluids with Body Substance Isolation guidelines.
- After selecting the site for injection, cleanse the skin. Most hospitals have a policy regarding the type of skin antiseptic used for cleansing the skin before parenteral drug administration. Cleanse the skin with a circular motion, starting at an inner point and moving outward.
- When administering medications such as penicillin, aspirate before injecting. After inserting the needle for IM administration, pull back the syringe barrel to aspirate the drug. Aspirate for 5 to 10 seconds. If blood is in a small vessel, it takes time for the blood to appear. If blood appears in the syringe, remove the needle so the drug is not injected. Discard the drug, needle, and syringe and prepare another injection. If no blood appears in the syringe, inject the drug. Aspiration is not necessary when injecting vaccines or immunizations IM or giving an intradermal or subcutaneous injection.
- After removing the needle from an IM, subcutaneous, or IV injection site, place pressure on the area. Patients with bleeding tendencies often require prolonged pressure on the area.
- Most hospitals use needles designed to prevent needle-stick injuries. This needle has a plastic guard that slips over the needle and locks in place as it is withdrawn from the injection site.
- Do not recap syringes, and dispose of them according to agency policy. Discard needles and syringes into clearly marked, appropriate containers to prevent needle-stick injuries. Most agencies have a "sharps" container located in each room for immediate disposal of needles and syringes after use. Proper disposal protects the nurse and others from injury and contamination.

Administration of Drugs by the Intradermal Route

Drugs given by the intradermal route are usually those for sensitivity tests (e.g., the tuberculin test or allergy skin testing; see Fig. 2.8A). Absorption is slow and allows for good results when testing for allergies.

Nursing Responsibilities

Observe the following points when administering drugs by the intradermal route:

- The inner part of the forearm and the upper back may be used for intradermal injections. The area should be hairless;

areas near moles or scars or pigmented skin areas should be avoided. Cleanse the area in the same manner as for subcutaneous and IM injections.
- A 1-mL syringe with a 25- to 27-gauge needle that is 1/4 to 5/8 inch long is best suited for intradermal injections. Small volumes (usually smaller than 0.1 mL) are used for intradermal injections and administered with the bevel up.
- Insert the needle at a 15-degree angle between the upper layers of the skin. Do not aspirate the syringe or massage the area. Injection produces a small wheal (raised area) on the outer surface of the skin. If a wheal does not appear on the outer surface of the skin, there is a good possibility that the drug entered the subcutaneous tissue, and any test results would be inaccurate.

Administration of Drugs by the Subcutaneous Route

A subcutaneous injection places the drug into the tissues between the skin and the muscle (see Fig. 2.8B). Drugs administered in this manner are absorbed more slowly than IM injections. Drugs for blood thinning and diabetes are commonly given by the subcutaneous route.

Nursing Responsibilities

Observe the following points when giving a drug by the subcutaneous route:

- A volume of 0.5 to 1 mL is used for subcutaneous injection. Larger volumes (e.g., more than 1 mL) are best given as IM injections. If a volume larger than 1 mL is ordered through the subcutaneous route, the injection is given in two sites, with separate needles and syringes.
- The sites for subcutaneous injection are the upper arms, the upper abdomen, and the upper thighs. The back is less frequently used (Fig. 2.9). Rotate injection sites to ensure proper absorption and minimize tissue damage.

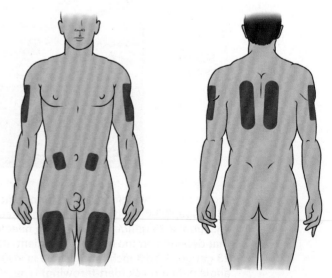

Figure 2.9 Sites on the body at which subcutaneous injections can be given.

• When giving a drug by the subcutaneous route, insert the needle at a 45-degree angle. However, to place the drug in the subcutaneous tissue, select the needle length and angle of insertion based on the patient's body weight. Obese patients have excess subcutaneous tissue, and it may be necessary to give the injection at a 90-degree angle. If the patient is thin or cachectic, there usually is less subcutaneous tissue. For such patients, the upper abdomen is the best site for injection. Generally, a syringe with a 23- to 25-gauge needle that is 3/8 to 5/8 inch in length is most suitable for a subcutaneous injection.

• When administering a subcutaneous medication, aspiration is not required. Should blood appear in the syringe, withdraw the needle, discard the syringe, and prepare a new injection.

Administration of Drugs by the Intramuscular Route

An IM injection is the administration of a drug into a muscle (see Fig. 2.8C). Drugs that are irritating to subcutaneous tissue can be given by IM injection. Drugs given by this route are absorbed more rapidly than drugs given by the subcutaneous route because of the rich blood supply in the muscle. In addition, a larger volume (1 to 3 mL) can be given at one site.

Nursing Responsibilities
The nurse should observe the following points when giving a drug by the IM route:

• If an injection is more than 3 mL, divide the drug and give it as two separate injections. Volumes larger than 3 mL will not be absorbed properly.
• A 22-gauge needle that is 1½ inches in length is most often used for IM injections.
• The sites for IM administration are the deltoid muscle (upper arm), the ventrogluteal or dorsogluteal sites (hip), and the vastus lateralis (thigh). See Figure 2.10 for IM injection sites. The vastus lateralis site is frequently used for infants and small children because it is more developed

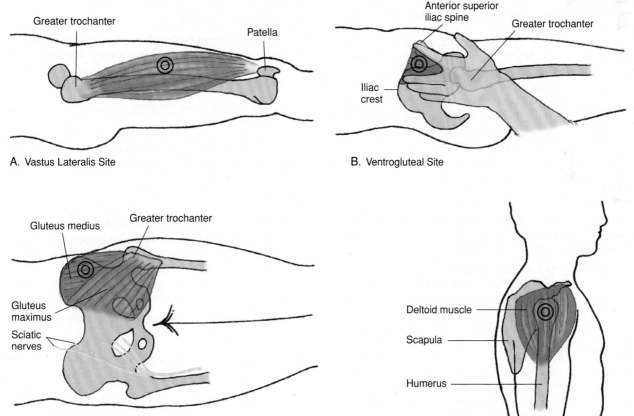

Figure 2.10 Sites for intramuscular administration. (**A**) Vastus lateralis site: the patient is supine or sitting. (**B**) Ventrogluteal site: your palm is placed on the greater trochanter and the index finger is placed on the anterior superior iliac spine; the injection is made into the middle of the triangle formed by your fingers and the iliac crest. (**C**) Dorsogluteal site: to avoid the sciatic nerve and accompanying blood vessels, choose an injection site above and lateral to a line drawn from the greater trochanter to the posterior superior iliac spine. (**D**) Deltoid site: the mid-deltoid area is located by forming a rectangle, the top of which is at the level of the lower edge of the acromion, and the bottom of which is at the level of the axilla; the sides are one third and two thirds of the way around the outer aspect of the patient's arm.

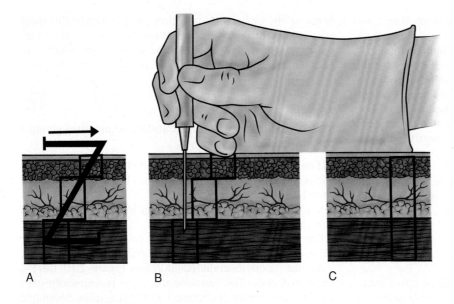

Figure 2.11 Z-track injection. (**A**) The tissue is tensed laterally at the injection site before the needle is inserted. This pulls the skin, subcutaneous tissue, and fat planes into a "Z" formation. (**B**) After the tissue has been displaced, the needle is thrust straight into the muscular tissue. (**C**) After injection, tissues are released while the needle is withdrawn. As each tissue plane slides by the other, the track is sealed.

than the gluteal or deltoid sites. In children who have been ambulating for more than 2 years, the ventrogluteal site may be used.

- When giving a drug by the IM route, insert the needle at a 90-degree angle. When injecting a drug into the ventrogluteal or dorsogluteal muscles, it is a good idea to place the patient in a comfortable position, preferably in a prone position with the toes pointing inward. When injecting the drug into the deltoid, a sitting or lying-down position may be used. Place the patient in a recumbent position for injection of a drug into the vastus lateralis.

Z-Track Technique

The *Z-track* technique of IM injection is used when a drug is highly irritating to tissues or has the ability permanently to stain the skin. The nurse should adhere to the following procedure when using the Z-track technique (Fig. 2.11):

- Draw the drug up into the syringe.
- Discard the needle and place a new needle on the syringe. This prevents any solution that may remain in the needle (that was used to draw the drug into the syringe) from contacting tissues as the needle is put into the muscle.
- Pull the plunger down to draw approximately 0.1 to 0.2 mL of air into the syringe. The air bubble in the syringe follows the drug into the tissues and seals off the area where the drug was injected, thereby preventing oozing of the drug up through the extremely small pathway created by the needle.
- Place the patient in the correct position for administration of an IM injection.
- Cleanse the skin.
- Pull the skin, subcutaneous tissues, and fat (that lie over the injection site) laterally, displacing the tissue to the side (approximately 1 inch).
- While holding the tissues in the lateral position, insert the needle at a 90-degree angle and inject the drug.
- After the drug is injected, wait 10 seconds to permit the medication to disperse into the muscle tissue, and then release the tissue while withdrawing the needle. This technique prevents the backflow of drug into the subcutaneous tissue.

Administration of Drugs by the Intravenous Route

A drug administered by the IV route is injected directly into the blood by a needle inserted into a vein. Drug action occurs almost immediately. Drugs administered by the IV route may be given:

- Slowly, over 1 or more minutes
- Rapidly (IV push)
- By piggyback/syringe pump infusions (drugs are mixed with 50 to 100 mL of compatible IV fluid and administered during a period of 30 to 60 minutes piggybacked onto the primary IV line)
- Into an existing IV line (the IV port)
- Into an intermittent venous access device called a *heparin or saline lock* (a small IV catheter in the patient's vein; the catheter is connected to a small fluid reservoir with a rubber cap through which the needle is inserted to administer the drug)
- By being added to an IV solution and allowed to infuse into the vein over a longer period

For explanation of the procedure and nursing responsibilities see Chapter 54.

Other Parenteral Routes of Drug Administration

The primary care provider may administer a drug by the intracardial, intra-arterial, or intra-articular routes. You may be responsible for preparing the drug for administration. If so, ask the primary health care provider what special materials will be required for administration.

Venous access ports are totally implanted ports with a self-sealing septum that is attached to a catheter leading to a large vessel, usually the vena cava. These devices are most commonly used for chemotherapy or other long-term therapy and require surgical insertion and removal. Drugs are administered through injections made into the portal through the skin. These drugs are administered by the primary health care provider or a registered nurse.

Administration of Drugs Through the Skin and Mucous Membranes

Drugs may be applied to the skin and mucous membranes using several routes: topically (on the outer layers of skin), transdermally through a patch on which the drug has been implanted, or inhaled through the membranes of the upper respiratory tract.

Administration of Drugs by the Topical Route

Most topical drugs act on the skin but are not absorbed through the skin. These drugs are used to soften, disinfect, or lubricate the skin. A few topical drugs are enzymes that have the ability to remove superficial debris, such as the dead skin and purulent matter present in skin ulcerations. Other topical drugs are used to treat minor, superficial skin infections. The various forms of topical applications and locations of use are described in Display 2.2.

Nursing Responsibilities

Consider the following points when administering drugs by the topical route:

- The primary care provider may write special instructions for the application of a topical drug—for example, to apply the drug in a thin, even layer or to cover the area after application of the drug to the skin.
- Other drugs may have special instructions provided by the manufacturer, such as to apply the drug to a clean, hairless area or to let the drug dissolve slowly in the mouth. All of these instructions are important because drug action may depend on correct administration of the drug.
- Ointments are sometimes used and come with a special paper marked in inches. Measure the correct length (onto

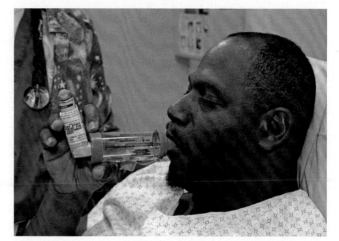

Figure 2.12 A respiratory inhalant is used to deliver a drug directly into the lungs. To deliver a dose of the drug, the patient takes a slow, deep breath while depressing the top of the inhaler's canister. (*Photo by Rick Brady.*)

the paper), place the paper with the drug ointment side down on the skin, and secure it with tape. Before the next dose, remove the paper and tape and cleanse the skin.

Administration of Drugs Through Inhalation

Drug droplets, vapor, and gas are administered through the mucous membranes of the respiratory tract using a face mask, nebulizer, or positive-pressure breathing machine. Examples of drugs administered through **inhalation** include bronchodilators, mucolytics, and some anti-inflammatory drugs. These drugs primarily produce a local effect in the lungs.

Nursing Responsibilities

The primary nursing responsibility with drugs administered by inhalation is to provide the patient with proper instructions for administering the drug. For example, many patients with asthma use a metered-dose inhaler to dilate the bronchi and make breathing easier. Without proper instruction on how to use the inhaler, much of the drug can be deposited on the tongue rather than in the respiratory tract. This decreases the therapeutic effect of the drug. Instructions may vary with each inhaler. To be certain that the inhaler is used correctly, refer the patient to the instructions accompanying each device. Figure 2.12 illustrates the proper use of one type of inhaler.

Administration of Drugs by the Transdermal Route

Drugs administered by the **transdermal** route are readily absorbed from the skin and provide systemic effects. This type of administration is called a *transdermal drug delivery system* (Fig. 2.13). The drug dosages are implanted in a small, patch-type bandage and the drug is gradually absorbed into the systemic circulation. This type of drug system maintains a relatively constant blood concentration and reduces the possibility of toxicity. In addition, the administration of drugs

---

Display 2.2 Topical Applications and Locations of Use

- Creams, lotions, or ointments applied to the skin with a tongue blade, gloved fingers, or gauze
- Sprays applied to the skin or into the nose or oral cavity
- Liquids inserted into body cavities, such as fistulas
- Liquids inserted into the bladder or urethra
- Solids (e.g., suppositories) or jellies inserted into the urethra
- Liquids dropped into the eyes, ears, or nose
- Ophthalmic ointments applied to the eyelids or dropped into the lower conjunctival sac
- Solids (e.g., suppositories, tablets), foams, liquids, and creams inserted into the vagina
- Continuous or intermittent wet dressings applied to skin surfaces
- Solids (e.g., tablets, lozenges) dissolved in the mouth
- Sprays or mists inhaled into the lungs
- Liquids, creams, or ointments applied to the scalp
- Solids (e.g., suppositories), liquids, or foams inserted into the rectum

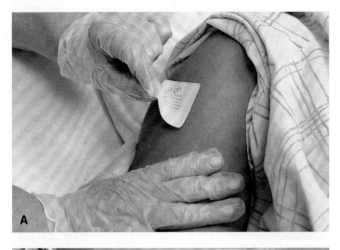
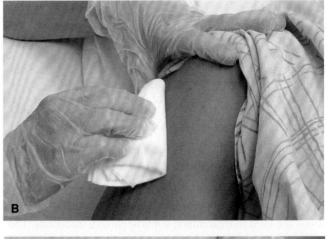
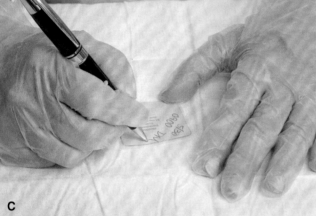
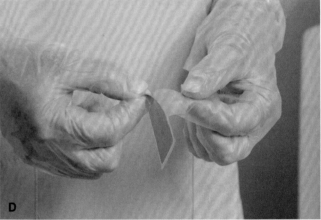
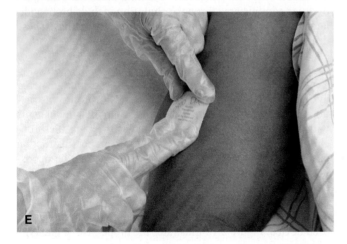

Figure 2.13 Transdermal drug delivery system. (**A**) Find and remove a previously placed patch. (**B**) Cleanse application site. (**C**) Record date, time, and initials on the new patch. (**D**) Remove protective covering. (**E**) Apply new patch to hairless area of skin.

transdermally causes fewer adverse reactions, and administration is less frequent than when the drugs are given by another route. Duragesic (used to treat severe pain) and Ortho Evra (used as birth control) are two drugs given frequently by the transdermal route. See Figure 2.13 for the application of transdermal medications.

Nursing Responsibilities

Observe the following points when administering drugs by the transdermal route:

• Wear gloves to prevent accidental exposure to the medication.

• Remove all old patches to prevent added dosing of the drug, fold sticky sides together, and discard in sharp container (if not available, flush down a toilet)—do not place in waste container.
• Choose a dry, hairless area of intact skin large enough for the patch to fit smoothly.
• Rotate sites for transdermal patches to prevent skin irritation. The chest, abdomen, buttocks, and upper arm are the most commonly used sites. Do not shave the area to apply the patch; shaving may cause skin irritation.
• Use the back between the shoulder blades for patients with dementia who are likely to remove the patch by themselves.

Nursing Responsibilities after Drug Administration

After the administration of any type of drug, you are responsible for the following:

- Record the administration of the drug. Complete this task as soon as possible. This is particularly important when PRN drugs (especially opioids) are given.
- Record (when necessary) any information concerning the administration of the drug. This includes information such as the IV flow rate, the site used for parenteral administration, problems with administration (if any), and vital signs taken immediately before administration.
- Evaluate and record the patient's response to the drug. Evaluation may include such facts as relief of pain, decrease in body temperature, relief of itching, and decrease in the number of stools passed.
- Observe for adverse reactions. The frequency of these observations depends on the drug administered. Record all suspected adverse reactions and report them to the primary care provider. Immediately report serious adverse reactions to the primary care provider.

Administration of Drugs in the Home

Often, drugs are not administered by the nurse in the home setting, but rather by the patient or family members serving as caregivers. When this is the case, it is important that the patient or caregivers understand the treatment regimen and are given an opportunity to ask questions concerning the drug therapy, such as why the drug was prescribed, how to administer the drug, and adverse reactions of the drug (see Chapter 5 for information concerning patient and family education). When a patient is taking a drug at home, special equipment or items may be needed in the home to administer the drug. Patient Teaching for Improved Patient Outcomes: Assessing the Home for Safe Drug Use gives some guidelines to follow when drugs are administered in the home by the patient or caregiver, rather than by the nurse.

Administration of Drugs (side tab)

Patient Teaching for Improved Patient Outcomes

Assessing the Home for Safe Drug Use

For most patients, drugs will be prescribed after discharge to be taken at home. Because the home is not a controlled environment like a health care facility, you should assess the patient's home environment carefully to ensure complete safety. It is important to keep in mind the following when making a home safety assessment:

- ✔ Does the home have a space for medicines that is relatively free of clutter and easily accessible to the patient or a caregiver?
- ✔ Do any small children live in or visit the home? If so, is there a place where drugs can be stored safely out of their reach?
- ✔ Does the drug require refrigeration? If so, does the refrigerator work?
- ✔ If the patient needs several drugs, can the patient or caregiver identify which drugs are used and when? Do they know how to use them and why?
- ✔ Does the patient need special equipment, such as needles and syringes? If so, where and how can the equipment be stored for safety and convenience? Does the patient have an appropriate disposal container? Will the refuse be safe from children and pets?
  - ■ Suggest using plastic storage containers with snap-on lids made especially for home syringe disposal.
  - ■ Advise the patient to use an impervious container with a properly fitting lid, such as a plastic milk jug, for safe disposal of needles.
  - ■ Advise the patient of Sharps Disposal Programs in the area. These may be at local pharmacies, police and fire stations, or local health care centers.

KEY POINTS

- The nurse administering the drug is responsible for all steps in preparing the drug including the right (correct) patient, drug, dose, route, and time. You will document the administration immediately upon giving the drug to prevent inadvertent drug errors.
- Standard practice is to use two identifiers (means to identify who the patient is) before administering a medication. The patient room number should never be used as one of the patient identifiers.
- Be aware that drug names may look or sound alike.
- When taking medication orders, confirm verbal orders with a "read back" confirmation and make efforts to get

the orders in writing before the drug is administered. Always question unclear orders before administration.

- Nurses are the last defense in preventing medication errors before the drug is administered. Using methods to reduce distraction and better identify patients and drugs helps to reduce errors.
- Automation and use of bar coding in the administration of medications helps reduce drug errors.
- Medications are given orally, parenterally, through the skin, or by inhalation. Many drugs can be given by multiple routes to best meet patient needs. Each method has specific steps associated with it to ensure the best absorption of the medication.

● Chapter Review
● Prepare for the NCLEX-PN

Build Your Knowledge

1. The nurse correctly documents administration of a drug
   _____.
   1. at the beginning of the shift
   2. when preparing to give the drug
   3. immediately after giving the drug
   4. at the end of the shift

2. The nurse is to administer aspirin 325 mg now. This is
   an example of what type of order?
   1. standing order
   2. single order
   3. PRN order
   4. STAT order

3. An IM injection is correctly administered by _____.
   1. displacing the skin to the side before making the
      injection
   2. using a 1-inch needle
   3. inserting the needle at a 90-degree angle
   4. using a 25-gauge needle

4. When preparing a drug for subcutaneous administration,
   the nurse should be aware that the usual volume of a
   drug injected by the subcutaneous route is _____.
   1. less than 0.5 mL
   2. 0.5 to 1 mL
   3. 2 to 5 mL
   4. 3 to 4 mL

5. The nurse explains to a client receiving an IV injection
   that the action of the drug occurs _____.
   1. in 5 to 10 minutes
   2. in 15 to 20 minutes
   3. within 30 minutes
   4. almost immediately

6. The best placement of a transdermal patch for a client
   with dementia is the _____.
   1. abdomen
   2. back
   3. chest
   4. upper arm

Apply Your Knowledge

7. A new long-term care center is being built and the nurse
   is requested to help in planning the medication administration system. Which is the best, most cost-effective
   system to use to prevent errors in this facility?
   1. automated dispensing medication carts
   2. bar-code identification bracelets
   3. "Do Not Distract" apparel
   4. two-identifier patient system

8. When administering a drug, the nurse _____.
   1. should check the drug label two times before admin-
      istration
   2. ask the client to identify him- or herself
   3. may administer a drug prepared by another nurse
   4. may crush any tablet that the patient is unable to
      swallow

Alternate-Format Questions

9. Identify selected items the nurse uses as part of the
   "five rights" of medication administration. **Select all
   that apply**.
   1. right language
   2. right route
   3. right patient
   4. right time

10. Identify which items you can use for client identifica-
    tion before giving a medication. **Select all that apply**.
    1. client room number
    2. medical record number
    3. date of birth
    4. maiden name of client

To check your answers, see Appendix G.

the**Point** *For more NCLEX-style questions, log on to
http://thepoint.lww.com to access more than 1000 questions.*

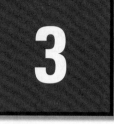

Making Drug Dosing Safer

LEARNING OBJECTIVES

On completion of this chapter, the student will:

1. Describe how safety is provided by the use of systematic processes in drug administration.
2. Identify information on a drug label used for calculating drug dosages.
3. Describe the importance of labeling numbers during the calculation process.
4. Accurately perform mathematical calculations when they are necessary to compute drug dosages.

KEY TERMS

denominator • part of a fraction representing the total number of parts (the number under the line)

dimensional analysis • newer method of calculating drug dosages based on fractions

dosage strength • amount of drug in the given form, such as tablet or capsule

gram • mass metric measure equivalent to one thousandth of a kilogram

liter • metric measure of volume, roughly equivalent to a quart in household measure

manual redundancy system • process of medication prescription and delivery in which each person checks the drug dosage for accuracy

meter • metric measure of distance

metric system • system of measurement based on units of 10

numerator • part of a fraction representing the number of parts taken (the number above the line)

solvent • fluid in which a solid dissolves; also called the diluent

Accurate dosage calculations are critical to the health of a patient who is receiving medications. When drugs are administered, it is important that the numbers used and the answers obtained are correct. Unlike an error on a math test in school, there is no partial credit for simple arithmetic errors or incomplete answers in dosage conversions and calculations. Harm, and even death, can result from an error in a drug dosage calculation.

Information about the process of drug preparation for administration and calculation is examined in this chapter. Many textbooks are designed to teach the methodology of dosage calculations; this chapter is meant to teach the process involved in obtaining and preparing the dose of the drug and includes math as a review and supplement to that instruction. Examples of drug dose calculations are provided throughout the ensuing chapters to test your ability to properly complete the math. Answers can be found in Appendix G.

Systematically Checking Accuracy

It has been estimated that 1 in 10,000 hospital deaths occur each year in the United States owing to mistakes made *specifically when calculating a drug dosage*. Often these miscalculations are because of human error. Factors in the work environment often contribute to errors made by people. These factors include poor lighting, noise, interruptions, and a taxing workload. We should be aware of all of these elements of our environment when preparing or calculating any drug regardless of how minor the dose or type of drug.

Technological changes such as computerized order entry and bar-coding systems can detect errors made by health care providers. However, the best method of error detection is the **manual redundancy system**. This is a system in which each person in the process of medication prescription and delivery checks the drug dosage for accuracy. Nurses use this system when they perform the "5 rights and 3 checks" to catch a potential error in drug administration. Although nurses may not be responsible for the initial mixing, packaging, or delivery of a medication, 95% of potential dose calculation errors are found during manual redundancy checks. When a nurse checks the dose calculation of a drug, during preparation or at the bedside, a serious error can be detected before it reaches the patient.

Calculating Drug Doses Safely

You should always systematically look at the process of drug delivery to calculate drug doses safely and do the following:

1. Recognize the way drugs are packaged and how to look for the information on the labels needed to calculate drug doses.
2. Look at the orders and how these are presented on the medication administration record (MAR).

The focus of this chapter is to help you learn to recognize essential information from drug labels. Basic mathematical calculations are provided in Appendix F if you need to review them.

Reading Drug Labels

Drug labels give important information used to obtain the correct dosage. Although labels contain a great amount of information about the drug being given, three specific items are needed to administer a drug: the name, form, and dosage strength.

Drug labels may contain two names: the trade (brand) name and the generic name (see Chapter 1). The trade name is usually capitalized, written first on the label, and identified by the registration symbol. The generic name is written in smaller print, often in parentheses, and usually located under the trade name. Drugs may be prescribed by either the trade name or the generic name. Often the generic drug is less expensive than the brand-name drug. If the primary health care provider does not specify that a substitution *cannot* be made, it is likely that a generic version of the drug will be dispensed to reduce the cost to the patient. Problems can arise if a patient recognizes the brand name of a drug but does not know the generic name and refuses the medication (companies that make generic-only drugs do not include a trade name on the label). Therefore, it is important to know the generic name of drugs and always check for brand-name versions if the patient questions the prescription.

QUESTION #1

Looking at the label in Figure 3.1, what are the brand and generic names of this drug? (*See Appendix G for answer.*)

The unit dose is the most common type of labeling seen in hospitals. The unit dose is a method of dispensing drugs in which each capsule or tablet is packaged separately. On the label, the type of preparation will be specified; in other words, it will list the drug as a capsule, tablet, or other form of the drug.

At times the drug will come to the nursing unit in a container with a number of capsules or tablets or as a solution. The nurse must then determine the number of capsules/tablets or the amount of solution to administer. Therefore, the nurse must know the amount of drug in each tablet or capsule (**dosage strength**). The dosage strength is also given on the container. The dosage strength is used to calculate the number of tablets or the amount of solution to administer.

QUESTION #2

Looking at the label in Figure 3.1, find the form of the drug and the dosage strength. (*See Appendix G for answer.*)

Mathematical Ability

Nurses find that mathematical calculations are performed using various methods to prepare drugs for administration. Sometimes the math is relatively simple, and a calculation can be done quickly in one's head. When distractions are present or if conversions are involved, the nurse may use a pen and paper to handwrite out the mathematical equations needed to determine the correct dose. A nurse may use a number of steps in the calculation of a medication and find that a calculator is helpful to hasten the process. When using any of these methods, it is important for the nurse to understand the basic concepts of the dose calculation to ensure the right answer is obtained.

In the remainder of this chapter a variety of calculation methods are presented. Try the calculations with the different formulas to discover the best way you calculate drug doses. See Appendix F for a review of basic mathematical concepts if you have difficulty understanding the math involved with the calculations.

Basic Formula Method of Dosage Calculation

Once the nurse has identified the basic information about the drug, the calculation can be performed to prepare the drug.

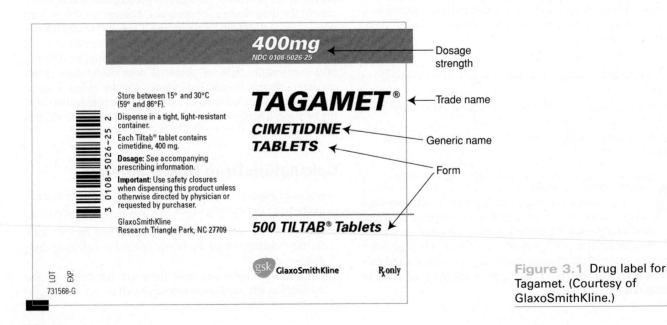

Figure 3.1 Drug label for Tagamet. (Courtesy of GlaxoSmithKline.)

CALCULATION #1

Looking at the label in Figure 3.1, use this information to solve the following dose problem:

The primary health care provider orders: 400 mg of cimetidine after each meal. How many tablets will the nurse administer following breakfast? (*See Appendix G for answer.*)

Although most hospital pharmacies dispense drugs as single doses or in a unit dose system, on occasion you must compute a drug dosage because it differs from the dose of the drug that is available. This is particularly true of long-term care facilities, of outpatient clinics, and in the home where the dose may be changed periodically or in situations in which having multiple dosage strengths of a particular drug for the patient would be costly.

CALCULATION #2

Looking at the label in Figure 3.1, use this information to solve the following dose problem:

The primary health care provider changes the order after late morning rounds: 800 mg of cimetidine after each meal. How many tablets will the nurse administer after meals? (*See Appendix G for answer.*)

Some nurses can do this type of calculation in their heads; others find it helpful to do the problem by hand on paper. This is especially helpful when the dosage ordered by the primary health care provider may not be available.

Basic Formula Method by Hand

To find the correct dosage of a solid oral preparation, the following formula may be used:

$$\frac{\text{dose desired}}{\text{dose on hand}} = \text{dose administered (the unknown or X)}$$

This formula may be abbreviated as:

$$\frac{D}{H} = X$$

When the dose ordered by the primary health care provider (dose desired) is written in the same *measurement* as the dose on the drug container (dose on hand) (e.g., they are both milligrams), then these two figures may be inserted into the formula without changes.

EXAMPLE

The primary health care provider orders cimetidine 800 mg (milligrams). The drug is available as cimetidine 400 mg (milligrams).

$$\frac{D}{H} = X$$

$$\frac{800\,\text{mg (dose desired)}}{400\,\text{mg (dose on hand)}} = 2 \text{ tablets of 400 mg cimetidine}$$

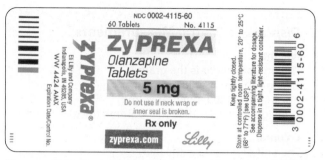

Figure 3.2 Drug label for Zyprexa. (Courtesy of Lilly Company.)

QUESTION #3

Use the label in Figure 3.2 to solve the following problem.

Looking at the label, find the drug name, form, and dosage strength. (*See Appendix G for answer.*)

CALCULATION #3

Looking at the label in Figure 3.2, use this information to solve the following dose problem:

The primary health care provider orders: 10 mg Zyprexa daily. How many tablets will the nurse administer? (*See Appendix G for answer.*)

Understanding the Metric System of Measurement

If the primary health care provider orders ascorbic acid (vitamin C) 0.5 g, and the drug container label reads ascorbic acid 250 mg, a *conversion of grams to milligrams* (because the drug container is labeled in milligrams) would be necessary before the basic formula can be used. Therefore, it is important for the nurse to understand the **metric system** of measurement.

There are three systems of measurement associated with drug dosing: (1) the metric system, (2) the apothecary system, and (3) household measurements.

The metric system is the most commonly used system of measurement in medicine. The metric system uses decimals (or the decimal system). In the metric system, the **gram** is the unit of weight, the **liter** the unit of volume, and the **meter** the unit of length. Display 3.1 lists the measurements used in the metric system. The abbreviations for the measurements are given in parentheses.

The apothecary system at one time was used for weight measurement. In 1994, recommendations were made by the Institute for Safe Medication Practices (ISMP) to eliminate this system due to the high rate of medication errors it produced (information about this system can be found in Appendix F). The household system is rarely used in a hospital setting but may be used to measure drug dosages in the home.

Making Drug Dosing Safer

Display 3.1 Metric Measurements

Weight
The unit of weight is the gram.
1 kilogram (kg) = 1000 grams (g)
1 gram (g) = 1000 milligrams (mg)
1 milligram (mg) = 1000 micrograms (mcg)

Volume
The unit of volume is the liter.
1 deciliter (dL) = 10 liters (L)
1 liter (L) = 1000 milliliters (mL)
1 milliliter (mL) = 0.001 liter (L)

Length
The unit of length is the meter.
1 meter (m) = 100 centimeters (cm)
1 centimeter (cm) = 0.01 meter (m)
1 millimeter (mm) = 0.001 meter (m)

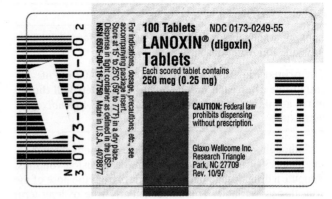

Figure 3.3 Drug label for Lanoxin. (Courtesy of GlaxoSmithKline.)

$$\frac{1000\,mg}{1\,g} = \frac{X\,mg}{0.5\,g}$$

$$X = 1000 \times 0.5$$
$$X = 500\ mg$$

Therefore, 0.5 gram (g) equals 500 milligrams (mg). After changing 0.5 g to 500 mg, use the basic method formula:

$$\frac{D}{H} = X$$

$$\frac{500\,mg}{250\,mg} = 2 \text{ tablets of 250 mg ascorbic acid}$$

Ratio and Proportion Method of Dosage Calculation

Converting Units for Calculation

When using the basic formula, the **numerator** and the **denominator** must be of like terms—for example, milligrams over milligrams or grams over grams. To set up a problem, a fraction must be stated in *like terms;* therefore, proportion may be used to convert grams to milligrams.

NURSING ALERT

Errors made by nurses in using this and other drug formulas will be reduced if the entire dose is labeled rather than just writing the numbers.

$$\frac{0.5\,g}{250\,mg} \text{ rather than } \frac{0.5}{250}$$

This will eliminate the possibility of using unlike terms in the fraction.

In the aforementioned example, where the order read ascorbic acid 0.5 g and the drug container was labeled ascorbic acid 250 mg, a conversion of grams to milligrams is necessary to perform the dose calculation. A nurse may be able to perform this calculation without writing it down. If it is done by hand, the proportion and a known equivalent are set up in a ratio and used for this type of conversion.

Ratio and Proportion Method by Hand

EXAMPLE

Convert 0.5 gram (g) to milligrams (mg); using proportion and the known equivalent 1000 mg = 1 g, set up the ratio:

$$1000\ mg : 1\ g :: X\ mg : 0.5\ g$$
$$X = 1000 \times 0.5$$
$$X = 500\ mg$$

or

Safeguard in Preventing Errors

To prevent dose calculation errors, many manufacturers include both levels of measurement (grams and milligrams) on the label if the drug is frequently ordered in doses different from the size dispensed (Fig. 3.3). This is very important when doses are in small amounts such as micrograms (mcg). Again, manufacturers typically include the dose strength in both units of measurement (milligrams and micrograms). Even when both are included, the nurse should perform the calculation to double check that the dose is correct.

Errors are a frequent problem when zeros (0) are involved. When there is no number to the left of the decimal, a zero is written, for example, 0.25. Although in general mathematics the zero may not be required, it should be used in the writing of all drug doses. *Use of the zero lessens the chance of drug errors,* especially when the dose of a drug is hurriedly written and the decimal point is indistinct.

For example, if a drug order is written as digoxin (Lanoxin) **.25 mg** instead of digoxin **0.25 mg**, the order might be interpreted as **25 mg**, which is 100 times the prescribed dose.

QUESTION #4

Use the label in Figure 3.3 to understand the following example.

Looking at the label, find the drug name, form, and dosage strength in both units of measurement. (*See Appendix G for answer.*)

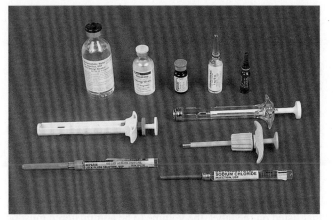

Figure 3.4 Drug preparations in solution form: (top row) vials and ampules; (middle/bottom rows) prefilled cartridges and holders.

CALCULATION #4

Looking at the label in Figure 3.3, use this information to solve the following dose problem:

The primary health care provider orders: 0.50 mg of digoxin daily. How many tablets will the nurse administer? (*See Appendix G for answer.*)

Drugs in Liquid Form

Drugs may be ordered in liquid form for many reasons: The patient is a child, the drug is to be put in a feeding tube or injected directly into the tissues or intravenous (IV) line, or the patient is too ill to swallow a solid form of the drug like a tablet. In these situations, the drug is made in a solution form.

Solutions

A solute is a substance dissolved in a **solvent** to make a solution. Usually, water is used as the solvent for preparing a solution unless another liquid is specified. Today, most solutions are prepared by a clinical pharmacist or the manufacturer and not by the nurse. It is important for the nurse to understand how the solutions will be prepared and labeled.

Examples of how solutions may be labeled include:

- 10 mg/mL—10 mg of the drug in each milliliter
- 1:1000—a solution denoting strength of 1 part of the drug per 1000 parts of solvent
- 5 mg/teaspoon—5 mg of the drug in each teaspoon of solution (home use)

Parenteral Drug Dosage Forms

Drugs for parenteral use must be in liquid form before they are administered. Parenteral drugs may be available in the following forms (Fig. 3.4):

1. As liquids in disposable cartridges or disposable syringes that contain a specific amount of a drug in a specific volume, for example, meperidine 50 mg/mL. After administration, the cartridge or syringe is discarded.
2. In ampules or vials that contain a specific amount of the liquid form of the drug in a specific volume. The vials may be single-dose vials or multidose vials. A multidose vial contains more than one dose of the drug.
3. In ampules or vials that contain powder or crystals, to which a liquid (called a diluent) must be added before the drug can be removed from the vial and administered. Vials may be single-dose or multidose vials.

Dose Calculations with Liquids

With drugs in liquid form, there is a specific amount of drug in a given volume of solution. Look at Figure 3.5. In this example, the dosage strength of Augmentin is 125 mg in 5 mL of solution (typically written as 125 mg/5 mL). Instead of labeling the drug in one unit of measure (tablet or capsule), the drug is written as a specific amount of drug in a specific *quantity* of solution. For example, if the label states that there is 125 mg/5 mL, 5 mL is the *quantity* (or volume) in which there is 125 mg of this drug.

 NURSING ALERT

Use "mL" instead of "ml" when writing the abbreviation for milliliters. This prevents the error of ml being misread as m 1 or meter 1.

The basic formula for computing the dosage of liquids is:

$$\frac{\text{dose desired}}{\text{dose on hand}} \times \text{quantity} = \text{volume administered}$$

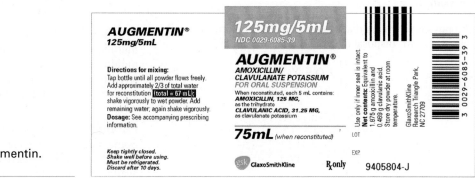

Figure 3.5 Drug label for Augmentin. (Courtesy of GlaxoSmithKline.)

Making Drug Dosing Safer

This may be abbreviated as

$$\frac{D}{H} \times Q = X$$

The quantity (or Q) in this formula is the amount of liquid in which the available drug is contained.

QUESTION #5

Use the label in Figure 3.5 to understand the following example. **Looking at the label, find the drug name, form, and dosage strength.** (*See Appendix G for answer.*)

CALCULATION #5

Looking at the label in Figure 3.5, use this information to solve the following dose problem:

The primary health care provider orders: Augmentin 125 mg – 4 times daily. How many mL (milliliters) will the nurse administer in each dose? (*See Appendix G for answer.*)

As with tablets and capsules, the prescribed dose of the drug may not be the same as what is on hand (or available). For example, the primary health care provider may order 500 mg Augmentin and the drug is labeled as 125 mg/5 mL. The 5 mL is the amount (quantity or Q) that contains 125 mg of the drug.

$$\frac{D}{H} \times Q = X \quad \text{(the liquid amount to be given)}$$

$$\frac{500\,mg}{125\,mg} \times 5 = X$$

$$\frac{4}{1} \times 5 = 20\,mL$$

Therefore, 20 mL contains the desired dose of 500 mg of Augmentin.

Parenteral Drugs in Disposable Syringes or Cartridges

In some instances specific dosage strength is not available and it will be necessary to administer less than the amount contained in the syringe.

EXAMPLE

The physician orders diazepam 5 mg IM. The drug is available as a 2-mL disposable syringe labeled 5 mg/mL.

$$\frac{D}{H} \times Q = X$$

$$\frac{5\,mg}{10\,mg} \times 2\,mL = X$$

$$X = \frac{1}{2} \times 2 = 1\,mL$$

Note that because the syringe contains 2 mL of the solution and that *each* mL contains 5 mg of the drug, there is a total of 10 mg of the drug in the syringe. Because there is 10 mg of the drug in the syringe, half of the liquid in the syringe (1 mL) is discarded, and the remaining half (1 mL) is administered to give the prescribed dose of 5 mg.

Parenteral Drugs in Ampules and Vials

If the drug is in liquid form in the ampule or vial, the desired amount is withdrawn from the ampule or vial. In some instances, the entire amount is used; in others, only part of the total amount is withdrawn from the ampule or vial and administered.

Whenever the dose to be administered is different from that listed on the label, the volume to be administered must be calculated. To determine the volume to be administered, the formula for liquid preparations is used. The calculations are the same as those given in the preceding section for parenteral drugs in disposable syringes or cartridges.

EXAMPLE

The physician orders chlorpromazine 12.5 mg IM.

The drug is available as chlorpromazine 25 mg/1 mL in a 1-mL ampule.

$$\frac{D}{H} \times Q = X$$

$$\frac{12.5\,mg}{25\,mg} \times 1\,mL = X$$

$$\frac{1}{2} \times 1\,mL = \frac{1}{2}\,mL\,(\text{or } 0.5\,mL)\,\text{volume to be administered}$$

In this example, 0.5 mL is the amount of solution that contains the dose 12.5 mg of the drug. Using a syringe, 0.5 mL of the solution is withdrawn. Because you cannot store medications once an ampule has been opened, the remainder of the drug is discarded.

EXAMPLE

The physician orders hydroxyzine 12.5 mg. The drug is available as hydroxyzine 25 mg/mL in 10-mL vials.

$$\frac{D}{H} \times Q = X$$

$$\frac{12.5\,mg}{25\,mg} \times 1\,mL = \frac{1}{2}\,mL\,(\text{or } 0.5\,mL)$$

Using a syringe, 0.5 mL is withdrawn from the 10-mL multidose vial and administered. The amount in this or any multidose vial is *not* entered into the equation. What is entered into the equation as quantity (Q) is the amount of the available drug that is contained in a specific volume.

Parenteral Drugs in Dry Form

Some parenteral drugs are available as a crystal or a powder. Because these drugs have a short life in liquid form, they are available in ampules or vials in dry form and must be made into a solution (reconstituted) before they are removed and administered. Often the drug is in a container with both the powder and liquid separated by a barrier that is broken right before mixing and administering. If the drug is not dispensed in this form, the product directions for reconstitution on the label or on the enclosed package insert should be included with the drug. The manufacturer may give the following information for reconstitution: (1) the name of the diluent(s) that must be used with the drug, or (2) the amount of diluent that must be added to the drug.

In some instances, the manufacturer supplies a diluent with the drug. If a diluent is supplied, no other stock diluent should be used. Before a drug is reconstituted, the label is carefully checked for instructions.

EXAMPLES

Methicillin: To reconstitute a 1-g vial, add 2 mL of sterile water for injection or sodium chloride injection. Each reconstituted milliliter contains approximately 500 mg of methicillin. If there is any doubt about the reconstitution of the dry form of a drug, and there are no manufacturer's directions, the clinical pharmacist should be consulted.

Once a diluent is added, the volume to be administered is determined. In some cases, the entire amount is given; in others, a part (or fraction) of the total amount contained in the vial or ampule is given.

After reconstitution of any multidose vial, the following information *must* be added to the label:

• Amount of diluent added
• Dose of drug in mL (500 mg/mL, 10 mg/2 mL, etc.)
• Date of reconstitution
• Expiration date (the date after which any unused solution is discarded)

Dosage Calculation Using Dimensional Analysis

Dimensional analysis (DA) is a method to perform calculations where the focus is on the units of measure, thereby eliminating the need to memorize equations. Because the units are set up in a specific order, it eliminates the need to be concerned about setting up proportions correctly. When using DA to calculate dosage problems, dosages are written as common fractions. For example:

$$\frac{1\,mL}{4\,mg} \quad \frac{5\,mL}{10\,mg} \quad \frac{1\,tablet}{100\,mg}$$

When written as common fractions, the numerator is the top number. In the example above, 1 mL, 5 mL, and 1 tablet are the numerators.

The numbers on the bottom are called denominators. In the example above, 4 mg, 10 mg, and 100 mg are denominators.

EXAMPLE

The primary health care provider orders 10 mg of diazepam. The drug comes in a dosage strength of 5 mg/mL. How many milliliters would the nurse administer?

Step 1. To work this problem using DA, always begin by identifying the unit of measure to be calculated. The unit to be calculated will be milliliters if the drug is to be administered parenterally. Another drug form is the solid, and the unit of measure would be a tablet or capsule. In this problem, the unit of measure to be calculated is milliliters.

Step 2. Write the identified unit of measure to be calculated, followed by an equal sign. In this problem, milliliters is the unit to be calculated, so the nurse writes:

$$mL =$$

Step 3. Next, the dosage strength is written with the numerator *always expressed in the same unit that was identified before the equal sign.* For example:

$$mL = \frac{1\,mL}{5\,mg}$$

Step 4. Continue by writing the next fraction with the numerator having the same unit of measure as the denominator in the previous fraction.

For example, our problem continues:

$$mL = \frac{1\,mL}{5\,mg} \times \frac{10\,mg}{X\,mL}$$

Step 5. The problem is solved by multiplication of the two fractions.

$$mL = \frac{1\,mL}{5\,mg} \times \frac{10\,mg}{X\,mL} = \frac{10\,mg}{5X\,mL} = 2\,mL$$

NOTE: Each alternate denominator and numerator cancel, with only the final unit remaining.

EXAMPLE

Ordered: 200,000 Units

On hand: Drug labeled 400,000 Units/mL

$$mL = \frac{1\,mL}{400,000\,U} \times \frac{200,000\,U}{X\,mL} = \frac{1}{2}\,mL\,or\,0.5\,mL$$

Metric Conversions Using Dimensional Analysis

Occasionally, the primary health care provider may order a drug in one unit of measure, whereas the drug is available in another unit of measure.

EXAMPLE

The physician orders 0.4 mg of atropine. The drug label reads 400 mcg per 1 mL. This dosage problem is solved by expanding the DA equation, by adding one step to the equation.

Step 1. As above, begin by writing the unit of measure to be calculated, followed by an equal sign.
Step 2. Next, express the dosage strength as a fraction with the numerator having the same unit of measure as the number before the equal sign.

$$mL = \frac{1 \, mL}{400 \, mcg}$$

Step 3. Continue by writing the next fraction with the numerator having the same unit of measure as the denominator in the previous fraction.

$$mL = \frac{1 \, mL}{400 \, mcg} \times \frac{mcg}{mg}$$

Step 4. Expand the equation by filling in the missing numbers using the appropriate equivalent. In this problem, the equivalent would be 1000 mcg = 1 mg. This will convert micrograms to milligrams.

$$mL = \frac{1 \, mL}{400 \, mcg} \times \frac{1000 \, mcg}{1 \, mg}$$

Repeat Steps 3 and 4. Continue with the equation by placing the next fraction, beginning with the unit of measure of the denominator of the previous fraction.

$$mL = \frac{1 \, mL}{400 \, mcg} \times \frac{1000 \, mcg}{1 \, mg} \times \frac{0.4 \, mg}{X \, mL}$$

When possible, cancel out the units, leaving only mL.

Step 5. Solve the problem by multiplication. Cancel out the numbers when possible.

$$mL = \frac{1 \, mL}{400 \, mcg} \times \frac{1000 \, mcg}{1 \, mg} \times \frac{0.4 \, mg}{X \, mL} = \frac{400}{400X} = 1 \, mL$$

Solve the following problems using DA. Refer to the equivalents table if necessary (see Display 3.1).

EXAMPLE

Ordered: 250 mg
On hand: Drug labeled 1 g per 1 mL

$$mL = \frac{1 \, mL}{1 \, g} \times \frac{1 \, g}{1000 \, mg} \times \frac{250 \, mg}{X \, mL} = \frac{1 \, mL}{4} = \text{or } 0.25 \, mL$$

Selected Methods Used in Calculation of Drug Dosages

Pediatric Dosages

The dosages of drugs given to children are usually less than those given to adults. The dosage may be based on age, weight, or body surface area (BSA). Today, most pediatric dosages are clearly given by the manufacturer, thus eliminating the need for formulas, except for determining the dosage of some drugs based on the child's weight or BSA.

Drug Dosages Based on Weight

The dosage of an oral or parenteral drug may be based on the patient's weight. In many instances, references give the dosage based on the weight in kilograms (kg) rather than pounds (lb) (to convert pounds to kilograms you need to know the conversion equivalent, 2.2 lb = 1 kg).

When the dosage of a drug is based on weight, the primary health care provider or clinical pharmacist, in most instances, computes and orders the dosage to be given. However, errors can occur for any number of reasons. The nurse should be able to calculate a drug dosage based on weight to detect any type of error that may have been made in the prescribing or dispensing of a drug whose dosage is based on weight.

EXAMPLE

To convert a known weight in pounds to kilograms, divide the known weight by 2.2.
Patient's weight in pounds is 135:

$$135/2.2 = 61.36 \text{ (or } 61.4) \, kg$$

CALCULATION #6

Determine the patient's weight in kilograms when the patient weighs 142 lb. (*See Appendix G for answer.*)

Determine the child's weight in kilograms when the child weighs 43 lb. (*See Appendix G for answer.*)

Once the weight is converted to pounds or kilograms, this information is used to determine drug dosage.

EXAMPLE

A drug dosage is 5 mg/kg/day. The patient weighs 135 lb, which is converted to 61.4 kg.

$$61.4 \, kg \times 5 \, mg = 307 \, mg$$

Proportions also can be used:

$$5 \, mg : 1 \, kg :: X \, mg : 61.4 \, kg$$

$$X = 307 \, mg$$

A drug dosage is 60 mg/kg/day in three equally divided doses. The patient weighs 143 lb, which is converted to 65 kg.

$$65 \, kg \times 60 \, mg = 3900 \, mg/day$$

$$3900 \, mg \div 3 \text{ (doses per day)} = 1300 \, mg \text{ each dose}$$

Body Surface Area

If the drug dosage is based on body surface area (m^2), the same method of calculation may be used.

Charts (called nomograms, see Appendix F) are used to determine the BSA in square meters according to the child's height and weight. Once the BSA is determined, the following formula is used:

$$\frac{\text{surface area of the child in square meters}}{\text{surface area of an adult in square meters}} \times \text{usual adult dose} = \text{pediatric dose}$$

EXAMPLE

A drug dosage is 60 mg/m^2 as a single IV injection.
The BSA of a patient is determined by means of a nomogram for estimating BSA and is found to be 1.8 m^2. The physician orders 60 mg/m^2.

$$60 \, mg \times 1.8 \, m^2 = 108 \, mg$$

Proportion can also be used:

$$60 \, mg : 1 \, m^2 :: X \, mg : 1.8 \, m^2$$

$$X = 108 \, mg$$

Display 3.2 Household Measurements

3 teaspoons = 1 tablespoon
2 tablespoons = 1 ounce
2 pints = 1 quart
4 quarts = 1 gallon

Temperatures

Two scales used in the measuring of temperatures are Fahrenheit (F) and Celsius (C) (also known as centigrade). On the Fahrenheit scale, the freezing point of water is 32°F, and the boiling point of water is 212°F. On the Celsius scale, 0°C is the freezing point of water and 100°C is the boiling point of water.

To convert from Celsius to Fahrenheit, the following formula may be used: F = 9/5 C + 32 (9/5 times the temperature in Celsius, then add 32).

EXAMPLE

Convert 38°C to Fahrenheit:

$$F = \frac{9}{5} \times 38° + 32$$
$$F = 68.4° + 32$$
$$F = 100.4°$$

To convert from Fahrenheit to Celsius, the following formula may be used: C = 5/9 (F − 32) (5/9 times the temperature in Fahrenheit minus 32).

EXAMPLE

Convert 100°F to Celsius:

$$C = \frac{5}{9} \times (100 - 32)$$
$$C = \frac{5}{9} \times 68$$
$$C = 37.77 \, or \, 37.8°$$

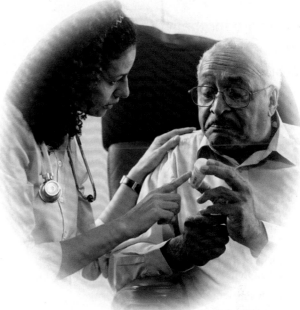

Figure 3.6 Nurses are primarily involved in the administration component of drug therapy, yet they hold great responsibility in helping the entire team provide safe patient care and correct calculation of drug doses.

Household Measurements

When used, household measurements are for liquids or powders to make solutions only. In the hospital, household measurements are rarely used because they are inaccurate when used to measure drug dosages. On occasion, the nurse may use the pint, quart, or gallon when ordering, irrigating, or sterilizing solutions or stock solutions. For the ease of a patient taking a drug at home, the physician may order a drug dosage in household measurements. Display 3.2 lists the more common household measurements.

KEY POINTS

- One in every 10,000 hospital deaths is a result of a drug calculation error.
- Nurses systematically and repeatedly check for drug accuracy by performing the "5 rights and 3 checks" when preparing to administer drugs to patients. Ninety-five percent of the time, an error will be found before the medication is given to the patient.
- Drug labels should always contain the name, form, and strength of a drug.
- The metric system is the preferred dose system. Household measures may be used to simplify administration by family members in the home, and the apothe-

cary system is rarely seen due to the higher rate of drug errors when used.
- Nurses use basic, dimensional analysis, and ratio/proportion formulas to calculate drug doses.
- Numbers are always labeled (0.25 mg) when doing a calculation, especially if conversion between units is done. For safety purposes zeros before decimal points (0.25) should be used, as well as "mL" for milliliters.
- Use specified diluents to make powders into solutions when needed, and always discard unused ampules. Vials should be dated when opened and solutions specified if mixed by the nurse.

● Chapter Review
● Prepare for the NCLEX-PN

Build Your Knowledge

1. Manual redundancy activities help the nurse provide:
   1. control over dangerous drugs
   2. safety by recognizing error
   3. reassurance to the patient
   4. feedback to other providers

2. What percentage of potential drug errors is found when nurses check medication calculations for accuracy?
   1. 25%
   2. 49%
   3. 67%
   4. 95%

3. Identify the portion of this drug label in **bold**:
   LANOXIN (digoxin) **Tablets**, 250 mcg (0.25 mg).
   1. dose strength
   2. trade name
   3. generic name
   4. form

4. Knowing both trade and generic drug names is important because:
   1. cost is reduced using generic drugs
   2. only one name is provided on the drug label
   3. primary health care providers do not know the differences
   4. clients may think the drug is incorrect

5. The ISMP discourages use of which measurement system?
   1. household
   2. metric
   3. apothecary
   4. body surface area

6. Which of the following is the correct abbreviation for milligram?
   1. mg
   2. gm
   3. mL
   4. mcg

7. If the nurse has 2 mL remaining in an ampule. It should be _____.
   1. labeled and dated
   2. placed in the refrigerator
   3. thrown in a sharps container
   4. returned to client medication storage

Apply Your Knowledge

8. Which of the following drug doses is written correctly?
   1. Lanoxin .25 mg orally
   2. Lanoxin .250 mg orally
   3. Lanoxin 0.25 mg orally
   4. Lanoxin 0.250 mg orally

9. One gram of ascorbic acid (vitamin C) is equivalent to:
   1. 10,000 milligrams of ascorbic acid
   2. 1000 milligrams of ascorbic acid
   3. 100 milligrams of ascorbic acid
   4. 0.1 milligrams of ascorbic acid

10. A child weighs 53 lb. How many kilograms would the child weigh? (Round to the nearest whole number.)
    1. 0.23 kg
    2. 24 kg
    3. 54 kg
    4. 117 kg

To check your answers, see Appendix G.

the**Point** *For more NCLEX-style questions, log on to http://thepoint.lww.com to access more than 1000 questions.*

The Nursing Process

LEARNING OBJECTIVES

On completion of this chapter, the student will:

1. List the five phases of the nursing process.
2. Discuss assessment, analysis, nursing diagnosis, planning, implementation, and evaluation as they apply to the administration of drugs.
3. Differentiate between objective and subjective data.
4. Identify common nursing diagnoses used in the administration of drugs and nursing interventions related to each diagnosis.

KEY TERMS

analysis • using data to determine patient need or nursing diagnosis

assessment • collection of subjective and objective data

evaluation • decision-making process determining the effectiveness of nursing actions or interventions

expected outcome • expected behavior and physical and mental state of the patient after a therapeutic intervention

implementation • carrying out of a plan of action

independent nursing actions • actions that do not require a physician's orders

initial assessment • gathering of baseline data

nursing diagnosis • description of a patient problem

nursing process • framework for nursing action, consisting of a series of problem-solving steps, which helps members of the health care team provide effective and consistent patient care

objective data • information obtained through a physical assessment or physical examination, lab tests, or scans

ongoing assessment • continuing assessment activities that proceed from the initial nursing assessment

planning • design of steps to carry out nursing actions

subjective data • information supplied by the patient or family

The **nursing process** is a framework for nursing action consisting of problem-solving steps that help members of the health care team provide effective patient care. It is a specific and orderly plan used to gather data, identify patient problems from the data, develop and implement a plan of action, and then evaluate the results of nursing activities, including the administration of drugs.

The five phases of the process are used not only in nursing but also in daily life. For example, when buying a computer, first think about what type of device is needed, shop in several different stores to find out more about computer types and brands (**assessment**), and then determine what each store has to offer (**analysis**). At this point, decide exactly what computer to buy and how to pay for the computer (**planning**); then purchase the computer (**implementation**). After purchase and use, make the decision to keep or upgrade the computer (**evaluation**).

Using the nursing process requires practice, experience, and a constant updating of knowledge. It is not within the scope of this textbook to list all of the assessments, nursing diagnoses, plans, implementations, and evaluations for the vast number of nursing problems associated with the illness that require the administration of a specific drug. The nursing process is used in this text only as it applies to drug administration.

The Five Phases of the Nursing Process

Although the nursing process can be described in various ways, it generally consists of five phases: assessment, analysis (or formation of the **nursing diagnosis**), planning, implementation, and evaluation. Each part is applicable, with modification, to the administration of medications. Figure 4.1 relates the nursing process to administration of medications.

Assessment

Assessment involves collecting objective and subjective data. **Objective data** are facts obtained by means of a physical assessment or physical examination. **Subjective data** are facts supplied by the patient or the patient's family.

Assessments are both initial and ongoing. An **initial assessment** is made based on objective and subjective data collected when the patient is first seen in a hospital, ambulatory setting (clinic or health care provider's office), or long-term care facility. The initial assessment usually is more thorough and provides a database (sometimes called a *baseline*) against which later data can be compared and decisions made. The initial assessment provides information that is analyzed to identify problems that can be resolved or alleviated by nursing actions.

Objective data are obtained during an initial assessment through activities such as examining the skin, obtaining vital

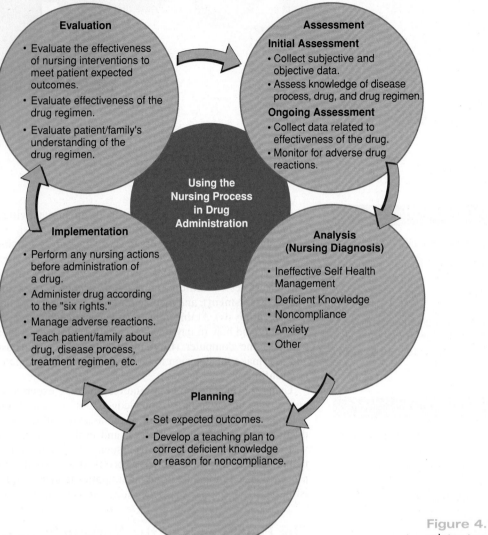

Figure 4.1 The nursing process as it relates to administration of medication.

signs, palpating a lesion, and auscultating the lungs. A review of the results of any recent laboratory tests and diagnostic studies also is part of the initial physical assessment. Subjective data are acquired during an initial assessment by obtaining information from the patient, such as a family history of disease, an allergy history, an occupational history, a description (in the patient's own words) of the current illness or chief complaint, a medical history, and a drug history. In addition to the prescription drugs that the patient may be taking, it is important to know the over-the-counter drugs, vitamins, or herbal therapies that the patient uses. For women of childbearing age, ask about the woman's pregnancy status and whether or not she is breastfeeding.

An **ongoing assessment** is one that is made at the time of each patient contact and may include the collection of objective data, subjective data, or both. The scope of an ongoing assessment depends on many factors, such as the patient's diagnosis, the severity of illness, the response to treatment, and the prescribed medical or surgical treatment.

The assessment phase (including the initial and ongoing assessment) of the nursing process can be applied to the administration of drugs, with objective and subjective data collected before and after to obtain a thorough baseline or initial assessment. This allows subsequent assessments to be compared with the baseline information. This comparison helps to evaluate the effectiveness of the drug and the presence of any adverse reactions. Ongoing assessments of objective and subjective data are equally important when administering drugs. Important objective data include blood pressure, pulse, respiratory rate, temperature, weight, appearance of the skin, appearance of an intravenous infusion site, and pulmonary status as assessed by auscultation of the lungs. Important subjective data include any statements made by the patient about relief or nonrelief of pain or other symptoms after administration of a drug.

The extent of the assessment and collection of objective and subjective data before and after a drug is administered depends on the type of drug and the reason for its use.

Analysis

Analysis is the way nurses cluster data into similar groupings to determine patient need. The data collected during assessment are examined for common threads; the nurse identifies the patient's needs (problems) and formulates one or more nursing diagnoses. A nursing diagnosis is not a medical diagnosis; rather, it is a description of the patient's problems and their probable or actual related causes based on the subjective and objective data in the database.

Nursing Diagnosis

A nursing diagnosis identifies problems that can be solved or prevented by **independent nursing actions**—actions that do not require a physician's order and may be legally performed by a nurse. Nursing diagnoses provide the framework and consistent language for selection of nursing interventions to achieve expected outcomes.

The North American Nursing Diagnosis Association-International (NANDA-I) was formed to standardize the terminology used for nursing diagnoses. NANDA-I continues to define, explain, classify, and research summary statements about health problems related to nursing. NANDA-I has approved a list of diagnostic categories to be used in formulating a nursing diagnosis. This list of diagnostic categories is periodically revised and updated.

In some instances, nursing diagnoses may apply to a specific group or type of drug or a particular patient. One example is Deficient Fluid Volume related to active fluid volume loss (diuresis) secondary to administration of a diuretic. Specific drug-related nursing diagnoses are highlighted in each chapter. However, it is beyond the scope of this book to individualize care and provide every nursing diagnosis that you may use for all patients you may encounter related to a drug or a drug class.

Some of the nursing diagnoses developed by NANDA-I may be used to identify patient problems associated with drug therapy and are more commonly used when administering drugs. The most frequently used nursing diagnoses related to the administration of drugs include:

- Effective Self Health Management
- Ineffective Self Health Management
- Deficient Knowledge
- Noncompliance
- Anxiety

Because these nursing diagnoses are commonly used when all types of drugs are administered, they will not be repeated for each chapter. Keep these nursing diagnoses in mind when administering any drug. Expansion of nursing actions corresponding to these nursing diagnoses is featured later in this chapter.

Planning

After the nursing diagnoses are formulated, a patient-oriented goal and expected outcomes are developed for each nursing diagnosis. The goal statement is a broad expectation that will indicate the problem is resolved. An **expected outcome** is a direct statement of how patient goals are to be achieved. The expected outcome describes the maximum level of wellness that is reasonably attainable for the patient. For example, common expected patient outcomes related to drug administration, in general, include:

- The patient will effectively manage the drug regimen.
- The patient will understand the drug regimen.
- The patient will comply with the drug regimen.

The expected outcomes define the behavior of the patient or family that indicates the problem is being resolved or that progress toward resolution is occurring.

Selecting the appropriate interventions is based on the expected outcomes that help to develop a plan of action or patient care plan. Planning for nursing actions specific to the drug to be administered can result in greater accuracy in drug administration, enhanced patient understanding of the drug regimen, and improved patient adherence to the prescribed drug therapy after discharge from the hospital. For example, during the initial assessment interview, the patient may report an allergy to penicillin. This information is important, and you must now plan the best methods of informing all members of the health care team of the patient's allergy to penicillin.

The planning phase describes the steps for carrying out nursing activities or interventions that are specific and that will meet the expected outcomes. Planning anticipates the implementation phase or the carrying out of nursing actions that are specific to the drug being administered. If, for example, the patient is to receive a drug by the intravenous route, you must plan for the materials needed and the patient instruction for administration of the drug by this route. In this instance, the planning phase occurs immediately before the implementation phase and is necessary to carry out the technique of intravenous administration correctly. Failing to plan effectively may result in forgetting to obtain all of the materials necessary for drug administration.

Implementation

Implementation is the carrying out of a plan of action and is a natural outgrowth of the assessment and planning phases of the nursing process. When related to the administration of drugs, implementation refers to the preparation and administration of one or more drugs to a specific patient. Before administering a drug, review the subjective and objective data obtained on assessment and consider any additional data, such as blood pressure, pulse, or statements made by the patient. The decision of whether to administer the drug is based on an analysis of all information. For example, a patient is hypertensive and is supposed to receive a drug to lower the blood pressure. Objective data obtained at the time of admission (baseline) included a blood pressure of 188/110. Additional objective data obtained immediately before the administration of the drug (ongoing) included a blood pressure of 182/110. A decision is made by the nurse to administer the drug because the change in the patient's blood pressure is minimal. However, if the patient's blood pressure is 132/84, and this is only the second dose of the drug, the nurse could decide to withhold the drug and contact the prescribing health care provider. Giving or withholding a drug and contacting the patient's health care provider are nursing activities related to the implementation phase of the nursing process.

The more common nursing diagnoses used when administering drugs are Effective Self Health Management, Ineffective Self Health Management, Deficient Knowledge, and Noncompliance. Nursing interventions applicable to each of these nursing diagnoses are discussed in the following sections. However, each patient is an individual, and nursing care must be planned on an individual basis after a careful collection and analysis of the data. In addition, each drug is different and may have various effects in the body. (For drugs discussed in subsequent chapters, some possible nursing diagnoses related to that specific drug are featured.)

Effective Self Health Management

This nursing diagnosis takes into consideration that the patient is willing to participate and integrate into daily living the treatment of an illness, such as the self-administration of medications. For this nursing diagnosis to be used, the patient verbalizes the desire to manage the medication schedule. When the patient is willing and able to manage the treatment activities, he or she may simply need information concerning the drug, method of administration, what type of reactions to expect, and what to report to the primary health care provider. A patient willing to take responsibility may need you to develop a teaching plan that gives the patient the information needed to manage the treatment activities properly (see Chapter 5 for more information on educating patients).

Ineffective Self Health Management

NANDA-I defines Ineffective Self Health Management as "a pattern of difficulty integrating into daily living a program for treatment of illness and the sequelae of illness." In the case of medication administration, the patient may not be taking the medication correctly or following the medication schedule prescribed by the primary health care provider.

The reasons for not following the drug routine vary (Display 4.1). For example, some people do not fill their prescriptions because they do not have enough money to pay for them. Other patients skip doses, take the drug at the wrong times, or take an incorrect dose. Some may simply forget to take the drug; others take a drug for a few days, see no therapeutic effect, and quit.

When working with a patient who is not managing the drug routine correctly, assess the patient's level of health literacy

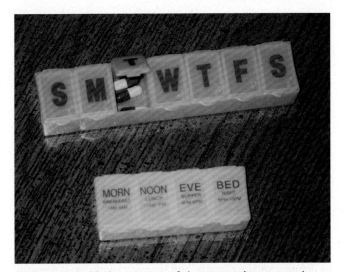

Figure 4.2 Various types of drug containers may be used to help individuals remember to take their medication at the correct time.

(see Chapter 5). If possible, allow the patient to administer the drug before the patient is dismissed from the health care facility. Determine if adequate funds are available to obtain the drug and any necessary supplies. For example, when a bronchodilator is administered by inhalation, a spacer or extender may be required for proper administration. This device is an additional expense. A referral to the social services department of the institution may help the patient when finances are a problem.

For those who need help to remember to take the drug, you may suggest the use of small compartmentalized boxes marked with the day of the week or time the drug is to be taken (Fig. 4.2). These containers can be obtained from the local pharmacy.

It is important to discuss the drug schedule with the patient, including the reason the drug is to be taken, the times, the amount, adverse reactions to expect, and reactions that should be reported. The patient needs a thorough understanding of the desired or expected therapeutic effect and the approximate time expected to attain that effect. For example, a patient may become discouraged after taking an antidepressant for 5 to 7 days and seeing no response. An explanation that 2 to 3 weeks is required before the depression begins to lift will, in many cases, promote adherence to the drug schedule.

It is important to provide ways to minimize adverse reactions if possible. For example, many anticholinergic drugs cause dry mouth. Instruct the patient to take frequent sips of water or suck on hard candy to help minimize the discomfort of a dry mouth.

Frequent follow-up sessions are needed to determine adherence to the drug schedule. If a follow-up visit is not feasible, consider a telephone call or home visit. It is vital that you strive to develop a caring and nurturing relationship with the patient. Adherence to the drug schedule is enhanced when a patient trusts you and feels comfortable confiding any problem encountered during drug therapy.

Display 4.1 Possible Causes of Ineffective Self-Health Management

- Extended therapy for chronic illness causes patient to become discouraged
- Troublesome adverse reactions
- Lack of understanding of the purpose for the drug
- Forgetfulness
- Misunderstanding of oral or written instructions on how to take the drug
- Weak nurse–patient relationships
- Lack of funds to obtain drug
- Mobility problems
- Lack of family support
- Cognitive deficits
- Visual or hearing defects

Reprinted with permission from Carpenito-Moyet, L. J. (2006). *Nursing diagnosis: Application to clinical practice* (11th ed., pp. 473–480). Philadelphia: Lippincott Williams & Wilkins.

Deficient Knowledge

Deficient Knowledge is the absence or deficiency of cognitive information on a specific subject. In the case of self-administration of drugs, the patient lacks sufficient knowledge to administer the drug regimen correctly. It may also relate to a lack of interest in learning, cognitive limitation, or inability to remember.

Most patients, at least in the initial treatment stages, lack knowledge about the drug, its possible adverse reactions, and the times and method of administration. At times, the patient may lack knowledge about the disease condition. In these situations, address the specific knowledge deficit (e.g., adverse reactions, disease process, method of administration) in words that the patient can understand. It is important to determine first what information the patient is lacking and then plan a teaching session that directly pertains to the specific area of need (see Chapter 5 for more information on patient education). If the patient lacks the cognitive ability to understand the information concerning self-administration of drugs, then one or more of the caregivers should be taught to administer the proper treatment regimen.

Noncompliance (Issue of Adherence)

Noncompliance is the behavior of a patient or caregiver that fails to coincide with the therapeutic plan agreed on by the patient and the prescribing health care provider. Patients are noncompliant (nonadherent to the therapeutic plan) for various reasons, such as a lack of information about the drug, the reason the drug is prescribed, or the expected or therapeutic results. Some patients find the adverse effects so bothersome that they discontinue taking the drug without notifying the prescribing health care provider. Display 4.1 identifies some reasons for this.

Noncompliance also can be the result of anxiety or bothersome side effects. Anxiety can be relieved by allowing the patient to express feelings or concerns, by actively listening as the patient verbalizes feelings, and by providing information so that the patient can be fully informed about the drug. Many patients have a tendency to discontinue use of the drug once the symptoms have been relieved. It is important to emphasize the importance of completing the prescribed course of therapy. For example, failure to complete a course of antibiotic therapy may result in recurrence of the infection. To combat noncompliance, find out the exact reason for the noncompliance, if possible. Factors related to noncompliance are similar to those listed in Display 4.1. The term *noncompliance* frequently has negative connotations for both patients and providers. You will see the term *adherence* is used in this book to support a positive outcome.

Anxiety

Anxiety is a vague uneasiness or apprehension that manifests itself in varying degrees, from expressions of concern regarding drug regimen to total lack of adherence to the drug routine. The anxiety experienced during drug administration depends on the severity of the illness, the occurrence of adverse reactions, and the knowledge level of the patient. When anxiety is high, the ability to focus on details is reduced. If the patient or caregiver is given information concerning the medication regimen during a high-anxiety state, the patient may not remember the information. This could lead to nonadherence to the regimen. Anxiety usually decreases with understanding of the treatment plan. To decrease anxiety before discussing the treatment plan with the patient, take time to talk with and actively listen to the patient. This helps to build a caring relationship and decrease patient anxiety. It is critical to allow time for a thorough explanation and to answer all questions and concerns in language the patient can understand (see Chapter 5).

It is important to identify and address the specific fear and, if possible, reassure the patient that the drug will alleviate the symptoms or, if possible, cure the disorder. Thoroughly explain any procedure. Actively listen and provide encouragement as the patient expresses fears and concerns. Reassurance and understanding on your part are required; the amount of reassurance and understanding depends on the individual patient.

Evaluation

Evaluation is a decision-making process that involves determining the effectiveness of the nursing interventions in meeting the expected outcomes. When related to the administration of a drug, this phase of the nursing process is used to evaluate the patient's response to drug therapy. Expected outcomes define the behavior of the patient or family that indicates that the problem is being resolved or that progress toward resolution is occurring. Expected outcomes serve as a basis for evaluating the effectiveness of nursing interventions. For example, if the nursing intervention is to "monitor the blood pressure every hour," the expected outcome is that "the patient experiences no further elevation in blood pressure."

The evaluation is complete if the expected outcomes are accomplished or if progress occurs. If the outcomes are not accomplished, different interventions are needed. During the administration of the drug the expected response is alleviation of specific symptoms or the presence of a therapeutic effect. Evaluation also may be used to determine if the patient or family member understands the drug schedule.

To evaluate the patient's response to therapy, and depending on the drug administered, check the patient's blood pressure every hour, inquire whether pain has been relieved, or monitor the patient's pulse every 15 minutes. After evaluation, certain other decisions may need to be made and plans of action implemented. For example, you may need to notify the primary health care provider of a marked change in a patient's pulse and respiratory rate after a drug was administered, or you may need to change the bed linen because sweating occurred after a drug used to lower the patient's elevated temperature was administered.

You can evaluate the patient's or family's understanding of the drug regimen by noting if one or both appear to understand the material that has been presented. Facial expression may indicate that one or both do or do not understand what has been explained. You also may ask questions about the information that has been given to evaluate further the patient's or family's understanding.

KEY POINTS

- Nursing process is the method of problem solving used in the nursing discipline. It consists of five phases: assessment, analysis, planning, implementation, and evaluation.

- Assessment involves the collection of patient data. The initial assessment provides baseline information for comparison later. It can be objective, that is, facts obtained from information sources such as the examination, lab tests, or other findings. It can also be subjective, data that is told to the nurse from the patient or the family. Ongoing assessment helps to update information about the patient's progress.

- Analysis involves the grouping of assessment data into like threads. Review of the data determines the patient needs and is described using consistent language, termed a *nursing diagnosis*. A nursing diagnosis is different from a medical diagnosis because interventions carried out are independent nursing actions, that is, those not requiring a health care provider's order.

- The planning phase is the formulation of the goals and expected outcomes to assist the patient to return to the maximum level of wellness. These should be reasonably attainable and patient oriented. The outcomes help to formulate the plan of action to be used during implementation and help to measure success during the evaluation phase.

- With most drug therapy routines there are typical patient problems to address: Self Health Management, Deficient Knowledge, Noncompliance, and Anxiety. Other specific problems are dependent upon illness type, drugs ordered, and patient knowledge and experience with the treatment routine.

Chapter Review

Prepare for the NCLEX-PN

Build Your Knowledge

1. When the nurse enters subjective data in the client's record, this information is obtained from _____.

   1. the primary health care provider
   2. other members of the health care team
   3. the client or family
   4. laboratory and x-ray reports

2. What is the name of the organization that approves and standardizes nursing diagnoses?

   1. ANA
   2. NLN
   3. NCSBN
   4. NANDA-I

3. A client states that he does not understand why he has to take a specific medication. The most accurate nursing diagnosis for this man would be _____.

   1. Self Health Management
   2. Anxiety
   3. Noncompliance
   4. Deficient Knowledge

4. Which of the following would be an appropriate expected outcome related to drug administration?

   1. The client will verbalize three ways to use crutches.
   2. The client will take an antibiotic pill daily.
   3. The client will understand the use of blood pressure medications.
   4. The client will demonstrate ways to prevent having to use insulin.

5. Which of the following is an independent nursing action?

   1. administering insulin
   2. withholding a drug according to physician standing orders
   3. client teaching about drug therapy
   4. asking respiratory care to come do an inhalation treatment

6. During the evaluation phase of the nursing process, the nurse _____.

   1. makes decisions regarding the effectiveness of nursing interventions based on the outcome
   2. ensures nursing procedures have been performed correctly
   3. makes notations regarding the client's response to medical treatment
   4. makes a list of all adverse reactions the patient may experience while taking the drug

Apply Your Knowledge

7. Which of the following is an example of objective client data?

   1. Daughter states, "Mom's BP is always 150/90."
   2. "My pain is about 7 out of 10 right now."
   3. "I think the doctor said my blood sugar was 105."
   4. The nurse's aide reports a BP of 132/78.

8. The nurse makes a note in the chart that the client's pain has lessened following a 14-day course of antibiotics. This is an example of which phase of the nursing process?

   1. assessment
   2. analysis
   3. implementation
   4. evaluation

Alternate-Format Questions

9. Arrange the following steps of the nursing process correctly:

   1. analysis
   2. assessment
   3. evaluation
   4. implementation
   5. planning

10. The nurse greets the new clinic client, saying, "Tell me about the pain you are having." This is an example of gathering data. Describe the type of data. **Select all that apply**.

   1. baseline assessment
   2. objective data
   3. ongoing assessment
   4. subjective data

To check your answers, see Appendix G.

the**Point** *For more NCLEX-style questions, log on to http://thepoint.lww.com to access more than 1000 questions.*

5

Patient and Family Teaching

On completion of this chapter, the student will:

1. Describe the steps of patient teaching about drug therapy.
2. Identify important aspects of the patient–nurse relationship.
3. Describe the three components of good health communication.
4. Identify important aspects of the teaching/learning process.
5. Describe how to use information about relationship and communication with the nursing process.
6. Discuss suggestions to make to the patient for adapting drug administration in the home.

KEY TERMS

cultural competency • the ability to understand, appreciate, and interact with persons from cultures different from our own

health communication • the use of communication strategies to inform and influence individual and community decisions that enhance health

health literacy • the ability to understand information about health and disease, then use the information to make decisions about health care

learning • acquisition of new knowledge or skills; outcome of learning is change in behavior, thinking, or both

motivation • desire for action or recognition of need

teaching • interactive process that promotes learning

Patient **teaching** is an integral part of nursing. When drugs are ordered by the primary health care provider, you are responsible for supplying the patient with accurate and up-to-date information about the drugs prescribed. The patient is educated about the drugs he or she has taken while in the hospital and any drugs to be taken after being discharged. By understanding the reason for the prescribed medications, the patient is more likely to be adherent to the treatment plan and get better.

Described as a sequential plan, patient teaching can logically be seen as an essential nursing task. To best accomplish the task of patient teaching, you need to optimize the relationship between the patient and you as well as use principles of learning.

Patient–Nurse Relationship

The relationship between a nurse and a patient is built upon trust and respect. Different factors can either support or block the ability to form positive relationships. Nurses use their knowledge of understanding changes in the health care system and emphasis on better health communication to build strong relationships.

Changes in Health Care

In the United States, we are about to go into an era of health care reform where all people are required to have insurance and some services will become the basic rights to all—no longer a privilege to only some. The Health Care and Education Reconciliation Act, which passed in 2010 and was upheld by the Supreme Court in 2012, may change health care as we know it.

As part of this new plan, individuals will be asked to assume greater responsibility not only in the decision making but also in the day-to-day management of their personal health care. This will change how patients and health care providers relate to one another. The ease with which this will transition is dependent on how well change is received by the patient and how we, the health care providers and nurses specifically, educate patients about their health, wellness, and illness concerns. Important factors that influence patients and their willingness to change include attitudes, the aging population, and chronic illness.

Attitudes

Traditional health care was practiced differently than care today. It was a *patriarchal relationship,* meaning the doctor gave the nurse an order, and then the nurse carried out the treatment on the patient. Previously, people were hospitalized for long periods and not responsible for schedules and treatments—everything was done to them. Relating to patients was very different. Doctors told patients what to do and they followed the instructions. If the patient questioned care, they were seen as "bad patients."

Currently, patients are frequently cared for on an outpatient basis or even at home. Treatments once done only in a hospital may be assumed by the patient or family members in the home. How health care providers address people has changed. Depending on the setting, we call people different titles—patient, client, or consumer. Despite the name we choose, they are all persons with a deviation from wellness caused by an acute disease, genetic affliction, or chronic condition worsening over time.

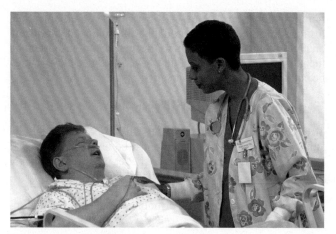

Figure 5.1 By 2030, the health care system will have to service 6% more older adults.

Aging Population

Older individuals grew up in the traditional health care system. They regard the doctor as an authoritative expert. This attitude is seen especially when a patient has an acute medical problem. Again, the patient waits for direction from the doctor and allows nurses to do the treatments to them.

This presents a problem because older people use more health care resources than others. People aged 65 and older presently make up 13% of the population, but they account for over 30% of the medications, hospital stays, and emergency responses. By 2030 it is estimated that 19% of our population will be over 65 (Fig. 5.1). If costs rise at the same rate, no one will be able to afford health care. You can help older people take a greater role in their own care by finding ways to empower them to help cut costs. One option is to help educate patients to direct their own care rather than relying on their health care providers.

Chronic Illness

As people with medical conditions live longer and our population ages, there will be increasing rates of chronic illnesses. This group of patients is thought to be the best group to handle the change from provider-directed care to patient-centered care. According to some researchers, patients with chronic illnesses exercise a great deal of control. No matter what health care providers do or say, when patients leave the hospital or clinic, it is the patient who determines what to do. Patients decide what they are going to eat, whether they will exercise, and to what extent they will take prescribed medications.

It is imperative that patients make wise and cost-conscious decisions in managing their own health care. You can support this by practicing good **health communication** with patients.

Health Communication

The quality of health communication has an impact on the outcome of patient–nurse interactions. Patients' ability to follow instructions is heavily influenced by your communication style.

Results of good health communication include better medication compliance. Rates of patient adherence to prescribed treatments increase when health care providers deliver clear and concise instructions. Bad health communication results in the inability to follow medication instructions.

To practice good health communication, remember that it involves understanding patients as well as talking to them. Three important factors include **health literacy**, **cultural competency**, and identifying limited English proficiency.

Health Literacy

Health literacy is the ability to understand information about health and disease, then use the information to make decisions about health care. Assessment is required to determine a patient's ability to understand health concepts and carry out health care instructions. Patients with limited health literacy can be difficult to identify. A person may speak well and appear well educated, yet fail to grasp disease concepts or understand how to follow medication dosage instructions properly.

 LIFESPAN CONSIDERATIONS
Health literacy is not the same thing as language or skill ability. One third of the adult population in the United States has limited health literacy.

Identifying Limited Health Literacy

Patients with limited health literacy often try to hide their literacy issues. Display 5.1 describes populations at risk or behaviors that may alert nurses to suspect limited health literacy. Identify potential limited health literacy by understanding which population groups are at higher risk for limited health literacy skills. Then you can be alert for certain behaviors that may indicate a limited health literacy problem exists.

> ### *Display 5.1* Identifying Limited Health Literacy
>
> Groups with higher rates of limited health literacy include:
>
> - Elderly
> - Low income
> - U.S. born but speak English as a second language
> - Deaf or hard of hearing
> - People who did not finish high school
> - Learning disabled
> - Immigrants who do not speak English
> - Unemployed
>
> Behaviors that may indicate a patient has limited health literacy include:
>
> - Medical forms incomplete or inaccurately completed
> - Frequently missed appointments
> - Not following medication directions
> - Inability to name or give purpose of medications
> - Inability to describe how to take medications
> - Lab tests do not change when patients say they are taking their medication

Improving Health Literacy

Using simple and clear language helps patients understand and follow instructions. People who are highly literate can have problems understanding language used in health care. The word *negative* is a positive finding when discussing an infection or cancer. This can be confusing to those who use negative in a different context. Avoid medical terms and instead use everyday language; for example, say "pain killer" instead of "analgesic" when talking to patients. Other examples include "wound" instead of "lesion" or "tumor" instead of "carcinoma."

Limit the amount of information at each interaction with a patient. Patients remember small pieces of information that are relevant to current needs or situations. This does not mean withholding information. Rather, focus communication on the one or two most important things the patient needs to know at that time.

 LIFESPAN CONSIDERATIONS
Up to 80% of patients forget instructions spoken to them. Of those who say they remember the instruction, 50% recall the instruction incorrectly.

Cultural Competency

Cultural competence is the ability to deal with people from different cultures. Many people fail to realize that the United States is a nation of immigrants and we have people from almost every country or culture of the world within our borders. There are many things that you need to take into account when working with a wide array of different people from different cultures. To care for different people, you need to be able to respect their traditions, norms, and other traits.

To become respectful, the first things you should consider are the different cultures served by the institution. Learning about the cultural norms of the people served will help you to identify certain behaviors that are acceptable. Health care providers gain the trust from patients and family members when their customs are respected or advocated for in the care setting.

Taking care not to stereotype patients because of their culture is another important concept. For example, when caring for an Asian patient, you may know that rice is a basic staple in many Asian diets. Do not assume that the patient would prefer rice for a meal. Instead, ask what the patient's preference is for diet choices. The important concept is to acknowledge cultural differences and to ask if the individual practices these traditions.

Limited English Proficiency

In recent years, the United States has become increasingly multilingual. During the past decade, the number of Spanish- and Asian-language speakers has grown by 50%. Almost 45 million people in the United States speak a language other than English; additionally, 17% of the nation's population speak a language other than English at home.

With the growing complexity of treatments and medication instructions, it is important to provide teaching resources for patients with limited English proficiency (LEP). Use written instructions that have been translated into the familiar language when teaching LEP patients. During conversations, use the service of professional interpreters to relay oral interactions. Avoid using family and friends for interpretation. Sometimes family members or friends will paraphrase communication, losing some important parts of the interaction. Do not rely on children for interpretation as this puts an unfair burden on them, because they may feel they have to tell bad news or may be embarrassed by the conversation.

Teaching/Learning Process

Teaching is an interactive process that promotes **learning**. Both the patient and the nurse must be actively involved if teaching is to be effective. You are better prepared to actively engage patients when you understand the principles of motivation, adult learning, and different learning styles. The patient's behavior, thinking, or both can change when learning occurs.

Motivation

A patient must be motivated (having a desire or seeing a need) to learn. **Motivation** depends on the patient's perception of the need to learn. Educating the patient about the disease process improves the patient's motivation to learn tasks to stay healthy. Encouraging patient participation in planning realistic and attainable goals also promotes motivation. Creating an accepting and positive atmosphere also enhances learning. If the patient has little or no motivation, he or she is likely to be nonadherent to therapy.

Adult Learning

Generally, adults learn only what they feel they need to learn. Adults learn best when they have a strong inner motivation to acquire a new skill or new knowledge. They will learn less if they are passive recipients of "canned" educational content. Adults have a vast array of experiences and knowledge to bring to a new learning experience. Nurses who use this experience will bring about the greatest behavior change. Most adults retain the information taught if they are able to "do" something with that new knowledge immediately. For example, in teaching a patient how to administer his or her own insulin, demonstrate the technique, allow time for supervised practice, and, as soon as he or she appears ready, allow the patient to prepare and inject the insulin. Most adults prefer an informal learning environment in which mutual exchange and freedom of expression prevail.

Learning Styles and Domains of Learning

Learning styles involve preferred ways to learn a concept and are frequently grouped as visual, auditory, or kinesthetic. Assessing a patient's learning style helps you to discover the best methods to use when providing patient teaching.

 LIFESPAN CONSIDERATIONS
Remember that 83% of adults are visual learners and only 11% learn by listening (auditory learners). When instructing patients, use props and visual materials as much as possible.

Learning occurs in what is known as three domains: cognitive, affective, and psychomotor. When developing a teaching plan for the patient, consider how a patient learns and what they are to learn. Display 5.2 describes both learning styles and domains of learning.

Combining Teaching Skills and the Nursing Process

Nurses are in the unique position of delivering health care and educating patients. Using the above concepts, teach patients to master skills and to assume self-care responsibilities. The empowered patient feels confident that he or she is part of a patient-centered relationship with you, and positive outcomes will occur.

A Framework for Patient Teaching

The nursing process is a systematic method of identifying patient health needs, devising a plan of care to meet the identified needs, initiating the plan, and evaluating its effectiveness. This process provides the necessary framework to develop an effective teaching plan. However, the teaching plan differs from the nursing process in that the nursing process encompasses all of the patient's health care needs, whereas the teaching plan focuses primarily on the patient's learning needs. The use of the nursing process as the framework and the concepts of relationships, health communication, and the learning process demonstrate ways to teach patients about taking drugs, the possibility of adverse reactions, and the signs and symptoms of toxicity (if applicable).

NURSING PROCESS
PATIENT TEACHING FOR MEDICATION INFORMATION

ASSESSMENT

Assessment is the data-gathering phase of the nursing process. Assessment assists you in choosing the best teaching methods and individualizing the teaching plan. To develop an effective teaching plan, first determine the patient's needs. Needs stem from three areas: (1) information the patient or family needs to know about a particular drug; (2) the patient's or family member's ability to learn, accept, and use information; and (3) any barriers or obstacles to learning.

Some drugs have simple uses and, therefore, relatively little patient teaching is needed. For example, applying a nonprescription ointment to the skin requires minimal teaching. Other drugs, such as insulin, require detailed information that may need to be given over several days.

Assessing an individual's ability to learn may be difficult. Using the concept of good *health communication*, you may find that not all adults have the same *health literacy* level. Information should be geared to the patient's level of understanding. Carefully assess the patient's ability to communicate, language preference, and health literacy skills. You may find that some patients do not read well. If the patient has a learning impairment, a family member or friend should be included in the teaching process. People may readily understand what is being taught, but some cannot. For example, a visually impaired patient may be unable to read a label or printed directions supplied by the primary health care provider, pharmacist, or nurse. Because patients can mimic instructions does not mean they understand them. Display 5.3 illustrates use of the "Brown Bag Method" to assess medication use and understanding.

Through assessment, you can determine what barriers or obstacles (if any) may prevent the patient or family member from fully understanding the material being presented. Use your skills of *cultural competence* to consider the patient's cultural background when planning a teaching session. For example, for some patients, an interpreter is needed. In other cultures, a certain individual (e.g., mother or grandmother) is the decision maker in the family. In such cases, it is important to include the decision maker and/or an interpreter with the patient in the teaching session.

NURSING DIAGNOSES (ANALYSIS)

The nursing diagnosis is formulated after analyzing the information obtained during the assessment phase. Examples of nursing diagnoses related to the administration of drugs are listed in the Nursing Diagnosis Checklist.

Nursing Diagnosis Checklist

- **Effective Self Health Management**
- **Ineffective Self Health Management** related to lack of knowledge
- **Deficient Knowledge** related to the drug regimen, possible adverse reactions, disease process, or other factors

The nursing diagnosis *Effective Self Health Management* generally describes a patient who is successfully managing the medication regimen. Use this nursing diagnosis to enhance the patient's management by teaching the patient possible adverse reactions that could affect his or her health and how to manage them or reduce the potential harmful effects.

The nursing diagnosis *Ineffective Self Health Management* is useful for discharge teaching, especially when you must teach the patient how to manage the medication tasks and schedules. Often, chronic illness or a variety of health problems may mean that the patient is taking as many as eight or more medications and may have difficulty managing a complicated medication regimen. This diagnosis describes individuals who are having difficulty achieving positive results.

Deficient Knowledge is a nursing diagnosis that may be used when the patient has a deficit in cognitive knowledge or psychomotor skills necessary to administer a medication properly. The defining characteristic would be that the patient would report deficient knowledge or request information, or the patient does not correctly perform a prescribed skill necessary to the medication task. It is sometimes difficult to know exactly when to use the nursing diagnosis of Deficient Knowledge because all nursing diagnoses have related patient teaching as part of their nursing interventions. If teaching is related directly to a nursing diagnosis, then incorporate the teaching into the plan.

PLANNING

Planning is the development of strategies to be used in the teaching plan and the selection of information to be taught. Planning begins with the development of a goal and the expected outcomes that the nurse will use to measure attainment of the goal. Display 5.4 identifies important basic information about any drug to include in any teaching plan.

Display 5.4 Important Information to Include in Any Medication Teaching Plan

1. Therapeutic response expected from the drug
2. Adverse reactions to expect when taking the drug
3. Adverse reactions to report to the nurse or primary health care provider
4. Dosage and route
5. Any special considerations or precautions associated with the particular drug prescribed
6. Additional education regarding special considerations for certain drugs, such as techniques for giving injections, applying topical patches, or instilling eye drops

---

Developing an Individualized Teaching Plan

Teaching plans are individualized because patients' needs are unique. Make use of the patient's cognitive abilities when information is given to the patient or caregivers about the disease process, medication regimen, and adverse reactions. The patient uses the *cognitive domain* to process the information, ask questions, and make decisions.

Areas covered in an individualized teaching plan vary depending on the drug prescribed, the primary health care provider's preference for including or excluding specific facts about the drug, and what the patient needs to know to take the drug correctly. Teaching strategies will reflect your knowledge of *limited English proficiency* of the patient. For example, a patient who speaks and reads only Spanish should be given materials prepared in Spanish and not discharge instructions written in English. If needed, ask for assistance in communicating through another nurse who is fluent in Spanish.

Develop strategies for the individualized teaching plan based on information gained during the assessment. For example, if during the assessment you discover that the patient is a *kinesthetic learner,* the teaching plan may focus on learning using the *psychomotor domain.* Plan to teach a task or skill using a step-by-step method. The patient will have hands-on practice under your supervision. Plan for a return demonstration by the patient to show mastery of the skill.

Selecting Relevant Information

Use concepts of *health literacy* to develop an individualized teaching plan for patients and their families by selecting information relevant to a specific drug, adapting teaching to the individual's level of understanding, and avoiding medical terminology unless terms are explained or defined.

It is important to remember that repetition enhances learning. Repeated teaching sessions help you to assess better what the patient is actually learning and provide time for clarification. Encourage the patient to ask questions and express feelings to build confidence in the care provided or the ability to engage in self-health strategies.

When individualized written material is provided, if the patient has *limited English proficiency,* be sure the material includes the basic information that a patient would receive in English. Display 5.5 identifies basic drug information for all patients regardless of language.

Display 5.5 Basic Considerations When Developing a Drug Teaching Plan

General information to consider when developing a teaching plan includes information on the dosage regimen and adverse reactions, issues relating to family members, and basic information about drugs, drug containers, and drug storage.

All patients should understand the following information before discharge:

- **Take with a full (8-ounce) glass of water:** capsules or tablets should be taken with water unless the primary health care provider or pharmacist directs otherwise (e.g., take with food, milk, or an antacid). Some liquids, such as coffee, tea, fruit juice, and carbonated beverages, may interfere with the action of certain drugs.
- **Do not crush or chew:** it is important not to chew capsules before swallowing; they must be swallowed whole. The patient also should not chew tablets unless they are labeled "chewable." This is because some tablets have special coatings that are required for specific purposes, such as proper absorption of the drug or prevention of irritation of the lining of the stomach.
- **Same dose, same time:** the dose (amount) of a drug or the time between doses is never increased or decreased unless directed by the primary health care provider.
- **Take all of it:** a prescription drug or nonprescription drug course of therapy recommended by a primary health care provider is not stopped or omitted except on the advice of the primary health care provider.
- **Call your primary health care provider:** if the symptoms for which a drug was prescribed do not improve or become worse, the primary health care provider must be contacted as soon as possible, because a change in dosage or a different drug may be necessary.
- **Do not change or add a dose:** if a dose of a drug is omitted or forgotten, the next dose must not be doubled or the drug taken at more frequent intervals unless advised to do so by the primary health care provider.
- **Tell all your providers:** all health care providers, including physicians, dentists, nurses, and health personnel, must always be informed of all drugs (prescription and nonprescription) currently being taken on a regular or occasional basis.
- **Keep a list:** the exact names of all prescription and nonprescription drugs currently being taken should be kept in a wallet or purse for instant reference when seeing a physician, dentist, or other health care provider.
- **Report differences:** check prescriptions carefully when obtaining refills from the pharmacy and report any changes in the prescribed drug (e.g., changes in color, size, shape) to the pharmacist or primary health care provider before taking the drug, because an error may have occurred.
- **Resources to learn more:** the Internet (or World Wide Web) is one of the most frequently used resources when taking responsibility to understand your care and medications. Be sure your sources are true and accurate by looking at who posts the site. As a general rule sites ending with .gov, .edu, or .org are reputable. Commercial sites end with .com; remember anyone can put those sites on the Internet. When in doubt, ask your health care provider about the source.

- **Wear a MedicAlert bracelet** or other type of medical identification when taking a drug for a long time. This is especially important for drugs such as anticoagulants, steroids, oral hypoglycemic agents, insulin, or digitalis. In case of an emergency, the bracelet ensures that medical personnel are aware of health problems and current drug therapy.

Adverse Drug Effects
- **All drugs cause adverse reactions** (side effects). Examples of some of the more common adverse reactions are nausea, vomiting, diarrhea, constipation, skin rash, dizziness, drowsiness, and dry mouth. Some effects may be mild and subside with time or when the primary health care provider adjusts the dosage. In some instances, mild reactions, such as dry mouth, may have to be tolerated. Some adverse reactions, however, are potentially serious and even life-threatening.
- **Report adverse reactions** to the primary health care provider as soon as possible.
- **Report drug allergies:** medical personnel must be informed of all drug allergies before any treatment or drug is given.

Family Members
Consider the following points concerning family members when developing a teaching plan:

- **Never take another person's drugs:** a drug prescribed for one family member is never given to another family member, relative, or friend unless directed to do so by the primary health care provider.
- **Tell your family:** make sure that all family members or relatives are aware of all drugs, prescription and nonprescription, that are currently being taken by the patient.

Drugs, Drug Containers, and Drug Storage/Disposal
- **A drug must be kept in the container in which it was dispensed or purchased:** some drugs require special containers, such as light-resistant (brown) bottles, to prevent deterioration that may occur on exposure to light.
- **Keep the original label on the drug container:** do not remove directions on the label (e.g., "shake well before using," "keep refrigerated," "take before meals"), as these must be followed to ensure drug effectiveness.
- **Never mix different drugs in one container,** even for a brief time, because one drug may chemically affect another. Mixing drugs can also lead to mistaking one drug for another, especially when the size and color are similar.
- **All drugs must be kept out of the reach of children and pets.**
- **Do not expose a drug** to excessive sunlight, heat, cold, or moisture, because deterioration may occur.
- **When traveling, always carry drugs in their original containers with proper labeling.**
- **Never save a prescription for later use** unless the primary health care provider so advises.
- **Dispose of unused drugs properly:** use containers provided, or plastic containers for sharp objects. Never flush unused drugs down a toilet; return them to your primary health care provider or an accepted disposal area.

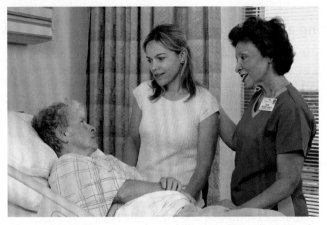

Figure 5.2 The nurse uses skills to build a therapeutic relationship to enhance learning.

IMPLEMENTATION

Implementation is the actual performance of the interventions identified in the teaching plan—putting the plan into action. Using knowledge of the *affective domain of learning*, develop a therapeutic relationship with the patient (a relationship that is based on trust and caring). When you take the time to develop a therapeutic relationship, the patient/family has confidence in you and more confidence in the information conveyed. As shown in Figure 5.2, approach the patient and caregivers with respect and encourage the expression of thoughts and feelings. Exploring the patient's beliefs about health and illness enhances your understanding of the patient's behavior.

Teaching at an appropriate time for each patient fosters learning. Plans for teaching should begin when a patient comes to the hospital, and sessions can begin at a time when the patient is alone, alert, and free of distractions. For example, do not perform patient teaching when there are visitors (unless they are to be involved in the administration of the patient's drugs), immediately before discharge from the hospital, or if the patient is sedated or in pain. Understand the principle of *motivation* and realize that physical discomfort negatively affects the patient's concentration and, thus, the ability to learn. A patient in pain is motivated to be pain-free, not educated about a medication.

Gear teaching to the patient's level of understanding and, when necessary, provide written as well as oral instructions. If a lot of information is given, it is often best to present the material in two or more sessions. Drug administration modifications may be necessary once the patient is at home (see Patient Teaching to Improved Patient Outcomes: Preparing the Patient and Family for Drug Administration in the Home). Keep these modifications in mind when teaching the patient.

EVALUATION

To determine the effectiveness of patient teaching, evaluate the patient's confidence in understanding the knowledge of the material presented. Evaluation can occur in several ways, depending on the nature of the information. For example, if the patient is being taught to administer

---

Patient Teaching for Improved Patient Outcomes

Preparing the Patient and Family for Drug Administration in the Home

Once the patient is at home, some modifications may be necessary to ensure safe drug administration. Provide written instructions using words that the patient and caregiver can understand. It is important to modify your teaching by using the following suggestions.

When you teach, make sure your patient understands the following:

✔ For patients taking more than one drug, develop a clear, easy-to-read drug schedule for the patient or caregiver to consult.
✔ Try using a daily calendar as an inexpensive, yet effective, means for scheduling.
✔ If the patient or caregiver has a problem with drug names, refer to the drug by shape or color only if other teaching has been unsuccessful. Another idea is to number bottles and use this number on the drug chart.
✔ Suggest the use of commercially available drug organizers.
✔ If your patient finds it helpful to keep all drugs together, suggest using a small box (fishing tackle box) to hold all the containers and keep it away from children and pets.
✔ Suggest conducting an inventory of medications early each week to ensure supply for weekends and holidays.
✔ If temporary refrigeration is necessary, suggest the use of a small cooler or insulated bag.
✔ If equipment items, such as needles and syringes, are used, suggest keeping all the supplies in one area. If the supplies came in a delivery box, suggest that the patient use it for storage.
✔ Advise the patient to use an approved container with a properly fitting lid for safe disposal of needles and syringes. Return used supplies to the hospital, pharmacy, or local health facility.
✔ Explain the importance of disposing any unused medication in the proper facility and not to flush items into the water supply through a toilet.

---

insulin, a return demonstration by the patient with you observing the patient's technique is an evaluation method.

Be knowledgeable about limited health literacy so you will know that questions such as "Do you understand?" or "Is there anything you don't understand?" should be avoided because the patient may feel uncomfortable admitting a lack of understanding. Or, the patient may not feel well enough to be aware of what he or she does not know. When factual material is being evaluated, periodically ask the patient to list or repeat some of the information presented.

KEY POINTS

- Patient teaching is an essential task in nursing. It involves both an established relationship and the use of teaching/learning principles. It involves supplying the patient with information and evaluating that understanding.

- Patient–nurse relationships are built upon mutual trust and respect. Nurses who understand the changing health care system and practice good health communication skills can empower patients, resulting in better outcomes.

- Good health communication includes assessment and interventions to enhance health literacy, having cultural competency, and providing resources for those with limited English proficiency.

- For learning to occur, one needs to be motivated. Adults learn best when they have an inner motivation. Most adults are visual learners, others learn hands-on, while only a few learn best by listening. You will use cognitive, affective, and psychomotor learning strategies to enhance learning by patients and families. All three domains of learning help to evaluate teaching effectiveness.

- As you assess health literacy, know that basic language literacy and understanding about health and disease are not the same thing. Analysis of data may indicate how motivated a patient is to learn. Learning style preferences help plan the best methods of patient teaching. Cultural competency and knowing if patients have limited English proficiency guide the choice of interventions used for patient teaching.

- Adapt basic drug information for the home setting to ensure safety of both the patient and other family members.

PHARMACOLOGY IN PRACTICE
THINK CRITICALLY

Because adults learn best by applying concepts familiar to them, this book uses a case study approach to help you learn about drug information. Here we introduce a number of patients to you so that you can become familiar with their health care needs. Throughout the various chapters, you will be introduced to pharmacology concepts in a case study approach by using a group of patients from Any Ambulatory Clinic.

MEET THE PATIENTS

 Lillian Chase is a 36-year-old woman who has had asthma for most of her childhood and adult life. After an accident, she suffered seizures and injuries to both her head and her leg; she now needs knee replacement surgery. Additionally, she is a smoker who has hypertension.

 Alfredo Garcia speaks little English. He is seen for an upper respiratory infection, and, upon examination, we discover he lives with hypertension.

 Mrs. Moore is 85 years of age and seems forgetful and confused at times. She was able to manage her heart failure until she had a urinary tract infection. Her chest pain is now worse, and she has lots of medications to manage.

 Mr. Park, aged 77 years, is staying in a long-term care facility following hip replacement surgery. The stress of the procedure has caused an outbreak of *Herpes zoster* (shingles).

 Betty Peterson lives in an apartment. She suffers from aches, pains, and depression.

 Mr. Phillip is a 72-year-old widower, and he lives alone. He has both diabetes and early-stage chronic kidney disease. His children do not live close; therefore, in addition to managing his own health care issues, he must learn to live alone and manage a household.

 Janna Wong is a 16-year-old high school gymnast. We learn from Janna's mother that she was recovering from mononucleosis before the school year. They both attribute her increased fatigue level to Janna's busy extracurricular schedule.

In each unit, information related to specific types of drugs is discussed. The aforementioned patients will present at the beginning of each chapter with both acute and chronic medical problems. Each selected patient in the chapter will challenge you to think critically about each case to achieve the best management approach. In the Pharmacology in Practice: Think Critically section at the end of each chapter, different patient scenarios are presented for discussion and reflection to explore the best way to meet patient needs.

This chapter describes good health communication. Picture yourself as the nurse obtaining vital signs in the clinic. Given the information you learned in this chapter, review the list of patients, identify any of them that you think may have limited health literacy, and prepare a list of questions you would want to ask to help you determine who has limited health literacy.

● Chapter Review

● Prepare for the NCLEX®

Build Your Knowledge

1. An interactive process that promotes learning is defined as:

   1. motivation
   2. cognitive ability
   3. psychomotor domain
   4. teaching

2. The patient–nurse relationship is built upon:

   1. communication
   2. cultural competency
   3. health literacy
   4. respect

3. Typically, what percentage of people remember instructions given by the primary health care provider?

   1. 80%
   2. 65%
   3. 20%
   4. 10%

4. When developing a teaching plan, the nurse assesses the affective learning domain, which means that the nurse considers the client's:

   1. attitudes, feelings, beliefs, and opinions
   2. ability to perform a return demonstration
   3. intellectual ability
   4. home environment

5. Actual development of the strategies to be used in the teaching plan and selection of the information to be taught occur in this phase of the nursing process:

   1. assessment
   2. planning
   3. implementation
   4. evaluation

Apply Your Knowledge

6. A client is preparing for discharge from the hospital tomorrow. She tells you that she has some questions about the medications that she will be taking at home. She explains that the regimen is complicated, and she is afraid she will not be able to remember when to take her medications. Which of the following nursing diagnoses would be most appropriate for this client?

   1. Effective Individual Self Health Management
   2. Ineffective Self Health Management
   3. Deficient Knowledge
   4. Risk for Impaired Home Maintenance

7. Unless the primary health care provider or clinical pharmacist directs otherwise, the nurse informs the client to take oral medications with:

   1. fruit juice
   2. milk
   3. water
   4. food

8. The nurse is teaching a mother of twin toddlers to give self-injections. She says, "I will see if we have anything at home to put needles in when I get there." The best action for the nurse to do is:

   1. compliment the woman for planning ahead
   2. obtain a sharps container from the pharmacy
   3. note her answer in the medical record
   4. request that she demonstrate the technique before going home ·

Alternate-Format Questions

9. Arrange the following steps of patient teaching correctly:

   1. provide drug information sheets in the preferred language
   2. call for an interpreter to attend the teaching session
   3. assess for health literacy and limited English proficiency
   4. have the client demonstrate how to give the medication

10. Identify high-risk populations for limited health literacy. **Select all that apply**.

   1. older persons
   2. high income
   3. unemployed
   4. hard of hearing

To check your answers, see Appendix G.

the**Point** *For more NCLEX-style questions, log on to http://thepoint.lww.com to access more than 1000 questions.*

Drugs Used to Fight Infections

The body is equipped with a natural defense system, our skin and bodily secretions. Infections occur when a pathogenic microorganism (which can cause a disease) breaches the defense system. Microbes enter the body in different ways, such as through a break in the skin or by ingestion, breathing, or contact with the mucous membranes of the body. This unit discusses drugs used to kill or retard the growth of microorganisms that invade the body. These are classed together as anti-infective drugs. They include drugs used to treat infections from bacteria, viruses, fungi, and protozoans.

The sulfonamides (Chapter 6) were the first antibiotic drugs developed to effectively treat bacterial infections. Since then, medications have been developed to target specific portions of a bacterial cell. These pathogens have select components that differ from human cells, such as specific enzymes and a cell wall instead of a cell membrane.

Chapters 7 to 9 discuss drugs, known as antibiotics, that target these bacterial cell differences. The mechanisms of action of the antibacterial drugs inhibit the following bacterial cell activities: cell wall synthesis, DNA or RNA synthesis, and protein synthesis. Drugs used to treat the bacterial infections associated with tuberculosis are included in Chapter 10.

Chapter 11 covers drugs that are used to treat viral infections. Viruses are organisms that do not have a typical cell structure and use host cells to grow and divide. Because viruses use the DNA or RNA of other cells, their ability to change has posed a problem in making drugs to treat viral infections. Scientific discoveries have led to the production of more effective antiviral drugs.

Fungal and protozoal infections have played a more prominent role in health issues in recent years because of advances in medical treatments that cause immunosuppression (a reduction in white blood cells). Infections that were minor at one time have become life-threatening in immunosuppressed patients because low numbers of infection-fighting white blood cells leave the body unable to resist the infection. These drugs are covered in Chapter 12.

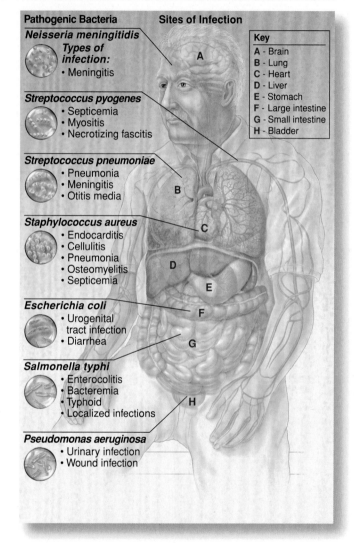

Pathogenic Bacteria

Sites of Infection

Neisseria meningitidis
Types of infection:
- Meningitis

Streptococcus pyogenes
- Septicemia
- Myositis
- Necrotizing fascitis

Streptococcus pneumoniae
- Pneumonia
- Meningitis
- Otitis media

Staphylococcus aureus
- Endocarditis
- Cellulitis
- Pneumonia
- Osteomyelitis
- Septicemia

Escherichia coli
- Urogenital tract infection
- Diarrhea

Salmonella typhi
- Enterocolitis
- Bacteremia
- Typhoid
- Localized infections

Pseudomonas aeruginosa
- Urinary infection
- Wound infection

Key
A - Brain
B - Lung
C - Heart
D - Liver
E - Stomach
F - Large intestine
G - Small intestine
H - Bladder

Antibacterial Drugs—Sulfonamides

LEARNING OBJECTIVES

On completion of this chapter, the student will:

1. Discuss the uses, general drug actions, and general adverse reactions, contraindications, precautions, and interactions for the sulfonamides.
2. Discuss important preadministration and ongoing assessment activities the nurse should perform on the patient taking sulfonamides.
3. List nursing diagnoses particular to a patient taking sulfonamides.
4. Discuss ways to promote an optimal response to therapy, how to manage adverse reactions, and important points to keep in mind when educating patients about the use of the sulfonamides.
5. Identify the rationale for increasing fluid intake when taking sulfonamides.
6. Describe the objective signs indicating that a severe skin reaction, such as Stevens-Johnson syndrome, is present.

KEY TERMS

anorexia • loss of appetite

antibacterial • active against bacteria

antibiotic • term used synonymously with antibacterial

aplastic anemia • blood disorder caused by damage to the bone marrow resulting in a marked reduction in the number of red blood cells and some white blood cells

bactericidal • drug or agent that destroys or kills bacteria

bacteriostatic • drug or agent that slows or retards the multiplication of bacteria

crystalluria • formation of crystals in the urine

leukopenia • decrease in the number of leukocytes (white blood cells)

pruritus • itching

Stevens-Johnson syndrome (SJS) • fever, cough, muscular aches and pains, headache, and lesions of the skin, mucous membranes, and eyes; the lesions appear as red wheals or blisters, often starting on the face, in the mouth, or on the lips, neck, and extremities

stomatitis • inflammation of a cavity opening, such as the oral cavity

thrombocytopenia • decreased number of platelets in the blood

toxic epidermal necrolysis (TEN) • toxic skin reaction with sloughing of skin and mucous membranes

urticaria • hives; itchy wheals on the skin resulting from contact with or ingestion of an allergenic substance or food

DRUG CLASSES

Single sulfonamide agents	Urinary anti-infective combinations
	Topical preparations

PHARMACOLOGY IN PRACTICE

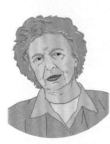

Each chapter in this book features a specific case study corresponding to the drug therapy in each chapter. In this chapter, the patient featured is Mrs. Moore. She is 85 years old and has been prescribed a sulfonamide for a urinary tract infection (UTI). She is to take the drug for 10 days. Mrs. Moore seems forgetful and a bit confused as you talk with her. As you begin learning about the preassessment interview, think about Mrs. Moore.

Drugs that are used against bacteria are either **bacteriostatic** (they slow or retard the multiplication of bacteria) or **bactericidal** (they destroy the bacteria). To choose the appropriate drug, the primary health care provider needs to know how sensitive the bacteria will be to the drugs.

Culture and Sensitivity Testing

To determine if a specific type of bacteria is sensitive to an **antibiotic** drug, culture and sensitivity tests are performed. A culture is performed by placing infectious material obtained from areas such as the skin, respiratory tract, and blood on a culture plate that contains a special growing medium. This growing medium is "food" for the bacteria. After a specified time, the bacteria are examined under a microscope and identified. The sensitivity test involves placing the infectious material on a separate culture plate and then placing small disks impregnated with various antibiotics over the area. After a specified time, the culture plate is examined. If there is little or no growth around a disk, the bacteria are considered sensitive to that particular antibiotic. Therefore, the infection will be controlled by this antibiotic. If there is considerable growth around the disk, then the bacteria are considered resistant to that particular antibiotic, and the infection will not be controlled by this antibiotic (Fig. 6.1).

SULFONAMIDES

Sulfonamides (commonly called sulfa drugs) are **antibacterial** agents, meaning they are active against bacteria. Sulfadiazine, sulfisoxazole, and sulfamethizole are examples of sulfonamide preparations. Although the use of sulfonamides began to decline after the introduction of more effective anti-infectives such as the penicillins and other antibiotics, these drugs remain important for the treatment of certain types of infections.

Actions

The sulfonamides are primarily *bacteriostatic* because of their ability to inhibit the activity of folic acid in bacterial cell metabolism. The sulfonamides are well absorbed by the gastrointestinal (GI) system and excreted by the kidneys (see Chapter 48). They are often used to control infections caused by both gram-positive and gram-negative bacteria, such as *Escherichia coli, Staphylococcus aureus,* and *Klebsiella* and *Enterobacter* species. Once the rate of bacterial multiplication is slowed, the body's own defense mechanisms (white blood cells) are able to rid the body of the invading microorganisms and therefore control the infection.

When sulfasalazine interacts with intestinal bacteria, it helps to inhibit the inflammatory process, which is how the drug works to treat ulcerative colitis.

Uses

The sulfonamides are often used according in the treatment of infections such as:

- Urinary tract infections (UTIs) and acute otitis media
- Ulcerative colitis
- Mafenide (Sulfamylon) and silver sulfadiazine (Silvadene) are topical sulfonamides used in the treatment and prevention of infections in second- and third-degree burns.

Additional uses of the sulfonamides are given in the Summary Drug Table: Sulfonamides.

Adverse Reactions

The sulfonamides are capable of causing a variety of adverse reactions. Some of these are serious or potentially serious; others are mild. **Anorexia** (loss of appetite) is an example of a mild adverse reaction.

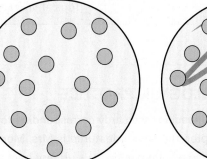

A. Culture plate with small disks containing various antibiotics.

B. Infectious material is spread on the culture plate.

C. After a specific time, the culture plate is inspected. If there is little or no growth around a disk, the bacteria is said to be sensitive to that antibiotic.

Figure 6.1 Culture and sensitivity tests indicate which drug is most effective against the bacteria on the culture plate.

Gastrointestinal System Reactions

- Nausea, vomiting, anorexia
- Diarrhea, abdominal pain
- **Stomatitis** (inflammation of the mouth)

In some instances, these may be mild. At other times they may cause serious problems, such as pronounced weight loss, requiring discontinuation of the drug.

Other Reactions

- Chills, fever
- **Crystalluria** (crystals in the urine)
- Photosensitivity

Various types of hypersensitivity (allergic) reaction may be seen during sulfonamide therapy, including **urticaria** (hives), **pruritus** (itching), generalized skin eruptions, or severe reactions leading to potentially lethal conditions such as **toxic epidermal necrolysis (TEN)** or **Stevens-Johnson syndrome (SJS)**.

> **NURSING ALERT**
>
> TEN and SJS are serious and sometimes fatal hypersensitivity reactions. Widespread sloughing of both the skin and mucous membranes can occur. Internal organ involvement can cause death. Patients with SJS may complain of fever, cough, muscular aches and pains, and headache, all of which are signs and symptoms of many other disorders. Be alert for the additional signs of lesions on the skin and mucous membranes, eyes, and other organs, a diagnostically important indicator of these problems. The lesions appear as red wheals or blisters, often starting on the face, in the mouth, or on the lips, neck, and extremities. These conditions may occur with the administration of other types of drugs. Notify the primary health care provider and withhold the next dose of the drug. In addition, exercise care to prevent injury to the involved areas.

The most frequent adverse reaction seen with the topical application of a sulfonamide is a burning sensation or pain when the drug is applied to the skin. Other possible allergic reactions include rash, itching, edema, and urticaria. Burning, rash, and itching may also be seen with the use of silver sulfadiazine. It may be difficult to distinguish between adverse reactions due to the use of mafenide or silver sulfadiazine and those that occur from a severe burn injury or from other agents used for the management of burns.

The following hematologic changes may occur during prolonged sulfonamide therapy:

- **Leukopenia**—decrease in the number of white blood cells
- **Thrombocytopenia**—decrease in the number of platelets
- **Aplastic anemia**—deficient red blood cell production in the bone marrow

These changes are examples of serious adverse reactions. If any of these occur, discontinuation of sulfonamide therapy may be required.

Contraindications

The sulfonamides are contraindicated in patients with hypersensitivity to the sulfonamides, during lactation, and in children younger than 2 years of age. The sulfonamides are not used near the end (at term) of pregnancy (pregnancy category D). If the sulfonamides are given near the end of pregnancy, significantly high blood levels of the drug may occur, causing jaundice or hemolytic anemia in the neonate. In addition, the sulfonamides are not used for infections caused by group A beta (β)-hemolytic streptococci because the sulfonamides have *not* been shown to be effective in preventing the complications of rheumatic fever or glomerulonephritis.

Precautions

The sulfonamides are used with caution in patients with renal impairment, hepatic impairment, or bronchial asthma.

These drugs are given with caution to patients with allergies. Safety for use during pregnancy has not been established (pregnancy category C, except at term; see above).

Interactions

The following interactions may occur when a sulfonamide is administered with another agent:

Interacting Drug	Common Use	Effect of Interaction
oral anticoagulants	Blood thinner; prevent clot formation	Increased action of the anticoagulant
methotrexate	Immunosuppression and chemotherapy	Increased bone marrow suppression
hydantoins	Anticonvulsants	Increased serum hydantoin level

 CHRONIC CARE CONSIDERATIONS

When diabetic patients are prescribed sulfonamides, assess for a possible hypoglycemic reaction. Sulfonamides may inhibit the (hepatic) metabolism of the oral hypoglycemic drugs tolbutamide and chlorpropamide (Diabinese).

HERBAL CONSIDERATIONS

Cranberries and cranberry juice are commonly used folk remedies for preventing and relieving symptoms of UTIs. The use of cranberries in combination with antibiotics has been recommended by physicians for the long-term suppression of UTIs. Cranberries are thought to prevent bacteria from attaching to the walls of the urinary tract. The suggested dose is 6 ounces of juice twice daily. Cranberry capsules are not recommended because the fluid for hydration may be as helpful as the berries (Brown, 2012). Extremely large doses can produce GI disturbances, such as diarrhea or abdominal cramping. Although cranberries may relieve symptoms or prevent the occurrence of a UTI, their use will not cure a UTI. If an individual suspects a UTI, medical attention is necessary.

NURSING PROCESS

PATIENT RECEIVING A SULFONAMIDE

ASSESSMENT

Preadministration Assessment

Before the initial administration of the drug, it is important to assess the patient's general appearance and take and record the vital signs. Obtain information regarding the symptoms experienced by the patient and the length of time these symptoms have been present. If an elderly patient appears distracted or the family notes sudden confusion, these may be signs of a genitourinary infection. Many infections are diagnosed and treated in ambulatory settings; therefore, it is important to ask about self-remedies the patient may have tried before seeing a primary health care provider. Depending on the type and location of the infection or disease, review the results of tests such as a urine culture, urinalysis, complete blood count, intravenous pyelogram, renal function tests, and examination of the stool.

Ongoing Assessment

During the course of therapy, evaluate the patient at periodic intervals for response to the drug—that is, a relief of symptoms and a decrease in temperature (if it was elevated before therapy started), as well as the occurrence of any adverse reactions.

If fever is present and the patient's temperature suddenly increases or if the temperature was normal and suddenly increases, instruct the patient to contact the primary health care provider immediately.

The ongoing assessment for patients receiving sulfasalazine for ulcerative colitis includes observation for evidence of the relief or intensification of the symptoms of the disease. Ask the patient to monitor when using the bathroom for changes in number or appearance of the stool. The patient should contact the primary health care provider regarding changes.

When administering a sulfonamide for a burn, inspect the burned areas every 1 to 2 hours, because some treatment regimens require keeping the affected areas covered with the mafenide or silver sulfadiazine ointment at all times. Any adverse reactions should be reported immediately to the primary health care provider.

NURSING DIAGNOSES

Drug-specific nursing diagnoses include the following:

- **Impaired Urinary Elimination** related to effect on the bladder from sulfonamides
- **Impaired Skin Integrity** related to burns
- **Impaired Skin Integrity** related to photosensitivity or severe allergic reaction to the sulfonamides
- **Risks for (Secondary) Infection** related to lowered white blood cell count resulting from sulfonamide therapy

Nursing diagnoses related to drug administration are discussed in Chapter 4.

PLANNING

The expected patient outcomes depend on the reason for administration of the sulfonamide but may include an optimal response to drug therapy, meeting patient needs related to the management of adverse drug reactions, and confidence in an understanding of the medication regimen.

IMPLEMENTATION

Promoting an Optimal Response to Therapy

The patient receiving a sulfonamide drug almost always has an active infection. Some patients may be receiving one of these drugs to prevent an infection (prophylaxis) or as part of the management of a disease such as ulcerative colitis.

Unless the primary health care provider orders otherwise, give sulfonamides to the patient whose stomach is empty—that is, 1 hour before or 2 hours after meals. If GI irritation occurs, give sulfasalazine with food or immediately after meals.

Sulfasalazine may cause the urine and skin to take on an orange-yellow color; this is normal. Crystalluria may occur during administration of a sulfonamide, although this problem occurs less frequently with some of the newer sulfonamide preparations. Often, this potentially serious problem can be prevented by increasing fluid intake during sulfonamide therapy. It is important to instruct the patient to drink a full glass (8 ounces) of water when taking an oral sulfonamide and to drink at least eight large glasses of water each day until therapy is finished.

Monitoring and Managing Patient Needs

Observe the patient for adverse reactions, especially an allergic reaction (see Chapter 1). If one or more adverse reactions should occur, withhold the next dose of the drug and notify the primary health care provider.

IMPAIRED URINARY ELIMINATION. Because one adverse effect of the sulfonamide drugs is altered elimination patterns, it is important to help the patient maintain adequate fluid intake and output. Encourage patients to increase fluid intake to 2000 mL or more per day to prevent crystalluria and stones (calculi) forming in the genitourinary tract, as well as to aid in removing microorganisms from the urinary tract. It is important to measure and record the patient's intake and output every 8 hours and notify the primary health care provider if the urinary output decreases or the patient fails to increase his or her oral intake (Fig. 6.2).

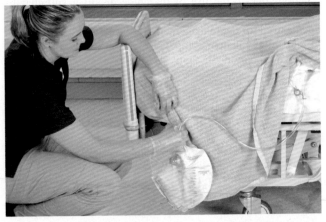

Figure 6.2 Nurses monitor for decreased urinary output and possible crystal formation in the patient receiving sulfonamides.

LIFESPAN CONSIDERATIONS
Gerontology

Because renal function diminishes normally as people age, administer the sulfonamides with great caution to the older patient. There is an increased danger of the sulfonamides causing additional renal damage when renal impairment is already present. An increase of fluid intake up to 2000 mL (if the older adult can tolerate this amount) decreases the risk of crystals and stones forming in the urinary tract. The older adult may be hesitant to increase oral fluid intake because of fear of incontinence. It is important to assess for this fear and teach the patient when to take fluids to maintain continence and reduce the risk of crystal formation.

IMPAIRED SKIN INTEGRITY: BURN INJURY. When mafenide or silver sulfadiazine is used in treating burns, the treatment regimen is outlined by the primary health care provider or the personnel in the burn treatment unit. There are various burn treatment regimens, such as débridement (removal of burned or dead tissue from the burned site), special dressings, and cleansing of the burned area (Display 6.1). The use of a specific treatment regimen often depends on the extent of the burned area, the degree of the burns, and the physical condition and age of the patient. Other concurrent problems, such as lung damage from smoke or heat or physical injuries that occurred at the time of the burn injury, also may influence the treatment regimen.

IMPAIRED SKIN INTEGRITY: PHOTOSENSITIVITY. The skin can become more sensitive to sunlight during sulfonamide therapy. Patients should be cautioned to wear protective clothing and sunscreen when outside. In areas where the climate is overcast, solar glare and indirect sunshine can cause a sunburn reaction. The skin should be inspected each shift when treatment is started for signs of sores or blisters indicating the possibility of a severe allergic reaction. The skin and mucous membranes should be inspected for up to 14 days after the end of therapy, the period of time during which reactions can still occur.

RISK FOR SECONDARY INFECTION. Lab results are scanned to monitor the patient for leukopenia and thrombocytopenia. Leukopenia may also present with physical signs and symptoms of an infection, such as fever, sore throat, and cough. Protect the patient with leukopenia from individuals who have an infection.

Thrombocytopenia is manifested by easy bruising and unusual bleeding after moderate to slight trauma to the skin or mucous membranes. The extremities of the patient with thrombocytopenia are handled with care to prevent bruising.

Display 6.1 Steps in Applying Topical Preparations to Burns

1. Clean and remove debris present on the surface of the skin.
2. Apply drug in a layer approximately 1/16 inch thick; thicker application is not recommended.
3. While wound is exposed, keep away from air draft because it can cause pain.
4. Warn the patient that stinging or burning may be felt during and for a short time after application.

Care is taken to prevent trauma when moving the patient. Inspect the skin daily for the extent of bruising and evidence of exacerbation of existing ecchymotic areas. It is important to encourage the patient to use a soft-bristled toothbrush to prevent any trauma to the mucous membranes of the oral cavity. Report any signs of leukopenia or thrombocytopenia immediately, because these are indications to stop drug therapy.

Educating the Patient and Family
Carefully planned patient and family education is important to foster adherence to the therapy, relieve anxiety, and

---

Patient Teaching for Improved Patient Outcomes

Taking Anti-Infectives

When you teach, make sure your patient understands the following:

✔ Take the drug at the prescribed time intervals. These time intervals are important because a certain amount of the drug must be in the body at all times for the infection to be controlled.
✔ Drink six to eight 8-ounce glasses of fluid while taking these drugs, and take each dose with a full glass of water.
✔ Do not increase or omit the dose unless advised to do so by the primary health care provider.
✔ Complete the entire course of treatment. Do not stop the drug, except on the advice of a primary health care provider, before the course of treatment is completed, even if symptoms improve or disappear. Failure to complete the prescribed course of treatment may result in a return of the infection.
✔ Follow the directions supplied with the prescription regarding taking the drugs with meals or on an empty stomach. Take drugs that must be taken on an empty stomach 1 hour before or 2 hours after a meal.
✔ Distinguish between immediate- and extended-release medications. Do not break, chew, or crush extended-release medications.
✔ Notify the primary health care provider if symptoms of the infection become worse or if original symptoms do not improve after 5 to 7 days of drug therapy.
✔ Avoid any exposure to sunlight or ultraviolet light (tanning beds, sunlamps) while taking these drugs and for several weeks after completing the course of therapy. Wear sunblock, sunglasses, and protective clothing when exposed to sunlight.
✔ Avoid tasks requiring mental alertness until response to the drug is known.

Specific Instructions Regarding Sulfonamides

✔ Take sulfasalazine (Azulfidine) with food or immediately after a meal.
✔ When taking sulfasalazine, the skin or urine may turn orange-yellow; this is *normal*. Soft contact lenses may acquire a permanent yellow stain. It is a good idea to seek the advice of an ophthalmologist regarding disposable lenses while taking this drug.

promote therapeutic effect. When a sulfonamide is prescribed for an infection, symptoms may diminish quickly and some outpatients have a tendency to discontinue the drug once symptoms are gone. When teaching the patient and family, emphasize the importance of completing the prescribed course of therapy to ensure all microorganisms causing the infection are eradicated. Help patients to understand that failure to complete a course of therapy may result in a recurrence of the infection. To increase adherence to the treatment recommendations, a teaching plan is developed to include the information that appears in the Patient Teaching for Improved Patient Outcomes: Taking Anti-Infectives.

EVALUATION

■ Therapeutic response is achieved, and there is no evidence of infection.

■ Adverse reactions are identified, reported to the primary health care provider, and managed successfully with appropriate nursing interventions:
  • Patient maintains an adequate fluid intake for proper urinary elimination.
  • Skin is intact and free of inflammation, irritation, infection, or ulcerations.

■ Patient and family express confidence and demonstrate an understanding of the drug regimen.

PHARMACOLOGY IN PRACTICE
THINK CRITICALLY

 Information from the preassessment can help you determine whether Mrs. Moore's confusion is an ongoing problem or due to her current illness. What questions will you ask her? What about other family members? Are there specific lab tests that will help you understand her confusion better? When her urinalysis comes back from the lab showing 3+ for bacteria, how does that influence your assessment?

KEY POINTS

• Infections occur when pathogenic microorganisms breach our natural defenses, such as the skin.

• Culture and sensitivity testing helps to identify the best drug for eradicating the bacterial infection.

• Sulfonamides are primarily bacteriostatic; they slow or retard the multiplication of bacteria, not destroy it.

• Sulfonamides are used primarily for urinary tract infections and as topical preparations.

• Persons taking sulfonamides need to increase fluid intake to at least 2000 mL to prevent genitourinary problems caused by the drug. Because kidney function diminishes as we age, there is an increased danger of renal damage and fluid increase is even more important with the elderly.

• Photosensitivity is an adverse reaction of sulfonamides; people taking these drugs should lessen outdoor activities or take care to protect their skin while outdoors.

Summary Drug Table SULFONAMIDES

Generic Name	Trade Name	Uses	Adverse Reactions	Dosage Ranges
Single Agents				
℞ sulfadiazine *sul-fah-dye'-ah-zeen*		UTIs, chancroid, acute otitis media, *Haemophilus influenzae* and meningococcal meningitis, rheumatic fever	Vomiting, headache, diarrhea, chills, fever, anorexia, crystalluria, stomatitis, urticaria, pruritus, hematologic changes, Stevens-Johnson syndrome, nausea	Loading dose: 2–4 g orally; maintenance dose: 2–4 g/day orally in 4–6 divided doses
sulfasalazine *sul-fah-sal'-ah-zeen*	Azulfidine, Azulfidine EN-tabs	UTI, acute otitis media, *Haemophilus influenzae,* meningococcal meningitis	Same as sulfadiazine; may cause skin and urine to turn orange-yellow	Initial therapy: 1–4 g/day orally in divided doses; maintenance dose: 2 g/day orally in evenly spaced doses (500 mg QID)
℞ sulfisoxazole *sul-fih-sox'-ah-zoll*		Same as sulfadiazine	Same as sulfadiazine	Loading dose: 2–4 g orally; maintenance dose: 4–8 g/day orally in 4–6 divided doses
Urinary Anti-Infective Combinations				
trimethoprim (TMP) and sulfamethoxazole (SMZ) *trye-meth'-oh-prim* *sul-fah-meth-ox'-ah-zoll*	Bactrim, Bactrim DS, Septra, Septra DS	Acute bacterial UTI, acute otitis media, traveler's diarrhea due to *Escherichia coli*	Headache, GI disturbances, allergic skin reactions, hematologic changes, Stevens-Johnson syndrome, anorexia, glossitis	160 mg TMP/800 mg SMZ orally q 12 hr; 8–10 mg/kg/day (based on TMP) IV in 2–4 divided doses
Topical Sulfonamide Preparations				
mafenide *maf'-eh-nyde*	Sulfamylon	Second- and third-degree burns	Pain or burning sensation, rash, itching, facial edema	Apply to burned area 1–2 times/day
silver sulfadiazine *sil'-ver sul-fah-dye'-ah-zeen*	Silvadene, Thermazene, SSD (cream)	Same as mafenide	Leukopenia, skin necrosis, skin discoloration, burning sensation	Same as mafenide

℞ This drug should be administered at least 1 hour before or 2 hours after a meal.

● Chapter Review

Know Your Drugs

Clients sometimes know a medication by the brand (or trade) name and not the generic name. To help you recognize both names, match the brand name with the generic name of the same medication

Generic Name	Brand Name
1. sulfasalazine	A. Bactrim
2. sulfamethoxazole/trimethoprim	B. Silvadene
3. silver sulfadiazine	C. Azulfidine

Calculate Medication Dosages

1. The primary health care provider prescribed sulfasalazine oral suspension 500 mg every 8 hours. The nurse has sulfasalazine oral suspension 250 mg/5 mL on hand. What dosage should the nurse give?

2. The primary health care provider orders sulfamethoxazole 2 g orally initially, followed by 1 g orally two times a day. The nurse has 1000-mg tablets on hand. How many tablets should the nurse give for the initial dose?

● Prepare for the NCLEX®

Build Your Knowledge

1. A nurse working in the clinic asks how the sulfonamides control an infection. The most accurate answer is that these drugs _____.
   1. encourage the production of antibodies
   2. inhibit folic acid metabolism
   3. reduce urine output
   4. make the urine alkaline, which eliminates bacteria

2. Clients receiving sulfasalazine for ulcerative colitis are told that the drug _____.
   1. is not to be taken with food
   2. rarely causes adverse effects
   3. may cause hair loss
   4. may turn the urine an orange-yellow color

3. On an overcast day, the nurse instructs the client taking sulfonamides to _____.
   1. wear sunscreen
   2. sunbathe without fear of skin reaction
   3. stay indoors with blinds shut
   4. protect feet from harm

4. A diabetic client who takes oral medications is receiving a sulfonamide for a UTI. The client is taught that compared to what the usual reading has been, the blood glucose level will be:
   1. higher
   2. the same
   3. lower
   4. unreadable due to the medication

5. The nurse observes a client receiving a sulfonamide for Stevens-Johnson syndrome. The signs and symptoms that might indicate this syndrome include _____.
   1. swelling of the extremities
   2. increased blood pressure and pulse rate
   3. lesions on the skin or mucous membranes
   4. pain in the joints

6. The nurse can evaluate the client's response to therapy by asking him if _____.
   1. he completed the entire course of therapy
   2. his symptoms have been relieved
   3. he has seen any evidence of blood in the urine
   4. he has experienced any constipation

Apply Your Knowledge

7. The nurse instructs Mrs. Moore to drink at least 2000 mL of fluid while taking a sulfa drug. The client states she cannot drink that much. The nurse should ask questions to assess which body system?
   1. respiratory
   2. genitourinary
   3. neurologic
   4. cardiac

8. When mafenide (Sulfamylon) is applied to a burned area, the nurse _____.
   1. first covers the burned area with a sterile compress
   2. irrigates the area with normal saline solution
   3. warns the client that stinging or burning may be felt
   4. instructs the client to drink two to three extra glasses of water each day

Alternate-Format Questions

9. Arrange the following steps of caring for a burn with Silvadene correctly:
   1. apply dressing material
   2. cleanse and remove debris on surface
   3. apply drug according to directions
   4. remove dressing

10. Identify the correct properties of sulfonamide drugs. **Select all that apply**.
    1. bacteriocidal
    2. reduces inflammation in colon
    3. inhibits folic acid in bacterial cells
    4. antibacterial

To check your answers, see Appendix G.

the**Point** *For more NCLEX-style questions, log on to http://thepoint.lww.com to access more than 1000 questions.*

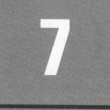

Antibacterial Drugs That Disrupt the Bacterial Cell Wall

LEARNING OBJECTIVES

On completion of this chapter, the student will:

1. Identify the uses, general drug actions, and general adverse reactions, contraindications, precautions, and interactions of antibacterial drugs that disrupt bacterial cell walls.
2. Identify important preadministration and ongoing assessment activities the nurse should perform on the patient taking an antibacterial drug that disrupts bacterial cell walls.
3. List nursing diagnoses particular to a patient taking an antibacterial drug that disrupts bacterial cell walls.
4. Discuss hypersensitivity reactions as they relate to antibiotic therapy.
5. Discuss ways to promote optimal response to therapy, nursing actions to minimize adverse effects, and important points to keep in mind when educating patients about the use of antibacterial drugs that disrupt bacterial cell walls.

KEY TERMS

anaphylactic reactions • unusual or exaggerated allergic reactions; see anaphylactic shock (Chapter 1)

angioedema • localized wheals or swellings in subcutaneous tissues or mucous membranes, which may be due to an allergic response

bacterial resistance • phenomenon by which a bacteria-produced substance inactivates or destroys an antibiotic drug

beta (β)-lactam ring • portion of the penicillin drug molecule that can break a bacterial cell wall

cross-sensitivity • allergy to drugs in the same or related groups

culture and sensitivity test • culture of bacteria to determine to which antibiotic the microorganism is sensitive

glossitis • inflammation of the tongue

malaise • discomfort, uneasiness

methicillin-resistant *Staphylococcus aureus* (MRSA) • bacterium that is resistant to methicillin

nephrotoxicity • damage to the kidneys by a toxic substance

otitis media • infection of the middle ear

pathogens • disease-producing microorganisms

penicillinase • enzyme produced by bacteria that deactivates penicillin

perioperative • pertaining to the preoperative, intraoperative, or postoperative period

phlebitis • inflammation of a vein

prophylaxis • prevention

pseudomembranous colitis • severe, life-threatening form of diarrhea that occurs when normal flora of the bowel is eliminated and replaced with *Clostridium difficile* (*C. diff*) bacteria

Stevens-Johnson syndrome (SJS) • fever, cough, muscular aches and pains, headache, and lesions of the skin, mucous membranes, and eyes; the lesions appear as red wheals or blisters, often starting on the face, in the mouth, or on the lips, neck, and extremities

stomatitis • inflammation of a cavity opening, such as the oral cavity

synthesis • combining or growing a number of different parts to make a new item

thrombophlebitis • inflammation of a vein with clot formation

DRUG CLASSES

Penicillins	Cephalosporins
• Natural penicillins	• First generation
• Aminopenicillins	• Second generation
• Extended-spectrum penicillins	• Third generation
	• Fourth generation
	Carbapenems

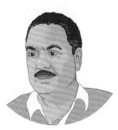

PHARMACOLOGY IN PRACTICE

Alfredo Garcia is seen in the outpatient clinic for an upper respiratory infection. The primary health care provider prescribes a cephalosporin and asks you to give the patient instructions for taking the drug. You note that Mr. Garcia appears to understand very little English.

69

The cellular content in a human being is contained by a cell membrane. Unlike the human cell, a bacterial cell has a wall, not a membrane. Penicillins, cephalosporins, carbapenems, and vancomycin all inhibit bacterial cell wall **synthesis** (growth and repair).

Enzymes known as penicillin-binding proteins (PBPs) are involved in bacterial cell wall synthesis and cell division. Antibiotics, which interfere with these processes, inhibit cell wall synthesis, causing rapid destruction of the bacterial cell. When penicillin was first used, these drugs worked very well because bacteria have a receptor on the cell wall that attracts the penicillin molecule. That is, when the drug attaches to the cell, a portion of the drug molecule (the **beta (β)-lactam ring**) breaks the cell wall and the cell dies (bactericidal action). Now, however, after many years of use of the penicillins, drug-resistant strains of microorganisms developed, making the penicillins less effective than some of the new antibiotics in treating a broad range of infections.

Cephalosporins are structurally and chemically related to penicillin. The cephalosporins are a valuable group of drugs that are effective in the treatment of infection with almost all of the strains of bacteria affected by the penicillins, as well as some strains of bacteria that have become resistant to penicillin. Carbapenems are a relatively new class of bacteriocidal drugs that have the largest spectrum of any antibiotic (Fig. 7.1).

Identifying the Appropriate Anti-Infective

Selection of Drugs

After a culture and sensitivity report is received, the strain of microorganisms causing the infection is known as well as which antibiotics will or will not kill the microorganisms (see Chapter 6). The primary health care provider then selects the antibiotic to which the microorganism is sensitive, because that is the antibiotic that will be effective in the treatment of the infection.

Drugs have bactericidal action provided there is an adequate concentration of the drug in the body. The concentration of any drug in the body is referred to as the *blood level.* An inadequate concentration (or inadequate blood level) of an antibiotic may produce bacteriostatic activity, which may or may not control the infection.

Resistance to Drugs

Bacterial resistance is the ability of bacteria to produce substances that inactivate or destroy the antibiotic. Because bacteria have this ability, many more drugs have been developed in addition to the sulfonamides and penicillins to fight bacterial infections. They include cephalosporins, the tetracycline group, and various other drugs.

When antibiotics are used by one person over time, or by a group of people who live in close proximity (as in a long-term care facility), drug resistance becomes an issue. Some bacteria may be naturally resistant to an antibiotic, or they may acquire a resistance to the drug. When the susceptible bacteria are destroyed, what remains are the resistant bacteria. As a result, strains of drug-resistant bacteria multiply. These can range from the penicillinase enzyme–producing bacteria to **methicillin-resistant *Staphylococcus aureus*** (**MRSA**).

MRSA is a type of bacteria that is resistant to certain antibiotics. These antibiotics include methicillin and other, more common antibiotics, such as oxacillin, penicillin, and amoxicillin. According to the Centers for Disease Control and Prevention (CDC), staphylococcal infections, including MRSA, occur most frequently among persons who are in hospitals and health care facilities (such as skilled nursing facilities and dialysis centers) and who have weakened immune systems. In recent years, outbreaks in the community have heightened

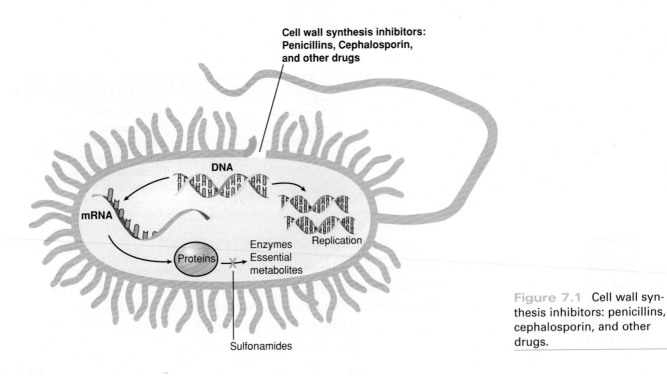

Figure 7.1 Cell wall synthesis inhibitors: penicillins, cephalosporin, and other drugs.

the public's awareness of MRSA. Also emerging is a new resistance associated with bacteria that have both natural and acquired resistance. An example is vancomycin-resistant enterococci (VRE). This drug resistance is affecting severely ill, immunocompromised patients in intensive care, transplant, and some cancer treatment units.

Patient education to increase behaviors that will prevent or diminish resistance is important when antibiotics are prescribed (see Patient Teaching for Improved Patient Outcomes: Preventing Anti-Infective Resistance at the end of this chapter).

PENICILLINS

The antibacterial properties of natural penicillins were discovered in 1928 and used clinically to treat infections by 1941. Although the sulfonamides were the first anti-infectives, the natural penicillins were the first large-scale antibiotics used to combat infection. Used for more than 70 years, the penicillins are still an important and effective group of antibiotics for the treatment of susceptible **pathogens** (disease-causing microorganisms).

Actions

There are four groups of penicillins: (1) natural penicillins, (2) penicillinase-resistant penicillins, (3) aminopenicillins, and (4) extended-spectrum penicillins, All work to inhibit the integrity of the bacterial cell wall. See the Summary Drug Table: Antibacterial Drugs That Inhibit Cell Wall Synthesis for a more complete listing of the penicillins.

The natural penicillins have a fairly narrow spectrum of activity, which means that they are effective against only a few strains of bacteria. Newer, chemically modified aminopenicillins were developed to combat this problem. Because of their chemical modifications, they are more slowly excreted by the kidneys and thus have a somewhat wider spectrum of antibacterial activity.

Various types of bacterial resistance have developed against the penicillins. One example of bacterial resistance is the ability of certain bacteria to produce **penicillinase**, an enzyme that inactivates penicillin. The penicillinase-resistant penicillins were developed to combat this problem.

Certain bacteria have developed the ability to produce enzymes called *β-lactamases,* which are able to destroy the β-lactam ring of the drug. Fortunately, chemicals were discovered that inhibit the activity of these enzymes. Penicillin–β-lactamase inhibitor combinations are a type of penicillin with a wider spectrum of antibacterial activity. Examples of these β-lactamase inhibitors are clavulanic acid, sulbactam, and tazobactam. When these chemicals are used alone, they have little antimicrobial activity. However, when combined with certain penicillins, they extend the spectrum of the penicillin's antibacterial activity. The β-lactamase inhibitors bind with the penicillin and protect the penicillin from destruction. Examples of combinations of penicillins with β-lactamase inhibitors are given in Display 7.1; also see the Summary Drug Table: Antibacterial Drugs That Inhibit Cell Wall Synthesis for more information on these combinations.

> ### *Display 7.1* **Penicillin–β-Lactamase Inhibitor Combinations**
>
> - Augmentin—combination of amoxicillin and clavulanic acid
> - Timentin—combination of ticarcillin and clavulanic acid
> - Unasyn—combination of ampicillin and sulbactam
> - Zosyn—combination of piperacillin and tazobactam

Extended-spectrum penicillins are effective against an even wider range of bacteria than the broad-spectrum penicillins. These penicillins are used to destroy bacteria such as *Pseudomonas.*

Uses

Infectious Disease

The natural and semisynthetic penicillins are used in the treatment of moderate to mildly severe bacterial infections. Penicillins may be used to treat infections such as:

- Urinary tract infections (UTIs)
- Septicemia
- Meningitis
- Intra-abdominal infections
- Sexually transmitted infections (syphilis)
- Pneumonia and other respiratory infections

Examples of infectious microorganisms (bacteria) that may respond to penicillin therapy include pneumococci and group A β-hemolytic streptococci. Because of the increasing resistance of staphylococci to penicillin G, the penicillinase-resistant penicillins are used as initial therapy for any suspected staphylococcal infection until culture and sensitivity results are known.

Prophylaxis

Because penicillin targets bacterial cells, it is of no value in treating viral or fungal infections. However, the primary health care provider occasionally prescribes penicillin as **prophylaxis** (prevention) against a potential secondary bacterial infection that can occur in a patient with a viral infection. In these situations the viral infection has weakened the body's defenses and the person is susceptible to other infections, particularly a bacterial infection. Penicillin also may be prescribed as prophylaxis for a potential infection in high-risk individuals, such as those with a history of rheumatic fever. Penicillin is taken several hours or in some instances days before and after an operative procedure, such as dental, oral, or upper respiratory tract procedures, that can result in bacteria entering the bloodstream. Taking penicillin before and after the procedure will usually prevent a bacterial infection in high-risk patients. Penicillin also may be given prophylactically on a continuing basis to those with rheumatic fever or chronic ear infections.

Adverse Reactions

Gastrointestinal System Reactions

- **Glossitis** (inflammation of the tongue) when given orally
- **Stomatitis** (inflammation of the mouth), dry mouth
- Gastritis
- Nausea, vomiting
- Diarrhea, abdominal pain

Administration route reactions include pain at the injection site when given intramuscularly (IM) and irritation of the vein and **phlebitis** (inflammation of a vein) when given intravenously (IV).

Hypersensitivity Reactions

A hypersensitivity (or allergic) reaction to a drug occurs in some individuals, especially those with a history of allergy to many substances. Signs and symptoms of a hypersensitivity to penicillin are highlighted in Display 7.2.

An **anaphylactic reaction**, which is a severe form of hypersensitivity, also can occur (see Chapter 1). Anaphylactic reactions occur more frequently after parenteral administration but can occur with oral use. This reaction is likely to be immediate and severe in susceptible individuals. Signs of anaphylactic reaction or shock include severe hypotension, loss of consciousness, and acute respiratory distress. If not immediately treated, anaphylactic shock can be fatal.

Once an individual is allergic to one penicillin, he or she is usually allergic to all of the penicillins. Those allergic to penicillin also have a higher incidence of allergy to the cephalosporins. Allergy to drugs in the same or related groups is called **cross-sensitivity**.

Other Reactions

Other adverse reactions associated with penicillin include hematopoietic (blood cell) changes:

- Anemia (low red blood cell count)
- Thrombocytopenia (low platelet count)

Display 7.2 Signs and Symptoms of Hypersensitivity to Penicillin and Other Antibiotics

- Skin rash
- Urticaria (hives)
- Sneezing
- Wheezing
- Pruritus (itching)
- Bronchospasm (spasm of the bronchi)
- Laryngospasm (spasm of the larynx)
- Angioedema (also called angioneurotic edema)—swelling of the skin and mucous membranes, especially around and in the mouth and throat
- Hypotension—can progress to shock
- Signs and symptoms resembling serum sickness—chills, fever, edema, joint and muscle pain, and malaise

---

- Leukopenia (low white blood cell count)
- Bone marrow depression

Contraindications and Precautions

Penicillins are contraindicated in patients with a history of hypersensitivity to penicillin or the cephalosporins.

Penicillins should be used cautiously in patients with renal disease, asthma, bleeding disorders, gastrointestinal (GI) disease, pregnancy (pregnancy category C) or lactation (may cause diarrhea or candidiasis in the infant), and history of allergies. Any indication of sensitivity is reason for caution.

Interactions

The following interactions may occur when a penicillin is administered with another agent.

Interacting Agent	Common Use	Effect of Interaction
oral contraceptives (with estrogen)	Contraception	Decreased effectiveness of contraceptive agent (with ampicillin, penicillin V).
tetracyclines	Anti-infective	Decreased effectiveness of penicillins
anticoagulants	Prevent blood clots	Increased bleeding risks (with large doses of penicillins)
β-adrenergic blocking drugs	Blood pressure control and heart problems	May increase the risk for an anaphylactic reaction

HERBAL CONSIDERATIONS

Goldenseal (*Hydrastis canadensis*) is an herb found growing in certain areas of the northeastern United States, particularly the Ohio River valley. Goldenseal has been used to wash inflamed or infected eyes and in making yellow dye. There are many more traditional uses of the herb, including as an antiseptic for the skin, as a mouthwash for canker sores, and in the treatment of sinus infections and digestive problems such as peptic ulcers and gastritis. In the 19th century, goldenseal was touted as an "herbal antibiotic" for treating gonorrhea and UTIs. Though used over time by American Indian tribes as an insect repellent, stimulant, and diuretic, there is no scientific evidence to support its benefit for these purposes. Another myth surrounding goldenseal's use is that taking the herb masks the presence of illicit drugs in the urine. Evidence does support the use of goldenseal to treat diarrhea caused by bacteria or intestinal parasites, such as *Giardia*. The herb is contraindicated during pregnancy and in patients with hypertension. Adverse reactions are rare when the herb is used as directed. However, this herb should not be taken for more than a few days to 1 week (DerMarderosian, 2003).

CEPHALOSPORINS

The cephalosporins are divided into first-, second-, third-, and fourth-generation drugs. In general, progression from the first-generation to the fourth-generation drugs shows an

> ### *Display 7.3* Examples of First-, Second-, Third-, and Fourth-Generation Cephalosporins
>
> - First generation—cephalexin (Keflex), cefazolin (Ancef)
> - Second generation—cefaclor (Raniclor), cefoxitin (Mefoxin), cefuroxime (Zinacef)
> - Third generation—cefoperazone (Cefobid), cefotaxime (Claforan), ceftriaxone (Rocephin)
> - Fourth generation—cefepime (Maxipime)

increase in the sensitivity of gram-negative microorganisms and a decrease in the sensitivity of gram-positive microorganisms. For example, a first-generation cephalosporin would be more useful against gram-positive microorganisms than would a third-generation cephalosporin. This scheme of classification is becoming less clearly defined as newer drugs are introduced. The fourth generation of cephalosporins has a broader spectrum and longer duration of resistance to β-lactamase. These drugs are used to treat urinary tract and skin infections and hospital-acquired pneumonias. Examples of first-, second-, third-, and fourth-generation cephalosporins are listed in Display 7.3. For a more complete listing, see the Summary Drug Table: Antibacterial Drugs That Inhibit Cell Wall Synthesis.

Actions

Cephalosporins have a β-lactam ring and target the bacterial cell wall, making it defective and unstable. This action is similar to the action of penicillin. The cephalosporins are usually bactericidal.

Uses

The cephalosporins are used in the treatment of infections caused by bacteria, including:

- Respiratory infections
- **Otitis media** (ear infection)
- Bone/joint infections
- Genitourinary tract and other infections caused by bacteria

Cephalosporins are used prophylactically to prevent infection when victims are treated following a sexual assault. The most frequent infections diagnosed following an assault include trichomoniasis, bacterial vaginitis, gonorrhea, and chlamydia. A cephalosporin drug is the primary drug in post–sexual assault medication protocols (see Appendix E).

This class of drugs also may be used throughout the **perioperative** period—that is, during the preoperative, intraoperative, and postoperative periods—to prevent infection in patients having surgery on a contaminated or potentially contaminated area, such as the GI tract or vagina. In some instances, a specific drug may be recommended for postoperative prophylactic use only.

Adverse Reactions

Gastrointestinal System Reactions

- Nausea
- Vomiting
- Diarrhea

Other Reactions

- Headache
- Dizziness
- **Malaise**
- Heartburn
- Fever
- **Nephrotoxicity**
- Hypersensitivity (allergic) reactions—may occur with administration of the cephalosporins and may range from mild to life-threatening. Mild hypersensitivity reactions include pruritus, urticaria, and skin rashes; the more serious reactions include **Stevens-Johnson syndrome** and hepatic and renal dysfunction.
- Aplastic anemia (deficient red blood cell production)
- Toxic epidermal necrolysis (death of the epidermal layer of the skin)

> **! NURSING ALERT**
>
> Because of the close relationship of the cephalosporins to penicillin, a patient who is allergic to penicillin also may be allergic to the cephalosporins. Approximately 10% of the people allergic to a penicillin drug are also allergic to a cephalosporin drug.

Administration route reactions include pain, tenderness, and inflammation at the injection site when given IM, and phlebitis or **thrombophlebitis** along the vein when given IV. Therapy with cephalosporins may result in a bacterial or fungal superinfection. Diarrhea may be an indication of **pseudomembranous colitis**, which is one type of bacterial superinfection (see Chapter 9).

Contraindications and Precautions

Do not administer cephalosporins if the patient has a history of allergies to cephalosporins.

Cephalosporins should be used cautiously in patients with renal disease, hepatic impairment, bleeding disorder, pregnancy (pregnancy category B), and known penicillin allergy.

Interactions

The following interactions may occur when a cephalosporin is administered with another agent:

Interacting Drug	Common Use	Effect of Interaction
aminoglycosides	Anti-infective	Increased risk for nephrotoxicity
oral anticoagulants	Blood thinner	Increased risk for bleeding
loop diuretics	Hypertension, reduce edema	Increased cephalosporin blood level

Probenecid (Benemid, used for gout pain) will increase the levels of most cephalosporins (*except* cefoperazone, ceftazidime, and ceftriaxone).

! NURSING ALERT

A disulfiram-like (Antabuse) reaction may occur if alcohol is consumed within 72 hours after administration of certain cephalosporins (i.e., cefamandole, cefoperazone, and cefotetan). Symptoms of a disulfiram-like reaction (associated with the use of disulfiram, a drug used to treat alcoholism) include flushing, throbbing in the head and neck, respiratory difficulty, vomiting, sweating, chest pain, and hypotension. Severe reactions may cause dysrhythmias and unconsciousness.

CARBAPENEMS AND MISCELLANEOUS DRUGS THAT INHIBIT CELL WALL SYNTHESIS

The carbapenems, vancomycin, and monobactam drugs all play a role in the inhibition of bacterial cell wall synthesis.

Actions

Carbapenems inhibit synthesis of the bacterial cell wall and cause the death of susceptible cells. Vancomycin and its synthetic derivative drug (telavancin) act against susceptible gram-positive bacteria by inhibiting bacterial cell wall synthesis and increasing cell wall permeability. Aztreonam has a β-lactam nucleus and therefore is called a *monobactam*. This is structurally different from the β-lactam ring of the penicillins, yet it still functions to inhibit bacterial cell wall synthesis.

Uses

Meropenem (Merrem IV) is used for intra-abdominal infections and bacterial meningitis. Imipenem-cilastatin (Primaxin) is used to treat serious infections, endocarditis, and septicemia. Doripenem (Doribax) is used to treat intra-abdominal and complicated urinary tract infections caused by bacteria. Telavancin (Vibativ) is used to treat complicated skin and skin structure infections. Vancomycin (Vancocin) is used in the treatment of serious gram-positive infections that do not respond to treatment with other anti-infectives. It also may be used in treating anti-infective–associated pseudomembranous colitis caused by *Clostridium difficile*. The monobactams have bactericidal action and are used to treat gram-negative microorganisms.

Adverse Reactions

The most common adverse reactions with these drugs include nausea, vomiting, diarrhea, and rash. As with many other anti-infectives, there is a risk of pseudomembranous colitis (see Chapter 9). Assess stools for blood when the patient has diarrhea.

Carbapenems also can cause an abscess or phlebitis at the injection site. An abscess is suspected if the injection site appears red or is tender and warm to the touch. Tissue sloughing at the injection site also may occur.

Nephrotoxicity (damage to the kidneys) and ototoxicity (damage to the organs of hearing) may be seen with the administration of vancomycin especially in patients with preexisting kidney disease. Additional adverse reactions include chills, fever, urticaria, and sudden fall in blood pressure with parenteral administration. For more information, see Summary Drug Table: Anti-infective Drugs That Inhibit Cell Wall Synthesis.

Contraindications, Precautions, and Interactions

Carbapenems, aztreonam, and telavancin are contraindicated in patients who are allergic to cephalosporins and penicillins and in patients with renal failure. These drugs are not recommended in children younger than 3 months or for women during pregnancy (pregnancy category B) or lactation. Carbapenems are used cautiously in patients with central nervous system (CNS) disorders, seizure disorders, or renal or hepatic failure. The excretion of carbapenems is inhibited when the drug is administered to a patient also taking probenecid (Benemid). Aztreonam should be used cautiously in patients with renal or hepatic impairment.

Vancomycin should not be used in patients with a known hypersensitivity to the drug and is used cautiously in patients with renal or hearing impairment and during pregnancy (pregnancy category C) and lactation. When administered with other ototoxic and nephrotoxic drugs, additive effects may occur. In other words, one drug alone may not cause the hearing or kidney problem, but when another drug with similar adverse effects is given with vancomycin, the patient is more likely to experience a problem.

NURSING PROCESS

PATIENT RECEIVING PENICILLIN, CEPHALOSPORIN, CARBAPENEMS, OR MISCELLANEOUS CELL WALL INHIBITORS

ASSESSMENT

Preadministration Assessment

Before administering the first dose of penicillin or a cephalosporin, obtain or review the patient's general health history. The health history includes an allergy history, a history of all medical and surgical treatments, a drug history, and the current symptoms of the infection. If the patient has a history of allergy—particularly a drug allergy—be sure to explore this area to ensure the patient is not allergic to penicillin or a cephalosporin.

Take and record vital signs. When appropriate, it is important to obtain a description of the signs and symptoms of the infection from the patient or family. Assess the infected area (when possible) and record findings on the patient's chart. It is important to describe accurately any signs and symptoms related to the patient's infection, such as color and type of drainage from a wound, pain, redness and inflammation, color of sputum, or presence of an odor. In addition, note the patient's general appearance. A culture and sensitivity test is almost always ordered, and you should obtain the results if possible, before giving the first dose of antibiotic. Liver and kidney function tests may be ordered by the primary health care provider; if so, check the results before administering the drug.

Ongoing Assessment

An ongoing assessment is important in evaluating the patient's response to therapy, such as a decrease in temperature, the relief of symptoms caused by the infection (e.g., pain or discomfort), an increase in appetite, and a change in the appearance or amount of drainage (when originally present). Notify the primary health care provider if signs of the infection appear to worsen.

Additional culture and sensitivity tests may be performed during therapy because microorganisms causing the infection may become resistant to the antibiotic, or a superinfection may occur. Check the patient's skin regularly for rash and be alert for any loose stools or diarrhea. A urinalysis, complete blood count, and renal and hepatic function tests also may be performed at intervals during therapy.

>
> **NURSING ALERT**
> Observe the patient closely for a hypersensitivity reaction, which may occur any time during therapy with the penicillins. If it does occur, it is important to contact the primary health care provider immediately and withhold the drug. Interventions below outline supportive care measures for hypersensitivity reactions while awaiting primary health care provider orders.

NURSING DIAGNOSES

Drug-specific nursing diagnoses include the following:

- **Impaired Skin Integrity** related to hypersensitivity to the drug
- **Risk for Impaired Gas Exchange** related to an allergic reaction to the drug
- **Impaired Urinary Elimination** related to nephrotoxic effects of cephalosporin
- **Diarrhea** related to a bacterial secondary infection or superinfection
- **Impaired Oral Mucous Membranes** related to a secondary bacterial or fungal infection
- **Impaired Comfort: Increased Fever** related to ineffectiveness of antibiotic against the infection

Nursing diagnoses related to drug administration are discussed in Chapter 4.

PLANNING

The expected outcomes for the patient depend on the reason for administering the antibiotic but may include an optimal response to drug therapy, meeting patient needs related to management of common adverse reactions, and confidence in an understanding of the medication regimen.

IMPLEMENTATION

Promoting Optimal Response to Therapy: Proper Administration

The results of a culture and sensitivity test may take a number of days, because time must be allowed for the bacteria to grow on the culture media. However, infections are treated

as soon as possible. The primary health care provider determines the treatment of choice until the results of the culture and sensitivity tests are known. In many instances, the primary health care provider selects a broad-spectrum antibiotic for initial treatment because of the many penicillin-resistant strains of microorganisms.

>
> **NURSING ALERT**
> Be sure to question the patient about allergy to penicillin or cephalosporins before administering the first dose, even when an accurate drug history has been taken. It is important to tell patients what drug they are receiving because information regarding a drug allergy may have been forgotten at the time the initial drug history was obtained. If a patient states he or she is allergic to penicillin or a cephalosporin, withhold the drug and contact the primary health care provider.

ORAL ADMINISTRATION. Adequate blood levels of the drug must be maintained for the agent to be effective. Accidental omission or delay of a dose results in decreased blood levels, which will reduce the effectiveness of the antibiotic. It is best to give oral penicillins on an empty stomach, 1 hour before or 2 hours after a meal. Penicillin V and amoxicillin may be given without regard to meals. Most cephalosporins may be taken on an empty stomach, especially ceftibuten (Cedax). However, if the patient experiences GI upset, you can administer the drugs with food. The absorption of oral cefuroxime and cefpodoxime is increased when given with food.

Some antibiotics are available as powder for a suspension and are reconstituted by a pharmacist or a nurse. Shake oral suspensions well before administering them. It is important to keep this form of the drug refrigerated until it is used.

> **CHRONIC CARE CONSIDERATIONS**
> People with phenylketonuria (PKU) need to be aware that the oral suspension cefprozil (Cefzil) contains phenylalanine, a substance that people with PKU cannot process. In addition, diabetic patients who use urine testing for determining diabetic medicine dosing and who are prescribed cephalosporins need to be aware that this drug may interfere with accurate test results. The primary care provider should be consulted before diet and drug changes are made.

PARENTERAL ADMINISTRATION. In most health care facilities, the drug is prepared in the pharmacy and delivered to the nurse for administration. When this service is not available in preparing a parenteral form of antibiotics, you should read the manufacturer's package insert for each drug for instructions regarding reconstitution of powder for injection, storage of unused portions, life of the drug after it is reconstituted, methods of IV administration, and precautions to be taken when the drug is administered.

> **NURSING ALERT**
> Administer each IV dose of vancomycin over 60 minutes. Too rapid an infusion may result in a sudden and profound fall in blood pressure and shock.

When giving vancomycin IV, closely monitor the infusion rate and the patient's blood pressure. Report any decrease in blood pressure or occurrence of throbbing neck or back pain. These symptoms could indicate a severe adverse reaction referred to as red-neck or red-man syndrome. Other symptoms of red-man syndrome include fever, chills, paresthesias, and erythema (redness) of the neck and back.

It is important to note that penicillin is often ordered in units; milligram equivalency may or may not be included. The exact equivalency usually is stated on the container or package insert. If there is any question regarding the reconstitution of any drug, consult with a clinical pharmacist.

 LIFESPAN CONSIDERATIONS
Gerontology
When a penicillin or cephalosporin is given IM, inject the drug into a large muscle mass, such as the gluteus muscle or lateral aspect of the thigh. If the patient has been nonambulatory for any length of time or has paralysis, assess the muscle carefully because the large muscle may be atrophied. It is important to rotate injection sites. Warn the patient that at the time the drug is injected into the muscle, there may be a stinging or burning sensation and the area may be sore for a short time. Inform the primary health care provider if previously used areas for injection appear red or if the patient reports continued pain in the area.

Monitoring and Managing Patient Needs

IMPAIRED SKIN INTEGRITY. Dermatologic reactions such as hives, rashes, and skin lesions can occur with the administration of penicillin or cephalosporin. Treatment of minor hypersensitivity reactions may include administration of an antihistamine such as diphenhydramine (Benadryl) for a rash or itching. In mild cases, or where the benefit of the drug outweighs the discomfort of skin lesions, administer frequent skin care. Emollients, antipyretic creams, or a topical corticosteroid may be prescribed to promote comfort. Harsh soaps and perfumed lotions are avoided. Instruct the patient to avoid rubbing the area and to wear clothing that is not rough or irritating. It is important to report a rash or hives to the primary health care provider because this may be a precursor to a severe anaphylactic reaction (see section on Hypersensitivity Reactions). In severe cases, the primary health care provider may discontinue the drug therapy.

RISK FOR IMPAIRED GAS EXCHANGE. Major hypersensitivity reactions, such as bronchospasm, laryngospasm, hypotension, and **angioedema**, require immediate treatment with drugs such as epinephrine, cortisone, or an IV antihistamine (Fig. 7.2). When respiratory difficulty occurs, a tracheostomy may need to be performed.

! NURSING ALERT
After administering penicillin IM in the outpatient setting, ask the patient to wait in the area for at least 30 minutes. Anaphylactic reactions are most likely to occur within 30 minutes after injection.

IMPAIRED URINARY ELIMINATION. Nephrotoxicity may occur with the administration of cephalosporins. An early sign of this adverse reaction may be a decrease in urine output. Measure and record the fluid intake and output and notify the primary health care provider if the output is less than 500 mL daily. Any changes in the fluid intake–output ratio or in the appearance of the urine also may indicate nephrotoxicity.

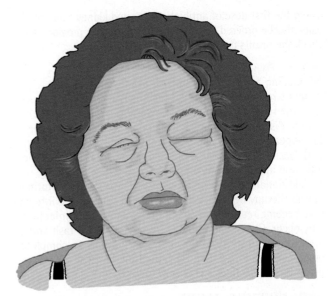

Figure 7.2 Example of person with an angioedema reaction to a drug.

It is important that you report these findings to the primary health care provider promptly.

 LIFESPAN CONSIDERATIONS
Gerontology
The older adult is more susceptible to the nephrotoxic effects of the cephalosporins, particularly if renal function is already diminished because of aging or disease. If renal impairment is present, a lower dosage and monitoring of blood creatinine levels are indicated. Blood creatinine levels greater than 4 mg/dL indicate serious renal impairment. In older patients with decreased renal function, a dosage adjustment may be necessary.

DIARRHEA. Diarrhea may be an indication of a superinfection of the GI tract or pseudomembranous colitis (see Chapter 9). Inspect all stools and notify the primary health care provider if diarrhea occurs, because it may be necessary to stop the drug. If diarrhea does occur and there appears to be blood and mucus in the stool, it is important to save a sample of the stool and test for occult blood using a test such as Hemoccult. If the stool tests positive for blood, save the sample for possible further laboratory analysis.

Observe the patient for other symptoms of a bacterial or fungal superinfection in the vaginal or anal area, such as pain or itching. It is important to report any signs and symptoms of a superinfection to the primary health care provider before administering the next dose of the drug. When symptoms are severe, additional treatment measures may be necessary, such as administration of an antipyretic drug for fever or an antifungal drug.

IMPAIRED ORAL MUCOUS MEMBRANES. The administration of oral penicillin may result in a fungal superinfection in the oral cavity. This condition is characterized by varying degrees of oral mucous membrane inflammation, swollen and red tongue, swollen gums, and pain in the mouth and throat.

To detect this problem early, inspect the patient's mouth daily for evidence of glossitis, sore tongue, ulceration, or a black, furry tongue. You may explain that, if the diet permits, yogurt, buttermilk, or *Acidophilus* capsules may be taken to reduce the risk of fungal superinfection.

Inspect the mouth and gums often and give frequent mouth care with a nonirritating solution. A soft-bristled toothbrush is used when brushing is needed. A nonirritating soft diet may be required. Monitor the dietary intake to ensure that the patient is receiving adequate nutrition. Antifungal agents or local anesthetics are sometimes recommended to soothe the irritated membranes.

IMPAIRED COMFORT: INCREASED FEVER. Take vital signs every 4 hours, or more often if necessary. It is important to report any increase in temperature to the primary health care provider, because additional treatment measures, such as administration of an antipyretic drug or change in the drug or dosage, may be necessary. An increase in body temperature several days after the start of therapy may indicate a secondary bacterial infection or failure of the drug to control the original infection. On occasion, the fever may be caused by an adverse reaction to the penicillin. In these cases, the fever can usually be managed by using an antipyretic drug.

Educating the Patient and Family
Any time a drug is prescribed for a patient, you are responsible for ensuring that the patient has a thorough understanding of the drug, the treatment regimen, and adverse reactions. Some patients do not adhere to the prescribed drug regimen for a variety of reasons, such as failure to comprehend the prescribed regimen or failure to understand the importance of continued and uninterrupted therapy. Describing the drug regimen and stressing the importance of continued and uninterrupted therapy when teaching the patient who is prescribed an antibiotic will help prevent drug resistance due to stopping the medication too early.

Provide the following information to patients who are prescribed an antibiotic:

■ Prophylaxis—Take the drug as prescribed until the primary health care provider discontinues therapy.

■ Infection—Complete the full course of therapy. Do not stop taking the drug, even if the symptoms have disappeared, unless directed to do so by the primary health care provider.

■ Take the drug at the prescribed times of day because it is important to keep an adequate amount of drug in the body throughout the entire 24 hours of each day.

■ Penicillin (oral)—Take the drug on an empty stomach either 1 hour before or 2 hours after meals (exceptions: penicillin V and amoxicillin).

■ Take each dose with a full 8-ounce glass of water.

■ Oral suspensions—Keep the container refrigerated (if so labeled), shake the drug well before pouring (if so labeled), and return the drug to the refrigerator immediately after pouring the dose. Drugs that require refrigeration lose their potency when kept at room temperature. A small amount of the drug may be left after the last dose is taken. Discard any remaining drug, because the drug (in suspension form) begins to lose its potency after a few weeks.

■ ⚠ Avoid drinking alcoholic beverages when taking the cephalosporins and for 3 days after completing the course of therapy, because severe reactions may occur.

■ To reduce the risk of superinfection during antibiotic therapy, take yogurt, buttermilk, or *Acidophilus* capsules.

■ If you are a woman who has been prescribed ampicillin and penicillin V and who takes birth control pills containing estrogen, use additional contraception measures.

■ Notify the primary health care provider immediately should one or more of the following occur: skin rash; hives (urticaria); severe diarrhea; vaginal or anal itching; black, furry tongue; sores in the mouth; swelling around the mouth or eyes; breathing difficulty; or GI disturbances such as nausea, vomiting, and diarrhea. Do not take the next dose of the drug until the problem has been discussed with the primary health care provider.

■ Never give this drug to another individual even though his or her symptoms appear to be the same as yours.

■ Notify the primary health care provider if the symptoms of the infection do not improve or if the condition becomes worse.

■ Never skip doses or stop therapy unless told to do so by the primary health care provider (see Patient Teaching for Improved Patient Outcomes: Preventing Anti-Infective

---

Patient Teaching for Improved Patient Outcomes

Preventing Anti-Infective Resistance

When you teach, make sure your patient understands the following:

✔ Review the reason for the drug and the prescribed drug regimen, including drug name, correct dose, and frequency of administration. Have the patient or family member tell you about the reason and drug in his or her own terms. Use the services of an interpreter if the patient has limited English proficiency.
✔ Stress the importance of continued and uninterrupted therapy, even if the patient feels better after a few doses and symptoms have disappeared.
✔ Give written materials to take home; find language-appropriate items if the patient has limited English proficiency.
✔ Instruct the patient to continue taking the drug until the drug is finished or the prescriber discontinues therapy.
✔ Urge the patient and family to discard any unused drug once therapy is discontinued or completed.
✔ Warn the patient not to use any leftover antibiotic or to take another family member's antibiotic as self-treatment for a suspected infection.
✔ Review the possible adverse reactions and the signs and symptoms of a new infection or of a worsening infection, both verbally and in writing.
✔ Instruct the patient and family to notify the health care provider at once should the patient experience any adverse reactions or signs and symptoms of infection.

Resistance). When a penicillin is to be taken for a long time for prophylaxis, you may feel well despite the need for long-term antibiotic therapy. There may be a tendency to omit one or more doses or even neglect to take the drug for an extended time.

EVALUATION

- Therapeutic response is achieved, and there is no evidence of infection.
- Adverse reactions are identified, reported to the primary health care provider, and managed successfully with appropriate nursing interventions:
  - Skin is intact and free of infection.
  - Patient maintains adequate gas exchange.
  - Patient maintains an adequate fluid intake for proper urinary elimination.
  - Patient reports adequate bowel movements.
  - Mucous membranes are moist and intact.
  - Patient reports comfort without fever.
- Patient and family express confidence and demonstrate understanding of the drug regimen.

PHARMACOLOGY IN PRACTICE
THINKING CRITICALLY

Mrs. Garcia also came to the clinic visit. She has been telling the staff members about the party they are giving this weekend and hopes that Mr. Garcia is well enough to be the bartender for the event. As you prepare to assess and teach Mr. Garcia, what do you know about limited health literacy? What teaching points should you emphasize after your discussion with Mrs. Garcia? What tools can you use to help you with his limited English proficiency?

KEY POINTS

- Penicillin, cephalosporin, carbapenem, and vancomycin are primarily bactericidal; they work by breaking or inhibiting the growth of the cell walls found in bacterial cells. Categories of penicillin drugs are defined by modifications for resistance, and cephalosporin generations tend to define the sensitivity of the drugs to microorganisms.

- These drugs are used to treat bacterial infections such as UTIs or otitis media or prophylactically to prevent secondary bacterial infections.

- People allergic to penicillin may also have an allergy to cephalosporins because they are structurally and chemically related drugs.

- Bacteria can become resistant to certain drugs. Drugs with modifications are created to combat resistance. One of the best methods to prevent resistance is to teach the patient to take the medication as instructed: take on time, no omissions, and for the length of the prescription.

- Adverse reactions are often times gastrointestinal, and superinfections can occur when normal flora is also killed by the drugs. Chronic use of cephalosporins may result in damage to the kidneys. Older patients using these drugs should be monitored closely for kidney function.

Summary Drug Table ANTIBACTERIAL DRUGS THAT INHIBIT BACTERIAL CELL WALL SYNTHESIS

Generic Name	Trade Name	Uses	Adverse Reactions	Dosage Ranges
Penicillins				
Narrow Spectrum Penicillins				
℞ penicillin G (aqueous) *pen-ih-sill'-in*	Pfizerpen	Infections due to susceptible microorganisms; meningococcal meningitis, septicemia	Glossitis, stomatitis, gastritis, furry tongue, nausea, vomiting, diarrhea, rash, fever, pain at injection site, hypersensitivity reactions, hematopoietic changes	Up to 20–30 million Units/day IV or IM; dosage may also be based on weight
℞ penicillin G benzathine *ben-zah-theen*	Bicillin C-R, Bicillin L-A, Permapen	Infections due to susceptible microorganisms, syphilis; prophylaxis of rheumatic fever or chorea	Same as penicillin G	Up to 2.4 million Units/day IM

Summary Drug Table — ANTIBACTERIAL DRUGS THAT INHIBIT BACTERIAL CELL WALL SYNTHESIS (continued)

Generic Name	Trade Name	Uses	Adverse Reactions	Dosage Ranges
® penicillin G procaine		Moderate to severe infections due to susceptible organisms	Same as penicillin G	600,000–2.4 million Units/day IM
penicillin V	Veetids	Infections due to susceptible organisms	Same as penicillin G	125–500 mg orally q 6 hr or q 8 hr
Semisynthetic Penicillins				
Penicillinase-Resistant Penicillins (Narrow Spectrum) ® dicloxacillin *dye-klox-ah-sill'-in*		Same as penicillin G	Same as penicillin G	125–250 mg orally q 6 hr
® nafcillin *naf-sill'-in*		Same as penicillin G	Same as penicillin G	500 mg IV q 4 hr
® oxacillin *ox-ah-sill'-in*	Bactocill	Same as penicillin G	Same as penicillin G	500 mg–1 g orally q 4–6 hr; 250 mg–1 g q 4–6 hr IM, IV
Aminopenicillins (Broad Spectrum) amoxicillin *ah-mox-ih-sill'-in*	Amoxil, Trimox	Same as penicillin G	Same as penicillin G	500–875 mg orally q 12 hr or 250 mg orally q 8 hr
® ampicillin *am-pih-sill'-in*	Principen	Same as penicillin G	Same as penicillin G	250–500 mg orally q 6 hr; 1–12 g/day IM, IV in divided doses q 4–6 hr
Extended-Spectrum Penicillins				
® carbenicillin indanyl *in-dah-nill*	Geocillin	UTIs caused by *Escherichia coli, Proteus, Enterobacter*	Same as penicillin G	382–764 mg orally QID
® piperacillin *pih-per-ah-sill'-in*		Same as penicillin G	Same as penicillin G	3–4 g q 4–6 hr IV or IM; maximum dosage, 24 g/day
® ticarcillin *tye-kar-sill'-in*	Ticar	Same as penicillin G	Same as penicillin G	150–300 mg/kg/day IV every 3, 4, or 6 hours; maximum dosage 2 g for IM injection
Penicillin–β-Lactamase Inhibitor Combinations				
® amoxicillin and clavulanate *ah-mox-ih-sill'-in/klah-vew-lan'-ate*	Augmentin	Same as penicillin G	Same as penicillin G	250 mg orally q 8 hr or 500 mg orally q 12 hr; for severe infections: up to 875 mg q 12 h
® ampicillin/sulbactam *am-pih-sill'-in/sull-bak'-tam*	Unasyn	Same as penicillin G	Same as penicillin G	1.5 g–3 g q 6 hr IM or IV
® piperacillin and tazobactam *pih-per-ah-sill'-in/tay-zoe-bak'-tam*	Zosyn	Same as penicillin G	Same as penicillin G	3.375 g–4.5 g q 6 hr IV
® ticarcillin and clavulanate *tye-kar-sill'-in klah-vew-lan'-ate*	Timentin	Same as penicillin G	Same as penicillin G	Up to 3.1 g IV q 4–6 hr or 200–300 mg/kg/day IV in divided doses q 4–6 hr

(table continues on page 80)

Antibacterial Drugs That Disrupt the Bacterial Cell Wall

Summary Drug Table ANTIBACTERIAL DRUGS THAT INHIBIT BACTERIAL CELL WALL SYNTHESIS (continued)

Generic Name	Trade Name	Uses	Adverse Reactions	Dosage Ranges
Cephalosporins				
First-Generation Cephalosporins				
cefadroxil *sef-ah-drox'-ill*		Infections due to susceptible microorganisms	Nausea, vomiting, diarrhea, hypersensitivity reactions, superinfection, nephrotoxicity, headache, Stevens-Johnson syndrome, pseudomembranous colitis	1–2 g/day orally in divided doses
cefazolin *she-fah'-zoe-lin*	Ancef, Kefzol	Same as cefadroxil; perioperative prophylaxis	Same as cefadroxil	250 mg–1 g IM, IV q 6–12 hr; perioperative: 0.5–1 g IM, IV
cephalexin *sef'-ah-lex-in*	Keflex	Same as cefadroxil	Same as cefadroxil	1–4 g/day orally in divided doses
Second-Generation Cephalosporins				
cefaclor *sef'-ah-klor*		Infections due to susceptible microorganisms	Nausea, vomiting, diarrhea, hypersensitivity reactions, nephrotoxicity, headache, hematologic reactions	250 mg orally q 8 hr
cefotetan *sef-oh-tee'-tan*		Same as cefaclor; perioperative prophylaxis	Same as cefaclor	1–2 g IM, IV q 12 hr for 5–10 days; perioperative: 1–2 g in a single dose IV
cefoxitin *sef-ox'-ih-tin*	Mefoxin	Same as cefaclor; perioperative prophylaxis	Same as cefaclor	1–2 g IV q 6–8 hr
cefprozil *sef-proe'-zil*		Same as cefaclor	Same as cefaclor	250–500 mg orally q 12 hr
cefuroxime *sef-yoor-ox'-eem*	Ceftin, Zinacef	Same as cefaclor; preoperative prophylaxis	Same as cefaclor	250 mg orally BID; 750 mg–1.5 g IM or IV q 8 hr
Third-Generation Cephalosporins				
cefdinir *sef'-din-eer*		Same as cefaclor	Same as cefaclor	300 mg orally q 12 hr or 600 mg orally q 24 hr
cefditoren *sef'-dih-tore-en*	Spectracef	Same as cefaclor	Same as cefaclor	200–400 mg orally BID
cefixime *she-fix'-eem*	Suprax	Same as cefaclor	Same as cefaclor	400 mg/day orally
cefotaxime *sef-oh-taks'-eem*	Claforan	Same as cefaclor; perioperative prophylaxis	Same as cefaclor	2–8 g/day IM, IV in equally divided doses q 6–8 hr; maximum 12 g/day
cefpodoxime *sef-poe-dox'-eem*		Same as cefaclor; sexually transmitted infection treatment	Same as cefaclor	100–400 mg/day orally in equally divided doses
ceftazidime *sef-taz'-ih-deem*	Fortaz	Same as cefaclor	Same as cefaclor	250 mg–2g IV, IM q 8–12 hr
® ceftibuten *sef-tah-byoo'-ten*	Cedax	Same as cefaclor	Same as cefaclor	400 mg/daily orally

Summary Drug Table — ANTIBACTERIAL DRUGS THAT INHIBIT BACTERIAL CELL WALL SYNTHESIS (continued)

Generic Name	Trade Name	Uses	Adverse Reactions	Dosage Ranges
ceftriaxone *sef-try-ax'-on*	Rocephin	Same as cefaclor; perioperative prophylaxis; gonorrhea	Same as cefaclor	1–2 g/day IM, IV q 12 hr, maximum 4 g/day; perioperative: 1 g IV; gonorrhea: 250 mg IM as a single dose
Fourth-Generation Cephalosporins				
cefepime *sef'-ah-pime*	Maxipime	Same as cefaclor; febrile neutropenia	Same as cefaclor	0.5–2 g IV, IM q 12 hr
Carbapenems				
doripenem *dor-ih-pen'-em*	Doribax	Complicated intra-abdominal or urinary tract infections	Headache, nausea, diarrhea, and anemia	500 mg IV q 8 hr
ertapenem *er-ta-pen'-em*	Invanz	Complicated intra-abdominal or urinary tract infections	Headache, nausea, diarrhea, and liver dysfunction	1 g IV daily, 3–14 days
imipenem-cilastatin *ih-mih-pen'-em/sye-lah-stat'-in*	Primaxin	Serious infections caused by *Staphylococcus* spp., *Streptococcus* spp., and *Escherichia coli*	Nausea, diarrhea	250 mg–1 g q 6 hr, not to exceed 4 g/day
meropenem *meh-row-pen'-em*	Merrem IV	Intra-abdominal and soft tissue infections caused by multiresistant gram-negative organisms	Headache, diarrhea, abdominal pain, nausea, pain and inflammation at injection site, pseudomembranous colitis	500 mg–1 g IV q 8 hr
Miscellaneous Drugs That Inhibit Bacterial Cell Wall Synthesis				
aztreonam *az'-tree-oh-nam*	Azactam	Gram-negative bacterial infections	Nausea, diarrhea, hypotension, rash, and headache	500 mg–1 g q 8–12 hr
telavancin *tel'-a-van'-sin*	Vibativ	Complicated skin infections	Nausea, vomiting, and altered taste	10 mg/kg IV daily, 4–7 days
vancomycin *van-koe-mye'-sin*	Vancocin	Serious susceptible gram-positive infections not responding to treatment with other antibiotics	Nausea; chills; fever; urticaria; sudden fall in blood pressure, with redness on face, neck, arms, and back; nephrotoxicity; ototoxicity	500 mg–2 g/day orally in divided doses; 500 mg IV q 6 hr or 1 g IV q 12 hr

Ⓡ This drug should be administered at least 1 hour before or two hours after a meal.

● Chapter Review

Know Your Drugs

Clients sometimes know a medication by the brand (or trade) name and not the generic name. To help you recognize both names, match the brand name with the generic name of the same medication

Generic Name	Brand Name
1. ceftriaxone	A. Augmentin
2. telavancin	B. Vancocin
3. amoxicillin/clavulanic acid	C. Rocephin
4. vancomycin	D. Vibativ

Calculate Medication Dosages

1. A client is prescribed amoxicillin in oral suspension. The drug is reconstituted to a solution of 250 mg/5 mL. The primary health care provider prescribes 500 mg of the amoxicillin. The caregiver insists on using a spoon to administer the drug. Answer the following questions: How much amoxicillin will 1 teaspoon contain? How many milliliters (mL) were ordered, and what is the conversion to teaspoons (how much should the nurse teach the caregiver to administer)?

2. The physician prescribes 1 g of cefoxitin (Mefoxin) for parenteral administration. Cefoxitin is available in a solution of 250 mg/1 mL. What amount of cefoxitin would the nurse prepare? Could this be given in one IM injection?

● Prepare for the NCLEX®

Build Your Knowledge

1. Bacterial cells are different from human cells because they:
   1. have a cell wall
   2. synthesize DNA and RNA
   3. contain a β-lactam ring
   4. contain proteins

2. Cephalosporins are divided into "generations" according to:
   1. when they were discovered
   2. their administration method
   3. manufacturer's preference
   4. sensitivity to microorganisms

3. A client taking oral penicillin reports he has a sore mouth. On inspection, the nurse notes a black, furry tongue and bright red oral mucous membranes. The primary care provider is notified immediately, because these symptoms may be caused by:
   1. a vitamin C deficiency
   2. a superinfection
   3. dehydration
   4. poor oral hygiene

4. The nurse correctly administers penicillin V:
   1. 1 hour before or 2 hours after meals
   2. without regard to meals
   3. with meals to prevent GI upset
   4. every 3 hours around the clock

5. When giving a cephalosporin by the IM route, the nurse tells the client that _____.
   1. a stinging or burning sensation and soreness at the site may be experienced
   2. the injection site will be red for several days
   3. all injections will be given in the same area
   4. the injection will not cause any discomfort

6. The nurse observes a client taking a cephalosporin for common adverse reactions, which include _____.
   1. hypotension, dizziness, urticaria
   2. nausea, vomiting, diarrhea
   3. skin rash, constipation, headache
   4. bradycardia, pruritus, insomnia

7. After administering penicillin in an outpatient setting, the nurse:
   1. asks the client to wait 10 to 15 minutes before leaving the clinic
   2. instructs the client to report any numbness or tingling of the extremities
   3. keeps pressure on the injection site for 10 minutes
   4. asks the client to wait in the area for at least 30 minutes

Apply Your Knowledge

8. When reviewing a client's culture and sensitivity test results, the nurse learns that the bacteria causing the infection are sensitive to penicillin. The nurse interprets this result to mean that:
   1. the client is allergic to penicillin
   2. penicillin will be effective in treating the infection
   3. penicillin will not be effective in treating the infection
   4. the test must be repeated to obtain accurate results

9. A nurse asks if the client is allergic to penicillin before the first dose of the cephalosporin is given. The rationale for this question is that persons allergic to penicillin _____.
   1. are usually allergic to most antibiotics
   2. respond poorly to antibiotic therapy
   3. require higher doses of other antibiotics
   4. have a higher incidence of allergy to the cephalosporins

Alternate-Format Questions

10. Which of the following are signs and symptoms of a drug hypersensitivity reaction? **Select all that apply**.
    1. skin rash
    2. wheezing
    3. hypertension
    4. angioedema
    5. urinary incontinence

To check your answers, see Appendix G.

the**Point** *For more NCLEX-style questions, log on to http://thepoint.lww.com to access more than 1000 questions.*

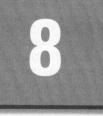

Antibacterial Drugs That Interfere With Protein Synthesis

LEARNING OBJECTIVES

On completion of this chapter, the student will:

1. Discuss the uses, general drug actions, adverse reactions, contraindications, precautions, and interactions of antibacterial drugs that interfere with protein synthesis.
2. Discuss important preadministration and ongoing assessment activities the nurse should perform on the patient taking an antibacterial drug that interferes with protein synthesis.
3. List nursing diagnoses particular to a patient taking an antibacterial drug that interferes with protein synthesis.
4. Discuss ways to promote an optimal response to therapy, how to manage adverse reactions, and important points to keep in mind when educating patients about the use of antibacterial drugs that interfere with protein synthesis.

KEY TERMS

adjunctive treatment • therapy used in addition to the primary treatment

blood dyscrasias • abnormality of blood cell structure

bowel preparation • treatment protocol to cleanse the bowel of bacteria before surgery or other procedures; also known as *bowel prep*

circumoral • encircling the mouth

enteric coated • special coating on drug that prevents absorption until drug reaches the small bowel

Helicobacter pylori • stomach bacterium that causes peptic ulcer; also known as *H. pylori*

hematuria • blood in the urine

hepatic coma • coma induced by liver disease

nephrotoxicity • damage to the kidneys by a toxic substance

neuromuscular blockade • acute muscle paralysis and apnea (absence of breathing)

neurotoxicity • damage to the nervous system by a toxic substance

ototoxicity • damage to the organs of hearing by a toxic substance

phenylketonuria (PKU) • a genetic birth defect causing the amino acid phenylalanine to build up to toxic levels in the body

proteinuria • protein in the urine

vancomycin resistant *Enterococcus faecium* (VREF) • bacteria resistant to the drug vancomycin

DRUG CLASSES

Tetracycline
• Glycylcycline
Aminoglycosides
• Spectinomycin

Macrolides
• Ketolide
Lincosamides
Miscellaneous agents
• Oxazolidinone

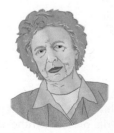

PHARMACOLOGY IN PRACTICE

When taking the drug history of Mrs. Moore, an 85-year-old patient in the outpatient clinic, you note that she has been taking 0.25 mg digoxin, one baby aspirin, and the tetracycline minocycline (Minocin). As you read, think about possible drug interactions.

The drugs in this chapter are antibacterial agents that interfere with the development of protein (*synthesis*) in the bacterial cell. To make protein, a message is made by messenger RNA (mRNA) that tells the cell how to build amino acids. The message is translated by the ribosomes to make the string of amino acids that becomes a protein. These drugs act on different areas of the cell, interfering with the process of protein synthesis.

This chapter discusses four classes of broad-spectrum antibiotics: the tetracyclines, the aminoglycosides, the macrolides, and the lincosamides. There are a number of newer antibacterial drugs that are a single drug in a class, and these are grouped as miscellaneous drugs. The Summary Drug Table: Antibacterial Drugs That Interfere With Protein Synthesis describes the broad-spectrum antibiotics discussed in this chapter (Fig. 8.1).

TETRACYCLINES

The tetracyclines are a group of antibacterial drugs composed of natural and semisynthetic compounds. They are useful in select infections when the organism shows sensitivity (see Chapter 6) to the tetracyclines, such as cholera, Rocky Mountain spotted fever, and typhus. These drugs are also useful when a patient is allergic to the penicillins or cephalosporins.

Actions

The tetracyclines are bacteriostatic and exert their effect by inhibiting bacterial protein synthesis, which is a process necessary for reproduction of the microorganism. Growing resistance to the drugs is a problem with the tetracyclines.

Tigecycline (Tygacil) is the first drug in the glycylcycline class of tetracycline-like drugs that is more bacteria resistant.

Uses

These antibiotics are effective in the treatment of infections caused by a wide range of gram-negative and gram-positive microorganisms. Tetracyclines are used as broad-spectrum antibiotics when penicillin is contraindicated, and also to treat the following infections:

- Rickettsial diseases (Rocky Mountain spotted fever, typhus fever, and tick fevers)
- Intestinal amebiasis
- Some skin and soft tissue infections
- Uncomplicated urethral, endocervical, or rectal infections caused by *Chlamydia trachomatis*
- Severe acne as an **adjunctive treatment**
- Infection with *Helicobacter pylori* in combination with metronidazole and bismuth subsalicylate

Adverse Reactions

Gastrointestinal System Reactions

- Nausea or vomiting
- Diarrhea
- Epigastric distress
- Stomatitis
- Sore throat

Other Reactions

- Skin rashes

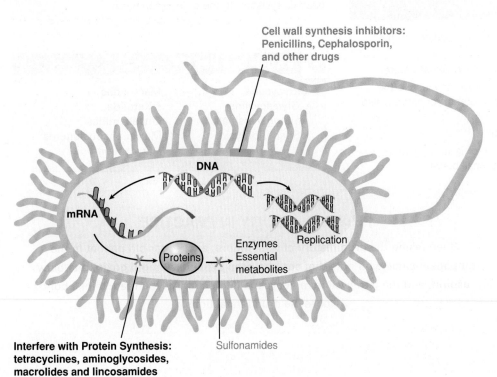

Cell wall synthesis inhibitors: Penicillins, Cephalosporin, and other drugs

DNA

mRNA

Replication

Proteins

Enzymes Essential metabolites

Interfere with Protein Synthesis: tetracyclines, aminoglycosides, macrolides and lincosamides

Sulfonamides

Figure 8.1 Action of bacterial protein synthesis inhibitors such as tetracycline, aminoglycosides, macrolides, and lincosamides.

- Photosensitivity reaction (demeclocycline seems to cause the most serious photosensitivity reaction, whereas minocycline is least likely to cause this type of reaction)

Contraindications

Tetracyclines are contraindicated in the patient known to be hypersensitive to any of the tetracyclines; during pregnancy, because of the possibility of toxic effects to the developing fetus (pregnancy category D); during lactation; and in children younger than 9 years of age.

LIFESPAN CONSIDERATIONS
Pediatric
Tetracyclines are not given to children younger than 9 years of age unless their use is absolutely necessary because these drugs may cause permanent yellow-gray-brown discoloration of the teeth. The use of tetracyclines, especially prolonged or repeated therapy, may result in overgrowth of nonsusceptible bacterial or fungal organisms.

Precautions

Tetracyclines should be used cautiously in patients with impaired renal function (when degradation of the tetracyclines occurs, the agents are highly toxic to the kidneys) and those with liver impairment (doses greater than 2 g/day can be extremely damaging to the liver).

CHRONIC CARE CONSIDERATIONS
Tetracyclines may reduce insulin requirements in patients with diabetes. Blood glucose levels should be monitored frequently during tetracycline therapy.

Interactions

The following interactions may occur when a tetracycline is administered with another agent:

Interacting Drug or Agent	Common Use	Effect of Interaction
antacids containing aluminum, zinc, magnesium, or bismuth salts	Relief of heartburn and gastrointestinal (GI) upset	Decreased effectiveness of tetracycline
oral anticoagulants	Blood thinner	Increased risk for bleeding
oral contraceptives	Contraception	Decreased effectiveness of contraceptive agent (breakthrough bleeding or pregnancy)
digoxin	Management of heart disease	Increased risk for digitalis toxicity (see Chapter 38)

LIFESPAN CONSIDERATIONS
Women
Women of childbearing age should be assessed for oral contraception use whenever tetracyclines are prescribed. The contraception effectiveness is decreased and women should always be taught and feel confident in the use of other forms of birth control during and after tetracycline treatment.

AMINOGLYCOSIDES

The aminoglycosides include amikacin, gentamicin, kanamycin, neomycin, streptomycin, and tobramycin.

Actions

The aminoglycosides exert their bactericidal effect by blocking the ribosome from reading the mRNA, a step in protein synthesis necessary for bacterial multiplication.

Uses

Aminoglycosides are used primarily in the treatment of infections caused by gram-negative microorganisms. In addition, the drugs may be used to reduce bacteria (normal flora) in the bowel when patients are having abdominal surgery or when a patient is in a **hepatic coma**. Because the oral aminoglycosides are poorly absorbed, they are useful in suppressing GI bacteria. For example, kanamycin and neomycin are used before surgery to reduce intestinal bacteria. It is thought this reduces the possibility of abdominal infection that may occur after surgery on the bowel. This drug treatment protocol is referred to as a portion of the surgical **bowel preparation** (bowel prep). By destroying bacteria in the gut and washing it out with laxatives or enemas, the surgical area becomes as clean as possible before the operation.

Kanamycin, neomycin, and paromomycin are used orally in the management of hepatic coma. In this disorder, liver failure results in an elevation of blood ammonia levels. By reducing the number of ammonia-forming bacteria in the intestines, blood ammonia levels may be lowered, thereby temporarily reducing some of the symptoms associated with this disorder.

Adverse Reactions

General system reactions include the following:

- Nausea
- Vomiting
- Anorexia
- Rash
- Urticaria

More serious adverse reactions may lead to discontinuation of the drug. These reactions include:

- **Nephrotoxicity**
- **Ototoxicity**
- **Neurotoxicity**

Signs and symptoms of nephrotoxicity may include **proteinuria** (protein in the urine)**, hematuria** (blood in the urine), an increase in the blood urea nitrogen (BUN) level, a decrease in urine output, and an increase in the serum creatinine concentration. Nephrotoxicity is usually reversible once the drug is discontinued.

Signs and symptoms of ototoxicity include tinnitus (ringing in the ears), dizziness, roaring in the ears, vertigo, and a mild to severe loss of hearing. If hearing loss occurs, it is usually permanent. Ototoxicity may occur during drug therapy or even after therapy is discontinued. The short-term administration of kanamycin and neomycin as a preparation for bowel surgery rarely causes these two adverse reactions.

Signs and symptoms of neurotoxicity include numbness, skin tingling, **circumoral** (around the mouth) paresthesia, peripheral paresthesia, tremors, muscle twitching, convulsions, muscle weakness, and **neuromuscular blockade** (acute muscular paralysis and apnea).

The administration of the aminoglycosides may result in a hypersensitivity reaction, which can range from mild to severe and, in some cases, be life-threatening. Mild hypersensitivity reactions may require only discontinuing the drug, whereas the more serious reactions require immediate treatment. When aminoglycosides are given, individual drug references, such as the package insert, should be consulted for more specific adverse reactions. As with other anti-infectives, bacterial or fungal superinfections and pseudomembranous colitis (see Chapter 9) may occur with the use of these drugs.

Contraindications

The aminoglycosides are contraindicated in patients with hypersensitivity to aminoglycosides, pre-existing hearing loss, myasthenia gravis, and parkinsonism. They are also contraindicated during lactation or pregnancy (pregnancy category C, except for neomycin, amikacin, gentamicin, kanamycin, and tobramycin, which are in pregnancy category D). Aminoglycosides are also contraindicated for long-term therapy, because of the potential for ototoxicity and nephrotoxicity.

Precautions

The aminoglycosides are used cautiously in older patients and patients with renal failure (dosage adjustments may be necessary) and neuromuscular disorders.

Interactions

The following interactions may occur when an aminoglycoside is administered with another agent:

Interacting Drug	Common Use	Effect of Interaction
cephalosporins	Anti-infective agent	Increased risk of nephrotoxicity
loop diuretics (water pills)	Management of edema and water retention	Increased risk of ototoxicity
Pavulon or Anectine (general anesthetics)	Anesthesia (e.g., for surgery)	Increased risk of neuromuscular blockade

MACROLIDES

The macrolides are effective against a variety of pathogenic organisms, particularly infections of the respiratory and genitourinary tract.

Actions

The macrolides are bacteriostatic or bactericidal in susceptible bacteria. The drugs act by causing changes in protein function and synthesis.

Uses

These antibiotics are effective as prophylaxis before dental or other procedures in patients allergic to penicillin and in the treatment of:

• A wide range of gram-negative and gram-positive infections
• Acne vulgaris and skin infections
• Upper respiratory infections caused by *Haemophilus influenzae* (with sulfonamides)

Adverse Reactions

GI reactions include the following:

• Nausea
• Vomiting
• Diarrhea
• Abdominal pain or cramping

As with almost all antibacterial drugs, pseudomembranous colitis may occur, ranging in severity from mild to life-threatening. Visual disturbances (associated with telithromycin) may also occur.

Contraindications

These drugs are contraindicated in patients with hypersensitivity to the macrolides and in patients with pre-existing liver disease. Telithromycin (Ketek) should not be ordered if a patient is taking cisapride (Propulsid) or pimozide (Orap).

Precautions

Macrolides should be used cautiously in patients who have liver dysfunction or myasthenia gravis (a disease that affects the myoneural junction in nerves and is manifested by extreme weakness and exhaustion of the muscles) or who are pregnant or lactating (azithromycin and erythromycin are in pregnancy category B; clarithromycin and telithromycin are in pregnancy category C).

Interactions

The following interactions may occur when a macrolide is administered with another agent:

Interacting Drug	Common Use	Effect of Interaction
antacids (kaolin, aluminum salts, or magaldrate)	Relief of GI upset, such as diarrhea	Decreased absorption and effectiveness of the macrolides
digoxin	Management of cardiac disorders	Increased serum levels
anticoagulants	Blood thinner	Increased risk of bleeding
clindamycin, lincomycin, or chloramphenicol	Anti-infective agent	Decreased therapeutic activity of the macrolides
theophylline	Management of respiratory problems, such as asthma	Increased serum theophylline level

LINCOSAMIDES

The lincosamides, another group of antibacterial drugs with a high potential for toxicity, are usually used only for treating serious infections in which penicillin or erythromycin (a macrolide) is not effective.

Actions

The lincosamides act by inhibiting protein synthesis in susceptible bacteria, causing cell death. They disrupt the functional ability of the ribosomes (which assemble amino acids in the cell), causing cell death.

Uses

These antibiotics are effective in the treatment of infections caused by a range of gram-negative and gram-positive microorganisms. Lincosamides are used for the more serious infections and may be used in conjunction with other antibiotics.

Adverse Reactions

Gastrointestinal System Reactions

- Abdominal pain
- Esophagitis
- Nausea
- Vomiting
- Diarrhea

Other Reactions

- Skin rash
- **Blood dyscrasias**

These drugs also can cause pseudomembranous colitis, which may range from mild to very severe. Discontinuing the drug may relieve mild symptoms of pseudomembranous colitis.

Contraindications

The lincosamides are contraindicated in infants younger than 1 month of age and in patients:

- Hypersensitive to the lincosamides
- Taking cisapride (Propulsid) or the antipsychotic drug pimozide (Orap)
- With minor bacterial or viral infections

Precautions

These drugs should be used cautiously in patients with a history of GI disorders, renal disease, liver impairment, or myasthenia gravis (lincosamides have neuromuscular blocking action).

Interactions

The following interactions may occur when a lincosamide is administered with another agent:

Interacting Drug	Common Use	Effect of Interaction
kaolin- or aluminum-based antacids	Relief of stomach upset	Decreased absorption of the lincosamides
neuromuscular blocking drugs	Anesthesia	Increased action of neuromuscular blocking drug, possibly leading to severe and profound respiratory depression

MISCELLANEOUS DRUGS INHIBITING PROTEIN SYNTHESIS

Actions

These drugs are unique and individually in their own classes, yet they all interfere with protein synthesis in the bacterial cell. Daptomycin is a member of a new category of antibacterial agents called *cyclic lipopeptides*. Linezolid (Zyvox) is the first drug in a new drug class, the oxazolidinones. Spectinomycin (Trobicin) is chemically related to but different from the aminoglycosides. Quinupristin/dalfopristin has bactericidal action against both methicillin-susceptible and methicillin-resistant staphylococci.

Uses

Daptomycin is used to treat complicated skin and skin structure bacterial infections as well as *Staphylococcus aureus* infections of the blood. Linezolid is used in the treatment of **vancomycin-resistant *Enterococcus faecium* (VREF)**, health care–and community-acquired pneumonias, and skin and skin structure infections, including those caused by methicillin-resistant *S. aureus* (MRSA). Spectinomycin is used for treating gonorrhea in patients who are allergic to penicillins, cephalosporins, or probenecid. Quinupristin/

dalfopristin is a bacteriostatic agent also used in the treatment of VREF.

Adverse Reactions

The most common adverse reactions include the following:

- Nausea
- Vomiting
- Diarrhea or constipation
- Headache and dizziness
- Insomnia
- Rash
- Chills

Less common adverse reactions include:

- Fatigue
- Depression
- Nervousness
- Photosensitivity

Pseudomembranous colitis and thrombocytopenia are the most serious adverse reactions caused by linezolid.

> **! NURSING ALERT**
>
> Quinupristin/dalfopristin is irritating to the vein. After peripheral infusion, the vein should be flushed with 5% dextrose in water (D₅W), because the drug is incompatible with saline or heparin flush solutions.

Contraindications and Precautions

Linezolid is contraindicated in patients who are allergic to the drug or who are pregnant (pregnancy category C) or lactating and in patients with **phenylketonuria (PKU)**. Daptomycin, spectinomycin, and quinupristin/dalfopristin are contraindicated in patients with a known hypersensitivity to the drug, and it should not be used during pregnancy (pregnancy category B) or lactation.

Linezolid is used cautiously in patients with bone marrow depression, hepatic dysfunction, renal impairment, hypertension, and hyperthyroidism. If another sexually transmitted infection (STI) is present with gonorrhea, anti-infectives (in addition to spectinomycin) may be needed to eradicate the infectious processes. Because prolonged use of anti-infectives can disrupt normal flora, the patient should be monitored for secondary bacterial or fungal infections.

Interactions

The following interactions may occur when linezolid is administered with another agent:

- Antiplatelet drugs (aspirin or the nonsteroidal anti-inflammatory drugs [NSAIDs])—increased risk of bleeding and thrombocytopenia
- Monamine oxidase inhibitor (MAOI) antidepressants—decreased effectiveness
- Large amounts of food containing tyramine (e.g., aged cheese, caffeinated beverages, yogurt, chocolate, red wine, beer, pepperoni)—risk of severe hypertension

Myopathy with elevated creatine phosphokinase (CPK) levels may occur if daptomycin is administered with statin drugs (cholesterol reduction). No significant drug or food interactions for spectinomycin are known. Daptomycin should be used cautiously in patients taking warfarin (Coumadin). When taking quinupristin/dalfopristin, the serum levels of the following drugs may increase: antiretrovirals, antineoplastic and immunosuppressant agents, calcium channel blockers, benzodiazepines, and cisapride.

NURSING PROCESS
PATIENT RECEIVING AN ANTIBACTERIAL INTERFERING WITH PROTEIN SYNTHESIS

ASSESSMENT

Preadministration Assessment

It is important to establish an accurate database before the administration of any antibiotic. Identify and record signs and symptoms of the infection. Signs and symptoms may vary and often depend on the organ or system involved and whether the infection is external or internal. Examples of some of the signs and symptoms of an infection in various areas of the body are pain, drainage, redness, changes in the appearance of sputum, general malaise, chills and fever, cough, and swelling.

Obtain a thorough allergy history, especially a history of drug allergies. Some antibiotics have a higher incidence of hypersensitivity reactions in those with a history of allergy to drugs or other substances. If the patient has a history of drug allergies and has not told the primary health care provider, do not administer the first dose of the drug; instead, immediately contact the primary health care provider to discuss the allergy history.

The primary health care provider may order culture and sensitivity tests, which should also be performed before the first dose of the drug is given. Other laboratory tests such as renal and hepatic function tests, complete blood count, and urinalysis may also be ordered by the primary health care provider. In persons with impaired hearing or at risk for hearing loss, a hearing test may be recommended.

When kanamycin or neomycin is given to a patient with altered consciousness for hepatic coma, evaluate the patient's ability to follow directions and to swallow.

Ongoing Assessment

An ongoing assessment is important during therapy with anti-bacterials that interfere with protein synthesis. Take vital signs every 4 hours or as ordered by the primary health care provider. Notify the primary health care provider if there are changes in the vital signs, such as a significant drop in blood pressure, an increase in the pulse or respiratory rate, or a sudden increase in temperature. When an aminoglycoside is being administered, it is important to monitor the patient's respiratory rate because neuromuscular blockade has been reported with the administration of these drugs. Report any changes in the respiratory rate or rhythm to the primary health care provider because immediate treatment may be necessary. When kanamycin or neomycin is given for hepatic coma, assess and record the patient's general condition and changes in mentation daily.

Each day, compare current signs and symptoms of the infection against the initial signs and symptoms and record any specific findings in the patient's chart.

When an antibiotic is ordered for prevention of a secondary infection (prophylaxis), observe the patient for signs and symptoms that may indicate the beginning of an infection despite the prophylactic use of the antibiotic. If signs and symptoms of an infection occur, report them to the primary health care provider.

NURSING DIAGNOSES

Drug-specific nursing diagnoses include the following:

- **Impaired Comfort: Increased Fever** related to ineffectiveness of anti-infective therapy
- **Acute Confusion** related to increased ammonia blood levels
- **Ineffective Tissue Perfusion: Renal** related to adverse drug reactions to aminoglycosides
- **Risk for Injury** related to visual disturbances from telithromycin treatment, paresthesia secondary to neurotoxicity, or auditory damage from aminoglycosides
- **Diarrhea** related to superinfection secondary to anti-infective therapy, adverse drug reaction

Nursing diagnoses related to drug administration are discussed in Chapter 4.

PLANNING

The expected outcomes for the patient may include an optimal response to therapy, which includes control of the infectious process or prophylaxis of bacterial infection, meeting of patient needs related to the management of adverse drug effects, and confidence in an understanding of the medication regimen.

IMPLEMENTATION

Promoting an Optimal Response to Therapy

These drugs are of no value in the treatment of infections caused by a virus or fungus. There may be times when a secondary bacterial infection has occurred or may occur when the patient has a fungal or viral infection. The primary health care provider may then order one of the broad-spectrum antibiotics, but its purpose is for preventing (prophylaxis) or treating a secondary bacterial infection that could potentially develop after the primary fungal or viral infection.

ORAL ADMINISTRATION. Adverse reactions to most anti-infective drugs include nausea, vomiting, or abdominal pain. Patients may want to eat foods when these drugs are administered to reduce GI problems. It is important for you to know how medications will be affected if taken with foods.

Tetracyclines. It is important to give tetracyclines on an empty stomach. The exceptions are minocycline (Minocin) and tigecycline (Tygacil), which may be taken with food. All tetracyclines should be given with a full glass of water (8 ounces).

> **NURSING ALERT**
>
> Do not give tetracyclines along with dairy products (milk or cheese), antacids, laxatives, or products containing iron. When the aforementioned drugs are prescribed, make sure they are given 2 hours before or after the administration of a tetracycline. Food or drugs containing calcium, magnesium, aluminum, or iron prevent the absorption of the tetracyclines if ingested concurrently.

Aminoglycosides. When kanamycin or neomycin is given to suppress intestinal bacteria before surgery, the primary health care provider's orders regarding the timing of the administration of the drug are extremely important. Omission of a dose or failure to give the drug at the specified time may result in inadequate suppression of intestinal bacteria. When neomycin is given, enteric-coated erythromycin may be given at the same time as part of surgical bowel preparation. Enteric-coated tablets have a special coating that prevents the drug from being absorbed in the stomach. Absorption takes place lower in the GI tract after the coating has dissolved.

Macrolides. Clarithromycin, fidaxomicin, and telithromycin may be taken without regard to meals, and clarithromycin may be taken with milk if desired. Azithromycin is given 1 hour or more before a meal or 2 hours or more after a meal. Erythromycin is given on an empty stomach (1 hour before or 2 hours after meals) and with 180 to 240 mL of water.

Lincosamides. Food impairs the absorption of lincomycin. The patient should take nothing by mouth (except water) for 1 to 2 hours before and after taking lincomycin. Clindamycin may be taken with food or a full glass of water.

PARENTERAL ADMINISTRATION. When these drugs are given intramuscularly, inspect previous injection sites for signs of pain or tenderness, redness, and swelling. Some antibiotics may cause temporary local reactions, but persistence of a localized reaction should be reported to the primary health care provider. It is important to rotate injection sites and record the site used for injection in the patient's chart.

When these drugs are given intravenously (IV), inspect the needle site and area around the needle site for signs of extravasation of the IV fluid or signs of tenderness, pain, and redness (which may indicate *phlebitis* or *thrombophlebitis*). If these symptoms are apparent, restart the IV in another vein and bring the problem to the attention of the primary health care provider.

Monitoring and Managing Patient Needs

Observe the patient at frequent intervals, especially during the first 48 hours of therapy. It is important to report to the primary health care provider the occurrence of any adverse reaction before the next dose of the drug is due.

> **NURSING ALERT**
>
> Always report serious adverse reactions, such as a severe hypersensitivity reaction, respiratory difficulty, severe diarrhea, or a decided drop in blood pressure, to the primary health care provider immediately, because a serious adverse reaction may require emergency intervention.

IMPAIRED COMFORT: INCREASED FEVER. Monitor the temperature at frequent intervals, usually every 4 hours unless the patient has an elevated temperature. When the patient has an elevated temperature, check the temperature, pulse, and respirations every hour until the temperature returns to normal, and administer an antipyretic medication if prescribed by the primary health care provider.

ACUTE CONFUSION: HEPATIC COMA.   Exercise care when the aminoglycosides kanamycin and neomycin are administered orally as treatment for hepatic coma. During the early stages of this disorder, various changes in the level of consciousness may be seen. At times, the patient may appear lethargic and respond poorly to commands. Because of these changes in the level of consciousness, the patient may have difficulty swallowing, and a danger of aspiration is present. If the patient appears to have difficulty taking an oral drug, withhold the drug and contact the primary health care provider.

INEFFECTIVE TISSUE PERFUSION: RENAL.   The patient taking an aminoglycoside is at risk for nephrotoxicity. Measure and record the intake and output and notify the primary health care provider if the output is less than 750 mL/day. It is important to keep a record of the fluid intake and output as well as the patient's daily weight to assess hydration and renal function. Encourage fluid intake to 2000 mL/day (if the patient's condition permits). Any changes in the intake–output ratio or in the appearance of the urine may indicate nephrotoxicity. Report these types of changes to the primary health care provider promptly. In turn, the primary health care provider may order daily laboratory tests (e.g., serum creatinine and BUN) to monitor renal function. Report elevations in the creatinine or BUN level to the primary health care provider because elevation may indicate renal dysfunction.

RISK FOR INJURY.   Telithromycin (Ketek), a drug related to the macrolides, can cause the patient's eyes to have difficulty focusing and accommodating to light. Patients should be cautioned regarding the potential for accidents and injury when driving, operating machinery, or engaging in other hazardous activities.

Be alert for symptoms such as numbness or tingling of the skin, circumoral paresthesia, peripheral paresthesia (numbness or tingling in the extremities), tremors, and muscle twitching or weakness. The nurse reports any symptom of neurotoxicity immediately to the primary health care provider. Convulsions can occur if the drug is not discontinued.

! NURSING ALERT

Neuromuscular blockade or respiratory paralysis may occur after administration of the aminoglycosides. Therefore, it is extremely important that any symptoms of respiratory difficulty be reported immediately. If neuromuscular blockade occurs, it may be reversed by the administration of calcium salts, but mechanical ventilation may be required.

The patient taking a prolonged course of aminoglycosides is at risk for ototoxicity. Instruct the patient to report any ringing in the ears, difficulty hearing, or dizziness to the primary health care provider. Changes in hearing may not be noticed initially by the patient, but when changes occur they usually progress from difficulty in hearing high-pitched sounds to problems hearing low-pitched sounds. Auditory changes are irreversible, usually bilateral, and may be partial

or total. The risk is greater in patients with renal impairment or those with pre-existing hearing loss.

! NURSING ALERT

To detect ototoxicity, carefully evaluate the patient's complaints or comments related to hearing, such as a ringing or buzzing in the ears. The patient may report a sensation of stuffiness in the ears or difficulty hearing. If hearing problems do occur, report this problem to the primary health care provider immediately. To monitor for damage to the eighth cranial nerve, an evaluation of hearing may be done by audiometry before and throughout the course of therapy.

DIARRHEA.   Diarrhea may be an indication of a superinfection or pseudomembranous colitis, both of which can be serious. Inspect all stools for blood or mucus. If diarrhea is dark or there is mucus in the stool, save a sample and test for occult blood using a test such as Hemoccult. If the stool tests positive for blood, save a sample of the stool for possible further laboratory analysis.

Encourage the patient to drink fluids to replace those lost with the diarrhea. It is also important to maintain an accurate intake and output record to help determine fluid balance.

Observe the patient for other signs and symptoms of a bacterial or fungal superinfection, such as vaginal or anal itching, sores in the mouth, diarrhea, fever, chills, and sore throat. It is important to report any new signs and symptoms occurring during antibiotic therapy to the primary health care provider, who determines if these problems are part of the original infection or if a superinfection is occurring.

Educating the Patient and Family
The patient and family should feel confident in their understanding of the prescribed drug regimen. It is not uncommon for patients to stop taking a prescribed drug because they feel better. A detailed plan of teaching helps to reduce the incidence of this problem.

Use principles to support health literacy and easy-to-understand terms when teaching about the adverse reactions associated with the specific prescribed antibiotic. Advise the patient to contact the primary health care provider if any potentially serious adverse reactions, such as hypersensitivity reactions, moderate to severe diarrhea, sudden onset of chills and fever, sore throat, or sores in the mouth, occur.

Develop a teaching plan that includes the following information:

- Take the drug at the prescribed time intervals. These intervals are important because a certain amount of the drug must be in the body at all times for the infection to be controlled.

- Do not increase or omit the dose unless advised to do so by the primary health care provider.

- Complete the entire course of treatment. Never stop the drug, except on the advice of a primary health care provider, before the course of treatment is completed even if symptoms improve or disappear. Failure to complete the prescribed course of treatment may result in a return of the infection.

- Take each dose with a full (8-ounce) glass of water. Follow the directions given by the clinical pharmacist regarding taking the drug on an empty stomach or with food (see Patient Teaching for Improved Patient Outcomes: Avoiding Drug–Food Interactions).

■ Notify the primary health care provider if symptoms of the infection become worse or there is no improvement in the original symptoms after about 5 days.

■ When a tetracycline has been prescribed, avoid exposure to the sun or any type of tanning lamp or bed. When exposure to direct sunlight is unavoidable, completely cover the arms and legs and wear a wide-brimmed hat to protect the face and neck. Application of a sunscreen may or may not be effective. Therefore, consult the primary health care provider before using a sunscreen to prevent a photosensitivity reaction.

EVALUATION

■ Therapeutic response is achieved, and there is no evidence of infection.

■ Adverse reactions are identified, reported to the primary health care provider, and managed successfully with appropriate nursing interventions:
  • Patient reports comfort without fever.
  • Orientation and mentation remain intact.
  • Patient has adequate renal tissue perfusion.
  • No evidence of injury is seen due to visual or auditory disturbances.
  • Patient does not experience diarrhea.

■ Patient and family express confidence and demonstrate an understanding of the drug regimen.

Patient Teaching for Improved Patient Outcomes

Avoiding Drug–Food Interactions

When you teach, make sure your patient understands the following:

✔ Drugs may be taken with food or milk to minimize the risk for GI upset. However, most tetracyclines, when given with foods containing calcium, such as dairy products, are not absorbed as well as when they are taken on an empty stomach. So, if the patient is to receive tetracycline at home, it is important to be sure he or she knows to take the drug on an empty stomach, 1 hour before or 2 hours after a meal.

✔ Demonstrate to the patient how to read labels in the grocery store and to beware of items (e.g., cereals) that may be fortified with calcium.

✔ In addition, teach the patient to avoid the following dairy products before or after taking tetracycline:
  ■ Milk (whole, low fat, skim, condensed, or evaporated) and milkshakes
  ■ Cream (half-and-half, heavy, light), sour cream, coffee creamers, and creamy salad dressings
  ■ Eggnog
  ■ Cheese (natural and processed) and cottage cheese
  ■ Yogurt and frozen yogurt
  ■ Ice cream, ice milk, and frozen custard

PHARMACOLOGY IN PRACTICE
THINKING CRITICALLY

 Based on your knowledge of the tetracyclines, determine whether there is any reason to be concerned about Mrs. Moore's drug regimen. Given her confusion, how will you teach her about potential interactions of the drugs?

KEY POINTS

• Tetracyclines are primarily bacteriostatic and are often used when the patient is allergic to penicillin or a cephalosporin.

• A larger number of bacteria are becoming resistant to this class of drug. A newer class, glycylcycline, is more resistant to bacteria. Aminoglycosides, macrolides, and lincosamides are primarily bactericidal; they work by preventing the bacterial cell from making protein (synthesis), causing cell death.

• These drugs are used to treat a wide range of both gram-negative and gram-positive microorganisms. Many of

these drugs are used to remove bacteria from the bowel as part of preparing the GI tract for surgical procedures. When used for other infections and indications, these drugs may still cause bowel issues, ranging from diarrhea to pseudomembranous colitis.

• Although some drugs can be taken with food, many have interactions with foods and fluids. Dairy and calcium products inhibit the absorption of the tetracyclines. Therefore, take these drugs at least 1 hour before or 2 hours after a meal.

• Hearing, neurologic status, and contraception should all be monitored when these drugs are taken.

Summary Drug Table ANTIBACTERIAL DRUGS THAT INTERFERE WITH PROTEIN SYNTHESIS

Generic Name	Trade Name	Uses	Adverse Reactions	Dosage Ranges
Tetracyclines				
℞ demeclocycline deh-meh-kloe-sye'-kleen	Declomycin	Treatment of infections due to susceptible microorganisms	Nausea, vomiting, diarrhea, dizziness, headache, hypersensitivity reactions, photosensitivity reactions, pseudomembranous colitis, hematologic changes, discoloration of teeth in fetus and young children	150 mg orally QID or 300 mg orally BID; gonorrhea: 600 mg orally initially then 300 mg orally q 12 hr for 4 days
doxycycline dox-ih-sye'-kleen	Atridox, Doryx, Monodox, Periostat, Oracea, Vibra-Tabs, Vibramycin	Same as demeclocycline	Same as demeclocycline	100 mg orally q 12 hr first day then 100 mg/day orally Severe infections: 100 mg q 12 hr
minocycline min-oh-sye'-kleen	Arestin, Dynacin, Minocin, Solodyn	Same as demeclocycline	Same as demeclocycline	200 mg orally initially then 100 mg orally q 12 hr
℞ tetracycline tet-rah-sye'-kleen		Same as demeclocycline	Same as demeclocycline	1–2 g/day orally in 2–4 divided doses
tigecycline tih-geh-sye'-kleen (glycylcycline class similar to tetracycline)	Tygacil	Complicated skin structures and complicated intra-abdominal infections	Nausea, vomiting, diarrhea	100 mg IV initially then 50 mg IV q 12 hr
Aminoglycosides				
amikacin am-ih-kay'-sin		Treatment of serious infections caused by susceptible strains of microorganisms	Nausea, vomiting, diarrhea, rash, ototoxicity, nephrotoxicity, hypersensitivity reactions, neurotoxicity, superinfections, neuromuscular blockade	15 mg/kg IM, IV, in divided doses, not to exceed 1.5 g/day
gentamicin jen-tah-mye'-sin		Same as amikacin	Same as amikacin	3 mg/kg/day in 3 divided doses IM or IV For life-threatening infection: 5 mg/kg/day in divided doses
kanamycin kan-ah-mye'-sin		Same as amikacin; for hepatic coma and for suppression of intestinal bacteria	Same as amikacin	7.5–15 mg/kg/day in divided doses IM, not to exceed 15 mg/kg/day in divided doses IV; not to exceed 1.5 g/day
neomycin nee-oh-mye'-sin		Same as amikacin	Preoperative prophylaxis: 1 g/day orally for 3 days	Hepatic coma: 4–12 g/day in divided doses
paromomycin pa-rah-mo-mye'-sin		Hepatic coma, intestinal amebiasis	Same as amikacin	25–35 mg/kg/day
streptomycin strep-toe-mye'-sin		Same as amikacin, treatment of tuberculosis	Same as amikacin	15 mg/kg/day IM or 25–30 mg/kg IM 2–3 times per week
tobramycin toe-bra-mye'-sin		Same as amikacin	Same as amikacin	3–5 mg/kg/day IM, IV in 3 equal doses

Summary Drug Table ANTIBACTERIAL DRUGS THAT INTERFERE WITH PROTEIN SYNTHESIS (continued)

Generic Name	Trade Name	Uses	Adverse Reactions	Dosage Ranges
Macrolides				
℞ azithromycin *ay-zith-roe-mye'-sin*	Zithromax, Zmax	Same as demeclocycline	Nausea, vomiting, diarrhea, abdominal pain, hypersensitivity reactions, pseudomembranous colitis	500 mg orally first day then 250 mg/day orally
clarithromycin *klar-ith-roe-mye'-sin*	Biaxin	Same as demeclocycline, *Helicobacter pylori* therapy	Same as azithromycin	250–500 mg orally q 12 hr
℞ erythromycin *er-ith-roe-mye'-sin*	E-Glades, Eryc, Ery-Ped, E.E.S.	Same as demeclocycline	Same as azithromycin	250 mg orally q 6 hr or 333 mg q 8 hr up to 4 g/day
fidaxomicin *fye-dax'-oh-mye'-sin*	Dificid	Treatment of diarrhea from *Clostridium difficile* (*C. diff*)	Nausea, vomiting, stomach pain, rash	200 mg orally q 24 hr
telithromycin *tell-ith-roe-mye'-sin*	Ketek	Same as demeclocycline	Visual disturbance, nausea, diarrhea, vomiting, headache, dizziness	800 mg orally q 24 hr
Lincosamides				
clindamycin *klin-dah-mye'-sin*	Cleocin	Same as demeclocycline	Abdominal pain, esophagitis, nausea, vomiting, diarrhea, skin rash, pseudomembranous colitis, hypersensitivity reactions	Serious infection: 150–450 mg orally q 6 hr; severe infection: 600–2700 mg/day in 2–4 equal doses; life-threatening infection: up to 4.8 g/day IV, IM
℞ lincomycin *lin-koe-mye'-sin*	Lincocin	Same as demeclocycline	Same as clindamycin	500 mg orally q 6–8 hr; 600 mg IM q 12–24 hr; up to 8 g/day IV in life-threatening situations
Miscellaneous Drugs That Interfere With Protein Synthesis				
℞ daptomycin *dap-toe-mye'-sin*	Cubicin	Complicated skin and skin structure infections, *Staphylococcus aureus* blood infections	Nausea, diarrhea, constipation, rash, vein irritation	4 mg/kg IV daily for 7–14 days
linezolid *lih-nez'-oh-lid*	Zyvox	Infections with VREF; pneumonia from *Staphylococcus aureus* and penicillin-susceptible *Streptococcus pneumoniae;* skin and skin structure infections	Nausea, diarrhea, headache, insomnia, pseudomembranous colitis	600 mg orally or IV q 12 hr
quinupristin-dalfopristin *kwin-yoo'-pris-tin*	Synercid	VREF	Vein inflammation, nausea, vomiting, diarrhea	7.5 mg/kg IV q 8 hr
spectinomycin *spek-tin-oh-mye'-sin*	Trobicin	Gonorrhea	Soreness at injection site, urticaria, dizziness, rash, chills, fever, hypersensitivity reactions	2 g IM as single dose; up to 4 g IM
telithromycin *tell-ith-roe-mye'-sin*	Ketek	Same as demeclocycline	Visual disturbance, nausea, diarrhea, vomiting, headache, dizziness	800 mg orally q 24 hr

℞ This drug should be administered at least 1 hour before or 2 hours after a meal.

● Chapter Review

Know Your Drugs

Clients sometimes know a medication by the brand (or trade) name and not the generic name. To help you recognize both names, match the brand name with the generic name of the same medication

Generic Name	Brand Name
1. doxycycline	A. Biaxin
2. tigecycline	B. Dificid
3. fidaxomicin	C. Tygacil
4. clarithromycin	D. Vibramycin

Calculate Medication Dosages

1. A client is prescribed 600 mg of lincomycin every 12 hours IM. The drug is available as 300 mg/mL. How many milliliters does the nurse administer?

2. A client is prescribed 200 mg of minocycline oral suspension now, followed by 100 mg orally every 12 hours. The minocycline is available as an oral suspension of 50 mg/5 mL. How many milliliters does the nurse administer as the initial dose?

● Prepare for the NCLEX®

Build Your Knowledge

1. A client asks the nurse why the primary health care provider prescribed an antibiotic when she was told that she has a viral infection. The correct response by the nurse is that the antibiotic may be used to prevent a _____.
   1. primary fungal infection
   2. repeat viral infection
   3. secondary bacterial infection
   4. breakdown of the immune system

2. A client is receiving erythromycin for an infection. The patient's response to therapy is best evaluated by _____.
   1. monitoring vital signs every 4 hours
   2. comparing initial and current signs and symptoms
   3. monitoring fluid intake and output
   4. asking the patient if he is feeling better

3. When asked to describe a photosensitivity reaction, the nurse correctly states that this reaction may be described as a(n) _____.
   1. tearing of the eyes on exposure to bright light
   2. aversion to bright lights and sunlight
   3. sensitivity to products in the environment
   4. exaggerated sunburn reaction when the skin is exposed to sunlight

4. When giving spectinomycin for gonorrhea, the nurse advises the client to _____.
   1. return for a follow-up examination
   2. limit fluid intake to 1200 mL/day while taking the drug
   3. return the next day for a second injection
   4. avoid drinking alcohol for the next 10 days

5. Which of the following complaints by a man taking tetracycline would be most indicative that he is experiencing ototoxicity?
   1. tingling of the extremities
   2. he is unable to hear the television
   3. changes in mental status
   4. short periods of dizziness

Apply Your Knowledge

6. When giving one of the macrolide antibiotics, the nurse assesses the client for the most common adverse reactions, which are _____.
   1. related to the GI tract
   2. skin rash and urinary retention
   3. sores in the mouth and hypertension
   4. related to the nervous system

7. Which of the following urinary output measurements should be reported to the primary health care provider immediately?
   1. 2400 mL in 24 hours
   2. 30 mL in 1 hour
   3. 750 mL in 1 hour
   4. 1000 mL in 1 day

8. Which of the following medications may be taken with food?
   1. erythromycin
   2. doxycycline
   3. demeclocycline
   4. tigecycline

Alternate-Format Questions

9. When a client is instructed not to take a drug with dairy products, what can the client drink when swallowing the medication? **Select all that apply**.
   1. water
   2. yogurt fruit smoothie
   3. iced tea
   4. cranberry juice
   5. milk

10. A client with limited health literacy is prescribed azithromycin for a lower respiratory tract infection. Azithromycin is available in 250-mg tablets. The primary health care provider has ordered 500 mg on the first day, followed by 250 mg on days 2 through 5. The nurse shows the client how many tablets to be taken on the first day? _____. On the last day of therapy? _____

To check your answers, see Appendix G.

the**Point** *For more NCLEX-style questions, log on to http://thepoint.lww.com to access more than 1000 questions.*

Antibacterial Drugs That Interfere With DNA/RNA Synthesis

As antibiotics become resistant to various microorganisms, researchers develop drugs that affect different portions of the bacterial cell. In Chapters 7 and 8 you read about how the cell wall and protein-building capabilities of the bacteria are targeted by antibacterial drugs. In this chapter, you will read about drugs that kill bacteria by interfering with the synthesis of DNA or RNA. When these processes are interrupted, the bacterial cell cannot reproduce and it dies (Fig. 9.1). Some of these drugs are used to treat a broad spectrum of infections, others only for the treatment of one type of infection, and still others may be limited to the treatment of serious infections not treatable by other anti-infectives. The Summary Drug Table: Antibacterial Drugs That Interfere With DNA/RNA Synthesis lists the drugs discussed in this chapter.

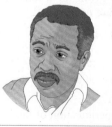

PHARMACOLOGY IN PRACTICE

Mr. Park, 77 years old, is a patient in a skilled nursing facility receiving gemifloxacin (Factive) for a lower respiratory infection over the last 9 days. Think about the adverse reactions experienced by patients as they end a course of antibacterial drug therapy.

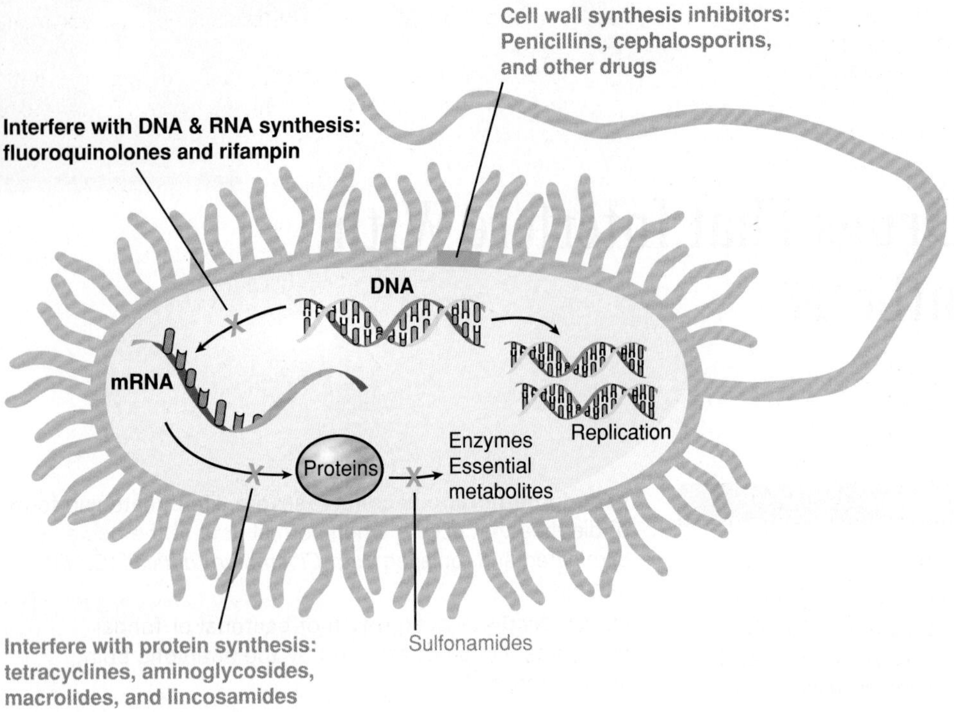

Cell wall synthesis inhibitors:
Penicillins, cephalosporins,
and other drugs

Interfere with DNA & RNA synthesis:
fluoroquinolones and rifampin

DNA

mRNA

Proteins

Enzymes
Essential
metabolites

Replication

Interfere with protein synthesis:
tetracyclines, aminoglycosides,
macrolides, and lincosamides

Sulfonamides

Figure 9.1 Action of bacterial DNA/RNA synthesis inhibitors such as the fluoroquinolones.

FLUOROQUINOLONES

The fluoroquinolone drugs include ciprofloxacin (Cipro), gemifloxacin (Factive), levofloxacin (Levaquin), moxifloxacin (Avelox), norfloxacin (Noroxin), and ofloxacin (Floxin).

Actions

The fluoroquinolones exert their bactericidal effect by interfering with the synthesis of bacterial DNA. This interference prevents cell reproduction, causing death of the bacterial cell (Fig. 9.1).

Uses

The fluoroquinolones are effective in treating infections caused by gram-positive and gram-negative microorganisms. They are primarily used in the treatment of the following:

- Lower respiratory infections
- Bone and joint infections
- Urinary tract infections
- Infections of the skin
- Sexually transmitted infections

Ciprofloxacin, norfloxacin, and ofloxacin are available in ophthalmic forms for infections in the eyes.

Adverse Reactions

Common adverse effects include the following:

- Nausea
- Diarrhea
- Headache
- Abdominal pain or discomfort

- Dizziness
- **Photosensitivity** (exaggerated skin reaction to sun exposure), which is a more serious adverse reaction seen with the administration of the fluoroquinolones, especially ofloxacin.

The administration of any drug may result in a hypersensitivity reaction, which can range from mild to severe and, in some cases, be life-threatening. Mild hypersensitivity reactions may require only discontinuing the drug, whereas the more serious reactions require immediate treatment. Bacterial or fungal superinfections and pseudomembranous colitis may occur with the use of these drugs.

Superinfections

A **superinfection** can develop rapidly and is potentially serious and even life-threatening. Antibiotics can disrupt the **normal flora** (nonpathogenic bacteria in the bowel), causing a secondary infection or superinfection. This new infection is "superimposed" on the original infection. The destruction of large numbers of nonpathogenic bacteria (normal flora) by the antibiotic alters the chemical environment. This allows uncontrolled growth of bacteria or fungal microorganisms that are not affected by the antibiotic being administered. A superinfection may occur with the use of any antibiotic, especially when these drugs are given for a long time or when repeated courses of therapy are necessary.

 LIFESPAN CONSIDERATIONS
Gerontology
Older adults who are debilitated, chronically ill, or taking oral antibiotics for an extended period are more likely to develop a superinfection.

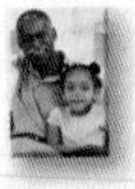

Symptoms of bacterial superinfection of the bowel include diarrhea or bloody diarrhea, rectal bleeding, fever, and abdominal cramping. **Pseudomembranous colitis** is one type of a bacterial superinfection. This potentially life-threatening problem develops because of an overgrowth of the microorganism *Clostridium difficile* (*C. diff*) in the bowel. This organism produces a toxin that affects the lining of the colon. Signs and symptoms include severe diarrhea with visible blood and mucus, fever, and abdominal cramps. This adverse reaction usually requires immediate discontinuation of the antibiotic. Mild cases may respond to drug discontinuation. Moderate to severe cases may require treatment with intravenous (IV) fluids and electrolytes, protein supplementation, and treatment with drugs such as fidaxomicin (Dificid) to eliminate the microorganism.

Candidiasis or moniliasis is a common type of fungal superinfection. Fungal superinfections commonly occur throughout the gastrointestinal (GI) and reproductive systems. Symptoms include lesions of the mouth or tongue, vaginal discharge, and anal or vaginal itching.

Vaginal yeast infections are frequent because a yeast-like fungus normally exists in small numbers in the vagina. The multiplication rate of these microorganisms is normally slowed and kept under control by a strain of bacteria (Döderlein's bacillus) in the vagina. If anti-infective therapy destroys these normal microorganisms of the vagina, the fungi become uncontrolled, multiply at a rapid rate, and cause symptoms of the fungal infection candidiasis (or moniliasis).

Contraindications and Precautions

Fluoroquinolones are contraindicated in patients with a history of hypersensitivity to the fluoroquinolones, in children younger than 18 years of age, and in pregnancy (pregnancy category C). These drugs also are contraindicated in patients whose lifestyles do not allow for adherence to the precautions regarding photosensitivity.

Tendonitis and tendon rupture risk increase when taking a fluoroquinolone. Although this can happen at any age, those older than 60 years who also take corticosteroids are at greater risk.

Fluoroquinolones are used cautiously in patients with diabetes, renal impairment, or a history of seizures; older patients; and patients on dialysis.

Interactions

The following interactions may occur when a fluoroquinolone is administered with another agent:

Interacting Drug	Common Use	Effect of Interaction
theophylline	Management of respiratory problems, such as asthma	Increased serum theophylline level
cimetidine	Management of GI upset	Interferes with elimination of the antibiotic
oral anticoagulants	Blood thinner	Increased risk of bleeding
antacids, iron salts, or zinc	Relief of heartburn and GI upset	Decreased absorption of the antibiotic
nonsteroidal anti-inflammatory drugs (NSAIDs)	Relief of pain and inflammation	Risk of seizure activity

There is also a risk of severe cardiac arrhythmias when the fluoroquinolones—moxifloxacin are administered with drugs that increase the QT interval (e.g., quinidine, procainamide, amiodarone, sotalol).

NURSING PROCESS
PATIENT RECEIVING A FLUOROQUINOLONE OR MISCELLANEOUS ANTI-INFECTIVE

ASSESSMENT

Preadministration Assessment
Before administering a fluoroquinolone or miscellaneous DNA/RNA inhibitors, identify and record the signs and symptoms of the infection, and also take and record vital signs. It is particularly important to obtain a thorough allergy history, especially any drug-related allergies. The primary health care provider may order culture and sensitivity tests, and the culture is obtained before the first dose of the drug is given. Other laboratory tests, such as renal and hepatic function tests, complete blood count, and urinalysis, also may be ordered before and during drug therapy for early detection of toxic reactions.

Ongoing Assessment
During drug therapy with the miscellaneous DNA/RNA inhibitors, it is important for you to perform an ongoing assessment. In general, compare the initial signs and symptoms of the infection, which were recorded during the initial assessment, with the current signs and symptoms. Document these findings in the patient's chart. Monitor the patient's vital signs every 4 hours or as ordered by the primary health care provider. Notify the primary health care provider if there are changes in the vital signs, such as a significant drop in blood pressure, an increase in the pulse or respiratory rate, or a sudden increase in temperature.

NURSING DIAGNOSES
Drug-specific nursing diagnoses include the following:

- **Risk for Impaired Comfort** related to fever
- **Risk for Impaired Skin Integrity** related to photosensitivity
- **Acute Pain** related to tissue injury during drug therapy
- **Diarrhea** related to superinfection secondary to antibiotic therapy, adverse drug reaction

Nursing diagnoses related to drug administration are discussed in Chapter 4.

PLANNING

The expected outcomes for the patient may include an optimal response to therapy, which includes control of the infectious process, meeting of patient needs related to the management of adverse drug reactions, and confidence in an understanding of the medication regimen.

IMPLEMENTATION

Promoting an Optimal Response to Therapy

A variety of adverse reactions can be seen with the administration of the fluoroquinolones. You should observe the patient, especially during the first 48 hours of therapy. It is important to report the occurrence of any adverse reaction to the primary health care provider before the next dose of the drug is due. If a serious adverse reaction, such as a hypersensitivity reaction, respiratory difficulty, severe diarrhea, or a decided drop in blood pressure, occurs, then contact the primary health care provider immediately. These adverse reactions can be distressing for the patient, so be sure to offer comfort measures, such as a warm blanket or gentle touch, while awaiting a response from the primary health care provider.

Always listen to, evaluate, and report any complaints the patient may have; certain complaints may be an early sign of an adverse drug reaction. Report all changes in the patient's condition and any new problems that occur (e.g., nausea or diarrhea) as soon as possible. The primary health care provider will determine if these changes or problems are a part of the patient's infectious process or the result of an adverse drug reaction.

Encourage patients who receive the fluoroquinolones to increase their fluid intake. Norfloxacin is given on an empty stomach (e.g., 1 hour before or 2 hours after meals). Some drugs are made so that they release the drug over time in the body; these formulations are known as extended-release (XR), sustained-release (SR), or controlled-release (CR) drugs. Because the amount of drug would be too great if released in the body at once, it is important to swallow these medications whole. Patients should not crush, chew, or break extended-release medications. If the patient is taking an antacid, ciprofloxacin and moxifloxacin should be administered 2 to 4 hours before or 6 to 8 hours after the antacid.

INTRAVENOUS ADMINISTRATION. When these drugs are administered intravenously, inspect the needle site and area around the needle at frequent intervals for signs of extravasation, or leakage into the soft tissue, of the IV fluid. More frequent assessments are performed if the patient is restless or uncooperative. Many of the miscellaneous anti-infectives irritate the vein when administered by the IV route.

The rate of infusion is checked every 15 minutes and adjusted as needed. Inspect the vein used for the IV infusion every 4 to 8 hours for signs of tenderness, pain, and redness (which may indicate phlebitis or thrombophlebitis). If these symptoms are apparent, the IV infusion is restarted in another vein and the problem is brought to the attention of the primary health care provider.

Monitoring and Managing Patient Needs

Although the drugs in this chapter are different, many of the patient problems are similar. Consider the commonalities of the drugs to look for common problems.

IMPAIRED COMFORT: INCREASED FEVER. The infectious process is accompanied by an elevation in temperature. Monitor the vital signs, particularly the body temperature, when patients have an infection. As the anti-infective works to rid the body of the infectious organism, the body temperature should return to normal. Monitoring the vital signs (temperature, pulse, and respiration) frequently aids in assessing the drug's effectiveness in eradicating the infection. Promptly notify the primary health care provider if a temperature rises over 101°F.

IMPAIRED SKIN INTEGRITY. The fluoroquinolone drugs cause severe photosensitivity reactions. Patients may experience "sunburn" reactions even when they use sunscreen or sunblock products. Caution patients to wear cover-up clothing with long sleeves and wide-brimmed hats when outside in addition to sunblock preparations. Remind patients that sunscreen needs to be applied repeatedly throughout the day or when going into water. Patients should be aware that glare during hazy or cloudy days can cause skin reactions as readily as direct sunlight on a clear day.

ACUTE PAIN: TISSUE INJURY. Many of these antibacterial drugs are irritating to the vein when administered IV. You should read instructions carefully for infusion rates. For intravenously administered fluoroquinolones, as with other caustic drugs, inspect the needle site and the area around the needle every hour for signs of extravasation of the IV fluid while the drug is infused. Inspect the vein used for the IV infusion every 4 hours for signs of tenderness, pain, and redness (which may indicate phlebitis or thrombophlebitis). Perform these assessments more frequently if the patient is restless or uncooperative. Be sure the proper flush solution is used after the infusion to keep the vein open and minimize irritation. If tissue or vein injury is apparent, the IV is stopped and restarted in another vein and the problem brought to the attention of the primary health care provider.

> **! NURSING ALERT**
> There is a risk with all fluoroquinolone drugs of causing pain, inflammation, or rupture of a tendon. The Achilles tendon is particularly vulnerable. Those 60 years of age and older who take corticosteroids are at greatest risk for tendon rupture.

DIARRHEA. Frequent liquid stools may be an indication of a superinfection or pseudomembranous colitis. If pseudomembranous colitis occurs, it is usually seen 4 to 10 days after treatment is started.

Teach the patient or family to feel confident in the ability to check bowel movements and immediately reporting to the primary health care provider the occurrence of diarrhea or loose stools containing blood and mucus. It may be necessary to discontinue drug therapy and institute treatment for diarrhea, a superinfection, or pseudomembranous colitis.

If blood and mucus appear to be in the stool, save a sample of the stool and test for occult blood using a test such as Hemoccult. If the stool tests positive for blood, the sample is saved for possible additional laboratory testing.

Educating the Patient and Family

When you teach the patient and family members, explain all adverse reactions associated with the specific prescribed antibiotic. Use written materials in the language of preference to describe the signs and symptoms of potentially serious adverse reactions, such as hypersensitivity reactions, moderate to severe diarrhea, and sudden onset of chills and fever. The patient should feel confident about when to contact the primary health care provider if such symptoms occur. Instruct the patient not to take the next dose of the drug until the problem is discussed with the primary health care provider (see Patient Teaching for Improved Patient Outcomes: Superinfections).

EVALUATION

- Therapeutic response is achieved, and there is no evidence of infection.
- Adverse reactions are identified, reported to the primary health care provider, and managed successfully with appropriate nursing interventions:
  - Patient reports comfort without fever.
  - Skin is intact and free of inflammation, irritation, infection, or ulcerations.
  - Patient reports no pain or injury.
  - Patient does not experience diarrhea.
- Patient and family express confidence and demonstrate an understanding of the drug regimen.

PHARMACOLOGY IN PRACTICE
THINK CRITICALLY

 Mr. Park complains about gas pains in his stomach and lots of "rumbling feelings." The nursing assistant reports that he has made multiple trips to the bathroom due to diarrhea for the past 2 days. He gets upset and says he can't wait for ambulation assistance; the nursing assistant is concerned he will get up at night by himself and fall. Analyze whether this matter should be investigated.

Patient Teaching for Improved Patient Outcomes
Superinfections

Antibiotics are one of the most commonly administered types of drug therapy in the home. Any patient taking antibacterial drugs is susceptible to superinfection. Make sure the patient knows the signs and symptoms of superinfection. A bacterial superinfection commonly occurs in the bowel.

When you teach, make sure your patient understands the following:
Report any of the following:

- ✔ Fever
- ✔ Burning sensation in the mouth or throat
- ✔ Localized redness, inflammation, and excoriation, particularly inside the mouth, in the groin, or in skin folds of the anogenital area
- ✔ Abdominal cramps
- ✔ Scaly, reddened, papular rash commonly in the breast folds, axillae, groin, or umbilicus
- ✔ Diarrhea, possibly severe with visible blood and mucus

A fungal superinfection commonly occurs in the mouth, vagina, and anogenital areas. Teach the patient to report any of the following:

- ✔ Creamy white, lace-like patches on the tongue, mouth, or throat
- ✔ White or yellow vaginal discharge
- ✔ Anal or vaginal itching

KEY POINTS

- Fluoroquinolones are the primary class of bactericidal drugs affecting the bacterial cell by interfering with the synthesis of DNA. These drugs are used to treat a wide range of both gram-negative and gram-positive microorganisms. Some drugs of this class come in ophthalmic solutions to treat infections of the eye.

- Some of these drugs are given in an oral form (extended-release form) so the drug is released into the body over time. When given IV, the vein needs to be monitored frequently because the medications can be irritating to the tissue.

- Photosensitivity can be a severe adverse reaction of this class of drugs. Sunscreen and lightweight clothing should be worn at all times when outdoors, even on overcast days.

- Tendon rupture has been noted, especially in those older than 60 years of age, when taking these drugs.

- When taking any antibacterial drug, overgrowth of other bacteria or elimination of normal flora can result in superinfection. Drugs may be stopped and supportive care with IV fluids, dietary supplement, and a different antibacterial drug can help.

Summary Drug Table ANTIBACTERIAL DRUGS THAT INTERFERE WITH DNA/RNA SYNTHESIS

Generic Name	Trade Name	Uses	Adverse Reactions	Dosage Ranges
Fluoroquinolones				
® ciprofloxacin *sih-proe'-flox-ah-sin*	Cipro	Treatment of infections due to susceptible microorganisms	Nausea, diarrhea, headache, abdominal discomfort, photosensitivity, superinfections, hypersensitivity reactions	250–750 mg orally q 12 hr; 200–400 mg IV q 12 hr
gemifloxacin *jem-ah-flox'-ah-sin*	Factive	Bronchitis and community-acquired pneumonia	Vomiting, diarrhea, stomach pain, restlessness, dizziness, confusion, taste changes, sleep disturbances	320 mg/day orally
levofloxacin *lee-voe-flox'-ah-sin*	Levaquin	Same as ciprofloxacin	Same as ciprofloxacin	250–750 mg/day orally, IV
moxifloxacin *mocks-ah-flox'-ah-sin*	Avelox	Same as ciprofloxacin	Same as ciprofloxacin	400 mg/day orally
® norfloxacin *nor-flox'-ah-sin*	Noroxin	Urinary tract infections, sexually transmitted infections (STIs), prostatitis	Same as ciprofloxacin	400 mg orally q 12 hr; 800 mg as single dose for STI
ofloxacin *oh-flox'-ah-sin*		Same as ciprofloxacin	Same as ciprofloxacin	200–400 mg orally, IV q 12 hr
Miscellaneous Drugs That Inhibit RNA/DNA Synthesis				
metronidazole *meh-troe-nye'-dah-zoll*	Flagyl	Treatment of anaerobic microorganisms in bone, skin, central nervous system, internal body cavity, respiratory system	Headache, nausea, peripheral neuropathy, disulfiram-like interaction with alcohol	Loading dose 15 mg/kg, then 7.5 mg/kg
rifaximin *rye-fax'-ah-min*	Xifaxan	Hepatic encephalopathy, irritable bowel syndrome, *C. diff* infection	Gas pains, headache	400–550 mg orally, 2–3 times daily

® This drug should be administered at least 1 hour before or 2 hours after a meal.

● Chapter Review

Know Your Drugs

Clients sometimes know a medication by the brand (or trade) name and not the generic name. To help you recognize both names, match the brand name with the generic name of the same medication

Generic Name	Brand Name
1. ciprofloxacin	A. Factive
2. gemifloxacin	B. Cipro
3. metronidazole	C. Flagyl

Calculate Medication Dosages

1. A client is prescribed 500 mg of ciprofloxacin orally every 12 hours for an acute sinus infection. The drug is available in 500-mg tablets. The nurse teaches the client to administer _____.

2. Metronidazole is available in 250-mg tablets. The client is instructed to take 750 mg once daily. How many tablets will the client take with each dose? _____

● Prepare for the NCLEX®

Build Your Knowledge

1. Fluoroquinolones kill bacterial cells by _____.

   1. inhibiting protein synthesis
   2. destroying the bacterial cell wall
   3. eliminating oxygen from the ribosome
   4. prohibiting DNA synthesis

2. Clients taking a fluoroquinolone are encouraged to _____.

   1. nap 1 to 2 hours daily while taking the drug
   2. eat a high-protein diet
   3. increase their fluid intake
   4. avoid foods high in carbohydrates

3. When taking levofloxacin the client is taught to _____.

   1. wear sun protection whenever outside
   2. assess for hearing loss
   3. carry an EpiPen at all times
   4. eat more fruits and vegetables

4. When monitoring the IV infusion of levofloxacin, the nurse makes sure the needle is in the vein because if not it can result in _____.

   1. irritation of the surrounding tissue
   2. a blood clot in the arm
   3. fluid deficit and dehydration
   4. a sudden and severe rise in blood pressure

5. To avoid a superinfection when taking fluoroquinolones, instruct the client to_____.

   1. eat a high-fiber diet
   2. wash with antibacterial soaps
   3. monitor for diarrhea
   4. use over-the-counter (OTC) creams on skin rashes

Apply Your Knowledge

6. A client is prescribed moxifloxacin. The nurse notes that the client is also taking an antacid. The nurse correctly administers moxifloxacin _____.

   1. once daily orally, 4 hours before the antacid
   2. twice daily orally, immediately after the antacid
   3. once daily IM without regard to the administration of the antacid
   4. every 12 hours IV without regard to the administration of the antacid

7. The client taking a fluoroquinolone plans to enter a marathon after treatment. The nurse is concerned about _____.

   1. prolonged QT interval cardiac changes
   2. spontaneous tendon rupture
   3. phlebitis at the IV site
   4. pseudomembranous colitis symptoms

8. Which of the following statements if made by the client would indicate that he understands to take the entire course of an antibacterial medication?

   1. "If it gets red, stop taking the medicine that is not working."
   2. "When the pain stops, stop the medicine."
   3. "Take this until you get diarrhea."
   4. "Take all the medicine in the bottle."

Alternate-Format Questions

9. Levofloxacin 500 mg IV is ordered for a client hospitalized with pneumonia. The drug is mixed in a syringe for an IV pump as a solution of 250 mg/15 mL. How many mL should be in the syringe? _____

10. Identify the interventions to use when taking drugs with photosensitive reactions. **Select all that apply**.

    1. wash the skin frequently
    2. use high SPF value sunscreen
    3. wear head coverings on overcast days
    4. clothing should be long sleeved

To check your answers, see Appendix G.

the**Point** *For more NCLEX-style questions, log on to http://thepoint.lww.com to access more than 1000 questions.*

10

Antitubercular Drugs

LEARNING OBJECTIVES

On completion of this chapter, the student will:

1. Discuss the drugs used in the treatment of mycobacteria for tuberculosis and leprosy.
2. Discuss the uses, general drug actions, contraindications, precautions, interactions, and general adverse reactions associated with the administration of the antitubercular drugs.
3. Discuss important preadministration and ongoing assessment activities the nurse should perform on the patient taking an antitubercular drug.
4. List nursing diagnoses particular to a patient taking an antitubercular drug.
5. Describe directly observed therapy (DOT).
6. Discuss ways to promote an optimal response to therapy, how to manage adverse reactions, and important points to keep in mind when educating patients about the use of the antitubercular drugs.

KEY TERMS

directly observed therapy (DOT) • drug dose taken in front of the administrator

extrapulmonary • occurring outside of the lungs in the respiratory system

gout • a metabolic disorder resulting in increased levels of uric acid and causing severe joint pain

leprosy • chronic, communicable disease caused by *Mycobacterium leprae;* also called *Hansen's disease*

Mycobacterium leprae • bacterium that causes leprosy (Hansen's disease)

Mycobacterium tuberculosis • bacterium that causes tuberculosis (TB)

optic neuritis • inflammation of the optic nerve, causing a decrease in visual acuity and changes in color perception

peripheral neuropathy • numbness and tingling of the extremities

prophylaxis • prevention

quiescent • having no symptoms

vertigo • feeling of a spinning or rotational motion; dizziness

DRUG CLASSES

Primary antitubercular
Secondary antitubercular

PHARMACOLOGY IN PRACTICE

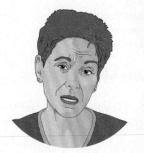

Betty Peterson has come into the clinic with complaints of a chronic cough. Ms. Peterson requests that a TB skin test be performed as well as a chest x-ray. She is concerned that she will be diagnosed with TB, telling you that she watched a TV show about the rise in TB in crowded areas. When questioned, she states that "a lot of people" live in the apartment next door. Should Betty Peterson be assessed for TB?

Tuberculosis (TB) is a major health problem throughout the world, especially in Asia and Sub-Saharan Africa; almost 1.5 million deaths each year are caused by TB. The World Health Organization (WHO) predicts that 8 million to 9 million people worldwide will contract this disease each year. Individuals living in crowded conditions, those with compromised immune systems, and those with debilitative conditions are especially susceptible to TB. People with human immunodeficiency virus (HIV) infection are especially at risk for TB because of their compromised immune systems.

Tuberculosis is an infectious disease caused by the *Mycobacterium tuberculosis* bacterium. The pathogen is also referred to as the tubercle bacillus. The disease is transmitted from one person to another by droplets dispersed in the air when an infected person coughs or sneezes. These droplets are then inhaled by noninfected persons. Although TB primarily affects the lungs, other organs may be involved.

NURSING ALERT

One quarter of all HIV-related deaths are caused by active TB. Yet, TB in patients infected with HIV can be difficult to diagnose. HIV patients' immune systems are deficient, so TB skin tests may not show a reaction even when the disease is present. X-ray studies, sputum analyses, or physical examinations may be needed to diagnose *M. tuberculosis* infection accurately in patients with HIV infection.

Extrapulmonary (outside of the lungs) tuberculosis is the term used to distinguish TB affecting other organs of the body from the infection located only in the lungs. Organs that can be affected include the liver, bones, spleen, and adrenal glands. Figure 10.1 illustrates the areas affected by TB and the drugs used in treatment.

Antitubercular drugs are classified as primary (first-line) and secondary (second-line) drugs. Primary drugs provide the foundation for treatment. Tuberculosis responds well to long-term treatment with a combination of three or more antitubercular drugs. Antitubercular drugs are also used as prophylactic therapy to prevent the spreading of TB. Secondary drugs are used for multidrug-resistant TB (MDR-TB), which are more costly and toxic than primary drugs.

Secondary drugs are also used to treat extrapulmonary TB. The primary antitubercular drugs are discussed in this chapter. Both primary and secondary antitubercular drugs are listed in the Summary Drug Table: Antitubercular Drugs. Certain fluoroquinolones such as ciprofloxacin, ofloxacin, and levofloxacin have proven effective against TB and are considered secondary drugs (see Chapter 9).

Actions

Many antitubercular drugs are bacteriostatic against the *M. tuberculosis* bacillus. These drugs usually act to inhibit bacterial cell wall synthesis, which slows the multiplication rate of the bacteria. Isoniazid is bactericidal, with rifampin and streptomycin having some bactericidal activity.

Uses

Antitubercular drugs are used in a protocol, called *Standard Treatment*, to treat active TB. Isoniazid (INH), however, may be used alone in preventive therapy (**prophylaxis**). For exam-

Display 10.1 **Prophylactic Uses for Isoniazid (INH)**

Isoniazid may be used in the following situations:

- Household members and other close associates of those recently diagnosed as having tuberculosis
- Those whose tuberculin skin test has become positive in the last 2 years
- Those with positive skin tests whose radiographic (x-ray) findings indicate nonprogressive, healed, or **quiescent** (causing no symptoms) tubercular lesions
- Those at risk for developing tuberculosis (e.g., those with Hodgkin's disease, severe diabetes mellitus, leukemia, and other serious illnesses and those receiving corticosteroids or drug therapy for a malignancy)
- All patients younger than 35 years (primarily children to age 7) who have a positive skin test
- Persons with acquired immunodeficiency syndrome (AIDS) or those who are positive for HIV and have a positive tuberculosis skin test *or a* negative tuberculosis skin test but have a history of a prior significant reaction to purified protein derivative (a skin test for tuberculosis)

ple, when a person is diagnosed with TB, family members of the infected individual must be given prophylactic treatment with isoniazid for 6 to 9 months. Display 10.1 identifies prophylactic uses for isoniazid.

Standard Treatment

Standard treatment for TB is divided into two phases: the initial phase, followed by a continuing phase. During the initial phase, drugs are used to kill the rapidly multiplying *M. tuberculosis* and to prevent drug resistance. The initial phase lasts approximately 2 months and the continuing phase approximately 4 months, with the total treatment regimen lasting for 6 to 9 months, depending on the patient's response to therapy.

The Centers for Disease Control and Prevention (CDC) recommends that treatment begin as soon as possible after the diagnosis of TB. The recommended treatment regimen is for the administration of the primary drugs—rifampin (Rifadin), isoniazid (INH), pyrazinamide, and ethambutol (Myambutol)—for a minimum of 2 months. The second or continuation phase includes only the drugs rifampin and isoniazid. The CDC recommends this phase for 4 months or up to 7 months in special populations. These special circumstances include the following:

- Positive sputum culture after completion of initial treatment
- Cavitary (hole or pocket of) disease and positive sputum culture after initial treatment
- When pyrazinamide was not included in the initial treatment
- Positive sputum culture after initial treatment in a patient with previously diagnosed HIV infection

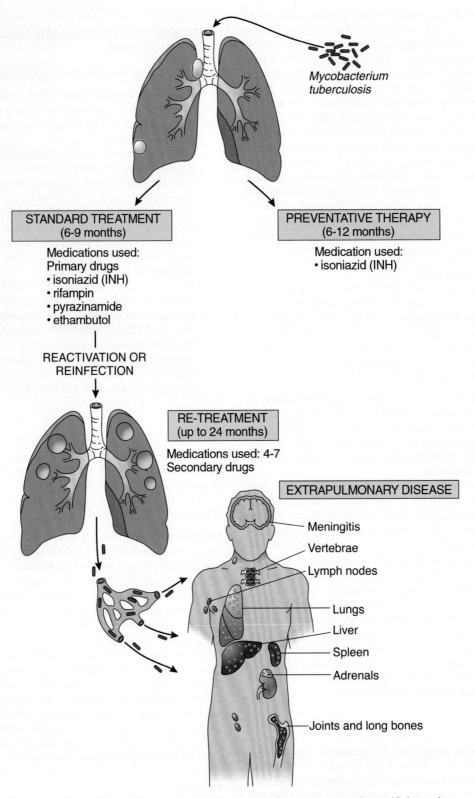

Figure 10.1 Sites of tuberculosis infection and treatment options. (Adapted from Rubin, E., & Farber, J. L. [1999]. *Pathology* [3rd ed.]. Philadelphia: Lippincott Williams & Wilkins.)

Retreatment

At times, treatment fails because of inadequate initial drug treatment or noncompliance with the drug regimen. When treatment fails, retreatment is necessary using the secondary drugs. Retreatment generally includes the use of four or more antitubercular drugs. Retreatment drug regimens most often consist of ethionamide (Trecator), aminosalicylic acid (Paser), cycloserine (Seromycin), and capreomycin (Capastat). Ofloxacin and ciprofloxacin (Cipro) may also be used in retreatment. Sometimes during retreatment, seven or more drugs may be used, with the ineffective drugs discontinued when susceptibility test results are available. Treatment is individualized based on the susceptibility of the microorganism. Up to 24 months of continued treatment after sputum cultures are no longer positive for TB can be part of the plan.

Resistance to the Antitubercular Drugs

Of increasing concern is MDR-TB. Bacterial resistance develops, sometimes rapidly, because of lack of adherence to lengthy drug dosing schedules. Treatment is individualized and based on laboratory studies that identify the drugs to which the organism is susceptible. The CDC recommends using three or more drugs with initial therapy, as well as in retreatment, because using a combination of drugs slows the development of bacterial resistance. Tuberculosis caused by drug-resistant organisms should be considered in patients who have no response to therapy and in patients who have been treated in the past.

This chapter discusses the following primary antitubercular drugs: ethambutol, isoniazid, pyrazinamide, and rifampin. Other primary and secondary drugs are listed in the Summary Drug Table: Antitubercular Drugs.

ETHAMBUTOL

Adverse Reactions

Generalized Reactions

- Dermatitis and pruritus (itching)
- Joint pain
- Anorexia
- Nausea and vomiting

Severe Reactions

- Anaphylactoid reactions (unusual or exaggerated allergic reactions)
- **Optic neuritis** (a decrease in visual acuity and changes in color perception); optic neuritis is dose related.

Contraindications, Precautions, and Interactions

Ethambutol is not recommended for patients with a history of hypersensitivity to the drug or children younger than 13 years. The drug is used with caution during pregnancy (category B), in patients with hepatic or renal impairment, and in patients with diabetic retinopathy or cataracts.

ISONIAZID

Adverse Reactions

The incidence of adverse reactions appears to be higher when larger doses of isoniazid are prescribed.

Generalized Reactions

- Nausea and vomiting
- Epigastric distress
- Fever
- Skin eruptions
- Hematologic changes
- Jaundice
- Hypersensitivity

Toxicity

- **Peripheral neuropathy** (numbness and tingling of the extremities) is the most common symptom of toxicity.
- Severe hepatitis has been associated with isoniazid therapy and may appear after many months of treatment and be fatal.

Contraindications and Precautions

Isoniazid is contraindicated in patients with a history of hypersensitivity to the drug. The drug is used with caution during pregnancy (category C) or lactation and in patients with hepatic and renal impairment.

Interactions

The following interactions may occur when isoniazid is administered with another agent:

Interacting Drug	Common Use	Effect of Interaction
antacids containing aluminum salts	Relief of heartburn and gastrointestinal upset	Reduced absorption of isoniazid
anticoagulants	Blood thinner	Increased risk for bleeding
phenytoin	Antiseizure drug	Increased serum levels of phenytoin
alcohol (in beverages)	Social situations	Higher incidence of drug-related hepatitis

When isoniazid is taken with foods containing tyramine, such as aged cheese and meats, bananas, yeast products, and alcohol, an exaggerated sympathetic-type response can occur (i.e., hypertension, increased heart rate, and palpitations).

PYRAZINAMIDE

Adverse Reactions

Generalized Reactions

- Nausea and vomiting
- Diarrhea
- Myalgia (aches)
- Rashes

Hepatotoxicity

Hepatotoxicity is the principal adverse reaction seen with pyrazinamide use. Symptoms of hepatotoxicity may range from none (except for slightly abnormal hepatic function test results) to a more severe reaction such as jaundice.

Contraindications and Precautions

Pyrazinamide is contraindicated in patients with a history of hypersensitivity to the drug, acute **gout** (a metabolic disorder resulting in increased levels of uric acid and causing severe joint pain), or severe hepatic damage.

Pyrazinamide should be used cautiously in patients during pregnancy (category C) and lactation and in patients with hepatic and renal impairment, HIV infection, and diabetes mellitus.

Interactions

When pyrazinamide is administered with the antigout medications allopurinol (Zyloprim), colchicine, or probenecid, its effectiveness decreases.

RIFAMPIN

Adverse Reactions

Generalized reactions include the following:

- Nausea and vomiting
- Epigastric distress, heartburn, fatigue
- **Vertigo** (dizziness)
- Rash
- Reddish-orange discoloration of body fluids (urine, tears, saliva, sweat, and sputum)
- Hematologic changes, renal insufficiency

Contraindications and Precautions

Rifampin is contraindicated in patients with a history of hypersensitivity to the drug. The drug is used with caution during pregnancy (category C) and lactation and in patients with hepatic or renal impairment.

Interactions

The following interactions may occur when rifampin is administered with another agent:

Interacting Drug	Common Use	Effect of Interaction
antiretrovirals (efavirenz, nevirapine)	HIV infection	Decreased serum levels of antiretrovirals
digoxin	Management of cardiac problems	Decreased serum levels of digoxin
oral contraceptives	Contraception	Decreased contraceptive effectiveness
isoniazid	Antitubercular agent	Higher risk of hepatotoxicity
oral anticoagulants	Blood thinner	Increased risk for bleeding
oral hypoglycemics	Antidiabetic agent	Decreased effectiveness of oral hypoglycemic agent
chloramphenicol	Anti-infective agent	Increased risk for seizures
phenytoin	Antiseizure agent	Decreased effectiveness of phenytoin
verapamil	Management of cardiac problems and blood pressure	Decreased effectiveness of verapamil

Leprosy, also referred to as *Hansen's disease*, is caused by the bacterium *Mycobacterium leprae*. Leprosy is a chronic, communicable disease that is not easily spread and has a long incubation period. Since 1985, the prevalence of leprosy has dropped by 90%. About 100 new cases are diagnosed yearly in the United States (primarily the southern states, Hawaii, and U.S. possessions).

Peripheral nerves are affected, causing sensory loss and muscle weakness. The traditional fear of leprosy relates to skin involvement, which may present with lesions confined to a few isolated areas or may be fairly widespread over the entire body. Dapsone, clofazimine (Lamprene), rifampin (Rifadin), and ethionamide (Trecator) are drugs currently used to treat leprosy. The leprostatic drugs are listed in the Summary Drug Table: Antitubercular Drugs.

NURSING PROCESS

PATIENT RECEIVING AN ANTITUBERCULAR DRUG

ASSESSMENT

Preadministration Assessment

Once the diagnosis of TB is confirmed, the primary health care provider selects the drugs that will best control the spread of the disease and make the patient noninfectious to others. Many laboratory and diagnostic tests may be necessary before starting antitubercular therapy, including radiographic studies, culture and sensitivity tests, and various types of laboratory tests, such as a complete blood count. It also is important to assess the family history and a history of contacts if the patient has active TB.

Depending on the severity of the disease, patients may be treated initially in the hospital and then discharged for supervised follow-up care, or they may have all treatment instituted on an outpatient basis.

Ongoing Assessment

When performing the ongoing assessment, teach the patient or caregiver to observe daily for the appearance of adverse reactions. These observations are especially important when a drug is known to be toxic to nerves or eyes. It is important to report any adverse reactions to the primary health care provider. In addition, carefully monitor vital signs daily or as frequently as every 4 hours when the patient is hospitalized.

NURSING DIAGNOSES

Drug administration–specific nursing diagnoses are the following:

- **Acute Pain** related to frequent injection of antitubercular drug
- **Imbalanced Nutrition: Less Than Body Requirements** related to gastric upset and general poor health status
- **Risk for Ineffective Self Health Management** related to indifference, lack of knowledge, long-term treatment regimen, other factors

The nursing diagnosis of Ineffective Self Health Management may be especially important with patients considering the long-term therapy required to treat TB. Refer to interventions discussed in Chapter 4 to deal with patient needs.

PLANNING

The expected outcomes for the patient may include an optimal response to antitubercular therapy, meeting patient needs related to the management of common adverse reactions, and confidence in an understanding of and adherence with the prescribed medication regimen.

IMPLEMENTATION

Promoting an Optimal Response to Therapy

The diagnosis of TB, along with the necessity of long-term treatment and follow-up, is often distressing to the patient. Patients with a diagnosis of TB may have many questions about the disease and its treatment. Health literacy may be low; patients may be unfamiliar with medical terms and treatment strategies. Try asking patients what they think is causing the illness. Cultural beliefs may play a role in the patient's understanding about the disease cause and treatment. Patients may have limited English proficiency, and education is important for the patient to remain compliant with long-term therapy. Use interpretative services and translated patient education tools in teaching sessions. Allow ample time for the patient and family members to ask questions. In some instances, it may be necessary to refer the patient to other health care professionals, such as a social service worker or a registered dietitian.

Monitoring and Managing Patient Needs

Managing adverse reactions in patients taking antitubercular drugs is an important nursing responsibility. Continuously observe for signs of adverse reactions and immediately report them to the primary health care provider.

Acute Pain: Frequent Parenteral Injections. When administering the antitubercular drug by the parenteral route, care is taken to rotate the injection sites. At the time of each injection, inspect previous injection sites for signs of swelling, redness, and tenderness. If a localized reaction persists or if the area appears to be infected, it is important to notify the primary health care provider.

Imbalanced Nutrition: Less Than Body Requirements. When TB affects patients who live in crowded and impoverished conditions, malnutrition may be prevalent. In some cases alcoholism may compound the patient's difficulties. This complicates the administration of drugs and compromises the general condition of the patient's gastrointestinal tract. Ethambutol should be given at the same time daily and may be given without regard to food. Pyrazinamide may also be given with food. Other antitubercular drugs are given by the oral route and on an empty stomach, unless epigastric upset occurs. If gastric upset occurs, it is important to notify the primary health care provider before the next dose is given. If a dose is missed, tell the patient *not* to double the dose the next day.

An alternative, twice-weekly dosing regimen has been developed to promote adherence on an outpatient basis. This may improve patient nutrition by decreasing the gastric upset of frequent dosing. Combination drugs (e.g., Rifater, which contains isoniazid, rifampin, and pyrazinamide) are being manufactured to promote adherence to medication regimens and reduce the need to take multiple drugs that produce gastric upset.

Teach the patient to minimize alcohol consumption due to the increased risk of hepatitis. Frequently, the inclusion of pyridoxine (vitamin B$_6$) is recommended to promote nutrition and prevent neuropathy.

It is helpful to explain to patients that their bodily fluids (urine, feces, saliva, sputum, sweat, and tears) may be colored reddish-orange from the different drugs and that this is normal. It is even more important to teach the patient that this is different from the skin and eye color changes that could indicate hepatic dysfunction (jaundice). Carefully monitor all patients at least monthly for any evidence of liver dysfunction. It is important to instruct patients to report any of the following symptoms: anorexia, nausea, vomiting, fatigue, weakness, yellowing of the skin or eyes, darkening of the urine, or numbness in the hands and feet.

 LIFESPAN CONSIDERATIONS
Gerontology

Older adults are particularly susceptible to a potentially fatal hepatitis when taking isoniazid, especially if they consume alcohol on a regular basis. Two other antitubercular drugs, rifampin and pyrazinamide, can cause liver dysfunction in the older adult as well. Careful observation and monitoring for signs of liver impairment are necessary (e.g., increased serum aspartate aminotransferase [AST], alanine aminotransferase [ALT], and bilirubin levels, and jaundice).

Ineffective Self Health Management. Because the antitubercular drugs must be taken for prolonged periods, adherence to the treatment regimen becomes a problem and increases the risk of development of MDR-TB. To help prevent the problem of nonadherence, directly observed therapy (DOT) is used to administer these drugs. With DOT, the patient makes periodic visits to the office of the primary care provider or the health clinic, where the drug is taken in the presence of the nurse. Nurses watch the patient swallow each dose of the medication treatment. In some cases, the nurse may travel to the patient's home, place of employment, or school to observe or administer medication. DOT may occur daily or two to three times weekly, depending on the patient's health care regimen. Studies indicate that taking the drugs intermittently does not cause a drop in the therapeutic blood levels of antitubercular drugs, even if the drugs are given only two or three times a week (Munsiff, 2006).

Educating the Patient and Family

Antitubercular drugs are given for a long time, and careful patient and family education and close medical supervision are necessary. Nonadherence to the medication regimen can be a problem whenever a disease or disorder requires long-term treatment. For this reason, the DOT method of administration is preferred. The patient and family must understand that short-term therapy is of no value in treating this disease. Remain alert for statements made by the patient or family that may indicate future nonadherence to the drug regimen necessary in controlling the disease. See Patient Teaching for Improved Patient Outcomes: Increasing Medication Adherence to Tubercular Drug Treatment Program for more information.

EVALUATION

- Therapeutic response is achieved, and there is no evidence of infection.

- Adverse reactions are identified, reported to the primary health care provider, and managed successfully with appropriate nursing interventions:
  - Patient manages injection pain.
  - Patient maintains an adequate nutritional status.
  - Patient manages the therapeutic regimen effectively.

- Patient and family express confidence and demonstrate an understanding of the drug regimen.

Patient Teaching for Improved Patient Outcomes

Increasing Medication Adherence to Tubercular Drug Treatment Program

When you teach, make sure your patient understands the following:

✔ Ask the patient what he or she thinks causes the symptoms; promote health literacy by integrating the patient's beliefs and fears into how the bacteria invades the body and how the drugs work to kill it.

✔ Discuss tuberculosis, its causes and communicability, and the need for long-term therapy for disease control using simple, nonmedical terms.

✔ Use visual props or educational materials to help emphasize that short-term treatment is ineffective.

✔ Review the drug therapy regimen, including the prescribed drugs, doses, and frequency of administration.

✔ Reassure the patient that various combinations of drugs are effective in treating tuberculosis.

✔ Urge the patient to take the drugs exactly as prescribed and not to omit, increase, or decrease the dosage unless directed to do so by the health care provider.

✔ Instruct the patient about possible adverse reactions and the need to notify the prescriber should any occur.

✔ Arrange for direct observation therapy with the patient and family.

✔ Instruct the patient in measures to minimize gastrointestinal upset.

✔ Advise the patient to avoid alcohol and the use of nonprescription drugs, especially those containing aspirin, unless use is approved by the health care provider.

✔ Reassure the patient and family that the results of therapy will be monitored by periodic laboratory and diagnostic tests and follow-up visits with the health care provider.

PHARMACOLOGY IN PRACTICE
THINK CRITICALLY

 After reading this chapter, what data would help you decide if Betty Peterson is at risk for TB? Determine what rationale and information to use in teaching Ms. Peterson about risks for TB.

KEY POINTS

- Tuberculosis is an infectious disease that continues to be a major health problem throughout the world. Crowded living conditions, especially where immune-compromised or debilitated people live, are sites of concern.

- Tuberculosis typically involves the lungs and other structures of the respiratory system. Other organs, such as the liver, bones, spleen, and even adrenal glands, can be affected by the bacterium.

- Treatment for active TB involves many months of multi-drug therapy. Standard treatment includes two phases, initial (about 2 months) and continuing (approximately 4 months). At least four different drugs are involved. Treatment failure may result in an additional four- to seven-drug course for 2 years. Bacterial resistance may occur, which is why multiple drugs are used. Combination drugs are being developed to include multiple drugs and to be given less frequently to increase adherence to continuing the entire course of treatment.

- Directly observed therapy (DOT) involves a patient being directly watched when taking the antitubercular drugs by a health provider.

- Preventive therapy (prophylaxis for those exposed but who do not have active disease) involves one drug taken for 6 months to 1 year.

- Body fluids may become orange in color; patient teaching needs to include the ability to differentiate this from liver involvement (hepatitis). Both gastrointestinal upset and hepatitis are adverse reactions to the antitubercular drugs.

Summary Drug Table ANTITUBERCULAR DRUGS

Generic Name	Trade Name	Uses	Adverse Reactions	Dosage Ranges
Primary (First-Line) Drugs				
ethambutol *eth-am'-byoo-toll*	Myambutol	Pulmonary TB	Optic neuritis, fever, pruritus, headache, nausea, anorexia, dermatitis, hypersensitivity, psychic disturbances	15–25 mg/kg/day orally
℞ isoniazid (INH) *eye-soe-nye'-ah-zid*		Active TB; prophylaxis for TB	Peripheral neuropathy, nausea, vomiting, epigastric distress, jaundice, hepatitis, pyridoxine deficiency, skin eruptions, hypersensitivity	*Active TB:* 5 mg/kg (up to 300 mg/day) orally or 15 mg/kg 2–3 times weekly *TB prophylaxis:* 300 mg/day orally
pyrazinamide *peer-ah-zin'-ah-mide*		Active TB	Hepatotoxicity, nausea, vomiting, diarrhea, myalgia, rashes	15–30 mg/kg/day orally, maximum 3 g/day orally; 50–70 mg/kg twice weekly orally
℞ rifabutin *rif-ah-byoo'-tin*	Mycobutin	*Mycobacterium avium*	Nausea, vomiting, diarrhea, rash, discolored urine	300 mg/day orally or 150 mg orally BID
℞ rifampin *rif-am'-pin*	Rifadin, Rimactane	Active TB, Hansen's disease	Heartburn, drowsiness, fatigue, dizziness, epigastric distress, hematologic changes, renal insufficiency, rash, body fluid discoloration	10 mg/kg (up to 600 mg/day) orally, IV
℞ rifapentine *rif-ah-pen'-teen*	Priftin	Active TB	Hyperuricemia, proteinuria, hematuria, rash, lymphopenia	600 mg twice weekly orally
Combination Drugs				
isoniazid 150 mg and rifampin 300 mg	Rifamate	TB	See individual drugs	1–2 tablets daily orally
isoniazid 50 mg, rifampin 120 mg, and pyrazinamide 300 mg	Rifater	TB	See individual drugs	1–2 tablets daily orally

(table continues on page 110)

Antitubercular Drugs

Summary Drug Table ANTITUBERCULAR DRUGS (continued)

Generic Name	Trade Name	Uses	Adverse Reactions	Dosage Ranges
Secondary (Second-Line) Drugs				
aminosalicylate *ah-meen-oh-sal'-sah-late* (*p*-aminosalicylic acid; 4-aminosalicylic acid)	Paser	TB	Nausea, vomiting, diarrhea, abdominal pain, hypersensitivity reactions	4 g (1 packet) orally TID
capreomycin *kap-ree-oh-mye'-sin*	Capastat	TB	Hypersensitivity reactions, nephrotoxicity, hepatic impairment, pain and induration at injection site, ototoxicity	1 g/day (maximum 20 mg/kg/day) IM
cycloserine *sye-kloe-ser'-een*	Seromycin	TB	Convulsions, somnolence, confusion, renal impairment, sudden development of congestive heart failure, psychoses	500 mg–1 g orally in divided doses
ethionamide *eh-thye-on-am'-ide*	Trecator	TB, Hansen's disease	Nausea, vomiting, diarrhea, headache	15–20 mg/kg/day orally
streptomycin *strep-toe-mye'-sin* (although still available, this drug is seldom used)		TB, infections due to susceptible microorganisms	Nephrotoxicity, ototoxicity, numbness, tingling, paresthesia of the face, nausea, dizziness	15 mg/kg but no more than 1 g IM daily (120 g therapeutic maximum)
Drugs to treat *M. leprae*				
clofazimine *kloe-fazz'-ih-meen*	Lamprene	Hansen's disease	Skin pigmentation (pink to brown), skin dryness, rash, abdominal/epigastric pain, nausea, vomiting, burning or itching of the eyes, dizziness, headache	100 mg/day orally
dapsone *dap'-sone*		Hansen's disease, dermatitis herpetiformis, *Pneumocystis carinii* pneumonia, rheumatic disorders (rheumatic arthritis, systemic lupus erythematosus), brown recluse spider bite	Hemolytic anemia, headache, insomnia, phototoxicity, nausea, vomiting, anorexia, rash, fever, jaundice, toxic epidermal necrolysis	50–300 mg/day orally

Ⓡ This drug should be administered at least 1 hour before or 2 hours after a meal.

● Chapter Review

Know Your Drugs

Clients sometimes know a medication by the brand (or trade) name and not the generic name. To help you recognize both names, match the brand name with the generic name of the same medication.

Generic Name	Brand Name
1. ethambutol	A. Myambutol
2. rifabutin	B. Mycobutin
3. rifampin	C. Priftin
4. rifapentine	D. Rifadin

Calculate Medication Dosages

1. A client is prescribed isoniazid syrup 300 mg. The isoniazid is available as 50 mg/mL. The nurse should administer _____.

2. Oral rifampin 600 mg is prescribed. The drug is available in 150-mg tablets. The nurse should administer _____.

● Prepare for the NCLEX

Build Your Knowledge

1. Which of the following drugs is the only antitubercular drug to be prescribed alone?

   1. rifampin
   2. pyrazinamide
   3. streptomycin
   4. isoniazid

2. The nurse monitors the client taking isoniazid for toxic symptoms. The most common symptom of toxicity is _____.

   1. peripheral edema
   2. circumoral edema
   3. peripheral neuropathy
   4. jaundice

3. Which of the following is a dose-related adverse reaction to ethambutol?

   1. peripheral neuropathy
   2. optic neuritis
   3. hyperglycemia
   4. fatal hepatitis

4. Which of the following antitubercular drugs is contraindicated in clients with gout?

   1. rifampin
   2. streptomycin
   3. isoniazid
   4. pyrazinamide

5. Hansen's disease (leprosy) is caused by which of the following bacteria?

   1. *Mycobacterium leprae*
   2. *Clostridium difficile*
   3. *Mycobacterium tuberculosis*
   4. *Pneumocystis carinii*

Apply Your Knowledge

6. A client reports orange stains on paper tissues when she urinates. Which of the following interventions should the nurse do first?

   1. notify the primary health care provider
   2. ask the client what she thinks is happening
   3. explain that this is an anticipated adverse reaction
   4. obtain a urine sample for lab studies

7. The nurse explains to the client that to prevent multidrug resistance to the antitubercular drugs, the primary health care provider may prescribe _____.

   1. at least three antitubercular drugs
   2. an antibiotic to be given with the drug
   3. vitamin B_6
   4. that the drug be given only once a week

8. Which of the following best describes DOT in the care of TB clients?

   1. The client takes at least four drugs daily
   2. The client calls the clinic once a week to describe adverse reactions
   3. The nurse involves family in client teaching activities
   4. The nurse observes the client swallow the TB drugs

Alternate-Format Questions

9. Identify which drugs are included in primary (first-line) treatment for TB. **Select all that apply**.

   1. ethambutol
   2. isoniazid
   3. ofloxacin
   4. pyrazinamide
   5. rifampin

10. Identify which culture plate (from culture and sensitivity testing) indicates the bacterium is resistant to all the drugs tested on the plate.

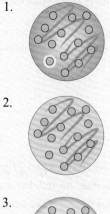

To check your answers, see Appendix G.

thePoint *For more NCLEX-style questions, log on to http://thepoint.lww.com to access more than 1000 questions.*

11

Antiviral Drugs

LEARNING OBJECTIVES

On completion of this chapter, the student will:

1. Discuss the uses, general drug actions, adverse reactions, contraindications, precautions, and interactions of antiviral drugs.
2. Discuss important preadministration and ongoing assessment activities the nurse should perform on the patient receiving an antiviral/antiretroviral drug.
3. List nursing diagnoses particular to a patient taking an antiviral drug.
4. List possible goals for a patient taking an antiviral/antiretroviral drug.
5. Discuss ways to promote an optimal response to therapy and manage adverse reactions, and special considerations to keep in mind when educating the patient and the family about the antiviral/antiretroviral drugs.

KEY TERMS

highly active antiretroviral therapy (HAART) • multiple drugs used together for treatment of human immunodeficiency virus (HIV) infection

retrovirus • virus that uses RNA as its primary component instead of DNA

unlabeled use • use of a drug to treat a condition that is not officially approved by the U.S. Food and Drug Administration (FDA)

DRUG CLASSES

Antivirals
Antiretrovirals
• Protease inhibitors
• Nucleoside/nucleotide reverse transcriptase inhibitors (NRTIs)
• Nonnucleoside reverse transcriptase inhibitors (NNRTIs)
• Entry inhibitors
• Integrase inhibitors

Compared with a fungus or bacterium, a virus is a very tiny infectious organism. A virus enters the body through various routes. It can be swallowed, inhaled, injected with a contaminated needle, or transmitted through the bite of an insect. To reproduce, the virus needs the cellular material of another living cell (the host cell). The virus attaches to a cell, enters it, and releases its DNA or RNA inside the cell. The viral material takes control of the cell and forces it to replicate the virus. The cell releases new viruses, which go on to infect other cells. The infected cell usually dies, because the virus keeps it from performing its normal functions.

More than 200 viruses have been identified as capable of producing disease. Common viral infections are those of the nose, throat, and respiratory system. An example is the common cold or influenza. A wart comes from a common virus that infects the skin. Other common viral infections are caused by the herpes viruses. Eight different herpes viruses infect people.

PHARMACOLOGY IN PRACTICE

Mr. Park, aged 77 years, lived alone at home. One day, as he was working in the garden, he fell. He lay in the garden with a fractured hip for about 2 hours before he was found. This event, compounded with other stressors of living alone, initiated an outbreak of herpes zoster (shingles). Consider this event as you read about medications that reduce the symptoms of viral disease.

Systemic viral infections occur when a virus attacks the nervous system (West Nile), liver (hepatitis C), or white blood cells (immunodeficiency diseases). The drugs used to treat viral infection are split into two categories: antiviral and antiretroviral agents. For a more complete listing, see the Summary Drug Table: Antiviral Drugs.

ANTIVIRALS

Actions

Drugs that combat viral infections are called *antiviral drugs*. Antiviral drugs work by interfering with the virus's ability to reproduce in a cell. Antiviral medications are limited in their ability to treat viral infections because viruses are tiny and replicate inside cells, changing how the cell works depending on the type of cell they invade. Antiviral drugs can be toxic to human cells, and viruses can develop resistance to antiviral drugs. These factors make antiviral drugs more difficult to develop. In comparison, a bacterial organism is relatively large and commonly reproduces outside of cells (e.g., in the bloodstream). Although antibiotics are not effective against viral infections, if a person has a bacterial infection in addition to a viral infection, an antibiotic is often needed.

Uses

Labeled Uses

Although infections caused by viruses are common, antiviral drugs have limited use because they are effective against only a small number of specific viral infections (Display 11.1). Antiviral drugs are used in the treatment or prevention of infections caused by:

- Cytomegalovirus (CMV) in transplant recipients
- Herpes simplex virus (HSV) 1 and 2 (genital) and herpes zoster
- Human immunodeficiency virus (HIV)
- Influenza A and B (respiratory tract illness)
- Respiratory syncytial virus (RSV; severe lower respiratory tract infection primarily affecting children)
- Hepatitis B and C

Unlabeled Uses

Because there are a limited number of antiviral drugs and more than 200 viral diseases, the primary health care provider may decide to prescribe an antiviral drug for an **unlabeled use** even though its effectiveness for that use is not documented. Approval by the U.S. Food and Drug Administration (FDA) is necessary for a drug to be prescribed. On occasion, the use of a drug for a specific disorder or condition may be under investigation, or it may be approved for use in another country. In this instance, the drug may be prescribed by the primary health care provider for the condition under investigation. The use of the drug for a specific disorder or condition that is not officially approved by the FDA is called an unlabeled use. Examples of unlabeled uses of the antiviral drugs include treatment of CMV and HSV infections after transplantation procedures and varicella pneumonia; the treatment of CMV retinitis in immunocompromised patients; and the use of ribavirin (in aerosol form) for influenza A and B, acute and chronic hepatitis, herpes genitalis, and measles (in oral form).

Adverse Reactions

Gastrointestinal System Reactions

- Nausea, vomiting
- Diarrhea

Other Reactions

- Headache
- Rash
- Fever
- Insomnia

Contraindications

Do not administer antivirals if the patient has a history of allergies to the drug or other antivirals. Cidofovir (Vistide) should not be given to patients who have renal impairment or in combination with medications that are nephrotoxic, such as aminoglycosides. Ribavirin should not be used in patients with unstable cardiac disease. These drugs should be used during pregnancy (pregnancy categories B and C) and lactation only when the benefit outweighs the risk to the fetus or child (ribavirin is a pregnancy category X).

Precautions

Antivirals should be used cautiously in patients with renal impairment, low blood cell counts, history of epilepsy (rimantadine), and history of respiratory disease (zanamivir).

Interactions

The following interactions may occur when an antiviral is administered with another agent:

Interacting Drug	Common Use	Effect of Interaction
probenecid	Gout treatment	Increased serum levels of the antivirals
cimetidine	Gastric upset, heartburn	Increased serum level of the antiviral valacyclovir
ibuprofen	Pain relief	Increased serum level of the antiviral adefovir
imipenem-cilastatin	Anti-infective agent	With ganciclovir only, increased risk of seizures
anticholinergic agents	Management of bladder spasms	With amantadine only, increased adverse reactions of anticholinergic agent
theophylline	Management of respiratory problems	With acyclovir only, increased serum level of theophylline

Display 11.1 Description of Viral Infections

Cytomegalovirus (CMV)

CMV, a virus of the herpes family, is a common viral infection. Healthy individuals may become infected yet have no symptoms. However, immunocompromised patients (such as those with HIV or cancer) may have the infection. Symptoms include malaise, fever, pneumonia, and superinfection. Infants may acquire the virus from the mother while in the uterus, resulting in learning disabilities and mental retardation. CMV can infect the eye, causing retinitis. Symptoms of CMV retinitis are blurred vision and decreased visual acuity. Visual impairment is irreversible and can lead to blindness if untreated.

Genital human Papillomavirus (HPV)

HPV is the most common sexually transmitted infection (STI). There are over 40 different HPV types that infect the genitals, mouth, and throat. However, symptoms can be minor enough that most people do not even know they are infected. HPV infection can lead to genital warts, cervical cancer, and rare forms of throat warts or cancers. Warts can appear weeks to months after contact with an infected partner. Cervical symptoms do not appear until late in the disease. Treatment includes removal of warts, yet HPV is best treated by prevention with vaccine (see Chapter 49).

Hepatitis B (HBV) and C (HCV) Virus

Hepatitis is an inflammation of the liver. HBV is spread by infected blood or body fluids. Sexual contact is the most frequent mode of transmission, followed by use of contaminated needles. Symptoms of infection include fever and joint pains. Acute HBV typically resolves; chronic HBV is treated to boost the immune system. HCV is related to the yellow fever virus and is primarily spread by exposure to infected blood. Most people show no signs or symptoms of HCV until the infection becomes chronic and lab results show persistent liver inflammation. Treatment is offered to reduce the chance of cirrhosis (final stages of liver disease). Late-stage cirrhosis due to HCV is currently the primary reason for liver transplant.

Herpes Simplex Virus (HSV)

HSV is divided into HSV-1, which causes oral, ocular, or facial infections, and HSV-2, which causes genital infection. However, either type can cause disease at either body site. HSV-1 causes painful vesicular lesions in the oral mucosa, on the face, or around the eyes. HSV-2 or genital herpes is usually transmitted by sexual contact and causes painful vesicular lesions on the mucous membranes of the genitalia. Vaginal lesions may appear as mucous patches with grayish ulcerations. The patient may appear irritable, lethargic, and jaundiced and may have difficulty breathing or experience seizures. The lesions usually heal within 2 weeks. Immunosuppressed patients may develop a severe systemic disease.

Herpes Zoster Virus (HZV)

Herpes zoster (shingles) is caused by the varicella (chickenpox) virus. It is highly contagious. The virus causes chickenpox in the child and is easily spread via the respiratory system. Recovery from childhood chickenpox results in the infection lying dormant in the nerve cells. The virus may become reactivated later in life as the older adult's immune system weakens or the individual becomes ill with other disorders. The lesions of herpes zoster appear as pustules along a sensory nerve route. Pain often continues for several months after the lesions have healed.

Human Immunodeficiency Virus (HIV)

HIV or AIDS is a type of viral infection transmitted through an infected person's bodily secretions, such as blood or semen. HIV destroys the immune system, causing the body to develop opportunistic infections such as Kaposi's sarcoma, *Pneumocystis carinii* pneumonia, or tuberculosis. Symptoms include chills and fever, night sweats, dry productive cough, dyspnea, lethargy, malaise, fatigue, weight loss, and diarrhea.

Influenza (flu)

Influenza, commonly called the "flu," is an acute respiratory illness caused by influenza viruses A and B. Symptoms include fever, cough, sore throat, runny or stuffy nose, headache, muscle aches, and extreme fatigue. Most people recover within 1 to 2 weeks. Influenza may cause severe complications such as pneumonia in children, the elderly, and other vulnerable groups. The viruses causing influenza continually change over time, which enables them to evade the immune system of the host. These rapid changes in the most commonly circulating types of influenza virus necessitate annual changes in the composition of the flu vaccine.

Respiratory Syncytial Virus (RSV)

RSV infection is highly contagious and affects mostly children, causing bronchiolitis and pneumonia. Infants younger than 6 months are the most severely affected. In adults, RSV causes colds and bronchitis, with fever, cough, and nasal congestion. When RSV affects immunocompromised patients, the consequences can be severe and sometimes fatal.

ANTIRETROVIRALS

Actions

HIV is called a **retrovirus**. When left untreated this viral infection can progress to acquired immunodeficiency syndrome (AIDS). Retroviruses attack the host cell just like a virus; the difference is that RNA is the primary component of the virus instead of DNA. Retroviruses also contain an enzyme called *reverse transcriptase* that is used to turn the RNA of the virus into DNA, helping to reproduce more of the virus. To control the disease effectively, a number of drugs are used that work at different portions of the life cycle of the virus. Figure 11.1 illustrates how HIV replicates in a human cell and where the antiretroviral drugs act. Using multiple antiretroviral drugs in therapy is called **highly active antiretroviral therapy (HAART)**. The first three categories of the following types of drugs are used in HAART (for more information see the Summary Drug Table: Antiviral Drugs):

- Protease inhibitors, which block the protease enzyme so the new viral particles cannot mature
- Reverse transcriptase inhibitors, which block the reverse transcriptase enzyme so the HIV material cannot change into DNA in the new cell, preventing new HIV copies from being created
- Nonnucleoside reverse transcriptase inhibitors, which latch on to the reverse transcriptase molecule to block the ability to make viral DNA
- Entry inhibitors, which prevent the attachment or fusion of HIV to a host cell for initial entry
- Integrase inhibitors, which prevent enzymes from inserting HIV genetic material into the cell's DNA

Uses

Antiretroviral drugs are used in the treatment of HIV infection and AIDS.

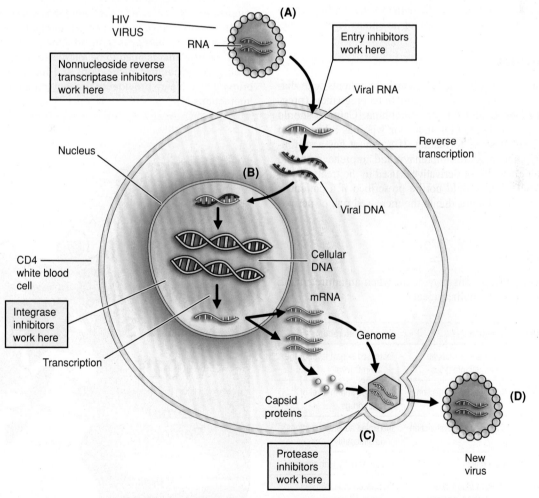

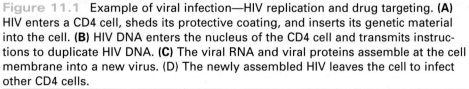

Figure 11.1 Example of viral infection—HIV replication and drug targeting. **(A)** HIV enters a CD4 cell, sheds its protective coating, and inserts its genetic material into the cell. **(B)** HIV DNA enters the nucleus of the CD4 cell and transmits instructions to duplicate HIV DNA. **(C)** The viral RNA and viral proteins assemble at the cell membrane into a new virus. **(D)** The newly assembled HIV leaves the cell to infect other CD4 cells.

Adverse Reactions

Gastrointestinal System Reactions

- Nausea, vomiting
- Diarrhea
- Altered taste

Other Reactions

- Headache, fever, and chills
- Rash
- Numbness and tingling in the circumoral area (around the mouth) or peripherally, or both

Contraindications

Do not administer antiretrovirals if the patient has a history of allergies to the drug or other antiretrovirals. Women who are lactating should not use antiretroviral drugs. Antiretrovirals should not be prescribed to the patient who is using cisapride, pimozide, triazolam, midazolam, or an ergot derivative. Ritonavir is contraindicated if the patient is taking bupropion (Wellbutrin), zolpidem (Ambien), or an antiarrhythmic drug.

Precautions

Antiretrovirals should be used cautiously in patients with diabetes mellitus, impaired hepatic function, pregnancy (pregnancy categories B and C), or hemophilia. Caution should be used for the patient taking indinavir who has a history of kidney or bladder stone formation. If a patient has a sulfonamide allergy, the drugs fosamprenavir and amprenavir should be used cautiously. Ergot derivatives (used in the treatment of migraine headaches) should not be prescribed if a patient is taking a protease inhibitor due to the increased risk of peripheral ischemia.

Interactions

The following interactions may occur when an antiretroviral is administered with another agent:

Interacting Drug	Common Use	Effect of Interaction
antifungals	Eliminate or manage fungal infections	Increased serum level of the antiretroviral
clarithromycin	Treat bacterial infection	Increased serum level of both drugs
sildenafil	Treat erectile dysfunction	Increased adverse reactions of sildenafil
opioid analgesics	Pain relief	Risk of toxicity with ritonavir
anticoagulant, anticonvulsant, antiparasitic agents	Prevent blood clots, seizures, parasitic infections, respectively	Decreased effectiveness when taking ritonavir

Interacting Drug	Common Use	Effect of Interaction
interleukins	Prevent severely low platelet counts usually related to chemotherapy	Risk of antiretroviral toxicity
fentanyl	Analgesia, used typically with procedures requiring anesthesia	Increased serum level of fentanyl
oral contraceptives	Birth control	Decreased effectiveness of the birth control agent
rifampin	Pulmonary tuberculosis	With efavirenz, nevirapine only; decreased serum levels of antivirals

HERBAL CONSIDERATIONS

Individuals have tried St. John's wort (Fig. 11.2) for both the antidepressive and antiviral effects of the supplement. Researchers have found that in patients with HIV infection who receive prescribed protease inhibitors, the effectiveness of drug therapy is reduced if the patient also takes St. John's wort. Patients need to be instructed to disclose the use of all over-the-counter medications and supplements to their primary health care provider to prevent potentially harmful interactions.

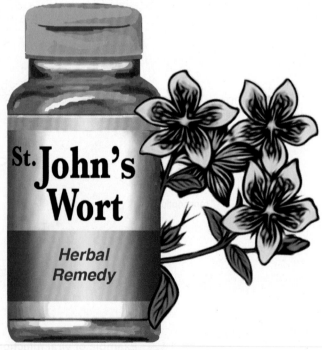

Figure 11.2 St. John's Wort, used for antidepressive and antiviral properties.

NURSING PROCESS

PATIENT RECEIVING AN ANTIVIRAL/ ANTIRETROVIRAL DRUG

ASSESSMENT

Preadministration Assessment

Preadministration assessment of the patient receiving an antiviral drug depends on the patient's symptoms or diagnosis. These patients may have a serious infection that weakens their natural defenses against disease. Before administering the antiviral drug, determine the patient's general state of health and resistance to infection. Record the patient's symptoms and complaints. In addition, take and record the patient's vital signs. Additional assessments may be necessary in certain types of viral infections or in patients who are acutely ill. For example, before treatment of patients with HSV-1 or HSV-2 infection, inspect the areas of the body affected with the lesions (e.g., the mouth, face, eyes, or genitalia) as a baseline for comparison during therapy. Many facilities have the capacity to take photographs of the area. This is helpful for comparison later in the treatment phase.

Ongoing Assessment

The ongoing assessment depends on the reason for giving the antiviral drug. It is important to make a daily assessment for improvement of the signs and symptoms identified in the initial assessment. Monitor for and report any adverse reactions from the antiviral drug. In addition, teach the patient or caregivers to feel confident in inspecting the intravenous (IV) infusion site several times a day for redness, inflammation, or pain and report any signs of phlebitis.

NURSING DIAGNOSES

Drug-specific nursing diagnoses include the following:

- **Risk for Imbalanced Nutrition: Less Than Body Requirements** related to adverse reaction of antiviral drugs
- **Risk for Impaired Skin Integrity** related to initial infection, adverse drug reactions, and administration of the antiviral drug
- **Risk for Injury** related to the patient's mental status, peripheral neuropathy, and generalized weakness
- **Body Image Disturbance** related to body fat redistribution
- **Acute Pain** related to kidney or bladder stones or inflammation caused by antiviral drugs

Nursing diagnoses that are related to drug administration are discussed in Chapter 4.

PLANNING

The expected outcomes for the patient depend on the reason for administration of the antiviral drug but may include an optimal response to therapy, meeting of patient needs related to the management of adverse reactions, and confidence in an understanding of the medication regimen.

IMPLEMENTATION

Promoting an Optimal Response to Therapy

Because these drugs may be used in the treatment of certain types of severe and sometimes life-threatening viral infections, the patient may be concerned about the diagnosis and prognosis. Allow the patient and family members time to talk and ask questions about treatment methods, especially when the drug is given IV. It is important to prepare the antiviral drugs according to the manufacturer's directions. The administration rate is ordered by the primary health care provider.

AMANTADINE. This drug is administered for the prevention or treatment of respiratory tract illness caused by influenza A virus. Some patients are prescribed this drug to manage extrapyramidal effects caused by drugs used to treat parkinsonism. Observe the patient for adverse effects similar to those associated with cholinergic blocking drugs (see Chapter 27).

RIBAVIRIN. Ribavirin is given by inhalation using a small particle aerosol generator (called a *SPAG-2 aerosol generator*). It is important to discard and replace the solution every 24 hours. This drug can worsen respiratory status. Sudden deterioration of respiratory status can occur in infants receiving ribavirin, and it is important to monitor respiratory function closely throughout therapy. Report immediately any worsening of respiratory function to the primary health care provider. Female caregivers should know that the drug is a pregnancy category X drug, and women of childbearing age should take care not to inhale the drug as they prepare or give the drug to the patient. In patients requiring mechanical ventilation, treatment should be provided only by health care providers familiar with the specific ventilator.

IV ADMINISTRATION. Rapid infusion or bolus administration of the antivirals has created toxicity in patients due to excessive plasma levels of the drug. You should always check the recommended infusion rate of the drug and not exceed the rate.

Monitoring and Managing Patient Needs

RISK FOR IMBALANCED NUTRITION: LESS THAN BODY REQUIREMENTS. The metabolic needs of patients with HIV infection are demanding. Because the antiviral drugs may cause anorexia, nausea, or vomiting, providing adequate nutrition becomes a real challenge. The gastrointestinal (GI) effects range from mild to severe. Many of the drugs can be given without regard to food. Two exceptions are didanosine (Videx) and entecavir (Baraclude). These drugs are provided in a buffered or enteric-coated form. Mix the buffered powder with 4 ounces of water (not juice), stir until it is dissolved, and give it to the patient to drink immediately. Avoid generating and inhaling the dust when preparing the medication.

The patient may be able to tolerate small, frequent meals with soft, nonirritating foods if nausea is mild. Frequent sips of carbonated beverages or hot tea may be helpful for others. It is important to keep the atmosphere clean and free of odors. Provide good oral care before and after meals. Sometimes daily-dose drugs can be given at bedtime to reduce the nausea. If nausea is severe or the patient is vomiting, notify the primary health care provider.

Antiviral Drugs

RISK FOR IMPAIRED SKIN INTEGRITY. Monitor any skin lesions carefully for worsening or improvement. Should the lesions not improve, inform the primary health care provider. Accurate observation and documentation are essential. If an antiviral drug is administered topically, use gloves when applying to avoid spreading the infection. These drugs may also cause a rash as an adverse reaction. Note and report any rash to the primary health care provider.

When administering the drug by the IV route, closely observe the injection site for signs of phlebitis. Take care to prevent trauma because even slight trauma can result in bruising if the platelet count is low. If injections are given, pressure is applied at the injection site to prevent bleeding. Occasionally, headache or a slight fever may occur in patients taking antiviral drugs. An analgesic may be prescribed to manage these effects. Depending on the patient's symptoms, monitor vital signs every 4 hours or as ordered by the primary health care provider.

RISK FOR INJURY. Some patients with a viral infection are acutely ill. Others may experience fatigue, lethargy, dizziness, or weakness as an adverse reaction to the antiviral/antiretroviral agent. Monitor these patients carefully. Call lights are placed in a convenient place for the patient and are answered promptly. If fatigue, dizziness, confusion, or weakness is present, the patient may require assistance with ambulation or activities of daily living. Plan activities to provide adequate rest periods. Other drugs can damage the peripheral nerves, especially when used with other neurotoxic agents. Watch for signs of peripheral neuropathy (numbness, tingling, or pain in the feet or hands). It is important to report these signs immediately to the primary health care provider.

DISTURBED BODY IMAGE. Patients taking the protease inhibitors (saquinavir, ritonavir, indinavir, nelfinavir, fosamprenavir, amprenavir, and atazanavir) have experienced redistribution of body fat. Movement is to the center of the body, so patients appear to have thinner arms and legs with a rounder abdomen or enlarged breasts. Sometimes body fat relocates to the area behind the neck (sometimes called a *buffalo hump*). Plan to spend time with these patients, encouraging them to verbalize their feelings regarding this change in appearance. It is also important to acknowledge these feelings as being both valid and important to the patient.

ACUTE PAIN. The drug indinavir (Crixivan) has been known to cause kidney or bladder stones in patients. Antiretroviral drugs have been known to cause acute pancreatitis. Patients should be assessed for pain. Any pain should be explored for location and intensity. When assessing the patient for GI problems such as nausea, vomiting, abdominal pain, and jaundice, be alert because these are symptoms of pancreatitis, and particular care should be taken in assessment of pain. Acute, sudden-onset pain should be reported to the primary health care provider for both treatment and further assessment for more involved disease.

⚠ NURSING ALERT

Patients receiving antiretroviral drugs for HIV infection may continue to contract opportunistic infections and other complications of HIV disease. Monitor all patients closely for signs of infection such as fever (even low-grade fever),

malaise, sore throat, or lethargy. All caregivers are reminded to use good hand hygiene technique.

Educating the Patient and Family

When an antiviral drug is given orally, explain the dosage schedule to the patient and family and instruct the patient to take the drug exactly as directed for the full course of therapy. If a dose is missed, the patient should take it as soon as remembered but should not double the dose at the next dosage time. Any adverse reactions should be reported to the primary health care provider or the nurse. Help the patient to understand that these drugs do not cure viral infections, but they can decrease symptoms and increase feelings of well-being.

Instruct patients to report any symptoms of infection, such as an elevated temperature (even a slight elevation), sore throat, difficulty breathing, weakness, or lethargy. Again, review possible signs of pancreatitis (nausea, vomiting, abdominal pain, jaundice) and peripheral neuropathy (tingling, burning, numbness, or pain in the hands or feet). Any indication of pancreatitis or peripheral neuropathy must be reported at once.

Include the following information in the teaching plan for antiviral drugs:

■ Antiviral drugs are not a cure for viral infections, but they will shorten the course of disease outbreaks and promote healing of the lesions. The drugs will not prevent the spread of the disease to others. Topical drugs should not be applied more frequently than prescribed but should be applied with a finger cot or gloves. All lesions should be covered. There should be no sexual contact while lesions are present. Notify the primary health care provider if burning, stinging, itching, or rash worsens or becomes pronounced.

■ Some drugs cause photosensitivity, so precautions should be taken when going outdoors, such as wearing sunscreen, head coverings, and protective clothing. Patients should also refrain from using tanning beds.

■ Some patients have experienced an acute exacerbation of the disease when medications used to treat hepatitis B are stopped. Hepatic function should be closely monitored in these patients.

■ Those taking antiretrovirals should be cautioned that there is an increased risk of adverse reactions (hypotension, visual disturbances, prolonged penile erection) when the drug sildenafil (Viagra) is used. Symptoms should be reported promptly to the primary health care provider.

■ Some drugs affect mental status. Activities requiring mental alertness, such as driving a car, should be delayed until the effect of the drug is apparent because vision and coordination can be affected. Patients should rise slowly from a prone to a sitting position to decrease the possibility of lightheadedness caused by orthostatic hypotension. Changes such as nervousness, tremors, slurred speech, or depression should be reported.

■ Some patients are on an alternate-dosage schedule. In this case, it is important to designate the days the drug is to be taken; calendars are helpful aids to track schedules.

■ Zanamivir (Relenza) is taken every 12 hours for 5 days using a "Diskhaler" delivery system. If a bronchodilator is also prescribed for use at the same time, the bronchodilator is used before the zanamivir. The drug may cause dizziness. The patient should use caution when driving an automobile or operating dangerous machinery. Treatment with this drug does not decrease the risk of transmission of influenza to others.

EVALUATION

■ Therapeutic response is achieved and there is management of the infection and viral load.

■ Adverse reactions are identified, reported to the primary health care provider, and managed successfully with appropriate nursing interventions:
- Patient maintains an adequate nutritional status.
- Skin is intact and free of inflammation, irritation, infection, or ulcerations.
- No evidence of injury is seen.
- Perceptions of body changes are managed successfully.
- Patient is free of pain.

■ Patient and family express confidence and demonstrate an understanding of the drug regimen.

PHARMACOLOGY IN PRACTICE
THINK CRITICALLY

 Mr. Park is staying in a long-term care facility following his hip replacement surgery. The primary health care provider prescribes acyclovir 200 mg every 4 hours during Mr. Park's waking hours for his outbreak of herpes zoster (shingles). Discuss what information you would give the skilled nursing facility staff concerning herpes zoster, the drug regimen, and the possible adverse reactions.

KEY POINTS

- A virus is smaller than a bacterium. To reproduce, the virus needs cellular material of another living cell. Viral infections range from the common cold to chronic systemic infections of the liver or immune system.

- Antiviral drugs work by interfering with the virus's ability to reproduce in a cell. These drugs are used to reduce the effects of viral infections such as HSV-1 and HSV-2, CMV, and RSV. The effectiveness of antivirals is limited based on how well the virus can mutate, which results in viral resistance to the drug.

- In most situations, antivirals have minor adverse reactions such as gastrointestinal disturbances or flu-like symptoms.

- Retroviruses attack cells and hamper the work of RNA in the cell. HIV is a retroviral disease.

- Antiretroviral drugs are used primarily to reduce viral load in patients with HIV. Multiple drugs are used to attack the virus at different parts of the life cycle; this is termed highly active antiretroviral therapy.

- Adverse reactions range from minor gastrointestinal issues to peripheral neuropathy or anaphylaxis. Shifts in body fat can be disturbing to patients taking these drugs.

Antiviral Drugs

Summary Drug Table ANTIVIRAL DRUGS

Generic Name	Trade Name	Uses	Adverse Reactions	Dosage Ranges
Antivirals				
acyclovir *ay-sye'-kloe-veer*	Zovirax	HSV, herpes zoster, varicella zoster	Nausea, vomiting, diarrhea, fever, headache, dizziness, confusion, rashes, myalgia	Oral: 200–800 mg q 4 hr for 5 doses per day, treat for 5–10 days; IV: 5–10 mg/kg q 8 hr; Topical: apply to lesions q 3 hr
adefovir dipivoxil *ah-def'-oh-veer*	Hepsera	Chronic hepatitis B	Asthenia, headache, abdominal pain	10 mg/day orally
amantadine *ah-man'-tah-deen*		Prevention and treatment of influenza A; Parkinson's disease	Nausea, diarrhea, dizziness, hypotension, insomnia	200 mg/day orally or 100 mg daily for patient older than age 65; begin before flu exposure and continue for 10 days postexposure
boceprevir *boe-se'-pre-veer*	Victrelis	Chronic hepatitis C	Fatigue, nausea, vomiting, taste changes	800 mg orally TID, at least 7 hr between doses
cidofovir *sih-doe'-foe-veer*	Vistide	CMV retinitis	Headache, nausea, vomiting, diarrhea, anorexia, dyspnea, alopecia, rash, neutropenia, fever, chills	5 mg/kg IV once a week for 2 wk, then once every 2 wk for maintenance
® entecavir *en-teh'-kah-veer*	Baraclude	Chronic hepatitis B	Dizziness, fatigue, headache	0.5–1 mg/day orally
famciclovir *fam-sih'-kloe-veer*	Famvir	Acute herpes zoster, HSV-2	Fatigue, fever, nausea, vomiting, diarrhea, sinusitis, constipation, headache	Herpes zoster: 500 mg orally q 8 hr for 7 days; HSV-2: 125 mg orally BID for 5 days
foscarnet *foss-kar'-net*	Foscavir	CMV retinitis; acyclovir-resistant HSV-1 and -2	Headache, seizures, nausea, vomiting, diarrhea, anemia, abnormal renal function test results	CMV retinitis: 90–120 mg/kg/day IV; HSV: 40 mg/kg IV q 8–12 hr
ganciclovir *gan-sih'-kloe-veer*	Cytovene	CMV prevention in transplant recipients	Anorexia, vomiting, diarrhea, fever, sweats, anemia, leukopenia	5 mg/kg IV q 12 hr for 14–21 days, then daily
oseltamivir *oh-sell-tam'-ih-veer*	Tamiflu	Prevention and treatment of influenza A and B	Nausea, vomiting, diarrhea	75 mg orally BID for 5 days
ribavirin (inhalation) *rye-bah-vye'-rin*	Virazole	RSV	Worsening of pulmonary status, bacterial pneumonia, hypotension	Administered by aerosol with special aerosol generator
ribavirin/ interferon combination	Copegus, Rebetol, Ribasphere	In combination with interferon for hepatitis C	Fatigue, headache, myalgia, anorexia, nausea, vomiting, insomnia, nervousness	800–1200 mg orally BID
rimantadine *rih-man'-tah-deen*	Flumadine	Influenza A	Lightheadedness, dizziness, insomnia, nausea, anorexia	100 mg/day orally BID
telaprevir *tel-ah-pre'-veer*	Incivek	Chronic hepatitis C	Fatigue, nausea, vomiting, rash, pruritus, anorectal discomfort, diarrhea	750 mg orally TID, at least 7 hr between doses
valacyclovir *val-ah-sye'-kloe-veer*	Valtrex	Herpes zoster; HSV-1 and -2	Nausea, headache	HSV-1: 2 g q 12 hr for 1 day HSV-2 initial: 1 g BID for 10 days Recurrent infection: 500 mg orally BID for 5 days Herpes zoster: 1 g orally TID for 7 days

Summary Drug Table ANTIVIRAL DRUGS (continued)

Generic Name	Trade Name	Uses	Adverse Reactions	Dosage Ranges
valganciclovir *val-gan-sih'-kloe-veer*	Valcyte	CMV retinitis, CMV prevention in transplant recipients	Headache, insomnia, diarrhea, nausea, vomiting, pancytopenia, fever	900 mg orally BID; transplant recipients: start 10 days before transplantation and continue 100 days after transplantation
zanamivir *zah-nam'-ah-veer*	Relenza	Prevention and treatment of influenza A, B	Nausea, headache, rhinitis	5-mg inhalation q 12 hr
Antiretrovirals				
Protease Inhibitors				
atazanavir *ah-taz'-ah-nah-veer*	Reyataz	HIV infection	Nausea, rash	300–400 mg/day
darunavir *dah-roon'-ah-veer*	Prezista	HIV infection	Headache, diarrhea, constipation, and pain	600 mg orally BID
fosamprenavir *foss-am-pren'-ah-veer*	Lexiva	HIV infection	Headache, nausea, vomiting, diarrhea, rash	1400 mg/day orally
indinavir *in-din'-ah-veer*	Crixivan	HIV infection	Headache, nausea, vomiting, diarrhea, kidney/bladder stones	800 mg orally q 8 hr
nelfinavir *nell-fin'-ah-veer*	Viracept	HIV infection	Diarrhea	750 mg orally TID or 1250 mg orally BID
ritonavir *rih-tonn'-ah-veer*	Norvir	HIV infection	Peripheral and circumoral paresthesias, nausea, vomiting, diarrhea, anorexia	600 mg orally BID
saquinavir *sah-kwin'-a-veer*	Invirase	HIV infection	Headache, nausea, diarrhea, heartburn, flatulence	Fortovase: Six 200-mg capsules orally TID Invirase: Three 200-mg capsules orally TID
tipranavir *tih-pran'-ah-veer*	Aptivus	HIV infection	Nausea, diarrhea, liver dysfunction, intracranial bleeding	500 mg orally BID
Nucleoside/Nucleotide Reverse Transcriptase Inhibitors (NRTIs)				
abacavir *ah-bak'-ah-veer*	Ziagen	HIV infection	Nausea, vomiting, diarrhea, anorexia, liver dysfunction	300 mg orally BID or 600 mg once daily
℞ didanosine (ddI) *dye-dan'-oh-seen*	Videx	HIV infection	Headache, nausea, rash, vomiting, peripheral neuropathy, abdominal pain, diarrhea	Oral: 400 mg/day or 200 mg BID; for patients weighing less than 60 kg, 250 mg/day or 125 mg BID
emtricitabine *em-trih-sih'-tah-been*	Emtriva	HIV infection	Headache, nausea, vomiting, diarrhea, rash	200 mg/day orally
lamivudine (3TC) *lam-ih-vew'-deen*	Epivir, Epivir-HB	HIV infection, chronic hepatitis B infection	Headache, nausea, diarrhea, nasal congestion, cough, fatigue	HIV: 150 mg orally BID HBV: 100 mg/day orally daily
rilpivirine *ril'-pi-veer'een*	Edurant	HIV infection	Headache, insomnia, depression, rash	25 mg orally daily
stavudine *stay-vew'-den*	Zerit	HIV infection	Headache, nausea, diarrhea, fever, rash, peripheral neuropathy	40 mg orally q 12 hr
telbivudine *tel-biv'-yew-deen*	Tyzeka	Chronic hepatitis B	Headache, abdominal pain, flu-like syndrome, fatigue, upper respiratory infection symptoms	600 mg/day orally

(table continues on page 122)

Summary Drug Table ANTIVIRAL DRUGS (continued)

Generic Name	Trade Name	Uses	Adverse Reactions	Dosage Ranges
tenofovir disoproxil *teh-noe'-foe-veer*	Viread	HIV infection, chronic hepatitis B	Nausea, vomiting, diarrhea, flatulence	300 mg/day orally
zalcitabine *zal-sit'-tah-been*	Hivid	HIV infection	Peripheral neuropathy, abnormal liver function	0.75 mg orally q 8 hr
zidovudine (AZT) *zye-doe'-vew-deen*	Retrovir	HIV infection, prevention of maternal–fetal HIV transmission	Asthenia, malaise, weakness, headache, anorexia, diarrhea, nausea, abdominal pain, dizziness, insomnia, anemia, agranulocytosis	600 mg/day orally in divided doses; 1 mg/kg IV q 4 hr
Nonnucleoside Reverse Transcriptase Inhibitors (NNRTI)				
delavirdine *dell-ah-veer'-deen*	Rescriptor	HIV infection	Headache, nausea, diarrhea	400 mg orally TID
efavirenz *ef-ah-veer'-enz*	Sustiva	HIV infection	Rash, pruritus, dizziness, insomnia, fatigue, nausea, vomiting	600 mg/day orally
etravirine *eh"-trah-veer'-een*	Intelence	HIV infection	Rash, nausea, diarrhea	200 mg orally BID
nevirapine *neh-veer'-ah-peen*	Viramune	HIV infection	Rash, fever, headache, nausea, stomatitis, liver dysfunction	200 mg orally BID
Entry Inhibitors				
maraviroc *mah-rah'-veer-ock*	Selzentry	HIV infection	Dizziness, cough, rash, abdominal and muscle pains	150–600 mg/day depending on other antiviral medications
enfuvirtide *en-foo-veer'-tide*	Fuzeon	HIV infection	Injection site discomfort, induration, erythema	90 mg subcutaneous injection BID
Integrase Inhibitors				
raltegravir *ral-teg'-rah-veer*	Isentress	HIV infection	Headache, nausea, diarrhea, fever	400 mg orally BID
Antiretroviral Combinations				
abacavir/ lamivudine	Epzicom	HIV infection	See individual drugs above	One tablet daily (600 mg/300 mg dose)
abacavir/ lamivudine/ zidovudine	Trizivir	HIV infection	See individual drugs above	One tablet orally twice daily (300 mg/150 mg/300 mg dose
efavirenz/ emtricitabine/ tenofovir disoproxil	Atripla	HIV infection	See individual drugs above	One tablet orally daily (600 mg/200 mg/300 mg)
emtricitabine/ rilpivirine/tenofovir disoproxil	Complera	HIV infection	See individual drugs above	One tablet orally daily (200 mg/25 mg/300 mg)
emtricitabine/ tenofovir disoproxil	Truvada	HIV infection	See individual drugs above	One tablet orally BID (200 mg/300 mg dose)
lamivudine/ zidovudine	Combivi	HIV infection	See individual drugs above	One tablet orally BID (150 mg/300 mg dose)
lopinavir/ ritonavir *low-pin'-ah-veer/ rih-tonn'-ah-veer*	Kaletra	HIV infection	See individual drugs above	One tablet orally BID (400 mg/100 mg dose)

Ⓡ This drug should be administered at least 1 hour before or 2 hours after a meal.

● Chapter Review

Know Your Drugs

Clients sometimes know a medication by the brand (or trade) name and not the generic name. To help you recognize both names, match the brand name with the generic name of the same medication.

Generic Name	Brand Name
1. acyclovir	A. prezista
2. darunavir	B. tamiflu
3. oseltamivir	C. valtrex
4. valacyclovir	D. zovirax

Calculate Medication Dosages

1. The client is prescribed amantadine 200 mg. The drug is available in 100-mg tablets. The nurse administers _____.

2. The nurse is to administer 100 mg of zidovudine orally. The drug is available as syrup 50 mg/5 mL. The nurse administers _____.

● Prepare for the NCLEX®

Build Your Knowledge

1. Which of the following statements about a virus is true?

   1. they are about the same size as a bacterium
   2. reproduction occurs by invading a host cell
   3. travel is exclusively by blood-borne routes
   4. there are only a limited number of viruses

2. How do a virus and a retrovirus differ?

   1. require cellular material of another (host) cell to reproduce
   2. viral content reprograms the cell to reproduce virus
   3. they attack the host cell RNA instead of DNA
   4. the infected cell goes back to the original function

3. Which of the following adverse reactions would the nurse expect in a client receiving acyclovir by the oral route?

   1. nausea and vomiting
   2. constipation and urinary frequency
   3. conjunctivitis and blurred vision
   4. nephrotoxicity

4. Which of the following would the nurse report immediately in a 3-month-old client receiving ribavirin?

   1. any worsening of the respiratory status
   2. refusal to take foods or fluids
   3. drowsiness
   4. constipation

5. The nurse is administering didanosine properly when _____.

   1. tablets are crushed and mixed thoroughly with 1 ounce of water
   2. the drug is prepared for subcutaneous injection
   3. the drug is given with meals
   4. the drug is given mixed with orange juice or apple juice

6. Administration of antiretrovirals can result in _____.

   1. abnormal hair growth
   2. body fat redistribution
   3. cardiac arrest
   4. discoloration of the skin

Apply Your Knowledge

7. As a nurse on a pediatric unit, you are making the assignment to care for an infant receiving aerosol ribavirin for RSV. Which of the following nurses should be assigned to care for this patient?

   1. Doris, a 22-year-old registered nurse
   2. Ariel, a female respiratory therapist
   3. Brad, a 26-year-old licensed practical nurse
   4. Vanessa, a 45-year-old pediatric certified nurse

8. Mr. Park is to begin acyclovir treatment for his outbreak of shingles. As the nurse initiating care for him, you will check the medication administration record (MAR) to see if he is taking which drug for potential interactions?

   1. cimetidine
   2. ibuprofen
   3. sildenafil
   4. theophylline

Alternate-Format Questions

9. A client is prescribed one inhalation of zanamivir every 12 hours. The drug is available as one 5-mg blister per inhalation and is to be given with a "Diskhaler" device. How many milligrams will the nurse administer in a 24-hour period?

10. Match the viral infection with its site of infection.

1. lies dormant in the nervous system	A. Hepatitis C
2. destroys the immune system	B. Genital human papillomavirus
3. inflammation of the liver	C. Herpes zoster virus
4. most common sexually transmitted infection (STI)	D. Respiratory syncytial virus
5. respiratory infection primarily in children	E. Human immunodeficiency virus

To check your answers, see Appendix G.

the**Point** *For more NCLEX-style questions, log on to http://thepoint.lww.com to access more than 1000 questions.*

Antifungal and Antiparasitic Drugs

LEARNING OBJECTIVES

On completion of this chapter, the student will:

1. Distinguish between superficial and systemic fungal infections.
2. Distinguish between helminthic infections, protozoal infections, and amebiasis.
3. Discuss the uses, general drug actions, adverse reactions, contraindications, precautions, and interactions of antifungal and antiparasitic drugs.
4. Discuss important preadministration and ongoing assessment activities the nurse should perform on the patient receiving an antifungal and antiparasitic drug.
5. List nursing diagnoses particular to a patient taking an antifungal and antiparasitic drug.
6. List possible goals for a patient taking an antifungal and antiparasitic drug.
7. Discuss ways to promote an optimal response to therapy, how to manage adverse reactions, and important points to keep in mind when educating the patient and family about antifungal and antiparasitic drugs.

KEY TERMS

candidiasis • infection of the skin or mucous membrane with the yeast *Candida albicans*

cinchonism • quinidine toxicity or poisoning

fungicidal • deadly to fungi

fungistatic • pertaining to agents that retard growth of fungi

fungus • single-cell, colorless plant that lacks chlorophyll, such as yeast or mold

helminthiasis • invasion by helminths (worms)

mycotic infections • infection caused by fungi

over the counter (OTC) • pertaining to drugs or other substances sold without a prescription; also known as *nonprescription*

parasite • organism living in or on another organism (host) without contributing to the survival or well-being of the host

thrush • candidiasis (candidal infection) of the mouth

DRUG CLASSES

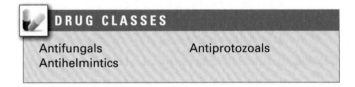

Antifungals	Antiprotozoals
Antihelmintics	

Fungal Infections

A **fungus** is a single-celled, colorless plant that lacks chlorophyll (Fig. 12.1). Fungi that cause disease in humans may be yeast-like or mold-like; the resulting infections are called fungal or **mycotic infections**.

Fungal infections range from superficial skin infections to life-threatening systemic infections. The superficial mycotic infections occur on the surface of, or just below, the skin or nails (see Chapter 52). Systemic fungal infections are serious infections that occur when fungi gain entrance into the interior of the body. These deep mycotic infections develop inside the body in sites such as in the lungs, brain, or gastrointestinal (GI) tract. Treatment for deep mycotic infections is often difficult and prolonged.

PHARMACOLOGY IN PRACTICE

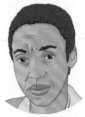

Lillian Chase, age 36, is caring for her two grandchildren. She calls the clinic because she thinks they are unusually fussy this visit. In asking about the children, there does not seem to be any indication they are ill; what you do learn is that they typically play in a large sand lot at home. Think about questions to ask about the children as you read this chapter.

Mold

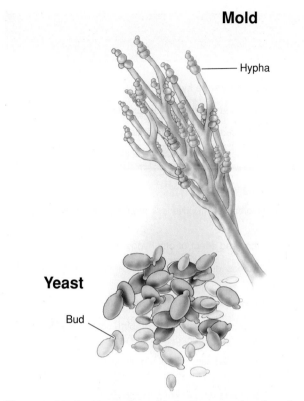

Hypha

Yeast

Bud

Figure 12.1 Examples of infection-causing fungi.

Yeast infections, such as those caused by *Candida albicans,* are known as **candidiasis**. Infection of the mouth by the microorganism *C. albicans* is commonly called **thrush**. Candidiasis also affects women in the vulvovaginal area and immunocompromised patients with chronic conditions in the perineum, the oral cavity, or systemically. Patients who are at increased risk for candidal infections are those who have diabetes, are pregnant, or are taking oral contraceptives, antibiotics, or corticosteroids such as posttransplant or surgical patients. The Summary Drug Table: Antifungal and Antiparasitic Drugs identifies drugs that are used to combat fungal infections.

ANTIFUNGAL DRUGS

Actions

Antifungal drugs may be **fungicidal** (able to destroy fungi) or **fungistatic** (able to slow or retard the multiplication of fungi). Amphotericin B (Fungizone IV), miconazole (Monistat), nystatin, voriconazole (Vfend), micafungin (Mycamine), and ketoconazole (Nizoral) are thought to have an effect on the cell membrane of the fungus. The fungicidal or fungistatic effect of these drugs appears to be related to their concentration in body tissues. Fluconazole (Diflucan) has fungistatic activity that appears to result from the depletion of sterols (a group of substances related to fats) in the fungus cells.

Griseofulvin (Grisactin) exerts its effect by being deposited in keratin precursor cells, which are then gradually lost (because of the constant shedding of top skin cells) and replaced by new, noninfected cells. The mode of action of flucytosine (Ancobon) is to inhibit DNA and RNA synthesis in the fungus. Clotrimazole (Lotrimin, Mycelex) binds with phospholipids in the fungal cell membrane, increasing permeability of the cell and resulting in loss of intracellular components.

Uses

Antifungal drugs are used prophylactically to prevent or to treat fungal infection in immunocompromised patients. They are also used to treat the following:

- Superficial and deep fungal infections
- Systemic infections such as aspergillosis, candidiasis, and cryptococcal meningitis
- Superficial infections of nail beds and oral, anal, and vaginal areas

The specific uses of antifungal drugs appear in the Summary Drug Table: Antifungal and Antiparasitic Drugs. Miconazole is an antifungal drug used to treat vulvovaginal "yeast" infections and is representative of all the vaginal antifungal agents. Fungal infections of the skin or mucous membranes may be treated with topical or vaginal preparations. A listing of the topical antifungal drugs appears in Table 12.1, and the vulvovaginal antifungal agents are listed in Table 12.2.

Table 12.1 Topical Antifungal Drugs

Generic Name (Form)	Trade Name(s)
butenafine HCl (cream)	Mentax
ciclopirox (cream, lotion)	Loprox, Penlac Nail Lacquer
clotrimazole (cream, solution, lotion)	Lotrimin
econazole (cream)	
miconazole (cream, solution, spray)	Monistat
naftifine (cream, gel)	Naftin
oxiconazole (cream, lotion)	Oxistat
sulconazole (cream, solution)	Exelderm

Table 12.2 Vaginal Antifungal Drugs

Generic Name	Select Trade Name(s)
clotrimazole	Lotrimin, Mycelex
miconazole	Monistat
nystatin	
terconazole	Terazol
tioconazole	Vagistat-1

Table 12.3 **Possible Interactions Between Antifungal and Other Drugs**

Interacting Drug	Common Use	Effect of Interaction
Amphotericin B corticosteroids	Reduce inflammation	Risk for severe hypokalemia
digoxin	Management of cardiac problems	Increased risk of digitalis toxicity
aminoglycosides	Anti-infective agent	Increased risk of nephrotoxicity
cyclosporine	Immunosuppressant (particularly for transplant recipients)	Increased risk of nephrotoxicity
flucytosine	Antifungal	Drug toxicity
miconazole	Antifungal for vaginal infections	Decreased effectiveness of amphotericin B
Fluconazole oral hypoglycemics	Diabetes control	Increased effect of oral hypoglycemic
phenytoin	Seizure control	Decreased effectiveness of phenytoin
Griseofulvin barbiturates	Sedation	Decreased effectiveness of sedative
oral contraceptives	Birth control	Decreased effectiveness of birth control (breakthrough bleeding, pregnancy, or amenorrhea)
salicylates	Analgesia, pain relief	Decreased serum level of pain reliever
Itraconazole digoxin and cyclosporine	See above	Elevated blood levels of itraconazole
phenytoin, histamine antagonists	Antiseizure drug and GI acid suppressant, respectively	Decreased blood levels of itraconazole
isoniazid and rifampin	Antitubercular drugs	Decreased blood levels of itraconazole
Ketoconazole histamine antagonists and antacids	Control of GI upset	Decreased absorption of ketoconazole
rifampin or isoniazid	Antitubercular drugs	May decrease the blood levels of ketoconazole
Posaconazole cimetidine	GI acid suppressant	May decrease the blood levels of posaconazole
phenytoin	Seizure control	Increased effectiveness of phenytoin
rifabutin	Antitubercular drugs	May decrease the blood levels of posaconazole
statins	Reduce cholesterol	Increased effectiveness of statins
Voriconazole methadone, tacrolimus, the statins, benzodiazepines, calcium channel blockers	Addiction control and pain relief, immunosuppressant, lipid-lowering agents, sedative hypnotics, and blood pressure or angina control, respectively	Increased effectiveness of voriconazole
sulfonylureas	Diabetes control	Hypoglycemia
vinca alkaloids	Antineoplastic (chemotherapy) agents	Increased risk of neurotoxicity
Micafungin sirolimus	Immunosuppression	Risk of greater immunosuppression
nifedipine	Management of angina (chest pain)	Risk of nifedipine toxicity
Terbinafine beta (β) blockers and antidepressants	Cardiac problems and depression, respectively	Increased effectiveness of the β blocker and antidepressant
Fluconazole, ketoconazole, itraconazole, voriconazole, or griseofulvin warfarin	Blood thinner	Increased risk of bleeding

Researchers have identified several antifungal herbs that are effective against skin infections, such as tea tree oil (*Melaleuca alternifolia*) and garlic (*Allium sativum*). Tea tree oil comes from an evergreen tree native to Australia. The herb has been used as a nonirritating antimicrobial for cuts, stings, wounds, burns, and acne. It can be found in shampoos, soaps, and lotions. Tea tree oil should not be ingested orally but is effective when used topically for minor cuts and stings. Topical application is most effective when used in a cream with at least 10% tea tree oil. Several commercially prepared ointments are available. The cream is applied to affected areas twice daily for several weeks.

Garlic is also used as an antifungal. A cream of 0.4% ajoene (the antifungal component of garlic) was found to relieve symptoms of athlete's foot and, like tea tree oil, is applied twice daily (DerMarderosian, 2003).

Adverse Reactions

Systemic Administration

- Headache
- Rash
- Anorexia and malaise
- Abdominal, joint, or muscle pain
- Nausea, vomiting, diarrhea

Contraindications

Antifungal drugs are contraindicated in patients with a history of allergy to the drug. Most of the systemic antifungal medications are contraindicated during pregnancy and lactation and are used only when the situation is life-threatening and outweighs the risk to the fetus.

Griseofulvin is not recommended for those with severe liver disease. Voriconazole is contraindicated when patients are taking the following medications: terfenadine, astemizole, sirolimus, rifampin, rifabutin, carbamazepine, ritonavir, ergot alkaloids, or long-acting barbiturates.

Both voriconazole and itraconazole are contraindicated in patients taking cisapride, pimozide, or quinidine. The systemic agent itraconazole should not be used to treat fungal nail infections in patients with a history of heart failure.

Precautions

Antifungals should be used cautiously in patients with renal dysfunction or hepatic impairment. Specific precautions include:

- Use amphotericin B cautiously in patients who have electrolyte imbalances or who currently use antineoplastic drugs (because severe bone marrow suppression can result).
- Administer griseofulvin cautiously with penicillin because of possible cross-sensitivity.
- Itraconazole should be used with caution in patients with human immunodeficiency virus (HIV) infection or hypochlorhydria (low levels of stomach acid).

Interactions

Possible interactions depend on the individual drugs, and many interactions can occur. See Table 12.3 for more drug interaction information.

NURSING PROCESS
PATIENT RECEIVING AN ANTIFUNGAL DRUG

ASSESSMENT

Preadministration Assessment
Assess the patient for signs of infection before giving the first dose of an antifungal drug. It is important to ask about pain and to describe white plaques or sore areas on mucous membranes of the oral or perineal areas, as well as any vaginal discharge. Take and record vital signs. When the patient is scheduled to receive amphotericin or flucytosine for a systemic fungal infection, be sure to weigh the patient because the dosage of the drug is determined according to the patient's weight.

Ongoing Assessment
The ongoing assessment involves careful observation of the patient every 2 to 4 hours for adverse drug reactions when the antifungal drug is given by the oral or parenteral route. When these drugs are administered topically or on an outpatient basis, instruct the patient in what to look for when gathering ongoing assessment data. This should include signs of improvement and adverse reactions, both minor and severe (requiring immediate notification of the primary health care provider).

NURSING DIAGNOSES
Drug-specific nursing diagnoses are the following:

- **Impaired Comfort** related to intravenous (IV) administration of amphotericin B
- **Risk for Ineffective Tissue Perfusion: Renal** related to adverse reactions of the antifungal drug

Nursing diagnoses related to drug administration are discussed in Chapter 4.

PLANNING
The expected outcomes for the patient depend on the reason for administering the antifungal drug but may include a therapeutic response to the antifungal drug, patient needs related to the management of adverse reactions, and confidence in an understanding of the medication regimen.

IMPLEMENTATION

Promoting an Optimal Response to Therapy: Administering Specific Antifungal Drugs
AMPHOTERICIN B. Amphotericin B is given only under close supervision in the hospital setting. Its use is reserved for serious and potentially life-threatening fungal infections. This drug is administered daily or every other day over several days or months.

The IV solution of amphotericin B is light sensitive and should be protected from exposure to light. If the solution is used within 8 hours, there is negligible loss of drug activity. Therefore, once the drug is reconstituted, administer the medication immediately, because the typical IV infusion is for a period of 6 hours or more. Consult the clinical pharmacist regarding whether to use a protective covering for the infusion container.

> **! NURSING ALERT**
>
> Renal damage is the most serious adverse reaction to the use of amphotericin B. Renal impairment usually improves with a modification of the dosage regimen (reduced dosage or increased time between doses). Serum creatinine levels and blood urea nitrogen (BUN) levels are checked frequently during the course of therapy to monitor kidney function. If the BUN exceeds 40 mg/dL or the serum creatinine level exceeds 3 mg/dL, the primary health care provider may discontinue the drug or reduce the dosage until renal function improves.

NONSYSTEMIC ANTIFUNGAL INFECTION PREPARATIONS. When a vaginal fungal infection is treated with miconazole during pregnancy, a vaginal applicator may be contraindicated. Manual insertion of the vaginal tablets may be preferred. Because small amounts of these drugs may be absorbed from the vagina, they are used only when essential during the first trimester.

Oral thrush infections (candidiasis) may be treated with oral solutions. Instruct the patient to swish and hold the solution in the mouth for several seconds (or as long as possible), gargle, and swallow the solution. Oral infections also may be treated with medication lozenges. Sometimes the vaginal troche preparation of an antifungal medication is prescribed for oral use. The patient needs specific instructions on how to use the medication to prevent confusion and improper use.

Monitoring and Managing Patient Needs

IMPAIRED COMFORT: MEDICATION ADMINISTRATION. When administering amphotericin B by IV infusion, be aware that immediate adverse reactions can occur. Nausea, vomiting, hypotension, tachypnea, fever, and chills (sometimes called *rigors*) may occur within 15 to 20 minutes of beginning the IV infusion. To prevent these adverse reactions, patients may be premedicated with antipyretics, antihistamines, or antiemetics. It is important to monitor the patient's temperature, pulse, respirations, and blood pressure carefully during the first 30 minutes to 1 hour of treatment. Monitor vital signs every 2 to 4 hours during therapy, depending on the patient's condition. Also check the IV infusion rate and the infusion site frequently during administration of the drug. This is especially important if the patient is restless or confused.

Patients should be taught before the drug is given that the side effects can be uncomfortable. Warm blankets should be provided for patient comfort. Reassure the patient that the medications administered before the antifungal will help to ease the adverse reactions. Instruction should include that the reactions decrease with ongoing therapy.

RISK FOR INEFFECTIVE TISSUE PERFUSION: RENAL. When the patient is taking a drug that is potentially toxic to the kidneys, carefully monitor fluid intake and output. If the patient is known to have renal compromise, perform hourly measurements of

urine output. Periodic laboratory tests are usually ordered to monitor the patient's response to therapy and detect toxic reactions. Serum creatinine and BUN levels are checked frequently during the course of therapy to monitor kidney function. If the BUN exceeds 40 mg/dL or if the serum creatinine level exceeds 3 mg/dL, the primary health care provider may discontinue the drug therapy or reduce the dosage until renal function improves.

LIFESPAN CONSIDERATIONS
Gerontology

Before administering fluconazole to an older adult or a patient with renal impairment, the primary health care provider may order a creatinine clearance test. Watch for and report the laboratory results to the primary health care provider because the dosage may be adjusted based on the test results.

Educating the Patient and Family

If the patient is being treated in the ambulatory care setting, include the following points in the teaching plan:

- Clean the involved area and apply the ointment or cream to the skin as directed by the primary health care provider.

- Do not increase or decrease the amount used or the number of times the ointment or cream should be applied unless directed to do so by the primary health care provider.

Drug-specific teaching points include:

- Flucytosine—Nausea and vomiting may occur with this drug. Reduce or eliminate these effects by taking a few capsules at a time during a 15-minute period. If nausea, vomiting, or diarrhea persists, notify the primary health care provider as soon as possible.

- Griseofulvin—Beneficial effects may not be noticed for some time; therefore, take the drug for the full course of therapy. Avoid exposure to sunlight and sunlamps because an exaggerated skin reaction (which is similar to severe sunburn) may occur even after a brief exposure to ultraviolet light. Notify the primary health care provider if fever, sore throat, or skin rash occurs.

- Ketoconazole—Complete the full course of therapy as prescribed by the primary health care provider. Do not take this drug with an antacid. In addition, avoid the use of nonprescription drugs unless use of a specific drug is approved by the primary health care provider. This drug may produce headache, dizziness, and drowsiness. If drowsiness or dizziness occurs, use caution while driving or performing other hazardous tasks. Notify the primary health care provider if pronounced abdominal pain, fever, or diarrhea occurs.

- Itraconazole—The drug is taken with food. Therapy continues for at least 3 months until infection is controlled. Report unusual fatigue, yellow skin, darkened urine, anorexia, nausea, and vomiting.

- Miconazole—If the drug (cream or tablet) is administered vaginally, insert the drug high in the vagina using the applicator provided with the product. Wear a pantiliner after insertion of the drug to prevent staining of the clothing and bed linen. Continue taking the drug during the menstrual period if the vaginal route is being used.

Do not have intercourse while taking this drug, or advise the partner to use a condom to avoid reinfection. To prevent recurrent infections, avoid nylon, thong underwear, and tight-fitting garments. If there is no improvement in 5 to 7 days, stop using the drug and consult the primary care provider, because a more serious infection may be present. If abdominal pain, pelvic pain, rash, fever, or offensive-smelling vaginal discharge is present, do not use the drug, but notify the primary health care provider.

EVALUATION

■ Therapeutic response is achieved and there is no evidence of infection.

■ Adverse reactions are identified, reported to the primary health care provider, and managed successfully with appropriate nursing interventions:

  • Patient reports comfort, without fever or chills.
  • Kidney perfusion is maintained.

■ Patient and family express confidence and demonstrate understanding of the drug regimen.

Parasitic Infections

A **parasite** is an organism that lives in or on another organism (the host) without contributing to the survival or well-being of the host. These infections are infrequent in most populations in the United States except the immunocompromised. **Helminthiasis** (invasion of the body by parasitic worms) and protozoal infections (invasion of the body by single-celled parasites or malaria) are worldwide health problems. What makes these diseases especially worthy of concern is the frequency of global air travel in modern society. Conditions once confined to specific parts of the world can now be spread in hours or days by air travel.

ANTHELMINTIC DRUGS

Roundworms, pinworms, whipworms, hookworms, and tapeworms are examples of helminths. The most common parasitic worm across the world is the roundworm. In the United States, the most common worm seen is the pinworm. *Anthelmintic* (against helminths) drugs are used to treat helminthiasis.

Actions and Uses

Although the actions of anthelmintic drugs vary, their primary purpose is to kill parasites.

Albendazole (Albenza) interferes with the synthesis of the parasite's microtubules, resulting in death of susceptible larvae. This drug is used to treat larval forms of pork tapeworm and to treat liver, lung, and peritoneum disease caused by the dog tapeworm.

Mebendazole blocks the uptake of glucose by the helminth, resulting in depletion of the helminth's own glycogen. This drug is used to treat whipworm, pinworm, roundworm, American hookworm, and the common hookworm.

The activity of pyrantel (Antiminth) is probably due to its ability to paralyze the helminth. Paralysis causes the helminth

to release its grip on the intestinal wall, after which it can be excreted in the feces. Pyrantel is used to treat roundworm and pinworm.

Adverse Reactions

Generalized adverse reactions include the following:

• Drowsiness, dizziness
• Nausea, vomiting
• Abdominal pain and cramps, diarrhea

Adverse reactions associated with the anthelmintic drugs, if they do occur, are usually mild when the drug is used in the recommended dosage. Rash is a serious adverse reaction to pyrantel, which is sold **over the counter** (without a prescription). As such, patients may begin self-treatment before notifying their primary health provider. Therefore, it is important to instruct the patient to notify the primary health care provider if this skin reaction occurs. For more information, see the Summary Drug Table: Antifungal and Antiparasitic Drugs.

Contraindications and Precautions

The anthelmintic drugs are contraindicated in patients with known hypersensitivity to the drugs and during pregnancy (pregnancy category C). They should be used cautiously in lactating patients, patients with hepatic or renal impairment, and patients with malnutrition or anemia.

Interactions

The following interactions may occur when a specific anthelmintic drug is administered with another agent:

Interacting Drug	Common Use	Effect of Interaction
albendazole (Albenza)		
dexamethasone	Inflammation or immunosuppression	Increased effectiveness of albendazole
cimetidine	Relief of GI problems, such as heartburn	Increased effectiveness of albendazole
mebendazole		
hydantoins and carbamazepine	Seizure control	Lower levels of mebendazole

ANTIPROTOZOAL DRUGS

One of the greatest protozoal problems worldwide is the treatment and prevention of malaria. Although rare in the United States, on a worldwide scale, 216 million cases of malaria occur yearly, with a yearly death rate of more than one-half million people. As global travel increases, more people may be at risk depending on where they go. The protozoal infections seen in the United States include giardiasis (contracted from contaminated food or water), trichomoniasis, toxoplasmosis, and opportunistic infections (such as pneumonia seen in immunocompromised patients). Examples of antiprotozoal drugs in use today are listed in the Summary Drug Table: Antifungal and Antiparasitic Drugs.

Actions

Protozoa are single-celled animals. The protozoan that causes malaria is *Plasmodium falciparum*. Malaria is transmitted from person to person by certain species of the *Anopheles* mosquito. Figure 12.2 illustrates the life cycle of malaria transmission and the drugs used in treatment. On the other hand, transmission of the more common protozoans (*Giardia, Trichomonas,* and *Toxoplasma* spp.) occurs through contaminated food or water, by fecal matter, or through sexual intercourse. In immunocompromised patients, the organism *Pneumocystis jiroveci* causes pneumonia. Antiprotozoal drugs interfere with, or are active against, the life cycle of the protozoan.

Uses

Infectious Disease

Antiprotozoal drugs may be used to treat infections such as:

- Malaria
- Giardiasis
- Toxoplasmosis
- Intestinal amebiasis
- Sexually transmitted infections (trichomoniasis)
- *Pneumocystis* pneumonia (PCP)

Prophylaxis

Antimalarial drugs are used for suppressing (i.e., preventing) malaria.

Adverse Reactions

GI reactions include the following:

- Anorexia
- Nausea, vomiting
- Abdominal cramping and diarrhea

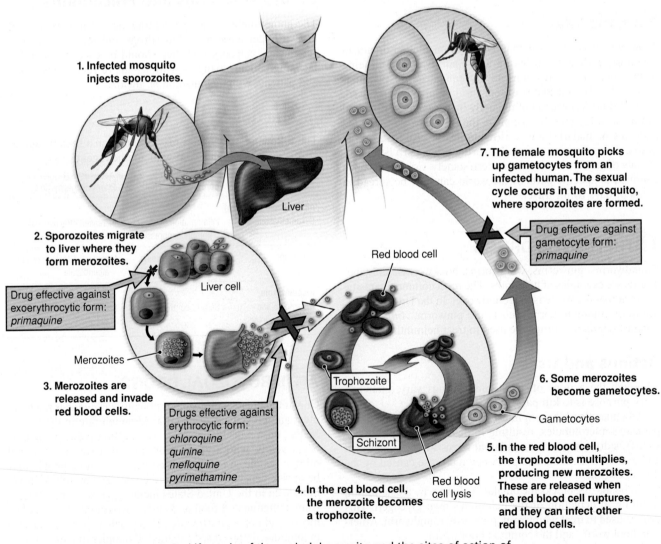

1. Infected mosquito injects sporozoites.

2. Sporozoites migrate to liver where they form merozoites.

Liver

Liver cell

Drug effective against exoerythrocytic form: *primaquine*

Merozoites

3. Merozoites are released and invade red blood cells.

Drugs effective against erythrocytic form: *chloroquine quinine mefloquine pyrimethamine*

4. In the red blood cell, the merozoite becomes a trophozoite.

Red blood cell

Trophozoite

Schizont

Red blood cell lysis

5. In the red blood cell, the trophozoite multiplies, producing new merozoites. These are released when the red blood cell ruptures, and they can infect other red blood cells.

6. Some merozoites become gametocytes.

Gametocytes

7. The female mosquito picks up gametocytes from an infected human. The sexual cycle occurs in the mosquito, where sporozoites are formed.

Drug effective against gametocyte form: *primaquine*

Figure 12.2 Life cycle of the malarial parasite and the sites of action of antimalarial drugs.

Other Reactions

- Headache and dizziness
- Visual disturbances or tinnitus
- Hypotension or changes detected on an electrocardiogram (ECG; associated with chloroquine)
- **Cinchonism**—a group of symptoms associated with quinine administration, including tinnitus, dizziness, headache, GI disturbances, and visual disturbances. These symptoms usually disappear when the dosage is reduced.
- Peripheral neuropathy (numbness and tingling of the extremities), with metronidazole
- Nephrotoxicity and ototoxicity, with paromomycin

Contraindications and Precautions

Antiprotozoal drugs are contraindicated in patients with known hypersensitivity. Many of the drugs are contraindicated during pregnancy (most are pregnancy category C; except metronidazole, nitazoxanide, pregnancy category B; doxycycline, pregnancy category D; quinine, pregnancy category X). Quinine should not be prescribed for patients with myasthenia gravis, because it may cause respiratory distress and dysphagia. Antiprotozoal drugs should be used cautiously in children, lactating patients, and those who have hepatic or renal disease or bone marrow depression. Pregnancy category B antiprotozoals should be used cautiously in patients during pregnancy and lactation (can be given during the second and third trimesters) and in patients with blood dyscrasias, seizure disorders, severe hepatic impairment (metronidazole), bowel disease (paromomycin use interferes with absorption causing ototoxicity and renal impairment), or history of alcohol dependency.

Interactions

Foods that acidify the urine (cranberries, plums, prunes, meats, cheeses, eggs, fish, and grains) may interact with chloroquine and increase its excretion, thereby decreasing the effectiveness of the antimalarial drug. The following interactions may also occur when an antiprotozoal is administered with another agent:

Interacting Drug	Common Use	Effect of Interaction
antacids	GI upset	Decreased absorption of the antimalarial
iron	Treat anemia	Decreased absorption of the antimalarial
digoxin	Treat cardiac disease	Increased risk of digoxin toxicity
cimetidine	Management of GI upset or heartburn	Decreased metabolism of metronidazole
phenobarbital	Sedative	Increased metabolism of metronidazole
Quinine warfarin	Blood thinner, prevents blood clots	Increased risk of bleeding

NURSING PROCESS

PATIENT RECEIVING AN ANTIPARASITIC DRUG

ASSESSMENT

Preadministration Assessment
Patients with parasitic infections may or may not be acutely ill. The acutely ill patient requires hospitalization, but many individuals with parasitic infections can be treated on an outpatient basis. Because a great number of infections are transmitted by the GI route, the diagnosis of a parasitic infection is often made by examination of the stool for parasites. Several stool specimens may be necessary before the parasite is seen and identified. The patient history also may lead to a suspicion of a parasitic infection, but some patients have no symptoms.

A relatively common infection, especially in pediatric populations, is the pinworm (helminth) infection. When a pinworm infection is suspected, instruct the parent on how to take a specimen from the anal area, preferably early in the morning before the patient gets out of bed. Specimens are taken by swabbing the perianal area with a cellophane tape–covered swab.

Ongoing Assessment
Unless ordered otherwise, instruct the parent to observe all stools that are passed after the drug is given. It is important to inspect each stool visually for passage of the helminth. If stool specimens are to be saved for laboratory examination, follow facility procedure for saving the stool and transporting it to the laboratory. If the patient is acutely ill or has a massive infection, it is important to monitor vital signs every 4 hours and measure and record fluid intake and output. Observe the patient for adverse drug reactions, as well as severe episodes of diarrhea. It is important to notify the primary health care provider if these occur.

NURSING DIAGNOSES

The nursing diagnoses depend on the patient and the type of parasitic infection. Drug-specific nursing diagnoses are the following:

- **Diarrhea** related to parasitic invasion of body
- **Risk for Deficient Fluid Volume** related to parasitic invasion of body
- **Imbalanced Nutrition: Less Than Body Requirements** related to adverse effects of drug therapy
- **Risk for Ineffective Airway Clearance** related to adverse effects of drug therapy

Nursing diagnoses related to drug administration are discussed in Chapter 4.

PLANNING

The expected outcomes for the patient depend on the reason for administering the antiparasitic but may include an optimal response to drug therapy, meeting patient needs related to management of common adverse reactions, and confidence in an understanding of the therapeutic regimen.

IMPLEMENTATION

Promoting an Optimal Response to Therapy: Proper Administration

When treating a patient for a parasitic infection, instruct the family on methods to prevent reinfection or passing the infection on to other persons. Instruct the family in frequent changing and washing of bed linens and undergarments. Caregivers need to also take care in obtaining or handling stool specimens. Instruct the patient to wash his or her hands thoroughly after personal care and before meals.

When taking the drug pentamidine, patients should be placed in a reclining or supine position to prevent adverse effects should a sudden decrease in blood pressure occur. The patient should be monitored for hypotension over a number of doses to be sure the patient remains stable during treatments.

When administering an antimalarial drug, such as chloroquine, for prophylaxis (prevention), therapy should begin 2 weeks before exposure and continue for 6 to 8 weeks after the client leaves the area where malaria is prevalent.

Monitoring and Managing Patient Needs

DIARRHEA AND RISK FOR FLUID VOLUME DEFICIT. Daily stool specimens may be ordered to be sent to the laboratory for examination. Keep a record of the number, consistency, color, and frequency of stools. Immediately deliver all stool specimens saved for examination to the laboratory because the organisms may die (and therefore cannot be seen microscopically). Inform laboratory personnel that the patient has a parasite, because the specimen must be kept at or near body temperature until examined under a microscope.

Also monitor fluid intake and output and symptoms of a fluid volume deficit, and make sure the patient is clean and the room free of odor. If dehydration is apparent, notify the primary health care provider. If the patient is or becomes dehydrated, oral or IV fluid and electrolyte replacement may be necessary.

IMBALANCED NUTRITION: LESS THAN BODY REQUIREMENTS. GI upset may occur, causing nausea, vomiting, abdominal pain, and diarrhea. Taking the drug with food often helps to alleviate the nausea. The patient may require frequent, small meals of easily digested food. A discussion of eating habits, food preferences, and food aversions assists in meal planning. Monitor body weight daily to identify any changes (increase or decrease). Make sure that meals are well balanced nutritionally, appetizing, and attractively served. Consult the registered dietitian if necessary.

RISK FOR INEFFECTIVE AIRWAY CLEARANCE. Bronchospasm or cough is more likely to occur when inhaled treatments of pentamidine are given. The primary health care provider may prescribe a bronchodilator to be given before the pentamidine treatment. Instruct the patient and caregivers in the proper methods of administration and care of the respiratory equipment used at home with pentamidine (see Patient Teaching for Improved Patient Outcomes: Administering Pentamidine at Home).

Patient Teaching for Improved Patient Outcomes

Administering Pentamidine at Home

The patient may be required to receive aerosol pentamidine at home. Before discharge, the nurse checks to make sure arrangements have been made to deliver the specialized equipment and supplies, such as nebulizer and diluent, to the home.

When you teach, make sure your patient and the caregiver understand the following:

✔ Prepare the solution immediately before use.
✔ Dissolve the contents in the proper amount of sterile water and protect the solution from light.
✔ Place the entire solution in the nebulizer's reservoir. Do not put any other drugs into the reservoir.
✔ Attach the tubing to the nebulizer and reservoir.
✔ Place the mouthpiece in your mouth and turn on the nebulizer.
✔ Breathe in and out deeply and slowly. The entire treatment should last 30 to 45 minutes.
✔ Tap the reservoir periodically to ensure that all of the drug is aerosolized.
✔ When the treatment is finished, turn off the nebulizer.
✔ Clean the equipment according to the manufacturer's instructions.
✔ Allow tubing, reservoir, and mouthpiece to air dry.
✔ Store the equipment in a clean plastic bag and put it away for the next dose.
✔ Use a calendar to mark the days you are to receive the drug and check off each time you've done the treatment.

Educating the Patient and Family

When an antiparasitic is prescribed on an outpatient basis, give the patient or family member complete instructions about taking the drug, as well as household precautions that should be followed until the parasite is eliminated from the intestine. Should the family have limited English proficiency, be sure to include language-appropriate written materials. When developing a patient education plan, be sure to include the following:

■ Follow the dosage schedule exactly as printed on the prescription container. It is absolutely necessary to follow the directions for taking the drug to eradicate the parasite.

■ Follow-up stool specimens will be necessary because this is the only way to determine the success of drug therapy.

■ When an infection is diagnosed, multiple members of the family may be infected, and all household members may need to be treated. Playmates of the infected child may also need to be treated.

■ It is important to wash all bedding and bed clothes once treatment has started.

■ Daily bathing (showering is best) is recommended. Disinfect toilet facilities daily, and disinfect the bathtub or shower stall immediately after bathing. Use the disinfectant recommended by the primary health care provider or use chlorine bleach. Scrub the surfaces thoroughly and allow the disinfectant to remain in contact with the surfaces for several minutes.

- During treatment for a ringworm infection, keep towels and facecloths for bathing separate from those of other family members to avoid the spread of the infection. It is important to keep the affected area clean and dry.
- Wash the hands thoroughly after urinating or defecating and before preparing and eating food. Clean under the fingernails daily and avoid putting fingers in the mouth or biting the nails.
- Food handlers should not resume work until a full course of treatment is completed and stools do not contain the parasite.
- Child care workers should be especially careful of diaper disposal and proper hand washing to prevent the spread of infections.
- Report any symptoms of infection (low-grade fever or sore throat) or thrombocytopenia (easy bruising or bleeding).
- Albendazole can cause serious harm to a developing fetus. Inform women of childbearing age of this. Explain that a

barrier contraceptive is recommended during the course of therapy and for 1 month after discontinuing the therapy.

When an antimalarial drug is used for preventing malaria and taken once a week, the patient also must take the drug on the same day each week. The prevention program is usually started 1 week before the individual departs to an area where malaria is prevalent.

EVALUATION

- Therapeutic response is achieved, and there is no evidence of infection.
- Adverse reactions are identified, reported to the primary health care provider, and managed successfully with appropriate nursing interventions:
  • Patient reports adequate bowel movements.
  • Adequate fluid volume is maintained.
  • Patient maintains an adequate nutritional status.
  • Lungs function effectively.
- Patient and family express confidence and demonstrate understanding of the drug regimen.

PHARMACOLOGY IN PRACTICE
THINK CRITICALLY

 While listening to Lillian Chase talk about her grandchildren, the primary health care provider suspects the children may have pinworms. Determine what you would include in teaching Lillian how to collect a specimen for examination and a teaching plan to prevent the spread of pinworms to other family members.

KEY POINTS

- A fungus is a single-celled plant that can cause yeast-like infections. These are called fungal or mycotic infections. Antifungal drugs slow the growth of or destroy fungi.
- Superficial fungal infections to the skin, nails, and genital area are bothersome and are treated topically or by oral preparations. Systemic infections happen when the fungi gain entry into the body; these are serious infections, especially for those who are immunocompromised.
- Most antifungals used for superficial infections cause minimal adverse reactions such as headache, rash, or minor GI disturbances. Antifungals used for systemic infections can cause greater adverse reactions. Patients are premedicated with antipyretics, antihistamines, and antiemetics due to the adverse reactions (chills, fever,

rigors, etc.) caused by amphotericin B. Renal function should be monitored when older adults and renal patients take these medications.
- Helminthiasis and protozoal infections are caused when a parasite invades a host organism. Though found infrequently in the United States, these infections are of concern because travelers can bring them back home. Because many more people travel worldwide, many travelers are treated prophylactically to prevent infection.
- Many of these infections are treated on an outpatient basis, so patient and caregiver confidence in managing the treatment and adverse reactions is important. Patients and caregivers need teaching to separate items of the infected person from those of other family members to prevent infection or reinfection.

Summary Drug Table ANTIFUNGAL DRUGS AND ANTIPARASITIC DRUGS

Generic Name	Trade Name	Uses	Adverse Reactions	Dosage Ranges
Antifungal Drugs				
amphotericin B *am-foe-ter'-ih-sin*	Abelcet, AmBisome, Amphotec, Fungizone	Systemic fungal infections, cryptococcal meningitis in patients with HIV infection	Headache, hypotension, fever, shaking, chills, malaise, nausea, vomiting, diarrhea, abnormal renal function, joint and muscle pain	Desoxycholate: 1–1.5 mg/kg/day IV Lipid-based: 3–6 mg/kg/day IV
anidulafungin *an"-ih-doo-la-fun'-jin*	Eraxis	Abdominal and esophageal candidiasis	Headache, rash, nausea, vomiting	100–200-mg loading dose IV, followed by 50–100 mg/day IV for at least 14 days
caspofungin *kass-poe-fun'-jin*	Cancidas	Invasive aspergillosis, hepatic insufficiency	Headache, rash, nausea, vomiting, abdominal pain, hematologic changes, fever	70-mg loading dose IV, followed by 50 mg/day IV for at least 14 days
fluconazole *floo-kon'-ah-zole*	Diflucan	Oropharyngeal and esophageal candidiasis, vaginal candidiasis, cryptococcal meningitis	Headache, nausea, vomiting, diarrhea, skin rash	50–400 mg/day orally, IV
flucytosine (5-FC) *floo-sye'-toe-seen*	Ancobon	Systemic fungal infections	Nausea, diarrhea, rash, anemia, leukopenia, thrombocytopenia, renal insufficiency	50–150 mg/kg/day orally q 6 hr
griseofulvin *griz-ee-oh-full'-vin*	Grifulvin V, Gris-PEG	Ringworm infections of the skin, hair, nails	Nausea, vomiting, diarrhea, oral thrush, headache, rash, urticaria	For ringworm and jock itch: 330–375 mg orally in a single or divided dose For athlete's foot: 660–750 mg/day orally in divided doses; take for 2–6 wk until the infection is completely gone
itraconazole *eye-trah-kon'-ah-zole*	Sporanox	Systemic fungal infections, may be used for nail infections	Nausea, vomiting, diarrhea, rash, abdominal pain, edema, hypokalemia in dosages over 600 mg/day	200–400 mg/day orally; IV as a single or divided dose Nail infections: 200 mg BID for 1 wk, then repeat in 3 wk
ketoconazole *kee-toe-kon'-ah-zole*	Nizoral	Treatment of systemic fungal infections	Nausea, vomiting, abdominal pain, headache, pruritus	200 mg/day orally; may increase to 400 mg/day orally
micafungin *mye-ka-fun'-jin*	Mycamine	Esophageal candidiasis, candidal infection prevention in stem cell transplantation	Rash, pruritus, facial swelling, vasodilation, flushing, headache, dizziness, anorexia, nausea, vomiting	150 mg/day IV
miconazole *my-kon'-ah-zole*	Oravig	Oropharyngeal candidiasis	Headache, nausea	50 mg oral cavity daily
nystatin, oral *nye-stat'-in*		Nonesophageal GI membrane candidiasis	Rash, diarrhea, nausea, vomiting	500,000–1 million units TID
posaconazole *poe'-sa-kon'-ah-zole*	Noxafil	Oral/pharyngeal candidiasis, prophylaxis of fungal infections	Headache; fever; abdominal pain; diarrhea; low potassium, red and white cells, and platelets	100–200 mg orally, 1–3 times daily

Summary Drug Table ANTIFUNGAL DRUGS AND ANTIPARASITIC DRUGS (continued)

Generic Name	Trade Name	Uses	Adverse Reactions	Dosage Ranges
terbinafine *ter-bin'-ah-feen*	Lamisil	Nail fungal infections	Headache, nausea, flatulence, diarrhea, rash	250 mg/day for 6–12 wk
voriconazole *vor-ih-kon'-ah-zole*	Vfend	Aspergillus systemic fungal infections	Visual disturbances, fever, rash, headache, anorexia, nausea, vomiting, diarrhea, peripheral edema, photosensitivity	Loading dose: 6 mg/kg q 12 hr for the first day Maintenance: If tolerated orally: 200 mg q 12 hr; if unable to take orally: 4 mg/kg q 12 hr IV until able to switch to oral drug

Antiparasitic Drugs

Anthelmintic Drugs

Generic Name	Trade Name	Uses	Adverse Reactions	Dosage Ranges
albendazole *al-ben'-dah-zole*	Albenza	Parenchymal neurocysticercosis due to pork tapeworms, hydatid disease (caused by the larval form of the dog tapeworm)	Abnormal liver function test results, abdominal pain, nausea, vomiting, headache, dizziness	Weight greater than or equal to 60 kg: 400 mg Weight less than 60 kg: 15 mg/kg/day
ivermectin *eye-ver-mek'-tin*	Stromectol	Treatment of threadworm	Pruritus, rash, lymph node tenderness	Single dose of 200 mcg/kg
mebendazole *meh-ben'-dah-zole*		Treatment of whipworm, pinworm, roundworm, common and American hookworm	Transient abdominal pain, diarrhea	100 mg orally morning and evening for 3 consecutive days Pinworm: 100 mg orally as a single dose
pyrantel *pye-ran'-tel*	Antiminth, Reese's Pinworm	Treatment of pinworm and roundworm	Anorexia, nausea, vomiting, abdominal cramps, diarrhea, rash (serious)	11 mg/kg orally as a single dose; maximum dose, 1000 mg

Antiprotozoal Drugs

Primary Antimalarial Drugs

Generic Name	Trade Name	Uses	Adverse Reactions	Dosage Ranges
chloroquine *klor'-oh-kween*	Aralen	Treatment and prevention of malaria, extraintestinal amebiasis	Hypotension, electrocardiographic changes, headache, nausea, vomiting, anorexia, diarrhea, abdominal cramps, visual disturbances	Treatment: 160–200 mg IM and repeat in 6 hr if necessary Prevention: 300 mg orally weekly; begin 1–2 wk before travel and continue for 4 wk after return from endemic area
doxycycline *dox-ih-sye'-kleen*	Monodox, Vibramycin, Vibra-Tabs	Short-term prevention of malaria	Photosensitivity, anorexia, nausea, vomiting, diarrhea, superinfection, rash	100 mg orally daily, 1–2 days before travel and for 4 wk after return from endemic area
quinine *kwi'-nine*	Qualaquin	Treatment of malaria	Nausea, vomiting, cinchonism, skin rash, visual disturbances	260–650 mg TID for 6–12 days

Other Antiprotozoal Drugs

Generic Name	Trade Name	Uses	Adverse Reactions	Dosage Ranges
artemether and lumefantrine *ar-tem'-e-ther* and *loo-me-fan'-treen*	Coartem	Treatment of malaria	Headache, nausea, anorexia, muscle aches	3-day treatment of 4 tablets twice daily
atovaquone *ah-toe'-vah-kwone*	Mepron	Prevention and treatment of PCP	Nausea, vomiting, diarrhea, headache, rash	750 mg orally BID for 21 days

(table continues on page 136)

Summary Drug Table **ANTIFUNGAL DRUGS AND ANTIPARASITIC DRUGS** (continued)

Generic Name	Trade Name	Uses	Adverse Reactions	Dosage Ranges
atovaquone and proguanil *ah-toe'-vah-kwone* and *pro-gwa'-nill*	Malarone	Prevention and treatment of malaria	Headache, fever, myalgia, abdominal pain, diarrhea	Prevention: 1–2 days before travel, 1 tablet orally per day during period of exposure and for 7 days after exposure Treatment: 4 tablets orally daily for 3 days
hydroxychloroquine *hye-drox-ee-klor'-oh-kwin*	Plaquenil	Prevention and treatment of malaria, systemic lupus erythematosus, and rheumatoid arthritis	Nausea, vomiting, diarrhea, headache	Prevention: begin 1–2 wk before travel, 310 mg/wk orally, continue for 4 wk after return from endemic area Treatment: 620 mg orally in 2 doses
mefloquine *meh'-flow-kwin*		Prevention and treatment of malaria	Vomiting, dizziness, disturbed sense of balance, nausea, fever, headache, visual disturbances	Prevention: begin 1 wk before travel, 250 mg/wk orally, continue for 4 wk after return from endemic area Treatment: 5 tablets orally as a single dose
metronidazole *meh-troe-nye'-dah-zole*	Flagyl	Treatment of intestinal amebiasis, trichomoniasis, anaerobic microorganisms	Headache, nausea, peripheral neuropathy, disulfiram-like interaction with alcohol	750 mg orally TID for 5–10 days
nitazoxanide *nye-tah-zocks'-ah-nide*	Alinia	Diarrhea caused by *Giardia lamblia*	Abdominal pain, nausea, vomiting, diarrhea, headache	500 mg orally q 12 hr with food
paromomycin *par-oh-moe-mye'-sin*		Treatment of intestinal amebiasis	Nausea, vomiting, diarrhea	25–35 mg/kg/day in 3 divided doses with meals for 5–10 days
pentamidine *pen-tah'-mih-deen*	Pentam, Nebupent	PCP	IM: pain at injection site; fatigue, metallic taste, anorexia, shortness of breath, dizziness, rash, cough	Injection: 4 mg/kg IM or IV daily, for 14 days Aerosol (preventative): 300 mg/wk for 4 wk by nebulizer
primaquine *prim'-ah-kween*		Treatment of malaria	Nausea, vomiting, epigastric distress, abdominal cramps	26.3. mg/day orally for 14 days
pyrimethamine *peer-ih-meth'-ah-meen*	Daraprim	Prevention and treatment of malaria	Nausea, vomiting, hematologic changes, anorexia	Prevention: 25 mg orally once weekly Treatment: 50 mg/day for 2 days
sulfadoxine and pyrimethamine *sul-fah-dox'-een* and *peer-ih-meth'-ah-meen*	Fansidar	Prevention and treatment of malaria	Hematologic changes, nausea, emesis, headache, hypersensitivity reactions, Stevens-Johnson syndrome	Prevention: 1 tablet orally weekly Treatment: 2–3 tablets orally as a single dose
tinidazole *tih-nye'-dah-zole*	Tindamax	*Giardia lamblia*, trichomoniasis	Nausea, vomiting, metallic taste	Single dose of 2 g orally

● Chapter Review

Know Your Drugs

Clients sometimes know a medication by the brand (or trade) name and not the generic name. To help you recognize both names, match the brand name with the generic name of the same medication.

Generic Name	Brand Name
1. terbinafine	A. Antiminth
2. pyrantel	B. Fungizone
3. doxycycline	C. Lamisil
4. amphotericin B	D. Vibramycin

Calculate Medication Dosages

1. The primary care provider has prescribed fluconazole 200 mg orally initially, followed by 100 mg orally daily. On hand are fluconazole 100-mg tablets. What should the nurse administer as the initial dose? _____

2. Pyrantel 360 mg is prescribed. The drug is available in 180-mg capsules. The nurse teaches the caregiver to administer _____.

● Prepare for the NCLEX®

Build Your Knowledge

1. Mycotic infections are caused by:
   1. bacteria
   2. fungi
   3. parasites
   4. viruses

2. A client asks how antimalarial drugs prevent or treat malaria. The nurse correctly responds that this group of drugs:
   1. kills the mosquito that carries the protozoa
   2. interferes with the life cycle of the protozoa causing the malaria
   3. ruptures the red blood cells that contain merozoites
   4. increases the body's natural immune response to the protozoa

3. Which of the following laboratory tests would the nurse monitor in clients receiving flucytosine?
   1. liver function tests
   2. complete blood count
   3. renal functions tests
   4. prothrombin levels

4. When discussing the adverse reactions of an anthelmintic, the nurse correctly states that:
   1. clients must be closely observed for 2 hours after the drug is given
   2. adverse reactions are usually mild when recommended doses are used
   3. most clients experience severe adverse reactions and must be monitored closely
   4. no adverse reactions are associated with these drugs

5. When preparing a client for pentamidine administration, the correct position is:
   1. lying on left side
   2. reverse Trendelenburg
   3. prone
   4. reclining position

Apply Your Knowledge

6. When giving one of the topical antifungals, the nurse assesses the client for the most common adverse reactions, which are _____.
   1. related to the GI tract
   2. urinary retention
   3. hypotension
   4. related to the nervous system

7. A client is receiving amphotericin B for a systemic fungal infection. Which of the following would most likely indicate to the nurse that the client is experiencing an adverse reaction to amphotericin B?
   1. fever and chills
   2. abdominal pain
   3. drowsiness
   4. flushing of the skin

8. The nurse is teaching preschool mothers about pyrantel treatment for pinworm infection. Which adverse reaction should the mothers report immediately to the primary health care provider?
   1. nausea
   2. rash
   3. diarrhea
   4. headache

Alternate-Format Questions

9. Identify the household precautions to prevent spread of parasitic infections. **Select all that apply**.
   1. wash all bedding in the home
   2. provide separate towels for bathing
   3. wash hands after using the bathroom or changing diapers
   4. sterilize toys with boiling water

10. A client weighs 140 lb. If amphotericin B 1.5 mg/kg/day is prescribed, what is the total daily dosage of amphotericin B for this client?

To check your answers, see Appendix G.

the**Point** *For more NCLEX-style questions, log on to http://thepoint.lww.com to access more than 1000 questions.*

Drugs Used to Manage Pain

The body uses pain to warn about potential or actual danger to body tissues. Typically, when danger is present the tissues send a signal to the brain to pull away from the harmful object or situation. The danger can be something outside the body, such as heat, or inside the body, such as a blood clot. Pain is a protective sensation; it lets our body know there is an injury.

The treatment of pain is important because when patients recover more slowly than expected from injury and illness, pain may be the key factor. In this unit, the basic concepts in understanding pain are introduced and many of the drugs used to reduce or alleviate pain are discussed. In Chapter 13 you will learn the basics of pain and about drugs typically purchased over the counter and taken without health care supervision; therefore, patient teaching and outpatient interactions are highlighted. Chapter 14 discusses assessment of patient pain. This is as vital as knowing the temperature, pulse, and respiration and is often termed the fifth vital sign.

Analgesics are drugs used to relieve pain. The nonopioid analgesics are a group of drugs used to relieve mild to moderate pain. They can be divided into three categories: salicylates, nonsalicylates (acetaminophen), and nonsteroidal anti-inflammatory drugs (NSAIDs). These drugs are discussed in Chapters 13 and 14. Drugs used to treat migraine headaches are also covered in Chapter 14; these drugs affect the nerve impulses controlling blood vessels in the brain.

Chapter 15 discusses the major uses of the opioid analgesics in the relief or management of moderate to severe acute and chronic pain. The ability of an opioid analgesic to relieve pain depends on several factors, such as the drug, the dose, the route of administration, the type of pain, the patient, and the length of time the drug has

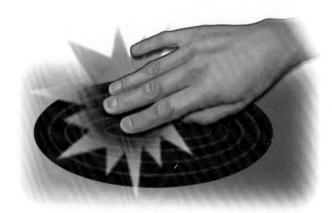

(From Premkumar K. *The Massage Connection Anatomy and Physiology*. Baltimore: Lippincott Williams & Wilkins, 2004.)

been administered. Treatment of moderate to severe pain may include both an opioid and a nonopioid analgesic. Manufacturers make products containing a combination of these drugs for ease of administration and standard selection of dosage combinations so the primary health care provider can prescribe the most effective pain relief. These combination products are listed in Chapter 15. If too much of an opioid is taken, opioid antagonists may be used; these drugs are discussed in Chapter 16. To complete this unit's discussion of pain management, Chapter 17 reviews the use of drugs for anesthesia—the elimination of sensation and the perception of pain.

Nonopioid Analgesics: Salicylates and Nonsalicylates

13

LEARNING OBJECTIVES

On completion of this chapter, the student will:

1. Discuss in general terms how pain is defined and the challenges of understanding the patient's pain experience.
2. Discuss the types, uses, general drug actions, common adverse reactions, contraindications, precautions, and interactions of the salicylates and acetaminophen.
3. Discuss important preadministration and ongoing assessment activities the nurse should perform for the patient taking salicylates or acetaminophen.
4. List nursing diagnoses particular to a patient taking salicylates or acetaminophen.
5. Discuss the ways to promote an optimal response to therapy, how to manage common adverse reactions, and important points to keep in mind when educating patients about the use of salicylates or acetaminophen.

KEY TERMS

aggregation • clumping of blood elements

analgesic • drug that relieves pain

antipyretic • fever-reducing agent

jaundice • yellow discoloration of the skin due to liver disease

pain • unpleasant sensory or emotional perception

pancytopenia • reduction in all cellular elements of the blood

prostaglandins • fatty acid derivative found in almost every tissue and fluid of the body that affects the uterus and other smooth muscles; also thought to increase the sensitivity of peripheral pain receptors to painful stimuli

Reye's syndrome • acute and potentially fatal disease of childhood; associated with a previous viral infection

salicylism • adverse reaction to a salicylate characterized by dizziness; impaired hearing; nausea; vomiting; flushing; sweating; rapid, deep breathing; tachycardia; diarrhea; mental confusion; lassitude; drowsiness; respiratory depression; and possibly coma

tinnitus • ringing in the ears

DRUG CLASSES

Salicylates
Acetaminophen

Pain can be described as "the unpleasant sensory and emotional perception associated with actual or potential tissue damage" (International Association for the Study of Pain, 1979). To treat pain, both opioid and nonopioid analgesics are used. This chapter discusses a simplistic understanding of pain as well as treating pain with the nonopioid analgesics: the salicylates and acetaminophen.

Understanding Pain

The nervous system is the mechanism involved in the recognition and perception of pain. The pain perception pathway in Figure 13.1 illustrates how pain signals that noxious stimuli has or may cause injury to the body tissues. Nerve fibers in

---

PHARMACOLOGY IN PRACTICE

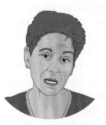

Betty Peterson is at the outpatient clinic with complaints of a cold, muscular aches, and pain. She is currently taking a nonprescription aspirin product. She states she is experiencing some gastric upset and tells you that she plans to begin taking Tylenol because she has heard that it does not cause upset stomach. As you read this chapter consider whether this is a good change for Betty.

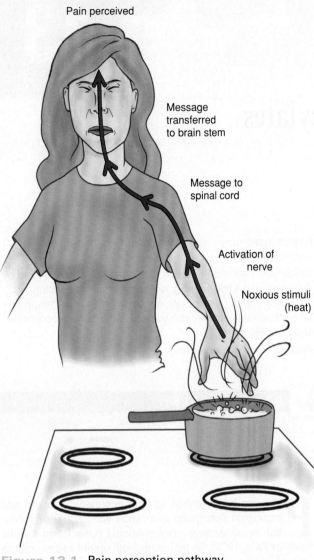

Pain perceived

Message transferred to brain stem

Message to spinal cord

Activation of nerve

Noxious stimuli (heat)

Figure 13.1 Pain perception pathway.

the tissue are stimulated by stretching (an example would be the swelling of a blood clot that would force the nerve to stretch) or a noxious substance, such as heat from a pan of steaming water. In the peripheral (outside or distal) tissues, the nerve endings (or receptors) are activated and send a message to the spinal cord. Here, the nerve impulses are transferred across different nerve pathways in the central nervous system and sent to the brainstem. From this area, the message goes to the brain cortex, where the perception of pain occurs, and the person should remove the hand from the heat to eliminate the pain sensation and prevent injury to the hand.

Defining Pain

There are several ways to define pain. Defining the duration and how the pain sensation is perceived will help you understand pain. Acute pain and chronic pain are used when discussing duration. *Acute pain* is brief and lasts less than 3 to 6 months. Causes range from a sunburn to postoperative, procedural, or

traumatic pain. Acute pain usually subsides when the injury heals. A finger burned by the steam of hot water (as illustrated in Fig. 13.1) is an example of acute pain.

Chronic pain lasts more than 6 months and is often associated with specific diseases, such as cancer, sickle cell anemia, and end-stage organ or system failure. Various neuropathic and musculoskeletal disorders, such as headaches, fibromyalgia, rheumatoid arthritis, and osteoarthritis, are also causes of chronic pain.

The *sensation* of pain can be modified at the site (peripherally) when the cause is treated or by modifying the signal in the brain (centrally). Pain, such as a burned finger, can be reduced when treated at the site of injury.

The Pain Experience

To treat pain effectively, you need a good understanding of the patient's pain experience. This is challenging, because sometimes patients feel the provider is too busy to worry about the pain, or a previous bad pain management situation will make the patient think you do not know how to treat the pain. In addition, patients sometimes offer only a vague or poor description of their pain experience. The sensation of pain is a complex phenomenon that is uniquely experienced by each individual. Therefore, the patient's report of pain should always be taken seriously.

Medications to treat pain deal with the sensation experienced—drugs correct or help to heal the site of tissue damage or nerve stimulation (peripherally) or change or modulate the brain's perception of the pain signal (centrally). Peripheral pain (such as a burned finger) can be treated using nonopioid analgesics. The nonopioid analgesics such as the salicylates and nonsalicylates are used for mild to moderate peripheral pain. Many of these products can be obtained without a prescription. This fact sometimes makes patients think they are harmless drugs. This chapter discusses both routine use and harmful adverse reactions of salicylates and nonsalicylate analgesics.

SALICYLATES

The salicylates are drugs derived from salicylic acid. Salicylates are useful in pain management because of their **analgesic** (pain-relieving), **antipyretic** (fever-reducing), and anti-inflammatory effects. Examples include aspirin (acetylsalicylic acid) and magnesium salicylate. Specific salicylates are listed in the Summary Drug Table: Nonopioid Analgesics: Salicylates and Nonsalicylates.

Actions

Salicylates lower body temperature by dilating peripheral blood vessels. The blood flows out to the extremities, resulting in the dissipation of the heat of fever, which in turn cools the body. The analgesic action of the salicylates is due to the inhibition of **prostaglandins.** Prostaglandins are found in almost every tissue of the body and body fluid. When prostaglandins are released, the sensitivity of pain receptors in the tissue increases, making the patient more likely to feel pain. Salicylates inhibit the production of prostaglandins, making pain receptors less likely to send the pain message to the brain. The reduction in prostaglandins is also thought to account for the anti-inflammatory activity of salicylates.

Aspirin more potently inhibits prostaglandin synthesis and has greater anti-inflammatory effects than other salicylates. In addition, aspirin prolongs the bleeding time by inhibiting the **aggregation** (clumping) of platelets. When bleeding time is prolonged, it takes a longer time for the blood to clot after a cut, surgery, or other injury to the skin or mucous membranes. Other salicylates do not have as great an effect on platelets as aspirin. This effect of aspirin on platelets is irreversible and lasts for the life of the platelet (7 to 10 days).

HERBAL CONSIDERATIONS

Willow bark has a long history of use as an analgesic. Willow trees or shrubs grow in moist places, often along river banks in temperate or cold climates. When used as a medicinal herb, willow bark is collected in early spring from young branches. In addition to its use as a pain reliever, the bark and leaves of various willow species have been used to lower fever and reduce inflammation. The salicylates were isolated from willow bark and identified as the most likely source of the bark's anti-inflammatory effects. The chemical structure was replicated in the laboratory and mass produced as synthetic salicylic acid. Years later, a modified version (acetylsalicylic acid) was first sold as aspirin. Aspirin became the most widely used pain reliever, fever reducer, and anti-inflammatory agent, leaving willow bark to be cast aside. The synthetic anti-inflammatory drugs work quickly and have a higher potency than willow bark. Willow bark takes longer to work and fairly high doses may be needed to achieve a noticeable effect. However, fewer adverse reactions are associated with willow bark than with the salicylates. Although adverse reactions are rare with willow bark, it should be used with caution in patients with peptic ulcers and medical conditions in which aspirin is contraindicated (DerMarderosian, 2003).

Uses

Salicylate nonopioid analgesics are used for:

- Relieving mild to moderate pain
- Reducing elevated body temperature
- Treating inflammatory conditions, such as rheumatoid arthritis, osteoarthritis, and rheumatic fever
- Decreasing the risk of myocardial infarction in those with unstable angina or previous myocardial infarction (aspirin only)
- Reducing the risk of transient ischemic attacks or strokes in men who have had transient ischemia of the brain due to fibrin platelet emboli (aspirin only). This use has been found to be effective in men (and women older than 65 years of age only).
- Helping maintain pregnancy in special at-risk populations (low-dose aspirin therapy). For example, it may be used to prevent or treat inadequate uterine–placental blood flow.

Adverse Reactions

Gastrointestinal (GI) system reactions include:

- Gastric upset, heartburn, nausea, vomiting
- Anorexia
- GI bleeding

Although salicylates are relatively safe when taken as recommended on the label or by the primary health care provider, their use can occasionally result in more serious reactions. Loss of blood through the GI tract may occur with salicylate use. The amount of blood lost is insignificant when a single dose is taken. However, use of these drugs over a long period, even in normal doses, can result in significant blood loss. Some individuals are allergic to aspirin and other salicylates. Allergy to salicylates may be manifested by hives, rash, angioedema, bronchospasm with asthma-like symptoms, and anaphylactoid (allergic) reactions.

Contraindications

Salicylates are contraindicated in patients with known hypersensitivity to salicylates or NSAIDs. Because salicylates prolong bleeding time, they are contraindicated in those with bleeding disorders or tendencies. These include patients with GI bleeding (from any cause), patients with blood dyscrasias (abnormalities), and patients receiving anticoagulant or antineoplastic drugs. Salicylates are classified as pregnancy category D (aspirin) and C drugs and should be used cautiously during pregnancy and lactation.

LIFESPAN CONSIDERATIONS
Pediatric

Children or teenagers with influenza or chickenpox should not take salicylates, particularly aspirin, because their use appears to be associated with **Reye's syndrome** (a life-threatening condition characterized by vomiting and lethargy progressing to coma).

Precautions

Salicylates should be used cautiously in patients during lactation and in those with hepatic or renal disease, preexisting hypoprothrombinemia (low levels of prothrombin, which hampers clotting ability), and vitamin K deficiency. The drugs are also used with caution in patients with GI irritation, such as peptic ulcers, and in patients with mild diabetes or gout.

CHRONIC CARE CONSIDERATIONS

Aspirin is an over-the-counter (OTC) medication that patients may use to self-treat for pain. Some may take more aspirin than the recommended dosage, and toxicity can then result in a condition called **salicylism**. Signs and symptoms of salicylism include dizziness; **tinnitus** (a ringing sound in the ear); impaired hearing; nausea; vomiting; flushing; sweating; rapid, deep breathing; tachycardia; diarrhea; mental confusion; lassitude; drowsiness; respiratory depression; and coma (from large doses). Mild salicylism usually occurs with repeated administration of large doses of a salicylate. This condition is reversible with reduction of the drug dosage.

Interactions

Foods containing salicylates (e.g., curry powder, paprika, licorice, prunes, raisins, and tea) may increase the risk of adverse reactions. The following interactions may occur when a salicylate is administered with another agent:

Interacting Drug	Common Use	Effect of Interaction
anticoagulant	Blood thinner	Increased risk for bleeding
NSAIDs	Pain relief	Increased serum levels of the NSAID
activated charcoal	Antidote (usually to poisons)	Decreased absorption of the salicylates
antacids	Relief of gastric upset, heartburn	Decreased effects of the salicylates
carbonic anhydrase inhibitors	Reduction of intraocular pressure; also used as diuretic	Increased risk for salicylism

NONSALICYLATES

The major drug classified as a nonsalicylate analgesic is acetaminophen. It is the most widely used aspirin substitute for patients who are allergic to aspirin or who experience extreme gastric upset when taking aspirin. Acetaminophen is also the drug of choice for treating children with fever and flu-like symptoms.

Actions

Acetaminophen is a nonsalicylate, nonopioid analgesic whose mechanism of action is unknown. The analgesic and antipyretic activity of acetaminophen is the same as salicylates. However, acetaminophen does not possess anti-inflammatory action and is of no value in the treatment of inflammation or inflammatory disorders (Table 13.1). Acetaminophen does not inhibit platelet aggregation; therefore, it is the analgesic of choice when bleeding tendencies are an issue.

Uses

Acetaminophen is used for:

- Treating mild to moderate pain
- Reducing elevated body temperature (fever)
- Managing pain and discomfort associated with arthritic disorders

The drug is particularly useful for those with aspirin allergy and bleeding disorders, such as bleeding ulcer or hemophilia; those receiving anticoagulant therapy; and those who have recently had minor surgical procedures.

Table 13.1 Comparison of Drug Properties		
Type of Analgesic	**Aspirin**	**Acetaminophen**
Analgesic (pain reliever)	Yes	Yes
Antipyretic (fever reducer)	Yes	Yes
Anti-inflammatory (reduce swelling)	Yes	No
Anticoagulant (blood thinner)	Yes	No

Adverse Reactions

Adverse reactions to acetaminophen are rare when the drug is used as directed. Adverse reactions associated with acetaminophen usually occur with chronic use or when the recommended dosage is exceeded. They include the following:

- Skin eruptions, urticaria (hives)
- Hemolytic anemia
- **Pancytopenia** (a reduction in all cellular components of the blood)
- Hypoglycemia
- **Jaundice** (yellow discoloration of the skin), hepatotoxicity (damage to the liver), and hepatic failure

Acute acetaminophen poisoning or toxicity can occur after a single 10- to 15-g dose of acetaminophen. Doses of 20 to 25 g may be fatal. With excessive doses, the liver cells undergo necrosis (die), and death can result from liver failure. The risk of liver failure increases in patients who drink alcohol habitually. Signs of acute acetaminophen toxicity include nausea, vomiting, confusion, liver tenderness, hypotension, cardiac arrhythmias, jaundice, and acute hepatic and renal failure.

Contraindications and Precautions

Hypersensitivity to acetaminophen is a contraindication to its use. Hepatotoxicity has occurred in habitual alcohol users after therapeutic dosages. The individual taking acetaminophen should avoid alcohol if taking more than an occasional dose of acetaminophen and avoid taking acetaminophen concurrently with the salicylates or the NSAIDs. Acetaminophen is classified as a pregnancy category B drug and is used cautiously during pregnancy and lactation. If an analgesic is necessary, it appears safe for short-term use. The drug is used cautiously in patients with severe or recurrent pain or high or continued fever because this may indicate a serious untreated illness. If pain persists for more than 5 days or if redness or swelling is present, the primary health care provider should be consulted.

LIFESPAN CONSIDERATIONS
Adolescents

Many people use acetaminophen for pain relief because it does not cause GI distress. Because acetaminophen is contained in many cold preparations, the 3-gram daily maximum can be unintentionally surpassed when combining cold and pain relievers. You should instruct parents to be aware of the different drug preparations being used especially when teens and adolescents may self-administer these drugs for cold or flu symptoms. Examples of nonpain relievers containing acetaminophen are Actifed, Benadryl, Cepacol, Dayquil, Formula 44, Nyquil, Robitussin, Sudafed, and Theraflu.

Interactions

The following interactions may occur when acetaminophen is administered with another agent:

Interacting Drug	Common Use	Effect of Interaction
barbiturates	Sedation, central nervous system depressants	Increased possibility of toxicity and decreased effect of acetaminophen
hydantoins	Anticonvulsants	Increased possibility of toxicity and decreased effect of acetaminophen
isoniazid and rifampin	Tuberculosis medications	Increased possibility of toxicity and decreased effect of acetaminophen
loop diuretics	Control of fluid imbalance	Decreased effectiveness of the diuretic

CHRONIC CARE CONSIDERATIONS

You should be aware of polypharmacy interactions when administering acetaminophen to diabetic patients; care needs to be taken when blood glucose testing is done. Acetaminophen may alter blood glucose test results, resulting in falsely lower blood glucose values. As a result, inaccurate and lower doses of antidiabetic medications may be given to the patient taking acetaminophen.

NURSING PROCESS

PATIENT RECEIVING A SALICYLATE OR A NONSALICYLATE

ASSESSMENT

Preadministration Assessment

Typically, a patient taking a nonopioid analgesic is not hospitalized. Because of this, it is important to ask how long the patient has taken the medication before seeing you or the primary health care provider. Ask if this pain or fever problem is different in any way from previous episodes of pain or discomfort. If the patient is receiving a nonopioid analgesic for an arthritic, musculoskeletal disorder or soft tissue inflammation, ask about or examine the joints involved.

NURSING ALERT

❗ Before administering acetaminophen, you should assess the overall health and alcohol usage of the patient. Patients who are malnourished or who consume alcohol habitually (more than 3 drinks per day on a regular basis) are at greater risk for developing hepatotoxicity (damage to the liver) with the use of acetaminophen.

Ongoing Assessment

As part of the ongoing assessment, monitor the patient for relief of pain and ask the patient to check the pain 30 to 60 minutes after administration of the drug. If pain persists, it is important to assess and document its severity, location, and intensity. (Examples of questions to ask the patient appear in Chapter 14.) When nonopioid analgesics are given for fever, ask the family to monitor the temperature every 4 hours or more frequently if necessary. Hot, dry, flushed skin and a decrease in urinary output may develop. If temperature elevation is prolonged, dehydration can occur. When given for any length of time, instruct the patient and family to report adverse reactions, such as unusual or prolonged bleeding or dark stools, to the primary care provider.

NURSING DIAGNOSES

Drug-specific nursing diagnoses are the following:

- **Impaired Comfort** related to fever of the disease process (e.g., infection or surgery)

- **Chronic** or **Acute Pain** related to peripheral nerve damage and/or tissue inflammation due to the disease process

- **Impaired Physical Mobility** related to muscle and joint stiffness

- **Risk for Poisoning** related to increased salicylate or acetaminophen use

Nursing diagnoses related to drug administration are discussed in Chapter 4.

PLANNING

The expected outcomes of the patient depend on the reason for administering a nonopioid analgesic but may include an optimal response to drug therapy, which includes relief of pain and fever; supporting patient needs related to the management of adverse drug reactions; and confidence in an understanding of the medication regimen.

IMPLEMENTATION

Promoting an Optimal Response to Therapy

SALICYLATES. The patient should be instructed to avoid salicylates for at least 1 week before any type of major or minor surgery, including dental surgery, because of the possibility of postoperative bleeding. In addition, the patient should not use salicylates after any type of surgery until complete healing has occurred because of the effects of salicylates on platelets. The patient may use acetaminophen or an NSAID after surgery or a dental procedure, when relief of mild pain is necessary.

You should observe the patient for adverse drug reactions. When high doses of salicylates are administered (e.g., to those with severe arthritic disorders), instruct how to observe for signs of salicylism. Should signs of salicylism occur, instruct the patient to notify the primary health care provider before the next dose is taken because a reduction in dose or determination of the plasma salicylate level may be necessary. Therapeutic salicylate levels are between 100 and 300 mcg/mL. See Table 13.2 for symptoms associated with salicylate poisoning.

Table 13.2 Symptoms of Salicylism	
Plasma Level of Salicylate	**Symptoms**
Levels greater than 150 mcg/mL (mild salicylism)	Tinnitus (ringing sound in the ear), difficulty hearing, dizziness, nausea, vomiting, diarrhea, mental confusion, central nervous system depression, headache, sweating, and hyperventilation (rapid, deep breathing)
Levels greater than 250 mcg/mL	Symptoms of mild salicylism plus headache, diarrhea, thirst, and flushing
Levels greater than 400 mcg/mL	Respiratory alkalosis, hemorrhage, excitement, confusion, asterixis (involuntary jerking movements especially of the hands), pulmonary edema, convulsions, tetany (muscle spasms), fever, coma, shock, and renal and respiratory failure

NURSING ALERT

Serious GI toxicity can cause bleeding, ulceration, and perforation and can occur at any time during therapy, with or without symptoms. Although minor GI distress may be common, remain alert for symptoms indicating ulceration and bleeding in patients receiving long-term therapy, even if no previous gastric symptoms have been experienced.

ACETAMINOPHEN. Acetaminophen should be taken with a full glass of water. The patient may take this drug with meals or on an empty stomach. Symptoms of overdosage include nausea, vomiting, diaphoresis, and generalized malaise.

NURSING ALERT

Studies suggest that the use of salicylates (especially aspirin) may be involved in the development of Reye's syndrome in children with chickenpox or influenza. This rare but life-threatening disorder is characterized by vomiting and lethargy, progressing to coma. Therefore, use of salicylates in children with chickenpox, fever, or flu-like symptoms is not recommended. Acetaminophen is recommended for managing symptoms associated with these disorders.

Monitoring and Managing Patient Needs

IMPAIRED COMFORT. If the patient is receiving the analgesic for reduction of elevated body temperature, teach caregivers to check the temperature immediately before and 45 to 60 minutes after administration of the drug. If a suppository form of the drug is used, it is important to check the patient after 30 minutes for retention of the suppository. If the drug fails to lower an elevated temperature, notify the primary health care provider because other means of temperature control, such as a cooling blanket, may be necessary. Patients can be made more comfortable by changing the clothing and bedding when it becomes damp because of the fluid loss during fever.

However, some health care providers may not prescribe an antipyretic for the patient with an elevated temperature because evidence suggests that fever is the result of the immune system's production of disease-fighting antibodies. The decision to treat an elevated temperature with an antipyretic is an individual one, based on the cause of the fever, the amount of discomfort to the patient, and the patient's physical condition.

PAIN. Teach the patient or caregiver to notify the primary health care provider if the salicylate or acetaminophen fails to relieve the patient's pain or discomfort. Give the salicylate with food, milk, or a full glass of water to prevent gastric upset. If gastric distress does not resolve with food or drink, you should notify the primary health care provider because other drug therapy may be necessary. An antacid may be prescribed to minimize GI distress. Ask the patient to check the color of the patient's stools. Black or dark stools or bright red blood in the stool may indicate GI bleeding. The patient should report any change in the color of stools to the primary health care provider.

LIFESPAN CONSIDERATIONS
Gerontology

Salicylates are prescribed for the pain and inflammation associated with arthritis. Because older adults have a higher incidence of both rheumatoid arthritis and osteoarthritis and may use the nonopioid analgesics on a long-term basis, they are particularly vulnerable to GI bleeding. Encourage the patient to take the drug with a full glass of water or with food because this may decrease the GI effects.

IMPAIRED PHYSICAL MOBILITY. The patient may have an acute or chronic disorder with varying degrees of mobility. The patient may be in acute pain or have long-standing mild to moderate pain. Along with the pain there may be skeletal deformities, such as the joint deformities seen with advanced rheumatoid arthritis. Considering the nature of the patient's condition, you may suggest physical therapy or occupational therapy consultation to recommend assistive devices to aid with ambulation or other activities of daily living.

RISK FOR POISONING. When patients contact you regarding fever, pain, or cold or flu symptoms, always ask what the patient has been using to treat the condition and for how long. Patients are not always aware of the medications that contain salicylates or acetaminophen that are not pain-relieving medications. By combining pain relievers and cold medications, a patient can inadvertently take more than the 3-gram maximum of acetaminophen for a couple of days before contacting the primary health care provider. Acute overdosage may be treated with administration of the drug acetylcysteine (Mucomyst) to prevent liver damage.

NURSING ALERT

Early diagnosis of acute acetaminophen toxicity is important because liver failure can be reversible. Toxicity is treated with gastric lavage, preferably within 4 hours of ingestion of the acetaminophen. Liver function studies are performed frequently. Acetylcysteine (Mucomyst) is an antidote to acetaminophen toxicity and acts by protecting liver cells and destroying acetaminophen metabolites. It is administered by nebulizer within 24 hours after ingestion of the drug and after the gastric lavage.

Teach the patient about the signs and symptoms of acute salicylate toxicity or salicylism when using aspirin. Initial treatment for an overdose of salicylates includes induction of emesis or gastric lavage to remove any unabsorbed drug from the stomach. Activated charcoal diminishes salicylate absorption if given within 2 hours of ingestion. Further therapy is supportive (reduce hyperthermia and treat severe convulsions with diazepam). Hemodialysis is effective in removing the salicylate but is used only in patients with severe salicylism.

Educating the Patient and Family

In some instances, a nonopioid analgesic may be prescribed for a prolonged period, such as when the patient has arthritis. Some patients may discontinue use of the drug, fail to take the drug at the prescribed or recommended intervals, increase the dose, or decrease the time interval between doses, especially if there is an increase or decrease in their symptoms. The patient and family should feel confident in their understanding of how the drug is to be taken. Instruct patients and family members on how to read and understand OTC medication labels (see Patient Teaching for Improved Patient Outcomes: Using Over-the-Counter Nonopioid Analgesic Drugs). Because patients frequently will begin use of OTC pain relievers before discussing with health care providers, develop teaching plans to include the following general points about these medications at any teaching session:

- Keep a record of when you take OTC pain relievers and notify the primary health care provider or dentist of use at your next office visit.
- Take the drug with food or a full glass of water unless indicated otherwise by the primary health care provider. If gastric upset occurs, take the drug with food or milk. If the problem persists, contact the primary health care provider.
- If the drug is used to reduce fever, contact the primary health care provider if the temperature continues to remain elevated for more than 24 hours.
- Do not self-treat chronic pain using an OTC nonopioid analgesic without first consulting the primary health care provider.
- All drugs deteriorate with age. Salicylates often deteriorate more rapidly than many other drugs. If there is a vinegar odor to the salicylate, discard the entire contents of the container.
- The ingredients of some OTC drugs include aspirin or acetaminophen. The name of the salicylate may not appear in the name of the drug, but it is listed on the label. Ask your health care provider before use of these products. Consult the clinical pharmacist about the product's ingredients if in doubt.
- If surgery or a dental procedure, such as tooth extraction or gum surgery, is anticipated, notify the primary health

care provider or dentist. Salicylates may be discontinued 1 week before the procedure because of the possibility of postoperative bleeding.
- If taking medication for arthritis, do not change from aspirin to acetaminophen without consulting the primary health care provider. Acetaminophen lacks the anti-inflammatory properties of aspirin.
- ♀ Avoid the use of alcoholic beverages.

Patient Teaching for Improved Patient Outcomes

Using Over-the-Counter Nonopioid Analgesic Drugs

Most nonopioid analgesics can be purchased without a prescription. A wide array of pain and fever reducers is readily available over-the-counter (OTC); therefore, a patient may be taking these medications for a period of time before consulting with a health care provider.

The potential for interaction with prescribed medications is high, especially when people view OTC preparations as harmless since they are readily available. This is why it is important for you to take any patient interaction as an opportunity to educate about these products.

When you teach, make sure your patient understands the following:

✔ Always read the label before you buy a product.
✔ What is the active ingredient? Are you taking that in any other drug?
✔ What is this drug supposed to do?
✔ Who should or should not take this drug?
✔ When should you consult your primary health care provider?
✔ Product tampering: Does the container still have a safety seal intact?
✔ How should this product be stored? Is it packaged in a safety container to prevent opening by children?

EVALUATION

- Therapeutic response is achieved, and pain is relieved.
- Adverse reactions are identified, reported to the primary health care provider, and managed successfully with appropriate nursing interventions:
  • Patient reports comfort without fever.
  • Discomfort is reduced or eliminated.
  • Patient maintains adequate mobility.
  • Toxic levels of medications are recognized before harm.
- Patient and family express confidence and demonstrate an understanding of the drug regimen.

PHARMACOLOGY IN PRACTICE
THINK CRITICALLY

 What assessments would be important for you to make regarding the aspirin product she is taking and her gastric complaints? What other medications should you ask Betty about that may contain either aspirin or acetaminophen? What questions would you ask and what information would you give Betty concerning Tylenol?

KEY POINTS

- Pain is the unpleasant sensory and emotional perception associated with actual or potential tissue damage.
- The sensation of pain is sent from the peripheral tissue to the brain where it is interpreted. Pain medications change the sensation in the tissues or modulate the signal in the brain.
- Acute pain has a short duration of less than 3 to 6 months, whereas chronic pain lasts more than 6 months.
- Salicylates and acetaminophen are used to treat mild to moderate pain and fever. Inflammation and blood thinning are additional properties of salicylates.
- Gastric distress is the primary adverse reaction of salicylates. Long-term users should be monitored for potential bleeding from the GI tract. Ringing in the ears (tinnitus) can be an early sign of salicylism (toxic reaction). Children should refrain from aspirin use due to Reye's syndrome.
- Acetaminophen is used because it has less gastric adverse reactions. The daily maximum amount is 3 grams and even less for those with liver function issues.
- Multiple OTC products contain salicylates or acetaminophen. Patients need confidence in understanding how to purchase and take these products since the majority of users do so without health care provider supervision.

Summary Drug Table NONOPIOID ANALGESICS: SALICYLATES AND NONSALICYLATES

Generic Name	Trade Name	Uses	Adverse Reactions	Dosage Ranges
Salicylates				
aspirin (acetylsalicylic acid) *ass'-purr-in*	Bayer, Ecotrin, Ecotrin (enteric coated), Empirin Buffered: Ascriptin, Asprimox, Bufferin, Alka-Seltzer with Aspirin	Analgesic, antipyretic, anti-inflammatory, stroke prevention in men (and women older than 65 only)	Nausea, vomiting, epigastric distress, gastrointestinal bleeding, tinnitus, allergic and anaphylactic reactions; salicylism with overuse	325–650 mg orally or rectally q 4 hr, up to 8 g/day
diflunisal *dye-floo'-ni-sal*		Same as aspirin	Same as aspirin	250–500 mg q 8–12 hr (maximum dose, 1.5 g/day)
magnesium salicylate *mag-nee'-see-um sal-ih'-sah-late*	Bufferin, Ecotrin	Same as aspirin	Same as aspirin	650 mg orally q 3 hr or 1090 mg TID
Nonsalicylate				
acetaminophen *a-sea-tah-min'-oh-fen*	Tempra, Tylenol (multiple trade names)	Analgesic, antipyretic	Rare when used as directed; skin eruptions, urticaria, hemolytic anemia, pancytopenia, jaundice, hepatotoxicity	325–650 mg/day orally q 4–6 hr; maximum dose, 3 g/day

● Chapter Review

Know Your Drugs

Clients sometimes know a medication by the brand (or trade) name and not the generic name. To help you recognize both names, match the brand name with the generic nonopioid pain reliever (either aspirin or acetaminophen) contained in the brand-name medication.

Generic Name	Brand Name
1. aspirin	A. Aspergum
2. acetaminophen	B. Cepacol
	C. Dayquil
	D. Pepto-Bismol
	E. Theraflu

Calculate Medication Dosages

1. The physician orders acetaminophen elixir 180 mg orally. Acetaminophen elixir is available in a 120-mg/mL solution. The nurse administers _____.

2. Aspirin 650 mg orally is prescribed. On hand is aspirin in 325-mg tablets. The nurse administers _____.

● Prepare for the NCLEX®

Build Your Knowledge

1. The best measurement of pain is:
   1. blood pressure
   2. medication plasma levels
   3. family observations
   4. client self-report

2. At a team conference, the nurse explains that the anti-inflammatory actions of the salicylates are most likely due to:
   1. a decrease in the prothrombin time
   2. a decrease in the production of endorphins
   3. the inhibition of prostaglandins
   4. vasodilation of the blood vessels

3. Which of the following symptoms would the nurse expect in a client experiencing salicylism?
   1. dizziness, tinnitus, mental confusion
   2. diarrhea, nausea, weight loss
   3. constipation, anorexia, rash
   4. weight gain, hyperglycemia, urinary frequency

4. When taking a salicylate, the drug is correctly administered:
   1. between meals
   2. with a carbonated beverage
   3. with food or milk
   4. dissolved in juice

5. While taking acetaminophen, clients who consume alcohol habitually are monitored by the nurse for symptoms of toxicity, which include:
   1. hypertension
   2. visual disturbances
   3. liver tenderness
   4. skin lesions

6. When hospitalized, which of the following drugs would the nurse most likely administer to a child with an elevated temperature?
   1. baby aspirin
   2. acetaminophen
   3. fenoprofen
   4. diflunisal

Apply Your Knowledge

7. A nurse instructs the client taking aspirin to avoid foods containing salicylates because this increases the risk of adverse reactions. Which foods should the client avoid?
   1. salt, soft drinks
   2. broccoli, milk
   3. prunes, tea
   4. liver, pepper

8. A client calls the clinic and tells the nurse a medication for aches smells like vinegar. The nurse's best response is:
   1. "Bring the medicine into the clinic"
   2. "Throw it away down your toilet"
   3. "Take it and let us know how your stomach feels in an hour"
   4. "Dispose of the drug where children and animals cannot get it"

Alternate-Format Questions

9. Teens seek cold remedies when visiting the school nurse's office. To assess for the amount of acetaminophen taken the nurse asks about which of the following products? **Select all that apply**.
   1. Actifed
   2. Alka-Seltzer Cold Tablets
   3. Bufferin
   4. Formula 44
   5. Sudafed

10. Look at the drug label provided; the maximum amount of drug would be met by how many tablets?

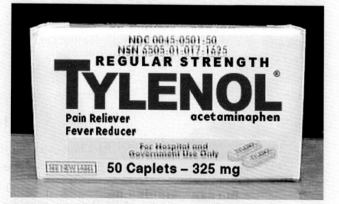

To check your answers, see Appendix G.

thePoint *For more NCLEX-style questions, log on to http://thepoint.lww.com to access more than 1000 questions.*

Nonopioid Analgesics: Nonsteroidal Anti-Inflammatory Drugs (NSAIDs) and Migraine Headache Medications

LEARNING OBJECTIVES

On completion of this chapter, the student will:

1. Discuss the importance of good pain assessment.
2. Describe standardized methods to assess pain in different patient populations.
3. Discuss the types, uses, general drug actions, common adverse reactions, contraindications, precautions, and interactions of the nonsteroidal anti-inflammatory drugs (NSAIDs).
4. Describe the types, general drug actions, common adverse reactions, contraindications, precautions, and interactions of drugs used to treat migraine headaches.
5. Discuss important preadministration and ongoing assessment activities the nurse should perform on the patient taking an NSAID.
6. List nursing diagnoses particular to a patient taking an NSAID.
7. Discuss the ways to promote an optimal response to therapy, how to manage common adverse reactions, and important points to keep in mind when educating patients about the use of NSAIDs.

KEY TERMS

cyclooxygenase • enzyme responsible for prostaglandin synthesis; contributes to integrity of stomach lining, pain, and inflammation

dysmenorrhea • painful cramping during menstruation

dysuria • painful or difficult urination

ecchymosis • bruise-like subcutaneous hemorrhage

fifth vital sign • inclusion of pain inquiry when temperature, pulse, respirations, and blood pressure readings are taken

jaundice • yellow discoloration of the skin due to liver disease

referred pain • pain felt in an area remote from the site of origin, possibly along the same dermatome

oliguria • reduced urine output

phenylketonuria (PKU) • a genetic birth defect causing the amino acid phenylalanine to build up to toxic levels in the body

polyuria • increased urination

purpura • excessive skin hemorrhage causing red-purple patches under the skin

somnolence • excessive drowsiness or sleepiness

stomatitis • inflammation of a cavity opening, such as the oral cavity

transient ischemic attack (TIA) • temporary interference with blood supply to the brain causing symptoms related to the portion of the brain affected (i.e., temporary blindness, aphasia, dizziness, numbness, difficulty swallowing, or paresthesias); may last a few moments to several hours, after which no residual neurologic damage is evident

DRUG CLASSES

Nonsteroidal anti-inflammatory	Selective serotonin agonists

PHARMACOLOGY IN PRACTICE

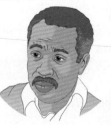

Mr. Park has osteoarthritis and has been taking buffered aspirin for almost a year. He is confused at times and has difficulty hearing; his hearing loss concerns his daughter, who is visiting from the coast. As you read about pain assessment and the NSAID drugs, consider whether changing to celecoxib for the osteoarthritis pain would be a consideration.

Because of the mode of action of nonsteroidal anti-inflammatory drugs (NSAIDs), some texts include the salicylates in the NSAID group. Although the chemical and physiologic effects are similar, this text discusses the salicylates in a separate chapter (see Chapter 13). Since NSAIDs are nonopioid analgesics like the salicylates, the NSAIDs have anti-inflammatory, antipyretic, and analgesic effects. The NSAIDs have emerged as important drugs in the treatment of the chronic pain and inflammation associated with disorders such as rheumatoid arthritis and osteoarthritis. Patients experiencing either acute or chronic pain are often undertreated because of an inadequate assessment. In this chapter pain assessment as well as general information on the NSAIDs is covered. NSAIDs are used for mild to moderate pain and are primarily taken on an outpatient basis; these drugs are listed in the Summary Drug Table: Nonsteroidal Anti-Inflammatory Drugs and Migraine Medications.

Pain Assessment

A key nursing role in administering pain relievers is a careful assessment of pain and the monitoring of the patient's response to the pain medications. Over time pain assessment has taken a prominent place in any basic patient encounter. It is often considered the "**fifth vital sign**" in nursing assessment. To perform this component of your vital sign routine, two basic measures are needed in any pain assessment: location and intensity. Assessment of location helps the primary health care provider prescribe drugs that target the pain peripherally or centrally. The strength of the analgesic is determined by the patient's report of the pain intensity.

The intensity of pain is subjective and individualized. Due to this subjectivity, it is sometimes difficult to measure objectively the signs of pain that match the level of distress reported by the patient. The patient's description of pain should always be taken seriously. Because failure to assess pain adequately is a major factor in the undertreatment of pain, guidelines to help you form questions to ask the patient about pain are listed in Display 14.1.

Barriers to Assessment and Treatment

Pain management in acute and chronic illness is an important responsibility in nursing. As pain managers, you need to be aware of and overcome the three main barriers to proper pain management having to do with assessment, intervention, and evaluation:

- Primary health care providers do not prescribe proper pain medicine doses.
- Nurses do not administer adequate medication for relief of pain.
- Patients do not report accurate levels of pain.

You can lessen these barriers to good pain management by showing sensitivity to patient needs and learning techniques to conduct a good assessment.

Assessment Technique

As noted earlier, to prescribe effective analgesics for pain, the primary health care provider needs two key assessments

---

> ### *Display 14.1* Guidelines and Questions for a Pain Assessment
>
> Known as the *fifth vital sign,* the assessment of pain is just as important as the assessment of temperature, pulse, respirations, and blood pressure. The following points help to guide your ability to assess pain.
>
> **Assessment Guidelines**
> - Patient's subjective description of the pain (What does the pain feel like?)
> - Location(s) of the pain
> - Intensity, severity, and duration
> - Any factors that influence the pain
> - Quality of the pain
> - Patterns of coping
> - Effects of previous therapy (if applicable)
> - Nurses' observations of patient's behavior
>
> **Sample Assessment Questions**
> Questions to include in the assessment of pain may include the following:
>
> - Does the pain keep you awake at night? Prevent you from falling asleep or staying asleep?
> - What makes your pain worse? What makes it better?
> - Can you describe what your pain feels like? Sharp, stabbing, burning, or throbbing?
> - Does the pain affect your mood? Are you depressed? Irritable? Anxious?
> - What over-the-counter or herbal remedies have you used for the pain?
> - Does the pain affect your activity level? Are you able to walk? Perform self-care activities?

about pain: location and intensity. To assess location, ask the patient to describe or point to where the pain is at; be cautious of labeling the pain, since pain on the jaw could be from either a tooth ache or **referred pain**. Help teach your patients to describe their pain (see Patient Teaching for Improved Patient Outcomes: Talking to Providers About Pain at the end of the chapter).

Standardized pain measurement tools are used to provide consistency in assessing intensity (see examples in Fig. 14.1). The most common method used is to have a patient rate the pain on a scale of 0 to 10, with 0 being "no pain" and 10 being the "most severe pain imagined" by the patient.

Some population groups are known to have difficulty in assigning a number value to pain. For these patients it is hard to think about their pain experience in a quantitative manner, like assigning a number to it. Display 14.2 gives examples of populations you should note may need alternate pain assessment tools. As with any group or individual suspected of limited health literacy, alternate ways to describe pain intensity are offered. All these tools help to assess the pain of patients no matter whether they are being treated with strong opioids or nonopioid analgesics such as the NSAIDs.

Pain intensity scales

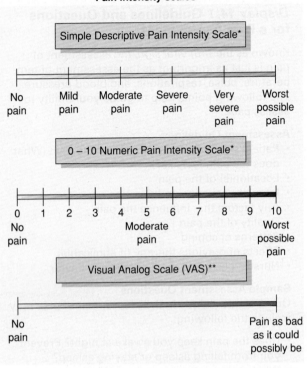

* If used as a graphic rating scale, a 10-cm baseline is recommended.
** A 10-cm baseline is recommended for VAS scales.

Figure 14.1 Examples of standardized pain assessment tools. (From Smeltzer SC, Bare BG. *Brunnar & Suddarth's textbook of medical-surgical nursing* [9th ed.]. Philadelphia: Lippincott Williams & Wilkins, 2000.)

NONSTEROIDAL ANTI-INFLAMMATORY DRUGS

Actions

The NSAIDs are so named because they have anti-inflammatory effects, but they do not belong to the steroidal group of substances and thus do not possess the adverse reactions

---

Display 14.2 Populations at Higher Risk for Poor Pain Assessment

Patients at risk for inadequate pain management are frequently those who are not assessed well. Consider using standardized visual analog tools to assess pain in these high-risk patient populations:

- Infants and children
- Older adults, especially those cognitively impaired
- Developmentally disabled children and adults
- Those with communication problems such as limited English proficiency or limited health literacy
- Those unable to communicate due to the illness or treatment process

---

associated with the steroids (see Chapter 43). In addition, NSAIDs have analgesic and antipyretic properties. Although their exact mechanisms of action are not known, the NSAIDs are thought to inhibit prostaglandin synthesis by blocking the action of the enzyme **cyclooxygenase**, an enzyme responsible for prostaglandin synthesis. The NSAIDs also inhibit the activity of two related enzymes:

- *cyclooxygenase-1* (COX-1), an enzyme that helps to maintain the stomach lining
- *cyclooxygenase-2* (COX-2), an enzyme that triggers pain and inflammation

The traditional NSAIDs, such as ibuprofen and naproxen, are thought to regulate pain and inflammation by blocking COX-2. However, these drugs also inhibit COX-1, the enzyme that helps maintain the lining of the stomach. When NSAIDs are taken they block the effects of COX-2, producing pain relief, but they also block the effects of COX-1, which in turn produces adverse reactions. This inhibition of COX-1 causes unwanted gastrointestinal (GI) reactions such as stomach irritation and ulcers. Combination drugs (that include a proton pump inhibitor) are being used to reduce the risk of gastric and duodenal ulcers.

The NSAID celecoxib (Celebrex) appears to work by specifically inhibiting the COX-2 enzyme without inhibiting the COX-1 enzyme. Celecoxib relieves pain and inflammation with less potential for GI adverse reactions.

> **! NURSING ALERT**
> Celecoxib is associated with an increased risk of serious cardiovascular thrombosis, myocardial infarction, and stroke, all of which can be fatal. All NSAIDs may carry a similar risk. Always question the patient regarding a history of risk for actual cardiovascular disease before administering NSAIDs. Because of this risk, celecoxib should not be used to relieve postoperative pain from a coronary artery bypass graft (CABG).

Uses

The NSAIDs are used for the treatment of the following:

- Pain associated with musculoskeletal disorders such as osteoarthritis and rheumatoid arthritis
- Mild to moderate pain
- Primary **dysmenorrhea** (menstrual cramps)
- Fever (reduction)

Adverse Reactions

Gastrointestinal System Reactions

- Nausea, vomiting, dyspepsia
- Anorexia, dry mouth
- Diarrhea, constipation
- Epigastric pain, indigestion, abdominal distress or discomfort, bloating
- Intestinal ulceration, **stomatitis**
- **Jaundice**

Central Nervous System Reactions

- Dizziness, anxiety, lightheadedness, vertigo
- Headache

- Drowsiness, **somnolence** (sleepiness), insomnia
- Confusion, depression
- Stroke, psychic disturbances

Cardiovascular System Reactions

- Decrease or increase in blood pressure
- Congestive heart failure, cardiac arrhythmias
- Myocardial infarction

Renal System Reactions

- **Polyuria** (excessive urination), **dysuria** (painful urination), **oliguria** (reduced urine output)
- Hematuria (blood in the urine), cystitis
- Elevated blood urea nitrogen (BUN)
- Acute renal failure in those with impaired renal function

Hematologic System Reactions

- Pancytopenia (reduction in blood cell components), thrombocytopenia (reduced platelet count)
- Neutropenia (abnormally few neutrophils), eosinophilia (low eosinophil count), leukopenia (reduced white blood cell count), agranulocytosis (reduced granulocyte count)
- Aplastic anemia

Integumentary System Reactions

- Rash, erythema (redness), irritation, skin eruptions
- **Ecchymosis** (subcutaneous hemorrhage), **purpura** (excessive skin hemorrhage causing red-purple patches under the skin)
- Exfoliative dermatitis, Stevens-Johnson syndrome

Metabolic/Endocrine System Reactions

- Decreased appetite, weight increase or decrease
- Flushing, sweating
- Menstrual disorders, vaginal bleeding
- Hyperglycemia or hypoglycemia (high or low blood sugar)

Sensory and Other Reactions

- Taste change
- Rhinitis (runny nose)
- Tinnitus (ringing in the ears)
- Visual disturbances, blurred or diminished vision, diplopia (double vision), swollen or irritated eyes, photophobia (sensitivity to light), reversible loss of color vision
- Thirst, fever, chills
- Vaginitis

Contraindications

The NSAIDs are contraindicated in patients with known hypersensitivity. There is a cross-sensitivity to other NSAIDs, meaning if a patient is allergic to one NSAID, there is an increased risk of an allergic reaction with any other NSAID. Hypersensitivity to aspirin is a contraindication for all NSAIDs. In general, NSAIDs are contraindicated during the third trimester of pregnancy and during lactation. Some NSAIDs are not used to treat rheumatoid arthritis or osteoarthritis; these include ketorolac, mefenamic, and meloxicam.

Celecoxib is contraindicated in patients who are allergic to sulfonamides or have a history of cardiac disease or stroke. Ibuprofen is contraindicated in those who have hypertension, peptic ulceration, or GI bleeding.

Precautions

The NSAIDs should be used cautiously during pregnancy (pregnancy category B), by older adults (increased risk of ulcer formation in patients older than 65 years), and by patients with bleeding disorders, renal disease, cardiovascular disease, or hepatic impairment.

Interactions

The following interactions may occur when an NSAID is administered with another agent:

Interacting Drug	Common Use	Effect of Interaction
anticoagulants	Blood thinner	Increased risk of bleeding
lithium	Antipsychotic drug used for bipolar disorder	Increased effectiveness and possible toxicity of lithium
cyclosporine	Antirejection agent (immunosuppressant)	Increased effectiveness of cyclosporine
hydantoins	Anticonvulsant	Increased effectiveness of anticonvulsant
diuretics	Excretion of extra body fluid	Decreased effectiveness of diuretic
antihypertensive drugs	Blood pressure control	Decreased effectiveness of antihypertensive drug
acetaminophen in long-term use	Pain relief	Increased risk of renal impairment

❦ HERBAL CONSIDERATIONS

Capsicum (hot pepper) has been cultivated in almost every society. Peppers are valued as a spice and flavoring for food. Capsaicin is the substance in peppers that, when applied topically, produces sensations varying from warmth to burning. For years, herbalists assumed that capsaicin worked by simply dilating blood vessels and increasing the supply of nutrients to injured joints. That may be a factor, but capsaicin actually works in a very different way.

People suffering from osteoarthritis have elevated levels of decapeptide substance P (DSP) in their blood and in the synovial fluid that bathes their joints. DSP has two undesirable functions. First, it breaks down the cartilage cushions in joints, contributing to osteoarthritis. Second, it serves as a pain neurotransmitter in both osteoarthritis and rheumatoid arthritis.

Researchers have discovered that capsaicin inhibits the activity of DSP. A cream containing capsaicin, when rubbed on the skin, penetrates to arthritic joints, where it stops the destruction of cartilage, relieves pain, and increases flexibility. Side effects include a localized burning sensation during the first few weeks of use, which diminishes with continued application.

People suffering from ulcers are usually warned to avoid spicy foods. But new research suggests that capsaicin produces the opposite effect—that capsaicin might actually protect against peptic ulcers. A number of experiments over the years have found that capsaicin protects the gastric mucosal membrane against damage from alcohol and aspirin (DerMarderosian, 2003).

DRUGS USED IN THE TREATMENT OF MIGRAINE HEADACHES

Pain associated with migraine headaches is believed to be caused by vascular spasms. Drugs used to treat migraine headaches are given (1) prophylactically to prevent the spasms or (2) to treat the acute pain when a migraine occurs. The mechanism of action and classification of the drugs to prevent migraine headaches are different from those used to treat the acute pain of the migraine attack. Prophylactic treatment may include drugs from the following categories: beta (β) blockers (see Chapter 25), calcium channel blockers (see Chapter 35), antidepressant medications (see Chapter 22), or anticonvulsant drugs (see Chapter 29). The selective serotonin (5-HT) agonists used to relieve the acute pain are covered in this chapter and are listed in the Summary Drug Table: Nonsteroidal Anti-Inflammatory Drugs and Migraine Medications.

Actions and Uses

The symptoms of migraine headaches are believed to be caused by local cranial vasodilation and stimulation of trigeminal nerves. Activation of the 5-HT receptors causes vasoconstriction and reduces the neurotransmission, which in turn produces pain relief. Selective serotonin drugs are used for the relief of moderate to severe pain and inflammation related to migraine headaches. Because reduced GI motility can happen during a migraine event, delayed absorption of oral drugs may occur and alternative routes of administration are needed: rectal, internasal, or subcutaneous injection.

Adverse Reactions

These agents are generally well tolerated, with most adverse reactions mild and transient. The most common are dizziness, nausea, fatigue, pain, dry mouth, and flushing.

Cardiovascular System Reactions

• Coronary artery vasospasm
• Cardiac arrhythmias and tachycardia
• Myocardial infarction

Contraindications and Precautions

These drugs are contraindicated in patients with a known hypersensitivity to selective serotonin agonists and should only be used when a clear diagnosis of migraine headache has been established. 5-HT agonists should not be used in patients with ischemic heart disease (such as angina or myocardial infarction), **transient ischemic attacks** (TIAs), or uncontrolled hypertension or those patients taking monoamine oxidase inhibitor (MAOI) antidepressants. These drugs should be used cautiously in patients with hepatic or renal function impairment, such as the elderly or patients requiring dialysis. Because these are pregnancy category C drugs, they should only be used during pregnancy when the benefit outweighs the risk to the fetus. Caution should be exercised when administering them to lactating mothers.

The ergot derivatives (see Summary Drug Table: Nonsteroidal Anti-Inflammatory Drugs and Migraine Medications) should not be used by HIV patients using protease inhibitors or patients taking macrolide antibiotics due to the risk of peripheral ischemia.

Interactions

The following interactions may occur when a selective serotonin drug is administered with another agent:

Interacting Drug	Common Use	Effect of Interaction
cimetidine	Decrease gastric secretions	Increased effectiveness of the 5-HT agonist
oral contraceptives	Birth control	Increased effectiveness of the 5-HT agonist

NURSING PROCESS

PATIENT RECEIVING A NONSTEROIDAL ANTI-INFLAMMATORY DRUG OR MIGRAINE MEDICATION

ASSESSMENT

Preadministration Assessment

Before administering an NSAID, you need to determine if the patient has any history of allergy to aspirin or any other NSAID. Determine if the patient has a history of GI bleeding, cardiovascular disease, stroke, hypertension, peptic ulceration, or impaired hepatic or renal function. If so, notify the primary health care provider before administering an NSAID.

Before giving an NSAID to a patient, assess and document the following information: type, onset, intensity, and location of the pain. Teach the patient how to rate their pain using one of the standardized pain scales. A visual analog tool known as the Wong-Baker FACES scale (shown in Fig. 14.2) can be used for those who find it difficult to quantify pain numerically. There are many of these visual tools that can be useful with scales made of colors or facial expressions. Reassure patients that health care providers want to know about the pain episode and consistent measurement makes it easier to treat (see Patient Teaching for Improved Patient Outcomes: Talking to Providers About Pain).

It is important to determine if this problem is different in any way from previous episodes of pain or discomfort. If the patient is receiving an NSAID for arthritis, a musculoskeletal disorder, or soft tissue inflammation, examine the

Figure 14.2 Wong-Baker FACES™ Pain Rating Scale. (© 1983, Wong-Baker FACES™ Foundation, www. WongBakerFACES.org. Used with permission, originally published in *Whaley & Wong's nursing care of infants and children.* © Elsevier Inc.)

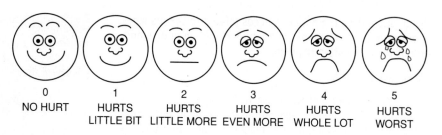

0	1	2	3	4	5
NO HURT	HURTS LITTLE BIT	HURTS LITTLE MORE	HURTS EVEN MORE	HURTS WHOLE LOT	HURTS WORST

joints or areas involved. The appearance of the skin over the joint or affected area or any limitation of motion is documented. Ask the patient about changes in the ability to carry out activities of daily living. This information is used to develop a care plan, as well as to evaluate the response to drug therapy.

Patient Teaching for Improved Patient Outcomes

Talking to Providers About Pain

Frequently patients are asked about pain, yet teaching the patient the essentials of measuring pain infrequently happens until the person is in a painful situation. Here are some principles to cover with a patient at any encounter so he or she is prepared to discuss pain when it happens.

When you teach, make sure your patient understands the following:

✔ Tell your provider where the pain is at. Not all pain originates from the area that hurts. Pain can be referred to a different area; for example, gallbladder inflammation might present as pain in the shoulder.

✔ Tell your provider how much it hurts. Intensity is measured using standardized scales so everyone treats your pain the same. Learn to rate your pain on a scale of 0 to 10, with 0 being "no pain" and 10 being the "most severe pain imagined" by the patient.

✔ Tell your provider what the most severe pain you can imagine is; this will help your health care provider gauge how well you handle pain.

✔ If you can't measure pain with a number, there are other ways you can show how much it hurts. There are many scales, called visual analog scales, you can use when you just don't think about pain as a number. You can use *mild*, *moderate*, or *severe pain* if those terms help you describe your pain. If you use a pain tool, bring it with you so your pain is measured consistently.

✔ How do you express that you are in pain? Some people are very stoic and may not show pain with moans or facial grimacing until the pain is hard to tolerate. How do you react when you hurt—do you withdraw or become irritable? Tell us what to look for when you have pain.

✔ What is your pain pattern? Are there times it hurts less or more? How does pain affect your activities?

✔ What helps? What do you do to make the pain tolerable? What have you tried that makes it worse? We don't want to do something to hurt you more.

LIFESPAN CONSIDERATIONS
Pediatric

Ibuprofen is available to individuals as an over-the-counter (OTC) drug that may be purchased without a prescription. When assessing patients with pain, you should ask what medications the patient is currently taking or has tried for pain relief already. Because of the risk of Reye's syndrome from aspirin, ibuprofen is used in treatment of children with juvenile arthritis and for fever reduction in children 6 months to 12 years of age.

Ongoing Assessment

Drugs used for mild to moderate pain are primarily administered at home or in long-term care settings. The responsibility of monitoring the relief of pain falls upon the patient or caregiver in these settings with follow-up made by a nurse. You should instruct the patient or caregiver to reassess the patient's pain 30 to 60 minutes after administration of the drug, and emphasize using the same pain rating tool the patient chooses to use. If pain persists, it is important to note its severity, location, and intensity and relay this information to the nurse or primary health care provider. Hot, dry, flushed skin and a decrease in urinary output may develop if temperature elevation is prolonged; consequently, dehydration can occur. Ask the patient or caregiver to make note if these problems arise and the patient is at risk for dehydration. Also instruct how to monitor joints for a decrease in inflammation and greater mobility. Provide instruction, using written materials in the preferred language to explain adverse reactions, such as unusual or prolonged bleeding or dark-colored stools, and when to report these observations to the primary health care provider.

NURSING DIAGNOSES

Drug-specific nursing diagnoses are the following:

■ **Acute or Chronic Pain** related to peripheral tissue damage caused by the disease process or GI bleeding or inflammation from NSAID therapy

■ **Impaired Physical Mobility** related to muscle and joint stiffness

■ **Risk for Injury** related to adverse reaction of NSAID causing damage to optical field

■ **Impaired Skin Integrity** related to photosensitivity when using 5-HT agonists

Nursing diagnoses related to drug administration are discussed in Chapter 4.

PLANNING

The expected outcomes for the patient depend on the reason for administration of the NSAID but may include an optimal response to drug therapy, which includes relief of pain and

Nonopioid Analgesics

fever; supporting the patient's needs related to the management of adverse reactions; and confidence in an understanding of the medication regimen.

IMPLEMENTATION

Promoting an Optimal Response to Therapy

A majority of the NSAID medications are taken in the outpatient setting; therefore, patient teaching is an important nursing task. Teach the patient to take the NSAID with food, milk, or antacids. Patients who do not experience adequate pain relief using one NSAID may have success using another NSAID. However, several weeks of treatment may be necessary to achieve full therapeutic response.

 CHRONIC CARE CONSIDERATIONS

Migraine headache sufferers with **phenylketonuria (PKU)** should be informed that rizatriptan (Maxalt) and zolmitriptan (Zomig) contain phenylalanine and should be avoided.

SUMATRIPTAN INJECTION FOR MIGRAINE HEADACHE PAIN. Administration of sumatriptan should be just below the skin in the subcutaneous tissue. This drug should be given at the onset of the headache but can be administered any time during the attack. A second injection can be delivered after 1 hour if pain has not been relieved. The drug is dispensed in prefilled syringes, which should be used for only one injection and disposed of properly, even if the entire amount in the syringe is not used. No more than two injections should be given in any 24-hour period. You should observe the patient administering his or her first dose of sumatriptan by subcutaneous injection to be sure proper technique is used.

Monitoring and Managing Patient Needs

PAIN. NSAIDs are prescribed for the pain and inflammation associated with arthritis. Because older adults have a higher incidence of both rheumatoid arthritis and osteoarthritis and may use the NSAID on a long-term basis, they are particularly vulnerable to GI bleeding. Encourage the patient to take the drug with a full (8-ounce) glass of water or with food, because this may decrease adverse GI effects.

 LIFESPAN CONSIDERATIONS
Gerontology

Age appears to increase the possibility of adverse reactions to the NSAIDs. The risk of serious ulcer disease in adults older than 65 years is increased with higher doses of the NSAIDs. Use greater care and begin with reduced dosages in older patients, increasing the dosage slowly.

IMPAIRED PHYSICAL MOBILITY. Teach caregivers to provide comfort measures to the patient with pain in the limbs or joints affected by the various musculoskeletal disorders. Support limbs with proper positioning; applications of heat or cold, joint rest, and avoidance of joint overuse are additional comfort measures. Various orthopedic devices, such as splints and braces, may be used to support inflamed joints. The use of assistive mobility devices, such as canes, crutches, and walkers, eases pain by limiting movement or stress from weight bearing on painful joints. Walking with a physically impaired patient gives you the opportunity to encourage ambulation

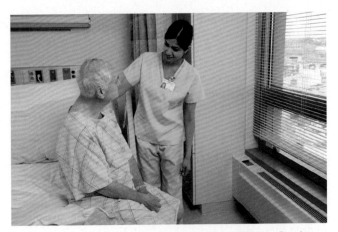

Figure 14.3 The nurse assesses the effects of pain medication while assisting the elderly patient with ambulation.

as well as assess the increase in function provided by the NSAIDs (Fig. 14.3). Patients with osteoarthritis using NSAIDs should exhibit an increased range of motion and a reduction in tenderness, pain, stiffness, and swelling.

It is important to teach the patient receiving an NSAID about adverse drug reactions throughout therapy. GI reactions are the most common and can be severe, especially in those prone to upper GI tract disease. Cardiovascular reactions can be severe and even lead to death. Because of the severity of some of these adverse drug reactions, instruct the patient to notify the primary health care provider of any complaints.

❗ NURSING ALERT

Instruct the patient and caregivers that sudden or extremely painful gastric or cardiac symptoms may indicate an emergent problem. In these situations, patients should contact emergency services immediately and withhold the next dose.

RISK FOR INJURY. NSAIDs may cause visual disturbances, which can lead to an injury. Report any complaints of blurred or diminished vision or changes in color vision to the primary health care provider. Corneal deposits and retinal disturbances may also occur. The primary health care provider may discontinue therapy if ocular changes are noted. Blurred vision may be significant and warrants thorough examination. Because visual changes may be asymptomatic, patients on long-term therapy require periodic eye examinations.

IMPAIRED SKIN INTEGRITY: PHOTOSENSITIVITY. The skin can become more sensitive to sunlight when a patient takes 5-HT agonists for migraine headache pain relief. Patients should be cautioned to wear protective clothing and sunscreen when outside. Teach patients that exposure to ultraviolet light in tanning salons can also cause a reaction; therefore, tanning should be discouraged when using these drugs until tolerance is determined.

Educating the Patient and Family

In many instances, an NSAID may be prescribed for a prolonged period, such as when the patient has arthritis. Some patients may discontinue their drug use, fail to take the drug at the prescribed or recommended intervals, increase the dose, or decrease the time interval between doses, especially if there is an increase or decrease in their symptoms. The patient and family should feel confident in understanding that the drug is to be taken even though symptoms have been relieved and the patient may be pain free. As you develop a teaching plan include the following information:

- Take the drug exactly as prescribed by the primary health care provider. Do not increase or decrease the dosage, and do not take aspirin, other salicylates, or any OTC drugs without first consulting the primary health care provider. Notify the primary health care provider or dentist if pain is not relieved.

- Take the drug with food or a full glass of water unless indicated otherwise by the primary health care provider. If gastric upset occurs, take the drug with food or milk. If the problem persists, contact the primary health care provider.

- Whether taking an NSAID on a regular or occasional basis, inform all health care providers, including dentists, that you are taking it.

- If the drug is used to reduce fever, contact the primary health care provider if the temperature remains elevated for more than 24 hours after beginning therapy. Severe or recurrent pain or high or continued fever may indicate serious illness. If pain persists more than 10 days in adults, or if fever persists more than 3 days, consult the primary health care provider.

- Do not self-treat chronic pain with an OTC nonopioid analgesic; consult your primary health care provider.

- The drug may take several days to produce an effect (relief of pain and tenderness). If some or all of the symptoms are not relieved after 2 weeks of therapy, continue taking the drug, but notify the primary health care provider.

- These drugs may cause drowsiness, dizziness, or blurred vision. Use caution while driving or performing tasks that require alertness.

- Notify the primary health care provider if any of the following adverse reactions occur: skin rash, itching, visual disturbances, weight gain, edema, diarrhea, black stools, nausea, vomiting, chest/leg pain, numbness, or persistent headache.

Instructions for using selective serotonin agonists for migraine headache pain include the following:

- These drugs are used to treat actual migraine headache pain; they will not prevent or reduce the number of migraine headaches.

- Administer the drug at the onset of migraine symptoms. Doses can be repeated one time after 1 hour (2 hours for nasal spray).

- Never take more than two doses in a 24-hour period. Notify the primary health care provider when the headache is not relieved.

EVALUATION

- Therapeutic response is achieved and discomfort is reduced.

- Adverse reactions are identified, reported to the primary health care provider, and managed successfully with appropriate nursing interventions:
  - Patient reports reduced or eliminated pain.
  - Patient reports improved mobility.
  - Patient is free of injury or uses adaptive devices for visual deficits.
  - Skin is intact and free of inflammation, irritation, or ulcerations.

- Patient and family express confidence and demonstrate an understanding of the drug regimen.

PHARMACOLOGY IN PRACTICE
THINK CRITICALLY

With the information learned about the patient pain experience and assessment of pain, discuss how you would perform a pain assessment with Mr. Park. What history of pain treatment is important for you to gather to help the primary health care provider determine the best pain management strategies for Mr. Park?

KEY POINTS

- A key component to good pain management is the pain assessment. Location and intensity are the basic components of an assessment.

- The sensation of pain is subjective—effort is taken with standardized pain measurement tools to help the patient relay information needed to provide pain relief.

- NSAIDs reduce inflammation differently than steroids by inhibiting prostaglandins. NSAIDs are used to treat mild to moderate pain, fever, and inflammation. They are used to treat a variety of chronic musculoskeletal disorders.

- These drugs also block an enzyme that maintains the stomach lining; therefore, GI adverse reactions are common. Patients also need to be monitored for serious cardiovascular problems such as thrombosis, myocardial infarction, and stroke.

- Migraine headaches are believed to be caused by vascular spasms. Selective serotonin agonists work to relieve the acute pain associated with the headache; they do not prevent the migraine attack.

Summary Drug Table NONOPIOID ANALGESICS: NONSTEROIDAL ANTI-INFLAMMATORY DRUGS AND MIGRAINE HEADACHE MEDICATIONS

Generic Name	Trade Name	Uses	Adverse Reactions	Dosage Ranges
diclofenac *dye-kloe'-fen-ak*	Cambia, Cataflam, Flector (transdermal), Voltaren, Zipsor	Acute or chronic pain of rheumatoid arthritis, osteoarthritis, ankylosing spondylitis, and dysmenorrhea	Nausea, gastric or duodenal ulcer formation, GI bleeding	50–200 mg orally divided into 2 or 3 doses
etodolac *ee-toe-doe'-lak*		Osteoarthritis, rheumatoid arthritis, and acute pain	Dizziness, nausea, dyspepsia, rash, constipation, bleeding, diarrhea, tinnitus	300–500 mg BID; maximum daily dose 1200 mg
fenoprofen *fen-oh-proe'-fen*	Nalfon	Same as etodolac	Same as etodolac	300–600 mg orally 3 or 4 times daily; maximum daily dose 3.2 g
flurbiprofen *flure-bih'-proe-fen*	Ansaid	Same as etodolac	Same as etodolac	Up to 300 mg/day orally in divided doses
ibuprofen *eye-byoo'-proe-fen*	Advil, Motrin, Nuprin	Mild to moderate pain, rheumatoid disorders, dysmenorrhea, fever	Nausea, dizziness, dyspepsia, gastric or duodenal ulcer, GI bleeding, headache	400 mg orally q 4–6 hr; maximum daily dose 3.2 g
indomethacin *in-doe-meth'-ah-sin*	Indocin	Rheumatoid disorders	Nausea, constipation, gastric or duodenal ulcer, GI bleeding, hematologic changes	25–50 mg orally, 3 to 4 times daily
ketoprofen *kee-toe-proe'-fen*		Mild to moderate pain, rheumatoid disorders, dysmenorrhea, aches and fever	Dizziness, visual disturbances, nausea, constipation, vomiting, diarrhea, gastric or duodenal ulcer formation, GI bleeding	12.5–75 mg orally TID
ketorolac *kee'-toe-roll-ak*		Moderate to severe acute pain	Dyspepsia, nausea, GI pain and bleeding	Single dose: 60 mg IM or 30 mg IV Multiple dosing: 10 mg q 4–6 hr; maximum daily dose 40 mg
meclofenamate *meh-kloe-fen-am'-ate*		Rheumatoid arthritis, mild to moderate pain, dysmenorrhea with heavy menstrual flow	Headache, dizziness, tiredness, insomnia, nausea, dyspepsia, constipation, rash, bleeding	50–400 mg orally q 4–6 hr, maximum dose 400 mg/day
mefenamic *meh-feh-nam'-ick*	Ponstel	Episodic acute mild to moderate pain (less than 1 wk duration)	Dizziness, tiredness, nausea, dyspepsia, rash, constipation, bleeding, diarrhea	250–500 mg q 6 hr
meloxicam *mel-ox'-ih-kam*	Mobic	Osteoarthritis	Nausea, dyspepsia, GI pain, headache, dizziness, somnolence, insomnia, rash	7.5–15 mg/day orally
nabumetone *nah-byoo'-meh-tone*		Rheumatoid arthritis and osteoarthritis	Dizziness, tiredness, nausea, dyspepsia, rash, constipation, bleeding, diarrhea	1000–2000 mg/day orally
naproxen *nah-prox'-en*	Aleve, Anaprox, Naprosyn, Naprelan	Rheumatoid arthritis, juvenile arthritis, osteoarthritis, mild to moderate pain, dysmenorrhea, general aches and fever	Dizziness, headache, nausea, vomiting, gastric or duodenal ulcer, GI bleeding	250–500 mg q 6–8 hr orally; maximum daily dose 1.25 g

Summary Drug Table NONOPIOID ANALGESICS: NONSTEROIDAL ANTI-INFLAMMATORY DRUGS AND MIGRAINE HEADACHE MEDICATIONS (continued)

Generic Name	Trade Name	Uses	Adverse Reactions	Dosage Ranges
oxaprozin *ox-ah-proe'-zin*	Daypro	Rheumatoid arthritis and osteoarthritis	Dizziness, nausea, dyspepsia, rash, constipation, GI bleeding, diarrhea	1200 mg/day orally
piroxicam *peer-ox'-ih-kam*	Feldene	Mild to moderate pain, rheumatoid arthritis and osteoarthritis	Nausea, vomiting, diarrhea, gastric or duodenal ulcer, GI bleeding	20 mg/day orally as a single dose or 10 mg orally BID
sulindac *soo-lin'-dak*		Mild to moderate pain, rheumatoid arthritis, ankylosing spondylitis, osteoarthritis, gouty arthritis	Nausea, vomiting, diarrhea, constipation, gastric or duodenal ulcer, GI bleeding	150–200 mg orally BID
tolmetin *toll'-meh-tin*		Rheumatoid arthritis, juvenile arthritis, and osteoarthritis	Nausea, vomiting, diarrhea, constipation, gastric or duodenal ulcer, GI bleeding	400 mg orally TID or BID; maximum daily dose 1800 mg
NSAID Combinations				
diclofenac/ misoprostol	Arthrotec	Same as diclofenac with gastric/duodenal ulcer protection	Nausea, heartburn, diarrhea	50 mg/200 mcg orally divided into 2 or 3 doses
ibuprofen/famotidine	Duexis	Same as ibuprofen with gastric/duodenal ulcer protection	Nausea, heartburn, diarrhea	1 tablet orally 3 times daily
naproxen/ esomeprazole	Vimovo	Same as naproxen with gastric/duodenal ulcer protection	Nausea, heartburn, diarrhea	1 tablet orally daily
naproxen/ lansoprazole	Prevacid NapraPAC	Same as naproxen with gastric/duodenal ulcer protection	Nausea, heartburn, diarrhea	Packet containing 1 capsule/2 tablets orally twice daily
Primarily COX-2 Inhibitor				
celecoxib *sell-ah-cok'-sib*	Celebrex	Acute pain, rheumatoid arthritis, ankylosing spondylitis, primary dysmenorrhea, and osteoarthritis; reduction of colorectal polyps in familial adenomatous polyposis	Headache, dyspepsia, rash, increased risk of cardiovascular events	100–200 mg orally BID
Agents for Migraines—Serotonin 5-HT Receptor Agonists				
almotriptan *al-moe-trip'-tan*	Axert	Acute migraine headache pain	Headache, dizziness, fatigue, somnolence, nausea, dry mouth, flushing, hot/cold sensations, pain in chest or neck, paresthesias	6.25–12.5 mg orally, may be repeated in 2 hr
eletriptan *el-ih-trip'-tan*	Relpax	Acute migraine headache pain	Same as almotriptan	20–40 mg orally at onset of symptoms, may be repeated in 2 hr, not to exceed 80 mg/day
frovatriptan *froe-vah-trip'-tan*	Frova	Acute migraine headache pain	Same as almotriptan	2.5 mg orally at onset of symptoms, may be repeated in 2 hr, not to exceed 7.5 mg/day

(table continues on page 160)

Nonopioid Analgesics

⬭ *Summary Drug Table* **NONOPIOID ANALGESICS: NONSTEROIDAL ANTI-INFLAMMATORY DRUGS AND MIGRAINE HEADACHE MEDICATIONS** (continued)

Generic Name	Trade Name	Uses	Adverse Reactions	Dosage Ranges
naratriptan *nar'-ah-trip-tan*	Amerge	Acute migraine headache pain	Same as almotriptan	1–2.5 mg orally at onset of symptoms, may be repeated in 4 hr, not to exceed 5 mg/day
rizatriptan *rye-zah-trip'-tan*	Maxalt	Acute migraine headache pain	Same as almotriptan	5–10 mg orally at onset of symptoms, may be repeated in 4 hr, not to exceed 30 mg/day
sumatriptan *soo-mah-trip'-tan*	Imitrex	Acute migraine and cluster headache pain	Same as almotriptan	25–100 mg orally; 20 mg nasally; 6 mg subcutaneously; 25 mg rectally; may be repeated in 2 hr, not to exceed 100 mg/day
zolmitriptan *zoll-mih-trip'-tan*	Zomig	Acute migraine headache pain	Same as almotriptan	2.5–5 mg orally; 5 mg nasally; may be repeated in 2 hr, not to exceed 10 mg/day
Ergotamine Derivatives				
dihydroergotamine *dye-hye-droe-er-got'-ah-meen*	DHE 45, Migranal	Acute migraine and cluster headache pain	Nausea, rhinitis, altered taste	Nasally: total dose of 2 mg; parenteral: no more than 3 mg injected in 24 hr
ergotamine *er-got'-ah-meen*	Ergomar	Vascular headaches	Nausea, rhinitis, altered taste	2 mg sublingually; may be repeated in 30 min, not to exceed 6 mg/day

● Chapter Review

Know Your Drugs

Patients sometimes know a medication by the brand (or trade) name and not the generic name. To help you recognize both names, match the brand name with the generic name of the same medication.

Generic Name	Brand Name
1. celecoxib	A. Advil
2. ibuprofen	B. Aleve
3. naproxen	C. Celebrex
4. zolmitriptan	D. Zomig

Calculate Medication Dosages

1. Naproxen (Naprosyn) oral suspension 250 mg is prescribed. The dosage on hand is oral suspension 125 mg/5 mL. The nurse administers _____.

2. The physician orders celecoxib (Celebrex) 200 mg orally. The nurse has celecoxib 100-mg tablets on hand. The nurse administers _____.

● Prepare for the NCLEX®

Build Your Knowledge

1. NSAIDs inhibit the action of _____.
   1. DNA synthesis
   2. prostaglandins
   3. cardiac muscles
   4. nerve fibers

2. The two basic measures of pain assessment are:
   1. time and intensity
   2. site and time
   3. duration and location
   4. location and intensity

3. The nurse monitors for which of the common adverse reactions when administering naproxen to a client?
   1. headache, dyspepsia
   2. blurred vision, constipation
   3. anorexia, tinnitus
   4. stomatitis, confusion

4. An older client is receiving sulindac. The nurse is aware that older adults taking NSAIDs are at increased risk for _____.
   1. ulcer disease
   2. stroke
   3. myocardial infarction
   4. gout

5. When a client is receiving an NSAID, the nurse must monitor the client for _____.
   1. agitation, which indicates nervous system involvement
   2. urinary retention, which indicates renal insufficiency
   3. decrease in white blood cell count, which increases the risk for infection
   4. GI symptoms, which can be serious and sometimes fatal

6. Which of the following statements would the nurse be certain to include in a teaching plan for the client taking an NSAID?
   1. If GI upset occurs, take this drug on an empty stomach.
   2. Avoid the use of aspirin or other salicylates when taking these drugs.
   3. These drugs can cause extreme confusion and should be used with caution.
   4. Relief from pain and inflammation should occur within 30 minutes after the first dose.

Apply Your Knowledge

7. The nurse teaches a client to self-administer sumatriptan; when is this injection contraindicated?
   1. at the onset of a migraine headache
   2. when a visual aura is seen
   3. 2 hours following a previous dose
   4. for weekly prophylactic use

8. Which of the following statements if made by the client taking an NSAID would indicate that he needs to see the primary health care provider immediately?
   1. "I'm able to walk around without my cane at the grocery store."
   2. "My wife has a fever so I gave her one of my pills."
   3. "That leg still hurts and now it is red, warm, and swollen."
   4. "I only have three pills left and the weekend is soon."

Alternate-Format Questions

9. Due to the nausea experienced during a migraine headache and reduced GI motility, migraine medications are available in forms other than oral pills and tablets for administration. In which forms are they available? **Select all that apply**.
   1. sublingual
   2. internasal
   3. subcutaneous
   4. rectal

10. Which pain assessment tool would be easiest to understand for a person with limited English reading ability? **Select all that apply**.
    1. Wong-Baker FACES Pain Rating Scale
    2. Simple descriptive pain intensity scale
    3. 0–10 numeric pain intensity scale
    4. visual analog scale

To check your answers, see Appendix G.

the**Point** *For more NCLEX-style questions, log on to http://thepoint.lww.com to access more than 1000 questions.*

15

Opioid Analgesics

KEY TERMS

adjuvant • therapy used in addition to the primary treatment

agonist • a drug that binds with a receptor and stimulates the receptor to produce a therapeutic response

agonist-antagonist • drug with both agonist and antagonist properties

cachectic • malnourished, in poor health, physically wasted

miosis • constriction of the pupil of the eye

opioid • drug having opiate properties but not necessarily derived from opium; used to relieve moderate to severe pain

opioid naive • no previous use or infrequent use of opioid medications

partial agonist • agent that binds to a receptor but produces a limited response

patient-controlled analgesia • drug pump and delivery system that allows patients to administer their own analgesic medication intravenously within a preset protocol

tolerance • the body's physical adaptation to a drug

DRUG CLASSES

Opioid agonists
Opioid agonist-antagonists

Pain and its treatment are universal issues. In this chapter the opioid drugs used for severe pain are discussed as well as how the intensity of pain determines the use of these drugs. The World Health Organization (WHO) developed a three-step analgesic protocol based on intensity as a guideline for treating pain. This "pain ladder" directs the use of both opioid and nonopioids in the treatment of pain using three steps (Fig. 15.1). For mild pain, a Step 1 nonopioid analgesic may be prescribed. If necessary, an **adjuvant** (extra helping) agent may be used to promote the pain-relieving effect. If pain persists or worsens even with appropriate dosage increases, a Step 2 or Step 3 analgesic is indicated. Step 2 and Step 3 analgesics contain opioid substances. Most patients with severe pain require a Step 2 or Step 3 analgesic.

Opioid is the general term used for the opium-derived or synthetic analgesics used to treat moderate to severe pain. The opioid analgesics are controlled substances (see Chapter 1). The analgesic properties of opium have been known for hundreds of years. These drugs do not change the tissues

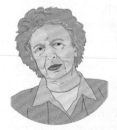

PHARMACOLOGY IN PRACTICE

Mrs. Moore is taking morphine sulfate to manage severe pain occurring as the result of heart failure. The primary health care provider has prescribed an around-the-clock dosage regimen. Mrs. Moore tells you that she is taking the pain drug 1 to 2 hours before the next dose is due. As you read this chapter, think about the appropriate response to her statement about taking her medicine on a more frequent schedule.

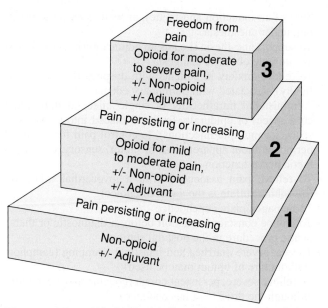

Figure 15.1 World Health Organization pain relief ladder. (Adapted with permission from WHO [2012].)

where the pain sensation originates; instead, they change how the patient perceives the pain.

OPIOID ANALGESICS

The opiates are natural substances and include morphine sulfate,* codeine, opium alkaloids, and tincture of opium. Synthetic opioids are those manufactured analgesics with properties and actions similar to the natural opioids. Examples of synthetic opioid analgesics are methadone, levorphanol, remifentanil, and meperidine. Morphine sulfate, when extracted from raw opium and treated chemically, yields the semisynthetic opioids hydromorphone, oxymorphone, oxycodone, and heroin.

Heroin is an illegal narcotic substance in the United States and is not used in medicine. *Narcotic* is a term referring to the properties of a drug to produce numbness or a stupor-like state. Although the terms *opioid* and *narcotic* were once interchangeable, law enforcement agencies have generalized the term *narcotic* to mean a drug that is addictive and abused or used illegally. Health care providers use the term *opioid* to describe drugs used in pain relief. Additional analgesics are listed in the Summary Drug Table: Opioid Analgesics.

Actions

Cells in the central nervous system (CNS) have receptor sites called *opiate receptors*. Although opiates are attracted to

---

*Numerous drug errors are attributed to using drug name suffixes (e.g., sulfate or HCl at the end of the drug name), according to the Institute for Safe Medicine Practices. Therefore, they have been removed from this book. Because morphine sulfate is considered a drug at greater risk for error when abbreviated, you will see it listed as such in this chapter (ISMP, 2012).

---

many different receptor sites, the mu (μ) and kappa (κ) receptors produce the analgesic, sedative, and euphoric effects associated with analgesic drugs.

Drugs that bind well to a receptor are called **agonist** agents. An opioid analgesic may be classified as an agonist, partial agonist, or mixed agonist-antagonist. The agonist binds to a receptor and causes a response. A **partial agonist** binds to a receptor, but the response is limited (i.e., is not as great as with the agonist). An **agonist-antagonist** has properties of both the agonist and antagonist. These drugs have some agonist activity at the receptor sites and some antagonist activity at the receptor sites. Antagonists bind to a receptor and cause no response. An antagonist can reverse the effects of the agonist. This reversal is possible because the antagonist competes with the agonist for a receptor site. Drugs that act as opioid antagonists are discussed in Chapter 16.

In addition to the pain-relieving effects, other, nonintended responses occur when the opiate receptor sites are stimulated. These include respiratory depression, decreased gastrointestinal (GI) motility, and **miosis** (pinpoint pupils). Table 15.1 identifies the responses in the body associated with three of the opiate receptors. The actions of the opioid analgesics on the various organs and structures of the body (also called *secondary pharmacologic effects*) are shown in Display 15.1. With long-term use, the patient's body adapts to these secondary effects. The only bodily system that does not adapt and compensate is the GI system. Slow GI motility and the resulting constipation are always a problem in opioid therapy.

The most widely used opioid, morphine sulfate, is an effective drug for moderately severe to severe pain. Morphine sulfate is considered the prototype (model) opioid. Morphine sulfate also is considered the gold standard in pain management—morphine sulfate's actions, uses, and ability to relieve pain are the standards against which other opioid analgesics are often compared. Charts called *equal-analgesic conversions* compare other opioid doses with the doses of morphine sulfate that would be used for the same level of pain control.

Other opioids, such as meperidine and levorphanol, are effective for the treatment of moderate to severe pain. For mild to moderate pain, the primary health care provider may order an opioid such as codeine or pentazocine.

Table 15.1	Bodily Responses Associated With Opioid Receptor Sites
Receptor	**Bodily Response**
Mu (μ)	Morphine-like supraspinal analgesia, respiratory and physical depression, miosis, reduced GI motility
Delta (δ)	Dysphoria, psychotomimetic effects (e.g., hallucinations), respiratory and vasomotor stimulations caused by drugs with antagonist activity
Kappa (κ)	Sedation and miosis (pinpoint pupils)

Display 15.1 Secondary Pharmacologic Effects of the Opioid Analgesics

- **Cardiovascular**—peripheral vasodilation, decreased peripheral resistance, inhibition of baroreceptors (pressure receptors located in the aortic arch and carotid sinus that regulate blood pressure), orthostatic hypotension, and fainting
- **Central nervous system**—euphoria, drowsiness, apathy, mental confusion, alterations in mood, reduction in body temperature, feelings of relaxation, dysphoria (depression accompanied by anxiety); nausea and vomiting are caused by direct stimulation of the emetic chemoreceptors located in the medulla. The degree to which these occur usually depends on the drug and the dose.
- **Dermatologic**—histamine release, pruritus, flushing, and red eyes
- **Gastrointestinal**—decrease in gastric motility (prolonged emptying time); decrease in biliary, pancreatic, and intestinal secretions; delay in digestion of food in the small intestine; increase in resting tone, with the potential for spasms, epigastric distress, or biliary colic (caused by constriction of the sphincter of Oddi). These drugs can cause constipation and anorexia.
- **Genitourinary**—urinary urgency and difficulty with urination, caused by spasms of the ureter. Urinary urgency also may occur because of the action of the drugs on the detrusor muscle of the bladder. Some patients may experience difficulty voiding because of contraction of the bladder sphincter.
- **Respiratory**—depressant effects on respiratory rate (caused by a reduced sensitivity of the respiratory center to carbon dioxide)
- **Cough**—suppression of the cough reflex (antitussive effect) by exerting a direct effect on the cough center in the medulla. Codeine has the most noticeable effect on the cough reflex.
- **Medulla**—Nausea and vomiting can occur when the chemoreceptor trigger zone located in the medulla is stimulated. To a varying degree, opioid analgesics also depress the chemoreceptor trigger zone. Therefore, nausea and vomiting may or may not occur when these drugs are given.

Uses

The opioid analgesics are used primarily for the treatment of moderate to severe acute and chronic pain and in the treatment and management of opiate dependence. Morphine sulfate is one of the primary drugs included in Hospice Comfort Care Medicine Packs (see Appendix E). In addition, the opioid analgesics may be used for the following reasons:

- To decrease anxiety and sedate the patient before surgery. Patients who are relaxed and sedated when an anesthetic agent is given are easier to anesthetize (requiring a smaller dose of an induction anesthetic), as well as easier to maintain under anesthesia.
- To support anesthesia (i.e., as an adjunct during anesthesia)
- To promote obstetric analgesia
- To relieve anxiety in patients with dyspnea (breathing difficulty) associated with pulmonary edema
- Administered intrathecally (a single injection into spinal cord space) or epidurally (catheter placed into spinal cord space for multiple injections), to control pain for extended periods without apparent loss of motor, sensory, or sympathetic nerve function
- To relieve pain associated with a myocardial infarction (morphine sulfate is the agent of choice)
- To manage opiate dependence
- To induce conscious sedation before a diagnostic or therapeutic procedure in the hospital setting
- To treat severe diarrhea and intestinal cramping (camphorated tincture of opium may be used)
- To relieve severe, persistent cough (codeine may be helpful, although the drug's use has declined)

Adverse Reactions

Central Nervous System Reactions

- Euphoria, weakness, headache
- Lightheadedness, dizziness, sedation
- Miosis, insomnia, agitation, tremor
- Increased intracranial pressure, impairment of mental and physical tasks

Respiratory System Reactions

- Depression of rate and depth of breathing

Gastrointestinal System Reactions

- Nausea, vomiting
- Dry mouth, biliary tract spasms
- Constipation, anorexia

Cardiovascular System Reactions

- Facial flushing
- Tachycardia, bradycardia, palpitations
- Peripheral circulatory collapse

Genitourinary System Reactions

- Urinary retention or hesitancy
- Spasms of the ureters and bladder sphincter

Allergic and Other Reactions

- Pruritus, rash, and urticaria
- Sweating, pain at injection site, and local tissue irritation

Contraindications

All opioid analgesics are contraindicated in patients with known hypersensitivity to the drugs. These drugs are contraindicated in patients with acute bronchial asthma, emphysema, or upper airway obstruction and in patients with head injury or increased intracranial pressure. The drugs are also contra-indicated in patients with convulsive disorders, severe renal or hepatic dysfunction, and acute ulcerative colitis. The opioid analgesics are pregnancy category C drugs (oxycodone is in pregnancy category B) and are not recommended for use during pregnancy or labor because they may prolong labor or cause respiratory depression in the neonate. The use of opioid analgesics is recommended during pregnancy only if the benefit to the mother outweighs the potential harm to the fetus.

Precautions

Opioid analgesics should be used cautiously in older adults and in patients considered **opioid naive**, that is, who have not been medicated with opioid drugs before and who are consequently at greatest risk for respiratory depression. The drugs should be administered cautiously in patients undergoing biliary surgery (because of the risk for spasm of the sphincter of Oddi, between the bile duct and small intestine; in these patients, meperidine is the drug of choice). Patients who are lactating should wait at least 4 to 6 hours after taking the drug to breastfeed the infant. Additional precautions apply to patients with undiagnosed abdominal pain, hypoxia, supraventricular tachycardia, prostatic hypertrophy, and renal or hepatic impairment.

Interactions

The following interactions may occur when an opioid analgesic is administered with another agent:

Interacting Drug	Common Use	Effect of Interaction
alcohol	Social occasions	Increased risk for CNS depression
antihistamines	Prevent or relieve allergic reactions	Increased risk for CNS depression

Interacting Drug	Common Use	Effect of Interaction
antidepressants	Alleviate depression	Increased risk for CNS depression
sedatives	Sedation	Increased risk for CNS depression
phenothiazines	Relief of agitation, anxiety, vomiting	Increased risk for CNS depression
opioid agonist-antagonist	Gynecologic or obstetric pain relief	Opioid withdrawal symptoms (if long-term opioid use)
barbiturates	Used in general anesthesia	Respiratory depression, hypotension, or sedation

HERBAL CONSIDERATIONS

The name passionflower denotes many of the approximately 400 species of herbs in the genus Passiflora. Passionflower has been used in medicine to treat pain, anxiety, and insomnia. Some herbalists use it to treat symptoms of parkinsonism. Passionflower is often used in combination with other natural substances, such valerian, chamomile, and hops, for promoting relaxation, rest, and sleep. Although no adverse reactions have been reported, large doses may cause CNS depression. The use of passionflower is contraindicated in pregnancy and in patients taking the monoamine oxidase inhibitors (MAOIs). Passionflower contains coumarin; the risk of bleeding may be increased in patients taking warfarin (Coumadin) and passionflower. The following are recommended dosages for passionflower:

- Tea: 1–4 cups per day (made with 1 tablespoon of the crude herb per cup)
- Tincture (2 g/5 mL): 2 teaspoons (10 mL) 3–4 times daily
- Dried herb: 2 g 3–4 times daily (DerMarderosian, 2003)

NURSING PROCESS

PATIENT RECEIVING AN OPIOID ANALGESIC FOR PAIN

ASSESSMENT

Preadministration Assessment
As part of the preadministration assessment, assess and document the type, onset, intensity, and location of the pain. Your documentation should include a description of the pain (e.g., sharp, dull, stabbing, throbbing) and an estimate of when the pain began. Treat each different pain like it is a new pain. Use the questions in Chapter 14 (Guidelines and questions for a pain assessment) if the pain is of a different type than the patient had been experiencing previously or if it is in a different area.

Review the patient's health history, allergy history, and past and current drug therapies. This is especially important when an opioid is given for the first time because data may be obtained during the initial history and physical assessment that require the nurse to contact the primary health care provider. For example, the patient may state that nausea and vomiting occurred when he or she was given a drug for pain several years ago. Further questioning of the patient is necessary because this information may influence the primary health care provider's decision to administer a specific opioid drug.

If promethazine (Phenergan) is used with an opioid to enhance the effects and reduce the dosage of the opioid, take the patient's blood pressure, pulse, and respiratory rate before giving the drug.

Ongoing Assessment
You can measure the effect of the opioid by taking the blood pressure, pulse and respiratory rate, and pain rating in 5 to 10 minutes if the drug is given intravenously (IV), 20 to 30 minutes if the drug is administered intramuscularly (IM) or subcutaneously (subcut), and 30 or more minutes if the drug is given orally. It is important to notify the primary health care provider if the analgesic is ineffective, because a higher dose or a different opioid analgesic may be required.

During the ongoing assessment, it is important for you to ask about the pain regularly and to accept the patient' and family's reports of pain. Nursing judgment must be exercised, because not all instances of a change in pain type, location, or intensity require notifying the primary health care provider. For example, if a patient recovering from recent abdominal surgery experiences pain in the calf of the leg (suggesting venous thrombosis), you should immediately notify the primary health care provider. However, it is not necessary to contact the primary health care provider for pain that is slightly worse because the patient has been moving in bed.

The opioid-naive patient who does not use opioids routinely and is being given an opioid drug for acute pain relief or a surgical procedure is at greatest risk for respiratory depression after opioid administration. Respiratory depression may occur in patients receiving a normal dose if the patient is vulnerable (e.g., in a weakened or debilitated state). Older, cachectic (malnourished/in general poor health), or debilitated patients should receive a reduced initial dose until their response to the drug is known. If the patient's respiratory rate is 10 breaths/min or less, monitor the patient at more frequent intervals and notify the primary health care provider immediately. Patients involved in long-term opioid therapy for pain relief build tolerance to the physical adverse effects of the drugs; respiratory depression is typically not seen in these patients.

When an opiate is used as an antidiarrheal drug, document each bowel movement, as well as its appearance, color, and consistency. Notify the primary health care provider immediately if diarrhea is not relieved or becomes worse, if the patient has severe abdominal pain, or if blood in the stool is noted.

NURSING DIAGNOSES

Drug-specific nursing diagnoses are the following:

- **Ineffective Breathing Pattern** related to pain and effects on breathing center by opioids
- **Risk for Injury** related to dizziness or lightheadedness from opioid administration
- **Constipation** related to the decreased GI motility caused by opioids
- **Imbalanced Nutrition: Less Than Body Requirements** related to anorexia caused by opioids

Nursing diagnoses related to drug administration are discussed in Chapter 4.

PLANNING

The expected outcomes of the patient may include relief of pain, supporting the patient needs related to the management of adverse reactions, an understanding of patient-controlled analgesia (PCA; when applicable), absence of injury, adequate nutrition intake, and confidence in an understanding of the medication regimen.

IMPLEMENTATION

Promoting an Optimal Response to Therapy

RELIEVING ACUTE PAIN. Acute pain can be severe following a surgical procedure. For acute pain, the goal is to control the pain, then reduce the dosage. Many postoperative patients require less opioid when they can self-administer the medicine for pain. PCA allows postsurgical patients to administer

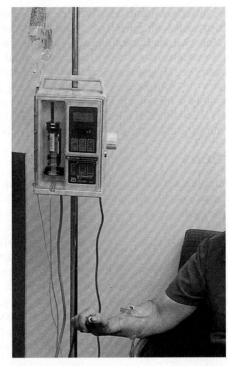

Figure 15.2 Patient-controlled analgesia (PCA) allows the patient to self-administer medication as necessary to control pain.

their own analgesic by means of an IV pump system (Fig. 15.2). Pumps are preset with small amounts of the opioid medication that the patient can administer by pushing a button on the pump. The medication can be delivered, for example, when the patient begins to feel pain or when the patient wishes to ambulate but wants some medication to prevent pain on getting out of bed. The patient does not have to wait for the nurse to administer the medicine. As a result, patients medicate before they cannot tolerate the pain, use less medication, and resume activity faster. When patients take less opioid, they also experience fewer unpleasant adverse reactions, such as nausea and constipation. Because the self-administration system is under the control of the nurse, who adds the drug to the infusion pump and sets the time interval (or lockout interval) between doses, the patient cannot receive an overdose of the drug.

RELIEVING CHRONIC SEVERE PAIN. Morphine sulfate is the most widely used drug in the management of chronic severe pain. The fact that this drug can be given orally, nasally, subcutaneously, IM, IV, and rectally in the form of a suppository makes it tremendously versatile. Medication for chronic pain should be scheduled around the clock and not given on a PRN (as-needed) basis. With any chronic pain medication, the oral route is preferred as long as the patient can swallow or can tolerate sublingual administration.

Using the concept of the WHO pain ladder for chronic pain, medications that work to relieve pain both peripherally and centrally are ordered. For ease of administration and to provide good pain relief based on the pain ladder, drugs that combine a nonopioid and an opioid analgesic are available. These drugs work well at dealing with the inflammation at

Table 15.2 Opioid/Nonopioid Combination Oral Analgesics		
Brand Name	**Opioid**	**Nonopioid**
Tylenol #3	codeine 30 mg	acetaminophen 300 mg
Lortab	hydrocodone 2.5 mg	acetaminophen 167 mg
Vicodin	hydrocodone 5 mg	acetaminophen 500 mg
Vicodin ES	hydrocodone 7.5 mg	acetaminophen 750 mg
Percodan	oxycodone 5 mg	aspirin 325 mg
Percocet	oxycodone 5 mg	acetaminophen 325 mg
Roxicet	oxycodone 5 mg	acetaminophen 325 mg

the peripheral site, as well as modifying the pain perception centrally in the brain. Table 15.2 lists many of these drugs and their combination ingredients.

Controlled-released forms of opioids are indicated for the management of moderate to severe pain when a continuous, around-the-clock analgesic is needed for an extended time. Examples of these drugs include oxycodone (OxyContin) and morphine sulfate (MS Contin). The medication is given once every 8 to 12 hours; the actual drug is slowly released over time so the patient does not get all the medication at once. Controlled-released drugs are not intended for use as a PRN analgesic. The patient may experience fewer adverse reactions with oxycodone products than with morphine sulfate, and the drug is effective and safe for older adults. Controlled-release tablets should be swallowed whole and are not to be broken, chewed, or crushed.

When long-acting forms of the opioids are used, a fast-acting form may be given for breakthrough pain. These are typically ordered on a PRN basis to be used between the long-acting doses for acute pain episodes. Morphine sulfate in oral or sublingual tablets is commonly used. Oral transmucosal fentanyl (Actiq) is also used to treat breakthrough pain for patients who cannot swallow a pill.

Fentanyl transdermal is a transdermal system that is effective in the management of severe pain associated with diseases like cancer. This drug should be used only when other opioids or routes are proven unsuccessful; it should never be used on an opiate-naive patient. The transdermal system allows for a timed-release patch containing the drug fentanyl to be activated over a 72-hour period. A small number of patients may require systems applied every 48 hours. When used, you should monitor for adverse reactions in the same manner as for other opioid analgesics.

LIFESPAN CONSIDERATIONS
Gerontology
The transdermal route should be used with caution in older adults, because the amount of subcutaneous tissue is reduced in the aging process. The transdermal route of drug administration for pain is used because it treats severe pain when other methods are not successful; it should not be used simply for the convenience of administration.

Sometimes pain is accompanied by symptoms such as anxiety or restlessness and is best relieved by a combination of drugs and not just the opioid analgesics alone. For better administration, especially if the patient is at home, a mixture of an oral opioid and other drugs may be used to obtain relief; this is referred to as compounding medications. Brompton's mixture is one of the most commonly used solutions. In addition to the opioid, such as morphine sulfate or methadone, other drugs may be used in the compounded preparation, including antidepressants, stimulants, aspirin, acetaminophen, and tranquilizers. The clinical pharmacist prepares the medication as a solution, salve, or suppository depending on the best method to administer the preparation to the specific patient. As the nurse, you are frequently required to teach the patient or caregivers how to store and self-administer these preparations. It is necessary to monitor for the adverse reactions of each drug contained in the preparation. The time interval for administration varies. Some primary health care providers may order the mixture on a PRN basis; others may order it given at regular intervals.

Over time, the patient taking an opioid analgesic develops a tolerance to the drug. This is different from *physical dependence*, where the body experiences adverse effects if the medicine is stopped. With tolerance, the body physically adapts to the drug, and greater amounts are needed to achieve the same effects. The rate at which tolerance develops varies according to the dosage, the route of administration, and the individual. Patients taking oral medications develop tolerance more slowly than those taking the drugs parenterally. Some patients develop tolerance quickly and need larger doses every few weeks, whereas others are maintained on the same dosage schedule throughout the course of the illness.

The fear of respiratory depression is a concern for many nurses when they administer an opioid, and some nurses may even hesitate to administer the drug. However, respiratory depression rarely occurs in patients using an opioid for chronic pain. In fact, these patients usually develop tolerance to the respiratory depressant effects of the drug very quickly. You should be more concerned about adverse effects on the GI system. The decrease in GI motility causes constipation, nausea, acute abdominal pain, and anorexia. It is important to provide a thorough, aggressive bowel program to patients when they are taking opioid medications.

! NURSING ALERT
When patients experience a drop in respiratory rate, sometimes you can increase the rate of respirations by coaching the patient to breathe. Should an antidote be needed, naloxone (Narcan) should be administered with great caution and only when necessary in patients receiving an opioid for severe pain. Naloxone removes all of the pain-relieving effects of the opioid and may lead to withdrawal symptoms or the return of intense pain.

USING TRANSDERMAL SYSTEM PAIN MANAGEMENT. When using a transdermal system, it is important to ensure that only one patch is on at a time to prevent additive effects of the drug. Find and remove the old patch before replacing it with a new one. To discard, fold the patch so the sticky side adheres to itself, and discard in the toilet or a "sharps" container. Before

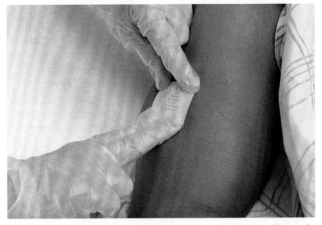

Figure 15.3 The nurse applies the transdermal patch securely.

the new transdermal patch is applied, date and initial the patch with a water-resistant pen. Use only water to cleanse the site before application, because soaps, oils, and other substances may irritate the skin. Rotate the site of application and do not apply over hair. To ensure complete contact with the skin surface, press for 10 to 20 seconds (Fig. 15.3). After 72 hours, remove the system and, if continuous therapy is prescribed, apply a new system.

> **NURSING ALERT**
>
> Heat can increase the absorption of the drug in a transdermal system, causing overdose of the drug. Caution patients and families never to place a heating blanket or pad over the patch. Also, teach patients to be aware of other heat sources as well such as tanning lamps, hot tubs, saunas, or hot baths.

USING EPIDURAL PAIN MANAGEMENT. Administration of morphine sulfate and fentanyl by the epidural route has provided an alternative to the IM or oral route. This approach was introduced with the idea that very small doses of opioid would provide long-lasting pain relief with significantly fewer systemic adverse reactions.

Epidural administration offers several advantages over other routes, including lower total dosages of the drug used, fewer adverse reactions, and greater patient comfort. This type of pain management is used for postoperative pain, labor pain, and intractable chronic pain. The administration of the opioid is either by bolus or by continuous infusion pump.

Patients experience pain relief with fewer adverse reactions; the adverse reactions experienced are those related to processes under direct CNS control. The most serious adverse reaction associated with the epidurally administered opioids is respiratory depression. Patients using epidural analgesics for chronic pain are monitored for respiratory problems with an apnea monitor. The patient may also experience sedation, confusion, nausea, pruritus, or urinary retention. Fentanyl is increasingly used as an alternative to morphine sulfate because patients experience fewer adverse reactions.

> **NURSING ALERT**
>
> Epidural analgesia should be administered only by those specifically trained in the use of IV and epidural anesthetics. Oxygen, resuscitative, and intubation equipment should be readily available.

Nursing care includes close monitoring of the patient for respiratory depression immediately after insertion of the epidural catheter and throughout therapy. Vital signs are taken every 30 minutes, apnea monitors are used, and an opioid antagonist, such as naloxone, is readily available.

Policies and procedures for administering, monitoring, and documenting drugs given through the epidural route must be specific to the nurse practice act in each state and in accordance with federal and state regulations. This type of analgesia is most often managed by registered nurses with special training in the care and management of epidural catheters.

Monitoring and Managing Patient Needs

You should contact the primary health care provider immediately if any of the following are present:

- Significant decrease in the respiratory rate or a respiratory rate of 10 breaths/min or less
- Significant increase or decrease in the pulse rate or a change in the pulse quality
- Significant decrease in blood pressure (systolic or diastolic) or a systolic pressure below 100 mm Hg

INEFFECTIVE BREATHING PATTERN. Opioids may depress the cough reflex. Encourage patients receiving an opioid, even for a few days, to cough and breathe deeply every 2 hours. This task prevents the pooling of secretions in the lungs, which can lead to hypostatic pneumonia and other lung problems. The patient may be fearful that exercise will cause even greater pain. Teach the patient that these activities are designed to help the body recover better. Performing tasks (such as getting out of bed) and therapeutic activities (such as deep breathing, coughing, and leg exercises) when the drug is producing its greatest analgesic effect, usually 1 to 2 hours after administering the opioid, aids in recovery. If the patient experiences nausea and vomiting, notify the primary health care provider. A different analgesic or an antiemetic may be necessary.

RISK FOR INJURY. Opioids may produce orthostatic hypotension, which in turn results in dizziness. Report any significant change in the patient's vital signs to the primary health care provider. Particularly vulnerable are postoperative patients and individuals whose ability to maintain blood pressure has been compromised. You should assist the patient with ambulatory activities and with rising slowly from a sitting or lying position to assess for hypotensive problems. Miosis (pinpoint pupils) may occur with the administration of some opioids and is most pronounced with morphine sulfate, hydromorphone, and opium alkaloids. Miosis decreases the ability to see in dim light. If miosis occurs, teach the patient and family to keep the room well lit during daytime hours and advise the patient to seek assistance when getting out of bed at night.

CONSTIPATION. Most patients should begin taking a stool softener or laxative with the initial dose of an opioid analgesic. Decreased GI motility due to the opioids, in addition to lower food and water intake and decreased mobility, causes the constipation. Teach the patient to keep a record of bowel movements and inform the primary health care provider if constipation appears to be a problem. Many patients need to continue taking a laxative for as long as they take an opioid analgesic. If the patient is constipated despite the use of a stool softener or laxative, the primary health care provider may prescribe an enema or other means of relieving constipation.

IMBALANCED NUTRITION: LESS THAN BODY REQUIREMENTS. When an opioid is prescribed for a prolonged time, anorexia (loss of appetite) may occur. Those receiving an opioid for pain relief caused by a terminal illness often have severe anorexia from the disease and the opioid. Note food intake after each meal. When anorexia is prolonged, weigh the patient as ordered by the primary health care provider. It is important to encourage caregivers to discuss with the primary health care provider treatment plans for continued weight loss and anorexia. Supplements may be ordered and administered orally, enterally, or parenterally. A decision may be made to support the terminal patient as he or she becomes anorexic and provide comfort measures without attempting to increase the weight or encourage eating.

OPIOID PHYSICAL DEPENDENCE IN ACUTE PAIN MANAGEMENT. Patients receiving the opioid analgesics for short-term, acute pain do not develop physical dependence. Delays in medication administration cause patients to ask repeatedly for pain medication. This behavior is sometimes interpreted as drug-seeking behavior, or it may be associated with the fear (of the nurse) of making a patient drug dependent. Nurses are also fearful that patients with a history of psychologic dependence might become dependent again when given pain medication. These individuals experience pain, too. They need to be provided adequate pain relief to *prevent* returning to dependency behaviors. Typically it is the behavior of the nurses and primary health care providers in delaying administration of opioids for good pain control that causes the problems associated with appearances of dependence.

Drug dependence can, however, occur in a newborn whose mother was dependent on opiates during pregnancy. Withdrawal symptoms in the newborn usually appear during the first few days of life. Symptoms include irritability, excessive crying, yawning, sneezing, increased respiratory rate, tremors, fever, vomiting, and diarrhea.

MANAGEMENT OF OPIOID DEPENDENCE. Two opioids are used in the treatment and management of opiate dependence: levomethadyl and methadone. Levomethadyl is given in an opiate dependency clinic to maintain control over the delivery of the drug. Because of its potential for serious and life-threatening prearrhythmic effects, levomethadyl is reserved for treating addicted patients who have had no response to other treatments. Levomethadyl is not taken daily; the drug is administered three times a week (Monday/Wednesday/Friday or Tuesday/Thursday/ Saturday). Daily use of the usual dose will cause serious overdose.

NURSING ALERT

If a patient is transferring from levomethadyl to methadone, the nurse should wait 48 hours after the last dose of levomethadyl before administering the first dose of methadone or other opioid.

Display 15.2 Symptoms of the Abstinence Syndrome

Early Symptoms
Yawning, lacrimation, rhinorrhea, sweating

Intermediate Symptoms
Mydriasis, tachycardia, twitching, tremor, restlessness, irritability, anxiety, anorexia

Late Symptoms
Muscle spasm, fever, nausea, vomiting, kicking movements, weakness, depression, body aches, weight loss, severe backache, abdominal and leg pains, hot and cold flashes, insomnia, repetitive sneezing; increased blood pressure, respiratory rate, and heart rate

Methadone, a synthetic opioid, may be used for the relief of pain, but it also is used in the detoxification and maintenance treatment of those dependent on opioids. Detoxification involves withdrawing the patient from the opioid while minimizing withdrawal symptoms. Maintenance therapy is designed to reduce the patient's desire to return to the drug that caused dependence, as well as to prevent withdrawal symptoms. Dosages vary with the patient, the length of time the individual has been dependent, and the average amount of drug used each day. Patients enrolled in an outpatient methadone program for detoxification or maintenance therapy on methadone must continue to receive methadone when hospitalized. In adults, withdrawal symptoms are known as the *abstinence syndrome* (see Display 15.2 for more information).

Educating the Patient and Family
Teach the patient about the drug he or she is receiving for pain. Provide written materials in the preferred language about how often the drug can be given, adverse reactions to monitor for, and what to do if the patient runs short of the drug.

If a patient is to receive drugs through a PCA infusion pump, the patient is taught how to use the machine during the preoperative visit rather than waiting until the patient is in pain in the postoperative unit (see Patient Teaching for Improved Patient Outcomes: Using Patient-Controlled Analgesia for Postoperative Pain). Notify the anesthesiologist or surgeon if the patient does not understand the PCA procedure so that an alternative method of pain relief can be ordered.

Opioids for outpatient use may be prescribed in the oral form or as a timed-release transdermal patch. In certain cases, such as when terminally ill patients are being cared for at home, the nurse may give the family instruction in the parenteral administration of the drug or use of an IV pump.

When an opioid has been prescribed, include the following points in the teaching plan:

- This drug may cause drowsiness, dizziness, and blurring of vision. Use caution when driving or performing tasks requiring alertness.

- ❗ Avoid the use of alcoholic beverages unless use has been approved by the primary health care provider. Alcohol may intensify the action of the drug and cause extreme drowsiness or dizziness. In some instances, the use of alcohol and an opioid can have extremely serious and even life-threatening consequences that may require emergency medical treatment.
- Take the drug as directed on the container label and do not exceed the prescribed dose. Contact the primary health care provider if the drug is not effective.
- If GI upset occurs, take the drug with food.
- Notify the primary health care provider if nausea, vomiting, and constipation become severe.

EVALUATION

- Therapeutic response is achieved and discomfort is reduced. If ordered, the patient demonstrates the ability to use PCA effectively.
- Adverse reactions are identified, reported to the primary health care provider, and managed successfully with appropriate nursing interventions:
  - An adequate breathing pattern is maintained.
  - No evidence of injury is seen.
  - Patient reports adequate bowel movements.
  - Patient maintains an adequate nutritional status.
- Patient and family express confidence and demonstrate an understanding of the drug regimen.

Patient Teaching for Improved Patient Outcomes

Using Patient-Controlled Analgesia for Postoperative Pain

In some situations, IV opioid analgesics may be ordered for pain relief following a surgical procedure. If the patient is able to participate, the anesthesiologist may offer PCA. The purpose of this is to allow the patient to manage pain to recuperate faster and return to daily activities of life sooner.

When you teach, make sure your patient understands the following:

- ✔ How the pump works; the machine regulates the dose of the drug as well as the time interval between doses.
- ✔ The location of the control button that activates the administration of the drug; the difference between the control button and the button to call the nurse (especially when both are similar in appearance and feel)
- ✔ Use the machine to prevent pain, such as when the patient feels the need for pain relief or is about to engage in an activity that might cause pain (e.g., coughing, exercises, or getting out of bed).
- ✔ Push the button once; the button does not need to be depressed to keep the drug flowing in the IV.
- ✔ The dose of drug is ordered by the primary health care provider and set by the nurse. If the control button is used too soon after the last dose, the machine will not deliver the drug until the correct time; therefore, the patient does not need to worry about taking too much drug.

PHARMACOLOGY IN PRACTICE
THINK CRITICALLY

 In discussing Mrs. Moore's medication changes, you would first do a pain assessment. Think about what you have learned about pain perception and assessment. What strategies would you use to determine her pain management needs that required more frequent dosing?

KEY POINTS

- The World Health Organization developed a three-step analgesic protocol based on intensity as a guideline for treating pain. The "pain ladder" directs the use of both opioids and nonopioids in the treatment of mild to severe pain.
- *Opioid* is a term used for drugs that change the pain sensation by attaching to receptor sites in the brain producing an analgesic, sedative, and euphoric effect. Most of these are derived from opium or a synthetic substance like opium.

- These drugs are used to treat moderate to severe pain.
- *Narcotic* is a term referring to the properties of a drug to produce numbness or a stupor-like state. Although the terms *opioid* and *narcotic* were once interchangeable, law enforcement agencies have generalized the term *narcotic* to mean a drug that is addictive and abused or used illegally. Health care providers use the term *opioid* to describe drugs used in pain relief.

- Morphine sulfate is a drug used through multiple routes for relief of chronic and acute pain. Other opioids are compared to this drug when attempting to determine dosing or conversion between drug types.

- Patient-controlled analgesia is a self-administered IV pump that patients use following painful procedures. By allowing patients to control administration, they tend to use less of the drug and recuperate faster.

- The more common non–pain relief effects (known as secondary effects) of these drugs include respiratory depression, decreased gastrointestinal motility, and miosis. Constipation is the one side effect to which the body does not build a tolerance.

Summary Drug Table OPIOID ANALGESICS

Generic Name	Trade Name	Uses	Adverse Reactions*	Dosage Ranges
Agonists				
alfentanil *al-fen'-tah-nil*	Alfenta	Anesthetic adjunct	Respiratory depression, skeletal muscle rigidity, constipation, nausea, vomiting	Individualize dosage and titrate to obtain desired effect
codeine *koe'-deen*		Moderate to severe pain, antitussive, anesthetic adjunct	Sedation, sweating, headache, dizziness, lethargy, confusion, lightheadedness	Analgesic: 15–60 mg q 4–6 hr orally, subcut, IM
fentanyl *fen'-tah-nil*	Abstral, Actiq, Fentora, Onsolis, Sublimaze	Severe pain, anesthetic adjunct, management of breakthrough cancer pain	Sweating, headache, vertigo, lethargy, confusion, nausea, vomiting, respiratory depression	Same as alfentanil 200–1600 mcg/dose, depending on pain severity
fentanyl transdermal systems	Duragesic	Chronic pain unmanaged by other opioids	Sedation, sweating, headache, vertigo, lethargy, confusion, lightheadedness, nausea, vomiting	Individualized dosage: 25–175-mcg transdermal patch (dose is amount absorbed per hour)
hydromorphone *hye-droe-mor'-fone*	Dilaudid, Exalgo	Moderate to severe pain	Sedation, vertigo, lethargy, confusion, lightheadedness, nausea, vomiting	2–4 mg orally q 4–6 hr; 3 mg rectally q 6–8 hr; 1–2 mg IM or subcut q 4–6 hr
levorphanol *lee-vor'-fah-noll*		Moderate to severe pain, preoperative sedation	Dizziness, nausea, vomiting, dry mouth, sweating, respiratory depression	2 mg orally q 3–6 hr; 1 mg IV q 3–8 hr
meperidine *meh-per'-ih-deen*	Demerol	Acute moderate to severe pain, preoperative sedation, anesthetic adjunct	Lightheadedness, constipation, dizziness, nausea, vomiting, respiratory depression	50–150 mg orally, IM, subcut q 3–4 hr
methadone *meth'-ah-doan*	Dolophine	Severe pain; treatment of opioid dependence	Lightheadedness, dizziness, sedation, nausea, vomiting, constipation	Analgesic: 2.5–10 mg orally, IM, subcut q 4 hr; detoxification: 10–40 mg orally, IV
morphine *mor'-feen*	Astramorph, Avinza, Kadian, Duramorph; timed release: MS Contin	Acute/chronic pain, preoperative sedation, anesthetic adjunct, dyspnea	Sedation, hypotension, increased sweating, constipation, dizziness, drowsiness, nausea, vomiting, dry mouth, somnolence, respiratory depression	Acute pain relief: 10–30 mg q 4 hr; chronic pain relief: individualized
oxycodone *ok-see-koe'-doan*	Roxicodone; timed release: OxyContin	Moderate to severe pain	Lightheadedness, sedation, constipation, dizziness, nausea, vomiting, sweating, respiratory depression	10–30 mg orally q 4 hr

(table continues on page 172)

Opioid Analgesics

Summary Drug Table OPIOID ANALGESICS (continued)

Generic Name	Trade Name	Uses	Adverse Reactions*	Dosage Ranges
oxymorphone *ok-see-mor'-fone*	Opana	Moderate to severe pain, preoperative sedation, obstetric analgesia	Lightheadedness, sedation, constipation, dizziness, nausea, vomiting, respiratory depression	1–1.5 mg subcut or IM q 4–6 hr
remifentanil *reh-mih-fen'-tah-nill*	Ultiva	Anesthetic adjunct	Lightheadedness, skeletal muscle rigidity, nausea, vomiting, respiratory depression, sweating	Same as alfentanil
sufentanil *suh-fen'-tah-nill*	Sufenta	Anesthetic adjunct	Same as alfentanil	Same as alfentanil
tramadol *tram'-ah-doll*	Ultram	Moderate to severe chronic pain	Same as morphine	Titrate individual dose starting at 25 mg up to 100 mg/day
Agonists-Antagonists				
buprenorphine *byoo-preh-nor'-feen*	Buprenex, Subutex, Suboxone (combo with naloxone)	Moderate to severe chronic pain, treatment of opioid dependence	Lightheadedness, sedation, dizziness, nausea, vomiting, respiratory depression	Parenteral: 0.03 mg q 6 hr IV or IM Sublingual: 12–16 mg/day
butorphanol *byoo-tor'-fah-noll*	Stadol	Acute pain, anesthetic adjunct	Lightheadedness, sedation, constipation, dizziness, nausea, vomiting, respiratory depression	1–4 mg IM, 0.5–2 mg IV; Nasal spray (NS): 1 mg (spray), repeat in 60–90 min; may repeat q 3–4 hr
nalbuphine *nal'-byoo-feen*		Moderate to severe chronic pain, anesthetic adjunct	Lightheadedness, sedation, constipation, dizziness, nausea, vomiting, respiratory depression	10 mg/70 kg subcut, IM, or IV q 3–6 hr
pentazocine *pen-taz'-oh-seen*	Talwin	Same as nalbuphine	Same as nalbuphine	30–60 mg IM, subcut, IV q 3–4 hr; maximum daily dose 360 mg

*Adverse reactions of opioid analgesics are discussed extensively in the chapter. Some of the reactions may be less severe or intense than others.

● Chapter Review

Know Your Drugs

Clients sometimes know a medication by the brand (or trade) name and not the generic name. To help you recognize both names, match the brand name with the generic name of the same medication.

Generic Name	Brand Name
1. fentanyl	A. Demerol
2. hydromorphone	B. Dilaudid
3. meperidine	C. Duragesic
4. oxycodone	D. OxyContin

Calculate Medication Dosages

1. A client is prescribed oral morphine sulfate 12 mg. The dosage available is 10 mg/mL. The nurse administers _____.

2. A client is prescribed oxycodone 10 mg for pain relief every 3 to 4 hours. The dosage available is 5 mg/capsule. The nurse administers _____.

● Prepare for the NCLEX®

Build Your Knowledge

1. The nurse explains to the client that some opioids may be used as part of the preoperative medication regimen to _____.

   1. increase intestinal motility
   2. facilitate passage of an endotracheal tube
   3. enhance the effects of the skeletal muscle relaxant
   4. lessen anxiety and sedate the patient

2. Each time the client requests an opioid analgesic, the nurse must _____.

   1. check the client's diagnosis
   2. talk to the client to see if he is awake
   3. determine the exact location and intensity of the pain
   4. administer the drug with food to prevent gastric upset

3. When administering opioid analgesics to an older client, the nurse monitors the client closely for _____.

   1. an increased heart rate
   2. euphoria
   3. confusion
   4. a synergistic reaction

4. When administering a timed-release medication to a client, the nurse must be aware that _____.

   1. it should not be crushed
   2. the medication is stronger
   3. serious cardiac arrhythmias may develop
   4. CNS stimulation is possible

Apply Your Knowledge

5. The client on opioid therapy complains of abdominal pain. What is the nurse's best response?

   1. "Let's see when you had your last pain medicine."
   2. "Can you rate your pain for me?"
   3. "Show me where on your tummy it hurts."
   4. "When was your last bowel movement?"

6. Which of the following drug combinations would follow Step 1 of the WHO pain ladder?

   1. morphine sulfate orally 10 mg every 4 hours and morphine sulfate sublingual 1 mg PRN
   2. hydrocodone orally 5 mg and acetaminophen 500 mg
   3. naproxen orally 200 mg twice daily and acetaminophen 325 mg at bedtime
   4. meperidine 20 mg with Phenergan IM

7. Which of the following findings requires the nurse to immediately contact the primary health care provider?

   1. pulse rate of 80 bpm
   2. complaint of breakthrough pain
   3. respiratory rate of 20 breaths/min
   4. systolic blood pressure of 140 mm Hg

Alternate-Format Questions

8. Which opiate receptors in the brain produce the analgesic, euphoric effects? **Select all that apply**.

   1. alpha
   2. delta
   3. kappa
   4. mu

9. A client is prescribed Vicodin for pain relief following a surgical procedure. If the client takes 1 tablet every 4 hours, how much acetaminophen will the client take in 24 hours?

10. A client is prescribed fentanyl (Sublimaze) 50 mcg IM 30 minutes before surgery. The nurse has available a vial with a dosage strength of 0.05 mg/1 mL. The nurse calculates the dosage and administers _____.

To check your answers, see Appendix G.

thePoint *For more NCLEX-style questions, log on to http://thepoint.lww.com to access more than 1000 questions.*

Opioid Antagonists

LEARNING OBJECTIVES

On completion of this chapter, the student will:

1. Discuss the uses, general drug actions, general adverse reactions, contraindications, precautions, and interactions of the opioid antagonists.
2. Discuss important preadministration and ongoing assessment activities the nurse should perform on the patient receiving an opioid antagonist.
3. List nursing diagnoses particular to a patient taking an opioid antagonist.
4. Discuss ways to promote optimal response to therapy, how to manage adverse reactions, and important points to keep in mind when educating patients about the use of opioid antagonists.

KEY TERMS

antagonist • substance that counteracts the action of something else

opioid naive • no previous use or infrequent use of opioid medications

DRUG CLASSES

Opioid antagonist

An **antagonist** is a substance that counteracts the action of something else. A drug that is an opioid antagonist has a greater affinity for a cell receptor than an opioid drug (agonist), and by binding to the cell it prevents a response to the opioid. Thus, an opioid antagonist reverses the actions of an opioid. One of the most severe adverse reactions to opioid treatment is respiratory depression. Specific antagonists have been developed to reverse the respiratory depression associated with the opioids. Naloxone is capable of restoring respiratory function within 1 to 2 minutes after administration. Naltrexone (another antagonist) is used primarily to treat alcohol dependence and to block the effects of suspected opioids if they are being used by a person undergoing treatment for alcohol dependence.

OPIOID ANTAGONISTS

Actions

Administration of an antagonist prevents or reverses the effects of opioid drugs. The antagonist reverses the opioid

PHARMACOLOGY IN PRACTICE

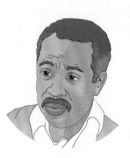

When Mr. Park came to the preoperative unit, he complained that the pain on his back (where the shingles rash was erupting) was greater than the pain in his broken hip and leg. On rounds before the surgical procedure to repair his femur, the primary health care provider assured him that the acyclovir would begin to alleviate some of the pain from the rash. Following the surgical procedure, the surgeon ordered meperidine (Demerol) for postoperative pain management. In assessing Mr. Park, he reported his pain is "8 out of 10" on a 0 to 10 pain scale. The nurse promptly gives the drug, and approximately 20 minutes after receiving an injection of meperidine, the nurse discovers Mr. Park's vital signs are as follows: blood pressure 80/50 mm Hg, pulse rate 130 bpm, and respiratory rate 8 breaths/minute. Now that you have read almost all the chapters in this unit, determine whether you could anticipate Mr. Park's risks for opioid toxicity and discuss what actions should be taken for a proper pain assessment and medication administration.

effects by competing for the opiate receptor sites and displacing the opioid drug (see Chapter 15). If the individual has taken or received an opioid, the effects of the opioid are reversed. An antagonist drug is not selective for specific adverse reactions. When an antagonist is given to reverse a specific adverse reaction, such as respiratory depression, it is important to remember the antagonist reverses *all* effects. Therefore, a patient who receives an antagonist to reverse respiratory effects will also experience a reversal of pain relief; that is, the pain will return. If the individual has not taken or received an opioid, an antagonist has no drug effect.

Uses

Opioid antagonists are used for the treatment of the following:

• Postoperative acute respiratory depression
• Opioid adverse effects (reversal)
• Suspected acute opioid overdosage

Adverse Reactions

Generalized reactions include:

• Nausea and vomiting
• Sweating
• Tachycardia
• Increased blood pressure
• Tremors

See the Summary Drug Table: Opioid Antagonists for more information.

Contraindications, Precautions, and Interactions

Antagonists are contraindicated in those with a hypersensitivity to the opioid antagonists. Antagonists are used cautiously in those who are pregnant (pregnancy category B), in infants of opioid-dependent mothers, and in patients with an opioid dependency or cardiovascular disease. These drugs also are used cautiously during lactation.

These drugs may produce withdrawal symptoms in individuals who are physically dependent on the opioid. Antagonists may prevent the action or intended use of opioid antidiarrheals, antitussives, and analgesics.

NURSING PROCESS

PATIENT RECEIVING AN OPIOID ANTAGONIST FOR RESPIRATORY DEPRESSION

ASSESSMENT

Preadministration Assessment
Patients involved in long-term opioid therapy for pain relief build tolerance to the physical adverse effects of the drugs. It is the patient who does not use opioids routinely and who is being given an opioid drug for acute pain relief or a surgical procedure who is at most risk for respiratory depression after opioid administration (Fig. 16.1). These patients are described as opioid naive.

Sometimes the somnolence and pain relief produced by the opioid drug will slow the patient's breathing pattern. This can be alarming if the respiratory rate you have been monitoring has been rapid because of anxiety and pain. The first step is to make efforts to arouse the patient and coach his or her breathing pattern if possible. Before administration of the antagonist, take the blood pressure, pulse, and respiratory rate, and review the record for the drug suspected of causing the symptoms of respiratory depression. If there is sufficient time, review the initial health history, allergy history, and current treatment modalities.

Ongoing Assessment
As part of the ongoing assessment during the administration of the antagonist, continue to monitor the blood pressure, pulse, and respiratory rate at frequent intervals, usually every 5 minutes, until the patient responds. This monitoring should be more frequent if respiratory depression occurs in the immediate postoperative setting. After the patient has shown a response to the drug, monitor vital signs every 5 to 15 minutes. Notify the anesthesiologist or primary health care provider if any adverse drug reactions occur because additional medical treatment may be needed. Continue to monitor the respiratory

rate, rhythm, and depth; pulse; blood pressure; and level of consciousness until the effects of the opioid wear off.

> **❗ NURSING ALERT**
> The effects of some opioids may last longer than the effects of naloxone (Narcan). A repeat dose of naloxone may be ordered if results obtained from the initial dose are unsatisfactory. The duration of close patient observation depends on the patient's response to the administration of the opioid antagonist.

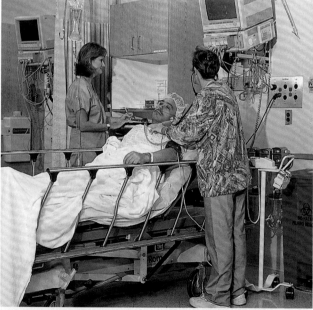

Figure 16.1 Patients who are in acute pain following a surgical procedure and do not use opioids routinely are more at risk for respiratory depression. (Photo by B. Proud.)

NURSING DIAGNOSES

Drug-specific nursing diagnoses are the following:

- **Impaired Spontaneous Ventilation** related to brain response to slow breathing induced by the opioid drug
- **Acute Pain** related to the antagonist drug displacing the opioid drug at cell receptor sites

Nursing diagnoses related to drug administration are discussed in Chapter 4.

PLANNING

The expected outcome for the patient with respiratory depression is an optimal response to therapy and support of patient needs related to the management of adverse drug effects. This is essentially a return to normal respiratory rate, rhythm, and depth. In this situation, you meet the patient's needs by providing adequate ventilation of the body as well as continued pain relief.

IMPLEMENTATION

Promoting an Optimal Response to Therapy

Frequently, the use of naloxone is in the controlled setting of the postanesthesia recovery unit (also called the *postanesthesia care unit* [PACU] or *surgical recovery room*). As the patient awakens from the deep operative sleep, you balance the need for continued pain relief against the person's ability to breathe independently after the procedure.

Monitoring and Managing Patient Needs

IMPAIRED SPONTANEOUS VENTILATION. Depending on the patient's condition, you may need to use cardiac monitoring, artificial ventilation (respirator), and other drugs during and after the administration of naloxone. It is important to keep suction equipment readily available because abrupt reversal of opioid-induced respiratory depression may cause vomiting. The goal is to maintain a patent airway, so you may need to turn and suction the patient to achieve this.

If naloxone is given by intravenous (IV) infusion, the anesthesiologist or primary health care provider orders the IV fluid and amount, the drug dosage, and the infusion rate. Giving the drug by IV infusion requires use of a secondary line, an IV piggyback, or an IV push (see Chapter 54).

> **! NURSING ALERT**
>
> When naloxone is used to reverse respiratory depression and the resulting somnolence, the drug is given by

slow IV push until the respiratory rate begins to increase and somnolence abates. Keep in mind that giving a rapid bolus will cause withdrawal and return of intense pain.

ACUTE PAIN. When the antagonist drug is given to patients, they experience pain abruptly, because the opioid no longer works in the body. Assess the pain level and begin to treat the pain again. As the patient's breathing returns, review the circumstances that led to the use of the antagonist as an opioid reversal drug. Steps can then be taken to resume pain relief without the adverse reaction.

If the patient is in a setting where family members may be present, it is your responsibility to educate the family about the action of the drug and what they will see happen. It can be distressing for others to see a person experience intense pain when the antagonist begins to work if they do not understand the reason for the intervention.

Monitor fluid intake and output and notify the primary health care provider of any change in the fluid intake–output ratio. Again, notify the primary health care provider if there is any sudden change in the patient's condition.

EVALUATION

- Therapeutic response is achieved and drug toxicity is reversed.
- Adverse reactions are identified, reported to the primary health care provider, and managed successfully with appropriate nursing interventions:
  - Patient's respiratory rate, rhythm, and depth are normal.
  - Pain relief is resumed.

PHARMACOLOGY IN PRACTICE
THINK CRITICALLY

 Determine whether you think Mr. Park could be considered *opiate naive* and more likely to experience respiratory depression. What factors were neglected during the pain assessment that resulted in his respiratory depression?

KEY POINTS

- An opioid antagonist reverses the effects of an opioid drug. This is used when patients experience extreme adverse reactions such as respiratory depression.
- These drugs reverse all effects of the opioids and the patient will experience pain.

- Patients who seldom use opioid pain relievers are termed opioid naive; they are at the greatest risk of experiencing respiratory depression when administered opioids.

⬤ *Summary Drug Table* OPIOID ANTAGONISTS

Generic Name	Trade Name	Uses	Adverse Reactions	Dosage Ranges
naloxone *nah-lox'-own*	Narcan	Complete or partial reversal of opioid effects after surgery or overdose	Nausea, vomiting, tachycardia, hypertension, return of postoperative pain, fever, dizziness	Postoperative opioid reversal: 0.1–0.2 mg IV at 2–3-min intervals Suspected opioid overdose: 0.4–2 mg IV at 2–3-min intervals

● Chapter Review

Calculate Medication Dosages

1. A client is prescribed 0.8 mg naloxone IV for postoperative respiratory depression caused by morphine. Available is a vial with 1 mg/mL. The nurse administers _____.

● Prepare for the NCLEX®

Build Your Knowledge

1. Which drug would most likely be prescribed for treatment of a client who is experiencing an opioid overdose?

1. naltrexone
2. naloxone
3. naproxen
4. nifedipine

2. What is the action when an opioid antagonist is administered?

1. increases renal clearance of the opioid drug
2. speeds up the cardiovascular system
3. displaces the opioid drug from the receptor site
4. causes the respiratory center to stop functioning

Apply Your Knowledge

3. Which client, given an opioid analgesic for acute pain, should the nurse monitor most closely for respiratory distress?

1. client with cancer taking morphine sulfate regularly
2. athlete who is taking Percocet for a leg injury
3. man who has never used an opioid pain medication
4. methadone client with a broken arm

Alternate-Format Questions

4. In the recovery room, the physician prescribes naloxone 0.4 mg by injection as the initial dose for opioid-induced respiratory depression; it may be followed in 5 minutes with 0.2 mg. Orders read that the nurse should contact the primary health care provider when a total of 1 mg is given. How many times can the nurse give the drug before contacting the primary health care provider?

5. Select the drugs that should be monitored for possible respiratory depression. **Select all that apply**.

1.

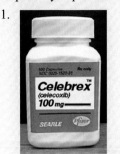

2.

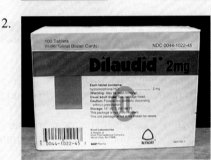

3.

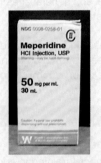

4.

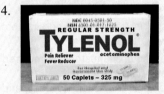

To check your answers, see Appendix G.

the**Point** *For more NCLEX-style questions, log on to http://thepoint.lww.com to access more than 1000 questions.*

17

Anesthetic Drugs

LEARNING OBJECTIVES

On completion of this chapter, the student will:

1. State the uses of local anesthesia, methods of administration, and nursing responsibilities when administering a local anesthetic.
2. Describe the purpose of a preanesthetic drug and the nursing responsibilities associated with the administration of a preanesthetic drug.
3. Identify several drugs used for local and general anesthesia.
4. List and briefly describe the four stages of general anesthesia.
5. Discuss important nursing responsibilities associated with caring for a patient receiving a preanesthetic drug and during the postanesthesia care (recovery room) period.

KEY TERMS

anesthesia • loss of feeling or sensation

anesthesiologist • physician with special training in administering anesthesia

anesthetist • nurse with special training who administers anesthesia; also called *nurse anesthetist*

conduction block • type of regional anesthesia produced by injection of a local anesthetic drug into or near a nerve trunk; examples include epidural, transsacral (caudal), and brachial

general anesthesia • sensation-free state of entire body

local anesthesia • provision of a pain-free state in a specific body area

neuroleptanalgesia • altered state of consciousness or sensation

preanesthetic drug • pertaining to status before administration of an anesthetic agent

regional anesthesia • injection of a local anesthetic around nerves to block sensation

spinal anesthesia • type of regional anesthesia produced by injection of a local anesthetic drug into the subarachnoid space of the spinal cord

DRUG CLASSES

Local anesthetics	General anesthetic
Preanesthetics	agents

nesthesia is a loss of feeling or sensation. Anesthesia may be induced by various drugs that can bring about partial or complete loss of sensation. There are two types of anesthesia: local anesthesia and general anesthesia. **Local anesthesia**, as the term implies, is the provision of a sensation-free state in a specific area (or region). With a local anesthetic, the patient is fully awake but does not feel pain in the area that has been anesthetized. However, some procedures performed under local anesthesia may require the patient to be sedated. Although not fully awake, sedated patients may still hear what is going on around them. **General anesthesia** is the provision of a sensation-free state for the entire body. When a general anesthetic is given, the patient loses consciousness and feels no pain. Reflexes, such as the swallowing and gag reflexes, are lost during deep general anesthesia (Fig. 17.1). Anesthetic drugs are included here because they eliminate the sensation of pain, which completes the spectrum of pain management in this unit.

Both physicians and nurses administer anesthesia. An **anesthesiologist** is a physician with special training in administering anesthesia. A nurse **anesthetist** is a nurse with at least a master's degree and special training who is qualified to administer anesthetics.

PHARMACOLOGY IN PRACTICE

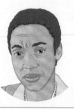

Lillian Chase has asked her primary health care provider to remove a mole on her arm. You are asked to draw up into a syringe the medication to numb the area. After reading this chapter, see if you can make the appropriate selection.

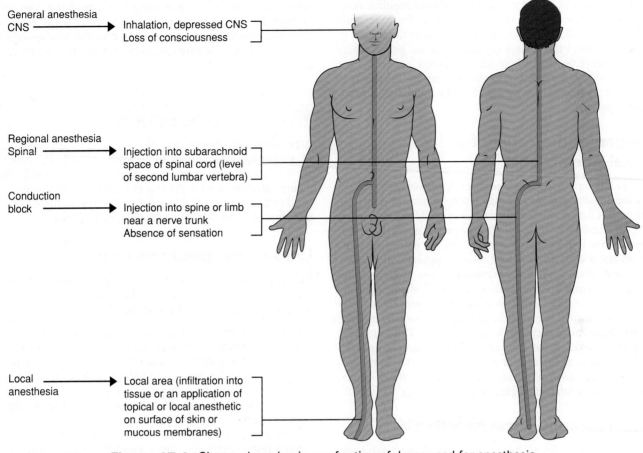

Figure 17.1 Sites and mechanisms of action of drugs used for anesthesia.

LOCAL ANESTHESIA

The various methods of administering a local anesthetic include topical application, local infiltration, and regional anesthesia.

Topical Anesthesia

Topical anesthesia involves the application of the anesthetic to the surface of the skin, open area, or mucous membrane. The anesthetic may be applied with a cotton swab or sprayed on the area. This type of anesthesia may be used to desensitize the skin or mucous membrane to the injection of a deeper local anesthetic. In some instances, topical anesthetics are dispensed in a transdermal form for chronic pain relief.

Local Infiltration Anesthesia

Local infiltration anesthesia is the injection of a local anesthetic drug into tissues. This type of anesthesia may be used for dental procedures, the suturing of small wounds, or making an incision into a small area, such as that required for removing a superficial piece of tissue for biopsy.

Regional Anesthesia

Regional anesthesia is the injection of a local anesthetic around nerves so that the area supplied by these nerves will not send pain signals to the brain. The anesthetized area is usually larger than the area affected by local infiltration anesthesia. Spinal anesthesia and conduction blocks are two types of regional anesthesia.

Spinal Anesthesia

Spinal anesthesia is a type of regional anesthesia that involves the injection of a local anesthetic drug into the subarachnoid space of the spinal cord, usually at the level of the second lumbar vertebra. There is a loss of feeling (anesthesia) and movement in the lower extremities, lower abdomen, and perineum.

Conduction Blocks

A **conduction block** is a type of regional anesthesia produced by injection of a local anesthetic drug into or near a nerve trunk. Examples of a conduction block include an epidural block (injection of a local anesthetic into the space surrounding the dura of the spinal cord), a transsacral (caudal) block (injection of a local anesthetic into the epidural space at the level of the sacrococcygeal notch), and a brachial plexus block (injection of a local anesthetic into the brachial plexus). Epidural—especially—and transsacral blocks are often used in obstetrics. A brachial plexus block may be used for surgery of the arm or hand.

The placement of the needle or a catheter requires strict aseptic technique by a skilled physician. Drug injected through the catheter spreads freely throughout the tissues in the space, interrupting pain conduction at the points where sensory nerve fibers exit from the spinal cord.

A catheter may be placed to give intermittent injections to maintain anesthesia over time such as the immediate postoperative period.

Preparing the Patient for Local Anesthesia

Depending on the procedure performed, preparing the patient for local anesthesia may or may not be similar to preparing the patient for general anesthesia. For example, administering a local anesthetic for dental surgery or for suturing a small wound may require that you explain to the patient how the anesthetic will be administered, take the patient's allergy history, and, when applicable, prepare the area to be anesthetized, which may involve cleaning the area with an antiseptic or shaving the area. Other local anesthetic procedures may require the patient to be fasting (taking in nothing by mouth), because a sedative may also be administered. This conscious sedation would include administering an intravenous (IV) sedative, such as the central nervous system (CNS) depressant drug midazolam, during some local anesthetic procedures, such as cataract surgery or a colonoscopy.

Administering Local Anesthesia

The physician or dentist administers a local injectable anesthetic. These drugs may be mixed with epinephrine to cause local vasoconstriction. The drug stays in the tissue longer when epinephrine is used. This is contraindicated, however, when the local anesthetic is used on an extremity. When preparing these medications, you should proceed cautiously and be aware of when epinephrine is to be used and when it should not be used. Table 17.1 lists the more commonly used local anesthetics.

Nursing Responsibilities

When caring for a patient receiving local anesthesia, you may be responsible for applying a dressing to the surgical area if

Table 17.1 Example of Local Anesthetics	
Generic Name	**Trade Name**
articaine	Septocaine
bupivacaine	Marcaine
chloroprocaine	Nesacaine
lidocaine	Xylocaine
mepivacaine	Carbocaine, Isocaine
prilocaine	Citanest
ropivacaine	Naropin

appropriate. Typically, when using local anesthesia, you will instruct the family or caregiver how to observe the area for bleeding, oozing, or other problems after the administration of the anesthetic and when to contact the primary health care provider.

PREANESTHETIC DRUGS

A **preanesthetic drug** is one given before the administration of anesthesia. These drugs are to relax or sedate the patient for the surgical procedure. They may be taken at home by the patient, given by a nurse in the preanesthesia unit, or administered right before general anesthesia. The preanesthetic agent may consist of one drug or a combination of drugs.

Uses of Preanesthetic Drugs

The general purpose, or use, of the preanesthetic drug is to prepare the patient for anesthesia. The more specific purposes of these drugs include the following:

- Opioid or antianxiety drug—to decrease anxiety and apprehension immediately before surgery. The patient who is calm and relaxed can be anesthetized more quickly, usually requires a smaller dose of an induction drug, may require less anesthesia during surgery, and may have a smoother recovery from the anesthesia period (awakening from anesthesia).
- Cholinergic blocking drug—to decrease secretions of the upper respiratory tract. Some anesthetic gases and volatile liquids are irritating to the lining of the respiratory tract and thereby increase mucous secretions. The cough and swallowing reflexes are lost during general anesthesia, and excessive secretions can pool in the lungs, resulting in pneumonia or atelectasis (lung collapse) during the postoperative period. The administration of a cholinergic blocking drug, such as glycopyrrolate (Robinul), dries up secretions of the upper respiratory tract and decreases the possibility of excessive mucus production.
- Antiemetic—to decrease the incidence of nausea and vomiting during the immediate postoperative recovery period

 LIFESPAN CONSIDERATIONS
Gerontology
Preanesthetic drugs may be omitted in patients who are 60 years or older because many of the medical disorders for which these drugs are contraindicated are seen in older individuals. For example, atropine and glycopyrrolate, drugs that can be used to decrease secretions of the upper respiratory tract, are contraindicated in certain medical disorders, such as prostatic hypertrophy, glaucoma, and myocardial ischemia. Other preanesthetic drugs that depress the CNS, such as opioids, barbiturates, and antianxiety drugs, with or without antiemetic properties, may be contraindicated in the older individual.

Selection of Preanesthetic Drugs

The preanesthetic drug is usually selected by the anesthesiologist and may consist of one or more drugs (Table 17.2). An

Table 17.2 Examples of Preanesthetic Drugs

Generic Name	Trade Name
Opioids	
fentanyl	Sublimaze
meperidine	Demerol
morphine	
Barbiturates	
pentobarbital	Nembutal
secobarbital	Seconal
Cholinergic Blocking Drugs	
atropine	
glycopyrrolate	Robinul
scopolamine	
Antianxiety Drugs With Antiemetic Properties	
hydroxyzine	Vistaril
Antianxiety Drugs	
chlordiazepoxide	Librium
diazepam	Valium
lorazepam	Ativan
midazolam	
Sedative Drugs	
droperidol	Inapsine

opioid (see Chapter 16) or antianxiety drug (see Chapter 20) may be given to relax or sedate the patient. A cholinergic blocking drug (see Chapter 27) is given to dry secretions in the upper respiratory tract. Scopolamine and glycopyrrolate also have mild sedative properties, and atropine may or may not produce some sedation. Antianxiety drugs have sedative action; when combined with an opioid, they allow a lowering of the opioid dosage because they also have the ability to potentiate (increase the effect of) the sedative action of the opioid. Diazepam (Valium), an antianxiety drug, is one of the more commonly used drugs for preoperative sedation.

Nursing Responsibilities

When caring for a patient receiving a preanesthetic drug, assess the patient's physical status and give an explanation of the anesthesia. In some hospitals, the anesthesiologist examines the patient at an outpatient visit, a few days or a week before surgery, although this may not be possible in emergency situations. Some hospitals use operating room or postanesthesia care unit (PACU) staff members to visit the patient before surgery to explain certain facts, such as the time of surgery, the effects of the preanesthetic drug, preparations for surgery, and the PACU. Proper explanation of anesthesia, the surgery itself, and the events that may occur in preparation for surgery, as well as care after surgery, requires

a team approach. As the nurse on the team, your responsibilities include the following:

- Describe or explain the preparations for surgery ordered by the physician. Examples of preoperative preparations include fasting from midnight (or the time specified by the physician), enema, shaving of the operative site, use of a hypnotic for sleep the night before, and the preoperative injection about 30 minutes before surgery.
- Describe or explain immediate postoperative care, such as that given in the PACU (also called the *recovery room*) or a special postoperative surgical unit, and the activities of the health care team during this period. Explain that the patient's vital signs will be monitored frequently and that other equipment, such as IV lines and fluids and hemodynamic (cardiac) monitors, may be used.
- Demonstrate, describe, and explain postoperative patient activities, such as deep breathing, coughing, and leg exercises.
- Emphasize the importance of pain control, and make sure the patient understands that relieving pain early on is better than trying to hold out, not take the medicine, and later attempt to relieve the pain. Teach the patient how to use the patient-controlled analgesia (PCA) pump.
- Tailor the preoperative explanations to fit the type of surgery scheduled. Not all of these teaching points may require inclusion in every explanation.
- Provide written instructions in the language of preference for the patient to take home and read to reinforce the teachings.

GENERAL ANESTHESIA

The administration of general anesthesia requires the use of one or more drugs. The choice of anesthetic drug depends on many factors, including:

- General physical condition of the patient
- Area, organ, or system being operated on
- Anticipated length of the surgical procedure

The anesthesiologist selects the anesthetic drugs that will produce safe anesthesia, analgesia (absence of pain), and, in some surgeries, effective skeletal muscle relaxation. General anesthesia is most commonly achieved when the anesthetic vapors are inhaled or administered IV. Volatile liquid anesthetics produce anesthesia when their vapors are inhaled. Volatile liquids are liquids that evaporate on exposure to air. Examples of volatile liquids include halothane, desflurane, and enflurane. Gas anesthetics are combined with oxygen and administered by inhalation. Examples of gas anesthetics are nitrous oxide and cyclopropane.

Drugs Used for General Anesthesia

Barbiturates and Similar Agents

Methohexital (Brevital), which is an ultrashort-acting barbiturate, is used for the following:

- Induction of anesthesia
- Short surgical procedures with minimal painful stimuli
- In conjunction with or as a supplement to other anesthetics

These types of drugs have a rapid onset and a short duration of action. They depress the CNS to produce hypnosis and anesthesia but do not produce analgesia. Recovery after a small dose is rapid.

Etomidate, a nonbarbiturate, is used for induction of anesthesia. Etomidate also may be used to supplement other anesthetics, such as nitrous oxide, for short surgical procedures. It is a hypnotic without analgesic activity.

Propofol (Diprivan) is used for induction and maintenance of anesthesia. It also may be used for sedation during diagnostic procedures and procedures that use a local anesthetic. This drug also is used for continuous sedation of intubated or respiratory-controlled patients in intensive care units.

Benzodiazepines

Midazolam, a short-acting benzodiazepine CNS depressant, is used as a preanesthetic drug to relieve anxiety; for induction of anesthesia; for conscious sedation before minor procedures, such as endoscopy; and to supplement nitrous oxide and oxygen for short surgical procedures. When the drug is used for induction anesthesia, the patient gradually loses consciousness over a period of 1 to 2 minutes.

Ketamine

Ketamine (Ketalar) is a rapid-acting general anesthetic. It produces an anesthetic state characterized by profound analgesia, cardiovascular and respiratory stimulation, normal or enhanced skeletal muscle tone, and occasionally mild respiratory depression. Ketamine is used for diagnostic and surgical procedures that do not require relaxation of skeletal muscles, for induction of anesthesia before the administration of other anesthetic drugs, and as a supplement to other anesthetic drugs.

Gases and Volatile Liquids

Nitrous oxide is the most commonly used anesthetic gas. It is a weak anesthetic and is usually used in combination with other anesthetic drugs. It does not cause skeletal muscle relaxation. The chief danger in the use of nitrous oxide is hypoxemia. Nitrous oxide is nonexplosive and is supplied in blue cylinders (oxygen tanks are green).

Enflurane (Ethrane) is a volatile liquid anesthetic that is delivered by inhalation. Induction and recovery from anesthesia are rapid. Muscle relaxation for abdominal surgery is adequate, but greater relaxation may be necessary and may require the use of a skeletal muscle relaxant. Enflurane may produce mild stimulation of respiratory and bronchial secretions when used alone. Hypotension may occur when anesthesia deepens.

Isoflurane (Forane) is a volatile liquid given by inhalation. It is used for induction and maintenance of anesthesia.

Desflurane (Suprane), a volatile liquid, is used for induction and maintenance of anesthesia. A special vaporizer is used to deliver this anesthetic, because delivery by mask results in irritation of the respiratory tract.

Sevoflurane (Ultane) is an inhalational analgesic. It is used for induction and maintenance of general anesthesia in adult and pediatric patients for both inpatient and outpatient surgical procedures.

Table 17.3 Examples of Muscle Relaxants Used During General Anesthesia

Generic Name	Trade Name
cisatracurium	Nimbex
pancuronium	
succinylcholine	Anectine

Opioids

The opioid analgesic fentanyl (Sublimaze) and the neuroleptic drug (major tranquilizer) droperidol (Inapsine) may be used together. The combination of these two drugs results in **neuroleptanalgesia**, which is characterized by general quietness, reduced motor activity, and profound analgesia. Complete loss of consciousness may not occur unless other anesthetic drugs are used. A combination of fentanyl and droperidol may be used for the tranquilizing effect and analgesia for surgical and diagnostic procedures. It may also be used as a preanesthetic for the induction of anesthesia and in the maintenance of general anesthesia.

The use of droperidol as a tranquilizer, as an antiemetic to reduce nausea and vomiting during the immediate postanesthesia period, as an induction drug, and as an adjunct to general anesthesia has decreased because of its association with fatal cardiac dysrhythmias. Fentanyl may be used alone as a supplement to general or regional anesthesia. It may also be administered alone or with other drugs as a preoperative drug and as an analgesic during the immediate postoperative period.

Remifentanil (Ultiva) is used for induction and maintenance of general anesthesia and for continued analgesia during the immediate postoperative period. This drug is used cautiously in patients with a history of hypersensitivity to fentanyl.

Skeletal Muscle Relaxants

The various skeletal muscle relaxants that may be used during general anesthesia are listed in Table 17.3. These drugs are administered to produce relaxation of the skeletal muscles during certain types of surgeries, such as those involving the chest or abdomen. They may also be used to facilitate the insertion of an endotracheal tube. Their onset of action is usually rapid (45 seconds to a few minutes), and their duration of action is 30 minutes or more.

Stages of General Anesthesia

General surgical anesthesia is divided into the following stages:

- Stage I—analgesia
- Stage II—delirium
- Stage III—surgical analgesia
- Stage IV—respiratory paralysis

Display 17.1 describes the stages of general anesthesia more completely. With newer drugs and techniques, the stages of

Display 17.1 Stages of General Anesthesia

Stage I
Induction is a part of stage I anesthesia. It begins with the administration of an anesthetic drug and lasts until consciousness is lost. With some induction drugs, such as the short-acting barbiturates, this stage may last only 5 to 10 seconds.

Stage II
Stage II is the stage of delirium and excitement. This stage is also brief. During this stage, the patient may move about and mumble incoherently. The muscles are somewhat rigid, and the patient is unconscious and cannot feel pain. During this stage, noises are exaggerated and even quiet sounds may seem extremely loud to the patient. If surgery were attempted at this stage, there would be a physical reaction to painful stimuli, yet the patient would not remember sensing pain. During these first two stages of anesthesia, you should avoid any unnecessary noise or motion in the room.

Stage III
Stage III is the stage of surgical analgesia and is divided into four parts, planes, or substages. The anesthesiologist differentiates these planes by the character of the respirations, eye movements, certain reflexes, pupil size, and other factors. The levels of the planes range from plane 1 (light) to plane 4 (deep). At plane 2 or 3, the patient is usually ready for the surgical procedure.

Stage IV
Stage IV is the stage of respiratory paralysis and is a rare and dangerous stage of anesthesia. At this stage, respiratory arrest and cessation of all vital signs may occur.

anesthesia may not be as prominent as those described in Display 17.1. In addition, movement through the first two stages is usually very rapid.

Anesthesia begins with a loss of consciousness. This is part of the induction phase (stage I). The patient is now relaxed and can no longer comprehend what is happening. After consciousness is lost, additional anesthetic drugs are administered. Some of these drugs are also used as part of the induction phase, as well as for deepening anesthesia. Depending on the type of surgery, an endotracheal tube also may be inserted to provide an adequate airway and to assist in administering oxygen and other anesthetic drugs. The endotracheal tube is removed during the postanesthesia period once the gag and swallowing reflexes have resumed. If an IV line was not inserted before the patient's arrival in surgery, it is inserted by the anesthesiologist before the administration of an induction drug.

Nursing Responsibilities

Preanesthesia

Before surgery, and during the administration of general anesthesia, as the nurse, you have the following responsibilities:

- Performing the required tasks and procedures as prescribed by the physician and hospital policy before surgery and documenting these tasks on the patient's chart. Examples of these tasks include administering a hypnotic agent before surgery, shaving the operative area, taking vital signs, seeing that the operative consent form is signed, checking that all jewelry or metal objects are removed from the patient, inserting a catheter, inserting a nasogastric tube, and teaching.
- Checking the chart for any recent abnormal laboratory test results. If a recent abnormal laboratory test finding was included in the patient's chart shortly before surgery, alert the surgeon and the anesthesiologist to the abnormality.
- Flagging the list of known or suspected drug allergies or idiosyncrasies
- Administering the preanesthetic (preoperative) drug
- Instructing the patient to remain in bed and placing the bed's side rails up once the preanesthetic drug has been given

> **NURSING ALERT**
> Preanesthetic drugs must be administered on time to produce their intended effects. Failure to give the preanesthetic drug on time may result in such events as increased respiratory secretions caused by the irritating effect of anesthetic gases and the need for an increased dose of the induction drug because the preanesthetic drug has not had time to sedate the patient.

Postanesthesia: Postanesthesia Care Unit (PACU)

After surgery, your responsibilities vary according to where you first come into contact with the postoperative patient:

- Admitting the patient to the unit according to hospital procedure or policy
- Checking the airway for patency, assessing the respiratory status, and giving oxygen as needed
- Positioning the patient to prevent aspiration of vomitus and secretions
- Checking blood pressure and pulse, IV lines, catheters, drainage tubes, surgical dressings, and casts
- Reviewing the patient's surgical and anesthesia records
- Monitoring the blood pressure, pulse, and respiratory rate every 5 to 15 minutes until the patient is discharged from the area
- Checking the patient every 5 to 15 minutes for emergence from anesthesia. Suctioning is provided as needed.
- Exercising caution in administering opioids. The nurse must check the patient's respiratory rate, blood pressure, and pulse before these drugs are given and 20 to 30 minutes after administration (see Chapter 16). The physician is contacted if the respiratory rate is below 10 breaths/min before the drug is given or if the respiratory rate falls below 10 breaths/min after the drug is given.
- Discharging the patient from the area to his or her room or other specified area. You should complete documentation of all drugs administered and nursing tasks performed before the patient leaves the PACU.

PHARMACOLOGY IN PRACTICE
THINK CRITICALLY

 Lillian Chase requires a local anesthetic to remove a mole on her arm. There are two vials sitting on the counter, lidocaine 2% solution and lidocaine 2% with epinephrine 1:100,000 in solution. After reading this chapter, can you determine the appropriate choice for the injection?

KEY POINTS

- Anesthesia is the loss of feeling or sensation. Local and general anesthesia is provided for pain relief and to perform otherwise painful procedures.

- Local anesthesia includes topical, local infiltration and regional pain relief and is used when dealing with a specific area of the body and the patient can remain conscious.

- General anesthesia requires multiple drugs and stages to achieve a state where surgical procedures can be performed without pain, movement, or memory.

- A greater number of body systems are involved when a general anesthetic is administered; patients need assistance and coaching to resume respiratory, gastrointestinal, and musculoskeletal function following the procedure.

- Nursing responsibility includes tasks to assist, maintain, and recover a patient who has been given an anesthetic.

● Chapter Review

Know Your Drugs

Clients sometimes know a medication by the brand (or trade) name and not the generic name. To help you recognize both names, match the brand name with the generic name of the same medication.

Generic Name	Brand Name
1. lidocaine	A. Demerol
2. meperidine	B. Diprivan
3. propofol	C. Marcaine
4. bupivacaine	D. Xylocaine

Calculate Medication Dosages

1. As a preoperative medication for a client going to surgery, the anesthesiologist prescribes meperidine (Demerol) 50 mg IM. Meperidine is available in a solution of 50 mg/mL. The nurse prepares to administer _____.

● Prepare for the NCLEX®

Build Your Knowledge

1. The type of anesthesia used when a small cut or wound is sutured is called _____.

   1. topical
   2. regional
   3. local infiltrate
   4. conduction block

2. When planning preoperative care, the nurse expects that a preanesthetic medication is given _____ before the client is transported to surgery.

   1. 20 minutes
   2. 30 minutes
   3. 40 minutes
   4. 60 minutes

3. Which of the following drugs is the most commonly used gas for general anesthesia?

   1. ethylene
   2. enflurane
   3. nitrous oxide
   4. sevoflurane

4. Neuroleptanalgesia is used to promote general quietness, reduce motor activity, and induce profound analgesia. Which of the following two drugs are used in combination to accomplish neuroleptanalgesia?

   1. fentanyl and droperidol
   2. morphine and glycopyrrolate
   3. atropine and meperidine
   4. fentanyl and midazolam

5. One use of skeletal muscle relaxants as part of general anesthesia is to:

   1. prevent movement during surgery
   2. facilitate insertion of the endotracheal tube
   3. allow for deeper anesthesia
   4. produce additional anesthesia

Apply Your Knowledge

6. Which group of individuals is at a higher risk for complications from preanesthetic drugs?

   1. infants
   2. adolescents and teens
   3. obese individuals
   4. older adults

7. Following general anesthesia, a client is rolled to the side during the recovery period to:

   1. assess respiratory status
   2. prevent the endotracheal tube from being swallowed
   3. assess vital signs better
   4. prevent aspiration during recovery

Alternate-Format Questions

8. Match the medication with its intended action related to anesthetic procedures.

1. opioid	A. decrease chance of nausea
2. antiemetic	B. depress the central nervous system
3. cholinergic blocker	C. relieve pain and decrease anxiety
4. benzodiazepine	D. decrease secretions

9. Arrange the following actions as they happen during the stages of general anesthesia:

   1. respiratory paralysis
   2. moving about and mumbling may occur
   3. consciousness is lost
   4. muscles become ridged and sounds exaggerated

10. Glycopyrrolate (Robinul) is prescribed for a client as part of the preoperative preparation for surgery. The drug dose recommendation is 0.002 mg/lb. The client weighs 150 lb. The nurse expects the anesthesiologist to prescribe _____.

To check your answers, see Appendix G.

the**Point** *For more NCLEX-style questions, log on to http://thepoint.lww.com to access more than 1000 questions.*

Drugs That Affect the Central Nervous System

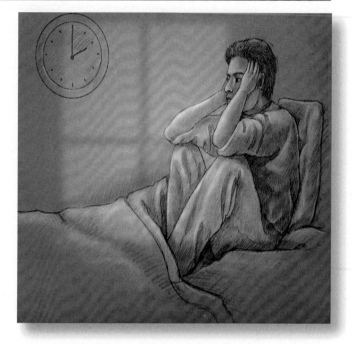

The nervous system is a complex part of the human body concerned with the regulation and coordination of body activities such as movement, behavior, digestion, and sleep. The nervous system has two main divisions: the central nervous system (CNS) and the peripheral nervous system (PNS). The CNS consists of the brain and the spinal cord. The CNS receives, integrates, and interprets nerve impulses, whereas the PNS connects all parts of the body with the CNS.

In this unit, drugs that affect the central nervous system are presented. Drugs that affect the CNS alter mood, sensation, and the interpretation of information in the brain. These drugs are used to enhance mental health well-being in both inpatient and outpatient settings.

Drugs that stimulate the CNS are presented in Chapter 18. CNS stimulants are used to reverse respiratory depression or to treat children with attention deficit hyperactivity disorder (ADHD).

Chapter 19 discusses the drugs used to enhance neurotransmission of certain substances to maintain and sometimes enhance the cognitive function of persons with dementia.

Currently, Alzheimer's disease (AD) is the ninth-leading cause of death in adults older than 65 years. Typically, an individual lives on average 8 years after diagnosis; yet, some people have been known to live up to 20 years after AD is discovered. Close to $200 billion is spent annually to care for people with AD (including both direct and indirect costs). Although a cure is not known for this degenerative disease, the dementia experienced can be slowed by the use of drugs called *cholinesterase inhibitors,* which are covered in Chapter 19. Drugs that have a depressing effect on neurotransmission in the CNS are used to treat anxiety (Chapter 20). The sedative/hypnotic drugs (Chapter 21) are used to treat insomnia or to produce a calming effect when patients are about to undergo a surgical or diagnostic procedure.

Drugs that act on the CNS are also used to change mood or behavior. These drugs may take many days or even weeks to produce a therapeutic response. Chapter 22 discusses drugs used to treat depression, which is one of the most common mental health disorders. Depression is characterized by impaired functioning and feelings of intense sadness, helplessness, and worthlessness. People experiencing major depressive episodes exhibit physical and psychological symptoms, such as appetite disturbances, sleep disturbances, and loss of interest in job, family, and other activities usually enjoyed.

A psychotic disorder, on the other hand, is characterized by extreme personality disorganization and the loss of contact with reality. Drugs given to patients with a psychotic disorder, such as schizophrenia, are called *antipsychotic drugs* or *neuroleptics.* The antipsychotic drugs are discussed in Chapter 23.

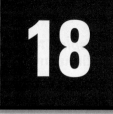

Central Nervous System Stimulants

LEARNING OBJECTIVES

On completion of this chapter, the student will:

1. List the three classes of central nervous system (CNS) stimulants.
2. Discuss the uses, general drug actions, general adverse reactions, contraindications, precautions, and interactions of CNS stimulants.
3. Discuss important preadministration and ongoing assessment activities the nurse should perform on the patient taking a CNS stimulant.
4. List nursing diagnoses particular to a patient taking a CNS stimulant.
5. Discuss ways to promote an optimal response to drug therapy, how to manage common adverse drug reactions, and important points to keep in mind when educating patients about the use of CNS stimulants.

KEY TERMS

attention deficit hyperactivity disorder (ADHD) • disorder characterized by inattention, hyperactivity, and impulsivity

euphoric • an intense feeling of excitement and happiness

narcolepsy • chronic disorder that results in recurrent attacks of drowsiness and sleep during daytime

sympathomimetic • drugs that mimic stimulation of the sympathetic nervous system

DRUG CLASSES

Amphetamines
Analeptics
Anorexiants

This chapter discusses the drugs that stimulate the central nervous system (CNS) and the nursing implications related to their administration. The three basic classes of stimulants are amphetamines, analeptics, and anorexiants. The definitions of these classes are presented in Display 18.1. These drugs are used with caution because the CNS stimulants have a high abuse potential due to their ability to produce euphoria and wakefulness.

CENTRAL NERVOUS SYSTEM STIMULANTS

Actions

The amphetamines are **sympathomimetic** (i.e., adrenergic) drugs, meaning they stimulate the CNS to speed up (see Chapter 24). Their drug action results in an elevation of blood pressure, wakefulness, and an increase or decrease in pulse rate. Amphetamines also produce a **euphoric** state; this pleasurable feeling is what increases their dependency potential.

One condition successfully treated by amphetamines is **attention deficit hyperactivitydisorder (ADHD)** in children. Amphetamines work by blocking the reuptake of norepinephrine and dopamine. This lessens the action of other neurotransmitters, thus helping to focus concentration and attention.

One of the most widely used CNS stimulants is caffeine. It is a mild to potent analeptic CNS stimulant. Analeptics

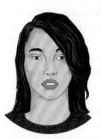

PHARMACOLOGY IN PRACTICE

Janna Wong is a 16-year-old high school gymnast. Mrs. Wong has brought her to the clinic after reading on the Internet about attention deficit hyperactivity disorder (ADHD). She is worried that Janna's lack of focus on training may be due to this disorder. She is here to have medications prescribed for her daughter.

Display 18.1 Central Nervous System Stimulants and Definitions

Analeptics. Drugs that stimulate the respiratory center of the brain and cardiovascular system, used with narcolepsy and as an adjuvant treatment for obstructive sleep apnea
Amphetamines. Drugs used to treat children with attention deficit hyperactivity disorder (ADHD)
Anorexiants. Drugs used to suppress the appetite

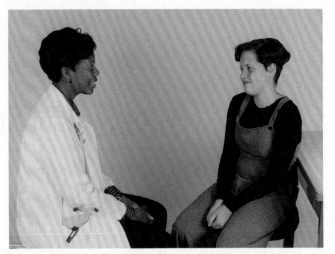

Figure 18.1 Children should always have a thorough examination before stimulants for attention deficit hyperactivity disorder (ADHD) are prescribed. (From Bickley, L. S., & Szilagyi, P. [2003]. *Bates' guide to physical examination and history taking* [8th ed.]. Philadelphia: Lippincott Williams & Wilkins.)

increase the depth of respirations by stimulating special receptors located in the carotid arteries and upper aorta. These special receptors (called *chemoreceptors*) are sensitive to the amount of oxygen in arterial blood. Stimulation of these receptors results in an increase in the depth of respirations. Caffeine is an analeptic that stimulates the CNS at all levels, including the cerebral cortex, the medulla, and the spinal cord. Caffeine also has mild diuretic activity. People take caffeine on their own in the form of coffee, tea, or even chocolate, yet caffeine's use as a therapeutic drug for stimulation in the neonatal setting is growing. Other actions of analeptics include cardiac stimulation (which may produce tachycardia), dilation of coronary and peripheral blood vessels, constriction of cerebral blood vessels, and skeletal muscle stimulation.

Modafinil (Provigil) and armodafinil (Nuvigil) are analeptics used to treat **narcolepsy** (a disorder that causes an uncontrollable desire to sleep during normal waking hours even though the individual has a normal nighttime sleeping pattern). The exact mechanism of action is not known, but the drugs are thought to bind to dopamine, thereby reducing the number of episodes. It does not cause cardiac and other systemic stimulatory effects like other CNS stimulants. These drugs are sometimes used in the treatment of obstructive sleep apnea to promote daytime wakefulness (not to replace continuous positive airway pressure during sleep).

The anorexiants are drugs pharmacologically similar to the amphetamines. Their ability to suppress the appetite is thought to be due to their action on the appetite center in the hypothalamus.

Uses

The CNS stimulants are used in the treatment of the following:

• ADHD
• Drug-induced respiratory depression
• Postanesthesia respiratory depression, without reduction of analgesia
• Narcolepsy
• Obstructive sleep apnea
• Exogenous obesity
• Fatigue (caffeine)

NURSING ALERT

ADHD is a condition of both children and adults and is characterized by inattention, hyperactivity, and impulsivity. Because these behaviors, when independently present, can be normal in any individual, it is important that the child receive

a thorough examination and appropriate diagnosis by a well-qualified professional before drug therapy is initiated (Fig. 18.1).

Adverse Reactions

Neuromuscular System Reactions

• Excessive CNS stimulation, headache, dizziness
• Apprehension, disorientation, hyperactivity

Other Reactions

• Nausea, vomiting, cough, dyspnea
• Urinary retention, tachycardia, palpitations

For more information on adverse reactions, see the Summary Drug Table: Central Nervous System Stimulants.

Contraindications

The CNS stimulants are contraindicated in patients with known hypersensitivity or convulsive disorders and in those with ventilation disorders (e.g., chronic obstructive pulmonary disease [COPD]). Do not administer CNS stimulants to patients with cardiac problems, severe hypertension, or hyperthyroidism. *CNS stimulants are not recommended as treatment for depression.* Amphetamines and anorexiants should not be taken concurrently or within 14 days of antidepressant medications. In addition, amphetamines are contraindicated in patients with glaucoma. Most anorexiants are classified as pregnancy category X and should not be used during pregnancy. Although armodafinil is considered a pregnancy category C drug, its safety has not been proven.

NURSING ALERT

Stimulants enhance dopamine transmission to areas of the brain that interpret well-being. To maintain pleasurable feelings, people continue the use of stimulants, which leads to their abuse and the potential for addiction.

Precautions

The CNS stimulants should be used cautiously in patients with respiratory illness, renal or hepatic impairment, and history of substance abuse. The CNS stimulants should be used cautiously in pregnant or lactating women.

Interactions

The following drugs may interact with a CNS stimulant when it is administered with them:

Interacting Drug	Common Use	Effect of Interaction
anesthetics	Anesthesia during surgical procedures	Increased risk of cardiac arrhythmias
theophylline	Respiratory problems, such as asthma	Increased risk of hyperactive behaviors
oral contraceptives	Birth control	Decreased effectiveness of oral contraceptive when taken with modafinil

NURSING PROCESS
PATIENT RECEIVING A CENTRAL NERVOUS SYSTEM STIMULANT

ASSESSMENT
Assessment of the patient receiving a CNS stimulant depends on the drug, the patient, and the reason for administration.

Preadministration Assessment
ATTENTION DEFICIT HYPERACTIVITY DISORDER. When an amphetamine is prescribed for any reason, weigh the patient and take the blood pressure, pulse, and respiratory rate before starting drug therapy. Work with the family to describe and document the observed behavior patterns the child with ADHD demonstrates for later comparison. If the child is hospitalized, ask the family for feedback and enter daily observations of the child's behavior into the patient's record. This provides a record of the results of therapy.

LIFESPAN CONSIDERATIONS
Pediatric
An increased risk of suicidal ideation in children and adolescents has been found when using the drug atomoxetine (Strattera). Patients with ADHD started on atomoxetine should be monitored carefully for suicidal thoughts or behaviors. Teach the family about specific behaviors to observe for and build confidence in how to ask their children about suicidal thinking that would indicate a need to contact the primary health care provider.

RESPIRATORY DEPRESSION. When a CNS stimulant is prescribed for respiratory depression, initial patient assessments include the blood pressure, pulse, and respiratory rate. It is important to note the depth of the respirations and any pattern to the respiratory rate, such as shallow respirations or alternating deep and shallow respirations. Review recent laboratory test results (if any), such as arterial blood gas studies. It is important to scan the chart to identify the drugs causing the respiratory depression.

OBESITY. When an anorexiant is used as part of obesity treatment, the drug is usually prescribed for outpatient use. Obtain and document the blood pressure, pulse, respiratory rate, and weight before therapy is started and at each outpatient visit.

Ongoing Assessment
RESPIRATORY DEPRESSION. After administering an analeptic, carefully monitor the patient's respiratory rate and pattern until the respirations return to normal. You should also monitor the level of consciousness, blood pressure, and pulse rate at 5- to 15-minute intervals or as ordered by the primary health care provider. Arterial blood gases may be drawn for analysis at intervals to determine the effectiveness of the analeptic, as well as the need for additional drug therapy. It is important to observe the patient for adverse drug reactions and to report their occurrence immediately to the primary health care provider.

NURSING DIAGNOSES
Drug-specific nursing diagnoses are the following:

- **Disturbed Sleep Pattern** related to CNS stimulation and hyperactivity, nervousness, insomnia, other (specify)
- **Ineffective Breathing Pattern** related to respiratory depression
- **Imbalanced Nutrition: Less Than Body Requirements** related to diminished appetite

Nursing diagnoses related to drug administration are discussed in Chapter 4.

PLANNING
The expected outcomes for the patient depend on the reason for administration of a CNS stimulant but may include an optimal response to therapy, support of patient needs related to management of adverse drug reactions, and confidence in an understanding of the medication regimen.

IMPLEMENTATION

Promoting an Optimal Response to Therapy
Stimulants are used long term for ADHD and may be used in the short-term treatment of exogenous obesity (obesity caused by a persistent calorie intake that is greater than needed by the body). However, their use in treating exogenous obesity has declined, because the long-term use of the amphetamines for obesity carries the potential for dependence and abuse.

Monitoring and Managing Patient Needs
DISTURBED SLEEP PATTERN. When CNS stimulant therapy causes insomnia, teach the caregiver to administer the drug early in the day (when possible) to diminish sleep disturbances. The primary health care provider may choose a long-acting form of the drug to be given daily in the morning to help reduce sleep pattern issues. Provide the patient with activities to distract him or her from napping during the day.

Other stimulants, such as coffee, tea, or cola drinks, are avoided. In some patients, nervousness, restlessness, and palpitations may occur. Check vital signs every 6 to 8 hours or more often if tachycardia, hypertension, or palpitations occur. The adverse drug reactions that may occur with amphetamine use may be serious enough to require discontinuation of the drug. In some instances, the adverse drug effects are mild and may even disappear during therapy as physical tolerance builds. Teach the patient to inform the primary care provider of all adverse reactions. An example would be if a patient tells you he or she can sleep without problem while on a stimulant. This would indicate the patient has built a tolerance to the drug, and in this case the dosage is not increased.

LIFESPAN CONSIDERATIONS
Gerontology
Older adults are especially sensitive to the effects of the CNS stimulants and may exhibit excessive anxiety, nervousness, insomnia, and mental confusion. Cardiovascular disorders, common in the older adult, may be worsened by the CNS stimulants. Careful monitoring is important because these reactions may result in the need to discontinue use of the drug.

These drugs may also be helpful in managing narcolepsy, a disorder manifested by an uncontrollable desire to sleep during normal waking hours even though the individual has a normal nighttime sleeping pattern. The individual with narcolepsy may fall asleep from a few minutes to a few hours many times in one day. The disorder begins in adolescence or young adulthood and persists throughout life.

INEFFECTIVE BREATHING PATTERN. Respiratory depression can be a serious event requiring administration of a respiratory stimulant. When an analeptic drug is administered, document the rate, depth, and character of the respirations before the drug is given. This provides a baseline for evaluating the effectiveness of drug therapy. Also before administering the drug, be sure that the patient has a patent airway. Oxygen is usually administered before, during, and after drug administration. After administration, monitor respirations closely and document the effects of therapy.

When respiratory depression occurs in the postsurgical setting, carefully assess the patient's level of pain. Respiratory depression can occur after a surgical procedure from the combination of drugs used to produce anesthesia. Opioid reversal drugs, such as naloxone (Narcan), that reverse the effects of opioid agents replace the pain relief drug at the receptor site of the cell. This means that the patient can experience a sudden and severe return of pain because the pain relief effect of the drug is eliminated along with the reversal of respiratory depression. Use of analeptic drugs for respiratory stimulation can enhance the breathing pattern without changing the effect of the opioid drug. Therefore, breathing improves and pain relief continues for the patient.

Nausea and vomiting may occur with the administration of an analeptic; therefore, you should keep a suction machine nearby in case the patient vomits. Urinary retention may result from doxapram administration; be sure to measure intake and output, and notify the primary health care provider if the patient cannot void or the bladder appears to be distended on palpation.

IMBALANCED NUTRITION: LESS THAN BODY REQUIREMENTS. One of the adverse reactions of CNS stimulant use in the child with ADHD is decreased appetite. Although decreased appetite is a desired effect when treating a patient with weight problems, it is not desirable when treating ADHD. This lack of appetite is thought to possibly retard growth in children because they do not eat (Manos, 2007). Therefore, it is important to monitor weight and growth patterns of children on long-term treatment with the CNS stimulant drugs.

Teach the parents to monitor the eating patterns of the child while he or she is taking CNS stimulants and to feel confident in preparing nutritious meals and snacks. A good breakfast is important to provide, because the drug will cause the child to possibly not feel hungry at lunchtime in school where the parent cannot monitor nutritional intake. The child should be checked frequently with height and weight measurements to monitor growth. During ADHD treatment, the drug regimen may be interrupted periodically under direction of the primary health provider to evaluate the effectiveness of drug management or to rest the body from the drug effects.

Educating the Patient and Family
The type of information included in the teaching plan depends on the drug and the reason for its use. The patient and family

---

Patient Teaching for Improved Patient Outcomes

Using Anorexiants for Weight Loss

When you teach, make sure your patient understands the following:

✔ These drugs are intended for patients with chronic weight management issues when used with an approved diet and physical activity program.
✔ These drugs should only be used for obesity (body mass index [BMI] of 30 or greater) or overweight (BMI of 27) when comorbid conditions exist, such as hypertension, type 2 diabetes, or dyslipidemia.
✔ Never take over-the-counter weight loss preparations with these drugs.
✔ If you have not achieved 5% weight loss in 12 weeks, contact your primary health care provider; never increase the dose to speed up or increase weight loss.
✔ Call your primary health care provider immediately if you experience mental changes (agitation or hallucinations), rapid heartbeat, dizziness, lack of coordination, or feelings of warmth. This may be a condition called neuroleptic malignant syndrome, which needs emergent treatment.
✔ Be aware of possible impairment in the ability to drive or perform hazardous tasks.
✔ Avoid other stimulants, including those containing caffeine such as coffee, tea, and cola drinks
✔ Read labels of foods and nonprescription drugs for possible stimulant content.
✔ Women: Use pregnancy protection and do not breastfeed when using these drugs.
✔ Men: Seek immediate medical treatment if you have an erection lasting more than 4 hours.

should feel confident in understanding what the purpose of the drug is and what possible adverse reactions may occur. It is important to emphasize the need to follow the recommended dosage schedule. As you develop the teaching plan, include the following additional teaching points:

- ADHD: Give the drug in the morning 30 to 45 minutes before breakfast and before lunch. Do not give the drug in the late afternoon. Keep a journal of the child's behavior, including the general patterns, socialization with others, and attention span. Bring this record to each primary health care provider or clinic visit, because this record may help the primary health care provider determine future drug dose adjustments or additional treatment modalities. The primary health care provider may prescribe drug therapy only on school days, when high levels of attention and performance are necessary.

- Narcolepsy: Keep a record of the number of times per day that periods of sleepiness occur, and bring this record to each visit to the primary health care provider or clinic.

- Amphetamines and anorexiants: These drugs are taken early in the day to avoid insomnia. Do not increase the dose or take the drug more frequently, except on the advice of the primary health care provider. These drugs may impair the ability to drive or perform hazardous tasks and may mask extreme fatigue. If dizziness, lightheadedness, anxiety, nervousness, or tremors occur, contact the primary care provider. Avoid or decrease the use of coffee, tea, and carbonated beverages containing caffeine (see Patient Teaching for Improved Patient Outcomes: Using Anorexiants for Weight Loss).

- Caffeine (oral, nonprescription): Over-the-counter caffeine preparations should be avoided if the individual has a history of heart disease, high blood pressure, or stomach ulcers. These products are intended for occasional use and should not be used if heart palpitations, dizziness, or lightheadedness occur.

EVALUATION

- Therapeutic response is achieved and respiratory depression is reversed; the child's behavior and school performance are improved; or the desired weight loss is achieved.

- Adverse reactions are identified, reported to the primary health care provider, and managed successfully with appropriate nursing interventions:
  - Patient reports fewer episodes of inappropriate sleep patterns.
  - Breathing pattern is maintained.
  - Patient maintains an adequate nutritional status.

- Patient and family express confidence and demonstrate an understanding of the drug regimen.

PHARMACOLOGY IN PRACTICE
THINK CRITICALLY

 What are some assessment questions you will ask Janna about her daily routine to determine if she has the behavior patterns described as ADHD? Are there other reasons that Janna's mother may want her to take stimulants?

KEY POINTS

- CNS stimulants enhance neurotransmission and stimulate receptors in different parts of the brain. These drugs are used for ADHD, narcolepsy, respiratory depression, and weight loss. They should not be used to treat clinical depression.

- There is a high degree of addiction potential with these drugs due to stimulation of the brain's pleasure centers with enhanced neurotransmission of dopamine.

- When used routinely, stimulants are offered in long-acting form or in the morning and at lunchtime to reduce the incidence of insomnia.

- Stimulants can affect other organs; adverse reactions include tachycardia, palpitations, headache, dizziness, apprehension, nausea, vomiting, and urinary retention.

Summary Drug Table CENTRAL NERVOUS SYSTEM STIMULANTS

Generic Name	Trade Name	Uses	Adverse Reactions	Dosage Ranges
Analeptics				
armodafinil *ar-moe-daf'-ih-nil*	Nuvigil	Narcolepsy, obstructive sleep apnea, sleepiness due to shift work	Headache, nausea, insomnia	150–250 mg/day orally in a single morning dose
caffeine *kah-feen'*	Cafcit, 5-hour Energy, Vivarin	Fatigue, drowsiness, as adjunct in analgesic formulation, respiratory depression	Palpitations, nausea, vomiting, insomnia, tachycardia, restlessness	Respiratory depression: 500 mg/1 g IM, IV

(table continues on page 194)

Summary Drug Table CENTRAL NERVOUS SYSTEM STIMULANTS (continued)

Generic Name	Trade Name	Uses	Adverse Reactions	Dosage Ranges
doxapram *dox'-ah-pram*	Dopram	Respiratory depression: postanesthesia, drug-induced, acute respiratory insufficiency superimposed on COPD	Dizziness, headache, apprehension, disorientation, nausea, cough, dyspnea, urinary retention	0.5–1 mg/kg IV
modafinil *moe-daf'-in-ill*	Provigil	Narcolepsy, obstructive sleep apnea	Headache, nausea	200–400 mg/day orally
Amphetamines				
amphetamine *am-fet'-ah-meen*		Narcolepsy, ADHD, exogenous obesity	Insomnia, nervousness, headache, tachycardia, anorexia, dizziness, excitement	Narcolepsy: 5–60 mg/day orally in divided doses ADHD: 5 mg BID, increase by 10 mg/wk until desired effect
amphetamine/ dextroamphetamine	Adderall XR	Narcolepsy, ADHD	Same as amphetamine	10–30 mg orally once daily
dexmethylphenidate *dex-meh-thill-fen'-ih-date*	Focalin	ADHD	Nervousness, insomnia, loss of appetite, abdominal pain, weight loss, tachycardia, skin rash	2.5 mg orally BID; maximum dosage, 20 mg/day
dextroamphetamine *dex-troe-am-fet'-ah-meen*	Dexedrine, DextroStat	Narcolepsy, ADHD	Same as amphetamine	Narcolepsy: 5–60 mg/day orally in divided doses ADHD: up to 40 mg/day orally
lisdexamfetamine *lis-dex'-am-fet-ah-meen*	Vyvanse	ADHD	Same as amphetamine	30–70 mg/day orally in one morning dose
methamphetamine *meth-am-fet'-ah-meen*	Desoxyn	ADHD, exogenous obesity	Same as amphetamine	ADHD: up to 25 mg/day orally Obesity: 5 mg orally 30 min before meals
methylphenidate *meh-thill-fen'-ih-date*	Concerta, Metadate, Ritalin, Methylin, Daytrana (transdermal patch)	ADHD, narcolepsy	Insomnia, anorexia, dizziness, headache, abdominal pain	5–60 mg/day orally
Anorexiants				
benzphetamine *benz-fet'-ah-meen*	Didrex	Obesity	Insomnia, nervousness, headache, dry mouth, palpitations, tachycardia, dizziness, excitement	25–50 mg orally 1–3 times/day
diethylpropion *dye-eth'-ill-proe-pee-on*	Tenuate, Tenuate Dospan	Obesity	Same as benzphetamine	Immediate release: 25 mg orally TID Sustained release: 75 mg once daily
lorcaserin *lor-cas'-er-een*	Belviq	Obesity	Low blood sugar, headache, dry mouth, constipation, dizziness	10 mg orally twice daily
phendimetrazine *fen'-dye-me'-tra-zeen*	Bontril	Obesity	Same as benzphetamine	35 mg orally 2–3 times/day
phentermine *fen-ter'-meen*	Adipex-P, Qsymia	Obesity	Same as benzphetamine	8 mg orally TID or 15–37.5 mg orally as a single daily dose
Miscellaneous Drugs				
atomoxetine *at'-oh-mox-eh-teen*	Strattera	ADHD (acts like antidepressant rather than stimulant)	Headache, decreased appetite, abdominal pain, vomiting, cough	Initial dose: 40 mg/day orally, may increase up to 100 mg/day orally
sodium oxybate *ox'-ih-bate*	Xyrem	Narcolepsy, excessive daytime sleepiness	Headache, dizziness, somnolence	4.5–9 g/night taken in 2 doses at least 2½ hr apart

Chapter Review

Know Your Drugs

Clients sometimes know a medication by the brand (or trade) name and not the generic name. To help you recognize both names, match the brand name with the generic name of the same medication.

Generic Name	Brand Name
1. methylphenidate	A. Adderall XR
2. lisdexamfetamine	B. Concerta
3. amphetamine/dextroamphetamine	C. Strattera
4. atomoxetine	D. Vyvanse

Calculate Medication Dosages

1. Adderall XR 30 mg daily in the morning is prescribed. The drug comes in 15-mg capsules. The parent will administer _____.

2. Modafinil 400 mg is prescribed. The drug is available in 200-mg tablets. The nurse administers _____.

Prepare for the NCLEX®

Build Your Knowledge

1. Which of the listed drug categories is not included as a class of CNS stimulants?

   1. amphetamines
   2. analeptics
   3. analgesics
   4. anorexiants

2. Initial assessment of the child with ADHD includes _____.

   1. assessing which stimuli the child responds to the most
   2. determining the child's intelligence
   3. obtaining a record of the child's behavior pattern
   4. obtaining vital signs

3. When assessing the client receiving doxapram for chronic pulmonary disease, the nurse observes the client for adverse drug reactions, which may include _____.

   1. headache, dizziness, variations in heart rate
   2. diarrhea, drowsiness, hypotension
   3. decreased respiratory rate, weight gain, bradycardia
   4. fever, dysuria, constipation

4. When teaching a client with narcolepsy who is receiving an amphetamine, the nurse instructs the client to _____.

   1. record the times of the day the medication is taken
   2. take the medication at bedtime as well as in the morning
   3. take the drug with meals
   4. keep a record of how often periods of sleepiness occur

5. When administering an amphetamine, the nurse first checks to see if the client is taking or has taken a monoamine oxidase inhibitor (MAOI) because _____.

   1. a lower dosage of the amphetamine may be needed
   2. a higher dosage of the amphetamine may be needed

   3. the amphetamine can be substituted as the antidepressant drug
   4. the amphetamine is not given within 14 days of the MAOI

Apply Your Knowledge

6. A child with ADHD is admitted to the pediatric unit for a fractured tibia. Dexmethylphenidate is prescribed 7.5 mg BID; when should these doses be given?

   1. 7 a.m. and 11 a.m.
   2. 7 a.m. and 5 p.m.
   3. 9 a.m. and 5 p.m.
   4. 9 a.m. and 9 p.m.

7. The parent of a child with ADHD asks why a stimulant is used on a child who is too stimulated already. The best answer is:

   1. the stimulation to the pleasure center relaxes the child
   2. the drug strengthens the nerve pathway to focus concentration
   3. the drug stimulates the child to wear him down enough to focus
   4. the drug is additive with the behavior to cancel out the bad behaviors

8. An obese client is weighed at the clinic. The starting weight was 370 lb; after 12 weeks the client now weighs 348 lb. The best action at this time is to:

   1. continue the anorexiant
   2. increase the anorexiant
   3. reduce the anorexiant
   4. stop the anorexiant

Alternate-Format Questions

9. An obese female client is starting an anorexiant for weight loss. Select all the points the nurse should emphasize in teaching this client about the drug. **Select all that apply**.

   1. You should modify your diet and exercise when taking these drugs.
   2. Never take over-the-counter diet pills when taking these drugs.
   3. You may take these drugs if your body mass index (BMI) is 22.
   4. Stop the anorexiant if you plan to get pregnant.

10. Phentermine 8 mg three times a day orally is prescribed as an adjunct for weight loss. The total amount of drug the patient will receive daily is _____. Is this an appropriate dose for this drug?

To check your answers, see Appendix G.

the Point *For more NCLEX-style questions, log on to http://thepoint.lww.com to access more than 1000 questions.*

19

Cholinesterase Inhibitors

LEARNING OBJECTIVES

On completion of this chapter, the student will:

1. Discuss the clinical manifestations of Alzheimer's disease (AD).
2. List the uses, general drug actions, general adverse reactions, contraindications, precautions, and interactions associated with the administration of cholinesterase inhibitors.
3. Discuss important preadministration and ongoing assessment activities the nurse should perform with the patient taking a cholinesterase inhibitor.
4. List nursing diagnoses particular to a patient taking a cholinesterase inhibitor.
5. Discuss ways to promote an optimal response to therapy, how to manage common adverse reactions, and important points to keep in mind when educating patients about the use of cholinesterase inhibitors.

KEY TERMS

acetylcholine • neurotransmitter that transmits impulses across the parasympathetic branch of the autonomic nervous system

Alzheimer's disease • progressive neurologic disorder that affects cognition, emotion, and movement

amyloid plaque • tangles of protein in nerve tissue

cholinesterase inhibitors • class of drugs that delays the breakdown of the neurotransmitter acetylcholine

delirium • an acute, temporary state of mental confusion

dementia • decrease in cognitive function

parasympathetic • pertaining to the part of the autonomic nervous system concerned with conserving body energy

DRUG CLASSES

Cholinesterase inhibitors

N-methyl-D-aspartate (NMDA) receptor antagonists

One of the greatest fears of aging is **dementia**. An overall term used in a variety of diseases and conditions, dementia involves the decrease in cognitive functioning, such as memory, attention, language or communication ability, and problem-solving skills. **Alzheimer's disease** (AD) is the cause of about 60% to 80% of these cases of dementia. The specific pathologic changes of AD occur in the cortex of the brain. These changes involve the degeneration of nerves by **amyloid plaques** and tangled nerve bundles (Fig. 19.1). When neurotransmission is impaired, the clinical symptoms of dementia result. **Cholinesterase inhibitors** and the newer *N*-methyl-D-aspartate (NMDA) receptor antagonists are used to strengthen neurotransmission and improve or maintain memory in those with dementia.

Approximately 5.4 million people in the United States are diagnosed with AD. Currently the Alzheimer's Association

PHARMACOLOGY IN PRACTICE

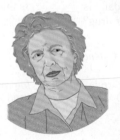

Mrs. Moore, 85 years of age, has been experiencing progressive forgetfulness for about a year. Her daughter was in town last week and accompanied her to the clinic. After an initial examination, the primary health care provider decided to try a cholinesterase inhibitor. Mrs. Moore has called the clinic today complaining of gastrointestinal distress symptoms. She tells you to order an x-ray and find the ulcer in her tummy. You ask her to come to the clinic and she agrees. What assessment questions do you need to ask to determine if this is an appropriate request?

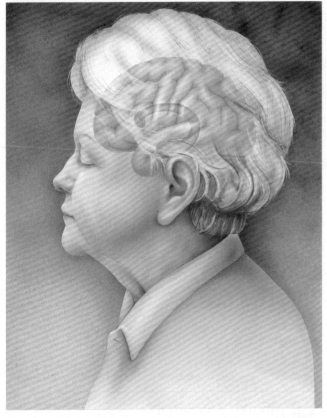

Figure 19.1 Alzheimer's disease and the resulting dementia occur when changes in the brain hamper neurotransmission.

Adapted from Jack, C. R. Jr., et al. (2011). Introduction to the recommendations from the National Institute on Aging—Alzheimer's Association workgroups on diagnostic guidelines for Alzheimer's disease. *Alzheimer's & Dementia: The Journal of the Alzheimer's Association, 7*(3), 257–262.

Display 19.1 Proposed Three Stages of Alzheimer's Disease (AD)

Preclinical AD (may occur 20 years before clinical symptoms)
- *Focus on research*
- Measureable changes are seen in the brain on magnetic resonance imaging
- Biomarkers may be present in blood or cerebrospinal fluid
- No changes in cognitive or functional ability

Mild Cognitive Impairment (MCI) Due to AD
- *Focus on limiting progression with medications*
- Changes in thinking ability noticeable to patient and family members
- Thinking or memory changes due to other causes ruled out
- Functional ability remains intact
- Mild to moderate anxiety noted by person

Dementia Due to AD
- *Focus on supporting function*
- Memory, thinking, and behavior limit ability to function
- Variable degrees of assistance needed for activities of daily living
- Reasoning and judgement impaired

and the National Institutes of Health are working to create a three-stage definition of the disease, which will aid in research of causes and ways to limit progression of symptoms. Display 19.1 identifies the stages of AD and their associated clinical manifestations.

Other diseases, such as Parkinson's disease, may have a dementia component, but cholinesterase inhibitors are approved primarily to treat mild to moderate dementia caused by AD. Drugs used to treat AD do not cure the disease but slow the progression of dementia. Examples of the cholinesterase inhibitors include donepezil (Aricept) and rivastigmine (Exelon). Other drug classes are used for symptomatic relief. For example, wandering, irritability, and aggression in people with AD are treated with antipsychotics, such as risperidone and olanzapine. Other drugs, such as antidepressants or antianxiety drugs, may be helpful in AD for symptoms of depression and anxiety; these drugs are all discussed in individual chapters.

Actions

Acetylcholine is the transmitter substance in the **parasympathetic** (or cholinergic) neuropathway. Individuals with AD experience reduction in nerve impulse transmission due to plaques and tangles as illustrated in Figure 19.2. As a result, the patient experiences problems with memory and thinking. The cholinesterase inhibitors act to increase the level of

acetylcholine in the central nervous system (CNS) by inhibiting its breakdown and slowing neural destruction. However, the disease is progressive, and although these drugs alter the progress of the disease, they do not stop it. Cholinesterase inhibitors are not frequently used in late-stage AD. A newer

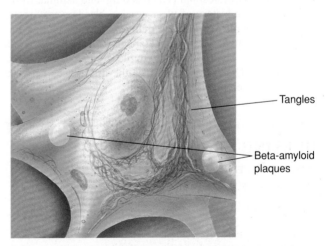

Figure 19.2 Amyloid plaques and nerve tangles clog neuropathways; cholinesterase inhibitors keep acetylcholine at the nerve junction longer to promote transmission.

Display 19.2 Differences Between Confusion of Delirium and Dementia

	Delirium	Dementia
Onset	Sudden change	Progressive change
Typical presentation	Affects senses (see, hear, feel)	Affects memory and judgment
Reversibility	Yes, when cause such as oxygen or chemical imbalances or infection is found and treated	No, can slow progression with drugs, need to change environment for patient to remain safe

group of drugs, NMDA receptor antagonists, is available. Memantine (Namenda) is thought to work by decreasing the excitability of neurotransmission caused by an excess of the amino acid glutamate in the CNS.

Uses

Cholinesterase inhibitors are used to treat early and moderate stages of dementia associated with AD. Their use for severe cognitive decline as well as other dementias, such as vascular or Parkinson's dementia, is being studied.

Adverse Reactions

Generalized adverse reactions include:

- Anorexia, nausea, vomiting, diarrhea
- Dizziness and headache

Additional adverse reactions are listed in the Summary Drug Table: Cholinesterase Inhibitors.

Contraindications and Precautions

Cholinesterase inhibitors are contraindicated in patients with hypersensitivity to the drugs and during pregnancy and lactation (pregnancy category B).

These drugs are used cautiously in patients with renal disease, bladder obstruction, seizure disorders, sick sinus syndrome, gastrointestinal (GI) bleeding, and asthma. In individuals with a history of ulcer disease, bleeding may recur. Some patients may experience **delirium** as well as their underlying dementia. These drugs are used to treat dementia and should not be used to treat confused patients experiencing delirium. Display 19.2 outlines the differences between delirium and dementia.

Interactions

The following interactions may occur when a cholinesterase inhibitor is administered with another agent:

Interacting Drug	Common Use	Effect of Interaction
anticholinergics	Decrease of bodily secretions	Decreased effectiveness of anticholinergics
nonsteroidal anti-inflammatory drugs	Pain relief	Increased risk of GI bleeding
theophylline	Breathing problems	Increased risk of theophylline toxicity

HERBAL CONSIDERATIONS

Ginkgo, one of the oldest herbs in the world, has many beneficial effects. It is thought to improve memory and brain function and enhance circulation to the brain, heart, limbs, and eyes. Conflicting research both supports and disputes ginkgo's ability to enhance memory. Medical studies in the United States and England (UM, 2008; Snitz, 2009) have not demonstrated increases in mental function. Despite this research, the "brain herb" is still taken by healthy adults hoping to retain their current memory and cognitive function. The recommended dose is 40 mg standardized extract ginkgo three times daily. The effects of ginkgo may not be evident until after 4 to 24 weeks of treatment. The most common adverse reactions include mild GI discomfort, headache, and rash. Excessively large doses have been reported to cause diarrhea, nausea, vomiting, and restlessness. Ginkgo is contraindicated in patients taking selective serotonin reuptake inhibitor (SSRI) or monoamine oxidase inhibitor (MAOI) antidepressants because of the risk of a toxic reaction. Moreover, individuals taking anticoagulants should take ginkgo only on the advice of a primary care provider.

NURSING PROCESS

PATIENT RECEIVING A CHOLINESTERASE INHIBITOR FOR DEMENTIA OF ALZHEIMER'S DISEASE

ASSESSMENT

Preadministration Assessment

A patient receiving a cholinesterase inhibitor may be treated in the hospital, long-term care facility, or outpatient setting. The patient's cognitive ability and functional ability are assessed before and during therapy. Cognition can be screened by using a tool called the Mini-Mental Status Examination (MMSE). Patients are assessed on items such as orientation, calculation, recall, and language. Scoring is done by comparison with a standardized answer sheet, and the likelihood of dementia is determined. You should also assess the patient for agitation, impulsive behavior, and functional ability, such as performing activities of daily living and self-care. These assessments are used not only for monitoring the patient's improvement (if any) after taking a cholinesterase inhibitor but also to determine appropriate living arrangements and level of care.

Before starting therapy, obtain a complete mental health and medical history. When the disease is advancing, patients with AD are not always able to give a reliable history of their illness. A family member or primary caregiver may be helpful in verifying or providing information needed for an accurate assessment. Ask the family about unusual behaviors, such as wandering or outbursts of anger or frustration. When taking the history, observe the patient for any behavior patterns that appear to deviate from normal. Examples of deviations include poor eye contact, failure to answer questions completely, inappropriate answers to questions, monotone speech pattern, and inappropriate laughter, sadness, or crying, signifying varying stages of decline. Using a standard assessment tool such as the MMSE, document the patient's cognitive ability.

Physical assessments include obtaining blood pressure measurements on both arms with the patient in a sitting position, the pulse, the respiratory rate, and weight. Assessing the patient's functional ability is also important.

Ongoing Assessment

Ongoing assessment of patients taking cholinesterase inhibitors includes both mental and physical assessments. Cognitive and functional abilities are assessed routinely for changes. Initial assessments will be compared with the ongoing assessments to monitor the patient's improvement (if any) after taking the cholinesterase inhibitors.

Using standardized tools to obtain an accurate description of the patient's behavior and cognitive ability aids the primary health care provider in planning therapy and thus becomes an important part of patient management. Patients with poor response to drug therapy may require dosage changes, discontinuation of the drug therapy, or the addition of other therapies to the treatment regimen. However, response to these drugs may take several weeks. The symptoms that the patient is experiencing may improve or remain the same, or the patient may experience only a small response to therapy. It is important to remember that a treatment that slows the progression of symptoms in AD is a successful treatment.

NURSING DIAGNOSES

Drug-specific nursing diagnoses include the following:

- **Imbalanced Nutrition: Less Than Body Requirements** related to anorexia, nausea, or vomiting
- **Risk for Injury** related to dizziness, syncope, clumsiness, or the disease process

Nursing diagnoses related to drug administration are discussed in Chapter 4.

PLANNING

The expected outcomes for the patient may include an optimal response to drug therapy, meeting patient needs related to the management of adverse reactions, an absence of injury, and confidence in an understanding of the medication regimen.

IMPLEMENTATION

Promoting an Optimal Response to Therapy

As you develop a care plan to meet the patient's individual needs, keep in mind this is a progressive disease. When the drugs no longer provide memory enhancement, environmental factors may need to change rather than modifying the patient's behavior.

If the patient is hospitalized, it is important to monitor vital signs and other assessments to determine if changes may be from the dementia or if the patient is experiencing delirium (acute confusion) due to reversible causes (see Display 19.2).

> **! NURSING ALERT**
>
> Should cholinesterase inhibitor therapy be discontinued, individuals lose any benefit they have received from the drugs within 6 weeks.

Rivastigmine (Exelon) is available in a transdermal form of the drug. The patches are changed on a daily basis and rotated to a clean, dry, and hairless area. Because the patient is experiencing dementia, the site for application should be where the patient is not able to pick at or remove the patch. The upper or lower portions of the back are recommended for the patch administration. Because the same site should not be used more than once every 2 weeks, document or teach the caregiver to make a chart of the back and indicate where patches have been applied during the last 14 days.

Monitoring and Managing Patient Needs

IMBALANCED NUTRITION: LESS THAN BODY REQUIREMENTS. When taking the cholinesterase inhibitors, patients may experience nausea and vomiting. Although this can occur with all of the cholinesterase inhibitors, patients taking rivastigmine (Exelon) appear to have more problems with nausea and severe vomiting. Attention to the dosing of medications can decrease adverse GI reactions and promote nutrition. The primary health care provider may discontinue use of the drug and then restart the drug therapy at the lowest dose possible. Restarting therapy at the lower dose helps to reduce nausea and vomiting.

The cholinesterase inhibitors can be taken with or without food. Although donepezil (Aricept) is administered orally once daily at bedtime, it can also be given with a snack. When administering rivastigmine as an oral solution, remove the oral dosing syringe provided in the protective container. The syringe provided is used to withdraw the prescribed amount. The dose may be swallowed directly from the syringe or first mixed with a small glass of water, cold fruit juice, or soda.

Weight loss and eating problems related to the inability to swallow are two major problems in the late stage of AD. These problems, coupled with anorexia and nausea associated with administration of cholinesterase inhibitors, present a challenge for caregivers. Typically these drugs are not administered during the late stage of dementia, but there may be a period of worsening symptoms before the drugs are stopped entirely.

Mealtime should be simple and calm. Offer the patient a well-balanced diet with foods that are easy to chew and digest. Frequent, small meals may be tolerated better than three regular meals. Offering foods of different consistency and flavor is important in case the patient can handle one form better than another. Fluid intake of six to eight glasses of water daily is encouraged to prevent dehydration.

Risk for Injury. Physical decline and the adverse reactions of dizziness and syncope place the patient at risk for injury. The patient may require assistance when ambulating. Assistive devices such as walkers or canes may reduce falls. To minimize the risk of injury, the patient's environment should be controlled and safe. Encouraging the use of bed alarms, keeping the bed in low position, and using night lights, as well as frequent monitoring, will reduce the risk of injury. The patient should wear medical identification, such as a MedicAlert bracelet, at all times.

Educating the Patient and Family

Early in the disease, the patient may be able to understand changes, yet suspicion and denial are classic symptoms of the disease; therefore, the patient may not be amenable to treatment. As cognitive abilities decrease, focus on educating the family and primary caregiver of the patient's needs. Depending on the degree of cognitive decline, discuss the drug regimen with the patient, family member, or caregiver. It is important to evaluate accurately the patient's ability to assume responsibility for taking drugs at home. The patient and family should feel confident in understanding that the drugs used do not cure but rather control symptoms of the disease. It is your task to help family members assume responsibility for medication administration when the patient appears to be unable to manage his or her own drug therapy in the home.

Teach and provide written handouts in the preferred language about the drugs and adverse reactions that may occur with a specific drug, and encourage the caregiver or family members to contact the primary health care provider immediately when a serious drug reaction occurs.

As you develop a teaching plan for the patient or family member, include the following points:

- Keep all appointments with the primary care provider or clinic, because close monitoring of therapy is essential. Dose changes may be needed to achieve the best results.

- Report any unusual changes or physical effects to the primary health care provider.

- Take the drug exactly as directed. Do not increase, decrease, or omit a dose or discontinue use of this drug unless directed to do so by the primary health care provider.

- Do not drive or perform other hazardous tasks if drowsiness occurs. Discuss with your primary health care provider when patients should be evaluated for their continued ability to drive.

- Do not take any nonprescription drug before talking to your primary health care provider.

- Keep track of when the drug is taken. Marking the calendar, cell phone alarms, or a pill counter that holds the medicine for each day of the week may be helpful tools to remind the patient to take the medication or determine whether the medication has been taken for the day.

- Notify the primary care provider if the following adverse reactions are experienced for more than a few days: nausea, diarrhea, difficulty sleeping, vomiting, or loss of appetite.

- Immediately report the occurrence of the following adverse reactions: severe vomiting, dehydration, or changes in neurologic functioning.

- Notify the primary health care provider if the patient has a history of ulcers, feels faint, experiences severe stomach pains, vomits blood or material that resembles coffee grounds, or has bloody or black stools.

- Remember that these drugs do not cure AD but slow the mental and physical degeneration associated with the disease. The drug must be taken routinely to slow the progression.

EVALUATION

- Therapeutic effect is achieved and cognitive function is maintained.

- Adverse reactions are identified, reported to the primary health care provider, and managed successfully through appropriate nursing interventions:
  - Patient maintains an adequate nutritional status.
  - No injury is evident.

- Patient (if able) and family express confidence and demonstrate an understanding of the drug regimen.

PHARMACOLOGY IN PRACTICE
THINK CRITICALLY

 While Mrs. Moore is putting on a patient gown at the clinic, you notice she appears to have multiple "bandages" all over her body. Upon closer examination, the bandage reads EXELON*PATCH*. Does this explain her GI distress?

KEY POINTS

- Alzheimer's disease is one of the conditions in which dementia is a major issue. This occurs due to the buildup of plaques and tangles in the neurons of the brain. Acetylcholine is reduced, resulting in symptoms of dementia.

- The progression of memory loss associated with dementia is treated with cholinesterase inhibitors. These drugs slow progression but do not cure dementia.

- Patients with dementia may at times experience acute confusion, known as delirium. These drugs do not treat delirium.

- Some of the most common adverse reactions of these drugs include dry mouth, nausea, and vomiting. Nutrition becomes a primary issue in treatment because patients with AD also may have reduced appetite and difficulty eating.

- Involvement of family members or caregivers is essential for the treatment and management of the patient with AD due to the cognitive and functional changes involved.

Summary Drug Table CHOLINESTERASE INHIBITORS

Generic Name	Trade Name	Uses	Adverse Reactions	Dosage Ranges
Cholinesterase Inhibitors				
donepezil *doe-nep'-eh-zill*	Aricept	Mild to severe dementia due to AD, memory improvement in dementia due to stroke, vascular disease, multiple sclerosis	Headache, nausea, diarrhea, insomnia, muscle cramps	5–10 mg/day orally
galantamine *gah-lan'-tah-meen*	Razadyne	Mild to moderate (AD) dementia	Nausea, vomiting, diarrhea, anorexia, dizziness	16–24 mg BID orally
rivastigmine *riv-ah-stig'-meen*	Exelon	Mild to moderate dementia of AD and Parkinson's disease	Nausea, vomiting, diarrhea, dyspepsia, anorexia, insomnia, fatigue, dizziness, headache	1.5–12 mg/day BID orally; 4.6, 9.5, 13.3 mg daily transdermal patch
NMDA Receptor Antagonist				
memantine *meh-man'-teen*	Namenda	Moderate to severe (AD) dementia	Dizziness, headache, confusion	5–10 mg BID orally

● Chapter Review

Know Your Drugs

Clients sometimes know a medication by the brand (or trade) name and not the generic name. To help you recognize both names, match the brand name with the generic name of the same medication.

Generic Name	Brand Name
1. donepezil	A. Aricept
2. galantamine	B. Exelon
3. memantine	C. Namenda
4. rivastigmine	D. Razadyne

Calculate Medication Dosages

1. Rivastigmine (Exelon) oral solution 6 mg is prescribed. The drug is available as an oral solution of 2 mg/mL. The nurse administers _____.

2. Oral memantine (Namenda) 10 mg is prescribed for a client with AD. On hand are 5-mg tablets. The nurse administers _____.

● Prepare for the NCLEX®

Build Your Knowledge

1. Alzheimer's disease involves protein plaques and nerve tangles that limit which neurotransmitter?
   1. acetylcholine
   2. dopamine
   3. norepinephrine
   4. serotonin

2. Adverse reactions that the nurse would assess for in a client taking rivastigmine (Exelon) include _____.
   1. occipital headache
   2. vomiting
   3. hyperactivity
   4. hypoactivity

3. When administering donepezil (Aricept) to a client with AD, the nurse would most likely expect which diagnostic test to be prescribed?
   1. complete blood count
   2. cholesterol levels
   3. brain scan
   4. electrolyte analysis

4. Which of the following nursing diagnoses would the nurse most likely place on the care plan of a client with AD that is related to adverse reactions of the cholinesterase inhibitors?
   1. Imbalanced Nutrition
   2. Confusion
   3. Risk for Suicide
   4. Bowel Incontinence

5. The nurse correctly administers donepezil (Aricept) _____.
   1. three times daily around the clock
   2. twice daily 1 hour before meals or 2 hours after meals
   3. once daily in the morning
   4. once daily at bedtime

Apply Your Knowledge

6. When a client's dementia causes him or her to pick at items, the rivastigmine transdermal patch should be placed:
   1. on the abdomen
   2. on the upper arms
   3. between the shoulder blades
   4. on the thigh

7. The nurse correctly disposes the rivastigmine transdermal patch by first:
   1. placing it in a tissue and discarding in trash can
   2. flushing the patch in the client's toilet
   3. folding it over so the adhesive side sticks together
   4. disposing in a sharps contaminated box in the client's room

8. Which of the following is a sign or symptom of delirium?
   1. progressive, insidious onset
   2. caused by bladder infection
   3. ongoing confusion
   4. problems with memory

Alternate-Format Questions

9. Which of the following are used to monitor progression of Alzheimer's disease? **Select all that apply**.
   1. Mini-Mental Status Examination
   2. brain scan
   3. blood studies
   4. urinalysis
   5. memory testing

10. Alzheimer's disease is now defined in three stages. Cholinesterase inhibitors are used during which stages? **Select all that apply**.
    1. stage 1
    2. stage 2
    3. stage 3

To check your answers, see Appendix G

thePoint *For more NCLEX-style questions, log on to http://thepoint.lww.com to access more than 1000 questions.*

Antianxiety Drugs

20

LEARNING OBJECTIVES

On completion of this chapter, the student will:

1. Discuss the uses, general drug actions, general adverse reactions, contraindications, precautions, and interactions associated with the administration of antianxiety drugs.
2. Discuss important preadministration and ongoing assessment activities the nurse should perform on the patient taking an antianxiety drug.
3. List nursing diagnoses particular to a patient taking an antianxiety drug.
4. Discuss ways to promote an optimal response to therapy, how to manage common adverse reactions, and important points to keep in mind when educating patients about the use of antianxiety drugs.

KEY TERMS

anxiety • feelings of apprehension, worry, or uneasiness

anxiolytics • drugs used to treat anxiety

ataxia • unsteady gait; muscular incoordination

gamma (γ)-aminobutyric acid (GABA) • a neurotransmitter inhibitor that is involved in the regulation of sleep and anxiety

physical dependence • habitual use of a drug, where negative physical withdrawal symptoms result from abrupt discontinuation

posttraumatic stress disorder (PTSD) • a mental health condition triggered by a terrifying event

psychological dependence • compulsion or craving to use a substance to obtain a pleasurable experience

tolerance • increasingly larger dosages of a drug are required to obtain the desired effect

DRUG CLASSES

Benzodiazepines
Nonbenzodiazepines

Anxiety is a feeling of apprehension, worry, or uneasiness that may or may not be based on reality. Anxiety may be seen in many types of situations, ranging from the "jitters" and excitement of a new job to the acute panic that may be seen during withdrawal from alcohol. Although a certain amount of anxiety is normal, excess anxiety interferes with day-to-day functioning and can cause undue stress in the lives of some individuals. Drugs used to treat anxiety are called *antianxiety drugs*. **Anxiolytics** is another term you may see referring to the antianxiety drugs.

Antianxiety drug classes include the benzodiazepines and the nonbenzodiazepines. Examples of the benzodiazepines include alprazolam (Xanax), chlordiazepoxide (Librium), diazepam (Valium), and lorazepam (Ativan). Long-term use of benzodiazepines can result in **physical** or **psychological dependence**, and as a result they are classified as schedule IV controlled substances (see Chapter 1). Due to the risk of dependence, benzodiazepines are used for short-term anxiety relief. Typically, long-term psychiatric anxiety disorders such as **posttraumatic stress disorder (PTSD)** are treated with antidepressant medications (Chapter 22). The nonbenzodiazepines useful in reducing anxiety include buspirone, doxepin, and hydroxyzine.

Actions

Anxiolytic drugs exert their tranquilizing effect by blocking certain neurotransmitter receptor sites. In turn, this prevents

---

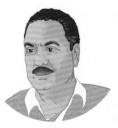

PHARMACOLOGY IN PRACTICE

Mr. Garcia, 55 years of age, is being seen in the clinic for an upper respiratory infection. Using an interpreter, he tells you that his shortness of breath makes him anxious. His respirations are 32 breaths/min, heart rate 98 beats/min, and blood pressure 161/92 mm Hg. The primary health care provider prescribes alprazolam (Xanax) 0.25 mg orally three times a day. As you read this chapter, determine if this is appropriate.

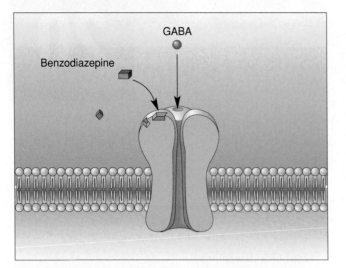

Figure 20.1 Benzodiazepine drugs bind to a site on the cell receptor, potentiating the effect of GABA (an inhibitory neurotransmitter) on the receptor. (Adapted from Bear, M. F., Connors, B. W., & Parasido, M. A. [2001]. _Neuroscience—exploring the brain_ [2nd ed.]. Philadelphia: Lippincott Williams & Wilkins.)

the neurotransmission of the anxious perception and the body's physical reaction to the anxiety. Benzodiazepines exert their tranquilizing effect by potentiating the effects of **gamma (γ)-aminobutyric acid (GABA)**, an inhibitory transmitter (Fig. 20.1). Nonbenzodiazepines exert their action in various ways. For example, buspirone is thought to act on the brain's serotonin receptors. Hydroxyzine (Vistaril) produces its antianxiety effect by acting on the hypothalamus and brainstem reticular formation.

Uses

Antianxiety drugs are used in the management of the following:

- Anxiety disorders and panic attacks
- Preanesthetic sedation and muscle relaxation
- Convulsions or seizures
- Alcohol withdrawal

Adverse Reactions

Frequent, early reactions include:

- Mild drowsiness or sedation
- Lightheadedness or dizziness
- Headache

Other adverse body system reactions include:

- Lethargy, apathy, fatigue
- Disorientation
- Anger
- Restlessness
- Nausea, constipation or diarrhea, dry mouth
- Visual disturbances

See the Summary Drug Table: Antianxiety Drugs for more information.

Dependence

Long-term use of benzodiazepines may result in physical dependence and **tolerance** (increasingly larger dosages required to obtain the desired effect). Withdrawal symptoms have occurred when the drug is stopped after as few as 4 to 6 weeks of therapy. When discontinuing a benzodiazepine a gradually decreasing dosage schedule (known as _tapering_) should be used.

> **! NURSING ALERT**
>
> Withdrawal symptoms are more likely to occur when the benzodiazepine is taken for 3 months or more and is abruptly discontinued. Therefore, antianxiety drugs must never be discontinued abruptly.

Symptoms of benzodiazepine withdrawal include increased anxiety, concentration difficulties, tremor, and sensory disturbances, such as paresthesias, photophobia, hypersomnia, and metallic taste. The onset of withdrawal symptoms usually occurs within 1 to 10 days after discontinuing the drug, with the duration of withdrawal symptoms from 5 days to 1 month. Symptoms of withdrawal are identified in Display 20.1.

The nonbenzodiazepine antianxiety drug buspirone is associated with less physical dependence potential and less effect on motor ability and cognition.

Contraindications

Do not administer antianxiety drugs to patients with known hypersensitivity, psychoses, and acute narrow-angle glaucoma. The benzodiazepines are contraindicated during pregnancy (pregnancy category D drugs) and labor. Reports of floppy infant syndrome manifested by sucking difficulties, lethargy, and hypotonia have been seen in the newborn. Lactating women should also avoid the benzodiazepines because of the effect on the infant (lethargy and weight loss). Due to a specific enzyme reaction, grapefruit or its juice should not be taken if the patient is on buspirone and diazepam.

Buspirone is a pregnancy category B drug and hydroxyzine is a pregnancy category C drug. Their safety is still questionable because adequate studies have not been performed in

---

Display 20.1 Symptoms of Withdrawal

- Increased anxiety
- Fatigue
- Hypersomnia
- Metallic taste
- Concentration difficulties
- Headache
- Tremors
- Numbness in the extremities
- Nausea
- Sweating
- Muscle tension and cramps
- Psychoses
- Hallucinations
- Memory impairment
- Convulsions (possible)

pregnant women. All of these drugs are contraindicated when patients are in a coma or shock, and if the vital signs of the patient in acute alcoholic intoxication are low.

Precautions

Antianxiety drugs are used cautiously in elderly patients and in patients with impaired liver function, impaired kidney function, or debilitation.

LIFESPAN CONSIDERATIONS
Gerontology

Recent studies link the chronic use of benzodiazepines by those older than 65 years of age to a greater chance of developing dementia (Billioti, 2012).

Interactions

The following interactions may occur when an anxiolytic is administered with another agent:

Interacting Drug	Common Use	Effect of Interaction
alcohol	Relaxation and enjoyment in social situations	Increased risk for central nervous system (CNS) depression or convulsions
analgesics	Pain relief	Increased risk for CNS depression

Interacting Drug	Common Use	Effect of Interaction
tricyclic antidepressants	Management of depression	Increased risk for sedation and respiratory depression
antipsychotics	Control of psychotic symptoms	Increased risk for sedation and respiratory depression
digoxin	Management of cardiac problems	Increased risk for digitalis toxicity

HERBAL CONSIDERATIONS

Kava is a popular herbal remedy thought to relieve stress, anxiety, and tension; promote sleep; and provide relief from menstrual discomfort. Kava's benefits are not supported by science, and the U.S. Food and Drug Administration (FDA) has issued an alert indicating that the use of kava may cause liver damage. Because kava-containing products have been associated with liver-related injuries (e.g., hepatitis, cirrhosis, and liver failure), the safest way to use kava is to take the herb occasionally for episodes of anxiety, rather than on a daily basis. It is important that individuals who use a kava-containing dietary supplement and experience signs of liver disease immediately consult their primary health care provider. Identifying kava-containing products can be difficult. Careful reading of the "Supplement Facts" information on the label may identify kava by any of the following names: kava, ava, ava pepper, awa, kava root, kava-kava, kew, *Piper methysticum* G. Forst, *Piper methysticum*, Sakau, tonga, or yanggona (FDA Consumer Advisory, 2009).

NURSING PROCESS
PATIENT RECEIVING AN ANTIANXIETY DRUG

ASSESSMENT

Preadministration Assessment

Individuals with mild anxiety or depression do not necessarily require inpatient care. These patients are usually seen at periodic intervals in the primary health care provider's office or in a mental health outpatient setting. Treatment for anyone in the hospital or in an outpatient setting may be anxiety provoking, especially if the individual has reduced health literacy (Fig. 20.2). Assessment of both patient groups is similar.

When an antianxiety drug is ordered, obtain as complete of a medical history as possible, including mental status and anxiety level. Because anxiety is a subjective feeling, you may ask the patient to rate his or her anxiety on a 0 to 10 scale, just as you would when asking about pain. When in a state of mild to moderate anxiety, patients may be able to give a reliable history of their illness.

Yet, when severe anxiety is present, the patient may be unable to communicate effectively. Therefore, it is important to seek information from a family member or friend when possible. During the intake exam, observe for behavioral signs indicating anxiety (e.g., inability to focus, extreme restlessness, facial grimaces, tense posture).

Physical assessment should include the blood pressure, pulse, respiratory rate, and weight. Physiologic manifestations of anxiety can include increased blood pressure and pulse rate, increased rate and depth of respiration, and increased muscle tension. An anxious patient may have cool and pale skin.

Be sure to obtain a history of any past drug or alcohol use. This information can help establish what the patient has used in the past as coping mechanisms to deal with anxiety. More accurate intake information is obtained when using questions

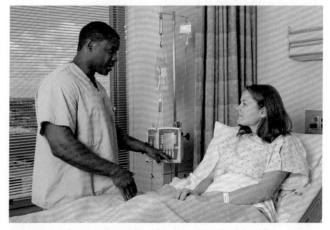

Figure 20.2 Hospitalization can be an anxious experience for patients. Anxiolytic medications can help the patient focus on patient teaching and activities of daily living to improve patient outcomes.

such as "How much alcohol do you drink daily?" or "Do you drink more or less than three alcohol beverages daily?"

Ongoing Assessment

An ongoing assessment is important for the patient taking an antianxiety drug. Ask the patient to rate the anxiety and compare this to the baseline rating. Check the patient's blood pressure before drug administration. If systolic pressure has dropped 20 mm Hg, withhold the drug because the patient is at greater risk to fall, and notify the primary health care provider. Periodically monitor the patient's mental status and anxiety level during therapy and assess for improvement or decline of behavioral and functional ability.

During follow-up in the ambulatory setting, ask the patient or a family member about adverse drug reactions or any other problems occurring during therapy. Flag these reactions or problems to be sure they come to the attention of the primary health care provider. Describe and document outward behavior and any complaints or problems in the patient's record. Compare your new information with previous notations and observations.

NURSING DIAGNOSES

Drug-specific nursing diagnoses are the following:

- **Risk for Injury** related to dizziness or hypotension and gait problems
- **Impaired Comfort** related to dryness in gastrointestinal (GI) tract from medications
- **Ineffective Individual Coping** related to situation causing anxiety

Nursing diagnoses related to drug administration are discussed in Chapter 4.

PLANNING

The expected patient outcomes may include an optimal response to drug therapy, support of patient needs related to the management of adverse drug reactions, and confidence in an understanding of the medication regimen.

IMPLEMENTATION

Promoting an Optimal Response to Therapy

During initial therapy, observe the patient closely for adverse drug reactions. Some adverse reactions, such as episodes of postural hypotension and drowsiness or dry mouth, may need to be tolerated because drug therapy must continue. The antianxiety drugs are not recommended for long-term use. When the antianxiety drugs are used for short periods (1 to 2 weeks), tolerance, dependence, or withdrawal symptoms usually do not develop. Should any signs of tolerance or dependence, such as the patient needing larger doses of drug or complaints of increased anxiety and agitation (see Display 20.1) develop, contact the primary health care provider.

Monitoring and Managing Patient Needs

RISK FOR INJURY. When these drugs are given in the outpatient setting, instruct both the patient and family about adverse reactions (dizziness, lightheadedness, or ataxia) that can cause a patient to fall and become injured. This is very important when the drugs are administered to older adults.

 LIFESPAN CONSIDERATIONS
Gerontology

Benzodiazepines are excreted more slowly in older adults, causing a prolonged drug effect. The drugs may accumulate in the blood, resulting in an increase in adverse reactions or toxicity.

Because antianxiety drugs stay in the body of older adults longer, the initial dose should be small, and the dose increased gradually until a therapeutic response is obtained. However, lorazepam and oxazepam are relatively safe for older adults when given in normal dosages. Buspirone also is a safe choice for older adults with anxiety, because it does not cause excessive sedation, and the risk of falling is not as great.

When the patient is hospitalized, develop a nursing care plan to meet the patient's individual needs regarding the anxious behavior. Vital signs should be monitored at frequent intervals, usually three or four times daily, when antianxiety medication doses are adjusted. Patients should be monitored for symptoms such as dizziness or lightheadedness. When antianxiety drugs are started or increased, instruct the patient to stay in bed and call for assistance to get up out of the bed or chair, and consider the need for supervision for any ambulatory activities. Provide assistance with activities of daily living to the patient experiencing any sedation effects. This includes help with eating, dressing, and ambulating. In some instances, such as when a hypotensive episode occurs, the vital signs are taken more often. Report any significant change in the vital signs to the primary health care provider. The sedation and drowsiness that sometimes occur with the use of an antianxiety drug may decrease as therapy continues.

Parenteral administration is indicated primarily in acute states when the patient's behavior makes it difficult to take the medication by mouth. Choose a large muscle mass, such as the gluteus muscle, when administering the drug by the intramuscular (IM) route. Then observe the patient closely for at least 3 hours after parenteral administration. The patient is kept lying down (when possible) for 30 minutes to 3 hours after the drug is given.

LIFESPAN CONSIDERATIONS
Gerontology

Parenteral (intravenous [IV] or IM) administration to older adults, the debilitated, and those with limited pulmonary reserve requires extreme care because the patient may experience apnea and cardiac arrest. Resuscitative equipment should be readily available during parenteral (particularly IV) administration. When administration of parenteral diazepam is advised, see Chapter 29 for specific information.

IMPAIRED COMFORT. Antianxiety drugs can cause both dryness of the mucous membranes and slower transit in the intestines, leading to constipation. Assess swallowing (because of a dry mouth) and give with lots of fluid, especially in the older, institutionalized adult. Nursing interventions to relieve some of these reactions may include offering frequent sips of water to relieve dry mouth and provide adequate hydration. The patient may also chew sugarless gum or suck on hard candy to reduce discomfort from dry mouth. Administer oral antianxiety drugs with food or meals to decrease the possibility of GI upset. Meals should include fiber, fruits, and vegetables to aid in preventing constipation.

INEFFECTIVE INDIVIDUAL COPING. When the patient is an outpatient, compare response to therapy at the time of each clinic visit. In some instances, question the patient or a family member about the response to therapy. The type of questions asked depends on the patient and the diagnosis, and may include open-ended questions such as "How are you feeling?" "Do you feel less nervous?" or "Would you like to tell me how everything is going?" Sometimes you may need to rephrase questions or direct the conversation toward other subjects until the patient feels comfortable enough to discuss his or her therapy.

Once the patient has reduced the anxious behavior, you may be able to help him or her identify what is precipitating the panic attacks or causing anxiety. It is important for you to help the patient understand that there are health care providers who can help him or her gain skills to cope with situations before the anxious behavior returns.

Although rare, benzodiazepine toxicity may occur from an overdose of the drug. Benzodiazepine toxicity causes sedation, respiratory depression, and coma. Flumazenil (Romazicon) is an antidote (antagonist) for benzodiazepine toxicity and acts to reverse the sedation, respiratory depression, and coma within 6 to 10 minutes after IV administration. Adverse reactions to flumazenil include agitation, confusion, seizures, and, in some cases, symptoms of benzodiazepine withdrawal. Adverse reactions to flumazenil, related to the symptoms of benzodiazepine withdrawal, are relieved by the administration of the benzodiazepine.

Educating the Patient and Family

Evaluate the patient's ability to assume responsibility for taking drugs at home. You should explain and provide written materials in the preferred language of any adverse reactions that may occur with a specific antianxiety drug and encourage the patient or family members to contact the primary health care provider immediately if a serious adverse reaction occurs. The patient and family should feel confident in understanding that the drugs prescribed will help to reduce anxiety on a short-term basis. If anxiety persists, notify the primary health care provider so that other therapy options can be explored. As you develop a teaching plan for the patient or family member, include the following:

- Take the drug exactly as directed. Do not increase, decrease, or omit a dose or discontinue use of this drug unless directed to do so by the primary health care provider.
- Do not discontinue use of the drug abruptly because withdrawal symptoms may occur.

- Avoid driving or performing other hazardous tasks if drowsiness occurs.
- Do not take any nonprescription drugs until discussing the specific drug with the primary health care provider.
- Inform physicians, dentists, and other health care providers of therapy with this drug.
- ❢ Do not drink alcoholic beverages while taking this medication.
- If dizziness occurs when changing position, rise slowly when getting out of bed or a chair. If dizziness is severe, always have help when changing positions.
- If dryness of the mouth occurs, relieve it by taking frequent sips of water, sucking on hard candy, or chewing gum (preferably sugarless).
- Prevent constipation by eating high-fiber foods, increasing fluid intake, and exercising if the condition permits.
- Keep all appointments with the primary health care provider because close monitoring of therapy is essential.
- Report any unusual changes or physical effects to the primary health care provider.

EVALUATION

- Therapeutic response is achieved and patient reports decrease in feelings of anxiety.
- Adverse reactions are identified, reported to the primary health care provider, and managed successfully with appropriate nursing interventions:
  - No evidence of injury is seen.
  - Patient reports comfort without increased GI distress.
  - Patient manages coping effectively.
- Patient and family express confidence and demonstrate an understanding of the drug regimen.

PHARMACOLOGY IN PRACTICE
THINK CRITICALLY

 Discuss what assessment findings in the beginning of the chapter would indicate increased anxiety. As part of the patient teaching, what precautions would you relay to Mr. Garcia about this medication? How will you determine if he understands the information correctly?

KEY POINTS

- Anxiety involves a feeling of apprehension, worry, or uneasiness that may or may not be based on reality. Anxiety is a normal feeling, yet as anxiety increases it can interfere with day-to-day functioning. Because it is a subjective feeling, patients can be asked to rate anxiety similar to rating pain.

- Benzodiazepines and nonbenzodiazepine anxiolytics are used to treat anxiety on a short-term basis. Physical and psychological dependence can occur with use of these drugs; typically psychiatric anxiety disorders (which need long-term treatment) use antidepressants for treatment instead of benzodiazepines.

- The anxiolytics work by blocking certain neurotransmitters, which in turn reduces anxiety; they additionally can reduce blood pressure, which can cause adverse reactions such as hypotension, dizziness, and drowsiness.
- Benzodiazepine doses should always be tapered and never stopped abruptly; withdrawal can occur with symptoms such as a return of anxiety, concentration problems, tremor, and sensory disturbances.
- Older adults do not eliminate these drugs as well as younger people and can experience adverse reactions with smaller doses than what younger people can tolerate.

Summary Drug Table ANTIANXIETY DRUGS

Generic Name	Trade Name	Uses	Adverse Reactions	Dosage Ranges
Benzodiazepines				
alprazolam *al-prah'-zoe-lam*	Niravam, Xanax	Anxiety disorders, short-term relief of anxiety, panic attacks	Transient mild drowsiness, lightheadedness, headache, depression, constipation, diarrhea, dry mouth	0.25–0.5 mg orally TID, may be increased to 4 mg/day in divided doses
chlordiazepoxide *klor-dye-az-eh-pox'-ide*	Librium	Anxiety disorders, short-term relief of anxiety, acute alcohol withdrawal	Same as alprazolam	Anxiety: 5–25 mg orally 3 or 4 times daily Acute alcohol withdrawal: 50–100 mg IM, then 25–50 mg IM
clonazepam *klon-az'-eh-pam*	Klonopin	Panic disorder, anticonvulsant	Same as alprazolam	0.25 mg orally BID
clorazepate *klor-az'-eh-pate*	Tranxene	Anxiety disorders, short-term relief of anxiety, acute alcohol withdrawal, anticonvulsant	Same as alprazolam	Anxiety: 15–60 mg/day orally in divided doses Acute alcohol withdrawal: up to 90 mg/day with taper-off schedule
diazepam *dye-az'-eh-pam*	Valium	Anxiety disorders, short-term relief of anxiety, acute alcohol withdrawal, anticonvulsant, preoperative muscle relaxant	Same as alprazolam	Individualize dosage: 2–10 mg IM, IV, or orally 2–4 times daily
lorazepam *lor-az'-eh-pam*	Ativan	Anxiety disorders, short-term relief of anxiety, preanesthetic	Same as alprazolam	1–10 mg/day orally in divided doses; when used as preanesthetic: up to 4 mg IM, IV
oxazepam *ox-az'-eh-pam*		Anxiety disorders, short-term relief of anxiety	Same as alprazolam	10–30 mg orally 3–4 times daily
Nonbenzodiazepines				
buspirone *byoo-spye'-rone*		Anxiety disorders, short-term relief of anxiety	Dizziness, drowsiness	15–60 mg/day orally in divided doses
doxepin *dox'-eh-pin*		Anxiety and depression	Same as buspirone	75–150 mg/day, up to 300 mg/day for those severely ill
hydroxyzine *hye-drox'-ih-zeen*	Vistaril	Anxiety and tension associated with psychoneurosis, pruritus, preanesthetic sedative	Dry mouth, transitory drowsiness, involuntary motor activity	25–100 mg orally QID Preanesthetic: 50–100 mg orally or 25–100 mg IM
meprobamate *meh-proe-bah'-mate*		Anxiety disorders, short-term relief of anxiety	Drowsiness, ataxia, nausea, dizziness, slurred speech, headache, weakness, vomiting, diarrhea	1.2–1.6 g/day orally in 3–4 doses, not to exceed 2.4 g/day
Benzodiazepine Antidote				
flumazenil *floo-maz'-e-nil*	Romazicon	Reverse sedation or drowsiness of benzodiazepines and some sleep aids, lessen benzodiazepine withdrawal symptoms	Tachycardia, panic	2 mg IV, may be repeated up to 4 doses

Chapter Review

Know Your Drugs

Clients sometimes know a medication by the brand (or trade) name and not the generic name. To help you recognize both names, match the brand name with the generic name of the same medication.

Generic Name	Brand Name
1. alprazolam	A. Ativan
2. clonazepam	B. Klonopin
3. diazepam	C. Valium
4. lorazepam	D. Xanax

Calculate Medication Dosages

1. Hydroxyzine (Vistaril) 100 mg IM is prescribed. Available is a vial with 100 mg hydroxyzine per milliliter. The nurse administers _____.

2. The client is prescribed 30 mg oxazepam three times a day orally. The drug is available in 15-mg tablets. The nurse administers _____.

Prepare for the NCLEX®

Build Your Knowledge

1. Benzodiazepines enhance which neurotransmitter?
   1. acetylcholine
   2. GABA
   3. norepinephrine
   4. serotonin

2. Alprazolam (Xanax) is contraindicated in clients with _____.
   1. glaucoma
   2. congestive heart failure
   3. diabetes
   4. hypertension

3. Which of the following drugs is a schedule IV controlled substance?
   1. hydroxyzine
   2. doxepin
   3. buspirone
   4. chlordiazepoxide

4. Which of the following is a sign of drug withdrawal and not an adverse reaction?
   1. dizziness
   2. metallic taste
   3. constipation
   4. sedation

5. The benzodiazepines are pregnancy category D drugs that should not be taken while lactating because the newborn may become _____.
   1. depressed
   2. excited and irritable
   3. lethargic and lose weight
   4. hypoglycemic

Apply Your Knowledge

6. Which condition is best treated with benzodiazepines?
   1. obsessive-compulsive anxiety disorder
   2. presurgical apprehension
   3. posttraumatic stress disorder
   4. grief reactions

7. A family member calls the nurse to report that the client taking an antianxiety medication is hypotensive. The nurse instructs the family member to:
   1. give oral fluids to increase the blood pressure
   2. have the client rise more slowly from a lying or sitting position
   3. take the client to a local fire station three times a week to check blood pressure
   4. stop the medication until the nurse checks with the primary health care provider

8. Antianxiety medications are used cautiously in older adults due to the:
   1. inability to absorb the drugs due to decreased acid production
   2. drug not being distributed as well due to poor circulation
   3. liver metabolizing the drug faster, making it ineffective
   4. reduced elimination, making it build up in the circulation

Alternate-Format Questions

9. Describe the feelings of anxiety. **Select all that apply**.
   1. apprehension
   2. panic
   3. uneasiness
   4. worry
   5. jitters

10. A client is restless as he is prepared for a gastric procedure in the outpatient clinic. The primary health care provider asks you to draw up 4 mg of lorazepam (Ativan). Looking at the photo, how many milliliters will you draw up in the syringe?

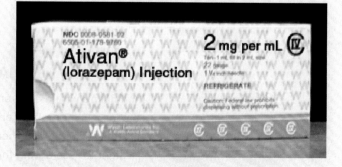

To check your answers, see Appendix G.

the**Point** *For more NCLEX-style questions, log on to http://thepoint.lww.com to access more than 1000 questions.*

Sedatives and Hypnotics

Sedatives and hypnotics are primarily used to treat insomnia. According to the National Sleep Foundation, insomnia affects nearly 70 million people in the United States. It may be caused by lifestyle changes, such as a new job, moving to a new town, or returning to school; jet lag; chronic pain; headaches; stress; or anxiety. Display 21.1 lists the criteria used to define insomnia.

In many cases insomnia is treated in the outpatient setting. Yet, one of the most frequent patient problems during hospitalization is insomnia. Patients are in unfamiliar surroundings that are unlike the home situation. Noises and lights at night often interfere with or interrupt sleep, as noted in Figure 21.1. An important part of meeting patient needs during illness is to help the patient gain rest and sleep. Sleep deprivation may interfere with the healing process; therefore, a **hypnotic** may be given. Also, these drugs may be prescribed for short-term use to promote sleep after discharge as a patient transitions to the home environment.

A hypnotic is a drug that induces drowsiness or sleep, meaning it allows the patient to fall asleep and stay asleep. Hypnotics are given at night or bedtime. A **sedative** is a drug that produces a relaxing, calming effect. Sedatives are usually given during daytime hours, and although they may make the patient drowsy, they usually do not produce sleep.

Sedatives and hypnotics are divided into two classes: barbiturates and nonbarbiturates. The nonbarbiturates are classified into two groups: benzodiazepines and nonbenzodiazepines. Barbiturates were once the drugs of choice to treat insomnia and anxiety; however, the side effects proved to be too harsh. Currently, barbiturates may be used in cases where a deep, nonwaking sleep is desired, such as the few states where assisted suicide is legal. The nonbarbiturates are now used as sedatives in place of barbiturates, because they are more effective in treating insomnia and the adverse reactions

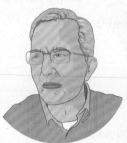

PHARMACOLOGY IN PRACTICE

Mr. Phillip's wife died in an automobile accident, and he has had trouble coping with the loss. He complains about sleeping difficulties, he wakes frequently through the night. The primary health care provider prescribes a hypnotic, 1 capsule per night for use during the next 3 weeks. Read in this chapter about the sedative and hypnotic drugs, and then see if this recommendation helped Mr. Phillip.

Display 21.1 Criteria for the Diagnosis of Insomnia

One or more of the following symptoms must occur

- Difficulty falling asleep
- Waking often and trouble going back to sleep at night
- Waking too early in the morning
- Feeling tired upon waking

are less than the barbiturates. Some of the benzodiazepines are also used as antianxiety drugs (see Chapter 20). The benzodiazepines used primarily for sedation rather than anxiety are discussed in this chapter and include temazepam (Restoril) and triazolam (Halcion).

The nonbenzodiazepines are a group of unrelated drugs. Examples include eszopiclone (Lunesta) and zolpidem (Ambien). Barbiturates, benzodiazepines, and nonbenzodiazepines are listed in the Summary Drug Table: Sedatives and Hypnotics.

Actions

Barbiturates

All barbiturates have essentially the same mode of action. These drugs are capable of producing central nervous system (CNS) depression and mood alterations ranging from mild excitation to mild sedation, hypnosis (sleep), and deep coma. These drugs also are respiratory depressants; the degree of depression usually depends on the dose taken.

Benzodiazepines and Nonbenzodiazepines

Nonbarbiturate sedatives and hypnotics have essentially the same mode of action as the barbiturates—that is, they depress the CNS. The benzodiazepine effect on gamma (γ)-aminobutyric acid (GABA) to potentiate neural inhibition is discussed in Chapter 20. However, these drugs have a lesser effect on the respiratory rate—another reason they are chosen over barbiturates for insomnia.

Figure 21.1 Noises and lights in the environment may cause insomnia for the hospitalized patient.

The nonbenzodiazepine effects diminish after approximately 2 weeks. Persons taking these drugs for longer than 2 weeks may have a tendency to increase the dose to produce the desired effects (e.g., sleep, sedation). Physical tolerance and psychological dependence may occur, especially after prolonged use of high doses. However, their addictive potential appears to be less than that of the barbiturates. Discontinuing use of a sedative or hypnotic after prolonged use may result in mild to severe withdrawal symptoms.

Uses

The sedative and hypnotic drugs are used in the treatment of:

- Insomnia
- Convulsions or seizures

They are also used as adjuncts for anesthesia and for:

- Preoperative sedation
- Conscious sedation

LIFESPAN CONSIDERATIONS
Gerontology
Older adult patients may require a smaller hypnotic dose, and in some instances, a sedative dose may act like a hypnotic and produce sleep.

Adverse Reactions

- Nervous system reactions include dizziness, drowsiness, and headache.
- A common gastrointestinal reaction is nausea.

Contraindications

These drugs are contraindicated in patients with known hypersensitivity to sedatives or hypnotics. Do not administer these drugs to comatose patients, those with severe respiratory problems, those with a history of drug and alcohol habitual use, or pregnant or lactating women. Due to a specific enzyme reaction, grapefruit or its juice should not be taken if the patient is on triazolam or zaleplon. The barbiturates are classified as pregnancy category D drugs.

Benzodiazepines (e.g., estazolam, quazepam, temazepam, triazolam) used for sedation are classified as pregnancy category X drugs. Most nonbenzodiazepines are pregnancy category B or C drugs.

LIFESPAN CONSIDERATIONS
Childbearing Women
Women taking benzodiazepines should be warned of the potential risk to the fetus so that contraceptive methods may be instituted, if necessary. A child born to a mother taking benzodiazepines may experience withdrawal symptoms during the postnatal period.

Precautions

Sedatives and hypnotics should be used cautiously in lactating patients and in patients with hepatic or renal impairment, habitual alcohol use, and mental health problems.

Interactions

The following interactions may occur when a sedative or hypnotic is administered with another agent:

Interacting Drug	Common Use	Effect of Interaction
antidepressants	Management of depression	Increased sedative effect
opioid analgesics antihistamines	Pain relief, relief of allergy symptoms (runny nose and itching)	Increased sedative effect
phenothiazines (e.g., Thorazine)	Management of agitation and psychotic symptoms	Increased sedative effect
cimetidine	Management of gastric upset	Increased sedative effect
alcohol	Relaxation and enjoyment in social situations	Increased sedative effect

Over-the-counter (OTC) sleep aids are abundant, and patients may not volunteer information regarding their use of these alternative or complementary remedies. Always inquire about use of herbal or OTC products. Although lab testing is not conclusive, medical reports indicate a possible interaction with eucalyptus products causing increased sedation.

HERBAL CONSIDERATIONS

Melatonin is a hormone produced by the pineal gland in the brain. Melatonin has been used in treating insomnia, overcoming jet lag, and improving the effectiveness of the immune system, and as an antioxidant. The most significant use—at low doses—is the short-term treatment of insomnia. Melatonin obtained from animal pineal tissue is not recommended for use because of the risk of contamination. The synthetic form of melatonin does not carry this risk. Supplements should be purchased from a reliable source to minimize the risk of contamination. Drowsiness may occur within 30 minutes after taking the supplement. The drowsiness may persist for an hour or more, affecting any activity that requires mental alertness, such as driving. Possible adverse reactions include headache and depression. Although uncommon, allergic reactions (difficulty breathing, hives, or swelling of the lips, tongue, or face) to melatonin have been reported (DerMarderosian, 2003).

NURSING PROCESS

PATIENT RECEIVING A SEDATIVE OR HYPNOTIC

ASSESSMENT

Preadministration Assessment

Before administering a sedative or hypnotic, document the patient's blood pressure, pulse, and respiratory rate. Changes in vital signs (especially hypotension) may occur after drug administration, so having baseline values is important for comparison. In addition to the vital signs, assess the patient's status by asking the following questions:

Hypnotic Drug Administration (for Sleep Disturbances)

- Is the patient uncomfortable? If the reason for discomfort is pain, an analgesic, rather than a hypnotic, may be required. A hypnotic may not be necessary because an analgesic can also induce drowsiness and sleep.

- When is the drug scheduled for administration? Is it too early for the patient to receive the drug—will they awaken early in the morning?

- Are there disturbances in the environment that may keep the patient awake and decrease the effectiveness of the drug?

Sedative Drug Administration (for Relaxing and Calming)

- Is the sedative for a surgical procedure, and is its administration correctly timed?

- Has a consent form for the procedure been signed before the medication is given? Informed consent cannot be established if the patient has medication in his or her system.

If the patient is receiving one of these drugs for daytime sedation, assess the patient's general mental state and level of consciousness. If the patient appears sedated and difficult to awaken, you should withhold the drug and contact the primary health care provider as soon as possible.

HERBAL CONSIDERATIONS

Valerian was originally used in Europe and was brought to North America on the *Mayflower* (Fig. 21.2). The herb is widely used for its sedative effects in conditions of mild anxiety or restlessness. It is particularly useful in individuals with insomnia. Valerian improves overall sleep quality by shortening the length of time it takes to fall asleep and decreasing the number of nighttime awakenings.

Formulated as a tea, tablet, capsule, or tincture, valerian is classified as "generally recognized as safe" (GRAS) for use in the United States. When used as an aid to sleep, valerian is taken approximately 1 hour before bedtime; less is used for anxiety. Valerian can be used in combination with other calming herbs, such as lemon balm or chamomile. It may take 2 to 4 weeks before the full therapeutic effect (i.e., improvement of mood and sleep patterns) occurs. Individuals have been known to experience withdrawal symptoms when they stop taking valerian abruptly (DerMarderosian, 2003).

Ongoing Assessment

Before administering the drug, perform an assessment that includes the patient's vital signs (temperature, pulse, respiration, and blood pressure) and level of consciousness (e.g., alert, confused, or lethargic). Ask the patient about the circumstances causing insomnia and whether other factors such as pain, lights, or disruptive activity are bothersome. After assessing the patient, make a decision regarding administration of the drug or if other interventions are more appropriate to try first.

Ask if the drug helped the patient sleep on previous nights. If not, a different drug or dose may be needed; consult the primary health care provider regarding the drug's ineffectiveness.

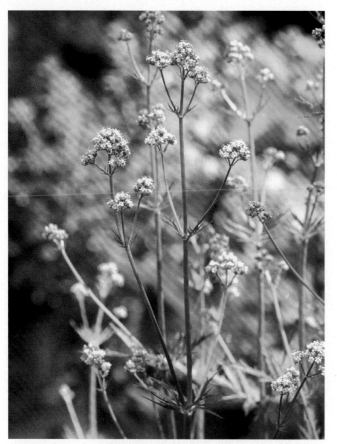

Figure 21.2 The root of the herb valerian is used medicinally. (From DerMarderosian, A., & Beutler, J. [Eds.]. [2003]. *Guide to popular natural products* [3rd ed.] St. Louis, MO: Lippincott Williams & Wilkins.)

If the patient has a given-as-needed (PRN) order for an opioid analgesic or other CNS depressant and a hypnotic, discuss with the primary health care provider regarding the time interval between administrations of these drugs. Usually, at least 2 hours should elapse between administration of a hypnotic and any other CNS depressant, but this interval may vary, depending on factors such as the patient's age and diagnosis.

NURSING ALERT

When giving a sedative or hypnotic, notify the primary health care provider if one or more vital signs significantly vary from the baseline, if the respiratory rate is 10 breaths/min or below, or if the patient appears lethargic.

NURSING DIAGNOSES
Drug-specific nursing diagnoses are the following:

■ **Risk for Injury** related to drowsiness or impaired memory

■ **Ineffective Breathing Pattern** related to respiratory depression

■ **Ineffective Individual Coping** related to excessive use of medication

Nursing diagnoses related to drug administration are discussed in Chapter 4.

PLANNING
The expected outcomes for the patient depend on the reason for administration of a sedative or hypnotic but may include an optimal response to drug therapy (e.g., sedation or sleep), support of patient needs related to management of adverse drug reactions, and confidence in an understanding of the medication regimen.

IMPLEMENTATION

Promoting an Optimal Response to Therapy
You should provide supportive care to promote the effects of the sedative or hypnotic drug. This includes interventions such as back rubs, night lights or a darkened room, and a quiet atmosphere. The patient is discouraged from drinking beverages containing caffeine, such as coffee, cola, or energy drinks, which can contribute to wakefulness.

Never leave hypnotics and sedatives at the patient's bedside to be taken at a later hour; hypnotics and sedatives are controlled substances (see Chapter 1). In addition, never leave these drugs unattended in the nurses' station, hallway, or other areas to which patients, visitors, or hospital personnel have direct access.

NURSING ALERT

Some sleep medicines (zolpidem) may cause memory loss or amnesia. A person may not remember getting up out of bed, driving, or eating. These drugs only should be taken when a person plans for 7 to 8 hours of sleep.

Monitoring and Managing Patient Needs
RISK FOR INJURY. It is important to observe the patient for adverse drug reactions. During periods when the patient is excited or confused, protect the patient from harm and provide supportive care and a safe environment. Assess the patient receiving a sedative dose and determine what safety measures must be taken. After administration of a hypnotic, such as before a procedure, raise the side rails of the bed and advise the patient to remain in bed and to call for assistance if it is necessary to get out of bed. Observe the patient receiving a hypnotic 1 to 2 hours after the drug is given to evaluate the effect of the drug. When used for insomnia, notify the primary health care provider if the patient fails to sleep, awakens one or more times during the night, or experiences an adverse drug reaction. In some instances, supplemental doses of a hypnotic may be ordered if the patient awakens during the night.

Excessive drowsiness and headache the morning after a hypnotic has been given (drug hangover) may occur in some patients. Report this problem to the primary health care provider because a smaller dose or a different drug may be necessary. Assist the patient, if groggy, with ambulation, if necessary. When getting out of bed, the patient is encouraged to rise to a sitting position first, wait a few minutes, and then rise to a standing position.

Patients using these drugs in an outpatient setting are taught about the hazards of operating machinery or involvement in other potentially hazardous tasks until they are sure that concentration and focus are not affected.

LIFESPAN CONSIDERATIONS
Gerontology

The older adult is at greater risk for oversedation, dizziness, confusion, or **ataxia** (unsteady gait) when taking a sedative or hypnotic. Also be aware of and check elderly and debilitated patients for a **paradoxical reaction**, such as marked excitement, or confusion. If excitement or confusion occurs, observe the patient at more frequent intervals (as often as every 5 to 10 minutes may be necessary) for the duration of this occurrence and institute safety measures to prevent injury. If oversedation, extreme dizziness, or ataxia occurs, notify the primary health care provider.

INEFFECTIVE BREATHING PATTERN. Sedatives and hypnotics depress the CNS and can cause respiratory depression. Carefully assess respiratory function (rate, depth, and quality) before administering a sedative, 30 minutes to 1 hour after administering the drug, and frequently thereafter.

Instruct the patient not to drink alcohol when taking sedatives or hypnotics. Alcohol is a CNS depressant, as are the sedatives and hypnotics. When alcohol and a sedative or hypnotic are taken together, there is an additive effect and an increase in CNS depression, which has, on occasion, resulted in death. Emphasize the importance of abstaining from alcohol use while taking this drug and stress that the use of alcohol and any one of these drugs can result in serious effects.

INEFFECTIVE INDIVIDUAL COPING. Sedatives and hypnotics are best given for no more than 2 weeks and preferably for a shorter time. Sedatives and hypnotics can become less effective after they are taken for a prolonged period. Thus, there may be a tendency for a patient to increase the dose without consulting the primary health care provider. To ensure compliance with the treatment regimen, emphasize the importance of not increasing or decreasing the dose unless a change in dosage is recommended by the primary health care provider. In addition, stress the importance of not repeating the dose during the night if sleep is interrupted or sleep lasts only a few hours, unless the primary health care provider has approved taking the drug more than once per night. There are time release medications that may be appropriate if insomnia remains; encourage the patient to talk to the primary health care provider about this option instead of changing dosing on his or her own.

Although the practice is not recommended, a patient with sleep disturbances may be taking one of these drugs for an extended period of time. A sedative or hypnotic can cause drug dependency. Teach the patient not to suddenly discontinue use of these drugs when there is a question of possible dependency. Patients who have been taking a sedative or hypnotic for several weeks should gradually withdraw from taking the drug to prevent withdrawal symptoms (see Chapter 20). Symptoms of withdrawal include restlessness, excitement, euphoria, and confusion. Withdrawal can result in serious consequences, especially in those with existing diseases or disorders.

Educating the Patient and Family

In educating the patient and family about sedatives and hypnotics, several general points must be considered. The patient and family should feel confident in understanding that the drug is to help promote sleep and is a time-limited solution. As you develop a teaching plan, be sure to include one or more of the following items of information:

- The primary health care provider usually prescribes these drugs for short-term use only.
- If the drug appears to be ineffective, contact the primary health care provider. Do not increase the dose unless advised to do so by the primary health care provider.
- Notify the primary health care provider if any adverse drug reactions occur.
- ⚠ Do not drink any alcoholic beverage 2 hours before, with, or 8 hours after taking the drug.
- When taking the drug as a sedative, be aware that the drug can impair the mental and physical abilities required for performing potentially dangerous tasks, such as driving a car or operating machinery.
- After taking a drug to sleep, observe caution when getting out of bed at night. Keep the room dimly lit and remove any obstacles that may result in injury when getting out of bed. Never attempt to drive or perform any hazardous task after taking a drug intended to produce sleep.
- Do not use these drugs if you are pregnant, considering becoming pregnant, or breastfeeding.
- Do not use OTC cold, cough, or allergy drugs while taking this drug unless their use has been approved by the primary health care provider. Some of these products contain antihistamines or other drugs that also may cause mild to extreme drowsiness. Others may contain an adrenergic drug, which is a mild stimulant, and therefore will defeat the purpose of the sedative or hypnotic.
- Do not take zolpidem with food. A high-fat meal or snack can interfere with the absorption of the following drugs: eszopiclone, ramelteon, or zaleplon.

EVALUATION

- Therapeutic response is achieved and sleep pattern is improved or the patient is calm and relaxed for a procedure.
- Adverse reactions are identified, reported to the primary health care provider, and managed successfully with appropriate nursing interventions:
  - No evidence of injury is seen.
  - An adequate breathing pattern is maintained.
  - Patient manages coping effectively.
- Patient and family express confidence and demonstrate an understanding of the drug regimen.

PHARMACOLOGY IN PRACTICE
THINK CRITICALLY

Two weeks following his initial prescription, Mr. Phillip calls the primary health care provider's office and asks for a refill of his prescription. Determine what questions you would ask Mr. Phillip. Explain why you would ask them.

KEY POINTS

- Sedatives produce a relaxing and calming effect. Hypnotic drugs produce sleep. These drugs work by depressing the CNS. Barbiturate use is lessening because of both dependency and harsh adverse reactions. The nonbarbiturates include both benzodiazepines and non-benzodiazepines.

- Insomnia affects nearly 70 million people in the United States. Although it is often treated in the outpatient setting, many hospitalized patients suffer from insomnia, too. These drugs are meant to treat insomnia for only a short period of time, such as 2 weeks. If continued longer dependency can occur.

- Patients should always be asked about sleep aids they have tried before, because both herbal and OTC products are abundant.

- Patients should be cautioned about activities requiring concentration and focus, such as driving, and be aware that blood pressure can drop, leading to dizziness and potential for injury. Doses should not be increased without consulting the primary health care provider.

- Sedatives and hypnotics can also cause respiratory depression. Other CNS depressants, such as alcohol, should not be used with these drugs.

Summary Drug Table SEDATIVES AND HYPNOTICS

Generic Name	Trade Name	Uses	Adverse Reactions	Dosage Ranges
Benzodiazepines				
estazolam *es-taz'-eh-lam*		Hypnotic	Headache, heartburn, nausea, palpitations, rash, somnolence, vomiting, weakness, body and joint pain	1–2 mg orally
flurazepam *flur-az'-eh-pam*		Hypnotic	Same as estazolam	15–30 mg orally
quazepam *kwa'-zeh-pam*	Doral	Hypnotic	Same as estazolam	7.5–15 mg orally
temazepam *teh-maz'-eh-pam*	Restoril	Hypnotic	Same as estazolam	15–30 mg orally
triazolam *trye-ay'-zoe-lam*	Halcion	Sedative, hypnotic	Same as estazolam	0.125–0.5 mg orally at bedtime
Nonbenzodiazepines				
dexmedetomidine *dex-med-eh-toe'-meh-deen*	Precedex	Sedation during intubation, procedural sedation	Hypotension, nausea, bradycardia	1 mcg/kg over 10 min IV
eszopiclone *es-zoe'-pih-kloan*	Lunesta	Insomnia	Headache, somnolence, taste changes, chest pain, migraine, edema	1–3 mg orally at bedtime
ramelteon *ram-el'-tee-on*	Rozerem	Insomnia	Dizziness, headache	8 mg orally at bedtime
zaleplon *zal'-ah-plon*	Sonata	Transient insomnia	Dizziness, headache, rebound insomnia, nausea, myalgia	10 mg orally at bedtime
℞ zolpidem *zoll'-pih-dem*	Ambien, Edluar, Intermezzo	Transient insomnia	Drowsiness, headache, myalgia, nausea	10 mg orally at bedtime
Barbiturates				
pentobarbital *pen-toe-bar'-bih-tall*	Nembutal	Sedative, hypnotic, preoperative sedation	Respiratory and CNS depression, nausea, vomiting, constipation, diarrhea, bradycardia, hypotension, syncope, hypersensitivity reactions, headache	Available only in parenteral form: 100 mg deep IM or IV, may titrate up to 200–500 mg
secobarbital *see-koe-bar'-bih-tall*	Seconal	Hypnotic, preoperative sedation	Same as pentobarbital sodium	Hypnotic: 100 mg orally at bedtime Sedation: 200–300 mg orally 1–2 hr before procedure

℞ This drug should not be administered with food (especially high-fat meals).

● Chapter Review

Know Your Drugs

Clients sometimes know a medication by the brand (or trade) name and not the generic name. To help you recognize both names, match the brand name with the generic name of the same medication.

Generic Name	Brand Name
1. eszopiclone	A. Ambien
2. zaleplon	B. Intermezzo
3. zolpidem	C. Lunesta
	D. Sonata

Calculate Medication Dosages

1. Halcion 0.125 mg is prescribed. The drug is available in 0.125-mg tablets. The nurse administers _____.

2. Eszopiclone (Lunesta) 2 mg is prescribed for insomnia. The drug is available in 1-mg tablets. The nurse administers _____.

● Prepare for the NCLEX®

Build Your Knowledge

1. Sedative and hypnotic drugs exert action to depress the _____.

   1. peripheral nervous system
   2. cardiovascular and respiratory systems
   3. musculoskeletal system
   4. central nervous system

2. Nonbarbiturates are used instead of barbiturates because they _____.

   1. produce better sleep patterns
   2. have fewer adverse reactions
   3. are newer formulas
   4. cause less amnesia

3. Which of these assessments should the nurse report immediately to the primary health provider?

   1. dizziness when arising from the chair
   2. heart rate of 80 bpm
   3. respiration rate of 8 breaths/min
   4. joint pain

4. When giving a hypnotic to an older client, the nurse is aware that _____.

   1. smaller doses of the drug are usually given to older clients
   2. older clients usually require larger doses of a hypnotic
   3. older adults excrete the drug faster than younger adults
   4. dosages of the hypnotic may be increased each night until the desired effect is achieved

5. Which of the following points should be included in a teaching plan for a client taking a sedative or hypnotic?

   1. An alcoholic beverage may be served 1 to 2 hours before a sedative is taken without any ill effects.
   2. Dosage of the sedative may be increased if sleep is not restful.
   3. These drugs may safely be used for 6 months to 1 year when given for insomnia.
   4. Do not use any OTC cold, cough, or allergy medications while taking a sedative or hypnotic.

6. Which of the following sedatives/hypnotics is a pregnancy category X drug?

   1. zolpidem (Ambien)
   2. amobarbital (Amytal)
   3. temazepam (Restoril)
   4. eszopiclone (Lunesta)

Apply Your Knowledge

7. An elderly woman has arthritis in her lower back, and the pain keeps her awake at night. She asks if she can have a "sleeping pill." In considering her request, the nurse must take into account that hypnotic medications might _____.

   1. not be the drug of choice when pain causes insomnia
   2. be given instead of an analgesic to relieve her pain
   3. increase the pain threshold
   4. be added to an analgesic to improve this situation

8. The clinic nurse prepares teaching materials to give a client about use of a hypnotic. Which statement would cause the nurse to contact the primary health care provider?

   1. "I plan to listen to some relaxing music tonight."
   2. "Stopping off at the tavern should help calm me before bedtime."
   3. "I will have a co-worker pick me up tomorrow morning."
   4. "A nutritious meal may help me sleep better."

Alternate-Format Questions

9. Criteria for diagnosing insomnia include which of the items below? **Select all that apply**.

   1. waking too early
   2. sleeping in the middle of the day
   3. difficulty falling asleep
   4. trouble returning to sleep at night

10. When teaching about the nonbenzodiazepine hypnotics, certain foods should not be taken because they interfere with absorption. **Select all of the foods that should not be taken with these drugs.**

    1. peanut butter and crackers
    2. ice cream
    3. apple pie with ice cream
    4. chocolate pudding

To check your answers, see Appendix G.

the**Point** *For more NCLEX-style questions, log on to http://thepoint.lww.com to access more than 1000 questions.*

22

Antidepressant Drugs

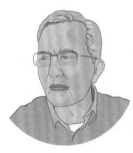

PHARMACOLOGY IN PRACTICE

Mr. Phillip has been severely depressed for about 2 months, following the death of his wife in a car accident. One week ago, the primary care provider prescribed Zoloft 100 mg orally daily. His family is concerned because he is still depressed. Mr. Phillip's daughter is concerned because he feels drowsy and can't seem to get up until 11 a.m. or noon on most days. They are requesting that the dosage be increased. Read about the antidepressants and determine what should happen next.

Depression may be described as feeling sad, unhappy, or "down in the dumps." Most of us feel this way at one time or another for short periods. Major depressive disorder is the medical diagnosis for one of the **mood disorders** (a spectrum of conditions that range from severe debilitation to an exhaustive elation). Also called clinical depression by many people, symptoms are not the result of normal bereavement, such as the loss of a loved one, or another disease, such as hypothyroidism. When the major depressive episode is a depressed or **dysphoric** (extreme or exaggerated sadness, anxiety, or unhappiness) mood that interferes with daily functioning, it is termed **unipolar depression**. For a diagnosis of major depressive disorder, five or more of the symptoms listed in Display 22.1 need to occur daily or nearly every day for a period of 2 weeks or more.

The depressive symptoms of mood disorders are treated with antidepressant drugs and psychotherapy. The four classes of antidepressants are:

- Selective serotonin reuptake inhibitors (SSRIs)
- Serotonin/norepinephrine or dopamine/norepinephrine reuptake inhibitors (SNRIs or DNRIs)
- Tricyclic antidepressants (TCAs)
- Monoamine oxidase inhibitors (MAOIs)

For several years it was thought that antidepressants blocked the reuptake of the **endogenous** (produced by the body) neurotransmitters norepinephrine and serotonin. This action resulted in stimulation of the central nervous system (CNS) and alleviation of the depressed mood. This theory is now being questioned. Research indicates that the effects of antidepressants are related to slow adaptive changes in norepinephrine and serotonin receptor systems (Fuller, 1985). Treatment with antidepressants is thought to produce complex changes in the sensitivities of both presynaptic and postsynaptic receptor sites. Antidepressants increase the sensitivity of postsynaptic alpha (α)-adrenergic and serotonin receptors and decrease the sensitivity of the presynaptic receptor sites. This enhances recovery from the depressive episode by making neurotransmission activity more effective, as visualized in Figure 22.1.

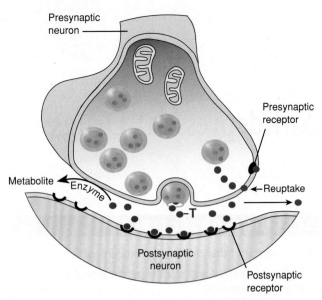

Figure 22.1   Antidepressant drugs inhibit the reuptake of the neurotransmitter (T), thus making it available to the postsynaptic neuron.

SELECTIVE SEROTONIN REUPTAKE INHIBITORS

Actions

The SSRIs inhibit CNS uptake of serotonin (a CNS neurotransmitter). The increase in serotonin levels is thought to act as a stimulant to reverse depression.

Uses

The SSRIs are used in the treatment of the following:

- Depressive episodes
- Obsessive-compulsive disorder (OCD)
- Bulimia nervosa

Unlabeled uses include panic disorders, premenstrual syndrome and posttraumatic stress disorders, generalized anxiety and social phobias, Raynaud's disease, migraine headaches, diabetic neuropathy, and hot flashes. These drugs may be used with psychotherapy in severe cases.

Adverse Reactions

Neuromuscular System Reactions

- Somnolence, dizziness
- Headache, insomnia
- Tremor, weakness

Gastrointestinal and Genitourinary System Reactions

- Constipation, dry mouth, nausea
- Pharyngitis and runny nose
- Urinary retention and abnormal ejaculation

Display 22.1 **Symptoms of Depression**

- Feelings of hopelessness or helplessness
- Diminished interest in activities of life
- Significant weight loss or gain (without dieting)
- Insomnia (inability to sleep) or hypersomnia (excessive sleeping)
- Agitation, restlessness, or irritability
- Fatigue or loss of energy
- Feelings of worthlessness
- Excessive or inappropriate guilt
- Diminished ability to think or concentrate, or indecisiveness
- Recurrent thoughts of death or suicide (or suicide attempt)

Contraindications

The SSRIs are contraindicated in patients with a hypersensitivity to the drugs and during pregnancy (pregnancy category C). Patients taking cisapride (Propulsid), pimozide (Orap), or carbamazepine (Tegretol) should not take fluoxetine (Prozac). Due to a specific enzyme reaction, grapefruit or its juice should not be consumed if the patient is on sertraline (Zoloft).

Precautions

The SSRI antidepressants should be used cautiously in patients with type 2 diabetes, cardiac disease, or impaired liver or kidney function and in those at risk for suicidal ideation or behavior. Patients should not be switched to an SSRI antidepressant drug within 2 weeks of stopping an MAOI antidepressant.

Interactions

The following interactions may occur when an SSRI is administered with another agent:

Interacting Drugs	Common Use	Effect of Interaction
other antidepressants	Treatment of depression	Increased risk of toxic effects
cimetidine	Relief of gastric upset	Increased anticholinergic symptoms (dry mouth, urinary retention, blurred vision)
nonsteroidal anti-inflammatory (NSAIDs) drugs	Relief of inflammation and pain	Increased risk for GI bleeding; decreased effectiveness of SSRI
lithium (interaction with fluoxetine)	Treatment of bipolar disorder	Increased risk of lithium toxicity

Note that the effectiveness of fluoxetine is decreased in patients who smoke cigarettes during administration of the drug.

SEROTONIN/NOREPINEPHRINE OR DOPAMINE/NOREPINEPHRINE REUPTAKE INHIBITORS

Actions

It is thought that the mechanism of action of most of the SNRIs/DNRIs is to affect neurotransmission of serotonin, norepinephrine, and dopamine. Examples in this group of drugs include venlafaxine (Effexor XR) and bupropion (Wellbutrin).

Uses

SNRIs/DNRIs may be used in conjunction with psychotherapy in severe cases or alone in the treatment of the following:

• Depressive episodes
• Depression accompanied by anxiety disorders
• Diabetic peripheral neuropathic pain

Unlabeled uses include enhancing weight loss and treating aggressive behaviors, neuropathic pain, menstrual disorders, cocaine withdrawal and alcohol cravings, fibromyalgia, and stress incontinence.

Adverse Reactions

Neuromuscular System Reactions

• Somnolence, migraine headache
• Hypotension, dizziness, lightheadedness, and vertigo
• Blurred vision, photosensitivity, insomnia, nervousness or agitation, and tremor

Gastrointestinal System Reactions

• Nausea, dry mouth, anorexia, thirst
• Diarrhea, constipation, bitter taste

Other System Reactions

• Fatigue, tachycardia, and palpitations
• Change in libido, impotence
• Skin rash, itching, vasodilation resulting in flushing and excessive sweating

Additional adverse reactions and adverse reactions associated with the use of all the antidepressant drugs are listed in the Summary Drug Table: Antidepressants.

Contraindications

SNRIs/DNRIs are contraindicated in patients with known hypersensitivity to the drugs. Among the SNRIs/DNRIs antidepressants, bupropion and maprotiline are pregnancy category B drugs. Other antidepressants discussed in this section are in pregnancy category C. Safe use of the antidepressants during pregnancy has not been established. They should be used during pregnancy only when the potential benefits outweigh the potential hazards to the developing fetus. Maprotiline should not be used with patients who have a seizure disorder or during the acute phase of a myocardial infarction. Patients taking cisapride, pimozide, or carbamazepine should not take nefazodone because of risk for hepatic failure. Due to a specific enzyme reaction, grapefruit or its juice should not be taken if the patient is on vilazodone or trazodone.

> **! NURSING ALERT**
> The smoking cessation product Zyban is a form of the antidepressant drug bupropion. Smokers should not use Zyban if they are currently taking bupropion for management of depression because of the possibility of bupropion overdose.

Precautions

SNRIs/DNRIs should be used cautiously in patients with cardiac disease, renal or hepatic impairment, or hyperthyroid disease or those who are at risk of suicidal ideation or behavior.

Interactions

The following interactions may occur when an SNRI/DNRI is administered with another agent:

Interacting Drug	Common Use	Effect of Interaction
sedatives and hypnotics, analgesics	Sedation and pain relief, respectively	Increased risk of respiratory and nervous system depression
warfarin	Anticoagulation (blood thinner)	Increased risk for bleeding
cimetidine	Gastrointestinal (GI) upset	Increased anticholinergic symptoms (dry mouth, urinary retention, blurred vision)
antihypertensive agents	Treatment of high blood pressure	Increased risk for hypotension
MAOIs	Antidepressant	Increased risk for hypertensive episodes, severe convulsions, and hyperpyretic episodes

Discovery of the role of dopamine in depression and the ability to be more selective in reuptake make the following classes of drugs less frequently prescribed than those already discussed.

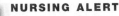

TRICYCLIC ANTIDEPRESSANTS

Actions

The TCAs, such as amitriptyline and doxepin, inhibit reuptake of norepinephrine or serotonin in the brain.

Uses

Tricyclic antidepressant drugs are used in the treatment of the following:

• Depressive episodes
• **Bipolar disorder**
• OCD
• Chronic neuropathic pain
• Depression accompanied by anxiety disorders
• Enuresis

Unlabeled uses include peptic ulcer disease, sleep apnea, panic disorder, bulimia nervosa, premenstrual symptoms, and some dermatologic problems. These drugs may be used with psychotherapy in severe cases.

Adverse Reactions

Generalized reactions include:

• Anticholinergic effects (e.g., sedation, dry mouth, visual disturbances, urinary retention)
• Constipation and photosensitivity

NURSING ALERT

Although the TCAs are not considered antipsychotic agents, the drug amoxapine has been associated with **tardive dyskinesia** and neuroleptic malignant syndrome (NMS). Tardive dyskinesia is a syndrome of involuntary movement that may be irreversible. Symptoms of NMS are similar and include muscle rigidity, altered mental status, and autonomic system problems, such as tachycardia or sweating. These syndromes tend to occur more readily in elderly women; the drug should be discontinued, the primary health care provider notified immediately, and treatment of adverse effects begun quickly.

Contraindications

The TCAs are contraindicated in patients with known hypersensitivity to the drugs. The TCAs are not given within 14 days of the MAOI antidepressants, to patients with a recent myocardial infarction, or to children or lactating mothers. These drugs are in pregnancy categories C and D, and the safety of their use during pregnancy has not been established. Doxepin is contraindicated in patients with glaucoma or in those with a tendency for urinary retention.

Precautions

The TCAs should be used cautiously in patients with cardiac disease, hepatic or renal impairment, hyperthyroid disease, history of seizure activity, narrow-angle glaucoma or increased intraocular pressure, or urinary retention and in those at risk of suicidal ideation or behavior.

NURSING ALERT

The TCAs can cause cardiac-related adverse reactions, such as tachycardia and heart block. Give these drugs with caution to older adults or the person with pre-existing cardiac disease.

Interactions

The following interactions may occur when a TCA is administered with another agent:

Interacting Drugs	Effect of Common Use	Interaction
sedatives and hypnotics, analgesics	Sedation and pain relief, respectively	Increased risk of respiratory and nervous system depression
cimetidine	Treatment of GI upset	Increased anticholinergic symptoms (dry mouth, urinary retention, blurred vision)
MAOIs	Antidepressant agents	Increased risk for hypertensive episodes, severe convulsions, and hyperpyretic episodes
adrenergic agents	Neuromuscular agents	Increased risk for arrhythmias and hypertension

MONOAMINE OXIDASE INHIBITORS

Actions

Drugs classified as MAOIs inhibit the activity of monoamine oxidase, a complex enzyme system responsible for inactivating certain neurotransmitters. Blocking monoamine oxidase results in an increase in *endogenous* epinephrine, norepinephrine, dopamine, and serotonin in the nervous system. An increase in these **neurohormones** (secreted rather than transmitted neurosubstances) stimulates the CNS.

Uses

The MAOI antidepressants are used in the treatment of depressive episodes and may be used in conjunction with psychotherapy in severe cases. Unlabeled uses include bulimia, night terrors, migraine headaches, seasonal affective disorder, and multiple sclerosis.

Adverse Reactions

• Neuromuscular reactions include **orthostatic hypotension**, dizziness, vertigo, headache, and blurred vision.
• GI and genitourinary system reactions include constipation, dry mouth, nausea, diarrhea, and impotence.
• A serious adverse reaction associated with MAOIs is hypertensive crisis (extremely high blood pressure), which may occur when foods containing **tyramine** (an amino acid) are eaten (see Display 22.2 for a list of foods containing tyramine).

Display 22.2 Foods Containing Tyramine to Be Avoided if Taking MAOI Antidepressant

• Aged cheese (e.g., blue, Camembert, cheddar, Emmenthaler, mozzarella, parmesan, Romano, Stilton, Swiss)
• Sour cream
• Yogurt
• Beef or chicken livers
• Pickled herring
• Fermented meats (e.g., bologna, pepperoni, salami, dried fish)
• Undistilled alcoholic beverages (e.g., imported beer; ale; red wine, especially Chianti and sherry)
• Caffeinated beverages (e.g., coffee, tea, colas)
• Chocolate
• Certain fruits and vegetables (e.g., avocado, bananas, fava beans, figs, raisins, sauerkraut)
• Yeast extracts
• Soy sauce

NURSING ALERT

One of the earliest symptoms of hypertensive crisis is headache (usually occipital), followed by a stiff or sore neck, nausea, vomiting, sweating, fever, chest pain, dilated pupils, and bradycardia or tachycardia. If a hypertensive crisis occurs, immediate medical intervention is necessary to reduce the blood pressure. Strokes (cerebrovascular accidents) and death have been reported.

Contraindications and Precautions

The MAOI antidepressants are contraindicated in the elderly and in patients with known hypersensitivity to the drugs, pheochromocytoma, liver and kidney disease, cerebrovascular disease, hypertension, history of headaches, or congestive heart failure. Safety has not been established for use in patients younger than 16 years or during pregnancy (pregnancy category C) or lactation.

The MAOIs should be used cautiously in patients with impaired liver function, history of seizures, parkinsonian symptoms, diabetes, or hyperthyroidism and in those at risk of suicidal ideation or behavior. Individuals on MAOIs should not take decongestants without the permission of their primary health care provider.

Interactions

The following interactions may occur when an MAOI antidepressant is administered with another agent:

Interacting Drugs or Agent	Common Use	Effect of Interaction
sedatives and hypnotics, analgesics	Sedation and pain relief, respectively	Increased risk for adverse reactions during surgery
thiazide diuretic	Relief of fluid retention	Increased hypotensive effects of the MAOI
meperidine	Pain relief	Increased risk for hypertensive episodes, severe convulsions, and hyperpyretic episodes
adrenergic agents	Neuromuscular agent	Increased risk for cardiac arrhythmias and hypertension
tyramine or tryptophan	Amino acids found in some foods	Hypertensive crisis, which may occur up to 2 weeks after the MAOI is discontinued
antitussives	Relieve cough	Hypotension, fever, nausea, jerking motions to the leg, and coma

HERBAL CONSIDERATIONS

Patients should be assessed for use of herbal preparations containing St. John's wort because of the potential for adverse reactions when taken with antidepressants (DerMarderosian, 2003).

LITHIUM

Although lithium is not a true antidepressant drug, it is grouped with the antidepressants because of its use in regulating the severe fluctuations of the manic phase of bipolar disorder (a mood disorder characterized by severe swings from extreme hyperactivity to depression). During the manic phase, the person experiences altered thought processes, which can lead to bizarre delusions. The drug diminishes the frequency and intensity of hyperactive (manic) episodes.

Lithium is rapidly absorbed after oral administration. The most common adverse reactions include tremors, nausea, vomiting, thirst, and polyuria. Toxic reactions may occur when serum lithium levels are greater than 1.5 mEq/L (Table 22.1). Because some of these toxic reactions are serious, lithium blood level measurements are usually obtained during therapy, and the dosage of lithium is adjusted accordingly.

Lithium is contraindicated in patients with hypersensitivity to tartrazine (commonly used yellow food dye), renal or cardiovascular disease, sodium depletion, and dehydration and in patients receiving diuretics. Lithium is a pregnancy category D drug and is contraindicated during pregnancy and lactation. For women of childbearing age, contraceptives may be prescribed while they are taking lithium.

Antacids will decrease the effectiveness of lithium. Lithium is monitored carefully in patients who sweat profusely,

Table 22.1 Lithium Toxicity	
Serum Lithium Level	**Signs of Toxicity**
1.5–2 mEq/L	Diarrhea, vomiting, nausea, drowsiness, muscular weakness, lack of coordination (early signs of toxicity)
2–3 mEq/L	Giddiness, ataxia, blurred vision, tinnitus, vertigo, increasing confusion, slurred speech, blackouts, myoclonic twitching or movement of entire limbs, choreoathetoid movements, urinary or fecal incontinence, agitation or manic-like behavior, hyperreflexia, hypertonia, dysarthria
More than 3 mEq/L	May produce a complex clinical picture involving multiple organs and organ systems, including seizures (generalized and focal), arrhythmias, hypotension, peripheral vascular collapse, stupor, muscle group twitching, spasticity, coma

experience diarrhea or vomiting, or have an infection or fever causing fluid loss. Patients taking diuretics or antipsychotic drugs should be monitored for lithium toxicity.

NURSING PROCESS
PATIENT RECEIVING AN ANTIDEPRESSANT DRUG

ASSESSMENT

Preadministration Assessment
A patient receiving an antidepressant drug may be treated in the hospital or in an outpatient setting. Before starting therapy, obtain a complete medical history. The patient should have thyroid function tested to rule out hypothyroidism before therapy is started. The patient's mental status can be assessed using standardized depression assessment tools or asking questions about *desire* to participate in activities, *withdrawal* from social interactions, and whether *dependency* on others has increased. A quick depression assessment involves asking the patient if in the last 2 weeks he or she has felt helpless or hopeless. Listen to the patient for comments about feelings of anxiety, sadness, guilt, or increased attachment to others. Document any changes in activity level or engagement with others as well as objective signs you see during the interview such as slowness to answer questions, a monotone speech pattern, or crying.

During the initial interview, it is important to assess the potential for self-harm or suicide. It is important to document the presence of suicidal thoughts. Providers sometimes think asking about suicidal thoughts is what causes patients to take their own lives; it does not. It is important to ask the questions in a straightforward manner using simple questions. See Display 22.3 for indications of who is at risk for suicidal behavior. Accurately document and immediately report any statements concerning suicide or the ability of the patient to carry out any suicidal intentions to the primary health care provider.

Ongoing Assessment
The therapeutic effects of the antidepressants may take 2 to 4 weeks to be seen. Therefore, many patients who are hospitalized when antidepressants are prescribed may be discharged before follow-up assessments are made. These patients are usually seen at periodic intervals in the primary health care provider's office or in a mental health outpatient setting.

Display 22.3 Indications of Suicidal Behavior

- Verbal cueing: statements of worthlessness or that a "situation" will be over soon
- *Coming out* of depressive mood: when a person is at the greatest risk for self-harm
- A "command" hallucination: when "voices" are telling a patient he or she is worthless and should die
- Lack of alternatives: when a person who has relatively few coping skills/support networks has the false belief that he or she has ruled out all resources available and death is now the only solution

Before the drug lifts the depressive mood, patients are monitored for the adverse reactions of the drugs, which can cause patients to stop taking them prematurely.

At the time of each visit to the primary health care provider or clinic, observe the patient for a response to therapy. Question the patient or family members about what they see or how they feel about the response to therapy. The type of questions asked depends on the patient and the diagnosis and may include questions such as:

- How are you feeling?
- How would you describe your depressed feelings?
- How would you rate your depression?
- Would you like to tell me how everything is going?

You may need to rephrase questions or direct conversation toward other subjects until the patient feels comfortable and can discuss therapy. Also, reinforce that it takes time for the patient to see results and praise the patient for continuing to take the medication even if he or she does not see a response yet.

NURSING DIAGNOSES

Drug-specific nursing diagnoses are the following:

- **Self-Care Deficit Syndrome** related to inability to participate in activities of daily living secondary to somnolence, drowsiness, and depressive state
- **Disturbed Sleep Pattern** related to depression and excessive drowsiness
- **Imbalanced Nutrition: Less Than Body Requirements** related to anorexia, constipation, and depression
- **Risk for Suicide** related to suicidal ideation and adverse reaction to antidepressive drug
- **Acute Pain** related to **priapism** (painful erection)
- **Imbalanced Fluid Volume** related to lithium toxicity

Nursing diagnoses related to drug administration are discussed in Chapter 4.

PLANNING

The expected outcomes of the patient depend on the reason for administration of an antidepressant but may include an optimal response to drug therapy, support of patient needs related to the management of adverse drug reactions, and confidence in an understanding of the medication regimen.

IMPLEMENTATION

Promoting an Optimal Response to Therapy

Response to antidepressant medications is not rapid. It can take a number of weeks for the drugs to take effect. Fluoxetine is an example of a drug that may take as long as 4 weeks to attain a full therapeutic effect. Some adverse reactions, such as dry mouth, episodes of orthostatic hypotension, and drowsiness, appear long before the intended effect of the antidepressant. The inability to deal with the unpleasantness of these adverse reactions is one of the greatest reasons patients stop taking antidepressants. The two adverse reactions that patients have the most trouble tolerating are somnolence and dry mouth. During initial therapy or whenever the dosage is increased or decreased,

instruct the patient what to expect in terms of the adverse reactions or behavioral changes. Teach the patient when to report change in behavior or the appearance of adverse reactions to the primary health care provider, because a further increase or decrease in dosage may be necessary or use of the drug may need to be discontinued.

When caring for hospitalized patients with depression, develop a nursing care plan to meet the patient's individual needs. Should patient behavior require the antidepressants to be given parenterally, give these drugs intramuscularly (IM) in a large muscle mass, such as the gluteus muscle. Keep the patient lying down (when possible) for about 30 minutes after administering the drug.

Monitoring and Managing Patient Needs

SELF-CARE DEFICIT SYNDROME. Initially, the patient may need assistance with self-care, because patients with depression often do not have the physical or emotional energy to perform self-care activities. This is complicated by the fact that many antidepressants cause excessive drowsiness during the initial stages of treatment, and patients may need assistance with ambulation and self-care activities. These problems usually subside as the depression lifts and tolerance to the adverse reactions builds with continued use of the antidepressant. To minimize the risk for injury, assist the patient when necessary and make the environment as safe as possible. When orthostatic hypotension is an effect of drug therapy, instruct the patient how to rise from a lying position to a sitting position. The patient remains in a sitting position for a few minutes before rising to a standing position. Position changes are made slowly, with assistance offered if necessary.

If the patient has a difficult time with self-care because of the depression or sedative effects of the antidepressants, arrange for total assistance with activities of daily living, including help with eating, dressing, and ambulating. However, encourage self-care whenever possible, allowing sufficient time for the patient to accomplish tasks to the fullest extent of his or her ability. It is important to provide positive feedback when appropriate. As a therapeutic effect of the drug is attained, the patient will be able to resume self-care (if no other physical conditions interfere).

Document behavioral observations at periodic intervals, the frequency of which depends on hospital or unit guidelines. An accurate assessment of the patient's behavior aids the primary health care provider in planning therapy and thus becomes an important part of nursing management. Patients with a poor response to drug therapy may require dosage changes, a change to another antidepressant drug, or the addition of other therapies to the treatment regimen.

DISTURBED SLEEP PATTERN. Many of the antidepressant drugs cause somnolence. This adverse reaction is one of the greatest reasons patients stop taking the medication. Teach the patient or care providers to administer the drug at night—the sedative effects promote sleep, and the adverse reactions appear less troublesome. An exception to this is the SSRIs; it is best to administer those medications in the morning.

Assess the environment to help promote sleep at night and wakefulness during the day. Drapes should be shut at night and opened in the day to let in light, and clocks should be available for the patient to see the time of day. These activities will help the patient to reorient to daytime and nighttime, thereby promoting an effective sleep pattern.

IMBALANCED NUTRITION: LESS THAN BODY REQUIREMENTS. Depressed patients may not feel like eating; therefore, they lose weight. This can be potentiated by the adverse reactions of anorexia and constipation. Monitor dietary intake and help the registered dietician in providing nutritious meals, taking into consideration foods that the patient likes and dislikes. Fluid intake and foods high in fiber are important for the patient to prevent constipation. Weighing the patient weekly is important for monitoring weight loss or gain. To minimize the dry mouth that frequently accompanies administration of antidepressants, teach good oral hygiene and provide frequent sips of fluids and sugarless gum or hard candy.

LIFESPAN CONSIDERATIONS
Pediatric
Studies show that children and adolescents with major depressive disorders have an increased risk of suicidal ideation when prescribed antidepressant medications.

RISK FOR SUICIDE. Patients with a high suicide potential require a well-supervised environment and protection from suicidal acts. For patients with severe depression, suicide precautions are important until a therapeutic effect is achieved. When the patient is hospitalized, policies of observation must be strictly followed for the patient's protection.

Of greatest concern is the depressed patient who has suicidal ideation but has not been identified as such (see Display 22.3 for indications of suicidal risk). Patients in a depressive state may lack the energy to carry out plans for ending their own life. Because the full therapeutic effect of the antidepressant may not be attained for 10 days to 4 weeks, patients have time to gain enough energy to carry out an injurious act upon themselves. Patients with suicidal ideation must be monitored closely. Report any expressions of guilt, hopelessness, or helplessness; insomnia; weight loss; and direct or indirect threats of suicide.

When suicidal ideation is suspected, oral administration of medications requires greater consideration. After administration of an oral drug, inspect the patient's oral cavity to be sure the drug has been swallowed. If the patient resists having his or her oral cavity checked, report this refusal to the primary health care provider. Patients planning suicide may try to keep the drug on the side of the mouth or under the tongue and not swallow in an effort to hoard or save enough of the drug to attempt suicide at a later time. Other patients may refuse to take the drug. If the patient refuses to take the drug, contact the primary health care provider regarding this problem because parenteral administration of the drug may be necessary.

LIFESPAN CONSIDERATIONS
Gerontology
Older men with prostatic enlargement are at increased risk for urinary retention when they take antidepressants.

ACUTE PAIN. An uncommon but potentially serious adverse reaction of trazodone is priapism (a persistent erection of the penis). This can be very painful and if not treated within a few hours, priapism can result in impotence. Because this can be an embarrassing adverse reaction, instruct the patient to report any prolonged or inappropriate penile erection. The drug is discontinued immediately and the primary care provider notified. Injection of α-adrenergic stimulants (e.g., norepinephrine) may be helpful in treating priapism. In some cases, surgical intervention may be required.

IMBALANCED FLUID VOLUME. Fluid volume determines the concentration of lithium in the blood. The dosage of lithium is individualized according to serum levels and clinical response to the drug. The desirable serum lithium level is between 0.6 and 1.2 mEq/L. Blood samples are drawn immediately before the next dose of lithium (8 to 12 hours after the last dose) when lithium levels are relatively stable.

Lithium toxicity is closely related to serum lithium levels and can occur even when the drug is administered at therapeutic doses. This can happen because during the acute manic phase, patients may be so active that they do not realize they need to eat or drink and are at greater risk of dehydration, resulting in a higher serum lithium level. Hospitalized patients may be required to take "fluid" breaks, where they are taught to stop and drink fluid at specified times. Patients should maintain an oral intake of approximately 3000 mL/day. Adverse reactions are seldom observed at serum lithium levels of less than I.5 mEq/L, except in the patient who is especially sensitive to lithium. See Table 22.1 for toxic symptoms that may occur. When patients are discharged, instruct them to notify the primary health care provider any time they experience fever, diarrhea, vomiting, or nausea to prevent dehydration and a possible increase in the serum lithium level.

LIFESPAN CONSIDERATIONS
Gerontology
Older adults are at increased risk for lithium toxicity because of a decreased rate of excretion. Lower dosages may be necessary to decrease the risk of toxicity.

Educating the Patient and Family
When some patients are discharged to the home setting, lack of adherence to drug therapy is a problem, due to unpleasant adverse drug effects. It is very important to educate the patient or family members thoroughly about the importance of managing the reactions so that the patient will continue the proper drug regimen. Evaluate the patient's ability to assume responsibility for taking drugs at home (see Patient Teaching for Improved Patient Outcomes: Empowering Patient Responsibility for Antidepressant Drug Therapy). The administration of antidepressant drugs becomes a family responsibility if the outpatient appears to be unable to manage his or her own drug therapy.

The patient and family should feel confident in understanding any adverse reactions that may occur with a specific antidepressant drug. Encourage the patient or family member to contact the primary health care provider immediately if a serious drug reaction occurs. As you develop a teaching plan, include the following points for the patient or family member:

■ Inform the primary health care provider, dentist, and other medical personnel of therapy with this drug.

■ If dizziness occurs when changing position, rise slowly when getting out of bed or a chair. If dizziness is severe, always have help when changing positions.

Patient Teaching for Improved Patient Outcomes

Empowering Patient Responsibility for Antidepressant Drug Therapy

Antidepressants are taken for long periods of time, requiring self-management on the part of the patient. When people feel empowered in decision making, they are more likely to remain adherent to a plan of care.

When you teach, make sure your patient understands the following:

✔ Explain the reason for drug therapy, including the type of antidepressant prescribed, drug name, dosage, and frequency of administration.
✔ Enlist the aid of family members to support adherence with therapy.
✔ Urge the patient to take the drug exactly as prescribed and not to increase or decrease dosage, omit doses, or discontinue use of the drug unless directed to do so by the health care provider.
✔ Advise that full therapeutic effect may not occur for several weeks.
✔ Instruct in the signs and symptoms of behavioral changes indicative of therapeutic effectiveness or increasing depression and suicidal tendencies.
✔ Review measures to reduce the risk for suicidal ideation.
✔ Instruct about possible adverse reactions with instructions to notify the health care provider should any occur.
✔ Reinforce safety measures such as changing positions slowly and avoiding driving or hazardous tasks.
✔ Advise avoidance of alcohol and use of nonprescription drugs unless discussed with the primary health care provider.
✔ Encourage the patient to inform other health care providers and medical personnel about drug therapy regimen.
✔ Instruct in measures to minimize dry mouth.
✔ Reassure results of therapy will be monitored by periodic laboratory tests and follow-up visits with the health care provider.
✔ Assist with arrangements for follow-up visits.

■ Relieve dry mouth by taking frequent sips of water, sucking on hard candy, or chewing gum (preferably sugarless gum).
■ Keep all clinic appointments or appointments with the primary health care provider because close monitoring of therapy is essential.
■ Do not take the antidepressants during pregnancy. Notify the primary health care provider if you are pregnant or wish to become pregnant.
■ Report any unusual changes or physical effects to the primary health care provider.
■ Avoid prolonged exposure to sunlight or sunlamps because an exaggerated reaction to the ultraviolet light may occur (photosensitivity), resulting in a burn.
■ For male patients who take trazodone and who experience prolonged, inappropriate, and painful erections, stop taking the drug and notify the primary care provider.
■ Remember to take lithium with food or immediately after meals to avoid stomach upset. Drink at least 10 large glasses of fluid each day and add extra salt to food if permissible. Prolonged exposure to the sun may lead to dehydration. If any of the following occurs, do not take the next dose and immediately notify the primary health care provider: diarrhea, vomiting, fever, tremors, drowsiness, lack of muscle coordination, or muscle weakness.

EVALUATION

■ Therapeutic response is achieved and the depressive mood is improved.
■ Adverse reactions are identified, reported to the primary health care provider, and managed successfully through appropriate nursing interventions:
• Patient resumes ability to care for self.
• Patient reports fewer episodes of inappropriate sleep patterns.
• Patient maintains an adequate nutritional status.
• Patient does not attempt suicide.
• Patient is free of pain.
• Adequate fluid volume is maintained.
■ Patient and family express confidence and demonstrate an understanding of the drug regimen.

PHARMACOLOGY IN PRACTICE
THINK CRITICALLY

What information do you need to give Mr. Phillip and his family regarding the action and adverse reactions of these drugs? How might this drug be interacting with other drugs prescribed in earlier chapters of this unit?

KEY POINTS

- Mood disorders are a spectrum of feelings that range from severe debilitation to an exhaustive elation.

- Major depressive disorder is also termed unipolar or clinical depression. This condition is characterized by a dysphoric mood lasting at least 2 weeks. Bipolar depression may or may not have the depressed component, yet it has the manic or energized portion.

- Drugs used to treat unipolar depression include those that modify the neurotransmission of one or more of the following: serotonin, norepinephrine, or dopamine. Currently the most frequently used drugs are from the SSRIs or the SNRIs/DNRIs.

- Antidepressants may take from 2 to 4 weeks for the intended response to occur. Unfortunately, adverse reactions can occur sooner, and patients may stop taking the drug before maximum benefit is obtained. These adverse reactions include drowsiness, dizziness and lightheadedness, dry mouth, thirst, and constipation.

- These drugs increase the risk of suicidal ideation and patients must be both questioned and observed for any suicidal behaviors.

- Patients taking drugs for mania have behaviors (energized) that put them at risk for dehydration—a condition that can increase serum levels of lithium, a drug used for bipolar depression, resulting in toxicity.

Summary Drug Table ANTIDEPRESSANTS

Generic Name	Trade Name	Uses	Adverse Reactions	Dosage Ranges
Selective Serotonin Reuptake Inhibitors (SSRIs)				
citalopram *sih-tal'-oh-pram*	Celexa	Depression, panic disorder, posttraumatic stress disorder (PTSD), premenstrual disorder	Nausea, dry mouth, sweating, somnolence, insomnia, anorexia, diarrhea	20–40 mg/day orally
escitalopram *es-sih-tal'-oh-pram*	Lexapro	Depression, generalized anxiety disorder, panic disorder	Headache, insomnia, somnolence, nausea	10–20 mg/day orally
fluoxetine *floo-ox'-eh-teen*	Prozac, Prozac Weekly, Sarafem	Depression, bulimia, OCD, panic disorder, premenstrual dysphoric disorder (Sarafem only)	Anxiety, nervousness, somnolence, insomnia, drowsiness, asthenia, tremor, headache, nausea, diarrhea, constipation, dry mouth, anorexia	20 mg/day orally in the morning or up to 80 mg/day (dose split between morning and at noon)
fluvoxamine *floo-vox'-ah-meen*	Luvox	OCD, depression	Headache, nervousness, somnolence, insomnia, nausea, diarrhea, dry mouth, constipation, dyspepsia, ejaculatory disturbances	50–300 mg/day orally in divided doses
paroxetine *par-ox'-eh-teen*	Paxil	Depression, OCD, panic disorder, general anxiety disorder, social anxiety disorder, PTSD	Headache, tremors, somnolence, nervousness, dizziness, insomnia, nausea, diarrhea, constipation, dry mouth, sweating, weakness, sexual dysfunction	20–50 mg/day orally
sertraline *sir'-trah-leen*	Zoloft	Depression, OCD, panic disorders, PTSD	Headache, drowsiness, anxiety, dizziness, insomnia, fatigue, nausea, diarrhea, dry mouth, ejaculatory disturbances, sweating	50–200 mg/day orally
vilazodone *vil-az'-oh-don*	Viibryd	Depression	Dry mouth, increased appetite, heartburn, dizziness, shakiness	40 mg daily orally

Summary Drug Table ANTIDEPRESSANTS (continued)

Generic Name	Trade Name	Uses	Adverse Reactions	Dosage Ranges
Serotonin/Norepinephrine and Dopamine/Norepinephrine Reuptake Inhibitors (SNRI/DNRI)				
bupropion *byoo-proe'-pee-on*	Aplenzin, Wellbutrin, Zyban (smok- ing cessation)	Depression, neuropathic pain, attention deficit hyper- activity disorder (ADHD), smoking cessation	Agitation, dizziness, dry mouth, insomnia, sedation, headache, nausea, vomiting, tremor, con- stipation, weight loss, anorexia, excess sweating	100–300 mg/day orally in divided doses; sustained release, 1 tablet BID orally
desvenlafaxine *des-ven'-la-fax-een*	Pristiq	Depression	Anxiety, constipation, decreased appetite, dizziness, insomnia, sexual dysfunction	50 mg daily orally
duloxetine *doo-lox'-eh-teen*	Cymbalta	Depression, diabetic periph- eral neuropathy, fibromyal- gia, stress incontinence	Insomnia, dry mouth, nausea, constipation	40–60 mg/day orally
maprotiline *mah-proe'-tih-leen*		Depression, anxiety associ- ated with depression	Sedation, dry mouth, constipa- tion, orthostatic hypotension	75–150 mg/day orally; for severe depression, dosage may increase to 225 mg/ day orally
milnacipran *mil-na'-si-pran*	Savella	Fibromyalgia	Constipation, dry mouth, tachy- cardia, hot flush, vomiting	12.5–50 mg twice daily orally
nefazodone *neh-faz'-oh-doan*		Depression	Somnolence, insomnia, dizzi- ness, nausea, dry mouth, con- stipation, headache, weakness	200–600 mg/day orally in divided doses
trazodone *traz'-oh-doan*	Oleptro	Depression, alcohol craving	Drowsiness, dizziness, priapism, dry mouth, nausea, vomiting, constipation, fatigue, nervousness	150–400 mg/day orally in divided doses, not to exceed 600 mg/day
venlafaxine *ven-lah-fax'-een*	Effexor XR	Depression, anxiety disor- ders, premenstrual disorder	Headache, insomnia, dizziness, nervousness, weakness, anorexia, nausea, constipation, dry mouth, somnolence, sweating	75–225 mg/day orally in divided doses
Tricyclic Antidepressants				
amitriptyline *am-ee-trip'-tih-leen*		Depression, neuropathic pain, eating disorders	Sedation, anticholinergic effects (dry mouth, dry eyes, urinary retention), constipation	Up to 150 mg/day orally in divided doses; 20–30 mg IM QID; severely depressed hospitalized patient: up to 300 mg/day orally. Do not administer IV
amoxapine *ah-mox'-ah-peen*		Depression accompanied by anxiety	Same as amitriptyline	50 mg orally 2–3 times daily up to 300 mg/day, if poor response may go up to 600 mg/day
clomipramine *kloe-mip'-rah-meen*	Anafranil	OCD	Same as amitriptyline, sexual dysfunction	25–250 mg/day orally in divided doses
desipramine *de-sip'-rah-meen*	Norpramin	Depression, eating disorders	Same as amitriptyline	100–200 mg/day orally, not to exceed 300 mg/day
doxepin *dox'-eh-pin*		Anxiety or depression, emo- tional symptoms accompa- nying organic disease	Same as amitriptyline	25–150 mg/day orally in divided doses

(table continues on page 228)

Antidepressant Drugs

Summary Drug Table ANTIDEPRESSANTS (continued)

Generic Name	Trade Name	Uses	Adverse Reactions	Dosage Ranges
imipramine *ih-mip'-rah-meen*	Tofranil	Depression, enuresis, eating disorders	Same as amitriptyline	100–200 mg/day orally in divided doses Childhood enuresis (older than 6 yr): 25 mg/day, 1 hr before bedtime, not to exceed 2.5 mg/kg/day
mirtazapine *mer-tah'-zah-peen*	Remeron	Depression	Sedation, dry mouth, constipation, orthostatic hypotension	15–45 mg/day orally
nortriptyline *nor-trip'-tih-leen*	Aventyl, Pamelor	Depression, premenstrual symptoms	Same as amitriptyline	25 mg orally 3–4 times/day; not to exceed 150 mg/day
protriptyline *proe-trip'-tih-leen*	Vivactil	Depression, sleep apnea	Same as amitriptyline	15–40 mg/day orally in 3–4 doses, not to exceed 60 mg/day
trimipramine *trye-mip'-rah-meen*	Surmontil	Depression, peptic ulcer disease	Same as amitriptyline	75–150 mg/day orally in divided doses, not to exceed 300 mg/day
Monoamine Oxidase Inhibitors				
phenelzine *fen'-el-zeen*	Nardil	Atypical depression	Orthostatic hypotension, vertigo, dizziness, nausea, constipation, dry mouth, diarrhea, headache, restlessness, blurred vision, hypertensive crisis	45–90 mg/day orally in divided doses
tranylcypromine *tran-ill-sip'-roe-meen*	Parnate	Atypical depression	Same as phenelzine	30–60 mg/day orally in divided doses
isocarboxazid *eye-so-car-box'-ah-zid*	Marplan	Depression	Same as phenelzine	10–40 mg/day orally
Mood Stabilizer				
lithium *lith'-ee-um*	Lithobid	Manic episodes of bipolar disorder	Headache, drowsiness, tremors, nausea, polyuria (see Table 22.1)	Based on lithium serum levels; average dose range is 900–1800 mg/day orally in divided doses

● Chapter Review

Know Your Drugs

Clients sometimes know a medication by the brand (or trade) name and not the generic name. To help you recognize both names, match the brand name with the generic name of the same medication.

Generic Name	Brand Name
1. bupropion	A. Celexa
2. citalopram	B. Paxil
3. paroxetine	C. Wellbutrin
	D. Zyban

Calculate Medication Dosages

1. The primary care provider prescribes trazodone 150 mg orally. Available are 50-mg tablets. The nurse administers _____.

2. The primary care provider prescribes oral paroxetine (Paxil) 50 mg/day. The drug is available as oral suspension with a strength of 10 mg/5 mL. The nurse administers _____.

● Prepare for the NCLEX®

Build Your Knowledge

1. A client exhibits high energy and disorganized behavior on the mental health unit. This is best termed _____.

   1. clinical depression
   2. unipolar disorder
   3. major depressive disorder
   4. bipolar disorder

2. Which of the following adverse reactions would the nurse expect to find in a client taking amitriptyline?

   1. constipation and abdominal cramps
   2. bradycardia and double vision
   3. sedation and dry mouth
   4. polyuria and hypotension

3. Clinical depression is suspected in which of the following clients?

   1. woman who is crying about her mastectomy performed yesterday
   2. line worker who lost his job in a manufacturing plant 3 months ago
   3. person diagnosed with hypothyroidism
   4. child who had a parent die from suicide

4. Which of the following antidepressants would be most likely to cause the client to have a seizure?

   1. amitriptyline
   2. bupropion
   3. sertraline
   4. venlafaxine

5. Which of the following symptoms would indicate to the nurse that a client taking lithium is experiencing toxicity?

   1. constipation, abdominal cramps, rash
   2. stupor, oliguria, hypertension
   3. nausea, vomiting, diarrhea
   4. dry mouth, blurred vision, difficulty swallowing

Apply Your Knowledge

6. The nurse instructs the client taking an MAOI not to eat foods containing _____.

   1. glutamine
   2. sugar
   3. tyramine
   4. large amounts of iron

7. In giving discharge instructions to a client taking lithium, the nurse stresses that the client should:

   1. eat a diet high in carbohydrates and low in proteins
   2. increase oral fluid intake to approximately 3000 mL/day
   3. have blood drawn before each dose of lithium is administered
   4. avoid eating foods high in amines

8. When administering an antidepressant to a client with suicidal ideation, it is most important for the nurse to _____.

   1. have the client remain upright for at least 30 minutes after taking the antidepressant
   2. assess the client in 30 minutes for a therapeutic response to the drug
   3. monitor the client for an occipital headache
   4. inspect the client's oral cavity to be sure the drug was swallowed

Alternate-Format Questions

9. A client with limited health literacy is prescribed fluoxetine for a depression. It will be prescribed to take one 90-mg capsule weekly. What methods should you use to help this client remember when to take the medication? **Select all that apply.**

   1. use a calendar on the wall
   2. ask a family member to call the client weekly
   3. set a cell phone to alarm weekly
   4. have the clinic receptionist call weekly

10. Antidepressant drugs prevent the reuptake of which neurotransmitter(s)? **Select all that apply.**

    1. acetylcholine
    2. dopamine
    3. norepinephrine
    4. serotonin

To check your answers, see Appendix G.

the**Point** *For more NCLEX-style questions, log on to http://thepoint.lww.com to access more than 1000 questions.*

23

Antipsychotic Drugs

LEARNING OBJECTIVES

On completion of this chapter, the student will:

1. List the uses, general drug actions, general adverse reactions, contraindications, precautions, and interactions associated with the administration of antipsychotic drugs.
2. Discuss important preadministration and ongoing assessment activities the nurse should perform on the patient taking an antipsychotic drug.
3. List nursing diagnoses for a patient taking an antipsychotic drug.
4. Discuss ways to promote an optimal response to therapy, how to manage common adverse reactions, and important points to keep in mind when educating patients about the use of antipsychotic drugs.

KEY TERMS

agranulocytosis • decrease or lack of granulocytes (a type of white blood cell)

akathisia • extreme restlessness and increased motor activity

alogia • inability to finish a sentence when communicating

anhedonia • lack of joy or pleasurable feelings

avolution • inability to determine and initiate goals and activities

blood dyscrasias • abnormal condition of the blood cells

delusions • false belief that cannot be changed with reason

dopamine • primary neurotransmitter in the sympathetic nervous system that deals with pleasure and reward in the brain

dystonia • prolonged muscle contractions that may cause twisting and repetitive movements of abnormal posture

extrapyramidal syndrome • group of adverse reactions involving the extrapyramidal portion of the nervous system causing abnormal muscle movements, especially akathisia and dystonia

hallucinations • false sensation or perception of reality

photophobia • intolerance to light

photosensitivity • abnormal sensitivity when exposed to light

psychosis • spectrum of disorders that affect mood and behavior

recidivism • act of repeating a behavior

tardive dyskinesia • rhythmic, involuntary movements of the tongue, face, mouth, or jaw and sometimes the extremities

💊 DRUG CLASSES

Conventional (first-generation) antipsychotics	Atypical (second-generation) antipsychotics

PHARMACOLOGY IN PRACTICE

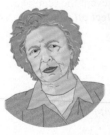

Mrs. Moore's daughter calls the clinic. She tells you that her mother has been up at night, wandering the house, listening and speaking to people who are not there. If she tries to stop her, Mrs. Moore gets agitated and has tried to hit the daughter. The daughter tells you that she volunteers at a long-term care facility back where she lives and there are a number of people like her mother taking Seroquel. She asks if she can get this drug for her mother. After reading this chapter, determine if this is an appropriate medication for Mrs. Moore.

Antipsychotic drugs are administered to patients experiencing a psychotic disorder. The term **psychosis** refers to a spectrum of disorders that affect mood and behavior, with schizophrenia being the most recognized disorder. Schizophrenia is characterized by disordered thinking, perceptual disturbance, behavioral abnormality, affective problems, and impaired socialization. Symptoms of the disease are known as positive or negative symptoms (Display 23.1). Antipsychotic medications are designed to diminish these behaviors so people can function in society.

Actions

Antipsychotic drugs act on the **dopamine** receptors of the brain. Neurobiologic theory suggests that it is higher levels of the neurotransmitter dopamine that cause problems. Positive symptoms result from misfiring at the nerve synapse. Anatomic changes coupled with misfiring cause the negative symptoms. Drugs work by inhibiting or blocking the release of the neurotransmitter dopamine in the brain and possibly regulate the firing of nerve cells in certain areas of the brain. These effects may be responsible for the ability of these drugs to suppress the symptoms of certain psychotic disorders (Fig. 23.1). The conventional or first-generation antipsychotics (FGAs) work to diminish the positive symptoms. But, because these drugs block dopamine transmission, they also produce unpleasant extrapyramidal effects (see Adverse Reactions). Examples of antipsychotic drugs include chlorpromazine, haloperidol (Haldol), and fluphenazine.

A newer group of antipsychotic drugs classified as atypical antipsychotics or second-generation antipsychotics (SGAs) is believed to act on serotonin receptors as well as on the dopamine

---

Display 23.1 Positive and Negative Symptoms in Schizophrenia

Positive (added to typical behavior)	Negative (removed from typical behavior)
• Agitation • Delusions (false beliefs) • Hallucinations (sensation without external stimuli—auditory are the most common)	• Affect (flat or blunt) • Alogia (poverty of speech) • Avolition (inability to set goals) • Anhedonia (no joy) • Concrete thinking (inability to abstract)

---

receptors in the brain. They are termed *atypical* because the typical extrapyramidal side effects are lessened, which in turn helps to both diminish the positive symptoms and enhance behaviors to reduce the negative symptoms. Examples of the atypical antipsychotic drugs include clozapine (Clozaril) and aripiprazole (Abilify). The Summary Drug Table: Antipsychotic Drugs gives a more complete listing of the antipsychotic drugs.

Uses

The antipsychotic drugs are used in the treatment of the following:

• Acute and chronic psychoses, such as schizophrenia
• Bipolar (manic-phase) illness
• Agitated behaviors associated with dementia

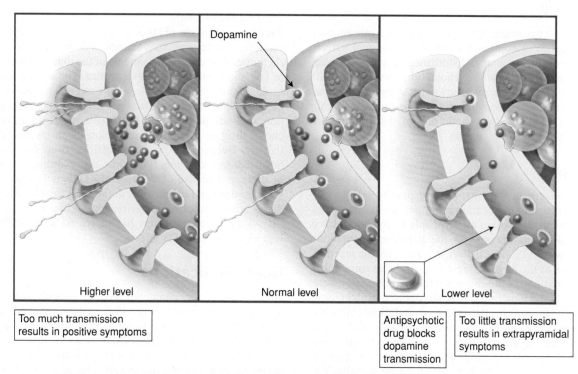

Higher level	Normal level	Lower level
Dopamine		Antipsychotic drug blocks dopamine transmission
Too much transmission results in positive symptoms		Too little transmission results in extrapyramidal symptoms

Figure 23.1 Psychotic disorders involve too much dopamine transmission. The antipsychotic drugs block dopamine.

Selected drugs may be used for their adverse effects to treat minor conditions; for example, chlorpromazine may be used to treat uncontrollable hiccoughs, and chlorpromazine and prochlorperazine are used as antiemetics.

Adverse Reactions

Generalized System Reactions

- Sedation, headache, hypotension
- Dry mouth, nasal congestion
- Urticaria, **photophobia** (intolerance to light), **photosensitivity** (abnormal sensitivity when exposed to light). Photosensitivity can result in severe sunburn when patients taking antipsychotic drugs are exposed to the sun or ultraviolet light, such as that in a tanning bed.

Behavioral Changes

- Possible increase in the intensity of the psychotic symptoms
- Lethargy, hyperactivity, paranoid reactions, agitation, and confusion

Endocrine Changes (SGA)

- Weight gain
- Increased cholesterol, triglyceride, and blood sugar levels

> **NURSING ALERT**
>
> Recent studies indicate there is a higher incidence of diabetes in patients with schizophrenia than in the general population (Llorente, 2006). This may be due to adverse reactions of the (SGA) medications or lifestyle behaviors of this patient population.

Neuroleptic malignant syndrome (NMS) is a rare reaction characterized by a combination of extrapyramidal effects, hyperthermia, and autonomic disturbance. It typically occurs within 1 month after the antipsychotic drugs are begun. NMS is potentially fatal and requires intensive symptomatic treatment and immediate discontinuation of the drug causing the syndrome. Once the antipsychotic drug is discontinued, recovery occurs within 7 to 10 days.

Recidivism

A major concern in the treatment of psychosis is adherence to a consistent medication regimen. Behaviors associated with the disease often cause people to be hospitalized. When medications are started the behavioral symptoms (see Display 23.1) diminish, yet in turn, adverse reactions occur. Some of the adverse reactions can be as uncomfortable to the patient as the disease itself. Additionally, these medications take time to produce the optimal affect (sometimes 6 to 10 weeks). Patients may independently stop using the drug because of the unpleasantness of the reactions, thus causing the psychotic symptoms to return. Once psychotic symptoms return the patient typically engages in the behaviors that caused him or her to be hospitalized. This becomes a "revolving door" of hospitalizations and discharges and is known as **recidivism**. The following sections

---

> ### *Display 23.2* Extrapyramidal Syndrome
>
> - Parkinson-like symptoms—fine tremors, muscle rigidity, mask-like appearance of the face, slowness of movement, slurred speech, and unsteady gait
> - Akathisia—extreme restlessness and increased motor activity
> - Dystonia—facial grimacing and twisting of the neck into unnatural positions

describe the adverse reactions that are typically unacceptable to patients.

Extrapyramidal Syndrome

Among the most significant adverse reactions associated with the antipsychotic drugs are the extrapyramidal effects. The term **extrapyramidal syndrome** (EPS) refers to a group of adverse reactions affecting the extrapyramidal portion of the nervous system as a result of antipsychotic drugs. This part of the nervous system affects body posture and promotes smooth and uninterrupted movement of various muscle groups. Antipsychotics disturb the function of the extrapyramidal portion of the nervous system, causing abnormal muscle movement. Extrapyramidal effects include Parkinson-like symptoms, **akathisia**, and **dystonia** (Display 23.2). Extrapyramidal effects usually diminish with a reduction in the dosage of the antipsychotic drug. Switching to an SGA antipsychotic medication is helpful in reducing symptoms.

Tardive Dyskinesia

Tardive dyskinesia (TD) is a syndrome consisting of irreversible, involuntary movements. TD is characterized by rhythmic, involuntary movements of the tongue, face, mouth, or jaw and sometimes the extremities. The tongue may protrude, and there may be chewing movements, puckering of the mouth, and facial grimacing. TD is a late-appearing reaction and may be observed in patients receiving an antipsychotic drug or after discontinuation of antipsychotic drug therapy. Because TD is nonreversible, drug therapy must be discontinued when symptoms occur during the course of therapy. Because of the risk of TD, it is best to use the smallest dose and the shortest duration of treatment that produces a satisfactory clinical response. The use of atypical (SGA) antipsychotic drugs has increased because they are less likely to cause TD effects.

Contraindications

Antipsychotics are contraindicated in patients with known hypersensitivity to the drugs, in comatose patients, in those who are severely depressed, and in those who have bone marrow depression, **blood dyscrasias**, Parkinson's disease (specifically, haloperidol), liver impairment, coronary artery disease, or severe hypotension or hypertension. Due to a specific enzyme reaction, grapefruit or its juice should not be taken if the patient is on the drug quetiapine.

Antipsychotic drugs are classified as pregnancy category C drugs (except for clozapine, which is pregnancy category B). Safe use of these drugs during pregnancy and lactation has not been clearly established. Antipsychotics should be used only when clearly needed and when the potential benefit outweighs any potential harm to the fetus.

Precautions

Antipsychotic drugs are used cautiously in patients with respiratory disorders, glaucoma, prostatic hypertrophy, epilepsy, decreased renal function, and peptic ulcer disease.

> **LIFESPAN CONSIDERATIONS**
> **Gerontology**
> Patients with dementia may exhibit agitated behaviors resulting in treatment using antipsychotic drugs. There is an association between increased cerebrovascular problems and mortality with the use of antipsychotic medications (especially SGAs) in this population.

Interactions

The following interactions may occur when an antipsychotic is administered with another agent:

Interacting Drug	Common Use	Effect of Interaction
anticholinergic drugs	Management of gastrointestinal (GI) problems such as peptic ulcer disease	Increased risk for TD and psychotic symptoms
immunologic drugs	Treatment of chronic illness such as cancer, arthritis, human immunodeficiency virus (HIV) infection	Increased severity of bone marrow suppression
alcohol	Relaxation and enjoyment in social situations	Increased risk for central nervous system depression

NURSING PROCESS

PATIENT RECEIVING AN ANTIPSYCHOTIC DRUG

ASSESSMENT

Preadministration Assessment
A patient receiving an antipsychotic drug may be treated in the hospital or in an outpatient setting. Assessment of the patient's mental status before and periodically throughout therapy should happen in any setting. Note the presence of both positive (hallucinations or delusions) and negative symptoms, documenting them accurately in the patient's record.

Before starting therapy for the hospitalized patient, attempt to obtain a complete mental health, social, and medical history. In the case of psychosis, patients often are unable to give a reliable history of their illness. When available, obtain this information from a family member or friend. As the history is taken, observe the patient for any behavior patterns that appear to be deviations from normal. Examples of deviations include poor eye contact, failure to answer questions completely, inappropriate answers to questions, a monotone speech pattern, and inappropriate laughter, sadness, or crying.

During the initial assessment, you may need to rely more on your own observation of the patient than actual physical assessment. Frequently, patients in a psychotic episode do not perceive reality in the same manner as other patients and touch may be thought of as a violent act against themselves instead of a therapeutic gesture as with other patient populations. The patient may strike out due to fear caused by the psychosis; therefore, touching can be perceived by the patient as a threatening gesture and should be avoided.

Some patients, such as those with controlled schizophrenia, do not require inpatient care. You may see these patients at periodic intervals in the mental health outpatient setting. The initial assessments of the outpatient are basically the same as those for the hospitalized patient. Obtain a medical history and a history of the symptoms of the mental disorder from the patient, a family member, or the patient's hospital documents.

Ongoing Assessment
Many antipsychotic drugs are administered for a long time, which makes the ongoing assessment an important part of determining therapeutic drug effects and monitoring for adverse reactions, particularly EPS (see Display 23.2) and TD. Your role is important in the administration of these drugs in both the inpatient and clinic settings for the following reasons:

- The patient's response to drug therapy on an inpatient basis requires around-the-clock assessments, because frequent dosage adjustments may be necessary during therapy.
- Accurate assessments for the appearance of adverse drug effects assume a greater importance when the patient may be unable to verbalize physical changes to the primary health care provider or nursing staff.

NURSING DIAGNOSES
Drug-specific nursing diagnoses are the following:

- **Risk for Injury** related to hypotension or sedation
- **Impaired Physical Mobility** related to impaired motor ability
- **Risk for Infection** related to agranulocytosis
- **Risk for Unstable Blood Glucose Level** related to medication and lifestyle

Nursing diagnoses related to drug administration are discussed in Chapter 4.

PLANNING
The expected outcomes for the patient depend on the reason for drug administration but may include an optimal response to drug therapy, meeting of patient needs related to management

of adverse drug reactions, an absence of injury, and confidence in an understanding of the medication regimen.

IMPLEMENTATION

Promoting an Optimal Response to Therapy

You should develop a nursing care plan that helps to empower the patient in dealing with the illness as well as meeting the patient's individual needs.

MANAGING CARE OF THE INPATIENT. Notations of patient behavioral patterns are written at periodic intervals (frequency depends on hospital or unit guidelines). An accurate description of the patient's behavior aids the primary health care provider in planning therapy and thus becomes an important part of nursing management. Patients with a poor response to drug therapy may require dosage changes, a change to another psychotherapeutic drug, or the addition of other therapies to the treatment regimen. However, it is important to know that full response to antipsychotic drugs takes several weeks.

If the patient's behavior is violent or aggressive, antipsychotic drugs may have to be given parenterally. You will require assistance in securing the patient and should give the drugs intramuscularly (IM) in a large muscle mass, such as the gluteus muscle. Keep the patient lying down (when possible) for about 30 minutes after administering the drug.

NURSING ALERT

In combative patients or those who have serious manifestations of acute psychosis (e.g., hallucinations or loss of contact with reality), parenteral administration may be repeated every 1 to 4 hours until the desired effects are obtained. Monitor the patient closely for cardiac arrhythmias or rhythm changes, or hypotension.

Antipsychotic drugs are typically given as a single oral daily dose. Oral administration, especially in the long-term care setting, requires special attention, because some patients have difficulty swallowing (due to dry mouth or other causes). After administration of an oral drug, inspect the patient's oral cavity to be sure the drug has been swallowed. If the patient resists having his or her oral cavity checked, report this refusal to the primary health care provider.

Other patients may refuse to take the drug altogether. Never force a patient to take an oral drug. If the patient refuses the drug, and you cannot reason with the patient to take the drug, contact the primary health care provider regarding this problem because parenteral administration of the medication may be necessary.

Oral liquid concentrates are available for patients who can more easily swallow a liquid. To aid in administration to debilitated or elderly patients, oral drugs can be mixed in liquids such as fruit juices, tomato juice, milk, or carbonated beverages. Semisolid foods, such as soups or puddings, may also be used.

MANAGING CARE OF THE OUTPATIENT. At the time of each visit of the patient to the primary health care provider's office or the clinic, observe and document the patient's behavior indicating a response to therapy. In some instances, you may question the patient or a family member about the response to

therapy. The questions asked depend on the patient and the diagnosis and may include:

■ Are you feeling nervous or restless?

■ Do you hear voices that others cannot hear?

■ How is everything going?

You may need to rephrase questions or direct conversation toward other subjects until the patient feels comfortable and is able to discuss therapy.

Ask the patient or a family member about adverse drug reactions or any other problems occurring during therapy. Document in the patient's record your observations of the patient's outward behavior and any complaints or problems. Compare these notations with previous documentation of behavior. Any reactions or problems should be brought to the attention of the primary health care provider.

Monitoring and Managing Patient Needs

The patient may need to tolerate some adverse reactions, such as dry mouth, episodes of orthostatic hypotension, and drowsiness during drug therapy. Nursing interventions to relieve some of these reactions may include offering frequent sips of water, reminders or offering assistance to the patient as he or she gets out of the bed or chair, and supervising ambulatory activities.

RISK FOR INJURY. Antipsychotic drugs may cause extreme drowsiness and sedation, especially during the first or second week of therapy. This reaction may impair mental or physical abilities. The patient may need assistance with activities of daily living due to the experience of extreme sedation. This includes cueing or help with eating, dressing, and ambulating. If hypotension or sedation occurs with these drugs, administration at bedtime helps to minimize the risk of injury. During hypotensive episodes, if possible it is important to monitor vital signs at least daily. Report any significant change in vital signs to the primary health care provider.

Drowsiness usually diminishes after 2 or 3 weeks of therapy. However, if the patient continues to be troubled by drowsiness and sedation, the primary health care provider may decide to prescribe a lower dosage or different drug.

IMPAIRED PHYSICAL MOBILITY. Patients can experience mobility problems if EPS occurs while taking the antipsychotic drugs. Extrapyramidal effects include muscular spasms of the face and neck, the inability to sleep or sit still, tremors, rigidity, or involuntary rhythmic movements. During initial therapy or whenever the dosage is increased or decreased, observe the patient closely for adverse drug reactions to prevent the development of EPS and TD. You will want to use a standardized tool, such as the Abnormal Involuntary Movement Scale (AIMS), to screen the patient for symptoms (Display 23.3) and any behavioral changes. Because these adverse effects are considered "late stage," be alert to their presence. Report immediately to the primary health care provider any change in behavior or the appearance of adverse reactions. An immediate decrease in dosage will not change the condition but may prevent further deterioration of the patient.

Display 23.3 Abnormal Involuntary Movement Scale Screening Tool

Client identification: _____ Date: _____

Rated by: _____

1. Either before or after completing the examination procedure, observe the patient unobtrusively at rest (e.g., in waiting room).
2. The chair to be used in this examination should be a hard, firm one without arms.
3. After observing the patient, he or she may be rated on a scale of 0 (none), 1 (minimal), 2 (mild), 3 (moderate), and 4 (severe) according to the severity of symptoms.
4. Ask the patient whether there is anything in his/her teeth (i.e., gum, candy, etc.) and, if there is, to remove it.
5. Ask patient about the current condition of his/her teeth. Ask patient if he/she wears dentures. Do teeth or dentures bother patient now?
6. Ask patient whether he/she notices any movement in mouth, face, hands, or feet. If yes, ask to describe and to what extent the movements currently bother patient or interfere with his/her activities.

0 1 2 3 4	Ask patient to tap thumb with each finger as rapidly as possible for 10–15 seconds, separately with right hand, then with left hand. (Observe facial and leg movements.)
0 1 2 3 4	Flex and extend patient's left and right arms (one at a time).
0 1 2 3 4	*Ask patient to stand up. (Observe in profile. Observe all body areas again, hips included.)
0 1 2 3 4	Have patient sit in chair with hands on knees, legs slightly apart, and feet flat on floor (look at entire body for movements while in this position).
0 1 2 3 4	Ask patient to sit with hands hanging unsupported: if male, hands between legs; if female and wearing a dress, hands hanging over knees. (Observe hands and other body areas.)
0 1 2 3 4	Ask patient to open mouth. (Observe tongue at rest within mouth.) Do this twice.
0 1 2 3 4	Ask patient to protrude tongue. (Observe abnormalities of tongue movement.) Do this twice.
0 1 2 3 4	Ask patient to extend both arms outstretched in front with palms down. (Observe trunk, legs, and mouth.)
0 1 2 3 4	*Have patient walk a few paces, turn, and walk back to chair. (Observe hands and gait.) Do this twice.

*Activated movements.

NURSING ALERT

Because there is no known treatment for TD and it is irreversible in patients, immediately report symptoms. These include rhythmic, involuntary movements of the tongue, face, mouth, jaw, or extremities.

RISK FOR INFECTION. The use of the drug clozapine has been associated with severe agranulocytosis, or decreased white blood cell (WBC) count. This bone marrow suppression can make the patient more susceptible to illness and infection. To ensure close monitoring for this adverse reaction, clozapine is available only through a patient management system (a program that combines WBC testing, patient monitoring, and pharmacy and drug distribution services). Only a 1-week supply of this drug is dispensed at a time. A weekly WBC count is done throughout therapy and for 4 weeks after therapy is discontinued. In addition, teach the patient to monitor for signs or symptoms indicating bone marrow suppression: lethargy, weakness, fever, sore throat, malaise, mucous membrane ulceration, or "flu-like" complaints.

RISK FOR UNSTABLE BLOOD GLUCOSE LEVEL. The tendency for diabetes and its risk factors (see Chapter 42) are greater for those patients with serious mental illness. These risk factors can include sedentary lifestyle, diet, or other factors such as obesity. The administration of atypical antipsychotic (SGA) drugs with the adverse reaction of weight gain can put the patient at higher risk of acquiring type 2 diabetes (clozapine and olanzapine users gain the most weight). Before starting treatment with an SGA, the patient should be weighed and a family history documented to indicate type 2 diabetes risk. Laboratory work for fasting blood sugar, total and low-density lipoprotein (LDL) cholesterol, and triglycerides should be taken and compared at periodic intervals.

Educating the Patient and Family

Adherence to routine medication use is a problem with some patients once they are discharged. It is important to evaluate accurately the patient's ability to assume responsibility for continuing to take the drugs. Some patients will have the benefit of family for assistance; others do not. The patient should feel confident in understanding that the drug has the benefit of reducing positive and negative symptoms. Also, reporting adverse reactions allows the primary health care provider to modify the doses to reduce problems while the patient still benefits from the drug.

As you develop a teaching plan for the patient or family member, include the following points:

- Keep all primary care provider and clinic appointments, because close monitoring of therapy is essential.

■ Report any unusual changes or physical effects to the primary health care provider.

■ Take the drug exactly as directed. Do not increase, decrease, or omit a dose or discontinue use of this drug unless directed to do so by the primary health care provider.

■ Do not drive or perform other hazardous tasks if drowsiness occurs.

■ Do not take any nonprescription drug unless use of a specific drug has been approved by the primary health care provider.

■ Inform physicians, dentists, and other medical personnel of therapy with this drug.

■ ♥ Do not drink alcoholic beverages unless approval is obtained from the primary health care provider.

■ If dizziness occurs when changing position, rise slowly when getting out of bed or a chair. If dizziness is severe, always have help when changing positions.

■ To relieve dry mouth, take frequent sips of water, suck on hard candy, or chew gum (preferably sugarless).

■ Notify your primary health care provider if you become pregnant or intend to become pregnant during therapy.

■ Immediately report the occurrence of the following adverse reactions: restlessness, inability to sit still, muscle spasms, mask-like expression, rigidity, tremors, drooling, or involuntary rhythmic movements of the mouth, face, or extremities.

■ Avoid exposure to the sun. If exposure is unavoidable, wear sunblock, keep arms and legs covered, and wear a sun hat.

■ Report increased thirst, urination, and weight gain to the primary health care provider.

■ Note that only a 1-week supply of clozapine is dispensed at a time. The drug is obtained through a special program designed to ensure the required blood monitoring. Weekly WBC laboratory tests are required. Immediately report any signs of weakness, fever, sore throat, malaise, or flu-like symptoms to the primary health care provider.

■ Note that olanzapine is available as a disintegrating tablet. If using the orally disintegrating tablet, peel back the foil on the blister packaging. Using dry hands, remove the tablet, and place the entire tablet in the mouth. The tablet will disintegrate immediately with or without liquid.

EVALUATION

■ Therapeutic effect is achieved and psychotic behavior is decreased.

■ Adverse reactions are identified, reported to the primary health care provider, and managed successfully through appropriate nursing interventions:
  • No evidence of injury is seen.
  • Patient maintains adequate mobility.
  • No evidence of infection is seen.
  • Blood glucose levels remain stable.

■ Patient and family express confidence and demonstrate an understanding of the drug regimen.

PHARMACOLOGY IN PRACTICE
THINK CRITICALLY

 The behaviors described by Mrs. Moore's daughter could be considered positive symptoms of a psychotic disorder. Are there other reasons or conditions that might be causing her to exhibit these behaviors? Mrs. Moore has been diagnosed with dementia and heart failure. From the information you learned, what class of drug is Seroquel, are there indications here for its use, and are there contraindications based on her history? If this drug is prescribed, what assessments need to be done on an ongoing basis?

KEY POINTS

• Psychosis is a spectrum of mood and behaviors, with schizophrenia being the most recognized. Symptoms of the disease are categorized as positive and negative. Antipsychotic medications are designed to diminish the behaviors so people can function in society.

• Conventional (first-generation) antipsychotics alleviate the positive symptoms such as agitation, delusions, and hallucinations. The newer atypical (second-generation) drugs reduce the negative symptoms—those that have an impact on affect, communication, initiative, thinking, and feeling.

• These drugs reduce the amount of dopamine for neurotransmission. Sometimes the reduction is too much, which results in extrapyramidal symptoms. If the medications are not stopped tardive dyskinesia (an irreversible

disorder) can result. The atypical medications affect both dopamine and serotonin, and EPS reactions are fewer.

• Although atypical (second-generation) antipsychotics have fewer extrapyramidal symptom reactions, caution needs to be exercised with patients with dementia because of the relationship between stroke and mortality. Additionally, the weight gain and other factors may predispose an individual to type 2 diabetes.

• Most medications need 6 to 10 weeks to demonstrate effect on the disorder. Unfortunately, adverse reactions begin much earlier; therefore, patients struggle with unpleasant symptoms of the disorder or reactions from the drugs. A revolving cycle of lack of adherence to therapy and rehospitalization occurs, called *recidivism.*

Summary Drug Table ANTIPSYCHOTIC DRUGS

Generic Name	Trade Name	Uses	Adverse Reactions	Dosage Ranges
Conventional Antipsychotics (First Generation)				
chlorpromazine *klor-proe'-mah-zeen*		Psychotic disorders, nausea, vomiting, intractable hiccoughs	Hypotension, drowsiness, TD, nasal congestion, dry mouth, dystonia, EPS, behavioral changes, photosensitivity	Psychiatric disorders: up to 400 mg/day orally in divided doses Nausea and vomiting: 10–25 mg orally, 25–50 mg IM, 50–100 mg rectally
fluphenazine *floo-fen'-ah-zeen*		Psychotic disorders	Drowsiness, tachycardia, EPS, dystonia, akathisia, hypotension	0.5–10 mg/day orally in divided doses, up to 20 mg/day; 1.25–10 mg/day IM in divided doses
haloperidol *hay-loe-per'-ih-dole*	Haldol	Psychotic disorders, Tourette's syndrome, hyperactivity, behavior problems in children	EPS, akathisia, dystonia, TD, drowsiness, headache, dry mouth, orthostatic hypotension	0.5–5 mg orally BID or TID with dosage up to 100 mg/day in divided doses; 2–5 mg IM Children: 0.05–0.075 mg/kg/day orally
loxapine *lox'-ah-peen*		Psychotic disorders	EPS, akathisia, dystonia, TD, drowsiness, headache, dry mouth, orthostatic hypotension	10–100 mg/day orally, not to exceed 250 mg/day
perphenazine *per-fen'-ah-zeen*		Psychotic disorders	Hypotension, postural hypotension, TD, photophobia, urticaria, nasal congestion, dry mouth, akathisia, dystonia, pseudoparkinsonism, behavioral changes, headache, photosensitivity	4–16 mg orally 2–4 times/day
pimozide *pih'-moe-zyde*	Orap	Tourette's syndrome	Parkinson-like symptoms, motor restlessness, dystonia, oculogyric crisis, TD, dry mouth, diarrhea, headache, rash, drowsiness	Initial dose: 1–2 mg/day orally Maintenance dose: up to 10 mg/day orally
prochlorperazine *proe-klor-per'-ah-zeen*		Psychotic disorders, nausea, vomiting, anxiety	EPS, sedation, TD, dry eyes, blurred vision, constipation, dry mouth, photosensitivity	Psychotic disorders: up to 150 mg orally, 10–20 mg IM Nausea, vomiting: 15–40 mg/day orally in divided doses Anxiety: 5 mg orally TID
thioridazine *thee-oh-rid'-ah-zeen*		Schizophrenia	Cardiac arrhythmias, drowsiness, TD, nausea, dry mouth, constipation, diarrhea	50–100 mg orally TID, not to exceed 800 mg/day
thiothixene *thye-oh-thick'-seen*	Navane	Schizophrenia	EPS, drowsiness, nausea, diarrhea, TD	6–30 mg/day orally, not to exceed 60 mg/day
trifluoperazine *trye-floo-oh-per'-ah-zeen*		Psychotic disorders, anxiety	Drowsiness, pseudoparkinsonism, dystonia, akathisia, TD, photophobia, blurred vision, dry mouth, salivation, nasal congestion, nausea, discolored urine (pink to red-brown)	Psychosis: 4–20 mg/day orally in divided doses Anxiety: 1–2 mg orally BID

(table continues on page 238)

Antipsychotic Drugs

Summary Drug Table ANTIPSYCHOTIC DRUGS (continued)

Generic Name	Trade Name	Uses	Adverse Reactions	Dosage Ranges
Atypical Antipsychotics (Second Generation)				
aripiprazole *ay-ri-pip'-rah-zoll*	Abilify	Schizophrenia, manic phase of bipolar disorders	Agitation, akathisia, anxiety, drowsiness, headache, constipation, dry mouth, nausea	10–30 mg/day orally
asenapine *a-sen'-a-peen*	Saphris	Schizophrenia, manic phase of bipolar disorders	Agitation, akathisia, anxiety, drowsiness, headache, constipation, dry mouth, nausea	5–10 mg orally twice daily
clozapine *kloe'-zah-peen*	Clozaril, FazaClo	Severely ill schizophrenic patients with no response to other therapies	Drowsiness, sedation, akathisia, tachycardia, nausea, agranulocytosis	Initial dose: 25–50 mg/day, titrate up to 300–400 mg/day orally, not to exceed 900 mg/day
olanzapine *oh-lan'-zah-peen*	Zyprexa	Schizophrenia, short-term treatment of manic episodes of bipolar disorder	Agitation, dizziness, nervousness, akathisia, constipation, fever, weight gain	5–20 mg/day orally
lurasidone *loo-ras'-i-done*	Latuda	Schizophrenia	Somnolence, nervousness, akathisia, nausea, weight gain	40–80 mg daily orally
iloperidone *eye'-loe-per'-i-done*	Fanapt	Schizophrenia	Agitation, dizziness, nervousness, akathisia, constipation, weight gain	12 mg twice daily orally
olanzapine/ fluoxetine *oh-lan'-zah-peen/floo-ox'-eh-teen*	Symbyax	Bipolar depressive episodes	Same as olanzapine	6-mg/25-mg combination tablet taken in the evening orally
paliperidone *pal-ee-per'-ih-doan*	Invega	Psychotic disorders	Dizziness, weakness, headache, dry mouth, increased saliva, weight gain, stomach pain	6–12 mg/day orally
quetiapine *kweh-tye'-ah-pyne*	Seroquel	Psychotic disorders, manic episodes of bipolar disorder	Orthostatic hypotension, dizziness, vertigo, nausea, constipation, dry mouth, diarrhea, headache, restlessness, blurred vision	150–750 mg/day orally in divided doses
risperidone *ris-per'-ih-doan*	Risperdal	Psychotic disorders; adolescent schizophrenia and mania	Agitation, dizziness, nervousness, akathisia, constipation, fever, weight gain	1–3 mg orally BID; adolescents: 0.5–6 mg orally once daily
ziprasidone *zih-pray'-sih-doan*	Geodon	Schizophrenia, bipolar mania, acute agitation	Somnolence, drowsiness, sedation, headache, arrhythmias, dyspepsia, fever, constipation, EPS	80 mg orally BID

● Chapter Review

Know Your Drugs

Clients sometimes know a medication by the brand (or trade) name and not the generic name. To help you recognize both names, match the brand name with the generic name of the same medication.

Generic Name	Brand Name
1. clozapine	A. Clozaril
2. haloperidol	B. Geodon
3. risperidone	C. Haldol
4. ziprasidone	D. Risperdal

Calculate Medication Dosages

1. A client is prescribed quetiapine (Seroquel) 100 mg BID. The drug is available in 50-mg tablets. The nurse would administer _____.

2. An agitated client is prescribed haloperidol 3 mg now. The drug is available in a 5 mg/1 mL preloaded syringe. How many milliliters will be administered?

● Prepare for the NCLEX®

Build Your Knowledge

1. Schizophrenia involves an overabundance of which neurotransmitter?

    1. acetylcholine
    2. dopamine
    3. norepinephrine
    4. serotonin

2. Which of the following is a negative symptom associated with schizophrenia?

    1. hallucinations
    2. delusions
    3. flat affect
    4. agitation

3. History of which disease is significant when administering a second-generation antipsychotic?

    1. hypertension
    2. liver failure
    3. type 2 diabetes
    4. cardiac failure

4. Which of the following behaviors would the nurse expect to see in a client experiencing TD?

    1. muscle rigidity, dry mouth, insomnia
    2. rhythmic, involuntary movements of the tongue, face, mouth, or jaw
    3. muscle weakness, paralysis of the eyelids, diarrhea
    4. dyspnea, somnolence, muscle spasms

5. Which of the following drugs is least likely to produce extrapyramidal effects?

    1. chlorpromazine
    2. haloperidol
    3. fluphenazine
    4. risperidone

Apply Your Knowledge

6. A client taking fluphenazine (Prolixin) for schizophrenia is also prescribed an antiparkinson drug. What is the best explanation for adding an antiparkinson drug to the regimen?

    1. prevents severe allergic reaction from sun exposure
    2. promotes the effects of fluphenazine
    3. reduces fine tremors, muscle rigidity, and slow movement
    4. decreases hallucinations and delusions

7. As a nurse on a mental health unit, you are ordering weekly lab draws for morning rounds. Three clients are taking the drug clozapine. Which of the following labs should be drawn on these clients?

    1. fasting blood glucose
    2. LDL
    3. complete blood count
    4. amylase

8. The nurse is leading a medication support group. Which is the best statement to make when a client says the drugs don't work?

    1. "They won't work if you don't take them."
    2. "I know it is hard to keep taking the medicine when you can't readily see the effects."
    3. "That's not appropriate to say in front of everyone else here."
    4. "Statements like that give me a headache."

Alternate-Format Questions

9. When administering a second-generation antipsychotic to a client, the nurse would most likely expect which diagnostic test(s) to be prescribed? **Select all that apply**.

    1. complete blood count
    2. fasting blood glucose levels
    3. cholesterol levels
    4. electrolyte analysis

10. Match the drug with its generation category:

1. Conventional (first generation)	A. aripiprazole
2. Atypical (second generation)	B. chlorpromazine
	C. Geodon
	D. quetiapine
	E. Zyprexa

To check your answers, see Appendix G.

the**Point** *For more NCLEX-style questions, log on to http://thepoint.lww.com to access more than 1000 questions.*

Drugs That Affect the Peripheral Nervous System

In the last unit, you learned how drugs affect the neurotransmitters working in the brain. In this unit you will learn about the drugs used to enhance or block the nerve impulses as they travel through the rest of the body in the peripheral nervous system (PNS). You will learn that because the nerves extend throughout the body, drugs that affect these nerves also affect many different body systems.

The peripheral nervous system connects all our body parts to one another. To understand how organs and tissues function you need first to understand how messages are sent via nerve transmission. Our senses are stimulated and a message is sent via the *afferent nerves* to the brain. The message is processed by the brain and then a command message is sent via the *efferent nerves* from the brain to the various organs or tissues of the body where an action is carried out.

To get from the brain to the tissue, the message (or nerve impulse) needs to travel over a network of nerves. At the end of every nerve is a terminal end, and the message "jumps" across the gap (or synapse) to a receptor on the beginning of the next nerve in the path. Substances called neurotransmitters are the elements that cross the synapse to keep the message conduction going.

The PNS is divided into the somatic nervous system and the autonomic nervous system. The somatic branch of the PNS is concerned with sensation and voluntary movement. The sensory part of the somatic nervous system sends messages to the brain concerning the internal and external environment, such as sensations of heat, pain, cold, and pressure. The movement part of the somatic nervous system is concerned with the voluntary movement of skeletal muscles, such as those used in walking, talking, or writing a letter.

Chapters in this unit focus on drugs that affect the autonomic branch of the peripheral nerves. The autonomic branch of the PNS is concerned with functions essential to the survival of the organism. Functional activity of the autonomic nervous system is not controlled consciously (i.e., the activity is automatic). This system controls blood pressure, heart rate, gastrointestinal activity, and glandular secretions.

A clear understanding of the autonomic branch makes learning about these drugs much easier. The autonomic nervous system is divided into the sympathetic

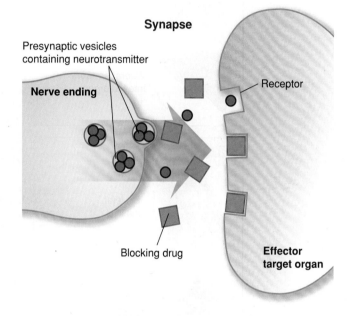

Synapse

Presynaptic vesicles containing neurotransmitter

Nerve ending

Receptor

Blocking drug

Effector target organ

and the parasympathetic branches. These two branches work as opposites to each other to make the body function properly. The sympathetic branch tends to regulate the expenditure of energy and activates when the organism is confronted with stressful situations. The sympathetic system is also called the *adrenergic branch.* Chapter 24 discusses drugs that mimic the effects of the sympathetic system—the adrenergic drugs. Again, these drugs have an impact on many different body systems and organs; therefore, the focus of Chapter 24 is on the drugs used in the prevention (responding to allergic reactions) and the treatment of shock. Drugs that block or inhibit the system are called *antiadrenergic drugs, adrenergic blocking drugs,* or *sympatholytics.* One of the major body systems affected by adrenergic blocking drugs is the heart and vascular system. Some of the drugs used to treat hypertension are featured in Chapter 25.

The parasympathetic branch of the autonomic nervous system, when activated, attempts to do the opposite actions from the sympathetic branch. The parasympathetic branch helps conserve body energy and is partly

(text continues on page 242)

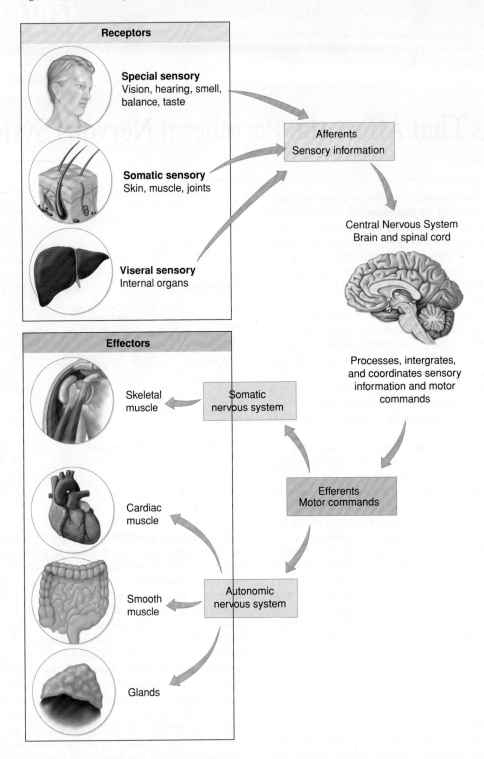

Receptors

Special sensory
Vision, hearing, smell, balance, taste

Somatic sensory
Skin, muscle, joints

Viseral sensory
Internal organs

Afferents
Sensory information

Central Nervous System
Brain and spinal cord

Processes, intergrates, and coordinates sensory information and motor commands

Effectors

Skeletal muscle

Cardiac muscle

Smooth muscle

Glands

Somatic nervous system

Autonomic nervous system

Efferents
Motor commands

responsible for such activities as slowing the heart rate, digesting food, and eliminating bodily wastes. The parasympathetic nervous system is known as the *cholinergic branch*. Drugs that enhance neurotransmission are discussed in Chapter 26; those that block transmission are covered in Chapter 27. The nerve pathways and the body tissues or organs they affect are illustrated in this unit. In each chapter you will learn about how these nerves work together or against each other to keep the body working smoothly.

Adrenergic Drugs

LEARNING OBJECTIVES

On completion of this chapter, the student will:

1. Discuss the activity of the autonomic nervous system, specifically the sympathetic branch.
2. Discuss the types of shock, physiologic responses of shock, and the use of adrenergic drugs in the treatment of shock.
3. Discuss the uses, general drug actions, contraindications, precautions, interactions, and adverse reactions associated with the administration of adrenergic vasopressor drugs.
4. Discuss important preadministration and ongoing assessment activities the nurse should perform on the patient taking an adrenergic drug.
5. List nursing diagnoses particular to a patient taking an adrenergic drug.
6. Discuss ways to promote an optimal response to therapy, how to manage common adverse reactions, and important points to keep in mind when educating patients about the use of adrenergic drugs.

KEY TERMS

adrenergic • pertaining to the sympathetic branch of the nervous system, which controls heart rate, breathing rate, and ability to divert blood to the skeletal muscles

autonomic nervous system • division of the peripheral nervous system concerned with functions essential to the life of the organism and not consciously controlled (e.g., blood pressure, heart rate, gastrointestinal activity)

extravasation • escape of fluid from a blood vessel into surrounding tissue

neurotransmitter • chemical substances released at the nerve ending that facilitate the transmission of nerve impulses

norepinephrine • neurotransmitter that transmits impulses across the sympathetic branch of the autonomic nervous system

parasympathetic • pertaining to the part of the autonomic nervous system concerned with conserving body energy (i.e., slowing the heart rate, digesting food, and eliminating waste)

peripheral nervous system • all nerves outside of brain and spinal cord

shock • inadequate blood flow to the bodily tissues

stroke volume • the volume of blood ejected (leaving) from a ventricle at each heart beat

sympathetic • pertaining to the sympathetic nervous system

sympathomimetic • drugs that mimic the actions of the sympathetic nervous system; see *adrenergic*

vasopressors • drugs that raise the blood pressure

DRUG CLASSES

Sympathomimetics	Optic agents (alpha 2
Short-acting beta (β)-2	agonists/
agonists	sympathomimetics)
Long-acting β_2 agonists	

PHARMACOLOGY IN PRACTICE

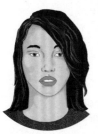

Janna Wong is brought into the clinic by her mother. Yesterday she was in the yard and came into the house crying after being stung by a bee. Later in the evening she complained of itching around her throat and what Janna called a "fat tongue." As you read this chapter, think about what type of reaction this might have been.

The component of the **peripheral nervous system** (PNS) studied in this unit is a system of nerves that automatically regulates bodily functions—the **autonomic nervous system**. This system is further divided into the **sympathetic** and the **parasympathetic** nervous system branches. In this unit you will learn about the sympathetic branch, which is regulated by involuntary control. In other words, a person does not have control over what this system does. Activation of this branch is often called the *fight-or-*

flight response. These nerves are activated when the body is confronted with stressful situations, such as danger, intense emotion, or severe illness. The sympathetic branch has control over a person's heart rate, breathing rate, and ability to divert blood to the skeletal muscles—to enable a person to run, for example. Figure 24.1 illustrates how specific organs respond when the sympathetic branch is activated throughout the body.

Norepinephrine is a **neurotransmitter** produced naturally by the body. It is the primary neurotransmitter in the sympathetic

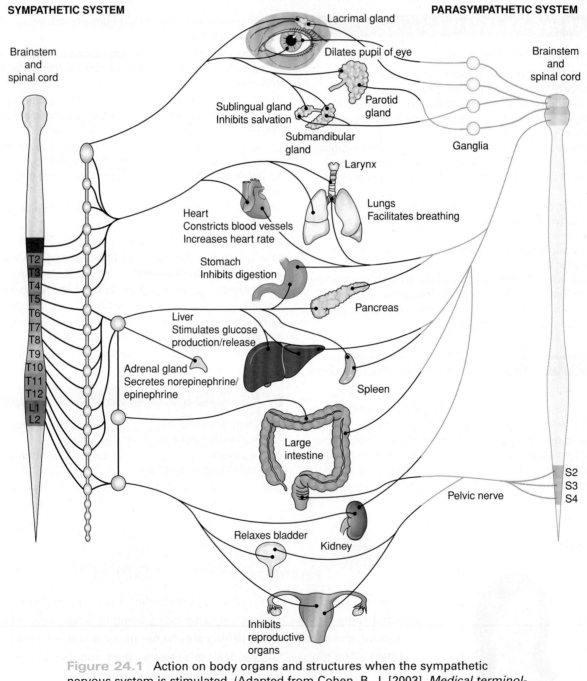

Figure 24.1 Action on body organs and structures when the sympathetic nervous system is stimulated. (Adapted from Cohen, B. J. [2003]. *Medical terminology* [4th ed.]. Philadelphia: Lippincott Williams & Wilkins.)

branch of the autonomic nervous system and the substance that keeps the nerve message (or impulse) going from the brain to the target organ. Because this system is activated by the precursor of epinephrine (adrenalin), another term for the sympathetic pathway is the **adrenergic** branch. Therefore, the medicines used that work like the adrenergic branch are termed adrenergic drugs.

In the sympathetic branch of the autonomic nervous system, adrenergic drugs produce activity similar to the neurotransmitter norepinephrine. Another name for these drugs is **sympathomimetic** (i.e., mimicking the actions of the sympathetic nervous system) drugs. The adrenergic drugs produce pharmacologic effects similar to the effects that occur in the body when the sympathetic nerves (norepinephrine) and the medulla (epinephrine) are stimulated. The primary effects of these drugs occur on the heart, the blood vessels, and the smooth muscles, such as the bronchi of the lung.

Actions

The purpose of stimulating the sympathetic (adrenergic) nerves is to divert blood flow to the vital organs so that the body can deal with a stressful situation (the fight-or-flight response). In general, adrenergic drugs produce one or more of the following responses in varying degrees:

- Central nervous system—wakefulness, quick reaction to stimuli, quickened reflexes
- Autonomic nervous system—relaxation of the smooth muscles of the bronchi, constriction of blood vessels, sphincters of the stomach, dilation of coronary blood vessels, decrease in gastric motility
- Heart—increase in the heart rate
- Metabolism—increased use of glucose (sugar) and liberation of fatty acids from adipose tissue

Receptor Selectivity

The degree to which any organ is affected by the sympathetic nervous system depends on which postsynaptic nerve receptor sites are activated (Fig. 24.2). Adrenergic nerves have

Table 24.1 Effects of the Adrenergic Receptors		
Receptor	**Site**	**Effect**
α_1	Peripheral blood vessels	Vasoconstriction of peripheral blood vessels
α_2	Presynaptic neuron	Regulates release of neurotransmitters; decreases tone, motility, and secretions of gastrointestinal tract
β_1	Myocardium	Increased heart rate, increased force of myocardial contraction
β_2	Peripheral blood vessels	Vasodilation of peripheral vessels
	Bronchial smooth muscles	Bronchodilation

either alpha (α) or beta (β) receptors. Drugs that act on the receptors are called *selective* or *nonselective*. Adrenergic drugs may be selective (act on α receptors or β receptors only) or nonselective (act on both α and β receptors). For example, isoproterenol acts chiefly on β receptors; it is considered a selective drug. Epinephrine is a nonselective drug and acts on both α and β receptors.

Whether an adrenergic drug acts on α, β, or α and β receptors accounts for the variation of responses to this group of drugs. Table 24.1 lists the type of adrenergic nerve receptor that corresponds with each action of the autonomic nervous system on the body. The α and β receptors can be further grouped as α_1- and α_2-adrenergic receptors and β_1- and β_2-adrenergic receptors.

Uses

Adrenergic drugs have a variety of uses and may be given for the treatment of the following:

- Hypovolemic and septic **shock**
- Moderate to severe episodes of hypotension
- Control of superficial bleeding during surgical and dental procedures of the mouth, nose, throat, and skin
- Cardiac decompensation and arrest
- Allergic reactions (anaphylactic shock, angioneurotic edema)
- Temporary treatment of heart block
- Ventricular arrhythmias (under certain conditions)
- Respiratory distress (as bronchodilators)
- Nasal congestion and glaucoma (topical formulation)

Patients at risk for life-threatening reactions to allergens, exercise, or unknown triggers may obtain and be instructed in the use of adrenergic drugs to lessen allergic reactions before emergency medical care is given.

Adrenergic drugs may also be used as a vasoconstricting adjunct to local anesthetics to prolong anesthetic action in the tissues. The adrenergic drugs used primarily as **vasopressors** (drugs that raise the blood pressure because of their ability to constrict blood vessels) are listed in the Summary Drug Table: Adrenergic Drugs. Sympathomimetics are also used as bronchodilators in the treatment of respiratory problems (see

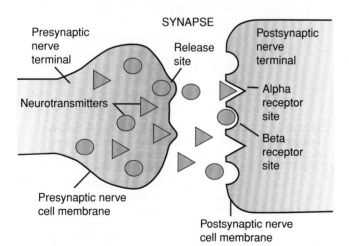

Figure 24.2 Neurotransmitter (e.g., norepinephrine), is released by the presynaptic nerve, crosses the synapse, and binds with α and β receptors in the cell membrane of the postsynaptic nerve, continuing the transmission of the nerve impulse.

Table 24.2 Respiratory and Ophthalmic Sympathomimetics

Short-Acting β₂ Agonists (SABAs—Used for Acute Respiratory Symptom Relief)*

albuterol	Proventil, Ventolin
epinephrine	Adrenalin, Epinephrine Mist, Primatene Mist
bitolterol	Tornalate
levalbuterol	Xopenex
metaproterenol	
pirbuterol	Maxair Autohaler
terbutaline	Brethine

Long-Acting β₂ Agonists (LABAs—Used for Long-Term Respiratory Management)*

arformoterol	Brovana
formoterol	Foradil
indacaterol	Arcapta
salmeterol	Serevent Diskus

α₂-Adrenergic Agonists (Optic Agents)†

brimonidine tartrate	Alphagan

Sympathomimetics†

apraclonidine	Iopidine
dipivefrin (dipivalyl epinephrine)	Propine, AKPro
epinephrine	Epifrin, Glaucon Solution

*See chapter 32 for detailed information.

†See chapter 53 for detailed information.

Chapter 32) or topically in the treatment of glaucoma (see Chapter 53). These drugs are listed in Table 24.2 by name only; more information is provided in the respective chapters.

Treating Shock

Adrenergic drugs are important in the care and treatment of patients in shock. Shock is a state of inadequate tissue perfusion. In shock, the supply of arterial blood and oxygen flowing to the cells and tissues is inadequate. To counteract the symptoms of shock, the body initiates physiologic mechanisms. The brain activates the hypothalamic-pituitary-adrenal (HPA) system. The HPA triggers the production of hormones and the release of epinephrine and norepinephrine. In some situations, the body is able to compensate, and blood pressure is maintained. However, if shock is untreated and compensatory mechanisms of the body fail, irreversible shock occurs and death follows. The three types of shock—hypovolemic shock, cardiogenic shock, and distributive shock—are described in Table 24.3.

Various clinical manifestations may be present in a patient in shock. For example, in the early stages of shock, the extremities may be warm because vasodilation is initiated, and blood flow to the skin and extremities is maintained. If the condition is untreated, blood flow to the vital organs, skin, and extremities is compromised. The patient becomes cool

and clammy, which is referred to as "cool" or "cold" shock. Regardless of the type, shock results in a decrease in cardiac output, decrease in arterial blood pressure (hypotension), reabsorption of water by the kidneys (causing a decrease in urinary output), decrease in the exchange of oxygen and carbon dioxide in the lungs, increase in carbon dioxide and decrease in oxygen in the blood, hypoxia (decreased oxygen reaching the cells), and increased concentration of intravascular fluid. This scenario compromises the functioning of vital organs such as the heart, brain, and kidneys. The various physiologic responses caused by shock are listed in Table 24.4.

Management of shock is aimed at providing basic life support (airway, breathing, and circulation) while attempting to correct the underlying cause. Antibiotics, inotropes, hormones (e.g., insulin, thyroid), and other drugs may be used to treat the underlying disease. However, the initial pharmacologic intervention is aimed at supporting the circulation with vasopressors.

Adrenergic drugs improve hemodynamic status by improving myocardial contractility and increasing heart rate, which results in increased cardiac output. Peripheral resistance is increased by vasoconstriction. In cardiogenic shock or advanced shock associated with low cardiac output, an adrenergic drug may be used with a vasodilating drug. A vasodilator, such as nitroprusside (see Chapter 35) or nitroglycerin (see Chapter 36), improves myocardial

Table 24.3 Types of Shock

Type*	Description
Hypovolemic	Occurs when the blood volume is significantly diminished. *Examples:* hemorrhage; fluid loss caused by burns, dehydration, or excess diuresis
Cardiogenic-obstructive shock	Occurs when cardiac output is insufficient and perfusion to the vital organs cannot be maintained. *Examples:* a result of acute myocardial infarction, ventricular arrhythmias, congestive heart failure, or severe cardiomyopathy
	Obstructive shock is categorized with cardiogenic shock. It occurs when obstruction of blood flow results in inadequate tissue perfusion. *Examples:* pericardial tamponade, restrictive pericarditis, and severe cardiac valve dysfunction
Distributive (vasogenic) shock	Occurs when there are changes to the blood vessels causing dilation, but no additional blood volume. The blood is redistributed within the body. This category is further differentiated: • Septic shock—circulatory insufficiency resulting from overwhelming infection (e.g., central line infection) • Anaphylactic shock—hypersensitivity resulting in massive systemic vasodilation (e.g., drug allergic reaction) • Neurogenic shock—interference with PNS control of blood vessels (e.g., spinal cord injury)

*Other causes of shock include hypoglycemia, hypothyroidism, and Addison's disease.

Bodily System	Possible Signs and Symptoms
Integumentary (skin)	Pallor, cyanosis, cold and clammy, sweating
Central nervous system	Agitation, confusion, disorientation, coma
Cardiovascular	Hypotension, tachycardia, arrhythmias, wide pulse pressure, gallop rhythm
Respiratory	Tachypnea, pulmonary edema
Renal	Urinary output less than 20 mL/hr
Metabolic (endocrine)	Acidosis

Table 24.4 Physiologic Manifestations of Shock

performance because the adrenergic drug maintains blood pressure.

Adverse Reactions

Adverse reactions associated with the administration of adrenergic drugs depend on the drug used, the dose administered, and individualized patient response. Some common adverse reactions include:

• Cardiac arrhythmias (bradycardia and tachycardia)
• Headache
• Nausea and vomiting
• Increased blood pressure (which may reach dangerously high levels)

Additional adverse reactions for specific adrenergic drugs are listed in the Summary Drug Table: Adrenergic Drugs.

LIFESPAN CONSIDERATIONS
Gerontology
The older adult is especially vulnerable to adverse reactions of adrenergic drugs, particularly epinephrine. In addition, older adults are more likely to have pre-existing cardiovascular disease that predisposes them to potentially serious cardiac arrhythmias. Closely monitor all older patients taking an adrenergic drug, and report any changes in the pulse rate or rhythm immediately. Also note, epinephrine may temporarily increase tremor and rigidity in older adults with Parkinson's disease.

Contraindications

Adrenergic drugs are contraindicated in patients with known hypersensitivity. Isoproterenol is contraindicated in patients with tachyarrhythmias, tachycardia, or heart block caused by digitalis toxicity, ventricular arrhythmias, and angina pectoris. Dopamine is contraindicated in those with pheochromocytoma (adrenal gland tumor), unmanaged arrhythmias, and ventricular fibrillation. Epinephrine is contraindicated in patients with narrow-angle glaucoma and as a local anesthetic adjunct in fingers and toes. Norepinephrine is contraindicated in patients who are hypotensive from blood volume

deficits. Midodrine causes severe hypertension in the patient who is lying down (supine).

NURSING ALERT
Supine hypertension is a potentially dangerous adverse reaction in the patient taking midodrine. The drug should be given only to patients whose lives are impaired despite standard treatment offered. This reaction is minimized by administering midodrine during the day while the patient is in an upright position. The suggested dosing schedule for the administration of midodrine is shortly before arising in the morning, midday, and late afternoon (not after 6:00 p.m.). Drug therapy should continue only in the patient whose orthostatic hypotension improves during the initial treatment.

Precautions

These drugs are used cautiously in patients with coronary insufficiency, cardiac arrhythmias, angina pectoris, diabetes, hyperthyroidism, occlusive vascular disease, or prostatic hypertrophy. Patients with diabetes may require an increased dosage of insulin. Adrenergic drugs are classified as pregnancy category C and are used with extreme caution during pregnancy.

Interactions

The following interactions may occur when an adrenergic drug is administered with another agent:

Interacting Drug	Common Use	Effect of Interaction
antidepressants	Treatment of depression	Increased sympathomimetic effect
oxytocin	Induction of uterine contractions	Increased risk of hypertension

There is an increased risk of seizures, hypotension, and bradycardia when dopamine is administered with phenytoin (Dilantin). Metaraminol is used cautiously in patients taking digoxin because of an increased risk for cardiac arrhythmias. There is an increased risk of hypertension when dobutamine is administered with the β-adrenergic blocking drugs.

HERBAL CONSIDERATIONS
Ephedra (Ma Huang) and the many substances of the *Ephedra* genus have been used medicinally (e.g., *E. sinica* and *E. intermedia*). Ephedra (ephedrine) preparations have traditionally been used to relieve cold symptoms and improve respiratory function, and as an adjunct in weight loss. Large doses may cause a variety of adverse reactions, such as hypertension and irregular heart rate. The use of ephedra has shifted from relief of respiratory problems to an aid to weight loss and enhanced athletic performance. Before taking this herb, the patient should consult a primary health care provider. Ephedra should not be used with the cardiac glycosides, halothane, guanethidine, monoamine oxidase inhibitor (MAOI) antidepressants, or oxytocin or by patients taking St. John's wort. The U.S. Food and Drug Administration (FDA) warns the public not to take ephedrine-containing dietary supplements. Stroke and heart attack have resulted from taking these products. Many producers of weight loss supplements are removing the ephedra component because of potential legal liability (DerMarderosian, 2003).

NURSING PROCESS
PATIENT RECEIVING AN ADRENERGIC DRUG

ASSESSMENT
Assessment of the patient receiving an adrenergic drug differs depending on the drug, the patient, and the reason for administration. For example, assessment of the patient in shock who is to be treated with norepinephrine is different from that for the patient receiving epinephrine with a local anesthetic while having a tooth cavity repaired. Both are receiving adrenergic drugs, but the circumstances are much different.

Preadministration Assessment
When a patient is to receive an adrenergic agent for shock, obtain the blood pressure, pulse rate and quality, and respiratory rate and rhythm. Assess the patient's symptoms, problems, or needs before administering the drug, and document any subjective or objective data on the patient's record. In emergencies, assessments are made quickly and accurately. This information provides an important database that is used during treatment.

A general survey of the patient also is necessary. It is important to look for additional symptoms of shock, such as cool skin, cyanosis, diaphoresis, and a change in the level of consciousness. Other assessments may be necessary if the hypotensive episode is due to trauma, severe infection, or blood loss.

Ongoing Assessment
During the ongoing assessment, observe the patient for the effect of the drug, such as improved breathing of the patient with asthma, or response of blood pressure to the administration of the vasopressor. During therapy, evaluate and document the drug effect and vital signs. Comparison of assessments made before and after administration may help the primary health care provider determine future use of the drug for this patient. It is important to report adverse drug reactions to the primary health care provider as soon as possible.

When a patient has self-administered a drug for a life-threatening allergic reaction, try to get as much information as possible from the patient about the incident leading up to using the drug. If the patient was with family or friends, gain subjective data from these people regarding the events leading up to the need for drug injection.

NURSING DIAGNOSES
Drug-specific nursing diagnoses are the following:

- **Risk for Allergy Response** related to response to substance trigger (insect sting, drug allergy, specific food)
- **Ineffective Tissue Perfusion** related to hypovolemia, blood loss, impaired distribution of fluid, impaired circulation, impaired transport of oxygen across alveolar and capillary bed, other (specify)
- **Decreased Cardiac Output** related to altered heart rate and/or rhythm
- **Disturbed Sleep Pattern** related to adverse reactions (nervousness) to the drug and the environment

Nursing diagnoses related to drug administration are discussed in Chapter 4.

PLANNING
The expected outcomes of the patient depend on the reason for administering an adrenergic agent but may include an optimal response to drug therapy, meeting patient needs related to management of adverse drug reactions, and confidence in an understanding of the medication regimen.

IMPLEMENTATION

Promoting an Optimal Response to Therapy
Management of the patient receiving an adrenergic agent varies and depends on the drug used, the reason for administration, and the patient's response to the drug. In most instances, adrenergic drugs are potent and potentially dangerous. Minimize distractions and exercise great care in the calculation and preparation of these drugs for administration. Although adrenergic drugs are potentially dangerous, proper supervision and management before, during, and after administration will minimize the occurrence of any serious problems. Report and document any complaint the patient may have while taking an adrenergic drug. However, nursing judgment is necessary when reporting adverse reactions. Report adverse effects, such as the development of cardiac arrhythmias, immediately, regardless of the time of day or night. Yet, other adverse effects, such as a nervous feeling, need not be dealt with on an emergent basis.

Monitoring and Managing Patient Needs
RISK FOR ALLERGY RESPONSE. Once a patient has experienced an allergic reaction, he or she is at risk for having another reaction. Triggers can include foods, stinging insects, latex, chemical or environmental items, and even exercise. Patients who have experienced an allergic reaction may be instructed in the use of epinephrine via the EpiPen (Fig. 24.3) so they may carry on normal daily activities. Sometimes patients are fearful and wonder if the situation calls for use of the drug, or if they should seek out care instead. During an allergic reaction,

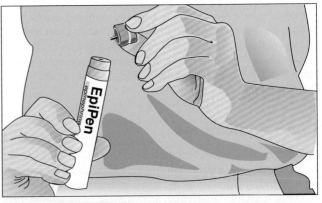

Figure 24.3 Example of preloaded auto-injection device for use in treating allergic reactions. (From Smeltzer, S. C., & Bare, B. G. [2000]. *Textbook of medical-surgical nursing* [9th ed.]. Philadelphia: Lippincott Williams & Wilkins.)

the drug should be administered first, then medical care obtained.

It is important that patients be taught how to recognize symptoms and use the device. Teach the patient to recognize the symptoms of an allergic reaction, which include hives, itching, flushing, and swelling of the lips, tongue, or inside of the mouth. Patients may feel tightness of the throat or chest if the airway is affected. Other symptoms can include chest pain, dizziness, and headache as the blood pressure gets lower. Specific instructions for using auto-injecting epinephrine are provided in Patient Teaching for Improved Patient Outcomes: Using an Auto-Injector for Allergic Reactions.

Patient Teaching for Improved Patient Outcomes

Using an Auto-Injector for Allergic Reactions

If an individual has experienced an allergic reaction or is at risk of having a reaction, he or she may be prescribed a self-administering antidote. It is important to carry this device at all times. It should not be exposed to extreme temperatures (e.g., do not store in refrigerator or put in glove box of car). The device is an auto-injector, meaning it is designed to inject the medication with minimal training, therefore minimizing fear of use. When the device is used it is still important to seek medical treatment as soon as possible. If alone, the patient should call the emergency number first, then administer the dose. Use of these devices should not be considered in place of medical care and advice; the patient should be taken to an emergency department as soon as possible.

When you teach, make sure your patient understands the following:

✔ Depending on the device, there is an orange or black tip on the small end of the auto-injector. NEVER put your fingers or hand over this, because this is where the needle comes out.
✔ Take off the activation cap only when you are ready to use the auto-injector, never when you do not plan to use it.
✔ Use only if the contents in the "window" of the auto-injector are clear.
✔ Hold the auto-injector in your fist with the orange or black tip pointing down. Pull off the activation cap (opposite end from the black tip) with your other hand.
✔ Hold the orange or black tip near the outer thigh of the person who is getting the injection. Most devices are designed to be used through clothing.
✔ Gently but FIRMLY swing and jab the black tip into the outer thigh so that the auto-injector is perpendicular to the thigh.
✔ Hold the auto-injector firmly in the thigh for 10 seconds.
✔ Remove the unit and massage the injection area for 10 seconds.
✔ Check the orange or black tip. If the needle is exposed, the dose was received. If not, repeat the steps.
✔ DO NOT THROW AWAY THE DEVICE. Be sure to take the used device to the emergency department with you.

INEFFECTIVE TISSUE PERFUSION. If the patient is being given an adrenergic drug for hypotension, there is already a problem with tissue perfusion. Administration of the adrenergic drug may correct the problem or, if the blood pressure becomes too high, tissue perfusion may again be a problem. By maintaining the blood pressure at the systolic rate prescribed by the primary health care provider, tissue perfusion will be maintained.

When a patient is in shock and experiencing ineffective tissue perfusion, there is a decrease in oxygen, resulting in an inability of the body to nourish its cells at the capillary level. If the patient has marked hypotension, the administration of a vasopressor is required. The primary health care provider determines the cause of the hypotension and then selects the best method of treatment. Some hypotensive episodes require the use of a less potent vasopressor, such as metaraminol; at other times, a more potent vasopressor, such as dobutamine, dopamine, or norepinephrine, is necessary.

Consider the following points when administering the potent vasopressors such as dopamine and norepinephrine:

■ Use an electronic infusion pump to administer these drugs.

■ Do not mix dopamine with other drugs, especially sodium bicarbonate or other alkaline intravenous (IV) solutions. Check with the clinical pharmacist before adding a second drug to an IV solution containing this drug.

■ Do not dilute norepinephrine or dopamine IV solutions before administration. The primary health care provider orders the IV solution, the amount of drug added to the solution, and the initial rate of infusion.

■ Blood pressure is monitored continuously from the beginning of therapy until the desired blood pressure is achieved, and until the patient is transferred to a less supervised unit.

■ Adjust the rate of drug administration according to the patient's blood pressure. The rate of administration of the IV solution is increased or decreased to maintain the patient's blood pressure at the systolic pressure ordered by the primary health care provider.

■ Readjustment of the rate of flow of the IV solution is often necessary. The frequency of adjustment depends on the patient's response to the vasopressor.

■ Inspect the needle site and surrounding tissues at frequent intervals for leakage (extravasation, infiltration) of the solution into the subcutaneous tissues surrounding the needle site. If leakage occurs, establish another IV line immediately, then discontinue the IV containing the vasopressor, and notify the primary health care provider. These drugs are particularly damaging when they leak into surrounding tissues. You should know the extravasation protocol and have orders signed by the primary health provider to implement the protocol whenever these drugs are used.

■ Never leave the patient receiving these drugs unattended.

Monitoring the patient in shock requires your vigilance. The patient's heart rate, blood pressure, and electrocardiogram are monitored continuously. Urine output is measured often (usually hourly), and accurate intake and output measurements are taken. Monitoring of central venous pressure by a central venous catheter provides an estimate of the patient's fluid status. Sometimes additional hemodynamic monitoring is necessary with a pulmonary artery catheter. The use of a pulmonary artery catheter allows nurses to monitor a number of parameters, such as cardiac output and peripheral vascular resistance. Therapy is adjusted according to the primary health care provider's instructions.

DECREASED CARDIAC OUTPUT. The heart rate and stroke volume (volume of blood leaving the heart) determine cardiac output. The stroke volume is determined in part by the contractile state of the heart and the amount of blood in the ventricle available to be pumped out. The interventions listed to support tissue perfusion also help to support cardiac output of the patient in shock.

When the patient is in shock, it is important to continually monitor vital signs (heart rate and rhythm, respiratory rate, and blood pressure) carefully to determine the severity of shock. For example, as cardiac output decreases, compensatory tachycardia (rapid heartbeat) develops to increase cardiac output. As shock deepens, the pulse volume becomes progressively weaker and assumes a "thready" feel. The heart rate increases and the heart rhythm may become irregular. Initially, the respiratory rate is rapid, as the patient experiences air hunger, but in profound shock, the respiratory rate decreases. Blood pressure decreases as shock progresses.

NURSING ALERT

Regardless of the actual numeric reading of the blood pressure, a progressive decrease in blood pressure is serious. Report any progressive decrease in blood pressure, a decrease in systolic blood pressure below 100 mm Hg, or any decrease of 20 mm Hg or more of the patient's normal blood pressure.

DISTURBED SLEEP PATTERN. Often adrenergic drugs are used in the critical care setting. These units can be as busy in the middle of the night as they are in the middle of the day. Patients can easily get confused regarding the time of day. This can cause a great deal of stress in the patient. It is helpful to identify circumstances that disturb sleep, such as when the nursing staff enter the room during the night or turn the overhead light on during the night (Fig. 24.4). Plan care with as few interruptions as possible or make modifications. For example, to filter light, curtains can be drawn over windows and between patients in critical care units. Weigh the importance of monitoring patient status and combine with comfort interventions when administering the adrenergic drugs. A thorough explanation of the reason for close monitoring of the vital signs is necessary, especially to family members who are present. In addition, caffeinated beverages are avoided, especially after 5:00 p.m. Other sleep aids may be used (e.g., warm milk, back rub, progressive relaxation, or bedtime snack).

Educating the Patient and Family

Specially trained health care providers give some adrenergic drugs, such as the vasopressors. Your responsibility focuses on monitoring for and teaching about the treatment and drug to the patient or family. Depending on the situation, you may include facts such as how the drug will be given (e.g., the route of administration) and what results are expected. Use your judgment regarding some of the information given to the patient or family regarding

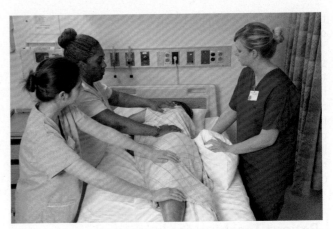
Figure 24.4 Nursing activities are clustered together to minimize the disruption in sleep patterns.

administration of an adrenergic drug in life-threatening situations, because certain facts, such as the seriousness of the patient's condition, are usually best explained by the primary health care provider.

When teaching the patient about self-administration of epinephrine, make sure the patient and family understand this is not to be used in place of medical treatment. It is an immediate intervention used while treatment is sought for the allergic reaction. After injection the patient may experience the following reactions: faster heartbeat, nausea, vomiting, sweating, dizziness, weakness, headache, and nervousness.

EVALUATION

- Therapeutic effect is achieved and perfusion is maintained.
- Adverse reactions are identified, reported to the primary health care provider, and managed successfully through appropriate nursing interventions:
  - Allergic response is minimized.
  - Adequate tissue perfusion is maintained.
  - Adequate cardiac output is maintained.
  - Patient reports fewer episodes of inappropriate sleep patterns.
- Patient (if able) and family express confidence and demonstrate an understanding of the drug regimen.

PHARMACOLOGY IN PRACTICE
THINK CRITICALLY

The primary health care provider has prescribed an auto-injector rescue drug for Janna to use. Her mother feels this is too much responsibility for a 16-year-old. How would you approach the mother to help her understand the significance of the reaction and ease of use of this device?

KEY POINTS

- The sympathetic branch of the autonomic nervous system regulates involuntary body functions. The neurotransmitter of the sympathetic branch is norepinephrine; activation of this system is often called the fight-or-flight response.

- The purpose is to divert blood flow to the vital organs so the body can deal with the stressful situation. A person becomes wakeful with quicker reflexes and pupils dilate. The smooth muscles of the bronchi relax as do the coronary vessels and the heart rate increases. Blood flow is constricted to areas such as the GI and genitourinary systems.

- Drugs that mimic the response are called sympathomimetic or adrenergic (because the primary transmitter is adrenalin or epinephrine). Actions in the body are modified depending on how the drug acts on different cell receptors. Drugs can be selective for α or β receptors. Drugs can also be nonselective.

- These drugs are used to treat shock, hypotension, allergic reactions, heart conditions, and bronchodilation. Topical formulas are used for glaucoma and nasal congestion. Older individuals are very susceptible to adverse reactions, especially to epinephrine.

- Adverse reactions include increased blood pressure, nausea, vomiting, headache, and cardiac arrhythmias.

● *Summary Drug Table* ADRENERGIC DRUGS

Generic Name	Trade Name	Uses	Adverse Reactions	Dosage Ranges
Adrenergic (Sympathomimetic) Drugs Used Primarily for Vasopressor Effects				
dobutamine *doe-byoo'-tah-meen*		Cardiac decompensation due to depressed contractility caused by organic heart disease or cardiac surgical procedures	Headache, nausea, increased heart rate, increase in systolic blood pressure, palpitations, anginal and nonspecific chest pain	2.5–10 mcg/kg/min IV (up to 40 mcg/kg/min); titrate to patient's hemodynamic and renal status
dopamine *doe'-pah-meen*		Shock due to myocardial infarction, trauma, open heart surgery, renal failure, and chronic cardiac decompensation in congestive heart failure	Nausea, vomiting, ectopic beats, tachycardia, anginal pain, palpitations, hypotension, dyspnea	2–50 mcg/kg/min IV (infusion rate determined by patient's response)
epinephrine *eh-pih-neh'-frin*	EpiPen	Ventricular standstill; treatment and prophylaxis of cardiac arrest, heart block; mucosal congestion and acute sinusitis; prolong regional/local anesthetics; anaphylactic reactions	Anxiety, restlessness, headache, lightheadedness, dizziness, nausea, dysuria, pallor	Cardiac arrest: 0.5–1.0 mg IV Respiratory distress (e.g., anaphylaxis): 0.1–0.25 mg of hay fever, rhinitis
isoproterenol *eye-soe-proe-tare'-eh-noll*	Isuprel	Shock, bronchospasm during anesthesia, cardiac standstill and arrhythmias	Anxiety, sweating, flushing, headache, lightheadedness, dizziness, nausea, vomiting, tachycardia	Shock: 4 mcg/mL diluted solution IV Cardiac arrhythmias, cardiac standstill: 0.02–0.06 mg of diluted solution IV, or 1:5000 solution intracardiac injection
metaraminol *meh-tah-ram'-ih-noll*		Hypotension with spinal anesthesia, hypotension due to hemorrhage, drug reactions, surgical complication, shock associated with brain damage	Headache, apprehension, palpitations, nausea, projectile vomiting, urinary urgency	2–10 mg IM, subcutaneously; 15–100 mg in 250- or 500-mL solution IV
midodrine *mid'-oh-dryne*	ProAmatine	Orthostatic hypotension, only when patient is considerably impaired	Paresthesias, headache, pain, dizziness, supine hypertension, bradycardia, piloerection, pruritus, dysuria, chills	10 mg orally TID during daylight hours when patient is upright
norepinephrine (levarterenol) *nor-ep-ih-nef'-rin*	Levophed	Shock, hypotension, cardiac arrest	Restlessness, headache, dizziness, bradycardia, hypertension	2–4 mcg/min, rate adjusted to maintain desired blood pressure

● Chapter Review

Know Your Drugs

Clients sometimes know a medication by the brand (or trade) name and not the generic name. To help you recognize both names, match the brand name with the generic name of the same medication.

Generic Name	Brand Name
1. epinephrine	A. Levophed
2. isoproterenol	B. Isuprel
3. norepinephrine	C. EpiPen

Calculate Medication Dosages

1. The physician orders 2 mg of 1:1000 epinephrine solution IV. The drug is available in 1:1000 solution 1 mg/mL. The nurse administers _____.

2. The physician orders 0.5 mg of 1:1000 epinephrine in a subcutaneous injection. The drug is available in 1:1000 solution 1 mg/mL. The nurse administers _____.

● Prepare for the NCLEX®

Build Your Knowledge

1. What is the transmitting substance in the sympathetic branch of the nervous system?

    1. serotonin
    2. norepinephrine
    3. dopamine
    4. acetylcholine

2. Shock is described as:

    1. result of blood loss
    2. compensation for bodily assault
    3. inadequate tissue perfusion
    4. the fight-or-flight response

3. The physician prescribes norepinephrine, a potent vasopressor, to be administered to a client in shock. The rate of the administration of the IV fluid containing the norepinephrine is:

    1. maintained at a set rate of infusion
    2. adjusted per protocol to maintain the patient's blood pressure
    3. given at a rate not to exceed 5 mg/min
    4. discontinued when the blood pressure is 100 mm Hg systolic

4. At what intervals would the nurse monitor the blood pressure of a client administered norepinephrine?

    1. continuously
    2. every 30 minutes
    3. every hour
    4. every 4 hours

5. Which of the following are the common adverse reactions the nurse would expect with the administration of the adrenergic drugs?

    1. bradycardia, lethargy, bronchial constriction
    2. increase in appetite, nervousness, drowsiness
    3. anorexia, vomiting, hypotension
    4. headache, nervousness, nausea

6. When dobutamine is administered with the β-adrenergic blocking drugs, the nurse is aware of an increased risk for_____.

    1. seizures
    2. arrhythmias
    3. hypotension
    4. hypertension

Apply Your Knowledge

7. If a client uses an auto-inject epinephrine device, the best disposal would be:

    1. container the injector is packaged in
    2. held until seen by emergency personnel
    3. hard plastic container
    4. sharps box or needle container

8. When norepinephrine is transmitted in the sympathetic nervous, which of the following occurs?

    1. heart rate slows
    2. blood pressure lowers
    3. GI system speeds up
    4. bronchi relax

Alternate-Format Questions

9. Select the terms that describe drugs that stimulate the sympathetic branch of the ANS. **Select all that apply**.

    1. sympathomimetic
    2. sympatholytic
    3. adrenergic
    4. cholinergic

10. An adult with an allergy to honeybees is stung and calls the nurse at the clinic. The client has two EpiPens at home. The solution is 1 mg/mL and each EpiPen contains 0.3 mL. What drug dose has the client taken if two injections were already given? _____

To check your answers, see Appendix G.

the**Point** *For more NCLEX-style questions, log on to http://thepoint.lww.com to access more than 1000 questions.*

Adrenergic Blocking Drugs

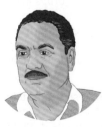

25

KEY TERMS

alpha (α)-adrenergic • α receptors of the adrenergic nerves that control the vascular system

antiadrenergic • blocks the neurotransmission of the sympathetic nervous system

beta (β)-adrenergic • β receptors of the adrenergic nerves that primarily control the heart

cardiac arrhythmia • abnormal rhythm of the heart, also known as cardiac *dysrhythmias*

first-dose effect • marked adverse reaction with the first dose

glaucoma • group of diseases of the eye characterized by increased intraocular pressure; results in changes within the eye, visual field defects, and eventually blindness (if left untreated)

heart failure (HF) • condition in which the heart cannot pump enough blood to meet the tissue needs of the body, commonly called *congestive heart failure (CHF)*

orthostatic hypotension • decrease in blood pressure occurring after standing in one place for an extended period

pheochromocytoma • tumor of the adrenal medulla characterized by hypersecretion of epinephrine and norepinephrine

postural hypotension • decrease in blood pressure after a sudden change in body position

sympatholytic • blocking the sympathetic nervous system

DRUG CLASSES

Alpha (α)-adrenergic blocking	α/β-adrenergic blocking
Beta (β)-adrenergic blocking	Centrally and peripherally acting antiadrenergic

Norepinephrine is a substance that transmits nerve impulses across the sympathetic branch of the autonomic nervous system. Activation of these nerves is sometimes called our *fight-or-flight response*. Drugs featured in Chapter 24 facilitate the transmission of norepinephrine. In this chapter drugs that prevent the response, called *adrenergic blocking,* are discussed. Figure 25.1 shows the organ responses when sympathetic nerve impulses are blocked. Also called **sympatholytic** drugs, these agents block the transmission of norepinephrine in the sympathetic system. Drugs blocking neurotransmission in the sympathetic nervous system work *directly* by blocking the receptor or *indirectly* by

---

PHARMACOLOGY IN PRACTICE

Alfredo Garcia is accompanied by his wife to the clinic. He came in with complaints of an upper respiratory infection. While taking vital signs you discover a blood pressure of 210/120. He has never been diagnosed with hypertension. As you read, think about what antiadrenergic drugs do to blood vessels and blood pressure.

SYMPATHETIC SYSTEM

PARASYMPATHETIC SYSTEM

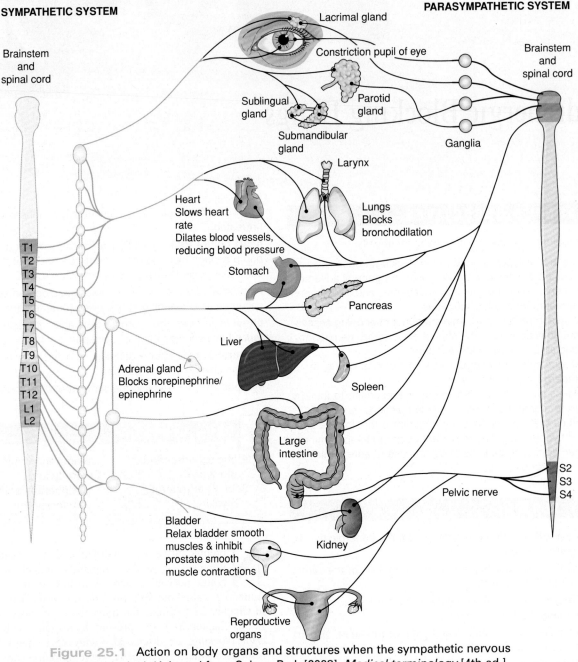

Brainstem
and
spinal cord

Lacrimal gland

Constriction pupil of eye

Brainstem
and
spinal cord

Sublingual
gland

Parotid
gland

Submandibular
gland

Ganglia

Larynx

Heart
Slows heart
rate
Dilates blood vessels,
reducing blood pressure

Lungs
Blocks
bronchodilation

Stomach

Pancreas

Liver

Adrenal gland
Blocks norepinephrine/
epinephrine

Spleen

Large
intestine

Pelvic nerve

S2
S3
S4

Bladder
Relax bladder smooth
muscles & inhibit
prostate smooth
muscle contractions

Kidney

Reproductive
organs

Figure 25.1 Action on body organs and structures when the sympathetic nervous system is blocked. (Adapted from Cohen, B. J. [2003]. *Medical terminology* [4th ed.]. Philadelphia: Lippincott Williams & Wilkins.)

preventing release of norepinephrine. They may be viewed as belonging to one of four different groups:

- **Alpha (α)-adrenergic blocking** drugs—drugs that block α-adrenergic receptors. These drugs produce their greatest effect on the α receptors of the adrenergic nerves that control the vascular system.
- **Beta (β)-adrenergic blocking** drugs—drugs that block β-adrenergic receptors. These drugs produce their greatest effect on the β receptors of adrenergic nerves, primarily the β receptors of the heart.

- α/β-Adrenergic-blocking drugs—drugs that block both α- and β-adrenergic receptors. These drugs act on both α and β nerve fibers.
- Centrally and peripherally acting **antiadrenergic** drugs—drugs that prevent the release of the neurotransmitter. These drugs block the adrenergic nerve impulse in both the central and peripheral nervous systems.

Each of these groups is discussed individually, followed by an example of the Nursing Process for the group as a whole. The focal group of drugs in this chapter is the β-adrenergic blocking drugs. See the Summary Drug Table: Adrenergic Blocking Drugs for a more complete listing of these drugs.

α-ADRENERGIC BLOCKING DRUGS

Actions

Stimulation of α-adrenergic nerves results in vasoconstriction. If stimulation of α-adrenergic nerves is interrupted or blocked, the result is vasodilation. This is the direct opposite of the effect of an adrenergic drug with α activity. The drug used in this category causes vasodilation by relaxing the smooth muscle of blood vessels. α-Adrenergic blockers used in ophthalmic preparations constrict the pupil and are discussed in Chapter 53.

Uses

α-Adrenergic blocking drugs are used in the treatment of the following:

- Hypertension caused by **pheochromocytoma** (a tumor of the adrenal gland that produces excessive amounts of epinephrine and norepinephrine)
- Hypertension during preoperative preparation

They are also used to prevent or treat tissue damage caused by extravasation of dopamine.

Adverse Reactions

Administration of an α-adrenergic blocking drug may result in weakness, orthostatic hypotension, cardiac arrhythmias, hypotension, and tachycardia. See the Summary Drug Table: Adrenergic Blocking Drugs for more information.

Contraindications, Precautions, and Interactions

α-Adrenergic blocking drugs are contraindicated in patients who are hypersensitive to the drugs and in patients with coronary artery disease. These drugs are used cautiously during pregnancy (pregnancy category C) and lactation, after a recent myocardial infarction (MI), and in patients with renal failure or Raynaud's disease. When phentolamine (Regitine) is administered with epinephrine, there is decreased vasoconstrictor and hypertensive action.

β-ADRENERGIC BLOCKING DRUGS

Actions

β-Adrenergic blocking drugs are also called *β blockers*. These drugs decrease the stimulation of the sympathetic nervous system on certain tissues. β-Adrenergic receptors are found mainly in the heart. Stimulation of β receptors of the heart results in an increase in the heart rate. Blocking the nerve impulse of β-adrenergic nerves decreases the heart rate and

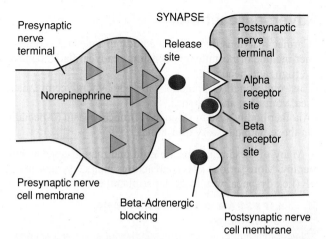

Figure 25.2 β-Adrenergic blocking drugs prevent epinephrine and norepinephrine from occupying receptor sites on cell membranes.

dilates the blood vessels (Fig. 25.2). These drugs decrease the heart's excitability, decrease cardiac workload and oxygen consumption, and provide membrane-stabilizing effects that contribute to the antiarrhythmic activity of the β-adrenergic blocking drugs. Examples of β-adrenergic blocking drugs used for cardiac purposes are esmolol (Brevibloc) and propranolol (Inderal).

β-Adrenergic blocking drugs such as betaxolol (Betoptic) and timolol (Timoptic) are used to treat glaucoma. **Glaucoma** is a narrowing or blockage of the drainage channels (canals of Schlemm) between the anterior and posterior chambers of the eye. This results in a buildup of pressure (increased intraocular pressure) in the eye. Blindness may occur if glaucoma is left untreated. When the aforementioned drugs are used topically as ophthalmic drops, they appear to reduce the production of aqueous humor in the anterior chamber of the eye, lessening the effects of glaucoma.

Uses

β-Adrenergic blocking drugs are used in the treatment of the following:

- Hypertension (first-choice drug for patients with stable angina)
- **Cardiac arrhythmia** (abnormal rhythm of the heart), such as ventricular or supraventricular tachycardia
- Migraine headaches
- **Heart failure (HF)**
- Angina pectoris
- Glaucoma (topical ophthalmic eye drops)

β-Adrenergic blockers are also used to prevent reinfarction in patients with a recent MI (1 to 4 weeks after the MI).

CHRONIC CARE CONSIDERATIONS

Hypertension research studies demonstrate better patient outcomes for African Americans when β blockers are used in combination with diuretics than other drugs alone to treat hypertension, such as angiotensin-converting enzyme (ACE) inhibitors (Ferdinand, 2007).

Adverse Reactions

- Cardiac reactions that affect the body in a generalized manner include orthostatic hypotension, bradycardia, dizziness, vertigo, and headache.
- Gastrointestinal (GI) reactions include hyperglycemia, nausea, vomiting, and diarrhea.
- Another bodily system reaction is bronchospasm (especially in those with a history of asthma).

Many of these reactions are mild and may disappear with therapy. More serious adverse reactions include symptoms of HF (i.e., dyspnea, weight gain, peripheral edema).

LIFESPAN CONSIDERATIONS
Gerontology
Older adults are at increased risk for adverse reactions when taking β-adrenergic blocking drugs. Monitor the older adult closely for confusion, HF, worsening of angina, shortness of breath, and peripheral vascular insufficiency (e.g., cold extremities, paresthesia of the hands, weak peripheral pulses).

Contraindications, Precautions, and Interactions

These drugs are contraindicated in patients with an allergy to β blockers; in patients with sinus bradycardia, second- or third-degree heart block, or HF; and in those with asthma, emphysema, and hypotension. The drugs are used cautiously in patients with diabetes, thyrotoxicosis, or peptic ulcer.

LIFESPAN CONSIDERATIONS
Pregnancy
β Blockers are recommended for pregnant women over other hypertensive drugs because the risk to the fetus is less with these drugs.

The following interactions may occur when a β-adrenergic blocker is administered with another agent:

Interacting Drug	Common Use	Effect of Interaction
antidepressants (monoamine oxidase inhibitors [MAOIs], selective serotonin reuptake inhibitors [SSRIs])	Management of depression	Increased effect of the β blocker, bradycardia
nonsteroidal anti-inflammatory drugs (NSAIDs), salicylates	Pain relief	Decreased effect of the β blocker
loop diuretics	Management of cardiovascular problems	Increased risk of hypotension
clonidine	Management of cardiovascular problems	Increased risk of paradoxical hypertensive effect
cimetidine	Management of GI problems	Increased serum level of the β blocker and higher risk of β blocker toxicity
lidocaine	Management of cardiac problems	Increased serum level of the β blocker and higher risk of β blocker toxicity

α/β-ADRENERGIC BLOCKING DRUGS

Actions

α/β-Adrenergic blocking drugs block the stimulation of both the α- and β-adrenergic receptors, resulting in peripheral vasodilation. The two drugs in this category are carvedilol (Coreg) and labetalol (Trandate).

Uses

Carvedilol is used to treat essential hypertension and in HF to reduce progression of the disease. Labetalol is used in the treatment of hypertension, either alone or in combination with another drug, such as a diuretic.

Adverse Reactions

Most adverse effects of α/β-adrenergic blocking drugs are mild and do not require discontinuation of therapy. General body system adverse reactions include fatigue, dizziness, hypotension, drowsiness, insomnia, weakness, diarrhea, dyspnea, chest pain, bradycardia, and skin rash.

Contraindications, Precautions, and Interactions

α/β-Adrenergic blockers are contraindicated in patients with hypersensitivity to the drugs, bronchial asthma, decompensated HF, and severe bradycardia. The drugs are used cautiously in patients with drug-controlled HF, chronic bronchitis, or impaired hepatic or cardiac function; in those with diabetes; and during pregnancy (pregnancy category C) and lactation.

The following interactions may occur when an α/β-adrenergic blocker is administered with another agent:

Interacting Drug	Common Use	Effect of Interaction
antidepressants (tricyclics and SSRIs)	Management of depression	Increased risk of tremors
cimetidine	Management of GI problems	Increased effect of the adrenergic blocker
clonidine	Management of cardiovascular problems	Increased effect of the clonidine
digoxin	Management of cardiac problems	Increased serum level of the digoxin and higher risk of digoxin toxicity

CENTRALLY AND PERIPHERALLY ACTING ANTIADRENERGIC DRUGS

Actions

One group of antiadrenergic drugs inhibits the release of norepinephrine from certain adrenergic nerve endings in the peripheral nervous system. This group is composed of *peripherally acting* (i.e., acting on peripheral structures) antiadrenergic drugs. An example of a peripherally acting antiadrenergic drug for treating hypertension is prazosin (Minipress). These drugs are also used to treat benign prostatic hypertrophy (BPH). Another group of antiadrenergic drugs are called *centrally acting* antiadrenergic drugs because they act on the central nervous system (CNS) rather than on the peripheral nervous system. This group affects specific CNS centers, thereby decreasing some of the activity of the sympathetic nervous system. Although the action of both types of antiadrenergic drugs is somewhat different, the results are basically the same. An example of a centrally acting antiadrenergic drug is clonidine (Catapres).

Uses

Antiadrenergic drugs are used mainly for the treatment of certain cardiac arrhythmias, hypertension, and BPH (see the Summary Drug Table: Adrenergic Blocking Drugs).

Adverse Reactions

• Dry mouth, drowsiness, sedation, anorexia, rash, malaise, and weakness are generalized reactions to antiadrenergic drugs that work on the CNS.
• Hypotension, weakness, lightheadedness, and bradycardia are adverse reactions associated with the administration of peripherally acting antiadrenergic drugs.

Contraindications, Precautions, and Interactions

Centrally acting antiadrenergic drugs are contraindicated in active hepatic disease, in antidepressant therapy using MAOIs, and in patients with a history of hypersensitivity to these drugs. The centrally acting antiadrenergic drugs are used cautiously in patients with a history of liver disease or renal impairment and during pregnancy and lactation.

The peripherally acting antiadrenergic drugs are contraindicated in patients with a hypersensitivity to any of the drugs. Reserpine (Serpasil) is contraindicated in patients who have an active peptic ulcer or ulcerative colitis and in patients who are mentally depressed. Reserpine is used cautiously in patients with a history of depression, in those with renal impairment or cardiovascular disease, and during pregnancy and lactation.

The following interactions may occur when an antiadrenergic drug is administered with another agent:

Interacting Drug	Common Use	Effect of Interaction
adrenergic drugs	Management of cardiovascular problems	Increased risk of hypertension
levodopa	Management of Parkinson's disease	Decreased effect of the levodopa, hypotension
anesthetic agents	Surgical anesthesia	Increased effect of the anesthetic
β blockers	Management of cardiovascular problems	Increased risk of hypertension
lithium	Treatment of psychosis	Increased risk of lithium toxicity
haloperidol	Treatment of psychosis	Increased risk of psychotic behavior

NURSING PROCESS
PATIENT RECEIVING AN ADRENERGIC BLOCKING DRUG

ASSESSMENT
Assessment depends on the drug, the patient, and the reason for administration.

Preadministration Assessment
Establish an accurate database before any adrenergic blocking drug is administered for the first time. If, for example, the patient has hypertensive disease, document the subjective and objective symptoms as well as vital signs during the initial assessment. Patients with hypertension have their blood pressure and pulse taken on both arms in sitting, standing, and supine positions before therapy is begun. If the patient has a cardiac arrhythmia, the initial assessment includes taking the pulse rate, determining the pulse rhythm, and noting the patient's general appearance.

If the drug is given for anginal pain, document the pain experience of the patient, and ask about the onset, type (e.g., sharp, dull, squeezing), radiation, location, intensity, and duration of anginal pain. Ask about any precipitating factors of the anginal pain, such as exertion or emotional stress. Once drug therapy is started, evaluation of the effects of therapy can be made by comparing the patient's current symptoms with the symptoms experienced before therapy was initiated. Additional diagnostic studies and laboratory tests, such as an electrocardiogram, also may be ordered.

If the drug is given to treat HF, the patient is assessed for evidence of the disease, such as dyspnea (especially on exertion), peripheral edema, distended neck veins, and cough.

Ongoing Assessment
It is important to perform an ongoing assessment of the patient receiving adrenergic blocking drug therapy. This assessment often depends on the reason the drug is administered. For all adrenergic blocking drugs, it is important to observe these patients continually for the appearance of adverse reactions. Some adverse reactions are mild, whereas others, such as diarrhea, may cause a problem, especially if the patient is older or debilitated.

Typically hypertensive patients will be asked to monitor their own blood pressures between clinic visits. This can be accomplished by obtaining equipment for the home or periodic visits to a local fire station or pharmacy. More in-depth information regarding care of the patient with hypertension is provided in Chapter 35.

NURSING DIAGNOSES

Drug-specific nursing diagnoses are the following:

- ■ **Impaired Comfort** related to drying of secretions secondary to medication
- ■ **Ineffective Tissue Perfusion: Peripheral** related to hypotension
- ■ **Risk for Injury** related to vertigo, dizziness, weakness, and syncope secondary to hypotension

Nursing diagnoses related to drug administration are discussed in Chapter 4.

PLANNING

The expected outcomes for the patient depend on the reason for administration of an adrenergic blocking drug but may include an optimal response to drug therapy, meeting of patient needs related to the management of adverse reactions, and confidence in an understanding of the medication regimen.

IMPLEMENTATION

Promoting an Optimal Response to Therapy

Most adrenergic blocking drugs may be given without regard to food. However, the drugs preventing release of neurotransmitters (antiadrenergics) should be taken at the same time each day because the fluctuation in blood level can affect blood pressure. Sotalol (Betapace) is given on an empty stomach because food may reduce absorption of the drug.

When adrenergic blocking drugs are given to patients to control hypertension, angina, or cardiac arrhythmias, it is important to communicate with the primary health care provider about the patient's response to therapy. When given for a cardiac arrhythmia, these drugs can provoke new or worsen existing ventricular arrhythmias. If angina worsens or does not appear to be controlled by the drug, the patient needs to feel confident to contact the primary health care provider immediately.

When the drug is administered for hypertension, the patient is monitored for a decrease in blood pressure. On the other hand, if there is a significant *increase* in blood pressure, administer the ordered dose and notify the primary health care provider immediately because additional drug therapy may be necessary.

When a β-adrenergic blocking ophthalmic preparation, such as timolol, is used by patients with glaucoma, it is important they continue periodic follow-up examinations with an ophthalmologist. At these examinations, the intraocular pressure is measured to determine the effectiveness of drug therapy.

Monitoring and Managing Patient Needs

IMPAIRED COMFORT. Some patients may experience one or more adverse drug reactions during treatment with adrenergic blocking drugs. Adverse reactions that pose no serious threat to the patient's well-being, such as dry mouth or mild constipation, are reactions that impair comfort.

Even minor adverse drug reactions can be distressing to the patient, especially when they persist for a long time. Therefore, when possible, you can relieve minor adverse reactions with simple nursing measures. For example, assist or teach the patient with dry mouth to take frequent sips of water or suck on a piece of hard candy (provided that the patient does not have diabetes or is not on a special diet that limits sugar intake) to relieve the dryness. Help relieve a patient's constipation by encouraging increased intake of high-fiber foods and fluids, unless extra fluids are contraindicated. The primary health care provider also may order a laxative or stool softener. It is important for you to maintain a daily record of bowel elimination for the hospitalized patient. Dryness, slower GI motility, and immobility all make constipation a greater risk for the hospitalized patient. Other GI side effects, such as anorexia, diarrhea, and constipation, can be minimized by administering drugs at a specific time in relation to meals, with food, or with antacids.

INEFFECTIVE TISSUE PERFUSION: PERIPHERAL. During therapy with an adrenergic blocking drug for hypertension, the patient's blood pressure is taken before each dose is given. Some patients have an unusual response to the drugs. In addition, some drugs may, in some individuals, decrease the blood pressure at a more rapid rate than other drugs. It is important to monitor the patient's blood pressure on both arms and in the sitting, standing, and supine positions for the first week or more of therapy. Once the patient's blood pressure has stabilized, take the blood pressure before each drug administration using the same arm and position for each reading until the patient is ready to return home. It is a good idea to make a notation on the medication administration record or care plan about the position and arm used for blood pressure determinations. Measuring the blood pressure near the end of the dosing interval or near the end of the day after the last dose of the day helps to determine if the blood pressure is controlled throughout the day.

> ### ! NURSING ALERT
>
> When administering a sympatholytic drug, such as propranolol (Inderal), take an apical pulse rate and blood pressure before giving the drug. If the pulse is below 60 beats/min, or if there is any irregularity in the patient's heart rate or rhythm, or if systolic blood pressure is less than 90 mm Hg, withhold the drug and contact the primary health care provider.

The patient with a life-threatening arrhythmia may receive an adrenergic blocking drug, such as propranolol, by the intravenous (IV) route. When these drugs are administered IV, cardiac monitoring is necessary. Patients not in a monitored unit are usually transferred to one as soon as possible. When administering these drugs for a life-threatening arrhythmia, it is important to monitor the patient continually with cardiac, blood pressure, and respiratory rate frequently.

When propranolol is administered orally for a less serious cardiac arrhythmia, cardiac monitoring is usually not necessary. Periodically monitor the patient's blood pressure and pulse rate and rhythm at varying intervals, depending on the length of treatment and the patient's response to the drug.

RISK FOR INJURY. Administration of the adrenergic blocking drugs may cause hypotension. If the drug is administered for hypertension, then a decrease in blood pressure is expected.

NURSING ALERT

If a significant decrease in blood pressure (a drop of 20 mm Hg systolic or a systolic pressure below 90 mm Hg) occurs after a dose of an adrenergic blocking drug, withhold the next drug dose and notify the primary health care provider immediately. A dosage reduction or discontinuation of the drug may be necessary. Some adrenergic blocking drugs (e.g., prazosin or terazosin) may cause a **first-dose effect**. A first-dose effect occurs when the patient experiences marked hypotension (or postural hypotension) and syncope with sudden loss of consciousness with the first few doses of the drug.

The first-dose effect may be minimized by decreasing the initial dose and administering the dose at bedtime. The dosage can then be slowly increased every 2 weeks until a full therapeutic effect is achieved. If the patient experiences syncope (lightheadedness or fainting), place the patient in a recumbent position and treat supportively. This effect is self-limiting and in most cases does not recur after the initial period of therapy. Lightheadedness and dizziness are more common than loss of consciousness. On occasion, patients receiving an adrenergic blocking drug may experience postural or orthostatic hypotension. Postural hypotension is characterized by a feeling of lightheadedness and dizziness when the patient suddenly changes from a lying to a sitting or standing position, or from a sitting to a standing position. Orthostatic hypotension is characterized by similar symptoms and occurs when the patient changes or shifts position after standing in one place for a long period. See Display 25.1 for tips on how to minimize these adverse reactions.

Display 25.1 **Minimizing the Effects of Adrenergic Blocking Drugs**

Assisting patients to minimize the uncomfortable effects of adrenergic blocking drugs can be challenging. The following measures may be useful:

- Instruct patients to rise slowly from a sitting or lying position.
- Provide assistance for the patient getting out of bed or a chair if symptoms of postural hypotension are severe. Place the call light nearby and instruct patients to ask for assistance each time they get in and out of bed or a chair.
- Assist the patient in bed to a sitting position and have the patient sit on the edge of the bed for about 1 minute before ambulating.
- Help seated patients to a standing position and instruct them to stand in one place for about 1 minute before ambulating.
- Remain with the patient while he or she is standing in one place, as well as during ambulation.
- Instruct the patient to avoid standing in one place for prolonged periods. This is rarely a problem in the hospital but should be included in the patient and family discharge teaching plan.
- Teach the patient to avoid taking hot showers or baths, which tend to increase vasodilation.

Symptoms of postural or orthostatic hypotension often lessen with time, and the patient may be allowed to get out of bed or a chair slowly without assistance. You should exercise good judgment in this matter. Allowing the patient to rise from a lying or sitting position without help is done only when the determination has been made that the symptoms have lessened and ambulation poses no danger of falling.

Educating the Patient and Family

Some patients do not adhere to the prescribed drug regimen for a variety of reasons, such as failure to comprehend the prescribed regimen, the cost of drug therapy, or failure to understand the importance of continued and uninterrupted therapy. If a stable patient has a sudden blood pressure increase, investigate the possibility of one of these factors causing the problem. In some instances, financial assistance may be necessary; in other instances, patients need to know why they are taking a drug and why therapy must be continuous to attain and maintain an optimal state of health and well-being.

Support your patient's health literacy by describing the drug regimen and stress the importance of continued and uninterrupted therapy when teaching the patient who is prescribed an adrenergic blocking drug. Patient education will differ according to the reason the adrenergic blocking drug was prescribed. If a β-adrenergic blocking drug has been prescribed for hypertension, cardiac arrhythmia, angina, or other cardiac disorders, the patient must be assisted in having a full understanding of the treatment regimen. In some instances, the primary health care provider may advise the hypertensive patient to lose weight or eat a special diet, such as the DASH (Dietary Approaches to Stop Hypertension) diet. A special diet also may be recommended for the patient with angina or a cardiac arrhythmia. When appropriate, enlist the help of a registered dietician to stress the importance of diet and weight loss in the therapy of hypertension.

It is important to include the following additional points in the teaching plan for the patient with hypertension, angina, or a cardiac arrhythmia:

- Do not stop taking the drug abruptly, except on the advice of the primary health care provider. Most of these drugs require that the dosage be gradually decreased to prevent precipitation or worsening of adverse effects.
- Notify the primary health care provider promptly if adverse drug reactions occur.
- Observe caution while driving or performing other hazardous tasks because these drugs (β-adrenergic blockers) may cause drowsiness, dizziness, or lightheadedness.
- Immediately report any signs of HF (weight gain, difficulty breathing, or edema of the extremities).
- Do not use any nonprescription drug (e.g., cold or flu preparations or nasal decongestants) unless you have discussed use of a specific drug with the primary health care provider.
- Inform dentists and other primary health care providers of therapy with this drug.
- Keep all primary health care provider appointments because close monitoring of therapy is essential.

■ Check with a primary health care provider or clinical pharmacist to determine if the drug is to be taken with food or on an empty stomach.

In addition, when an adrenergic blocking drug is prescribed for hypertension, the primary health care provider may want the patient to monitor his or her own blood pressure between office visits (see Patient Teaching for Improved Patient Outcomes: Monitoring Blood Pressure at Home).

EVALUATION

■ Therapeutic effect is achieved and hypertension or other disease is controlled.
■ Adverse reactions are identified, reported to the primary health care provider, and managed successfully through appropriate nursing interventions.
 • Dryness is managed and comfort maintained.
 • Peripheral tissue perfusion is maintained.
 • No evidence of injury is seen.
■ Patient and family express confidence and demonstrate an understanding of the drug regimen.

PHARMACOLOGY IN PRACTICE
THINK CRITICALLY

 Mr. Garcia is prescribed metoprolol 100 mg after breakfast daily. His wife is concerned about him getting up early in the mornings to urinate. When is he most likely to have hypotensive reactions and when is he least likely? How will you teach him to deal with the possibility of orthostatic hypotension?

KEY POINTS

• The sympathetic branch of the autonomic nervous system regulates involuntary body functions. The antiadrenergic drugs block the neurotransmitter norepinephrine in the sympathetic branch.
• The purpose of adrenergic blocking drugs is to block or interrupt the signals that divert blood flow to the vital organs. Instead, the blood vessels dilate and relax smooth muscle. The heart rate decreases and the blood pressure is lowered.

• Drugs that block the sympathetic system are called sympatholytic or antiadrenergic. Actions in the body are modified depending on how the drug acts on different cell receptors. Drugs can be selective for α or β receptors. Drugs can also be nonselective.
• These drugs are used to treat hypertension, cardiac arrhythmias, BPH, glaucoma, and a rare condition called pheochromocytoma. As with the adrenergic drugs, older

individuals are very susceptible to adverse reactions with these drugs.

- Adverse reactions include decreased blood pressure, weakness, increased heart rate, nausea, vomiting, headache, and bronchospasm in those with asthma.

- When starting therapy with antiadrenergic drugs, patients should be monitored and taught about orthostatic hypotension—the sudden drop in blood pressure when going from a lying to a sitting or standing position. This information can help prevent falls and injury.

Summary Drug Table ADRENERGIC BLOCKING DRUGS

Generic Name	Trade Name	Uses	Adverse Reactions	Dosage Ranges
α-Adrenergic Blocking Drugs				
phentolamine *fen-toll'-ah-meen*	Regitine	Diagnosis of pheochromocytoma, hypertensive episodes before and during surgery, prevention/treatment of dermal necrosis after IV administration of norepinephrine or dopamine	Weakness, dizziness, flushing, nausea, vomiting, orthostatic hypotension	5 mg IV, IM Tissue necrosis: 5–10 mg in 10 mL saline solution infiltrated into affected area
β-Adrenergic Blocking Drugs (β Blockers)				
acebutolol *ay-seh-byoo'-toe-loll*	Sectral	Hypertension, ventricular arrhythmias	Bradycardia, dizziness, weakness, hypotension, nausea, vomiting, diarrhea, nervousness	Hypertension: 400 mg orally in 1–2 doses Arrhythmias: 400–1200 mg/day orally in divided doses
atenolol *ay-ten'-oh-loll*	Tenormin, Tenoretic	Hypertension, angina, acute MI	Bradycardia, dizziness, fatigue, weakness, hypotension, nausea, vomiting, diarrhea, nervousness	Hypertension/angina: 50–200 mg/day orally Acute MI: 5 mg IV over 5 min, may be repeated
bisoprolol *bye-soe'-proe-loll*	Zebeta	Hypertension	Same as acebutolol	2.5–10 mg orally daily; maximum dose: 20 mg orally daily
esmolol *ess'-moe-loll*	Brevibloc	Supraventricular tachycardia, noncompensatory tachycardia	Hypotension, weakness, lightheadedness, urinary retention	50–200 mcg/kg/min IV, loading dose may be as high as 500 mcg/kg over 1 min
metoprolol *meh-toe'-proe-loll*	Lopressor, Toprol-XL	Hypertension, angina, MI, HF	Dizziness, hypotension, HF, cardiac arrhythmia, nausea, vomiting, diarrhea	Hypertension/angina: 100–450 mg/day orally Extended release: 50–100 mg/day orally HF: 25–200 mg/day orally Acute MI: 3 bolus doses of 5 mg IV
nadolol *nay-doe'-loll*	Corgard	Hypertension, angina	Dizziness, hypotension, nausea, vomiting, diarrhea, HF, cardiac arrhythmia	Hypertension: 40–80 mg/day orally Angina: 40–80, may go to 240 mg/day orally
nebivolol *neh-biv'-oh-loll*	Bystolic	Hypertension	Dizziness, headache, nausea, diarrhea, tingling extremities	5–40 mg/daily
penbutolol *pen-byoo'-toe-loll*	Levatol	Hypertension	Bradycardia, dizziness, hypotension, nausea, vomiting, diarrhea	20 mg orally daily
pindolol *pin'-doe-loll*		Hypertension	Bradycardia, dizziness, hypotension, nausea, vomiting, diarrhea	5–60 mg/day orally BID

(table continues on page 262)

Summary Drug Table ADRENERGIC BLOCKING DRUGS (continued)

Generic Name	Trade Name	Uses	Adverse Reactions	Dosage Ranges
propranolol *proe-pran'-oh-loll*	Inderal	Cardiac arrhythmias, MI, angina, hypertension, migraine prophylaxis, hypertrophic subaortic stenosis, pheochromocytoma, essential tremor	Bradycardia, dizziness, hypotension, nausea, vomiting, diarrhea, bronchospasm, hyperglycemia, pulmonary edema	Arrhythmias: 10–30 mg orally TID, QID Hypertension: 120–240 mg/day orally in divided doses Angina: 80–320 mg/day orally in divided doses Migraine: 160–240 mg/day orally in divided doses
℞ sotalol *soh'-tah-loll*	Betapace, Betapace AF	Ventricular arrhythmias (maintain normal sinus rhythm—Betapace AF only)	Dizziness, hypotension, nausea, vomiting, diarrhea, respiratory distress	160–320 mg/day orally in divided doses
timolol *tih'-moe-loll*		Hypertension, MI, migraine prophylaxis	Dizziness, hypotension, nausea, vomiting, diarrhea, pulmonary edema	Hypertension: 10–40 mg/day orally in divided doses MI: 10 mg orally BID Migraine: 20 mg/day orally
Topical Preparations				
betaxolol (ophthalmic) *beh-tax'-oh-loll*	Betoptic	Glaucoma	Brief ocular discomfort, tearing	1 gtt BID
timolol (ophthalmic) *tih'-moe-loll*	Timoptic	Glaucoma	Ocular irritation, tearing	1 gtt BID
α/β-Adrenergic Blocking Drugs				
carvedilol *car-veh'-dih-loll*	Coreg	Hypertension, HF, left ventricular dysfunction	Bradycardia, hypotension, cardiac insufficiency, fatigue, dizziness, diarrhea	6.25–25 mg orally BID
labetalol *lah-bet'-ah-loll*	Trandate	Hypertension	Fatigue, drowsiness, insomnia, hypotension, impotence, diarrhea	200–400 mg/day orally in divided doses IV: 20 mg over 2 min with blood pressure monitoring, may repeat
Antiadrenergic Drugs: Centrally Acting				
clonidine *klon'-nih-deen*	Catapres, Catapres-TTS (transdermal)	Hypertension, severe pain in patients with cancer	Drowsiness, dizziness, sedation, dry mouth, constipation, syncope, dreams, rash	100–600 mcg/day orally Transdermal: release rate 0.1–0.3 mg/24 hr
guanabenz *gwah'-nah-benz*		Hypertension	Dry mouth, sedation, dizziness, headache, weakness, arrhythmias	4–32 mg orally BID
guanfacine *gwan'-fah-sine*	Tenex	Hypertension	Dry mouth, somnolence, asthenia, dizziness, headache, constipation, fatigue	1–3 mg/day orally at bedtime
methyldopa or methyldopate *meh'-thill-doe-pah,* *meh'-thill-doe-pate*		Hypertension, hypertensive crisis	Bradycardia, aggravation of angina pectoris, HF, sedation, headache, rash, nausea, vomiting, nasal congestion	250 mg orally BID or TID; maintenance dose: 2 g/day; 250–500 mg q 6 hr IV

Summary Drug Table ADRENERGIC BLOCKING DRUGS (continued)

Generic Name	Trade Name	Uses	Adverse Reactions	Dosage Ranges
Antiadrenergic Drugs: Peripherally Acting				
alfuzosin *al-foo-zoe'-sin*	Uroxatral	BPH	Headache, dizziness	10 mg orally daily
doxazosin *dok-say-zoe'-sin*	Cardura	Hypertension, BPH	Headache, dizziness, fatigue	Hypertension: 1–8 mg orally daily BPH: 1–16 mg orally daily
prazosin *pray-zoe'-sin*	Minipress	Hypertension	Dizziness, postural hypotension, drowsiness, headache, loss of strength, palpitation, nausea	1–20 mg orally daily in divided doses
reserpine *reh-sir'-pyne*	Serpalan	Hypertension, psychosis	Bradycardia, dizziness, nausea, vomiting, diarrhea, nasal congestion	Hypertension: 0.1–0.5 mg orally daily Psychosis: 0.1–1 mg orally daily
silodosin	Rapaflo	BPH	Dizziness, lightheadedness, headache, diarrhea, nasal congestion	8 mg orally daily
tamsulosin *tam-soo-loe'-sin*	Flomax	BPH	Headache, ejaculatory dysfunction, dizziness, rhinitis	0.4 mg orally daily
terazosin *tare-ah'-zoe-sin*	Hytrin	Hypertension, BPH	Dizziness, postural hypotension, headache, dyspnea, nasal congestion	Hypertension: 1–20 mg orally daily BPH: 1–10 mg orally daily

Ⓡ This drug should be administered at least 1 hour before or 2 hours after a meal.

● Chapter Review

Know Your Drugs

Clients sometimes know a medication by the brand (or trade) name and not the generic name. To help you recognize both names, match the brand name with the generic name of the same medication.

Generic Name	Brand Name
1. carvedilol	A. Cardura
2. clonidine	B. Catapres
3. doxazosin	C. Coreg
4. nadolol	D. Corgard

Calculate Medication Dosages

1. A client in long-term care is ordered 50 mg of atenolol. The drug bubble pack card comes in 25-mg tablets per dose. How many tablets does the nurse remove from the bubble pack card?

2. The physician orders 0.4 mg of tamsulosin (Flomax) daily before breakfast. The drug is available in 0.4-mg capsules. The nurse instructs the client to take _____.

● Prepare for the NCLEX®

Build Your Knowledge

1. Antiadrenergic drugs block which of the following transmitters?
   1. serotonin
   2. norepinephrine
   3. dopamine
   4. acetylcholine

2. A client is to receive a β-adrenergic drug for hypertension. Before the drug is administered, the most important assessment the nurse performs is _____.
   1. weighing the client
   2. obtaining blood for laboratory tests
   3. taking a past medical history
   4. taking the blood pressure on both arms

3. When an adrenergic blocking drug is given for a life-threatening cardiac arrhythmia, which of the following activities would the nurse expect to be a part of client care?
   1. daily electrocardiograms
   2. fluid restriction to 1000 mL/day
   3. daily weights
   4. cardiac monitoring

4. To prevent complications when administering a β-adrenergic blocking drug to an elderly client, the nurse would be particularly alert for _____.
   1. vascular insufficiency (e.g., weak peripheral pulses and cold extremities)
   2. complaints of an occipital headache
   3. insomnia
   4. hypoglycemia

5. The client with glaucoma will likely receive a(n) _____.
   1. α/β-adrenergic blocking drug
   2. α-adrenergic blocking drug
   3. β-adrenergic blocking drug
   4. antiadrenergic drug

Apply Your Knowledge

6. When norepinephrine is blocked in the sympathetic nervous system, which of the following occurs?
   1. heart rate increase
   2. blood pressure lowers
   3. GI system slows
   4. bronchi constrict

7. Mr. Garcia was seen with a blood pressure of 210/120 and has taken one dose of metoprolol and returned for a blood pressure reading. Which of the following blood pressures should be reported to the primary health care provider immediately?
   1. 150/100
   2. 200/100
   3. 250/130
   4. 170/80

Alternate-Format Questions

8. The primary health care provider prescribes 60 mg propranolol to be given via the GI tube. The drug is available in an oral solution of 5 mg/mL. The nurse uses a total of 30 mL of warm water to flush before and after administering the drug. The total volume of fluid for this procedure was:
   1. 35 mL of water and drug solution
   2. 42 mL of water and drug solution
   3. 65 mL of water and drug solution
   4. 72 mL of water and drug solution

9. Select the terms that describe drugs that block the sympathetic branch of the ANS. **Select all that apply**.
   1. sympathomimetic
   2. sympatholytic
   3. antiadrenergic
   4. anticholinergic

10. A client has just had a dose increase to 12.5 mg of carvedilol. The client has a bottle with 3.125-mg tablets and insists on finishing the bottle before buying a different strength. The nurse tells the client to take_____.

To check your answers, see Appendix G.

the Point *For more NCLEX-style questions, log on to http://thepoint.lww.com to access more than 1000 questions.*

Cholinergic Drugs

LEARNING OBJECTIVES

On completion of this chapter, the student will:

1. Discuss important aspects of the parasympathetic nervous system.
2. Discuss the uses, drug actions, general adverse reactions, contraindications, precautions, and interactions of cholinergic drugs.
3. Identify important preadministration and ongoing assessment activities the nurse should perform on the patient taking a cholinergic drug.
4. List nursing diagnoses particular to a patient taking a cholinergic drug.
5. Discuss ways to promote an optimal response to therapy, how to manage common adverse reactions, and important points to keep in mind when educating the patient about the use of cholinergic drugs.

KEY TERMS

acetylcholine • neurotransmitter that transmits impulses across the parasympathetic branch of the autonomic nervous system

acetylcholinesterase • enzyme that can inactivate the neurotransmitter acetylcholine

cholinergic crisis • cholinergic drug toxicity

micturition • voiding of urine

miosis • constriction of the pupil of the eye

muscarinic receptors • neurologic receptors that stimulate smooth muscle in the parasympathetic branch of the autonomic nervous system

myasthenia gravis • neuromuscular condition characterized by weakness and fatigability of the muscles

nicotinic receptors • neurologic receptors that stimulate skeletal muscles in the parasympathetic branch of the autonomic nervous system

parasympathomimetic • mimic the activity of the parasympathetic nervous system; also called *cholinergic drugs*

synergistic • the effect is greater than that of each of the two drugs separately

DRUG CLASSES

Direct acting
Indirect acting (anticholinesterase)

Acetylcholine (ACh) is the substance that transmits nerve impulses across the parasympathetic branch of the autonomic nervous system. There are two types of receptors in the parasympathetic nervous branch: **muscarinic receptors** (which stimulate smooth muscle) and **nicotinic receptors** (which stimulate skeletal muscle). Stimulation of this pathway results in the opposite reactions to those triggered by the adrenergic system: blood vessels dilate, sending blood to the gastrointestinal (GI) tract; secretions and peristalsis are activated and salivary glands increase production; the heart slows and pulmonary bronchioles constrict; the smooth muscle of the bladder contracts and the pupils of the eyes constrict (Fig. 26.1). Activation of these nerves is sometimes called the *rest-and-digest* response.

PHARMACOLOGY IN PRACTICE

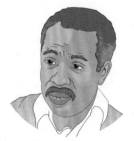

Mr. Park is in the perioperative area, having just been given his preoperative medications for hip surgery. He is very concerned about the function of his bladder and bowels, because after falling in the garden he was unable to get up to urinate and needed to be straight-catheterized in the emergency room. Mr. Park is fearful that the surgery will lead to more retention issues and another infection, this time in his bladder.

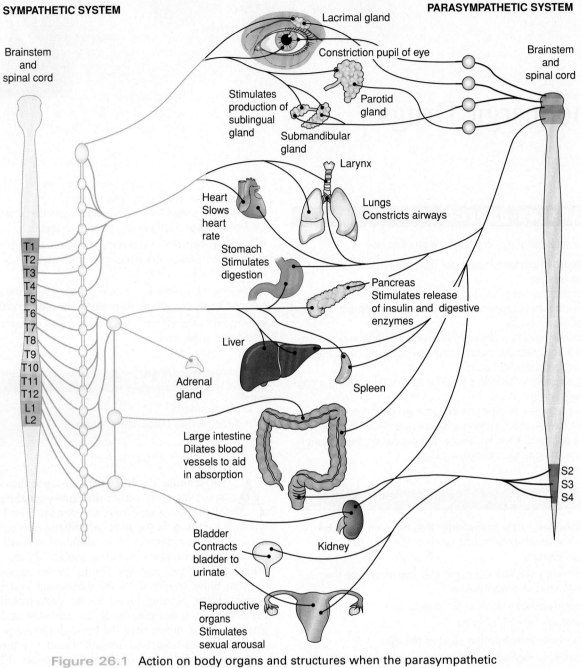

SYMPATHETIC SYSTEM

PARASYMPATHETIC SYSTEM

Brainstem
and
spinal cord

Lacrimal gland

Constriction pupil of eye

Brainstem
and
spinal cord

Stimulates
production of
sublingual
gland

Parotid
gland

Submandibular
gland

Larynx

Heart
Slows
heart
rate

Lungs
Constricts airways

T1
T2
T3
T4
T5
T6
T7
T8
T9
T10
T11
T12
L1
L2

Stomach
Stimulates
digestion

Pancreas
Stimulates release
of insulin and digestive
enzymes

Liver

Adrenal
gland

Spleen

Large intestine
Dilates blood
vessels to aid
in absorption

S2
S3
S4

Bladder
Contracts
bladder to
urinate

Kidney

Reproductive
organs
Stimulates
sexual arousal

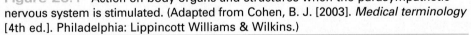

Figure 26.1 Action on body organs and structures when the parasympathetic nervous system is stimulated. (Adapted from Cohen, B. J. [2003]. *Medical terminology* [4th ed.]. Philadelphia: Lippincott Williams & Wilkins.)

Cholinergic drugs mimic the activity of the parasympathetic nervous system. They also are called **parasympathomimetic** drugs. What makes the parasympathetic system function differently is the enzyme **acetylcholinesterase**. Acetylcholinesterase (AChE) is an enzyme that can inactivate the neurotransmitter ACh, thereby preventing the nerve synapse from continuing the nerve impulse. This interruption in neurotransmission can diminish cognitive function, which is seen in illnesses such as Alzheimer's disease. Drugs that inhibit the enzyme AChE are called *anticholinesterases* or *acetylcholinesterase inhibitors*. These drugs are discussed specifically in Chapter 19.

Actions

Cholinergic drugs that act like the neurotransmitter ACh are called *direct-acting cholinergics*. The parasympathetic branch of the autonomic nervous system partly controls the process of **micturition** (voiding of urine) by constricting the detrusor muscle and relaxing the bladder sphincter (see Fig. 26.1). Micturition is both a voluntary and an involuntary act. Urinary retention (not caused by a mechanical obstruction, such as a stone in the bladder) results when micturition is impaired. Treatment of urinary retention with direct-acting cholinergic drugs causes contraction of the bladder smooth muscles and passage of urine.

Myasthenia gravis is a disease that involves rapid fatigue of skeletal muscles because of the lack of ACh released at the nerve endings of parasympathetic nerves. Cholinergic drugs that prolong the activity of ACh by inhibiting the release of AChE are called *indirect-acting cholinergics* or *anticholinesterase muscle stimulants*. Drugs used to treat this disorder act indirectly to inhibit the activity of AChE and promote muscle contraction.

Treatment of glaucoma with an indirect-acting cholinergic drug produces **miosis** (constriction of the iris). Although used for many years, these drugs are rarely used today due to frequency of dosing and side effects experienced. See the Summary Drug Table: Cholinergic Drugs for a more complete listing of these drugs.

Uses

Major uses of the cholinergic drugs are in the treatment of the following:

• Urinary retention
• Myasthenia gravis

Adverse Reactions

Topical administration usually produces few adverse effects, but a temporary reduction of visual acuity (sharpness) and headache may occur. With the exception of those applied topically, cholinergic drugs are not selective in action. General adverse reactions include the following:

• Nausea, diarrhea, abdominal cramping
• Salivation
• Flushing of the skin
• Cardiac arrhythmias and muscle weakness

Contraindications

These drugs are contraindicated in patients with known hypersensitivity to the drugs, asthma, peptic ulcer disease, coronary artery disease, and hyperthyroidism. Bethanechol is contraindicated in those with mechanical obstruction of the GI or genitourinary tracts. Patients with secondary glaucoma, iritis, corneal abrasion, or any acute inflammatory disease of the eye should not use the ophthalmic cholinergic preparations.

Precautions

These drugs are used cautiously in patients with hypertension, epilepsy, cardiac arrhythmias, bradycardia, recent coronary occlusion, and megacolon. The safety of these drugs has not been established for use during pregnancy (pregnancy category C) or lactation, or in children.

Interactions

The following interactions may occur when a cholinergic drug is administered with another agent:

Interacting Drug	Common Use	Effect of Interaction
aminoglycoside antibiotics	Anti-infective agent	Increased neuromuscular blocking effect
corticosteroids	Treatment of inflammation/ respiratory problems	Decreased effect of the cholinergic

When cholinergic drugs are administered with other cholinergics, there is a **synergistic** effect of the drugs and greater risk for toxicity. Concurrent use of more than one anticholinergic drug antagonizes the effects of cholinergic drugs. Because of this property, atropine is considered an antidote for overdosage of cholinergic drugs.

NURSING PROCESS
PATIENT RECEIVING A CHOLINERGIC DRUG

ASSESSMENT

Preadministration Assessment
The preadministration assessment depends on the drug and the reason for administration.

URINARY RETENTION. If a patient receives a cholinergic drug for the treatment of urinary retention, palpate the abdomen in the pelvic area and scan the bladder to determine if urine retention is present. A rounded swelling over the pelvis usually indicates retention and a distended bladder. The patient may also complain of discomfort in the lower abdomen. In addition, take and document the patient's blood pressure and pulse rate.

MYASTHENIA GRAVIS. Before giving a cholinergic drug to a patient with myasthenia gravis, the primary health care provider performs a complete neurologic assessment. Assessment is made for signs of muscle weakness, such as drooling (i.e., the lack of ability to swallow), inability to chew and swallow,

drooping of the eyelids, inability to perform repetitive movements (e.g., walking, combing hair, using eating utensils), difficulty breathing, and extreme fatigue.

Ongoing Assessment
While the patient is receiving a cholinergic drug, it is important to monitor for drug toxicity or cholinergic crisis.

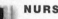 **NURSING ALERT**

Cholinergic crisis (cholinergic drug toxicity) symptoms include severe abdominal cramping, diarrhea, excessive salivation, muscle weakness, rigidity and spasm, and clenching of the jaw. Patients exhibiting these symptoms require immediate medical treatment. In the case of drug overdose, an antidote such as atropine (0.4 to 0.6 mg intravenously [IV]) is administered.

URINARY RETENTION. The ongoing assessment for a patient with urinary retention includes measuring and documenting fluid intake and output. If the amount of each voiding is insufficient or the patient fails to void, palpate the bladder to determine its size, use the bladder scanner after the patient attempts to void, and measure for urine residual. Notify the primary health care provider of the amount of urine the patient is unable to eliminate or if the patient fails to void after drug administration.

MYASTHENIA GRAVIS. Once therapy is under way, document any increase in symptoms of the disease or adverse drug reactions before giving each dose of the drug. Assess the patient for the presence or absence of the symptoms of myasthenia gravis before each drug dose. In patients with severe myasthenia gravis, carry out these assessments between drug doses as well as immediately before drug administration. Document each symptom as well as the patient's response or lack of response to drug therapy.

Assessment is important because the dosage frequently is increased or decreased early in therapy, depending on the patient's response. Regulation of dosage is important in keeping the symptoms of myasthenia gravis from incapacitating the patient. For many patients, the symptoms are fairly well controlled with drug therapy once the optimal drug dose is determined.

NURSING DIAGNOSIS
Drug-specific nursing diagnosis includes:

- **Diarrhea** related to adverse drug reaction

Nursing diagnoses related to drug administration are discussed in Chapter 4.

PLANNING
The expected outcomes of the patient depend on the reason for administration of the cholinergic drug but may include an optimal response to therapy, meeting patient needs related to the management of adverse reactions, and confidence in an understanding of the medication regimen.

IMPLEMENTATION

Promoting an Optimal Response to Therapy
The care of a patient receiving a cholinergic drug depends on the drug used, the reason for administration, and the patient's response to the drug.

MANAGING URINARY RETENTION. Voiding usually occurs in 5 to 15 minutes after subcutaneous drug administration and 30 to 90 minutes after oral administration. For hospitalized patients, place the call light and any other items the patient might need, such as the urinal or the bedpan, within easy reach. However, should the patient feel a sense of urinary urgency and not be able to handle these aids easily, promptly answer the patient's call light.

MANAGING MYASTHENIA GRAVIS. At the start of therapy, determining the dosage that will control symptoms may be difficult. In many cases, the dosage must be adjusted upward or downward until optimal drug effects are obtained. Patients with severe symptoms of the disease require the drug every 2 to 4 hours, even during the night. Sustained-release tablets are available that allow less frequent dosing and help the patient to have longer undisturbed periods during the night.

NURSING ALERT

Because of the need to make frequent dosage adjustments, observe the patient closely for symptoms of

drug overdosage or underdosage. Signs of drug overdosage include muscle rigidity and spasm, salivation, and clenching of the jaw. Signs of drug underdosage are signs of the disease itself, namely, rapid fatigability of the muscles, drooping of the eyelids, and difficulty breathing. If symptoms of drug overdosage or underdosage develop, contact the primary health care provider immediately.

Monitoring and Managing Patient Needs
When a cholinergic drug is given by the oral or parenteral route, adverse drug reactions may affect many systems of the body, such as the heart, respiratory and GI tracts, and central nervous system. Observe the patient closely for the appearance of adverse drug reactions, such as a change in vital signs or an increase in symptoms. You should document any complaints the patient may have and notify the primary health care provider.

DIARRHEA. When these drugs are used orally, they occasionally result in excessive salivation, abdominal cramping, flatus, and sometimes diarrhea. Inform the patient that these reactions will continue until tolerance develops, usually within a few weeks. Until tolerance develops, you need to ensure that proper facilities, such as a bedside commode, bedpan, or bathroom, are readily available. The patient is encouraged to ambulate to assist the passing of flatus. If needed, a rectal tube may be used to assist in the passing of flatus. Document fluid intake and output and track the number, consistency, and frequency of stools if diarrhea is present. The primary health care provider is informed if diarrhea is excessive because this may be an indication of toxicity.

Educating the Patient and Family
Patients required to take a drug over a long period may incur lapses in their drug schedule. For some, it is a matter of occasionally forgetting to take a drug; for others, a lapse may be caused by other factors, such as failure to understand the importance of drug therapy, the cost of the drug, or unfamiliarity with the consequences associated with discontinuing the drug therapy.

When developing a teaching plan for the patient and family, emphasize the importance of uninterrupted drug therapy. Allow the patient and family time to ask questions, especially when dealing with patients who are older or for whom English is not their first language. Explore any problems that appear to be associated with the prescribed drug regimen and then report them to the primary health care provider. Be sure confidence in understanding the purpose of the drug therapy is evident from the patient and family, as well as an understanding of the adverse reactions that may occur.

MYASTHENIA GRAVIS. Patients with myasthenia gravis learn to adjust their drug dosage according to their needs, because dosage needs may vary slightly from day to day. Teach the patient and family members to feel confident in recognizing symptoms of overdosage and underdosage, as well as what steps the primary health care provider wishes them to take if either occurs. The dosage regimen is explained and instruction is given in how to adjust the dosage upward or downward.

Be sure that written or printed descriptions of the signs and symptoms of drug overdosage or underdosage are in the preferred language if the patient does not understand

English. Demonstrate for the patient how to keep a record of the response to drug therapy (e.g., time of day, increased or decreased muscle strength, fatigue) and to bring this to each primary health care provider or clinic visit until the symptoms are well controlled and the drug dosage is stabilized. Make sure these patients have identification (such as a Medic Alert tag) indicating that they have myasthenia gravis.

EVALUATION

- Therapeutic effect is achieved.
- Adverse reactions are identified, reported to the primary health care provider, and managed successfully through appropriate nursing interventions:
  - Patient reports adequate bowel movements.
- Patient and family express confidence and demonstrate an understanding of the drug regimen.

PHARMACOLOGY IN PRACTICE
THINK CRITICALLY

 Urinary retention can lead to placement of a urinary catheter, putting the patient at risk for infection. With the information learned about the cholinergic drugs, what can you tell Mr. Park that will help calm him before surgery?

KEY POINTS

- The parasympathetic branch of the autonomic nervous system functions the opposite of the sympathetic branch. The neurotransmitter of the parasympathetic branch is acetylcholine; activation of this system is often called the rest-and-digest response. What makes this system different is the enzyme acetylcholinesterase. This enzyme inactivates acetylcholine in the nerve synapse.
- The purpose of cholinergic drugs is to send blood flow to the digestive tract, stimulating secretions and peristalsis. The heart rate slows and lung bronchi constrict. Smooth muscle of the bladder contracts and voiding is made possible.

- Drugs that mimic the response are called parasympathomimetic or cholinergic (because the primary transmitter is acetylcholine). Actions in the body are modified depending on how the drug acts on different cell receptors. Drugs can be selective for muscarinic or nicotinic receptors. Drugs can be direct acting or indirect acting.
- These drugs are used to treat urinary retention, the disease myasthenia gravis, and infrequently glaucoma. Adverse reactions are typically GI in nature, ranging from nausea to diarrhea and abdominal cramping.

Summary Drug Table CHOLINERGIC DRUGS

Generic Name	Trade Name	Uses	Adverse Reactions	Dosage Ranges
See Chapter 19 for Cholinesterase Inhibitors				
Direct-Acting Cholinergics				
bethanechol *beh-than'-eh-koll*	Duvoid, Urecholine	Acute nonobstructive urinary retention, neurogenic atony of urinary bladder with urinary retention	Abdominal discomfort, headache, diarrhea, nausea, salivation, urgency	10–50 mg orally BID to QID; 2.5–5 mg subcutaneously TID to QID
Indirect-Acting (Anticholinesterase) Muscle Stimulants				
ambenonium *am-beh-noe'-nee-um*	Mytelase	Myasthenia gravis	Increased bronchial secretions, cardiac arrhythmias, muscle weakness, urinary frequency	5–75 mg orally TID, QID
edrophonium *ed-roe-foh'-nee-yum*	Tensilon	Diagnosis of myasthenia gravis	Increased bronchial secretions, cardiac arrhythmias, muscle weakness, urinary frequency	2–10 mg IV, look for cholinergic reaction (muscle weakness)
guanidine *goo-wan'-eh-deen*		Myasthenic syndrome (Eaton-Lambert disease)	Palpitations, numbness in lips/extremities, dry mouth, nausea, abdominal cramping	10–30 mg/kg/day, titrate until adverse reaction occurs
pyridostigmine *peer-ih-doe-stig'-meen*	Mestinon, Regonol	Myasthenia gravis	Increased bronchial secretions, cardiac arrhythmias, muscle weakness	Average dose is 600 mg/day orally at spaced intervals

● Chapter Review

Know Your Drugs

Clients sometimes know a medication by the brand (or trade) name and not the generic name. To help you recognize both names, match the brand name with the generic name of the same medication.

Generic Name	Brand Name
1. bethanechol	A. Duvoid
2. edrophonium	B. Tensilon
	C. Urecholine

Calculate Medication Dosages

1. The primary care provider prescribes 2.5 mg of bethanechol subcutaneously. The drug is available in a solution of 5 mg/mL. The nurse administers _____.

● Prepare for the NCLEX®

Build Your Knowledge

1. What is the transmitting substance in the parasympathetic branch of the nervous system?

   1. serotonin
   2. norepinephrine
   3. dopamine
   4. acetylcholine

2. In which condition are drugs used to stop the enzyme that prevents neurotransmission?

   1. urinary retention
   2. myasthenia gravis
   3. glaucoma
   4. Alzheimer's disease

3. A client has received a diagnosis of myasthenia gravis and begins a regimen of ambenonium. The nursing assessment is important because the dose of the drug _____.

   1. usually must be increased every 4 hours early in therapy
   2. frequently is increased or decreased early in therapy
   3. is titrated according to the client's blood pressure
   4. is gradually decreased as a therapeutic response is achieved

Apply Your Knowledge

4. When acetylcholine is transmitted in the parasympathetic nervous system, which of the following occurs?

   1. heart rate increases
   2. pupils of the eye dilate
   3. digestion is stimulated
   4. bronchi relax

Alternate-Format Questions

5. Select the terms that describe drugs that stimulate the parasympathetic branch of the ANS. **Select all that apply**.

   1. parasympathomimetic
   2. parasympatholytic
   3. adrenergic
   4. cholinergic

6. The dosage of pyridostigmine bromide (Mestinon) is 600 mg/day. How many 60-mg tablets will the patient take?

To check your answers, see Appendix G.

the**Point** *For more NCLEX-style questions, log on to http://thepoint.lww.com to access more than 1000 questions.*

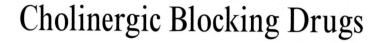

Cholinergic Blocking Drugs

LEARNING OBJECTIVES

On completion of this chapter, the student will:

1. Discuss the uses, general drug actions, general adverse reactions, contraindications, precautions, and interactions of the cholinergic blocking drugs (also called anticholinergic drugs and cholinergic blockers).
2. Discuss important preadministration and ongoing assessment activities the nurse should perform on the patient taking a cholinergic blocking drug.
3. List nursing diagnoses particular to the patient taking a cholinergic blocking drug.
4. Discuss ways to promote an optimal response to therapy, how to manage common adverse reactions, and important points to keep in mind when educating patients taking cholinergic blocking drugs.

KEY TERMS

anticholinergic • blocks the neurotransmission of the parasympathetic nervous system

cholinergic blocking • blocks the affect of the parasympathetic branch of the autonomic nervous system; also called anticholinergics

cycloplegia • paralysis of the ciliary muscle, resulting in an inability to focus the eye

drug idiosyncrasy • any unusual or abnormal response that differs from the response normally expected to a specific drug and dosage

mydriasis • dilation of the pupil

parasympatholytic • blocking the parasympathetic nervous system

xerostomia • drying of oral secretions

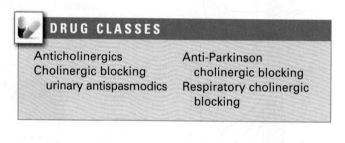

DRUG CLASSES

Anticholinergics	Anti-Parkinson
Cholinergic blocking	cholinergic blocking
urinary antispasmodics	Respiratory cholinergic blocking

Like adrenergic blocking drugs, the **cholinergic blocking** drugs have an effect on the autonomic nervous system. Cholinergic blocking drugs are also called **anticholinergic** drugs, *cholinergic blockers,* or **parasympatholytic** drugs.

Acetylcholine (ACh) is the primary neurotransmitter in the parasympathetic branch of the autonomic nervous system. Cholinergic blocking drugs block the action of the neurotransmitter ACh in the parasympathetic nervous system. Because parasympathetic nerves influence many areas of the body, the effects of the cholinergic blocking drugs are numerous.

Actions

Cholinergic blocking drugs inhibit the activity of ACh at the parasympathetic nerve synapse. When the activity of ACh is inhibited, impulses traveling along the parasympathetic nerve cannot pass from the nerve ending to the effector organ or structure.

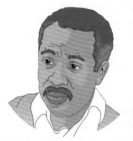

PHARMACOLOGY IN PRACTICE

Mr. Park is in the perioperative area having just been given his preoperative medications for hip surgery. He is very concerned about the function of his bladder and bowels. His stomach feels "rumbly" and he is very concerned that he will be incontinent of stool in the bed. After reading this chapter, decide whether his concerns are valid.

SYMPATHETIC SYSTEM

PARASYMPATHETIC SYSTEM

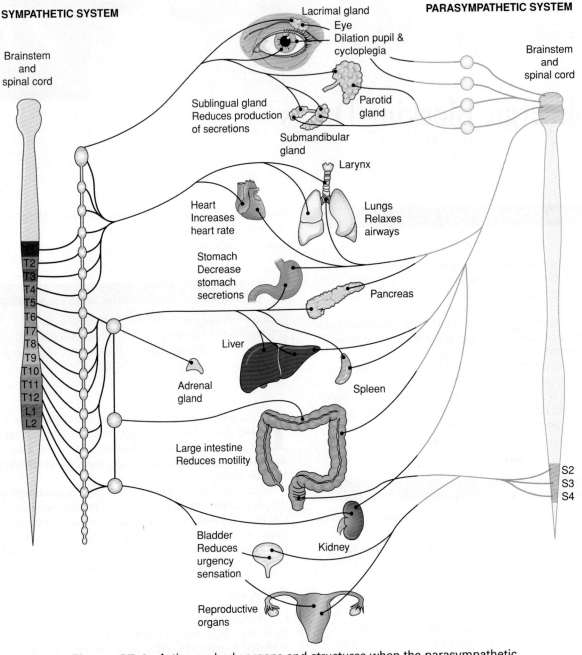

Figure 27.1 Action on body organs and structures when the parasympathetic nervous system is blocked. (From Cohen, B. J. [2003]. *Medical terminology* [4th ed.]. Philadelphia: Lippincott Williams & Wilkins.)

Two types of receptors are found in the parasympathetic nerve branch: muscarinic and nicotinic receptors. Cholinergic blocking drugs can specifically target one of these types of receptors. For example, antispasmodic drugs used to treat an overactive urinary bladder work by inhibiting the action of the muscarinic receptors in the parasympathetic nervous system. As a result, the detrusor muscle of the bladder does not contract, which prevents the sensations of urinary urgency. Yet, an antispasmodic drug has no effect on skeletal muscles, because it does not inhibit the nicotinic receptors in the parasympathetic nervous system.

Because of the wide distribution of parasympathetic nerves, some of these drugs that inhibit nerve impulses at both muscarinic and nicotinic receptors affect many organs and structures of the body, including the eyes, the respiratory and gastrointestinal (GI) tracts, the heart, and the bladder (Fig. 27.1).

However, responses to administration of a cholinergic blocking drug vary and often depend on the drug and the dose used. For example, scopolamine may occasionally cause excitement, delirium, and restlessness. This reaction is considered a **drug idiosyncrasy** (an unexpected or unusual drug effect).

Uses

The primary uses of cholinergic blocking drugs are in the treatment of the following:

- Pylorospasm and peptic ulcer
- Ureteral or biliary colic and bladder overactivity
- Vagal nerve–induced bradycardia
- Parkinsonism

In addition, the cholinergic blocking drugs are administered for the preoperative reduction of oral secretions. The Summary Drug Table: Cholinergic Blocking Drugs lists the uses of specific cholinergic blocking drugs.

Adverse Reactions

The severity of many adverse reactions is often dose dependent—that is, the larger the dose, the more intense the adverse reaction. Bodily system adverse reactions that may occur with the administration of a cholinergic blocking drug are listed in the following sections.

Gastrointestinal System Reactions

- Dry mouth, nausea, vomiting
- Difficulty in swallowing, heartburn
- Constipation

Central Nervous System Reactions

- Headache, flushing, nervousness
- Drowsiness, weakness, insomnia
- Nasal congestion, fever

Visual Reactions

- Blurred vision
- **Mydriasis** (dilation of the pupil)
- Photophobia
- **Cycloplegia** (paralysis of accommodation or inability to focus the eye)
- Increased ocular tension

Genitourinary System Reactions

- Urinary hesitancy and retention
- Dysuria

Cardiovascular System Reactions

- Palpitations
- Bradycardia (after low doses of atropine)
- Tachycardia (after higher doses of atropine)

Other Reactions

- Urticaria
- Decreased sweat production
- Anaphylactic shock
- Rash

Sometimes a secondary adverse reaction, such as drowsiness, is desirable. For example, when atropine is used before surgery to reduce the production of secretions in the respiratory tract, drowsiness is part of the desired response.

 LIFESPAN CONSIDERATIONS
Gerontology
Older patients receiving a cholinergic blocking drug may exhibit symptoms such as excitement, agitation, mental confusion, drowsiness, urinary retention, or other adverse effects. These effects may be seen even with small doses. If any should occur, withhold the next dose of the drug and contact the primary health care provider.

During hot summer months, patients receiving a cholinergic blocking drug should be instructed to watch for signs of heat prostration (e.g., fever; tachycardia; flushing; warm, dry skin; mental confusion) because these drugs decrease sweating.

Contraindications

Cholinergic blocking drugs are contraindicated in patients with known hypersensitivity to the drugs or glaucoma. Other patients for whom cholinergic blocking drugs are contraindicated are those with myasthenia gravis, tachyarrhythmias, myocardial infarction, and heart failure (unless bradycardia is present).

Precautions

These drugs are used with caution in patients with GI infections, benign prostatic hypertrophy, urinary retention, hyperthyroidism, hepatic or renal disease, and hypertension. Use atropine with caution in patients with asthma. Cholinergic blocking drugs are classified as pregnancy category C drugs and are used only when the benefit to the woman outweighs the risk to the fetus.

This caution also applies to over-the-counter (OTC) preparations available for the relief of allergy and cold symptoms and as aids to induce sleep. Some of these products contain atropine, scopolamine, or other cholinergic blocking drugs. Although this warning is printed on the container or package, many users fail to read drug labels carefully.

Interactions

The following interactions may occur when a cholinergic blocking drug is administered with another agent:

Interacting Drug	Common Use	Effect of Interaction
antibiotics/antifungals	Fight infection	Decreased effectiveness of anti-infective drug
meperidine, flurazepam, phenothiazines	Preoperative sedation	Increased effect of the cholinergic blocker
tricyclic antidepressants	Management of depression	Increased effect of the cholinergic blocker
haloperidol	Antianxiety/antipsychotic agent	Decreased effectiveness of the antipsychotic drug
digoxin	Management of cardiac problems	Increased serum levels of digoxin

NURSING PROCESS
PATIENT RECEIVING A CHOLINERGIC BLOCKING DRUG

ASSESSMENT

Preadministration Assessment
Before administering a cholinergic blocking drug to a patient for the first time, obtain a thorough health history as well as a history of the signs and symptoms of the current disorder. The focus of the initial physical assessment depends on the reason for administering the drug. In most instances, obtain the blood pressure, pulse, and respiratory rate. Additional assessments may include checking the stool of the patient who has a peptic ulcer for color and signs of occult blood, determining visual acuity in the patient with glaucoma, and looking for signs of dehydration and weighing the patient if prolonged diarrhea is one of the patient's symptoms.

Ongoing Assessment
When administering a cholinergic blocking drug, check vital signs, observe for adverse drug reactions, and evaluate the symptoms and complaints related to the patient's diagnosis. For example, question the patient with a peptic ulcer regarding current symptoms, and then make a comparison of these symptoms with the symptoms present before the start of therapy. Document any increase in the severity of symptoms and notify the primary health care provider.

NURSING DIAGNOSES
Drug-specific nursing diagnoses include:

- **Impaired Comfort** related to xerostomia
- **Constipation** related to slowing of peristalsis in the GI tract
- **Risk for Injury** related to dizziness, drowsiness, mental confusion, impaired vision, or heat prostration
- **Ineffective Tissue Perfusion** related to impaired heart pumping action

Nursing diagnoses related to drug administration are discussed in Chapter 4.

PLANNING
The expected outcomes for the patient depend on the reason for administration of a cholinergic blocking drug but may include an optimal response to therapy, meeting patient needs related to the management of adverse reactions, and confidence in an understanding of and adherence to the prescribed medication regimen.

IMPLEMENTATION

Promoting an Optimal Response to Therapy
If a cholinergic blocking drug is administered before surgery, be sure to give it at the exact time prescribed because the drug must be given time to produce the greatest effect (i.e., the drying of upper respiratory and oral secretions) before the administration of a general anesthetic. Before administration, instruct the patient to void. Inform the patient and family members that drowsiness and extreme dryness of the mouth and nose will occur about 20 to 30 minutes after the drug is

given. This is normal, and fluid is not to be taken. The side rails of the bed are raised, and the patient is instructed to remain in bed after administration of the preoperative drug.

LIFESPAN CONSIDERATIONS
Gerontology
Cholinergic blocking drugs are usually not included in the preoperative drugs of patients older than 60 years because of the effects of these drugs on the eye and the central nervous system.

Monitoring and Managing Patient Needs
IMPAIRED COMFORT: XEROSTOMIA. When taking these drugs on a daily basis, mouth dryness may be severe and extremely uncomfortable. The patient may complain of a "cottonmouth" sensation, in which oral dryness feels like a mouthful of cotton. The patient may have moderate to extreme difficulty swallowing drugs and food. The patient's speech may be impeded and hard to understand because of the dry mouth.

Encourage the patient to take a few sips of water before and while taking an oral drug and to sip water at intervals during meals. If allowed, hard candy slowly dissolved in the mouth and frequent sips of water during the day may help relieve persistent oral dryness. Check the oral cavity frequently for soreness or ulcerations. Refer to the Patient Teaching for Improved Patient Outcomes: Combating Dry Mouth for suggestions on diminishing the discomfort.

CONSTIPATION. Constipation caused by decreased gastric motility can be a problem with cholinergic blocking drugs. Encourage the patient to increase fluid intake up to 2000 mL

Patient Teaching for Improved Patient Outcomes
Combating Dry Mouth

One of the most common and uncomfortable adverse effects occurring with the use of cholinergic blocking drugs is a dry mouth. There are strategies to help both reduce the discomfort and maintain a healthy oral cavity.

When you teach, make sure your patient understands the following:

- ✔ Perform frequent mouth care, including brushing, rinsing, and flossing.
- ✔ Keep a glass or sports bottle filled with fluid on hand at all times.
- ✔ Sip small amounts of cool water or fluids throughout the day and with meals.
- ✔ Try one of the flavor additives or a slice of lemon, lime, or cucumber in the water.
- ✔ Take a few sips of water before taking any oral drugs.
- ✔ Suck on ice chips or frozen ices, such as popsicles.
- ✔ Chew gum, preferably sugarless.
- ✔ Suck on sugar-free hard candies.
- ✔ Avoid alcohol-based mouthwashes.

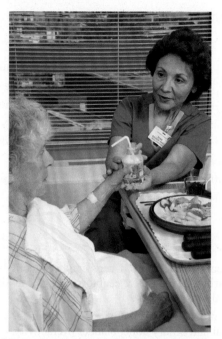

Figure 27.2 Due to the reduction in secretions caused by anticholinergic drugs, encouraging fluids is emphasized during all patient interactions.

daily (if health conditions permit), eat a diet high in fiber, and engage in adequate exercise. Patients being treated for an overactive bladder may be hesitant to increase fluids because of fear of an episode of urinary incontinence. Reassure the patient that increasing fluids will help minimize the adverse reactions of constipation and dry mouth, whereas the cholinergic blocking drug helps to eliminate the sensations of urinary frequency and urgency (Fig. 27.2). The primary health care provider may prescribe a stool softener, if necessary, to prevent constipation.

RISK FOR INJURY. These drugs may cause drowsiness, dizziness, and blurred vision. Patients (especially older adults) may require assistance with ambulation. Blurred vision and photophobia are commonly seen with the administration of a cholinergic blocking drug. The severity of this adverse reaction is commonly dose dependent; that is, the larger the dose, the more intense the adverse reaction.

Monitor the patient for any disturbance in vision. If photophobia is a problem, the patient may need to wear shaded glasses when going outside, even on cloudy days. Rooms are kept dimly lit and curtains or blinds closed to eliminate bright sunlight in the room. Those with photophobia may be more comfortable in a semi-darkened room, especially on sunny days. It is a good idea to use overhead lights as little as possible.

Mydriasis (prolonged pupillary dilation) and cycloplegia (difficulty focusing resulting from paralysis of the ciliary muscle), if they occur, may interfere with reading, watching television, and similar activities. If these drug effects upset the patient, discuss the problem with the primary health care provider. At times, these visual impairments will have to be tolerated because drug therapy cannot be changed or discontinued. Encourage the patient to engage in other forms of

diversional therapy, such as interaction with others or listening to the radio.

 LIFESPAN CONSIDERATIONS
Gerontology
Discuss with the family of an older patient possible visual and mental impairments (blurred vision, confusion, agitation) that may occur during therapy with these drugs. Objects or situations that may cause falls, such as throw rugs, footstools, and wet or newly waxed floors, are removed or avoided whenever possible. Show the family how to place against the walls any items of furniture (e.g., footstools, chairs, stands) that obstruct walkways. Alert the family to the dangers of heat prostration and explains the steps to take to avoid this problem.

In hot weather, sweating may decrease and may be followed by heat prostration. Make sure the patient is observed at frequent intervals for signs of heat prostration, especially if the patient is older or debilitated. Avoid going outside on hot, sunny days; use fans to cool the body if the day is extremely warm; sponge the skin with cool water if other cooling measures are not available; and wear loose-fitting clothes in warm weather. In cases of suspected heat prostration, the next dose of the drug is withheld and the primary health care provider contacted immediately. The older adult patient receiving a cholinergic blocking drug is also observed at frequent intervals for excitement, agitation, mental confusion, drowsiness, urinary retention, or other adverse effects. If any of these should occur, the next dose of the drug should be withheld and the primary health care provider contacted. Patient safety must be ensured until these adverse reactions subside.

INEFFECTIVE TISSUE PERFUSION. The patient receiving atropine for third-degree heart block is placed on a cardiac monitor during and after administration of the drug. The monitor is watched for a change in pulse rate or rhythm. Tachycardia, other cardiac arrhythmias, or failure of the drug to increase the heart rate is reported to the primary health care provider immediately because other drugs or medical management may be necessary.

Educating the Patient and Family
A cholinergic blocking drug may be prescribed for a prolonged period. Some patients may discontinue drug use, especially if their original symptoms have been relieved. Make sure that the patient and family understand that the prescribed drug is to be continued even though symptoms have been relieved.

When a cholinergic blocking drug is prescribed for outpatient use, teach the patient about the more common adverse reactions associated with these drugs, such as dry mouth, drowsiness, dizziness, and visual impairments. Warn the patient that if drowsiness, dizziness, or blurred vision occurs, caution must be observed while driving or performing other tasks requiring alertness and clear vision.

Some of the adverse reactions associated with the cholinergic blocking drugs may be uncomfortable or distressing. Encourage the patient to discuss these problems with the primary health care provider. You can offer suggestions to lessen the intensity of some of these adverse reactions.

EVALUATION

■ Therapeutic effect is achieved.

■ Adverse reactions are identified, reported to the primary health care provider, and managed successfully through appropriate nursing interventions:
- Mucous membranes remain moist.
- Patient reports adequate bowel movements.
- No evidence of injury is seen.
- Vision remains intact.
- Tissue perfusion is maintained.

■ Patient and family express confidence and demonstrate an understanding of the drug regimen.

PHARMACOLOGY IN PRACTICE
THINK CRITICALLY

 A nurse assistant comes to you because she is having difficulty with Mr. Park. The nursing assistant is frustrated with his continual struggles to get out of bed and asks you about the purpose of preoperative drugs and why patients cannot get out of bed after receiving a preoperative drug. Describe how you would explain this to the nurse assistant.

KEY POINTS

- The parasympathetic branch of the autonomic nervous system regulates both involuntary body functions and skeletal muscles. The anticholinergic drugs block the neurotransmitter acetylcholine in the parasympathetic branch.

- The purpose of cholinergic blocking drugs is to block or interrupt the signals that divert blood flow to the vital organs. Instead, the blood vessels dilate and smooth muscle relaxes. The heart rate decreases and lowers the blood pressure.

- Drugs that block the parasympathetic system are called parasympatholytic or anticholinergic. Actions in the body are modified depending on how the drug acts on

different cell receptors. Drugs can be selective for muscarinic or nicotinic receptors. Drugs can also affect skeletal muscles.

- These drugs are used to treat gastric sphincter spasm, ureteral and biliary colic, bladder overactivity, bradycardia, and Parkinson's disease.

- Adverse reactions include decreased oral secretions, slower GI motility, constipation, nasal congestion, vision problems, and urinary retention. Mental reactions of excitement, agitation, confusion, and drowsiness may occur, especially in the older patient.

Summary Drug Table CHOLINERGIC BLOCKING DRUGS

Generic Name	Trade Name	Uses	Adverse Reactions	Dosage Ranges
atropine *ah'-troe-peen*	AtroPen	Pylorospasm, reduction of bronchial and oral secretions, excessive vagal-induced bradycardia, ureteral and biliary colic	Drowsiness, blurred vision, tachycardia, dry mouth, urinary hesitancy	0.4–0.6 mg orally, IM, subcut, IV
belladonna *bel-lah-doan'-ah*		Adjunctive therapy for peptic ulcer, digestive disorders, diverticulitis, pancreatitis, diarrhea	Same as atropine	0.25–0.5 mg orally TID
dicyclomine *dye-sye'-kloe-meen*	Bentyl	Functional bowel/irritable bowel syndrome	Same as atropine	80–160 mg orally QID
glycopyrrolate *glye-koe-pye'-roe-late*	Robinul	Oral: peptic ulcer Parenteral: in conjunction with anesthesia to reduce bronchial and oral secretions, to block cardiac vagal inhibitory reflexes during induction of anesthesia and intubation; protection against the peripheral muscarinic effects of cholinergic agents (e.g., neostigmine)	Blurred vision, dry mouth, altered taste perception, nausea, vomiting, dysphagia, urinary hesitancy and retention	Oral: 1–2 mg BID or TID Parenteral: peptic ulcer, 0.1–0.2 mg IM, IV, TID, QID Preanesthesia: 0.002 mg/lb IM Intraoperative: 0.1 mg IV
mepenzolate *meh-pen'-zoe-late*	Cantil	Adjunctive treatment of peptic ulcer	Same as atropine	25–50 mg orally TID or QID with meals and at bedtime
methscopolamine *meth-scoe-pol'-ah-meen*	Pamine	Adjunctive therapy for peptic ulcer	Same as atropine	2.5 mg 30 min before meals and 2.5–5 mg orally at bedtime
propantheline *proe-pan'-theh-leen*		Adjunctive therapy for peptic ulcer	Dry mouth, constipation, hesitancy, urinary retention, blurred vision	15 mg orally 30 min before meals and at bedtime

Summary Drug Table CHOLINERGIC BLOCKING DRUGS (continued)

Generic Name	Trade Name	Uses	Adverse Reactions	Dosage Ranges
scopolamine *scoe-pol'-ah-meen*	.	Preanesthetic sedation, motion sickness	Confusion, dry mouth, constipation, urinary hesitancy, urinary retention, blurred vision	0.32–0.65 mg IM, subcut, IV, diluted with sterile water for injections Transdermal: apply 1 patch 4 hr before travel q 3 days
trimethobenzamide *trye-meth-oh-ben'-zah-mide*	Tigan	Control of nausea and vomiting	Hypotension (IM use), Parkinson-like symptoms, blurred vision, drowsiness, dizziness	250 mg orally or 200 mg IM, rectal suppository TID or QID
Cholinergic Blocking Urinary Antispasmodics				
darifenacin *dah-ree-fen'-ah-sin*	Enablex	Overactive bladder	Dry mouth, constipation	7.5 mg orally daily
fesoterodine *fes-oh-ter'-oh-deen*	Toviaz	Overactive bladder	Dry mouth, constipation	4–8 mg orally daily
flavoxate *flah-vox'-ate*		Urinary symptoms caused by cystitis, prostatitis, and other urinary problems	Dry mouth, drowsiness, blurred vision, headache, urinary retention	100–200 mg orally 3–4 times/day
oxybutynin *ox-see-byoo-tye'-nin*	Ditropan XL	Overactive bladder, neurogenic bladder	Dry mouth, nausea, headache, drowsiness, constipation, urinary retention	5 mg orally, 2–3 times/day; 3.9 mg transdermal, use 3–4 days
solifenacin *sole-ih-fen'-ah-sin*	Vesicare	Overactive bladder	Dry mouth, constipation, blurred vision, dry eyes	5 mg orally daily
tolterodine *toll-tare'-oh-dyne*	Detrol, Detrol LA (long acting, extended release)	Overactive bladder	Dry mouth, constipation, headache, dizziness	2 mg orally, TID; extended release: 4 mg daily
Ⓡ trospium *troz'-pee-um*	Sanctura	Overactive bladder	Dry mouth, constipation, headache	20 mg orally TID
Cholinergic Blocking Drugs for Parkinson's Disease				
benztropine mesylate *benz'-troe-peen*	Cogentin	Parkinson's disease, drug-induced extrapyramidal syndrome (EPS)	Dry mouth, blurred vision, dizziness, nausea, nervousness, skin rash, urinary retention, dysuria, tachycardia, muscle weakness, disorientation, confusion	0.5–6 mg/day orally Acute dystonia: 1–2 mL IM or IV
biperiden *bye-pare'-ih-den*	Akineton	Parkinson's disease, drug-induced EPS	Same as benztropine mesylate	2 mg orally TID or QID; maximum dose 16 mg/24 hr
diphenhydramine *dye-fen-hye'-dra-meen*	Benadryl	Drug-induced EPS, allergies	Same as benztropine mesylate	25–50 mg orally TID or QID
trihexyphenidyl *trye-hex-see-fen'-ih-dill*		Parkinsonism symptoms, drug-induced EPS	Same as benztropine mesylate	1–15 mg/day orally in divided doses
Cholinergic Blocking Drug (for Acute Respiratory Symptom Relief)				
ipratropium *ih-prah-troe'-pee-um*	Atrovent	Bronchospasm associated with chronic obstructive pulmonary disease, chronic bronchitis and emphysema, rhinorrhea	Dryness of the oropharynx, nervousness, irritation from aerosol, dizziness, headache, GI distress, dry mouth, exacerbation of symptoms, nausea, palpitations	Aerosol: 2 inhalations QID, not to exceed 12 inhalations; Solution: 500 mg (1 unit dose vial) TID, QID by oral nebulization Nasal spray: 2 sprays per nostril BID, TID of 0.03%, or 2 sprays per nostril TID, QID of 0.06%
tiotropium *tee-oh-troe'-pee-um*	Spiriva	Same as ipratropium	Same as ipratropium, increased stroke potential	1 capsule per day using inhalation device, not for oral use

Ⓡ This drug should be administered at least 1 hour before or 2 hours after a meal.

● Chapter Review

Know Your Drugs

Clients sometimes know a medication by the brand (or trade) name and not the generic name. To help you recognize both names, match the brand name with the generic name of the same medication.

Generic Name	Brand Name
1. benztropine mesylate	A. Cogentin
2. fesoterodine	B. Ditropan XL
3. oxybutynin	C. Tigan
4. trimethobenzamide	D. Toviaz

Calculate Medication Dosages

1. A client is prescribed glycopyrrolate (Robinul) 0.1 mg intramuscularly (IM). The drug is available in a solution of 0.2 mg/mL. The nurse administers _____.

2. Oral trihexyphenidyl 4 mg is ordered. The drug is available as an elixir with a strength of 2 mg/5 mL. The nurse administers _____.

● Prepare for the NCLEX®

Build Your Knowledge

1. Anticholinergic drugs block which of the following transmitters?
   1. acetylcholine
   2. dopamine
   3. norepinephrine
   4. serotonin

2. A client taking solifenacin (Vesicare) for an overactive bladder complains of dry mouth. The nurse should _____.
   1. consider this to be unusual and contact the primary health care provider
   2. encourage the client to take frequent sips of water
   3. give the client salt-water mouth rinses
   4. ignore this reaction because it is only temporary

3. Which of the following adverse reactions would the nurse expect after the administration of atropine as part of a client's preoperative medication regimen?
   1. enhanced action of anesthesia
   2. reduced secretions of the upper respiratory tract
   3. prolonged action of the preoperative opioid
   4. increased gastric motility

4. Because of the effect of cholinergic blocking drugs on intestinal motility, the nurse must monitor the client taking these drugs for the development of _____.
   1. esophageal ulcers
   2. diarrhea
   3. heartburn
   4. constipation

5. Cholinergic blocking drugs are contraindicated in clients with _____.
   1. gout
   2. glaucoma
   3. diabetes
   4. bradycardia

6. A cholinergic blocking drug is administered and the client becomes acutely confused this is an example of _____.
   1. synergism
   2. agonist–antagonist effect
   3. drug idiosyncrasy
   4. sympathetic nervous system response

Apply Your Knowledge

7. When acetylcholine is blocked in the parasympathetic nervous system, which of the following occurs?
   1. pupils constrict
   2. heart rate decreases
   3. GI system becomes active
   4. salivary glands secrete less

8. The nurse has administered a presurgical anticholinergic drug about 30 minutes ago. Which of the following responses would be of concern and should be reported immediately?
   1. "Nurse, my throat is dry."
   2. "I'm feeling a bit anxious. When will the surgeon be here?"
   3. "I need to leave. I have important business to do!"
   4. "My nose is suddenly stuffy. I wonder if I have a cold."

Alternate-Format Questions

9. Select the terms that describe drugs that block the parasympathetic branch of the ANS. **Select all that apply**.
   1. parasympathomimetic
   2. parasympatholytic
   3. antiadrenergic
   4. anticholinergic

10. A client says he is stopping the anticholinergic drug because of dry mouth and constipation. What are some teaching tips the nurse can offer to reduce these adverse reactions? **Select all that apply**.
    1. Add more fiber to diet
    2. Limit fluid intake
    3. Swish mouth with water periodically
    4. Add a cucumber to drinking water
    5. Brush and floss teeth regularly

To check your answers, see Appendix G.

thePoint *For more NCLEX-style questions, log on to http://thepoint.lww.com to access more than 1000 questions.*

Drugs That Affect the Neuromuscular System

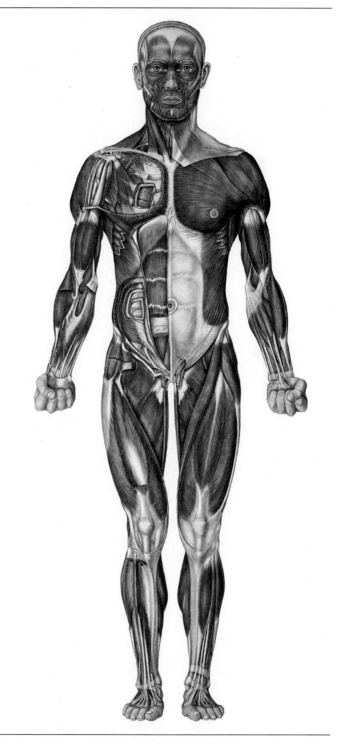

Previous units in this book have examined both the central and peripheral nervous systems of our bodies and how drugs affect function both in those systems and in other selected bodily systems. The focus of Unit VI is on how the nervous system connects with the muscles in our bodies to help produce movement based on the direction given by our brains.

The musculoskeletal system comprises the bones, joints, and muscles that provide the body with movement. Although separate from the nervous system, they work together as the neuromuscular system to provide our bodies with the ability to live, work, and play. A number of degenerative diseases (Alzheimer's disease, Parkinson's disease, and fibromyalgia) affect both the musculoskeletal and neurologic systems.

Many drugs are designed to strengthen or diminish motor messages from the brain to the muscles and other tissues. Some of these categories include antiparkinson, anticonvulsant (or antiseizure), and muscle relaxant drugs.

Parkinson's disease is seen in approximately 1% of those older than 60 years of age. This disease affects the messages sent from the central nervous system (CNS) to the muscles of the body. The disease is caused by an imbalance of dopamine and acetylcholine in the CNS. An area of the brain, the substantia nigra, loses cells and the supply of the neurotransmitter dopamine is decreased. As a result, too much acetylcholine affects this area of the brain, which controls muscle movement, causing such symptoms as trembling, rigidity, difficulty walking, and problems with balance. In earlier chapters you learned about drugs that can have adverse reactions similar to the symptoms of Parkinson's disease. Select drugs can reduce the symptoms that impact the neuromuscular system when caused by the disease or by other drugs. These drugs are covered in Chapter 28 and relieve the symptoms of both Parkinson's disease and adverse reactions of other drugs that assist in maintaining the patient's mobility and functioning capability for as long as possible.

Neurotransmission of the brain can be overexcited by injury or disease. When this happens, seizures (or convulsions) occur. Chapter 29 discusses the drugs used to depress abnormal brain activity and lessen or prevent seizure activity.

The promotion of mobility and function of bones and joints are the focus of Chapter 30. Drugs used to prevent injury or fracture from osteoporosis or to treat conditions such as rheumatoid arthritis and the use of relaxants for muscle spasm are discussed.

Drugs That Affect the Neuromuscular System

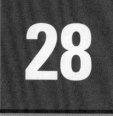

Antiparkinson Drugs

KEY TERMS

achalasia • failure to relax; usually referring to the smooth muscle fibers of the gastrointestinal (GI) tract, especially failure of the lower esophagus to relax, causing difficulty swallowing and a feeling of fullness in the sternal region

agonist • a drug that binds with a receptor and stimulates the receptor to produce a therapeutic response

akathisia • extreme restlessness and increased motor activity

blood–brain barrier • ability of the nervous system to prohibit large and potentially harmful molecules from crossing from the blood into the brain

bradykinesia • slow movement

choreiform movements • involuntary muscular twitching of the limbs or facial muscles

dystonic • muscular spasms most often affecting the tongue, jaw, eyes, and neck

extrapyramidal symptoms (EPS) • group of adverse reactions involving the extrapyramidal portion of the nervous system causing abnormal muscle movements, especially akathisia and dystonia

on-off phenomenon • fluctuation in levodopa therapy where inconsistent absorption causes alternating improved status and loss of therapeutic effect

parkinsonism • referring to a cluster of symptoms associated with Parkinson's disease (i.e., fine tremors, slowing of voluntary movements, muscular weakness)

Parkinson's disease • degenerative disorder caused by an imbalance of dopamine and acetylcholine in the CNS

restless leg syndrome • disorder with an irresistible urge to move the legs; urge lessens with movement but worsens with rest

DRUG CLASSES

Dopaminergic agents	COMT (catechol-O-methyltransferase) inhibitors
Monoamine oxidase inhibitors (MAOIs)	
Dopamine receptor agonists	Cholinergic blocking agents (anticholinergic drugs)

PHARMACOLOGY IN PRACTICE

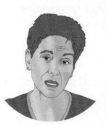

A woman in the clinic waiting room comes to the front desk and says, "That lady over there is odd. She looks like she is keeping tune to a song with her hand and her head, but there is no music playing. I don't feel comfortable sitting here in the waiting area." The patient is Betty Peterson, and she been taking amitriptyline for depression.

The drugs featured in this chapter are used to treat both disease and adverse reactions of other medications. **Parkinsonism** is a general term that refers to a group of symptoms involving motor movement. The name comes from **Parkinson's disease**, a progressive neurologic disease with symptoms that worsen over time. The cardinal signs of Parkinson's disease include tremors, rigidity, and slow movement (**bradykinesia**).

Other symptoms of Parkinson's disease include slurred speech, the face taking on a mask-like and emotionless appearance, and the patient possibly having difficulty chewing and swallowing. The patient assumes a rigid, bent-forward posture and the gait becomes unsteady and shuffled. All these Parkinson-like symptoms may be seen with the use of certain drugs, head injuries, and encephalitis. These movements are also termed **extrapyramidal symptoms (EPS)**.

Drugs used to treat parkinsonism (or more frequently called Parkinson-like symptoms) are called *antiparkinson drugs*. These drugs either supplement the dopamine in the brain or block excess acetylcholine (ACh) so that better transmission of nerve impulses occurs. The Summary Drug Table: Antiparkinson Drugs provides a listing of the drugs used to treat Parkinson's disease and EPSs.

DOPAMINERGIC DRUGS

Dopaminergics are drugs that affect the dopamine content of the brain. These drugs include levodopa, carbidopa (Lodosyn), amantadine, and carbidopa/levodopa combination (Sinemet). Other drugs that work to enhance dopamine include agonists such as bromocriptine (Parlodel) or monoamine oxidase inhibitors (MAOIs) such as selegiline (Eldepryl) (see Summary Drug Table: Antiparkinson Drugs).

Actions

The Parkinson-like symptoms are caused by a depletion of dopamine in the central nervous system (CNS). Supplementing dopamine is difficult due to a structure called the **blood–brain barrier**. The blood–brain barrier is a meshwork of tightly packed cells in the walls of the brain's capillaries that work to protect the brain by screening out certain substances. This unique meshwork of cells in the CNS prohibits large and potentially harmful molecules from leaving the blood and crossing into the brain. This ability to screen out certain substances has important implications for drug therapy, because different drugs can pass through the blood–brain barrier more easily than others. Therefore, dopamine is not easy to supplement because it is one that does not easily cross the blood–brain barrier.

Levodopa is a chemical formulation found in plants and animals and is converted into dopamine by the body. Dopamine, in the form of levodopa, crosses the blood–brain barrier but only in small quantities. At one time, levodopa, used alone, caused severe adverse reactions because too much dopamine stayed in the peripheral nervous system. Combining levodopa with another drug (carbidopa) allows more levodopa to reach the brain, which in turn permits the drug to have a better pharmacologic effect in patients with Parkinson's disease

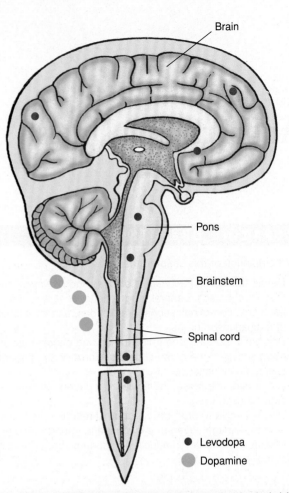

Figure 28.1 The blood–brain barrier selectively inhibits certain substances from entering the brain and spinal fluid. Cells in the brain form tight junctions that prevent or slow the passage of certain substances. Levodopa can pass the blood–brain barrier, whereas dopamine cannot.

(Fig. 28.1). Carbidopa has no effect when given alone. Therefore, the combination makes more levodopa available to the brain and, as a result, the dosage of levodopa may be reduced, decreasing peripheral effects. Combination tablets of carbidopa and levodopa are available in several strengths of the two drugs and as a timed-release medication.

Drugs that work to stimulate the dopamine receptors are called **agonists**. An example of this drug category includes bromocriptine. The action of amantadine is to make more of the dopamine available at the receptor site. Rasagiline (Azilect) and selegiline inhibit monoamine oxidase type B, again making more dopamine available.

Uses

Dopaminergic drugs are used to treat the Parkinson-like symptoms of the following:

- Parkinson's disease
- Parkinson-like symptoms (extrapyramidal) as a result of injury, drug therapy, or encephalitis

- **Restless leg syndrome** (RLS)
- Viral infections (amantadine)

Adverse Reactions

During early treatment with levodopa/carbidopa, adverse reactions are usually not a problem, because of the resolution of Parkinson-like symptoms. As the medication's effectiveness lessens, generalized adverse reactions include the following:

- Dry mouth and difficulty in swallowing
- Anorexia, nausea, and vomiting
- Abdominal pain and constipation
- Increased hand tremor
- Headache and dizziness

The most serious adverse reactions seen with levodopa include **choreiform movements** (involuntary muscular twitching of the limbs or facial muscles) and **dystonic** movements (muscular spasms most often affecting the tongue, jaw, eyes, and neck). Less common but still serious reactions include mental changes such as dementia, depression, psychotic episodes, paranoia, and suicidal tendencies, (covered in Unit IV—Drugs that effect the Central Nervous System).

Contraindications and Precautions

The dopaminergic drugs are contraindicated in patients with known hypersensitivity to the drugs. Levodopa is contraindicated in patients with narrow-angle glaucoma and those receiving MAOI antidepressants. The patient should be screened for unusual skin lesions, because levodopa can activate malignant melanoma. Levodopa is used cautiously in patients with cardiovascular or pulmonary diseases, peptic ulcer disease, renal or hepatic disease, and psychosis. Levodopa and combination antiparkinson drugs (e.g., carbidopa/levodopa) are classified in pregnancy category C and are used with caution during pregnancy and lactation.

> **! NURSING ALERT**
>
> The dopamine agonists selegiline and rasagiline should not be used with the opioid meperidine (Demerol) because of antimetabolite conversion. Caution should be taken with any other opioid used with these antiparkinson drugs.

Interactions

The following interactions may occur when a dopaminergic drug is administered with another agent:

Interacting Drug	Common Use	Effect of Interaction
tricyclic antidepressants	Management of depression	Increased risk of hypertension and dyskinesia
antacids	Relief of GI upset and heartburn	Increased effect of levodopa
anticonvulsants	Seizure control	Decreased effect of levodopa

Foods high in pyridoxine (vitamin B_6) or vitamin B_6 preparations reduce the effect of levodopa. However, when carbidopa is used with levodopa, pyridoxine has no effect on the action of levodopa. In fact, when levodopa and carbidopa are given together, pyridoxine may be prescribed to decrease the adverse effects associated with levodopa.

DOPAMINE RECEPTOR AGONISTS

Actions

It is thought that nonergot dopamine receptors act directly on postsynaptic dopamine receptors of nerve cells in the brain, mimicking the effects of dopamine in the brain.

Uses

Dopamine receptor agonists are used for the treatment of the signs and symptoms of Parkinson's disease. It is also used in the treatment of RLS, a disorder where the patient has an irresistible urge to move the legs, which lessens with movement but worsens with rest. The symptoms of this disorder worsen in the evening, causing difficulty with sleep. The drug apomorphine (Apokyn) is used for the **on-off phenomena** of Parkinson's disease. Antiemetic therapy must be initiated with this drug.

Adverse Reactions

The most common adverse reactions include the following:

- Nausea, dizziness, vomiting
- Somnolence, hallucinations, confusion, visual disturbances
- Postural hypotension, abnormal involuntary movements
- Headache

Contraindications and Precautions

Dopamine receptor agonists are contraindicated in patients with known hypersensitivity to the drugs. Dopamine receptor agonists are used with caution in patients with dyskinesia, orthostatic hypotension, hepatic or renal impairment, cardiovascular disease, and a history of hallucinations or psychosis. Both ropinirole and pramipexole are pregnancy category C drugs, and safety during pregnancy has not been established.

There is an increased risk of CNS depression when the dopamine receptor agonists are administered with other CNS depressants. When administered with levodopa, dopamine receptor agonists increase the effects of levodopa (a lower dosage of levodopa may be required). In addition, when dopamine receptor agonists are administered with levodopa, there is an increased risk of hallucinations. When administered with ciprofloxacin, there is an increased effect of the dopamine receptor agonist.

Interactions

The following interactions may occur when a dopamine receptor agonist is administered with another agent:

Interacting Drug	Common Use	Effect of Interaction
cimetidine, ranitidine	Management of GI problems	Increased dopamine agonist effectiveness
verapamil, quinidine	Management of cardiac problems	Increased dopamine agonist effectiveness
estrogen	Female hormonal supplement	Increased dopamine agonist effectiveness
phenothiazines	Antipsychotic agent	Decreased dopamine agonist effectiveness

COMT INHIBITORS

Another classification of antiparkinson drugs is the catechol-O-methyltransferase (COMT) inhibitors. Examples of the COMT inhibitors are entacapone (Comtan) and tolcapone (Tasmar).

Actions

These drugs are thought to prolong the effect of levodopa by blocking an enzyme, COMT, which eliminates dopamine. When given with levodopa, the COMT inhibitors increase the plasma concentrations and duration of action of levodopa.

Uses

The COMT inhibitors are used as adjuncts to levodopa/carbidopa in treating Parkinson's disease. Entacapone is a mild COMT inhibitor and is used to help manage fluctuations in the response to levodopa in individuals with Parkinson's disease. Tolcapone is a potent COMT inhibitor that easily crosses the blood–brain barrier. However, the drug is associated with liver damage and liver failure. Because of the danger to the liver, tolcapone is reserved for people who are not responding to other therapies.

Adverse Reactions

Adverse reactions most often associated with the administration of COMT inhibitors include the following:

- Dizziness
- Dyskinesias, hyperkinesias, **akathisia**
- Nausea, anorexia, and diarrhea
- Orthostatic hypotension, sleep disorders, excessive dreaming
- Somnolence and muscle cramps

Contraindications and Precautions

These drugs are contraindicated in patients with hypersensitivity to the drugs and during pregnancy and lactation (pregnancy category C). Tolcapone is contraindicated in patients with liver dysfunction. The COMT inhibitors are used with caution in patients with hypertension, hypotension, and decreased hepatic or renal function.

Interactions

The following interactions may occur when a COMT inhibitor is administered with another agent:

Interacting Drug	Common Use	Effect of Interaction
MAOI antidepressants	Management of depression	Increased risk of toxicity of both drugs
adrenergic drugs	Treatment of cardiac and blood pressure problems	Increased risk of cardiac symptoms

CHOLINERGIC BLOCKING DRUGS (ANTICHOLINERGICS)

Actions

ACh, a neurotransmitter, is produced in excess in Parkinson's disease. Drugs with cholinergic blocking activity block ACh in the CNS, enhancing dopamine transmission. Drugs with cholinergic blocking activity are generally less effective than levodopa in treating parkinsonism and are limited in dose by peripheral adverse reactions. Antihistamines, such as diphenhydramine (Benadryl), are used in older adult patients because they produce fewer adverse effects.

Uses

Drugs with cholinergic blocking activity are used as adjunctive therapy in all forms of Parkinson-like symptoms and in the control of drug-induced extrapyramidal disorders (Display 28.1).

Adverse Reactions

Adverse reactions to drugs with cholinergic blocking activity include the following:

- Dry mouth
- Blurred vision
- Dizziness, mild nausea, and nervousness

Display 28.1 Drugs With Parkinson-Like Adverse Reactions

The following drugs can produce symptoms similar to Parkinson's disease, also known as extrapyramidal symptoms (EPS), which may be treated with similar drugs to reduce the adverse reactions:

Antidepressants
Antiemetics
Antipsychotics—first generation
Lithium
Stimulants

These reactions may become less pronounced as therapy progresses. Other adverse reactions may include:

- Skin rash, urticaria (hives)
- Urinary retention, dysuria
- Tachycardia, muscle weakness
- Disorientation and confusion

If any of these reactions are severe, the drug may be discontinued for several days and restarted at a lower dosage, or a different antiparkinson drug may be prescribed.

Contraindications and Precautions

These drugs are contraindicated in those with a hypersensitivity to the anticholinergic drugs, glaucoma (angle-closure glaucoma), pyloric or duodenal obstruction, peptic ulcers, prostatic hypertrophy, **achalasia** (failure of the muscles of the lower esophagus to relax, causing difficulty swallowing), myasthenia gravis, and megacolon.

These drugs are used with caution in patients with tachycardia, cardiac arrhythmias, hypertension, or hypotension; those with a tendency toward urinary retention; those with decreased liver or kidney function; and those with obstructive disease of the urinary system or GI tract. The cholinergic blocking drugs are given with caution to the older adult.

LIFESPAN CONSIDERATIONS
Gerontology

Individuals older than 60 years frequently develop increased sensitivity to anticholinergic drugs and require careful monitoring. Confusion and disorientation may occur. Lower doses may be required.

Interactions

The following interactions may occur when a cholinergic blocking drug is administered with another agent:

Interacting Drug	Common Use	Effect of Interaction
amantadine	Treatment of parkinsonism	Increased anticholinergic effects
digoxin	Management of cardiac disease	Increased digoxin serum levels
haloperidol	Antipsychotic agent	Increased psychotic behavior
phenothiazines	Antipsychotic agent	Increased anticholinergic effects

NURSING PROCESS

PATIENT RECEIVING AN ANTIPARKINSON DRUG

ASSESSMENT

Preadministration Assessment
Because of memory impairment and alterations in thinking in some patients with Parkinson-like symptoms, a history obtained from the patient may be unreliable. When able, supplement the health history from a family member. Important data to include are information regarding the symptoms of the disorder, the length of time the symptoms have been present, the ability of the patient to carry on activities of daily living, and the patient's current mental condition (e.g., impairment in memory, signs of depression, or withdrawal).

Before starting the drug therapy, a physical assessment of the patient is preformed to provide a baseline for future evaluations of drug therapy. It also is important to include an evaluation of the patient's neuromuscular status. Display 28.2 describes the assessments used when evaluating the neurologic and musculoskeletal status.

Ongoing Assessment
Evaluate the patient's response to drug therapy by observing the patient or asking about various neuromuscular signs (see Display 28.2). Compare these observations with the data obtained during the initial physical assessment. For example, the patient is assessed for clinical improvement of the symptoms of the disease, such as improvement of tremor of head or hands at rest, muscular rigidity, mask-like facial expression, and ambulation stability. Although drug response may occur slowly in some patients, these observations aid the primary health care provider in adjusting the dosage to obtain the desired therapeutic results.

A serious and potentially fatal adverse reaction to tolcapone is hepatic injury. Regular blood testing to monitor liver function is usually prescribed. Testing of serum aminotransferase levels is ordered at frequent intervals (e.g., every 2 weeks for the first year and every 8 weeks thereafter). Treatment is discontinued if the alanine aminotransferase (ALT; previously, serum glutamic pyruvic transaminase [SGPT]) exceeds the upper normal limit or signs or symptoms of liver failure develop. The patient is

Display 28.2 Neuromuscular Assessment

The neuromuscular assessment includes observation for the following:

- Tremors of the hands or head while the patient is at rest
- Mask-like facial expression
- Changes (from normal) in walking
- Type of speech pattern (halting, monotone)
- Postural deformities
- Muscular rigidity
- Drooling, difficulty in chewing or swallowing
- Changes in thought processes
- Ability of the patient to carry out any or all of the activities of daily living (e.g., bathing, ambulating, dressing)

Antiparkinson Drugs

observed for indicators of liver dysfunction such as persistent nausea, fatigue, lethargy, anorexia, jaundice, dark urine, pruritus, and right upper quadrant tenderness.

NURSING DIAGNOSES
Drug-specific nursing diagnoses include the following:

- **Imbalanced Nutrition: Less Than Body Requirements** related to nausea, dry mouth
- **Constipation** related to neurologic changes in the bowel
- **Risk for Injury** related to dizziness, lightheadedness, orthostatic hypotension, loss of balance
- **Impaired Physical Mobility** related to alterations in balance, unsteady gait, dizziness
- **Disturbed Sleep Pattern** related to involuntary movement at rest

Nursing diagnoses related to drug administration are discussed in Chapter 4.

PLANNING
The expected outcomes for the patient may include an optimal response to drug therapy, meeting patient needs related to the management of adverse reactions, absence of injury, and confidence in an understanding of the medication regimen.

IMPLEMENTATION

Promoting an Optimal Response to Therapy
Effective management of the patient with Parkinson's disease requires careful monitoring of the drug therapy. Optimal response to these drugs often requires titration of doses based on patient activities. To accomplish this requires psychological support, with emphasis on patient and family teaching. Often patients and family members may be given a range of drug dosages to administer to find the best response with the fewest adverse reactions.

The antiparkinson drugs also may be used to treat the Parkinson-like symptoms that occur with the administration of some of the psychotherapeutic drugs. When used for this purpose, antiparkinson drugs may exacerbate mental symptoms and precipitate a psychotic event. Review Chapter 23 for intervention strategies and monitoring.

Monitoring and Managing Patient Needs
Teach the patient or a family member how to journal daily for the development of adverse reactions. By using a chart or journal describing adverse reactions, these can be reported in an easier fashion to the primary health care provider, because a dosage adjustment or change to a different antiparkinson drug may be necessary with the occurrence of more serious adverse reactions. Teach the patient or family how to describe movements and to be alert for those such as facial grimacing, protruding tongue, exaggerated chewing motions and head movements, and jerking movements of the arms and legs. If these occur, the patient should not take the next dose of the drug and should notify the primary health care provider immediately.

IMBALANCED NUTRITION: LESS THAN BODY REQUIREMENTS. Patients may experience multiple adverse reactions that can affect their dietary intake and cause them to lose weight. Some adverse reactions, although not serious, may be uncomfortable. An example of a less serious but uncomfortable adverse reaction is dryness of the mouth. Teach the patient to relieve dry mouth by taking frequent sips of water, ice chips, or hard candy (if allowed). If dry mouth is so severe that there is difficulty in swallowing or speaking, or if loss of appetite and weight loss occur, the dosage of the antiparkinson drug may be reduced.

Some patients taking the antiparkinson drugs experience GI disturbances such as nausea, vomiting, or constipation. This can affect the patient's nutritional status. Help the family to learn to create a calm environment; serve small, frequent meals; and serve foods the patient prefers to help improve nutrition. For those with eating issues, monitor the patient's weight daily. GI disturbances are sometimes helped by taking the drug with meals. Severe nausea or vomiting may necessitate discontinuing the drug and changing to a different antiparkinson drug. With continued use of the drug, nausea usually decreases or resolves.

CONSTIPATION. Neurologic changes cause changes in peristalsis and dilation of the bowel, leading to chronic constipation. Also, some patients with Parkinson's disease may have difficulty communicating and are not able to tell the caregiver or nurse that bodily urges are occurring. Observe the patient with Parkinson's disease for outward changes that may indicate the need to eliminate. For example, a sudden change in the facial expression or changes in posture may indicate abdominal pain or discomfort, which may be caused by urinary retention, paralytic ileus, or constipation. If constipation is a problem, stress the need for a diet high in fiber and increasing fluids in the diet. A stool softener may be needed to help prevent constipation.

RISK FOR INJURY. Minimizing the risk for injury is an important aspect in the care of the patient with Parkinson's disease. The patient with visual difficulties may need assistance with ambulation. Visual difficulties (e.g., adverse reactions of blurred vision and diplopia) may be evidenced only by the patient's sudden refusal to read or watch television or by the patient bumping into objects when ambulating. Lack of balance is an issue for those with Parkinson's disease. Research indicates a reduction in injury when patients participate in activities to improve balance, such as Tai Chi (Li, 2012). You can refer patients to occupational or activity directors who may have listings of exercise programs that cater to individuals with balance issues.

Carefully evaluate any sudden changes in the patient's behavior or activity and report them to the primary health care provider. Sudden changes in behavior may indicate hallucinations, depression, or other psychotic episodes.

LIFESPAN CONSIDERATIONS
Gerontology

Hallucinations occur more often in the older adult than in the younger adult receiving antiparkinson drugs. This is especially likely when taking dopamine receptor agonists.

Adverse reactions such as dizziness, muscle weakness, and ataxia (lack of muscular coordination) may further increase difficulty with ambulatory activities. Patients with Parkinson's disease are especially prone to falls and other accidents because of the disease process and possible adverse drug reactions. The patient should learn to ask for assistance in getting out of the bed or a chair, walking, and other self-care activities. In addition, assistive devices such as a cane or walker may help with ambulation (Fig. 28.2). You may suggest

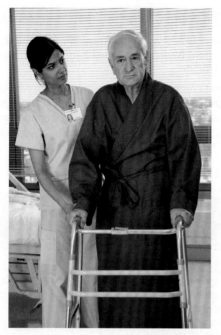

Figure 28.2 Nurses promote patient safety by providing ambulatory assistance to the patient with Parkinson-like (extrapyramidal) symptoms.

that the patient wear shoes with rubber soles to minimize the possibility of slipping. The room should be kept well lighted, the use of scatter or throw rugs should be avoided, and any small pieces of furniture or objects that might increase the risk of falling should be removed. Carefully assess the environment and make necessary adjustments to ensure the patient's safety.

Patients who are prone to orthostatic hypotension as a result of the drug regimen are instructed to arise slowly from a sitting or lying position, especially after sitting or lying for a prolonged time.

IMPAIRED PHYSICAL MOBILITY. The on-off phenomenon may occur in patients taking levodopa. In this condition, the patient may suddenly alternate between improved clinical status and loss of therapeutic effect. This effect is associated with long-term levodopa treatment. Low doses of the drug, reserving the drug for severe cases, or the use of a *drug holiday* may be prescribed. Should symptoms occur, the primary health care provider may order a drug holiday that includes complete withdrawal of levodopa for 5 to 14 days, followed by gradually restarting drug therapy at a lower dose. Patients on a drug holiday need to be monitored for complications.

DISTURBED SLEEP PATTERN. Patients with RLS have difficulty in sleeping due to leg movements that increase during periods of rest. To facilitate sleep, teach the patient to engage in activities to promote rest as he or she prepares for sleep. Bedtime rituals such as a hot bath, engaging the mind in a pleasant activity (crossword puzzle or reading), and leg massage may help to improve the ability to sleep.

Educating the Patient and Family

Provide a referral to the discharge planning coordinator or social worker if you find issues with the patient's ability to understand the therapeutic drug regimen, ability to perform self-care in the home environment, or ability to adhere to the prescribed drug therapy.

If the patient requires supervision or help with daily activities and the drug regimen, encourage the family to create a home environment that is least likely to result in accidents or falls. Changes such as removing throw rugs, installing a hand rail next to the toilet, and moving obstacles that can result in tripping or falling can be made at little or no expense to the family. As you develop a teaching plan for the patient or family member, include the following points:

- If dizziness, drowsiness, or blurred vision occurs, avoid driving or performing other tasks that require alertness.

- ⚠ Avoid the use of alcohol unless use has been approved by the primary health care provider.

- Relieve dry mouth by sucking on hard candy (unless the patient has diabetes) or taking frequent sips of water. Consult a dentist if dryness of the mouth interferes with wearing, inserting, or removing dentures or causes other dental problems.

- Keep all appointments with the primary health care provider or clinic personnel because close monitoring of therapy is necessary.

- Ask your primary health care provider before buying vitamin supplements when taking levodopa. Vitamin B$_6$ (pyridoxine) may interfere with the action of levodopa.

EVALUATION

- Therapeutic effect is achieved and the Parkinson-like symptoms are controlled.

- Adverse reactions are identified, reported to the primary health care provider, and managed successfully through appropriate nursing interventions.
  - Patient maintains an adequate nutritional status.
  - Patient has adequate bowel movements.
  - No evidence of injury is seen.
  - Patient maintains adequate mobility.
  - Patient reports restful sleep.

- Patient and family express confidence and demonstrate an understanding of the drug regimen.

PHARMACOLOGY IN PRACTICE
THINK CRITICALLY

You ask Betty to follow you into an exam room. There you assess a repetitive hand tremor, and she appears to open her mouth frequently with a dry, sticky sound. What do you think she is experiencing, and how will you document these findings for the primary health care provider?

KEY POINTS

- Parkinson's disease is a progressive neurologic disease caused by reduction in dopamine in the brain. Cardinal signs include tremors, rigidity, and bradykinesia.

- When drugs or other illnesses cause adverse reactions like the cardinal symptoms of Parkinson's disease, this is termed Parkinson-like or extrapyramidal symptoms.

- The drugs used to treat Parkinson's disease and Parkinson-like symptoms either supplement dopamine or

block excess acetylcholine to enhance neurotransmission. Blood–brain barrier issues make supplementing dopamine difficult.

- The most common adverse reactions are dry mouth and GI distress such as nausea, vomiting, and constipation. When combined with other drugs less common reactions such as involuntary muscle twitching and spasm can occur.

Summary Drug Table ANTIPARKINSON DRUGS

Generic Name	Trade Name	Uses	Adverse Reactions	Dosage Ranges
Dopaminergic Drugs				
amantadine *ah-man'-tah-deen*		Parkinson's disease/drug-induced extrapyramidal symptoms, prevention and treatment of infection with influenza A virus	Lightheadedness, dizziness, insomnia, confusion, nausea, constipation, dry mouth, orthostatic hypotension, depression	200–400 mg/day orally in divided doses
bromocriptine *broe-moe-krip'-teen*	Parlodel, Parlodel Snap Tabs	Parkinson's disease, female endocrine imbalances	Drowsiness, sedation, dizziness, faintness, epigastric distress, anorexia	10–40 mg/day orally
carbidopa *kar'-bih-doe-pah*	Lodosyn	Used with levodopa in the treatment of Parkinson's disease	None by itself; adverse reactions are those of levodopa	70–100 mg/day orally
carbidopa/levodopa *kar'-bih-doe-pah/lee'-voe-doe-pah*	Sinemet, Sinemet CR, Parcopa	Parkinson's disease	Anorexia, nausea, vomiting, abdominal pain, dysphagia, dry mouth, mental changes, headache, dizziness, increased hand tremor, choreiform or dystonic movements	Begin with 10 mg/100 mg tablet orally TID, titrated dose combination to minimize symptoms
levodopa *lee'-voe-doe-pah*		Parkinson's disease	Same as carbidopa/levodopa	0.5–1 g/day orally initially, not to exceed 8 g/day
Dopaminergic Drugs—MAOIs				
rasagiline *rah-sah'-jih-leen*	Azilect	Parkinson's disease	Headache, arthralgia, depression, dyspepsia, flu syndrome	0.5–1 mg/day orally
selegiline *seh-leh'-geh-leen*	Eldepryl, Emsam, Zelapar	Agonist for levodopa/carbidopa in Parkinson's disease	Nausea, dizziness	5 mg orally at breakfast and lunch
Dopamine Receptor Agonists, Nonergot				
apomorphine *ay-poe-more'-feen*	Apokyn	Parkinson's disease "off" episode	Profound hypotension, nausea, vomiting	0.2 mL as needed for "off" episode
pramipexole *pram-ih-pek'-sole*	Mirapex	Parkinson's disease, RLS	Dizziness, somnolence, insomnia, hallucinations, confusion, nausea, dyspepsia, syncope	0.125–1.5 mg orally TID
ropinirole *roe-pin'-oh-roll*	Requip	Parkinson's disease, RLS	Dizziness, somnolence, insomnia, hallucinations, confusion, nausea, dyspepsia, syncope	0.25–1 mg orally TID

Summary Drug Table ANTIPARKINSON DRUGS (continued)

Generic Name	Trade Name	Uses	Adverse Reactions	Dosage Ranges
COMT Inhibitors				
entacapone *en-tah-kap'-own*	Comtan	As adjunct to levodopa/carbidopa in Parkinson's disease	Dyskinesia, hyperkinesia, nausea, diarrhea, urine discoloration	200–1600 mg/day orally
tolcapone *toll-kap'-own*	Tasmar	Parkinson's disease when refractory to levodopa/carbidopa	Orthostatic hypotension, dyskinesia, sleep disorders, dystonia, excessive dreaming, somnolence, dizziness, nausea, anorexia, muscle cramps, liver failure	100–200 mg orally TID
Cholinergic Blocking Drugs (Anticholinergics)				
benztropine *benz'-troe-peen*	Cogentin	Parkinson's disease, drug-induced EPS	Dry mouth, blurred vision, dizziness, nausea, nervousness, skin rash, urinary retention, dysuria, tachycardia, muscle weakness, disorientation, confusion	0.5–6 mg/day orally Acute dystonia: 1–2 mL IM or IV
biperiden *by-pare'-ih-den*	Akineton	Parkinson's disease, drug-induced EPS	Same as benztropine	2 mg orally TID or QID; maximum dose 16 mg/24 hr
diphenhydramine *dye-fen-hye'-drah-meen*	Benadryl	Drug-induced EPS, allergies	Same as benztropine	25–50 mg orally TID or QID
trihexyphenidyl *trye-hex-see-fen'-ih-dill*		Parkinson's disease, drug-induced EPS	Same as benztropine	1–15 mg/day orally in divided doses
Combination Drugs				
carbidopa, levodopa, entacapone	Stalevo	Parkinson's disease	See individual drugs	Titrated to individual need of assorted drugs

Antiparkinson Drugs

● Chapter Review

Know Your Drugs

Clients sometimes know a medication by the brand (or trade) name and not the generic name. To help you recognize both names, match the brand name with the generic name of the same medication.

Generic Name	Brand Name
1. bromocriptine	A. Eldepryl
2. carbidopa	B. Lodosyn
3. pramipexole	C. Mirapex
4. selegiline	D. Parlodel

Calculate Medication Dosages

1. Oral levodopa 0.75 g is prescribed. The drug is available in 100-mg tablets, 250-mg tablets, and 500-mg tablets. The nurse administers _____.

2. Oral ropinirole 6 mg is prescribed. The drug is available in 2-mg tablets. The nurse administers _____.

● Prepare for the NCLEX®

Build Your Knowledge

1. Parkinson's disease or parkinsonism occurs because of the lack of which neurotransmitter?

   1. acetylcholine
   2. dopamine
   3. serotonin
   4. GABA

2. The most serious adverse reactions seen with levodopa include _____.

   1. choreiform and dystonic movements
   2. depression
   3. suicidal tendencies
   4. paranoia

3. Older clients prescribed one of the dopamine receptor agonists are monitored closely for which of the following adverse reactions?

   1. occipital headache
   2. hallucinations
   3. paralytic ileus
   4. cardiac arrhythmias

4. Clients should be monitored for EPS when taking which class of drugs?

   1. anticoagulants
   2. vitamins
   3. antidepressants
   4. antihypertensives

5. The client taking tolcapone for Parkinson's disease is monitored closely for _____.

   1. kidney dysfunction
   2. liver dysfunction
   3. agranulocytosis
   4. the development of an autoimmune disease

Apply Your Knowledge

6. The nurse reports which of the following as a diminished response to antiparkinson drug treatment rather than an adverse reaction?

   1. dry mouth and difficulty in swallowing
   2. anorexia, nausea, and vomiting
   3. abdominal pain and constipation
   4. increased hand tremor

7. When taking a cholinergic blocking drug for Parkinson-like symptoms, the client would mostly experience which of the following adverse reactions?

   1. constipation, urinary frequency
   2. muscle spasm, convulsions
   3. diarrhea, hypertension
   4. dry mouth, dizziness

8. A family member asks the nurse which exercise is best to help a client with Parkinson's disease maintain balance. Which is the best response?

   1. swimming
   2. Tai Chi
   3. jogging
   4. mind puzzles

Alternate-Format Questions

9. Identify the interventions to use to help promote sleep for the client with RLS. **Select all that apply**.

   1. Take a hot bath
   2. Watch a fast-paced show on television
   3. Do a crossword puzzle
   4. Take a brisk walk in the night air
   5. Take vitamin B_6

10. Arrange the following steps of dopamine distribution to a client with Parkinson's disease:

    1. Levodopa targets the nerve to complete neurotransmission
    2. The tablet(s) are swallowed
    3. The carbidopa allows the levodopa to cross the blood–brain barrier
    4. The levodopa and carbidopa combine together and are absorbed into the circulation

To check your answers, see Appendix G.

thePoint *For more NCLEX-style questions, log on to http://thepoint.lww.com to access more than 1000 questions.*

Anticonvulsants

LEARNING OBJECTIVES

On completion of this chapter, the student will:

1. List the different types of drugs used as anticonvulsants.
2. Discuss the general drug actions, uses, adverse reactions, contraindications, precautions, and interactions of anticonvulsants.
3. Discuss important preadministration and ongoing assessment activities the nurse should perform with the patient receiving an anticonvulsant.
4. List nursing diagnoses particular to a patient taking an anticonvulsant.
5. Discuss ways to promote an optimal response to therapy, how to manage common adverse reactions when administering the anticonvulsants, and important points to keep in mind when educating a patient about the use of anticonvulsants.

KEY TERMS

ataxia • unsteady gait; muscular incoordination

atonic • generalized seizure with loss of muscle tone; person suddenly drops

convulsion • paroxysm (occurring suddenly) of involuntary muscular contractions and relaxations

epilepsy • chronic, recurring seizure disorder

generalized seizures • loss of consciousness during seizure

gingival hyperplasia • overgrowth of gum tissue

myoclonic • sudden, forceful muscular contraction

nystagmus • involuntary and constant movement of the eyeball

pancytopenia • reduction in all cellular elements of the blood

partial seizures • localized seizure in the brain, with no impaired consciousness

precipitation • condensation of a solid from a solution during a chemical reaction

seizure • cluster of symptoms resulting from abnormal electrical activity in the brain

status epilepticus • emergency situation characterized by continual seizure activity

Stevens-Johnson syndrome (SJS) • fever, cough, muscular aches and pains, headache, and lesions of the skin, mucous membranes, and eyes; the lesions appear as red wheals or blisters, often starting on the face, in the mouth, or on the lips, neck, and extremities

tonic-clonic • generalized seizure activity consisting of alternating contraction (tonic) and relaxation of muscles (clonic)

DRUG CLASSES

Hydantoins	Oxazolidinediones
Carboxylic acid	Benzodiazepines
derivatives	Miscellaneous drugs
Succinimides	

PHARMACOLOGY IN PRACTICE

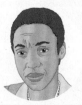

Lillian Chase was in a car accident last year and had a seizure on the way to the hospital. As you review her medication list and ask about her drugs, she tells you that since she has been taking phenytoin she has had no seizures.

The term **convulsion** refers to a sudden, involuntary contraction of the muscles of the body, often accompanied by loss of consciousness. A **seizure** may be defined as periodic disturbances of the brain's electrical activity. The terms *convulsion* and *seizure* are often used interchangeably, having basically the same meaning. Seizure disorders are generally categorized as idiopathic, hereditary, or acquired. Idiopathic seizures have no known cause; hereditary seizure disorders are passed from parent to child in their genetic makeup; and acquired seizure disorders have a known cause—causes include high fever, electrolyte imbalances, uremia, hypoglycemia, hypoxia, brain tumors, and some drug withdrawal reactions. The primary goal is to treat the underlying pathologic process to stop the seizures. Sometimes the cause is not clear, and the seizures cannot be stopped; rather, the activity needs to be controlled.

Seizures caused by disease, such as in epilepsy, may not be easy to eliminate. **Epilepsy** is defined as a permanent, recurrent seizure disorder. Examples of the known causes of epilepsy include brain injury at birth, head injuries, and inborn errors of metabolism. In some patients, the cause of epilepsy is never determined. Epileptic seizures are classified according to an international system (Fig. 29.1). Each different type of seizure disorder is characterized by a specific pattern of events, as well as a different pattern of motor or sensory manifestation.

Drugs used for managing seizure disorders are called anticonvulsants. Most anticonvulsants have specific uses; that is, they are of value only in treating certain types of

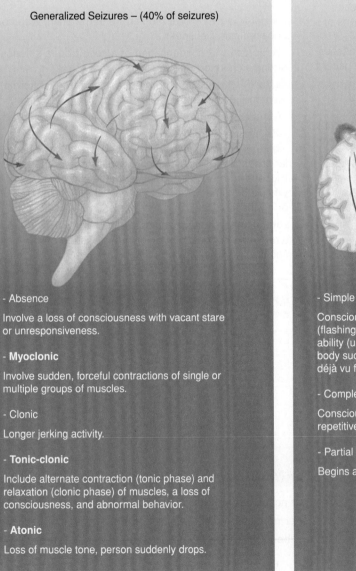

Generalized Seizures – (40% of seizures)

- Absence

Involve a loss of consciousness with vacant stare or unresponsiveness.

- **Myoclonic**

Involve sudden, forceful contractions of single or multiple groups of muscles.

- Clonic

Longer jerking activity.

- **Tonic-clonic**

Include alternate contraction (tonic phase) and relaxation (clonic phase) of muscles, a loss of consciousness, and abnormal behavior.

- **Atonic**

Loss of muscle tone, person suddenly drops.

Partial Seizures – (60% of seizures)

- Simple

Consciousness is not impaired, can involve senses (flashing lights or a change in taste or speech) or motor ability (uncontrolled stiffening or jerking in one part of the body such as the finger, mouth, hand, or foot), nausea, déjà vu feeling.

- Complex

Consciousness is impaired and variable (unconscious repetitive actions), staring gaze, hallucination/delusion.

- Partial evolving to generalized

Begins as partial seizure and becomes generalized.

Figure 29.1 Classification of seizures. (International League Against Epilepsy [ILAE], 1998, Courtesy of the Anatomical Chart Co.)

seizure disorders. The drug categories used as anticonvulsants are the hydantoins, carboxylic acid derivatives, succinimides, oxazolidinediones, and benzodiazepines. In addition, several adjunct drugs are used as anticonvulsants. All possess the ability to depress abnormal neural discharges in the central nervous system (CNS), thereby inhibiting seizure activity. The Summary Drug Table: Anticonvulsants provides a listing of the drugs used to treat seizure disorders.

Actions

Anticonvulsants depress abnormal nerve impulse discharges in the CNS. The six categories of anticonvulsants achieve this effect through different modes of action:

1. **Hydantoins** stabilize the hyperexcitability postsynaptically in the motor cortex of the brain.
2. **Carboxylic acid derivatives** increase levels of gamma (γ)-aminobutyric acid (GABA), which stabilizes cell membranes.
3. **Succinimides** depress the motor cortex, creating a higher threshold before nerves react to the convulsive stimuli.
4. **Oxazolidinediones** decrease repetitive synaptic transmissions of nerve impulses.
5. **Benzodiazepines** elevate the seizure threshold by decreasing postsynaptic excitation.
6. **Miscellaneous drugs** have differing properties; for example, gabapentin is a GABA agonist, and topiramate blocks the seizure activity rather than raising the threshold.

Seizures are theoretically reduced in intensity and frequency of occurrence or, in some instances, are virtually eliminated. For some patients, only partial control of the seizure disorder may be obtained with anticonvulsant drug therapy.

Uses

Anticonvulsants are used prophylactically to prevent seizures after trauma or neurosurgery or in patients with a tumor and in the treatment of the following:

- Seizures of all types
- Neuropathic pain
- Bipolar disorders
- Anxiety disorders

Occasionally, **status epilepticus** (an emergency characterized by continual seizure activity with no interruptions) can occur. Lorazepam (Ativan) is the drug of choice for this condition. However, because the effects of lorazepam last less than 1 hour, longer-lasting anticonvulsants such as phenytoin (Dilantin) are given to continue to control the seizure activity.

Adverse Reactions

Adverse reactions that may occur with the administration of an anticonvulsant drug include the following:

Central Nervous System Reactions

- Drowsiness, weakness, dizziness
- Headache, somnolence

- **Nystagmus** (constant, involuntary movement of the eyeball)
- **Ataxia** (loss of control of voluntary movements, especially gait)
- Slurred speech

Gastrointestinal System Reactions

- Nausea, vomiting
- Anorexia
- Constipation, diarrhea
- **Gingival hyperplasia** (overgrowth of gum tissue)

Other Reactions

- Skin rashes, pruritus, urticaria
- Urinary frequency; ezogabine (Potiga) has been associated with urinary retention and pain.
- Serious skin reactions, such as **Stevens-Johnson syndrome**, have been associated with the use of lamotrigine (Lamictal).
- Hematologic changes, such as **pancytopenia** (decrease in all the cellular components of the blood), leukopenia, aplastic anemia, and thrombocytopenia, have occurred with administration of selected drugs, including carbamazepine (Tegretol), felbamate (Felbatol), and trimethadione (Tridione). See the Summary Drug Table: Anticonvulsants for more information.

LIFESPAN CONSIDERATIONS
Women

Research suggests an association between the use of anticonvulsants by pregnant women with epilepsy and an increased incidence of birth defects. The use of anticonvulsants is not discontinued in pregnant women with a history of major seizures because of the danger of precipitating status epilepticus. However, when seizure activity poses no serious threat to the pregnant woman, the primary health care provider may consider discontinuing use of the drug during pregnancy.

Contraindications

All categories of anticonvulsants are contraindicated in patients with known hypersensitivity to the drugs. Phenytoin is contraindicated in patients with sinus bradycardia, sinoatrial block, Adams-Stokes syndrome, and second- and third-degree atrioventricular (AV) block; it also is contraindicated during pregnancy and lactation (ethotoin and phenytoin are pregnancy category D drugs). Ethotoin (Peganone) is contraindicated in patients with hepatic abnormalities. The oxazolidinediones have been associated with serious adverse reactions and fetal malformations. They should be used only when other, less toxic drugs are not effective in controlling seizures. The succinimides are contraindicated in patients with bone marrow depression or hepatic or renal impairment. A higher incidence of systemic lupus erythematosus has been found in patients taking succinimides.

Carbamazepine should not be given within 14 days of monoamine oxidase inhibitor (MAOI) antidepressants. Carbamazepine is contraindicated in patients with bone marrow depression or hepatic or renal impairment and during pregnancy (pregnancy category D). Valproic acid (Depakote) is not administered to patients with renal impairment or during pregnancy (pregnancy category D). Oxcarbazepine (Trileptal), a miscellaneous anticonvulsant, may exacerbate dementia.

Precautions

Anticonvulsants should be used cautiously in patients with liver or kidney disease and those with neurologic disorders. The benzodiazepines are used cautiously during pregnancy (pregnancy category D) and in patients with psychoses, patients with acute narrow-angle glaucoma, and older or debilitated patients. Phenytoin and lacosamide are used cautiously in patients with hypotension, severe myocardial insufficiency, and hepatic impairment. Trimethadione is used with caution in patients with eye disorders (e.g., retinal or optic nerve disease).

Miscellaneous anticonvulsants are used cautiously in patients with glaucoma or increased intraocular pressure; a history of cardiac, renal, or liver dysfunction; and psychiatric disorders. In addition to hepatic failure and birth defects, valproic acid is associated with an increased risk for pancreatitis.

Interactions

The following interactions may occur when an anticonvulsant is administered with another agent:

Interacting Drug	Common Use	Effect of Interaction
antibiotics/ antifungals	Fight infection	Increased effect of the anticonvulsant
tricyclic antidepressants	Manage depression	Increased effect of the anticonvulsant
salicylates	Pain relief	Increased effect of the anticonvulsant
cimetidine	Control gastrointestinal (GI) upset	Increased effect of the anticonvulsant
theophylline	Treatment of respiratory problems	Decreased serum levels of the anticonvulsant
antiseizure medications	Reduce seizure activity	May increase seizure activity
protease inhibitors	Treatment of human immunodeficiency virus (HIV) infection	Increased carbamazepine levels, resulting in toxicity
oral contraceptives	Birth control	Decreased effectiveness of birth control, resulting in breakthrough bleeding or pregnancy
analgesics or alcohol	CNS depressants	Increased depressant effect
antidiabetic medications	Manage diabetes mellitus	Increased blood glucose levels

NURSING PROCESS

PATIENT RECEIVING AN ANTICONVULSANT

ASSESSMENT

Preadministration Assessment

Seizures that occur in the outpatient setting are almost always seen first by family members or friends, rather than by a member of the health care profession. The occurrence of abnormal behavior patterns or convulsive movements usually prompts the patient to visit the primary health care provider's office or a neurologic clinic. A thorough patient history is necessary to identify the type of seizure disorder. In addition to the patient's report of seizure activity, the type of information that should be obtained from those who have observed the seizure is listed in Display 29.1.

Patient information should include a family history of seizures (if any) and recent drug therapy (all drugs currently being used). Depending on the type of seizure disorder, other information may be needed, such as a history of a head or other injury or a thorough medical history.

Take and document the vital signs at the time of the initial assessment to provide baseline data. The primary health care provider may order laboratory and diagnostic tests, such as an electroencephalogram (EEG), computed axial tomography (CAT) scan, and magnetic resonance imaging (MRI) scan. A complete blood count, lumbar puncture (LP), and hepatic and renal function tests are drawn to confirm the diagnosis and

identify a possible cause of the seizure disorder as well as to provide a baseline during therapy with anticonvulsants.

Ongoing Assessment

Anticonvulsants control, but do not cure, epilepsy. An accurate ongoing assessment is important for obtaining the desired effect of the anticonvulsant. The dosage of the anticonvulsant may require frequent adjustments during the initial treatment period. Dosage adjustments are based on the patient's response to therapy (e.g., the control of the seizures) as well as the occurrence of adverse reactions.

Display 29.1 General Assessment of Seizure Activity

- Description of the seizures (the motor or psychic activity occurring during the seizure)
- Frequency of the seizures (approximate number per day)
- Average length of a seizure
- Description of the aura (a subjective sensation preceding a seizure), if any has occurred
- Description of the degree of impairment of consciousness
- Description of what, if anything, appears to bring on the seizure

Depending on the patient's response to therapy, a second anticonvulsant may be added to the therapeutic regimen, or one anticonvulsant may be changed to another. Regularly, serum plasma levels of the anticonvulsant are measured to monitor for toxicity.

The patient's seizures, along with response to drug therapy, should be observed when a hospitalized patient is receiving an anticonvulsant. Most seizures occur without warning, and others may not see the patient until after the seizure has begun or after the seizure is over. A bedside assessment should include the following questions: What is your name? What are you feeling? Hold up two fingers and ask the patient, what do you see? Ask, where are you and where do you live? Ask the patient to touch his or her left ear. Show the patient an item, like your pen, and ask, what is this? Document the patient's responses.

Any observations made during and after the seizure are important and may aid in the diagnosis of the type of seizure, as well as assist the primary health care provider in evaluating the effectiveness of drug therapy.

NURSING DIAGNOSES

Drug-specific nursing diagnoses include the following:

- **Risk for Injury** related to seizure disorder, drowsiness, ataxia, and vision disturbances
- **Risk for Impaired Skin Integrity** related to adverse reactions (rash)
- **Risk for Infection** related to immunosuppression secondary to drug therapy
- **Impaired Oral Mucous Membranes** related to gum overgrowth secondary to hydantoins

Nursing diagnoses related to drug administration are discussed in Chapter 4.

PLANNING

The expected outcomes for the patient depend on the type and severity of the seizure but may include an optimal response to therapy (control of seizure), meeting patient needs related to the management of adverse reactions, and confidence in an understanding of the medication regimen.

MPLEMENTATION

Promoting an Optimal Response to Therapy

When administering an anticonvulsant, do not omit or miss a dose (except by order of the primary health care provider).

> **NURSING ALERT**
>
> Recurrence of seizure activity may result from abrupt discontinuation of the drug, even when the anticonvulsant is being administered in small daily doses.

Document and flag in the care plan anticonvulsant administration. If the primary health care provider discontinues the anticonvulsant therapy, the dosage is gradually withdrawn or another drug is gradually substituted.

SPECIAL CONSIDERATIONS FOR HYDANTOINS. Phenytoin is the most commonly prescribed anticonvulsant because of its effectiveness and relatively low toxicity. However, a genetically linked inability to metabolize phenytoin has been identified. For this reason, it is important to monitor serum concentrations of the drug on a regular basis to detect signs of toxicity (slurred speech, ataxia, lethargy, dizziness, nausea, and vomiting). Phenytoin plasma levels between 10 and 20 mcg/mL give optimal anticonvulsant effect. However, many patients achieve seizure control at lower serum concentration levels. Levels greater than 20 mcg/mL are associated with toxicity. Patients with plasma levels greater than 20 mcg/mL may exhibit nystagmus, and at concentrations greater than 30 mcg/mL, ataxia and mental changes are common. Phenytoin can be administered orally and parenterally. When taken orally, the drug should be taken with meals to avoid GI upset. If the drug is administered parenterally, the intravenous (IV) route is preferred over the intramuscular (IM) route, because erratic absorption of phenytoin causes pain and muscle damage at the injection site.

SPECIAL CONSIDERATIONS FOR BENZODIAZEPINES. The dosage of a benzodiazepine is highly individualized; increase the dose cautiously to avoid adverse reactions, particularly in older and debilitated patients. IV lorazepam may bring seizures under control quickly. However, for some patients, seizure activity may resume because of the short duration of the drug's effects. Drug precipitation can occur when diazepam (Valium) is administered IV. Never mix diazepam with other drugs. When used to control seizures, diazepam is administered by IV pushed slowly as close as possible to the IV site, allowing at least 1 minute for each 5 mg of drug.

LIFESPAN CONSIDERATIONS
Gerontology

Apnea and cardiac arrest have occurred when diazepam is administered to older adults, very ill patients, and individuals with limited pulmonary reserve. Older or debilitated adults may require a decreased dosage of diazepam to reduce ataxia and oversedation.

Monitoring and Managing Patient Needs

RISK FOR INJURY. Drowsiness is a common adverse reaction to anticonvulsant drugs, especially early in therapy. Assist the patient with all ambulatory activities until the patient is stable. Remind the patient to rise from the bed slowly and sit for a few minutes before standing. Drowsiness decreases with continued use.

Use caution when giving an oral preparation because aspiration of the tablet, capsule, or liquid may occur if the patient experiences drowsiness. Test the patient's swallowing ability by offering small sips of water before giving the drug. If the patient has difficulty swallowing, withhold the drug and notify the primary health care provider as soon as possible. A different route of administration may be necessary. Because injury may occur when the patient has a seizure, take precautions to prevent falls and other injuries until seizures are controlled by the drug.

Visual disturbances may occur with anticonvulsant therapy. Permanent vision loss has been associated with vigabatrin, and patients on this medication and other drugs causing visual disturbances should be regularly evaluated by an ophthalmologist. The patient with a visual disturbance is assisted with ambulation and oriented carefully to the environment. The patient may be especially sensitive to bright lights and want the room light dimmed. Because photosensitivity can occur, the patient should stay out of the sun if possible and wear sunscreens and protective clothing as needed until the individual effects of the drug are known.

RISK FOR IMPAIRED SKIN INTEGRITY. A severe and potentially fatal rash can occur in patients taking lamotrigine, and phenytoin also can produce a hypersensitivity rash. Should a rash occur, notify the primary health care provider immediately because the primary health care provider may discontinue the drug. If the rash is exfoliative (red rash with scaling of the skin), purpuric (small hemorrhages or bruising on the skin), or bullous (skin vesicle filled with fluid, i.e., blister), use of the drug is not resumed. If the rash is milder (e.g., acne/sunburn-like), therapy may be resumed after the rash completely disappears. As the rash heals, keep the patient's nails short, apply an antiseptic cream (if prescribed), and instruct the patient to avoid using soap until the rash subsides.

RISK FOR INFECTION. You should be alert for the signs of pancytopenia, such as sore throat, fever, general malaise, bleeding of the mucous membranes, epistaxis (bleeding from the nose), and easy bruising. Anticonvulsants such as carbamazepine and phenytoin may cause aplastic anemia and agranulocytosis. The succinimides are also particularly toxic. Routine laboratory tests, such as complete blood counts and differential counts, should be performed periodically. If bone marrow depression is evident (e.g., the patient's platelet count and white blood cell count decrease significantly), the primary health care provider may discontinue or change anticonvulsant drugs. When pancytopenia is present and blood cell counts are low, using a soft-bristled toothbrush may protect the mucous membranes from bleeding and easy bruising. The extremities also need to be protected from trauma or injury.

⚠ NURSING ALERT

Hematologic changes (e.g., aplastic anemia, leukopenia, and thrombocytopenia) need to be reported immediately. Teach the patient how to identify signs of thrombocytopenia (bleeding gums, easy bruising, increased menstrual bleeding, tarry stools) or leukopenia (sore throat, chills, swollen glands, excessive fatigue, or shortness of breath) and to contact the primary health care provider.

IMPAIRED ORAL MUCOUS MEMBRANE. Long-term administration of hydantoins can cause gingivitis and gingival hyperplasia (overgrowth of gum tissue). It is important to inspect periodically the mouth, teeth, and gums of patients in a hospital or long-term clinical setting who are receiving one of these drugs. Any changes in the gums or teeth are reported to the primary health care provider. Teach the patient to perform oral care after each meal.

Educating the Patient and Family

When the patient receives a diagnosis of epilepsy, you can assist the patient and the family in adjustment to the diagnosis. Instruct family members in the care of the patient before, during, and after a seizure. Explain the importance of restricting some activities until the seizures are controlled by drugs. Restriction of activities often depends on the age, sex, and occupation of the patient. For some patients, the restriction of activities may create problems with such activities as employment, management of the home environment, or child care. For example, the patient may be prohibited from driving while the primary health care provider attempts to control the seizure activity. You may assist the patient to look for other modes of transportation to continue typical activities or employment. If a problem is recognized, a referral to a social worker, discharge planning coordinator, or public health nurse may be needed.

Review adverse drug reactions associated with the prescribed anticonvulsant with the patient and family members. The patient and family members are instructed to contact the primary health care provider if any adverse reactions occur before the next dose of the drug is due. The patient must not stop taking the drug until the problem is discussed with the primary health care provider.

Some patients, once their seizures are under control (e.g., stop occurring or occur less frequently), may have a tendency to stop the drug abruptly or begin to omit a dose occasionally. The drug must never be abruptly discontinued or doses omitted. If the patient experiences drowsiness during initial therapy, a family member should be responsible for administering the drug. As you develop a teaching plan for the patient or family member, include the following points:

- Do not omit, increase, or decrease the prescribed dose.
- Anticonvulsant blood levels must be monitored at regular intervals, even if the seizures are well controlled.
- This drug should never be abruptly discontinued, except when recommended by the primary health care provider.
- Do not attempt to put anything in the mouth of a person having a seizure.
- If the primary health care provider finds it necessary to stop the drug, another drug usually is prescribed. Start taking this drug immediately (at the time the next dose of the previously used drug was due).
- Anticonvulsant drugs may cause drowsiness or dizziness. Observe caution when performing hazardous tasks. Do not drive unless the adverse reactions of drowsiness, dizziness, or blurred vision are not significant. Driving privileges will be approved or reinstated by the primary health care provider based on seizure control.
- ⚠ Avoid the use of alcohol unless use has been approved by the primary health care provider.
- Wear medical identification, such as a Medic Alert tag or bracelet, indicating drug use and the type of seizure disorder.
- Do not use any nonprescription drug unless the preparation has been approved by the primary health care provider.
- Keep a record of all seizures (date, time, length), as well as any minor problems (e.g., drowsiness, dizziness, lethargy), and take the record to each clinic or office visit.
- Contact the local branches of agencies, such as the Epilepsy Foundation of America, for information and assistance with problems, such as legal matters, insurance, driver's license, low-cost prescription services, and job training or retraining.

HYDANTOINS

- Inform the dentist and other primary health care providers of use of this drug.
- Brush and floss the teeth after each meal and make periodic dental appointments for oral examination and care.

- Take the medication with food to reduce GI upset.
- Thoroughly shake a phenytoin suspension immediately before use.
- Do not take capsules that are discolored.
- Notify the primary health care provider if any of the following occurs: skin rash, bleeding, swollen or tender gums, yellowish discoloration of the skin or eyes, unexplained fever, sore throat, unusual bleeding or bruising, persistent headache, malaise, or pregnancy.

SUCCINIMIDES

- If GI upset occurs, take the drug with food or milk.
- Notify the primary health care provider if any of the following occurs: skin rash, joint pain, unexplained fever, sore throat, unusual bleeding or bruising, drowsiness, dizziness, blurred vision, or pregnancy.

OXAZOLIDINEDIONES

- This drug may cause photosensitivity. Take protective measures (e.g., wear sunscreens and protective clothing) when exposed to ultraviolet light or sunlight until tolerance is determined.
- Notify the primary health care provider if the following reactions occur: visual disturbances, excessive drowsiness or dizziness, sore throat, fever, skin rash, pregnancy, malaise, easy bruising, epistaxis, or bleeding tendencies.
- Avoid pregnancy while taking trimethadione; the drug has caused serious birth defects.

EVALUATION

- Therapeutic effect is achieved and convulsions are controlled.
- Adverse reactions are identified, reported to the primary health care provider, and managed successfully through appropriate nursing interventions:
  - No injury is evident.
  - Skin remains intact.
  - No evidence of infection is seen.
  - Mucous membranes are moist and intact.
- Patient and family express confidence and demonstrate an understanding of the drug regimen.

PHARMACOLOGY IN PRACTICE
THINK CRITICALLY

 As you talk with Lillian she tells you that she has omitted one or two doses over the last month because she is "doing so well." How would you respond to Ms. Chase's statement?

KEY POINTS

- *Convulsion* and *seizure* are terms often used interchangeably to describe sudden, involuntary muscle contractions due to changes in brain electrical activity. Seizures may be caused by disease, injury, or metabolic changes or be inherited at birth.
- Anticonvulsant drugs are used to depress the abnormal nerve impulses discharged in the brain. When discontinued, the drugs should be tapered down or seizure activity may return.

- The most common adverse reactions are GI distress such as nausea, vomiting, constipation, or diarrhea, as well as drowsiness, dizziness, sleepiness, or headache. Prolonged use of the hydantoins can cause overgrowth of gum tissue.
- Monitoring for the more serious adverse reactions such as life-threatening skin rashes and decreased blood counts should be done regularly.

Summary Drug Table ANTICONVULSANTS

Generic Name	Trade Name	Uses	Adverse Reactions	Dosage Ranges
Hydantoins				
ethotoin *eth'-ih-toe-in*	Peganone	Tonic-clonic seizures	Ataxia, CNS depression, headache, hypotension, nystagmus, mental confusion, slurred speech, dizziness, drowsiness, nausea, vomiting, gingival hyperplasia, rash	2–3 g/day orally in 4–6 divided doses
fosphenytoin *fos-fen'-ih-toe-in*		Status epilepticus	Same as ethotoin	Loading dose: 15–20 mg/kg IV Maintenance dose: 4–6 mg/kg/day IV

(table continues on page 298)

Summary Drug Table ANTICONVULSANTS (continued)

Generic Name	Trade Name	Uses	Adverse Reactions	Dosage Ranges
phenytoin *fen'-ih-toe-in*	Dilantin	Tonic-clonic seizures, status epilepticus, prophylactic seizure prevention	Same as ethotoin	Oral: loading dose: 1 g divided into three doses prevention (400 mg, 300 mg, 300 mg) orally q 2 hr Maintenance dose: started 24 hr after loading dose, 300–400 mg/day Parenteral: 10–15 mg/kg IV
Carboxylic Acid Derivatives				
valproic acid *val-proe'-ik* **(divalproex)**	Depakote, Depakene	Epilepsy, migraine headache, mania	Headache, somnolence, dizziness, tremor, nausea, vomiting, diplopia	10–60 mg/kg/day orally; if dosage is more than 250 mg/day, give in divided doses
Succinimides				
ethosuximide *eth-oh-sux'-ih-mide*	Zarontin	Partial seizures	Drowsiness, ataxia, dizziness, nausea, vomiting, urinary frequency, pruritus, urticaria, gingival hyperplasia	Up to 1.5 g/day orally in divided doses; children, 250 mg/day orally
methsuximide *meth-sux'-ih-mide*	Celontin	Partial seizures	Same as ethosuximide	300–1200 mg/day orally
Oxazolidinediones				
trimethadione *trye-meth-ah-dye'-own*	Tridione	Epilepsy	Dizziness, drowsiness, nausea, vomiting, photosensitivity, personality changes, increased irritability, headache, fatigue	900 mg–2.4 g/day orally in equally divided doses
Benzodiazepines				
clonazepam *kloh-nay'-zeh-pam*	Klonopin	Seizure disorders, panic disorders	Drowsiness, depression, ataxia, anorexia, diarrhea, constipation, dry mouth, palpitations, visual disturbances, rash	Initial dose: do not exceed 1.5 mg/day orally in 3 divided doses; increase in increments of 0.5–1 mg q 3 day; do not exceed 20 mg/day
clobazam *klo-ba'-zam*	Onfi	Seizure disorders	Lethargy, somnolence, ataxia, aggression, fatigue, insomnia	Initial dose: 5–10 mg orally, titrate to no more than 40 mg
clorazepate *klore-az'-eh-pate*	Tranxene	Partial seizures, anxiety disorders, alcohol withdrawal	Same as clonazepam	Initial dose: 7.5 mg orally TID, maximum dose 90 mg/day
diazepam *dye-az'-eh-pam*	Valium	Status epilepticus, seizure disorders (all forms), anxiety disorders, alcohol withdrawal	Same as clonazepam	Seizure control: 2–10 mg/day orally BID to QID Status epilepticus: 5–10 mg IV initially, maximum dose 30 mg Rectally: 0.2–0.5 mg/kg
lorazepam *lor-az'-eh-pam*	Ativan	Status epilepticus, preanesthetic	Same as clonazepam	Status epilepticus: 4 mg IV over 2 min
Miscellaneous Preparations				
acetazolamide *ah-see-tah-zoll'-ah-myde*		Epilepsy, altitude sickness	Drowsiness, dizziness, nausea, diarrhea, constipation, visual disturbances	8–30 mg/kg/day in divided doses
carbamazepine *kar-bah-maz'-eh-peen*	Tegretol, Carbatrol, Epitol, Equetro	Epilepsy, bipolar disorder, trigeminal/postherpetic neuralgia	Dizziness, nausea, drowsiness, unsteady gait, aplastic anemia and other blood cell abnormalities	Maintenance: 800–1200 mg/day orally in divided doses

Summary Drug Table ANTICONVULSANTS (continued)

Generic Name	Trade Name	Uses	Adverse Reactions	Dosage Ranges
ezogabine *e-zog'-a-been*	Potiga	Partial seizures (adults)	Somnolence, fatigue, dizziness, confusion	100–400 mg orally in 3 divided doses
felbamate *fell'-bah-mate*	Felbatol	Partial seizures in patients who fail other drug therapy first	Insomnia, headache, anxiety, acne, rash, dyspepsia, vomiting, constipation, diarrhea, upper respiratory tract infection, fatigue, rhinitis, aplastic anemia, hepatic disorders	1200–3600 mg/day orally in divided doses
gabapentin *gab-ah-pen'-tin*	Gralise, Neurontin	Partial seizures (adults), postherpetic neuralgia	Somnolence, dizziness, ataxia	900–1800 mg/day orally in 3–4 divided doses
lacosamide *la-koe'-sa-mide*	Vimpat	Partial seizures (adults)	Dizziness, headache, nausea	100–400 mg orally in 2 divided doses
lamotrigine *lah-moe'-trih-geen*	Lamictal	Partial seizures (used with other anticonvulsants), bipolar disorder	Dizziness, insomnia, somnolence, ataxia, nausea, vomiting, diplopia, headache, Stevens-Johnson syndrome rash	50–500 mg/day orally in 2 divided doses
levetiracetam *lee-veh-tye-rah'-seh-tam*	Keppra	Partial seizures, tonic-clonic seizures, bipolar disorder, migraine headache	Headache, dizziness, asthenia, somnolence, infection	500 mg BID orally, increasing dose every 2 wk until reach 3,000 mg daily
magnesium *mag-nee'-ze-um*		Hypomagnesemia, seizures associated with eclampsia and acute nephritis (children)	Flushing, sweating, hypothermia, depressed reflexes, hypotension, cardiac and CNS depression	Nephritis: 20–40 mg/kg IM in a dilute solution Eclampsia: 4 g IV in dilute solution, titrate continued infusion per serum level
oxcarbazepine *ox-car-baz'-eh-peen*	Trileptal	Epilepsy	Headache, dizziness, fatigue, somnolence, ataxia, diplopia, nausea, vomiting, abdominal pain	600–1200 mg orally BID
pregabalin *preg'-ah-bal-in*	Lyrica	Partial seizures (adults), neuropathic pain, postherpetic neuralgia	Dizziness, somnolence	Seizure activity: 150 mg/day in 2–3 divided doses
primidone *prih'-mih-doan*	Mysoline	Epilepsy	Dizziness, somnolence, nausea, vomiting	Up to 500 mg orally QID
rufinamide *roo-fin'-a-mide*	Banzel	Seizures (associated with Lennox-Gastaut syndrome)	Dizziness, fatigue, headache, somnolence, nausea	400 mg–3200 mg orally BID
tiagabine *tye-ag'-ah-been*	Gabitril	Partial seizures	Dizziness, somnolence, asthenia, nervousness, nausea	4–56 mg/day orally
topiramate *toe-pye'-rah-mate*	Topamax	Partial/tonic-clonic seizures, migraine headache	Fatigue, concentration problems, somnolence, anorexia	Seizure activity: 200–400 mg/day orally in divided doses
vigabatrin *vye-ga'-ba-trin*	Sabril	Partial seizures, infantile spasms	Somnolence, fatigue, dizziness, headache, weight gain, upper respiratory infection symptoms	1.5 g orally twice daily, titrated for infants by body weight
zonisamide *zoe-niss'-ah-mide*	Zonegran	Partial seizures of epilepsy	Somnolence, anorexia, dizziness, headache, rash, heat stroke	100–400 mg/day orally

● Chapter Review

Know Your Drugs

Clients sometimes know a medication by the brand (or trade) name and not the generic name. To help you recognize both names, match the brand name with the generic name of the same medication.

Generic Name	Brand Name
1. carbamazepine	A. Dilantin
2. diazepam	B. Lyrica
3. phenytoin	C. Tegretol
4. pregabalin	D. Valium

Calculate Medication Dosages

1. Zonisamide 200 mg is prescribed. The drug is available in 100-mg tablets. The nurse administers _____.

2. The primary health care provider prescribes ethosuximide syrup 500 mg for a client with absence seizures. The drug is available in a strength of 250 mg/5 mL. The nurse administers _____.

● Prepare for the NCLEX®

Build Your Knowledge

1. A convulsion is best described as _____.
   1. loss of consciousness
   2. disturbances in brain electrical activity
   3. sudden, involuntary contractions
   4. disrupted CNS neurologic impulses

2. Partial seizures make up what percentage of total seizures?
   1. 20%
   2. 40%
   3. 60%
   4. 100%

3. A client is prescribed phenytoin for a recurrent convulsive disorder. The nurse teaches the client that the most common adverse reactions are _____.
   1. related to the gastrointestinal system
   2. associated with the reproductive system
   3. associated with kidney function
   4. related to the CNS

4. When administering diazepam to an older client, the nurse should monitor the client for unusual effects of the drug such as _____.
   1. marked excitement
   2. excessive sweating
   3. heart arrhythmias
   4. agitation

5. Some anticonvulsants may cause birth defects. The nurse should instruct the female client regarding:
   1. birth control methods
   2. prenatal vitamins and supplements
   3. alternative therapy for seizure control
   4. how to stop taking the drugs to get pregnant

Apply Your Knowledge

6. When caring for a client taking a succinimide for seizure control, the nurse monitors the client for blood dyscrasias. Which of the following symptoms would indicate that the client may be developing a blood dyscrasia?
   1. constipation, blood in the stool
   2. diarrhea, lethargy
   3. sore throat, general malaise
   4. hyperthermia, excitement

7. Which statement would be included when educating the client taking trimethadione for seizures?
   1. Take this drug with milk to enhance absorption.
   2. Wear a sunscreen and protective clothing when exposed to sunlight.
   3. To minimize adverse reactions, take this drug once daily at bedtime.
   4. Visit a dentist frequently because this drug increases the risk of gum disease.

8. Which of the following adverse reactions, if observed in a client prescribed phenytoin, would indicate that the patient may be developing phenytoin toxicity?
   1. severe occipital headache
   2. ataxia
   3. hyperactivity
   4. somnolence

Alternate-Format Questions

9. The nurse is preparing to administer an anticonvulsant for status epilepticus. The primary health care provider prescribes lorazepam (Ativan) 4 mg IV. Look at the package provided. The nurse will administer _____.

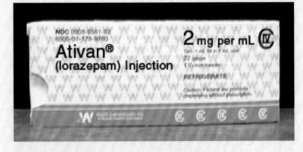

10. Look at the image provided. Which drug is most likely to cause gingival hyperplasia?

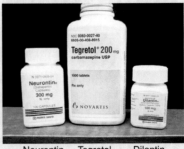

Neurontin   Tegretol   Dilantin

To check your answers, see Appendix G.

the**Point** *For more NCLEX-style questions, log on to http://thepoint.lww.com to access more than 1000 questions.*

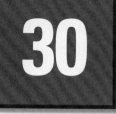

Skeletal Muscle, Bone, and Joint Disorder Drugs

LEARNING OBJECTIVES

On completion of this chapter, the student will:

1. List the types of drugs used to treat musculoskeletal disorders.
2. Discuss the uses, general drug actions, adverse reactions, contraindications, precautions, and interactions of the drugs used to treat musculoskeletal disorders.
3. Discuss important preadministration and ongoing assessment activities the nurse should perform on the patient taking a drug used to treat musculoskeletal disorders.
4. List nursing diagnoses particular to a patient taking a drug for the treatment of musculoskeletal disorders.
5. Discuss ways to promote an optimal response to therapy, how to manage adverse reactions, and important points to keep in mind when educating the patient about drugs used to treat musculoskeletal disorders.

KEY TERMS

alopecia • abnormal loss of hair; baldness

autoimmune • a response where antibodies are formed against one's own body

dyspepsia • fullness or epigastric discomfort

gout • a metabolic disorder resulting in increased levels of uric acid and causing severe joint pain

hypercalcemia • abnormally high level of serum calcium

musculoskeletal • pertaining to the bones and muscles

osteoarthritis • noninflammatory degeneration of joints and cartilage

Paget's disease • condition where bones grow too large and become weak

rheumatoid arthritis (RA) • inflammatory changes in connective tissue

Stevens-Johnson syndrome (SJS) • fever, cough, muscular aches and pains, headache, and lesions of the skin, mucous membranes, and eyes; the lesions appear as red wheals or blisters, often starting on the face, in the mouth, or on the lips, neck, and extremities

DRUG CLASSES

Disease-modifying antirheumatic drugs (DMARDs)

Bone resorption inhibitors—bisphosphonates

Skeletal muscle relaxants

Uric acid inhibitors

A variety of drugs are used in treating **musculoskeletal** (bone and muscle) injuries and disorders. When muscles are injured, typically rest, exercise, and physical therapy are used to heal the injury. Skeletal muscle relaxants are used to assist in relaxing certain muscle groups, as strains and sprains are repaired.

Chronic disease may also affect skeletal muscles, causing limitations in function. Drugs are frequently used to maintain

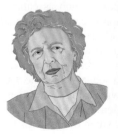

PHARMACOLOGY IN PRACTICE

A call has been taken at the clinic from Mrs. Moore's daughter, who lives out of town. When you contact her, she expresses concern about her mother's balance and possible risk for falls. She asks if she (Mrs. Moore) should be taking a pill to strengthen her bones. Consider this request as you read this chapter.

Table 30.1 Selected Musculoskeletal Disorders

Disorder	Description
Synovitis	Inflammation of the synovial membrane of a joint resulting in pain, swelling, and inflammation. It occurs in disorders such as rheumatic fever, RA, and gout.
Arthritis	Inflammation of a joint. The term is frequently used to refer to any disease involving pain or stiffness of the musculoskeletal system.
Osteoarthritis or degenerative joint disease (DJD)	Noninflammatory DJD marked by degeneration of the articular cartilage, changes in the synovial membrane, and hypertrophy of the bone at the margins.
Rheumatoid arthritis	Chronic systemic disease that produces inflammatory changes throughout the connective tissue in the body. It affects joints and other organ systems of the body. Destruction of articular cartilage occurs, affecting joint structure and mobility. RA primarily affects individuals between 20 and 40 years of age.
Gout	Form of arthritis in which uric acid accumulates in increased amounts in the blood and often is deposited in the joints. The deposit or collection of urate crystals in the joints causes the symptoms (pain, redness, swelling, joint deformity).
Osteoporosis	Loss of bone density occurring when the loss of bone substance exceeds the rate of bone formation. Bones become porous, brittle, and fragile. Compression fractures of the vertebrae are common. This disorder occurs most often in postmenopausal women but can occur in men as well.
Hypercalcemia of malignancy	Advanced-stage malignant disease. It can occur with 10%–50% of tumors. It is associated with parathyroid hormone production and can be difficult to manage. Symptoms include lethargy, anorexia, nausea, vomiting, thirst, polydipsia, constipation, and dehydration. If untreated, it may lead to cognitive difficulties, confusion, obtundation (extreme dullness, near-coma), and coma.
Paget's disease (osteitis deformans)	Chronic bone disorder characterized by abnormal bone remodeling. The disease disrupts the growth of new bone tissue, causing the bone to thicken and become soft. This weakens the bone, which increases susceptibility to fracture or collapse of the bone (e.g., the vertebrae) even with slight trauma.

function due to chronic illness. Examples of the drugs discussed for musculoskeletal disorders in this chapter include disease-modifying antirheumatic drugs (used to treat **rheumatoid arthritis [RA]**), bone resorption inhibitors (used to treat osteoporosis), and uric acid inhibitors (used to treat **gout**). A description of these and other musculoskeletal disorders is given in Table 30.1. The drug selected is based on the musculoskeletal disorder being treated, the severity of the disorder, and the patient's positive or negative response to past therapy. For example, early cases of RA may respond well to the nonsteroidal anti-inflammatory drugs (NSAIDs), whereas advanced RA not responding to other drug therapies may require the use of corticosteroids or immunosuppressive drugs.

Salicylates and NSAIDs are important agents used in treating arthritic conditions. For example, salicylates and NSAIDs are used for RA (a chronic disease characterized by inflammatory changes in the body's connective tissue) and **osteoarthritis** (a noninflammatory joint disease resulting in degeneration of the articular cartilage and changes in the synovial membrane), as well as for relief of pain or discomfort resulting from musculoskeletal injuries such as sprains.

DISEASE-MODIFYING ANTIRHEUMATIC DRUGS

RA, a chronic disorder involving the inflammation and accumulation of fluid in joints, is considered an **autoimmune** disease. This condition is typically treated using three classifications of drugs: NSAIDs, corticosteroids, and disease-modifying antirheumatic drugs. This section describes the disease-modifying antirheumatic drugs, frequently called DMARDs. The NSAIDs and corticosteroids are discussed in Chapters 14 and 43, respectively.

Actions and Uses

RA is an autoimmune disorder, in which antibodies are formed against one's own body. As a defense mechanism, white blood cells are mobilized and lodge in the joints, causing swelling, pain, and inflammation (Fig. 30.1). When the immobility and pain of RA can no longer be controlled by pain relief agents and anti-inflammatory drugs, DMARDs are used. These drugs have properties to produce immunosuppression, which in turn decreases the body's autoimmune response. Therefore, in RA treatment, DMARDs are useful for their immunosuppressive ability. Other autoimmune diseases treated with DMARDs include Crohn's disease and fibromyalgia. (DMARDs may also be used for other purposes, such as cancer therapy, in which the immunosuppression is considered an adverse reaction rather than an intended effect.)

Cytotoxic drugs, such as azathioprine (Imuran), cyclophosphamide (Cytoxan), and cyclosporine, are reserved for life-threatening problems (such as systemic vasculitis) because they are associated with a high rate of toxic adverse reactions. Gold salts and penicillamine are considered extremely toxic and used only when other drugs fail to achieve remission.

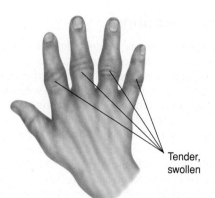

Tender,
swollen

Figure 30.1 Example of acute rheumatoid arthritis in the joints of the wrist and hand. (From Bickley, L. S., & Szilagyi, P. [2003]. *Bates' guide to physical examination and history taking* [8th ed.]. Philadelphia: Lippincott Williams & Wilkins.)

Adverse Reactions

Immunosuppressive drugs can cause the following adverse reactions:

• Nausea
• Stomatitis
• **Alopecia** (hair loss)

The adverse reactions to sulfa-based drugs, such as sulfasalazine, include ocular changes, gastrointestinal (GI) upset, and mild pancytopenia. The most common adverse reaction to the drugs given by injection is skin irritation. For more information, see the Summary Drug Table: Drugs Used to Treat Musculoskeletal, Bone, and Joint Disorders.

Contraindications

All categories of DMARDs are contraindicated in patients with known hypersensitivity to the drugs. Patients with renal insufficiency, liver disease, alcohol abuse, pancytopenia, or folate deficiency should not take methotrexate. Etanercept (Enbrel), adalimumab (Humira), and infliximab (Remicade) should not be used in patients with congestive heart failure or neurologic demyelinating diseases. Anakinra (Kineret) should not be used in combination with etanercept, adalimumab, or infliximab.

Precautions

These drugs should be used with caution in patients with obesity, diabetes, and hepatitis B or C. Women should not become pregnant, and sexual partners should use barrier contraception to prevent transmission of the drug by semen.

Sulfasalazine is selected over methotrexate for patients with liver disease. Patients taking etanercept, adalimumab, or infliximab should be screened for pre-existing tuberculosis because of the increase in opportunistic infections presenting after treatment.

Interactions

The following interactions may occur when a DMARD, such as methotrexate, is administered with another agent:

Interacting Drug	Common Use	Effect of Interaction
sulfa antibiotics	Fight infection	Increased risk of methotrexate toxicity
aspirin and NSAIDs	Pain relief	Increased risk of methotrexate toxicity

NURSING ALERT

Because DMARDs are designed to produce immunosuppression, patients need to be monitored routinely for infections. Instruct patients to report any problem, no matter how minor, such as a cold or open sore—even these can become life-threatening.

BONE RESORPTION INHIBITORS: BISPHOSPHONATES

Bisphosphonates are drugs used to treat musculoskeletal disorders such as osteoporosis and **Paget's disease** (bone growth and weakening). Osteoporosis involves the loss of bone mass, seen typically in postmenopausal women. As the skeleton deteriorates there is a larger risk for fracture of the bones.

Actions

Bisphosphonates act primarily on the bone by inhibiting normal and abnormal bone resorption. This results in increased bone mineral density, reversing the progression of osteoporosis.

Uses

Bisphosphonates are used in the treatment of the following:

• Osteoporosis in postmenopausal women and men (caused by glucocorticoid use)
• **Hypercalcemia** (increased serum calcium) of malignant diseases and bony metastasis of some solid tumors
• Paget's disease of the bone

Adverse Reactions

Adverse reactions with bisphosphonates include:

• Nausea, diarrhea
• Increased or recurrent bone pain
• Headache
• **Dyspepsia** (GI discomfort), acid regurgitation, dysphagia
• Abdominal pain

Contraindications and Precautions

These drugs are contraindicated in patients who are hypersensitive to the bisphosphonates. Alendronate (Fosamax) and risedronate (Actonel) are contraindicated in patients with hypocalcemia. Alendronate is a pregnancy category C drug and is contraindicated during pregnancy. These drugs are also contraindicated in patients with delayed esophageal emptying or renal impairment. Concurrent use of these drugs with hormone replacement therapy is not recommended.

Although these drugs have not been studied, if a pregnant woman presents with malignancy, their use during the pregnancy may be justified if the potential benefit outweighs the potential risk to the fetus.

Interactions

The following interactions may occur when a bisphosphonate is administered with another agent:

Interacting Drug	Common Use	Effect of Interaction
calcium supplements or antacids with magnesium and aluminum	Relief of gastric upset	Decreased effectiveness of bisphosphonates
aspirin	Pain relief	Increased risk of GI bleeding
theophylline	Alleviation of breathing problems	Increased risk of theophylline toxicity

SKELETAL MUSCLE RELAXANTS

Actions

The mode of action of many skeletal muscle relaxants, such as carisoprodol (Soma), baclofen (Lioresal), and chlorzoxazone (Parafon Forte), is not clearly understood. Many of these drugs do not directly relax skeletal muscles, but their ability to relieve acute painful musculoskeletal conditions may be due to their sedative action. Cyclobenzaprine appears to have an effect on muscle tone, thereby reducing muscle spasm.

The exact mode of action of diazepam (Valium), an antianxiety drug (see Chapter 20), in the relief of painful musculoskeletal conditions is unknown. The drug does have a sedative action, which may account for some of its ability to relieve muscle spasm and pain.

Uses

Skeletal muscle relaxants are used in various acute painful musculoskeletal conditions, such as muscle strains and back pain.

Adverse Reactions

Drowsiness is the most common reaction seen with the use of skeletal muscle relaxants. Additional adverse reactions are given in the Summary Drug Table: Drugs Used to Treat Musculoskeletal, Bone, and Joint Disorders. Some of the adverse reactions that may occur with the administration of diazepam include drowsiness, sedation, sleepiness, lethargy, constipation or diarrhea, bradycardia or tachycardia, and rash.

Contraindications

Skeletal muscle relaxants are contraindicated in patients with known hypersensitivity to the drugs. Baclofen is contraindicated in skeletal muscle spasms caused by rheumatic disorders. Carisoprodol is contraindicated in patients with a known hypersensitivity to meprobamate. Cyclobenzaprine is contraindicated in patients with a recent myocardial infarction, cardiac conduction disorders, and hyperthyroidism. In addition, cyclobenzaprine is contraindicated within 14 days of the administration of a monoamine oxidase inhibitor (MAOI). Oral dantrolene is contraindicated during lactation and in patients with active hepatic disease and muscle spasm caused by rheumatic disorders.

Precautions

Skeletal muscle relaxants are used with caution in patients with a history of cerebrovascular accident, cerebral palsy, parkinsonism, or seizure disorders and during pregnancy and lactation (pregnancy category C). Carisoprodol is used with caution in patients with severe liver or kidney disease and during pregnancy (category unknown) and lactation. Cyclobenzaprine is used cautiously in patients with cardiovascular disease and during pregnancy and lactation (pregnancy category B). Dantrolene, a pregnancy category C drug, is used with caution during pregnancy.

Interactions

The following interactions may occur when a skeletal muscle relaxant is administered with another agent:

Interacting Drug	Common Use	Effect of Interaction
central nervous system (CNS) depressants, such as alcohol, antihistamines, opiates, and sedatives	Promote a calming effect or provide pain relief	Increased CNS depressant effect
cyclobenzaprine MAOIs	Manage depression	Risk for high fever and convulsions
orphenadrine haloperidol	Treat psychotic behavior	Increased psychosis
tizanidine antihypertensives	Reduce blood pressure	Increased risk of hypotension

URIC ACID INHIBITORS

Gout is a type of arthritis in which uric acid accumulates in increased amounts in the blood and often is deposited in the joints. The deposit or collection of urate crystals in the joints causes the symptoms (pain, redness, swelling, joint deformity) of gout.

Actions

Allopurinol (Zyloprim) reduces the production of uric acid, thereby decreasing serum uric acid levels and the deposit of urate crystals in joints. This probably accounts for its ability to relieve the severe pain of acute gout. Febuxostat (Uloric), a newer drug, is used to reduce serum uric acid levels, preventing gout attacks.

The exact mechanism of action of colchicine is unknown, but it does reduce the inflammation associated with the deposit of urate crystals in the joints. Colchicine has no effect on uric acid metabolism.

In people with gout, the serum uric acid level is usually elevated. In an acute attack, pegloticase, an IV infusion, may be used to decrease the amount of uric acid in the body. Probenecid works in the same manner and may be given alone or with colchicine as combination therapy when there are frequent, recurrent attacks of gout. Probenecid also has been used to prolong the plasma levels of penicillins and cephalosporins.

Uses

Drugs indicated for treatment of gout may be used to manage acute attacks of gout or in preventing acute attacks of gout (prophylaxis).

Adverse Reactions

Gastrointestinal System Reactions

- Nausea, vomiting, diarrhea
- Abdominal pain

Other Reactions

- Headache
- Urinary frequency

One adverse reaction associated with allopurinol is skin rash, which in some cases has been followed by serious hypersensitivity reactions, such as exfoliative dermatitis and **Stevens-Johnson syndrome**. Colchicine administration may result in severe nausea, vomiting, and bone marrow depression; therefore, it is used as a second line of treatment when other drugs fail.

Contraindications

The drugs used for gout are contraindicated in patients with known hypersensitivity. Colchicine is contraindicated in patients with serious GI, renal, hepatic, or cardiac disorders and those with blood dyscrasias. Probenecid is contraindicated in patients with blood dyscrasias or uric acid kidney stones, and in children younger than 2 years. If patients are taking azathioprine (Imuran), mercaptopurine, or theophylline they should not be prescribed febuxostat.

Precautions

Uric acid inhibitors are used cautiously in patients with renal impairment and during pregnancy; these agents are either pregnancy category B or C drugs. Allopurinol is used cautiously in patients with liver impairment. Probenecid is used cautiously in patients who are hypersensitive to sulfa drugs or have peptic ulcer disease. Colchicine is used with caution in older adults.

Anaphylactic reactions have been seen with pegloticase infusions; therefore, antihistamines and corticosteroids are used to premedicate patients.

Interactions

The following interactions may occur when a uric acid inhibitor is administered with another agent:

Interacting Drug	Common Use	Effect of Interaction
allopurinol and febuxostat		
ampicillin	Anti-infective agent	Increased risk of rash
theophylline	Alleviation of breathing problems	Increased risk of theophylline toxicity
aluminum-based antacids	Relief of gastric upset	Decreased effectiveness of allopurinol
probenecid		
penicillins, cephalosporins, acyclovir, rifampin, and the sulfonamides	Anti-infective agent	Increased serum level of anti-infective
barbiturates and benzodiazepines	Sedation	Increased serum level of sedative
NSAIDs	Pain relief	Increased serum level of NSAID
salicylates	Pain relief	Decreased effectiveness of probenecid

HERBAL CONSIDERATIONS

Glucosamine and chondroitin are used, in combination or alone, to treat arthritis, particularly osteoarthritis. Chondroitin acts as the flexible connecting matrix between the protein filaments in cartilage. Chondroitin can be produced in the laboratory or can come from natural sources (e.g., shark cartilage). Some studies suggest that if chondroitin is available to the cell matrix, synthesis of tissue can occur. For this reason, it is used to treat arthritis. Although there is little information on chondroitin's long-term effects, it is generally not considered to be harmful.

Glucosamine theoretically provides a building block for regeneration of damaged cartilage. The absorption of oral glucosamine is 90% to 98%, making it widely accepted for use. Glucosamine is generally well tolerated, and no adverse reactions have been reported with its use (DerMarderosian, 2003).

NURSING PROCESS
PATIENT RECEIVING A DRUG FOR A MUSCULOSKELETAL DISORDER

ASSESSMENT

Preadministration Assessment

Obtaining the patient's history will be variable depending on whether the drug is used to prevent a problem or to stop a problem—that is, if preventative there may not be an onset, symptoms or current treatment. In some instances, it may be necessary to question patients regarding their ability to carry out activities of daily living, including employment when applicable; at other times it may not be affected.

During the physical assessment, describe the patient's physical condition and limitations. If the patient has arthritis (any type), examine the affected joints in the extremities for appearance of the skin over the joint, evidence of joint deformity, and mobility of the affected joint. Patients with osteoporosis are assessed for pain, particularly in the upper and lower back or hip. If the patient has gout, note the appearance of the skin over the joints, the pain experience, and any joint enlargement. Vital signs and weight are taken to provide a baseline for comparison during therapy.

The primary health care provider may order laboratory tests and bone scans to measure bone density. This is especially important for use as baseline data when a bone resorption inhibitor is prescribed for the patient.

> **! NURSING ALERT**
>
> When bisphosphonates are administered, serum calcium levels are monitored before, during, and after therapy.

Ongoing Assessment

Periodic evaluation is an important part of therapy for musculoskeletal disorders. With some disorders, such as acute gout, the patient can be expected to respond to therapy in hours. Therefore, it is important to inspect and document the joints involved every 1 to 2 hours to identify immediately a response or nonresponse to therapy. Also, question the patient regarding the relief of pain, as well as adverse drug reactions.

In other disorders, response is gradual and may take days, weeks, and even months of treatment. Depending on the drug administered and the disorder being treated, the evaluation of therapy may be daily or yearly. These documented evaluations help the primary health care provider plan current and future therapy, including dosage changes, changes in the drug administered, and institution of physical therapy.

NURSING DIAGNOSES

Drug-specific nursing diagnoses include the following:

- **Readiness for Enhanced Fluid Balance** related to need for increased fluid intake to promote excretion of urate crystals
- **Impaired Comfort: Gastric Distress** related to irritation of gastric lining from medication administration

- **Risk for Injury** related to medication-induced drowsiness and associated risk for imbalance and falls
- **Risk for Allergy Response** related to response to substance trigger (drug allergy)

Nursing diagnoses related to drug administration are discussed in Chapter 4.

PLANNING

The expected outcomes for the patient depend on the reason for administration but may include an optimal response to therapy, meeting patient needs related to the management of adverse reactions, and confidence in an understanding of the medication regimen.

IMPLEMENTATION

Promoting an Optimal Response to Therapy

The patient with a musculoskeletal disorder may have long-standing chronic pain, which can be just as difficult to tolerate as acute pain. Along with pain, there may be skeletal deformities, such as the joint deformities seen with advanced RA. For many musculoskeletal conditions, drug therapy is a major treatment modality. In addition to drug therapy, rest, physical therapy, and other measures may be part of treatment. Including drugs as a major part of the treatment plan may keep the disorder under control (e.g., therapy for gout), improve the patient's ability to carry out activities of daily living, or make the pain and discomfort tolerable.

Patients with a musculoskeletal disorder may have negative or self-defeating feelings related to the symptoms and the chronicity of the disorder. In addition to physical care, these patients often require emotional support, especially when a disorder is disabling and chronic. Be encouraging as you explain to the patient that therapy may take weeks or longer before any benefit is noted. When this is explained before therapy starts, the patient is less likely to become discouraged over slow results.

It is important to be alert to reactions such as skin rash, fever, cough, or easy bruising. Listen carefully for specific patient complaints that may seem unrelated to drug therapy, such as visual changes, tinnitus, or hearing loss. Be sure to immediately report these adverse reactions; the primary health care provider may need to change doses or even drugs. Particular attention is paid to visual changes because irreversible retinal damage may occur.

Administration of allopurinol may result in skin rash. A rash should be monitored carefully because it may precede a serious adverse reaction, such as Stevens-Johnson syndrome. Immediately report any rash to the primary health care provider.

Gold compounds and methotrexate are potentially toxic. Therefore, monitor labs closely for development of adverse reactions, such as thrombocytopenia and leukopenia. Hematology, liver, and renal function studies are monitored every 1 to 3 months with methotrexate therapy. Notify the primary health care provider of abnormal hematology, liver function, or kidney function findings.

Monitoring and Managing Patient Needs

READINESS FOR ENHANCED FLUID BALANCE. When the patient is using the uric acid inhibitors, encourage liberal fluid intake. The patient can tell if he or she is getting adequate fluids when the daily urine output is about 2 liters. An increase in urinary output is necessary to excrete the urates (uric acid) and prevent urate acid stone formation in the genitourinary tract. Discuss ways to provide adequate fluids and remind the patient frequently of the importance of increasing fluid intake. If the patient fails to increase fluid intake, contact the primary health care provider. In some instances, it may be necessary to administer intravenous fluids to supplement the oral intake when the patient fails to drink about 3000 mL of fluid per day.

IMPAIRED COMFORT: GASTRIC DISTRESS. Adequate drug absorption and metabolism can depend on timing with meals. To facilitate delivery of the bone resorption inhibitor to the stomach and minimize adverse GI effects, instruct the patient to take the drug upon arising in the morning, with 6 to 8 ounces of water, and remain in an upright position. Specific instructions to help patients remember the routine are provided in Patient Teaching for Improved Patient Outcomes: Taking Bisphosphonates for Best Results. The patient is instructed to remain upright (avoid lying down) for at least 30 minutes after taking the drug. Etidronate is not administered within 2 hours of food, vitamin and mineral supplements, or antacids.

Many bisphosphonates are available in both once-a-week and once-a-month dosing forms. Although there is a once-a-year drug, the patient has to come to the ambulatory clinic for intravenous administration. DMARDs, uric acid inhibitors, and skeletal muscle relaxants are taken with, or immediately after, meals to minimize gastric distress.

RISK FOR INJURY. Many of these drugs may cause drowsiness. In addition, pain or deformity may hamper mobility. These two factors place the patient at risk of injury. Therefore, teach the family to monitor the patient carefully before allowing the patient to ambulate alone. If drowsiness does occur, assistance with ambulatory activities is necessary. If drowsiness is severe, instruct the patient or family to contact the primary health care provider before the next dose is due.

The patient with an arthritis disorder may experience much pain or discomfort and may require assistance with activities, such as ambulating, eating, and grooming. Patients on bed rest require position changes and skin care every 2 hours. Patients with osteoporosis may require a brace or corset when out of bed.

RISK FOR ALLERGIC RESPONSE. When first-line treatments for gout are not successful, sometimes drugs that are more toxic may be prescribed such as the pegloticase infusion. During the infusion the patient is closely monitored for the development of adverse reactions. Should an anaphylactic reaction occur, the infusion center staff members are prepared to start resuscitative measures as emergency personnel are notified.

Educating the Patient and Family

The dosing schedule for these drugs may be variable. Dosing schedules may require taking medications on alternate days, at specific times of the day, or weekly or even monthly. The patient may not see a therapeutic response until 3 to 6 weeks

---

Patient Teaching for Improved Patient Outcomes

Taking Bisphosphonates for Best Results

Bone resorption inhibitors work to not only build bone density but also prevent bone fractures (sometimes by as much as 50%). You may have heard both good and bad issues from friends and family taking these drugs. Here is how to learn what is best for you. When you teach, make sure your patient understands the following:

When to treat. Diagnosis for osteoporosis treatment is made by your T-score (from the bone mineral density scan). You may not be a candidate for treatment if you have gastroesophageal problems, kidney disease, or severe vitamin D deficiency. Some preparations are taken daily and others as infrequently as monthly. Research shows good results when taken for 5 to 10 years—so correct administration is important.

Supplements. These drugs work by using the building blocks of bone formation. You need an intake of 1500 mg of calcium and 400 to 800 units of vitamin D daily. The drug you take may or may not have this supplement in the preparation. Check with your primary health care provider and follow the vitamin supplement recommended.

Specific drug administration routine. These drugs are absorbed slowly from the stomach and can cause severe irritation of the esophagus. You must take the pill with 6 to 8 ounces of plain water and cannot eat or drink for 30 minutes after taking the drug, and you must be in an upright position during that time. Here are suggestions to make taking this drug easier and build it into your weekly routine:

✔ Use a calendar or cell phone alert to remember your monthly dose.
✔ Do not prepare your coffee maker the night before you are to take the drug. This will prevent you from drinking your morning cup of coffee before you realize you should have taken the medication.
✔ Put the medication out the night before in a place you will see it when you first get up out of bed.
✔ Take your medication and then do a distracting activity, such as taking your morning shower or sitting in a chair and watching the morning news on television, listening to music on the radio, or looking at or answering e-mail.
✔ Make this morning's breakfast special with foods you especially like to eat; use breakfast as a reward for having taken your medication correctly!
✔ Make a habit of calling your primary health care provider at least every 6 months (if taking monthly) to talk about whether you are or are not having any GI changes (belching, pressure, heartburn)—it could be from the medication.

of therapy and become discouraged. In some cases, a patient may stop treatment. To ensure adherence with the treatment regimen, the patient must feel confidence in understanding the importance of the prescribed therapy and taking the drug exactly as directed to obtain the best results. To meet this goal, develop an effective plan of patient and family teaching. The following points are included in the teaching plan:

- Explain carefully that treatment for the disorder includes drug therapy, as well as other medical management, such as diet, exercise, limitations or specifications of activity, and periodic physical therapy treatments.
- Teach the importance of asking the primary health care provider before taking any nonprescription drugs or supplements.
- Some drugs used for RA require self-administered subcutaneous injections. Teach the patient and family proper injection and disposal techniques.
- Teach about site rotation, and have the patient demonstrate proper injection technique before this becomes a self-administered procedure.
- Patients need to be taught how to manage the discomfort to the site of injection and to report redness, pain, and swelling to the primary health care provider.

    When using drugs to treat RA:

- When taking methotrexate, use a calendar or some other memory device to remember to take the drug on the same day each week.
- Notify the primary health care provider immediately if any of the following occur: sore mouth or sores in the mouth, diarrhea, fever, sore throat, easy bruising, rash, itching, or nausea and vomiting.
- Women of childbearing age should use an effective contraceptive during therapy with methotrexate and for 8 weeks after therapy.

    When using drugs to treat gout:

- Drink at least 10 glasses of water a day until the acute attack has subsided.
- Take this drug with food to minimize GI upset.
- If drowsiness occurs, avoid driving or performing other hazardous tasks.

- Acute gout—notify the primary health care provider if pain is not relieved in a few days.
- Notify the primary health care provider if a skin rash occurs.

    When using drugs for muscle spasm and cramping:

- This drug may cause drowsiness. Do not drive or perform other hazardous tasks if drowsiness occurs.
- This drug is for short-term use. Do not use the drug for longer than 2 to 3 weeks.
- ⚕ Avoid alcohol or other CNS depressants while taking this drug.

EVALUATION

- Therapeutic drug effect is achieved, pain is decreased, and mobility is improved or maintained.
- Adverse reactions are identified, reported to the primary health care provider, and managed using appropriate nursing interventions:
  - Patient improves fluid balance.
  - GI comfort is maintained.
  - No evidence of injury is seen.
  - Allergic response is minimized.
- Patient and family express confidence and demonstrate an understanding of the drug regimen.

PHARMACOLOGY IN PRACTICE
THINK CRITICALLY

Based on your understanding of drugs to improve bone density and the requirements of these drugs, is Mrs. Moore an appropriate candidate for this medication?

KEY POINTS

- Musculoskeletal disorders that use drug therapy include arthritis (both rheumatoid and osteoarthritis), increased uric acid causing gout, and bone diseases such as osteoporosis. These are chronic and require long-term therapy.
- A variety of drugs are used to treat musculoskeletal injuries and disorders; they include DMARDs, bone resorption inhibitors, skeletal muscle relaxants, and uric acid inhibitors.

- The most common adverse reactions include GI distress, hair loss, and drowsiness.
- Patients using DMARDs should be monitored carefully for infection. Those taking bisphosphonates have specific drug routines to follow to prevent gastroesophageal irritation. When using uric acid inhibitors severe rashes should be monitored.

Summary Drug Table DRUGS USED TO TREAT MUSCULOSKELETAL, BONE, AND JOINT DISORDERS

Generic Name	Trade Name	Uses	Adverse Reactions	Dosage Ranges
Disease-Modifying Antirheumatic Drugs (DMARDs)				
abatacept *a-ba-ta'-sept*	Orencia	RA	Headache, nasal congestion, upper respiratory infection (URI) symptoms, nausea	500–750 mg IV every 4 wk
adalimumab *ah-dah-lim'-mu-mab*	Humira	RA; other autoimmune disorders (e.g., Crohn's disease)	Irritation at injection site, increased risk of infections	40 mg subcut every other week
anakinra *an-ah-kin'-rah*	Kineret	RA	Headache, irritation at injection site, pancytopenia	100 mg subcut daily
certolizumab *ser'-toe-liz'-oo-mab*	Cimzia	RA, Crohn's disease	URI and urinary tract infection (UTI) symptoms	400 mg subcut every 2 wk or monthly
etanercept *ee-tah-ner'-sept*	Enbrel	RA	Headache, rhinitis, irritation at injection site, increased risk of infections	25 mg subcut twice weekly, or 50 mg subcut weekly
golimumab *goe-lim'-oo-mab*	Simponi	RA	URI symptoms, rhinitis, irritation at injection site, increased risk of infections	50 mg subcut weekly
hydroxychloroquine *hye-drox-see-klor'-oh-kwin*	Plaquenil	RA, antimalarial	Irritability nervousness, retinal and corneal changes, anorexia, nausea, vomiting, hematologic effects	400–600 mg/day orally
infliximab *in-flick'-see-mab*	Remicade	RA in combination with methotrexate, Crohn's disease	Fever, chills, headache	3–10 mg/kg IV infusion at specified weekly intervals
leflunomide *leh-floo'-noe-mide*	Arava	RA	Hypertension, alopecia, rash, nausea, diarrhea	Initial dose: 100 mg for 3 days Maintenance dose: 20 mg/day orally
methotrexate (MTX) *meth-oh-trex'-sate*		RA, cancer chemotherapy	Nausea, stomatitis, alopecia	7.5–20 mg orally once weekly
sulfasalazine *sul-fah-sal'-ah-zeen*	Azulfidine	RA, ulcerative colitis	Nausea, emesis, abdominal pains, crystalluria, hematuria, Stevens-Johnson syndrome, rash, headache, drowsiness, diarrhea	2–4 g/day orally in divided doses
tocilizumab *toe'-si-liz'-oo-mab*	Actemra	RA	Headache, nasal congestion, URI symptoms, increased blood pressure, elevated alanine aminotransferase (liver function)	4 mg/kg IV every 4 wk

(table continues on page 310)

Summary Drug Table DRUGS USED TO TREAT MUSCULOSKELETAL, BONE, AND JOINT DISORDERS (continued)

Generic Name	Trade Name	Uses	Adverse Reactions	Dosage Ranges
Bone Resorption Inhibitors: Bisphosphonates				
℞ alendronate *ah-len'-droe-nate*	Fosamax	Treatment and prevention of postmenopausal osteoporosis, glucocorticoid-induced osteoporosis, osteoporosis in men, Paget's disease	Abdominal pain, esophageal reflux	5–10 mg orally, in daily or (70-mg) weekly doses
℞ etidronate *eh-tid'-roh-nate*	Didronel	Hypercalcemia of malignancy, Paget's disease, prevent bone spurs after total hip replacement or spinal cord injury	Nausea, fever, fluid overload	5–20 mg/kg/day orally (treatment not to exceed 6 mo)
℞ ibandronate *ih-ban'-droe-nate*	Boniva	Postmenopausal osteoporosis	Abdominal pain, nausea, diarrhea	2.5 mg/day orally, available in 150-mg tablet taken once monthly; 3-mg IV form available for dose once every 3 mo
pamidronate *pah-mid'-roh-nate*	Aredia	Hypercalcemia of malignancy, Paget's disease	Anxiety, headache, insomnia, nausea, vomiting, diarrhea, constipation, dyspepsia, pancytopenia, fever, fatigue, bone pain	60–90 mg in a single IV dose infused over 2–24 hr
℞ risedronate *rih-sed'-roh-nate*	Actonel, Atelvia	Treatment and prevention of postmenopausal osteoporosis, glucocorticoid-induced osteoporosis, osteoporosis in men, Paget's disease	Headache, abdominal pain, arthralgia, recurrent bone pain, nausea, diarrhea	5–75 mg orally, in daily or (75-mg) weekly doses
℞ tiludronate *tih-loo'-droe-nate*	Skelid	Paget's disease	Headache, nausea, diarrhea, arthralgia, pain	400 mg/day orally for no more than 3 mo
zoledronic acid *zole-eh-drone'-ik*	Zometa, Reclast	Zometa: Hypercalcemia of malignancy, solid tumor bone metastases Reclast: Postmenopausal osteoporosis, Paget's disease	Hypotension, confusion, anxiety, agitation, nausea, diarrhea, constipation, fatigue	Zometa: 4 mg in a single IV dose infused over 15 min every 3–4 wk Reclast: 5 mg IV once per year
Skeletal Muscle Relaxants				
baclofen *bak'-loe-fen*	Lioresal	Spasticity due to multiple sclerosis, spinal cord injuries (intrathecal administration for severe spasticity)	Drowsiness, dizziness, nausea, weakness, hypotension	15–80 mg/day orally in divided doses
carisoprodol *kare-eye-soe-proe'-doll*	Soma	Relief of discomfort due to acute, painful musculoskeletal conditions	Dizziness, drowsiness, tachycardia, nausea, vomiting	350 mg orally TID or QID
chlorzoxazone *klore-zox'-ah-zone*	Parafon Forte DSC	Same as carisoprodol	GI disturbances, drowsiness, dizziness, rash	250–750 mg orally TID or QID
cyclobenzaprine *sye-kloe-ben'-zah-preen*	Amrix	Same as carisoprodol	Drowsiness, dizziness, dry mouth, nausea, constipation	10–60 mg/day orally in divided doses

Summary Drug Table DRUGS USED TO TREAT MUSCULOSKELETAL, BONE, AND JOINT DISORDERS (continued)

Generic Name	Trade Name	Uses	Adverse Reactions	Dosage Ranges
dantrolene *dan'-troe-leen*	Dantrium	Spasticity due to spinal cord injury, stroke, cerebral palsy, multiple sclerosis	Drowsiness, dizziness, weakness, constipation, tachycardia, malaise	Initial dose: 25 mg/day orally, then 50–400 mg/day orally in divided doses
diazepam *dye-az'-eh-pam*	Valium	Relief of skeletal muscle spasm, spasticity due to cerebral palsy, epilepsy, paraplegia, anxiety	Drowsiness, sedation, sleepiness, lethargy, constipation, diarrhea, bradycardia, tachycardia, rash	2–10 mg orally BID–QID; 2–20 mg IM, IV Sustained release: 15–30 mg/day orally
metaxalone *me-tax'-ah-lone*	Skelaxin	Same as carisoprodol	Drowsiness, dizziness, headache, nausea, rash	800 mg orally TID or QID
methocarbamol *meth-oh-kar'-bah-moll*	Robaxin	Relief of discomfort due to musculoskeletal disorders	Drowsiness, dizziness, lightheadedness, confusion, headache, rash, blurred vision, GI upset	1–1.5 g QID orally; limit IM, IV dose to 3 g/day
orphenadrine *ore-fen'-ah-dreen*	Norflex	Discomfort due to musculoskeletal disorders	Drowsiness, dizziness, lightheadedness, confusion, headache, rash, blurred vision, GI upset	100 mg BID orally; 60 mg IV or IM q 12 hr
tizanidine *tih-zan'-ih-deen*	Zanaflex	Spasticity due to spinal cord injury, multiple sclerosis	Somnolence, fatigue, dizziness, dry mouth, UTIs	4–8 mg orally up to TID
Uric Acid Inhibitors				
allopurinol *al-oh-pyoor'-ih-noll*	Zyloprim	Management of symptoms of gout	Rash, exfoliative dermatitis, Stevens-Johnson syndrome, nausea, vomiting, diarrhea, abdominal pain, hematologic changes	100–800 mg/day orally
colchicine *koll'-chih-seen*		Relief of acute attacks of gout, prevention of gout attacks	Nausea, vomiting, diarrhea, abdominal pain, bone marrow depression	Prophylaxis: 0.5–0.6 mg/day orally Acute attack: initial dose 0.5–1.2 mg orally or 2 mg IV, then 0.5–1.2 mg orally q 1–2 hr or 0.5 mg IV q 6 hr until attack is aborted or adverse effects occur
febuxostat *feb-ux'-oh-stat*	Uloric	Hyperuricemia	Nausea, rash, arthralgia	40–80 mg orally daily
pegloticase *peg-loe'-ti-kase*	Krystexxa	Management of symptoms of gout	Disease flare-up, infusion reaction, nausea, bruising	8 mg IV every 2 wk
probenecid *proe-ben'-eh-sid*		Treatment of hyperuricemia of gout and gouty arthritis; adjuvant to antibiotics	Headache, anorexia, nausea, vomiting, urinary frequency, flushing, dizziness	0.25 g orally BID for 1 wk, then 0.5 g orally BID

Ⓡ This drug should be administered at least 1 hour before or 2 hours after a meal.

● Chapter Review

Know Your Drugs

Clients sometimes know a medication by the brand (or trade) name and not the generic name. To help you recognize both names, match the brand name with the generic name of the same medication.

Generic Name	Brand Name
1. alendronate	A. Amrix
2. allopurinol	B. Enbrel
3. cyclobenzaprine	C. Fosamax
4. etanercept	D. Zyloprim

Calculate Medication Dosages

1. A client is to receive allopurinol 300 mg orally for gout. The nurse has 100-mg tablets available. How many tablets would the nurse administer? _____

2. The physician prescribes 1.5 g methocarbamol (Robaxin) orally for a musculoskeletal disorder. Available for administration are 500-mg tablets. The nurse administers _____.

● Prepare for the NCLEX®

Build Your Knowledge

1. Bisphosphonates work by _____.
   1. inhibiting calcium digestion
   2. inhibiting abnormal bone resorption
   3. eliminating more phosphorus
   4. prohibiting vitamin D absorption

2. When administering a skeletal muscle relaxant, the nurse observes the client for the most common adverse reaction, which is _____.
   1. drowsiness
   2. GI bleeding
   3. vomiting
   4. constipation

3. When alendronate (Fosamax) is prescribed for osteoporosis, the nurse teaches the client to take the drug _____.
   1. with food or milk
   2. by injection
   3. 30 minutes before breakfast
   4. at bedtime

4. When allopurinol (Zyloprim) is used for treating gout, the nurse _____.
   1. administers the drug with juice or milk
   2. administers the drug after the evening meal
   3. restricts fluids during evening hours
   4. encourages liberal fluid intake

5. What teaching points would the nurse include when educating the client who will begin taking risedronate?
   1. The drug is administered once weekly.
   2. Take a daily laxative, because the drug will likely cause constipation.
   3. Take the drug with antacids to decrease gastric distress.
   4. After taking the drug, remain upright for at least 30 minutes.

Apply Your Knowledge

6. When giving one of the uric acid inhibitors, the nurse assesses the client for the most common adverse reactions, which are _____.
   1. related to the GI tract
   2. urinary retention
   3. hypertension
   4. related to the nervous system

7. When administering a DMARD subcutaneously, the nurse should:
   1. use a 5-mL syringe
   2. inject tissue close to the umbilicus
   3. massage the area to increase blood flow to the muscles
   4. rotate sites to minimize tissue irritation

8. Which of the following statements if made by the client would indicate that she understands how to take a bone resorption medication properly?
   1. "If I get sleepy after taking my med it is okay to lie down."
   2. "If I get a pain in the stomach, it means the medicine is working."
   3. "Take this until you get diarrhea."
   4. "Take a nice shower after taking the med, before I eat."

Alternate-Format Questions

9. Identify which drugs are included in therapy for rheumatoid arthritis. **Select all that apply**.
   1. NSAIDs
   2. DMARDs
   3. anti-infectives
   4. corticosteroids
   5. immunosuppressives

10. A client weighs 63 kilograms. If tocilizumab 4 mg/kg is prescribed, what is the total dosage of tocilizumab for this client?

To check your answers, see Appendix G.

thePoint *For more NCLEX-style questions, log on to http://thepoint.lww.com to access more than 1000 questions.*

Drugs That Affect the Respiratory System

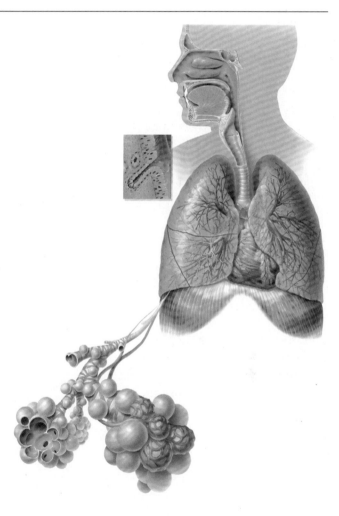

The respiratory system consists of the upper and lower airways, the lungs, and the thoracic cavity. The respiratory system provides a mechanism for the exchange of oxygen and carbon dioxide in the lungs. Any change in the respiratory status has the potential to affect every other bodily system, because all cells need an adequate supply of oxygen for optimal functioning. This unit focuses on drugs used to treat some of the more common disorders affecting the respiratory system. Drugs in this unit are presented in two groups: those that are used for upper respiratory problems and those used for lower respiratory problems.

Among the most common conditions of the upper respiratory system are infections, allergic rhinitis, coughs, the common cold, and congestion. Typically, upper respiratory infections are treated with an antibiotic if bacteria are involved. When the condition is viral, then comfort measures are used to tolerate the course of the illness. These measures include (1) antihistamines to relieve allergy symptoms, (2) decongestants to reduce nasal edema, and (3) antitussives, mucolytics, and expectorants to treat accompanying cough. These drugs are discussed in Chapter 31. Many of these drugs are available as non-prescription (over-the-counter [OTC]) drugs, whereas a few are available only by prescription.

Disorders of the lower respiratory tract include asthma (chronic inflammatory disease of the airways), emphysema (lung disorder in which the alveoli become enlarged and plugged with mucus), and chronic bronchitis (chronic inflammation and possible infection of the bronchi). These conditions are collectively termed chronic obstructive pulmonary disease (COPD). COPD is a slowly progressive disease of the airways characterized by a gradual loss of lung function. The symptoms of COPD range from chronic cough and sputum production to severe, disabling shortness of breath. There is no known cure for COPD; the treatment is usually supportive and designed to relieve symptoms and improve quality of life.

In Chapter 32, drugs used to treat disorders of the lower respiratory tract are discussed. These drugs include the bronchodilating drugs, which are the beta (β)$_2$-adrenergic agonists (which have sympathomimetic properties) and the xanthine derivatives. Along with the bronchodilating drugs, the antiasthma drugs include the corticosteroids, leukotriene modifiers, and mast cell stabilizers.

Asthma is a chronic inflammatory condition of the lower airway with airway constriction caused by broncho-spasm and bronchoconstriction. This condition is featured in Chapter 32. Patients with asthma may experience periods of exacerbation alternating with periods of normal lung function. Environmental exposure to such allergens as house dust mites, tobacco smoke, pets and pet dander, mold, and cockroach wastes and physical exercise are "triggers" for an asthma attack. Anti-inflammatory drugs play an important role in treating individuals with asthma. These drugs prevent asthma attacks by decreasing the swelling and mucous production in the airways, thereby making the airways less sensitive to asthma triggers. Drug therapy for asthma is aimed at preventing attacks and reducing swelling and mucous production in the airways.

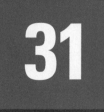

Upper Respiratory System Drugs

LEARNING OBJECTIVES

On completion of this chapter, the student will:

1. Describe the classes of medications used for upper respiratory system problems.
2. Discuss the uses, general drug actions, adverse reactions, contraindications, precautions, and interactions of antitussives, mucolytics, expectorants, antihistamines, and decongestants.
3. Discuss important preadministration and ongoing assessment activities that should be performed on the patient receiving an antitussive, mucolytic, expectorant, antihistamine, or decongestant.
4. List nursing diagnoses particular to a patient taking an antitussive, mucolytic, expectorant, antihistamine, or decongestant.
5. Discuss ways to promote an optimal response to therapy, manage common adverse reactions, and educate the patient about the use of an antitussive, mucolytic, expectorant, antihistamine, or decongestant.

KEY TERMS

anticholinergic action • blockage of parasympathetic nervous system

histamine • substance found in various parts of the body (i.e., liver, lungs, intestines, skin) and produced from the amino acid histidine in response to injury to trigger the inflammatory response

nonproductive cough • dry, hacking cough that produces no secretions

productive cough • cough by which secretions from the respiratory tract are expelled

urticaria • hives, itchy wheals on the skin resulting from contact with or ingestion of an allergenic substance or food

DRUG CLASSES

Antihistamine	Expectorant
Decongestant	Mucolytic
Antitussive	

This chapter focuses on drugs used to treat some of the more common disorders affecting the upper respiratory system, particularly allergies and the congestion associated with certain respiratory disorders. The drugs used to treat the discomfort associated with an upper respiratory disorder include antihistamines, decongestants, antitussives, and expectorants. Many of these drugs are available as nonprescription (over-the-counter [OTC]) drugs, whereas others are available only by prescription.

The buildup of secretions in the lower respiratory system is treated with mucolytics. These agents break down the thickness of the secretions for easier removal.

ANTIHISTAMINES

Histamine is produced in response to an allergic reaction or tissue injury. The release of histamine produces an inflammatory response. Dilation of small arterioles results in localized

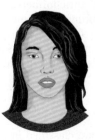

PHARMACOLOGY IN PRACTICE

Janna Wong, a 16-year-old gymnast, is experiencing nasal congestion. She has been prescribed a combination antihistamine and nasal decongestant. A number of antihistamines have anticholinergic effects. Think about the teaching points you will want to cover with Janna.

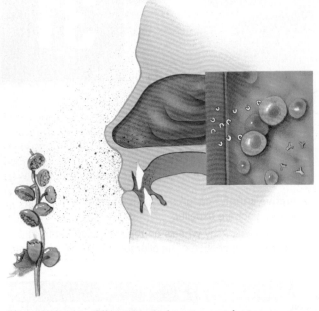

Table 31.1 Intranasal Steroids

Drug	Indication
beclomethasone (Beconase AQ)	Nasal polyps and rhinitis (perennial, seasonal, and vasomotor)
budesonide (Rhinocort Aqua)	Rhinitis (perennial and seasonal)
flunisolide (Nasarel)	Rhinitis (perennial and seasonal)
fluticasone (Flonase, Veramyst)	Rhinitis (perennial, seasonal, and vasomotor)
mometasone (Nasonex)	Nasal polyps, rhinitis (perennial and seasonal)
triamcinolone (Nasacort AQ and HFA)	Rhinitis (perennial and seasonal)

Figure 31.1 Allergens and upper respiratory system inflammation. (Courtesy of Anatomical Chart Co.)

redness. An increase in the permeability of small blood vessels promotes an escape of fluid from these blood vessels into the surrounding tissues, which produces localized swelling. This reaction is illustrated in Figure 31.1. Histamine is also released from mast cells in allergic reactions or hypersensitivity reactions, such as anaphylactic shock.

Actions

Antihistamines (or H_1 receptor antagonists) block most, but not all, of the effects of histamine. They do this by competing at the histamine receptor sites throughout the body, thereby preventing histamine from entering these receptor sites and producing an effect on body tissues. First-generation antihistamines bind *nonselectively* to central and peripheral H_1 receptors and may result in central nervous system (CNS) stimulation or depression. CNS depression usually occurs with higher doses and explains why some of these agents are used for sedation. Other first-generation drugs may have additional effects, such as antipruritic (anti-itching) or antiemetic (antinausea) effects. Second-generation antihistamines are selective for peripheral H_1 receptors and, as a group, are less sedating.

Desloratadine, loratadine, and fexofenadine minimally penetrate the blood–brain barrier, which means that little of the drug is distributed in the CNS so that fewer of the sedating effects are felt. Topical corticosteroid nasal sprays, such as fluticasone (Flonase) or triamcinolone (Nasacort), are also used to reduce the inflammation of nasal allergy symptoms; these are listed in Table 31.1.

Uses

The general uses of the antihistamines include the following:

- Relief of the symptoms of seasonal and perennial allergies
- Allergic and vasomotor rhinitis
- Allergic conjunctivitis
- Mild and uncomplicated angioneurotic edema and urticaria
- Relief of allergic reactions to drugs, blood, or plasma
- Relief of coughs caused by colds or allergies
- Adjunctive therapy in anaphylactic shock
- Treatment of Parkinson-like symptoms
- Relief of nausea and vomiting
- Relief of motion sickness
- Sedation
- Adjuncts to analgesics

Each antihistamine may be used for one or more of these reasons. The more specific uses of the various antihistamine preparations are given in the Summary Drug Table: Upper Respiratory System Drugs.

Adverse Reactions

Central Nervous System Reactions

- Drowsiness or sedation
- Disturbed coordination

Respiratory System Reactions

Anticholinergic actions of antihistamines affect the respiratory system and include the following:

- Dryness of the mouth, nose, and throat
- Thickening of bronchial secretions

Second-generation preparations (e.g., loratadine) cause less drowsiness and fewer anticholinergic effects than some of the other antihistamines. Although these drugs are sometimes used to treat allergies, a drug allergy can occur with the use of an antihistamine. Symptoms that may indicate an allergy to these drugs include skin rash or **urticaria**.

Contraindications

Although the antihistamines are classified in pregnancy category B (chlorpheniramine, cetirizine, dexchlorpheniramine, clemastine, diphenhydramine, and loratadine) and C (brompheniramine, desloratadine, fexofenadine, hydroxyzine, and promethazine), they are contraindicated during pregnancy and lactation.

The first-generation antihistamine drugs are contraindicated in patients with known hypersensitivity to the drugs, newborns, premature infants, and nursing mothers. These drugs are also contraindicated in individuals taking monoamine oxidase inhibitor (MAOI) antidepressants or who have one of the following conditions: angle-closure glaucoma, peptic ulcer, symptomatic prostatic hypertrophy, and bladder neck obstruction.

The second-generation antihistamines are contraindicated in patients with known hypersensitivity. Cetirizine is contraindicated in patients who are sensitive to hydroxyzine.

Precautions

The antihistamines are used cautiously in patients with bronchial asthma, cardiovascular disease, narrow-angle glaucoma, hypertension, impaired kidney function, urinary retention, pyloroduodenal obstruction, and hyperthyroidism.

NURSING ALERT

During the winter and spring seasons beware of a potential name mix-up between the antihistamine ZyRTEC and the antipsychotic ZyPREXA. Tracking reports note that these two drugs are easily misread due to similarity of brand names (ISMP, 2007).

Interactions

The following interactions may occur when an antihistamine is administered with another agent:

Interacting Drug	Common Use	Effect of Interaction
rifampin	Antitubercular agent	May reduce the absorption of the antihistamine (e.g., fexofenadine)
MAOIs	Antidepressant agent	Increased anticholinergic and sedative effects of the antihistamine
CNS depressants (e.g., opioid analgesics or alcohol)	Pain relief	Possible additive CNS depressant effect
beta (β) blockers	Management of cardiovascular disease	Risk for increased cardiovascular effects (e.g., with diphenhydramine)
aluminum- or magnesium-based antacids	Relief of gastrointestinal (GI) problems and upset	Decreased concentrations of drug in blood (e.g., fexofenadine)

DECONGESTANTS

A decongestant is a drug that works directly on blood vessels to reduce swelling of the nasal passages, which, in turn, opens clogged nasal passages and enhances drainage of the sinuses. These drugs are used for the temporary relief of nasal congestion caused by the common cold, hay fever, sinusitis, and other respiratory allergies.

Actions

The nasal decongestants are sympathomimetic, in that they produce localized vasoconstriction of the small blood vessels of the nasal membranes like adrenergic drugs. Vasoconstriction reduces swelling in the nasal passages (decongestive activity). Nasal decongestants may be applied topically, and a few are available for oral use. Examples of nasal decongestants include phenylephrine (Neo-Synephrine) and oxymetazoline (Afrin), both of which are available as nasal sprays or drops, and pseudoephedrine (Sudafed), which is taken orally. Additional nasal decongestants are listed in the Summary Drug Table: Upper Respiratory System Drugs.

Uses

Decongestants are used to treat the congestion associated with the following conditions:

• Common cold
• Hay fever
• Sinusitis
• Allergic rhinitis
• Congestion associated with rhinitis

Adverse Reactions

When used topically in prescribed doses, there are usually minimal systemic effects in most individuals. On occasion, nasal burning, stinging, and dryness may be seen. When the topical form is used frequently or if the liquid is swallowed, the same adverse reactions seen with the oral decongestants may occur. Use of oral decongestants may result in the following adverse reactions:

• Tachycardia and other cardiac arrhythmias
• Nervousness, restlessness, insomnia
• Blurred vision
• Nausea and vomiting

Contraindications

The decongestants are contraindicated in patients with known hypersensitivity and in patients taking MAOI antidepressants. Sustained-released pseudoephedrine is contraindicated in children younger than 12 years.

Precautions

Decongestants are used cautiously in patients with the following:

• Thyroid disease
• Diabetes mellitus
• Cardiovascular disease
• Prostatic hypertrophy
• Coronary artery disease

• Peripheral vascular disease
• Hypertension
• Glaucoma

Safe use of the decongestants during pregnancy (pregnancy category C) and lactation has not been established. Pregnant women should consult with their primary health care provider before using these drugs.

Interactions

The following interactions may occur when a decongestant is administered with another agent:

Interacting Drug	Common Use	Effect of Interaction
MAOIs	Antidepressant	Severe headache, hypertension, and possibly hypertensive crisis
β-adrenergic blocking drugs	Management of cardiovascular disease	Initial hypertension episode followed by bradycardia

ANTITUSSIVES, EXPECTORANTS, AND MUCOLYTICS

Coughing is the forceful expulsion of air from the lungs. A cough may be productive or nonproductive. A **nonproductive cough** is a dry, hacking one that produces no secretions. An antitussive drug is used to relieve coughing.

With a **productive cough**, secretions are made in the respiratory tract. An expectorant is a drug that thins respiratory secretions to remove them more easily from the respiratory system. Many *cough and cold* preparations are a combination such as an antihistamine, antitussive, and/or expectorant, and sold OTC as a nonprescription cough medicine. Other antitussives, either alone or in combination with other drugs, are available by prescription only. A mucolytic is a drug that breaks down thick, tenacious mucus in the lower portions of the lungs for better elimination from the respiratory system.

Actions

Most antitussives depress the cough center located in the medulla and are called centrally acting drugs. Codeine and dextromethorphan are examples of centrally acting antitussives. Benzonatate (Tessalon) is the exception; it works peripherally by anesthetizing stretch receptors in the respiratory passages, thereby decreasing cough.

Expectorants increase the production of respiratory secretions, which in turn appears to decrease the viscosity of the mucus. This helps to raise secretions from the respiratory passages. An example of an expectorant is guaifenesin. Drugs with mucolytic activity reduce the viscosity (thickness) of respiratory secretions by direct action on the mucus. An example of a mucolytic drug is acetylcysteine. One other mucolytic drug is on the market, dornase alfa (Pulmozyme). This agent is used for the treatment of cystic fibrosis.

Uses

Antitussives are used to relieve a nonproductive cough. Expectorants are used to help bring up respiratory secretions. The mucolytic acetylcysteine is used to treat the following:

• Acute bronchopulmonary disease (pneumonia, bronchitis, tracheobronchitis)
• Tracheostomy care
• Pulmonary complications of cystic fibrosis
• Pulmonary complications associated with surgery and during anesthesia
• Posttraumatic chest conditions
• Atelectasis due to mucous obstruction
• Acetaminophen overdosage

This drug is also used for diagnostic bronchial studies, such as bronchograms and bronchial wedge catheterizations. It is primarily given by nebulizer but also may be directly instilled into a tracheostomy to liquefy (thin) secretions.

Adverse Reactions

When used as directed, nonprescription cough medicines produce few adverse reactions. However, those that are combined with an antihistamine may cause:

• Lightheadedness
• Dizziness
• Drowsiness or sedation

Contraindications

Antitussives, expectorants, and mucolytics are contraindicated in patients with known hypersensitivity to the drugs. The opioid antitussives (those with codeine) are contraindicated in premature infants or during labor when delivery of a premature infant is anticipated. Mucolytics are not recommended for use by patients with asthma. The expectorant potassium iodide is contraindicated during pregnancy (pregnancy category D).

Precautions

Antitussives are given with caution to patients with a persistent or chronic cough or a cough accompanied by excessive secretions, a high fever, rash, persistent headache, and nausea or vomiting.

Antitussives containing codeine are used with caution during pregnancy (pregnancy category C) and labor (pregnancy category D) and in patients with COPD, acute asthmatic attack, pre-existing respiratory disorders, acute abdominal conditions, head injury, increased intracranial pressure, convulsive disorders, hepatic or renal impairment, and prostatic hypertrophy.

The expectorants are used cautiously during pregnancy and lactation (guaifenesin is a pregnancy category C drug and acetylcysteine is a pregnancy category B drug); in patients with persistent cough, severe respiratory insufficiency, or asthma; and in older adults or debilitated patients.

Interactions

Other CNS depressants and alcohol may cause additive depressant effects when administered with antitussives containing codeine. When dextromethorphan is administered with the MAOI antidepressants (see Chapter 22), patients may experience hypotension, fever, nausea, jerking motions to the leg, and coma. No significant interactions have been reported when the expectorants are used as directed. The exception is iodine products. If used concurrently with iodine products, lithium and other antithyroid drugs may potentiate the hypothyroid effects of these drugs. When potassium-containing medications and potassium-sparing diuretics are administered with iodine products, the patient may experience hypokalemia, cardiac arrhythmias, or cardiac arrest. Thyroid function test results may also be altered by iodine.

HERBAL CONSIDERATIONS

Eucalyptus is used as a decongestant and expectorant and is found as a component in OTC products used for the treatment of sinusitis and pharyngitis. The plant is grown throughout the world and the leaves and oil are used to treat various respiratory conditions, such as asthma and chronic bronchitis. The lozenges are useful to soothe sore throats and as cough drops. Eucalyptus can also be used as a vapor bath for asthma or other bronchial conditions. Scientific evidence is inconclusive regarding the respiratory benefit of the herb, yet people feel a sense of well-being from its use. The herb is available in many forms, including an essential oil, a fluid extract, and an aqueous solution in alcohol, as well as a component of various OTC products. Eucalyptus should not be used during pregnancy and lactation and in children younger than 2 years of age. Eucalyptus may be used topically on children and adults in combination with menthol and camphor. Individuals with hypersensitivity to eucalyptus should avoid its use (DerMarderosian, 2003).

NURSING PROCESS
PATIENT RECEIVING AN UPPER RESPIRATORY SYSTEM DRUG

ASSESSMENT

Preadministration Assessment
Patients most commonly self-prescribe what is frequently termed a *cough and cold* preparation (an antihistamine, decongestant, antitussive, and/or expectorant medication). Should the patient contact a health care provider, it is because the patient's own actions or home remedies used to treat the cough have not been successful. As you take and record vital signs, ask the patient about signs or symptoms suggesting an upper respiratory infection or a productive cough.

A hospitalized patient may occasionally have one of these preparations prescribed, due to an existing respiratory disorder or if coughing prevents a surgical patient from getting up and about or causes pain at the incisional site when coughing.

Ongoing Assessment
Effectiveness of the preparation is measured by the patient's self-report of diminishing symptoms (e.g., ability to sleep better due to less coughing). If the patient returns to the ambulatory setting or is monitored daily, lung sounds are auscultated and vital signs are taken periodically. When a patient has a cough, describe in your documentation the type of cough (productive or nonproductive of sputum) and the frequency of coughing. Note and record whether the cough interrupts activities of daily living such as sleep and whether it causes pain in the chest or other parts of the body.

NURSING DIAGNOSES
Drug-specific nursing diagnoses include the following:

- **Risk for Injury** related to drowsiness, dizziness, or sedation
- **Ineffective Airway Clearance** related to pooling of or thick secretions

- **Impaired Oral Mucous Membranes** related to dry mouth, nose, and throat

Nursing diagnoses related to drug administration are discussed in Chapter 4.

PLANNING
The expected outcomes for the patient depend on the reason for administration but may include an optimal response to therapy, support of patient needs related to managing adverse reactions, and confidence in an understanding of the medication regimen.

IMPLEMENTATION

Promoting an Optimal Response to Therapy
Problems can arise from the use of a nonprescription upper respiratory system medication for self-treatment of a chronic cough. Indiscriminate use of these products by the general public may prevent early diagnosis and treatment of serious disorders, such as lung cancer and emphysema. Patients should be advised that if a cough lasts more than 10 days or is accompanied by fever, chest pain, severe headache, or skin rash, the patient should consult the primary health care provider.

When you do have contact with patients taking upper respiratory system medications, be sure to reinforce teaching points such as the following:

- Loratadine or other rapidly disintegrating tablets can be administered with or without water and are placed on the tongue, where the tablet dissolves almost instantly.
- Fexofenadine is not administered within 2 hours of an antacid.
- Chewing benzonatate tablets may result in a local anesthetic effect (oropharyngeal anesthesia) with possible choking as a result.
- Acetylcysteine has a distinctive, disagreeable odor. The medication may smell like "rotten eggs." Although this odor may be nauseating, the smell dissipates quickly.

Upper Respiratory System Drugs

Monitoring and Managing Patient Needs
RISK FOR INJURY. If drowsiness is severe or if other problems such as dizziness or a disturbance in muscle coordination occur, the patient may require assistance with ambulation and other activities. If the patient is in an institution, be sure he or she is oriented to the surroundings, and that pathways to the bathroom are free of equipment and supervision is provided if there is a cognitive issue. Place call lights within easy reach and instruct the patient to call before attempting to get out of bed or ambulate. When the drug is taken in the home environment, caution the patient to refrain from activities that require a clear mind or operating equipment that requires attentive detail. Tell the patient that this adverse reaction may decrease with continued use of the drug.

LIFESPAN CONSIDERATIONS
Gerontology
Older adults are more likely to experience injury from dizziness because with age comes an increased risk for falls. Sensorimotor deficits, such as hearing loss, visual impairments, or balance problems, increase the older adult's risk for injury. Codeine may cause orthostatic hypotension when a patient rises too quickly from a sitting or lying position. Patients should not take codeine preparations for persistent or chronic cough, such as occurs with smoking, asthma, or emphysema, or when the cough is accompanied by excessive secretions, except when under the supervision of the health care provider.

INEFFECTIVE AIRWAY CLEARANCE. One problem associated with the use of an antitussive is related to its drug action. Although not an adverse reaction, depression of the cough reflex can cause secretions to pool in the lungs. Pooling of the secretions that are normally removed by coughing may result in more serious problems, such as pneumonia and atelectasis. For this reason, using an antitussive for a *productive cough* is contraindicated in many situations. Patients should be encouraged to increase fluids and change position frequently to facilitate removal of secretions.

For the patient with thick sputum, encourage a fluid intake of up to 2000 mL per day if this amount is not contraindicated by the patient's condition or disease process. Instruction is provided to help the patient with deep, diaphragmatic breathing. As sputum is expelled from the respiratory system monitor color, amount, and consistency.

Overuse of the topical form of decongestants can cause "rebound" nasal congestion. This means that the congestion becomes worse with the use of the drug. Although congestion may be relieved briefly after the drug is used, it recurs within a short time, which prompts the patient to use the drug at more frequent intervals, perpetuating the rebound congestion. Teach the patient to take the drug exactly as prescribed. A simple but uncomfortable solution to rebound congestion is to withdraw completely from the topical medication. The primary health care provider may recommend an oral decongestant. An alternative method to minimize the occurrence of rebound nasal congestion is to discontinue the drug therapy gradually by initially discontinuing the medication in one nostril, followed by withdrawal from the other nostril. You may suggest saline irrigation of nasal passages using a "neti pot" in place of using a decongestant. A neti pot, originally from the yogic tradition and now a part of Ayurvedic medicine, is a container that is filled with distilled or sterile water (not tap water) for flushing out the nasal sinuses. These can often be purchased at natural food stores.

IMPAIRED ORAL MUCOUS MEMBRANES. Dryness of the mouth, nose, and throat may occur when antihistamines are taken. Offer the patient frequent sips of water or ice chips to relieve these symptoms. Sugarless gum or sugarless hard candy may also relieve these symptoms.

LIFESPAN CONSIDERATIONS
Gerontology
Older adults are more likely to experience anticholinergic effects (e.g., dryness of the mouth, nose, and throat), dizziness, sedation, hypotension, and confusion from the antihistamines.

Educating the Patient and Family
During any patient encounter you can teach patients the proper use of OTC upper respiratory system medications, especially when coughing produces sputum. Advise the patient to read the label carefully, follow the dosage recommendations, and consult the primary health care provider if the cough persists for more than 10 days, the color of sputum changes, or fever or chest pain occurs.

Acetylcysteine usually is administered in the hospital but may be prescribed for the patient being discharged. Typically, the respiratory therapist gives the patient or a family member full instruction in the use and maintenance of the equipment, as well as the technique of administration of acetylcysteine. As the nurse, your responsibility is to be sure the patient or family member understands the instruction and has all questions addressed before use.

As you develop a teaching plan for the patient or family member, include the following points:

- Do not exceed the recommended dose.
- Avoid irritants, such as cigarette smoke, dust, or fumes, to decrease irritation to the throat.
- Drink plenty of fluids (if not contraindicated by disease process). A fluid intake of 1500 to 2000 mL is recommended.
- If taking oral capsules, do not chew or break open the capsules; swallow them whole.
- If taking a lozenge, avoid drinking fluids for 30 minutes after use to avoid losing effectiveness of the drug.
- Antihistamines may cause dryness of the mouth and throat. Frequent sips of water, sucking on hard candy, or chewing gum (preferably sugarless) may relieve this problem.
- Do not drive or perform other hazardous tasks if drowsiness occurs. This effect may diminish with continued use.
- ♥ Avoid the use of alcohol, as well as other drugs that cause sleepiness or drowsiness, while taking these drugs.
- Understand that overuse of topical nasal decongestants can make the symptoms worse, causing rebound congestion.
- Nasal burning and stinging may occur with the topical decongestants. This effect usually disappears with use. If burning or stinging becomes severe, discontinue use and discuss this problem with the primary health care provider, who may prescribe or recommend another drug.
- If using a spray, do not allow the tip of the container to touch the nasal mucosa and do not share the container with other people.

- If the cough is not relieved or becomes worse, contact the primary health care provider.
- If chills, fever, chest pain, or sputum production occurs, contact the primary health care provider as soon as possible.

EVALUATION

- Therapeutic response is achieved and coughing is relieved.
- Adverse reactions are identified, reported to the primary health care provider, and managed successfully with appropriate nursing interventions:
  - No evidence of injury is seen.
  - Patient has a clear airway.
  - Mucous membranes are moist and intact.
- Patient and family express confidence and demonstrate an understanding of the drug regimen.

PHARMACOLOGY IN PRACTICE
THINK CRITICALLY

 You know that Janna is an active teenager. Describe important teaching points that should be included in developing a teaching plan for her. What limitations might these drugs have on her activity? What other OTC products should she avoid?

KEY POINTS

- Cough, cold, congestion, and allergies are common problems in the upper respiratory system.
- Antihistamines are used to reduce inflammation, decongestants are used to reduce edema and swelling, and antitussives are used to eliminate cough. When congestion produces secretions in either the respiratory passages or the lungs, expectorants or mucolytics are used, respectively.
- Many of these products are obtained OTC, not requiring a prescription. Therefore, assessment of use and proper instruction are important nursing actions to remember because patients may not readily think to offer information about use.
- Antihistamines can produce drowsiness; other medications typically do not have bothersome adverse reactions unless the effects are potentiated by interaction with prescription drugs (especially extrapyramidal symptoms).

Summary Drug Table UPPER RESPIRATORY SYSTEM DRUGS

Generic Name	Trade Name	Uses	Adverse Reactions	Dosage Ranges
First-Generation Antihistamines				
brompheniramine *brome-fen-ear'-ah-meen*	LoHist, Bidhist, Lodrane, VaZol, Lodrane, BroveX	Temporary relief of sneezing, itchy, watery eyes, itchy nose or throat, and runny nose caused by hay fever or other respiratory allergies; VaZol also used for symptoms of the common cold; treatment of allergic reactions to blood or plasma and anaphylactic reactions	Drowsiness, sedation, dizziness, disturbed coordination, hypotension, headache, blurred vision, thickening of bronchial secretions	Adults and children 12 yr and older: 6–12 mg orally q 12 hr Sustained release: 8–12 mg orally q 12 hr Oral liquid: 4 mg QID
chlorpheniramine *klore-fen-ear'-ah-meen*	Aller-Chlor, Chlor-Trimeton	Temporary relief of sneezing, itchy, watery eyes, itchy throat, and runny nose caused by hay fever, other upper respiratory allergies, and the common cold	Drowsiness, sedation, hypotension, palpitations, blurred vision, dry mouth, urinary hesitancy	Adults and children 12 yr and older: 4 mg q 4–6 hr, maximum dose 24 mg in 24 hr Extended release: 8–12 mg orally q 8–12 hr
clemastine *klem'-ah-steen*	Tavist, Dayhist-1	Allergic rhinitis, urticaria, angioedema	Drowsiness, sedation, hypotension, palpitations, blurred vision, dry mouth, urinary hesitancy	Allergic rhinitis: 1.34 mg orally BID (not to exceed 8.04 mg/day for the syrup and 2.68 mg for the tablets) Urticaria and angioedema: 2.68 mg BID orally (not to exceed 4.02 mg/day)

(table continues on page 322)

Summary Drug Table   UPPER RESPIRATORY SYSTEM DRUGS (continued)

Generic Name	Trade Name	Uses	Adverse Reactions	Dosage Ranges
diphenhydramine *dye-fen-hye'-drah meen*	Benadryl, Banophen, Genahist, Tusstat, Dytan	Allergic symptoms; hypersensitivity reactions, including anaphylaxis and transfusion reactions; motion sickness; sleep aid; antitussive and Parkinson-like effects	Drowsiness, dry mouth, anorexia, blurred vision, urinary frequency	25–50 mg orally q 4–6 hr, maximum daily dose 300 mg; 10–400 mg IM, IV
promethazine *proe-meth'-ah-zeen*		Antiemetic, hypersensitivity reactions, motion sickness, sedation	Excessive sedation, drowsiness, dry mouth, confusion, disorientation, dizziness, fatigue, blurred vision	Individualize dosage to smallest effective dose Allergy: 12.5–25 mg orally, 25 mg IM, IV Antiemetic: 12.5–25 mg orally, IM, IV Motion sickness: 25 mg BID Preoperative: 50 mg IM or orally the night before surgery
Second-Generation Antihistamines				
azelastine *ah-zel'-as-teen*	Astelin	Seasonal and vasomotor rhinitis	Dizziness, drowsiness, glossitis, nose bleeds	2 sprays per nostril twice daily
cetirizine *seh-teer'-ih-zeen*	Zyrtec	Seasonal or perennial rhinitis, chronic urticaria	Sedation, dry mouth, pharyngitis, somnolence, dizziness	5–10 mg/day orally; maximum dosage 20 mg/day
desloratadine *des-loe-rah'-tah-deen*	Clarinex	Seasonal or perennial allergic rhinitis	Headache; fatigue; drowsiness; dry mouth, nose, and throat; flu-like symptoms	Adults and children 12 yr and older: 5 mg/day orally
fexofenadine *fex-oh-fen'-ah-deen*	Allegra	Seasonal rhinitis, urticaria	Headache, nausea, drowsiness, dyspepsia, fatigue, back pain, upper respiratory infection	30–60 mg orally BID; maximum dosage 180 mg/day
levocetirizine *lee'-voe-seh-teer-ih-zeen*	Xyzal	Allergic rhinitis, urticaria	Dizziness, drowsiness	5 mg orally in evening
loratadine *lor-ah'-tah-deen*	Claritin, Tavist ND, Alavert	Allergic rhinitis	Dizziness, headache, tremors, insomnia, dry mouth, fatigue	10 mg/day orally
Decongestants				
epinephrine *ep-ih-nef'-rin*	Adrenalin Chloride	Nasal congestion	Anxiety, restlessness, anorexia, arrhythmias, nervousness	2–3 drops or spray in each nostril q 4–6 hr
fexofenadine and pseudoephedrine	Allegra-D	Allergic rhinitis and nasal congestion	See separate drugs	1 tablet every 12 hr
naphazoline *nah-faz'-oh-leen*	Privine	Nasal congestion	Same as epinephrine	1–2 drops or sprays in each nostril no more than q 6 hr
oxymetazoline *ox-see-meh-taz'-oh-leen*	Afrin 12 Hour, Dristan 12-Hour Nasal, Vicks Sinex	Nasal congestion	Same as epinephrine	2–3 drops or sprays q 10–12 hr
phenylephrine *fen-ill-ef'-rin*	Neo-Synephrine	Nasal congestion	Same as epinephrine	2–3 sprays of 0–25% solution q 3–4 hr
pseudoephedrine *soo-doe-eh-fed'-rin*	Sudafed	Nasal congestion	Anxiety, restlessness, anorexia, arrhythmias, nervousness, nausea, vomiting, blurred vision	60 mg orally q 4–6 hr

Summary Drug Table UPPER RESPIRATORY SYSTEM DRUGS (continued)

Generic Name	Trade Name	Uses	Adverse Reactions	Dosage Ranges
tetrahydrozoline *tet-trah-hye-draz'-oh-leen*	Tyzine	Nasal congestion	Same as pseudoephedrine	2–4 drops in each nostril or 3–4 sprays in each nostril q 3 hr
xylometazoline *zye-loe-meh-taz'-oh-leen*	Otrivin, Natru-Vent	Nasal congestion	Same as epinephrine	2–3 drops or sprays in each nostril q 8–10 hr
Antitussives				
Opioid Antitussives				
codeine *koe'-deen*		Suppression of nonproductive cough, relief of mild to moderate pain	Sedation, nausea, vomiting, dizziness, constipation, CNS depression	10–20 mg orally q 4–6 hr; maximum dosage 120 mg/day
Nonopioid Antitussives				
benzonatate *ben-zoe'-nah-tate*	Tessalon Perles	Symptomatic relief of cough	Sedation, headache, mild dizziness, constipation, nausea, GI upset, pruritus, nasal congestion	Adults and children older than 10 yr: 100–200 mg TID (up to 600 mg/day)
dextromethorphan *dex-troe-meh-thore'-fan*	Benylin, DexAlone, Robitussin, Delsym, Formula 44 Cough	Symptomatic relief of cough	Drowsiness, dizziness, GI upset	Adults and children older than 12 yr: 10–30 mg q 4–8hr; sustained-release (SR) 60 mg q 12 hr orally Children 6–12 yr: 5–10 mg q 4 hr or 15 mg q 6–8 hr; SR 30 mg q 12 hr orally Children 2–5 yr: 2.5–7.5 mg q 4–8 hr; SR 15 mg q 12 hr orally
dextromethorphan and benzocaine *ben'-zoe-cane*	Cough-X	Symptomatic relief of cough and bronchial irritation	Same as dextromethorphan HBr	Varies, depending on formulation; take as directed on package orally
diphenhydramine *dye-fen-hye'-drah-meen*	ZzzQuil, AllerMax, Hydramine Cough	Symptomatic relief of cough caused by colds, allergy, or bronchial irritation	Drowsiness, dizziness, GI upset	Adults: 25 mg q 4 hr orally, not to exceed 150 mg/day Children 6–12 yr: 12.5 mg orally q 4 hr, not to exceed 75 mg/day Children 2–5 yr: 6.25 mg q 4 hr, not to exceed 25 mg/day
Mucolytics				
acetylcysteine *ah-seh-teel-sis'-tay-een*		Reduction of viscosity of mucus in acute and chronic bronchopulmonary diseases and diagnostic bronchial studies, acetaminophen toxicity	Stomatitis, nausea, vomiting, fever, drowsiness, bronchospasm, irritation of the trachea and bronchi	1–10 mL of 20% solution by nebulization or 2–20 mL of 10% solution q 2–6 hr PRN Acetaminophen toxicity: initially 140 mg/kg orally, then 70 mg/kg orally q 4 hr for 17 doses (total)
Expectorants				
guaifenesin (glyceryl guaiacolate) *gwye-fen'-eh-sin*	Hytuss, Organidin NR, Robitussin	Relief of cough associated with respiratory tract infection (sinusitis, asthma, bronchitis, pharyngitis), especially when the cough is dry and nonproductive	Nausea, vomiting, dizziness, headache, rash	Adults and children 12 yr and older: 200–400 mg orally q 4 hr Children 6–12 yr: 100–200 mg q 4 hr orally Children 2–6 yr: 50–100 mg q 4 hr
potassium iodide *poe-tah'-see-um eye-oh-dyde*	SSKI	Symptomatic relief of chronic pulmonary disease complicated by tenacious mucus	Iodine sensitivity or iodism (sore mouth, metallic taste, increased salivation, nausea, vomiting, epigastric pain, parotid swelling, and pain)	300–1000 mg orally after meals BID or TID, to 1.5 g orally TID

Upper Respiratory System Drugs

● Chapter Review

Know Your Drugs

Clients sometimes know a medication by the brand (or trade) name and not the generic name. To help you recognize both names, match the brand name with the generic name of the same medication:

Generic Name	Brand Name
1. dextromethorphan	A. Robitussin
2. diphenhydramine	B. Nasonex
3. loratadine	C. Claritin
4. mometasone	D. Benadryl

Calculate Medication Dosages

1. A client is prescribed 200 mg of guaifenesin syrup. The drug is available in syrup of 200 mg/5 mL. The nurse administers _____.

2. Loratadine 10 mg is prescribed. The drug is available in 5-mg tablets. The nurse instructs the client to take _____.

● Prepare for the NCLEX®

Build Your Knowledge

1. Antitussives are medications that _____.
   1. loosen respiratory secretions
   2. depress the cough center in the brain
   3. increase production of mucous secretion
   4. fight microbial infections of the lungs

2. Which of these drugs is classified as an expectorant?
   1. guaifenesin
   2. codeine
   3. dextromethorphan
   4. diphenhydramine

3. Which of the following is a common adverse reaction seen when administering an antihistamine?
   1. sedation
   2. blurred vision
   3. headache
   4. hypertension

4. When antihistamines are administered to clients receiving CNS depressants, the nurse monitors the client for _____.
   1. an increase in anticholinergic effects
   2. excessive sedation
   3. seizure activity
   4. loss of hearing

5. A client receives a prescription for phenylephrine (Neo-Synephrine). The nurse explains that overuse of this drug may _____.
   1. result in hypotensive episodes
   2. decrease sinus drainage
   3. cause rebound nasal congestion
   4. dilate capillaries in the nasal mucosa

Apply Your Knowledge

6. Which of the following statements is appropriate for the nurse to include in discharge instructions for a client taking an antitussive?
   1. Increase the dosage if the drug does not relieve the cough.
   2. Limit fluids to less than 1000 mL each day.
   3. Expect the cough to worsen during the first few days of treatment.
   4. Frequent sips of water may diminish coughing.

7. The nurse is to administer a mucolytic agent. Which of the following nursing actions is appropriate to take to promote an effective airway?
   1. Increase fluid intake to 2000 mL per day
   2. Limit fluids to 200 mL per day
   3. Monitor intake and output every 8 hours
   4. Have the client take the mucolytic after each coughing episode

8. Which of the following interactions would most likely occur when diphenhydramine is administered with a β blocker drug such as propranolol (Inderal)?
   1. increased risk for cardiovascular effects
   2. increased risk for seizures
   3. decreased risk for cardiovascular effects
   4. decreased risk for seizures

Alternate-Format Questions

9. Which of these drugs would mostly likely be used to bring up deep mucous plugs in the lungs of a client with a tracheostomy? **Select all that apply**.
   1. acetylcysteine
   2. guaifenesin
   3. benzonatate
   4. dextromethorphan

10. A client with limited health literacy is prescribed an antihistamine for an upper respiratory tract allergy. You want to be sure the client does not use other cold remedies with antihistamines included. What is the best way to relay this information? **Select all that apply**.
    1. Tell the client which drugs not to use
    2. Give the client a list of medicines that include antihistamines
    3. Show the client where to look on the medicine label for the ingredients
    4. Make a poster for your clinic with drugs that contain antihistamines for teaching

To check your answers, see Appendix G.

the**Point** *For more NCLEX-style questions, log on to http://thepoint.lww.com to access more than 1000 questions.*

Lower Respiratory System Drugs

LEARNING OBJECTIVES

On completion of this chapter, the student will:

1. Describe the uses, general drug actions, general adverse reactions, contraindications, precautions, and interactions of the bronchodilators and antiasthma drugs.
2. Discuss important preadministration and ongoing assessment activities the nurse should perform on the patient taking a bronchodilator or an antiasthma drug.
3. List nursing diagnoses particular to a patient taking a bronchodilator or an antiasthma drug.
4. Discuss ways to promote an optimal response to therapy, how to manage common adverse reactions, and important points to keep in mind when educating a patient about the use of bronchodilators or antiasthma drugs.

KEY TERMS

asthma • respiratory disorder characterized by bronchospasm and difficulty in breathing, especially exhaling

dyspnea • feelings of shortness of breath, labored or difficult breathing

leukotrienes • inflammatory substance that is released by mast cells during an asthma attack

rhinitis • inflammation of the mucous membranes of the nose

tachypnea • rapid breathing

theophyllinization • delivery of a high enough dose of theophylline to bring blood levels to a therapeutic range more quickly than over several days

DRUG CLASSES

Bronchodilators
- Short-acting beta-2 (β_2) (adrenergic) agonists (SABAs)
- Long-acting beta-2 (β_2) (adrenergic) agonists (LABAs)
- Xanthine derivative

- Cholinergic blocking (anticholinergic)

Antiasthma
- Inhaled corticosteroids (ICSs)
- Mast cell stabilizer
- Leukotriene modifier and immunomodulator

The term *chronic obstructive pulmonary disease* (COPD) includes the disorders of **asthma**, chronic bronchitis, chronic obstructive bronchitis, and emphysema, or a combination of these conditions. The patient with COPD experiences **dyspnea** (difficulty breathing) with physical exertion, has difficulty inhaling and exhaling, and may have a chronic cough. All of these disorders interfere with the exchange of gases in the lung alveoli.

More than 22 million Americans have asthma, which is a chronic inflammatory disease causing spasmodic constriction of the bronchi. It is one of the most common chronic diseases of childhood, affecting an estimated 6 million children.

During the inflammatory process, a large amount of histamine is released from the mast cells of the respiratory tract. The lung bronchi constrict, becoming hyperresponsive to the bronchoconstriction, and edema occurs. With asthma, the airways become narrow, the muscles around the airways tighten, the inner lining of the bronchi swell, and extra mucus clogs the smaller airways (Fig. 32.1). Characterized by recurrent attacks

---

PHARMACOLOGY IN PRACTICE

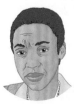

Lillian Chase, a 36-year-old woman who had a breathing problem over the weekend, was seen in the emergency department of the local hospital. You are seeing her in the clinic for her follow-up visit. At the end of the chapter, review the medication order and compare it with the established guidelines for her self-management of asthma.

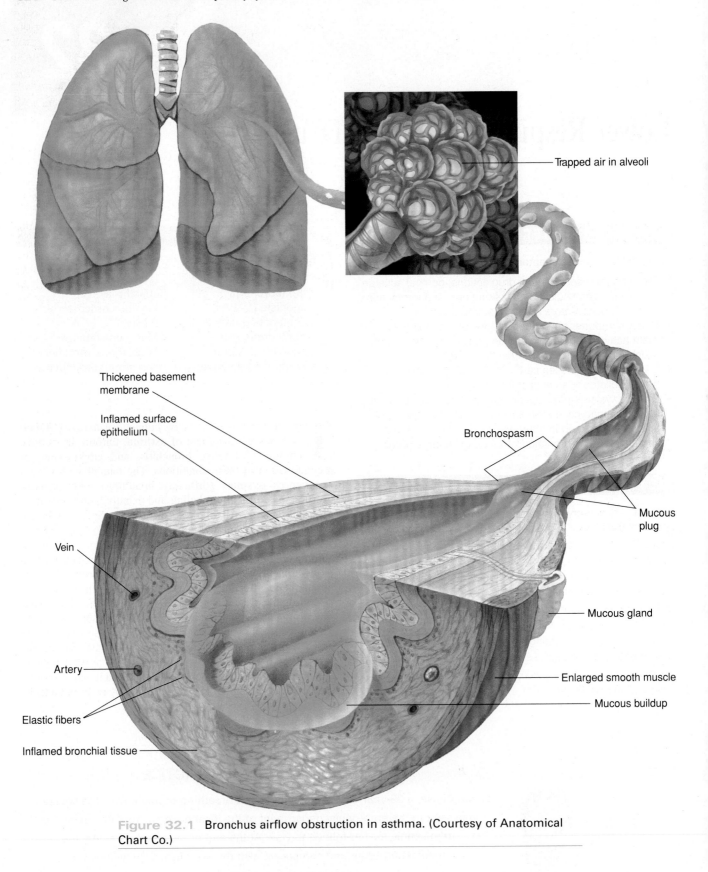

Trapped air in alveoli

Thickened basement membrane

Inflamed surface epithelium

Bronchospasm

Mucous plug

Vein

Mucous gland

Artery

Enlarged smooth muscle

Mucous buildup

Elastic fibers

Inflamed bronchial tissue

Figure 32.1 Bronchus airflow obstruction in asthma. (Courtesy of Anatomical Chart Co.)

of dyspnea and wheezing, this breathlessness causes the patient to experience anxiety.

Patients with asthma may experience periods of exacerbation of symptoms alternating with periods of normal respiratory function. The period of exacerbation may begin abruptly, often triggered by exercise or cold air, but usually is preceded by increasing symptoms over the previous several days:

- Cough (worse at night or early morning)
- Generalized wheezing (a whistle or squeaking sound on inspiration or expiration)
- Generalized chest tightness (may feel like someone is sitting on the chest)
- Dyspnea (shortness of breath or feeling of breathlessness)
- **Tachypnea** (rapid breathing)

These symptoms indicate that inflammation is occurring in the lungs. Stimulation of the sympathetic nervous system, the fight-or-flight response (as described in Chapter 24), is the body's reaction to the inflammation.

Asthma medications are categorized into two major groups: (1) long-term control medications and (2) quick-relief medications used to treat acute air flow obstruction. The long-term management of asthma uses a stepwise approach (Display 32.1), meaning that medications and their frequency of administration are adjusted according to the severity of the patient's asthma. The most effective long-term control medications are those that reduce inflammation, with inhaled corticosteroids (ICSs) being the first-line intervention. Quick-relief medications include inhaled short-acting beta-2 (β_2) (adrenergic) agonists (SABAs) and oral steroids.

Bronchodilators are the mainstay of treatment for many chronic pulmonary disorders. SABA bronchodilators are drugs used to relieve bronchospasm associated with respiratory disorders, such as bronchial asthma, chronic bronchitis, and emphysema. These conditions are progressive disorders characterized by a decrease in the inspiratory and expiratory

capacity of the lung. Examples of β_2 agonist bronchodilators include albuterol (Ventolin), epinephrine (Adrenalin), salmeterol (Serevent), and terbutaline. Along with the bronchodilators, several types of drugs are effective in treating asthma. These include ICSs, mast cell stabilizers, leukotriene formation inhibitors, leukotriene receptor agonists, and immunomodulators.

BRONCHODILATORS

The two major types of bronchodilators are the β_2-adrenergic agonists (or sympathomimetics) and the xanthine derivatives. The cholinergic blocking drug ipratropium bromide (Atrovent) is used for bronchospasm associated with COPD, chronic bronchitis, and emphysema in emergent situations. Ipratropium is featured in the Summary Drug Table: Lower Respiratory System Drugs. Chapter 27 provides specific information concerning the cholinergic blocking (anticholinergic) drugs.

Adrenergic Bronchodilators

When alpha (α)-adrenergic receptors (the sympathetic system) in the lungs are stimulated, bronchoconstriction results. The opposite, *bronchodilation,* occurs when β-adrenergic receptors are stimulated. Some theories propose that asthma is a lack of β-adrenergic stimulation. Many of the adrenergics used as bronchodilators have the subclassification of β_2 receptor agonists, which are either *short acting* (e.g., albuterol and terbutaline) or *long acting* (e.g., salmeterol). Additional information concerning the various adrenergic drugs is given in the Summary Drug Table: Lower Respiratory System Drugs.

Display 32.1 Step Care Approach for Managing Asthma in Adults and Youth 12 Years and Older

Asthma Classification	Daily Medications	Rescue Drugs
Step 1: intermittent asthma	No daily medications	SABA
Step 2: mild persistent asthma	Low-dose ICS	SABA
	Alternative: cromolyn sodium or zafirlukast for patient aged younger than 12 years or sustained-release theophylline	SABA SABA
Step 3: mild to moderate persistent asthma	Low-dose ICS *plus* LABA *or* medium-dose ICS **Alternative:**	SABA
	Low-dose ICS and zafirlukast or theophylline or zileuton	SABA
Step 4: moderate persistent asthma	Medium-dose ICS *plus* LABA	
Step 5: moderately severe persistent asthma	Daily combined use of a high-dose ICS *and* LABA, and consider immunomodulator	
Step 6: severe persistent asthma	High-dose ICS *and* LABA *plus* oral corticosteroid, and consider immunomodulator	

Expert Panel Report 3: Guidelines for the Diagnosis and Management of Asthma, National Heart, Lung, and Blood Institute, 2007.

Actions

When bronchospasm occurs, there is a decrease in the lumen (or inside diameter) of the bronchi, which decreases the amount of air taken into the lungs with each breath. A decrease in the amount of air taken into the lungs results in respiratory distress. Use of a bronchodilating drug opens the bronchi by relaxing the smooth muscles and allows more air to enter the lungs, which, in turn, completely or partially relieves respiratory distress.

Uses

The β_2-adrenergic drugs (which mimic the sympathetic nervous system) are used in the treatment of chronic respiratory problems due to bronchoconstriction, such as:

- Bronchospasm associated with acute and chronic bronchial asthma
- Exercise-induced bronchospasm (EIB)
- Bronchitis
- Emphysema
- Bronchiectasis (chronic dilation of the bronchi and bronchioles)
- Other obstructive pulmonary diseases

Adverse Reactions

Cardiovascular System Reactions

- Tachycardia, palpitations, or cardiac arrhythmias
- Hypertension

Other Reactions

- Nervousness, anxiety
- Insomnia

When these drugs are taken by inhalation, excessive use (e.g., more than the recommended dose times) may result in paradoxical bronchospasm.

 NURSING ALERT

Long-acting β_2 (adrenergic) agonists (LABAs; e.g., salmeterol) may increase the risk of asthma-related death. ICSs should be considered first for long-term control of asthma.

Contraindications

The adrenergic bronchodilators are contraindicated in patients with known hypersensitivity to the drug, cardiac arrhythmias associated with tachycardia, organic brain damage, cerebral arteriosclerosis, and narrow-angle glaucoma. Salmeterol is contraindicated during acute bronchospasm.

Precautions

The adrenergics are used cautiously in patients with hypertension, cardiac dysfunction, hyperthyroidism, glaucoma, diabetes, prostatic hypertrophy, and a history of seizures. The adrenergic drugs are also used cautiously during pregnancy and lactation (all are in pregnancy category C, except terbutaline, which is a pregnancy category B drug).

Interactions

The following interactions may occur when an adrenergic drug is used concurrently with another agent:

Interacting Drug	Common Use	Effect of Interaction
adrenergic drugs	Treatment of hypotension and shock	Possible additive adrenergic effects
tricyclics	Treatment of depression	Possible hypotension
β-adrenergic blockers	Treatment of hypertension	Inhibition of the cardiac, bronchodilating, and vasodilating effects of the adrenergic
methyldopa	Treatment of hypertension	Possible hypotension
oxytocic drugs	Uterine stimulant	Possible severe hypotension
theophylline	Treatment of asthma and COPD	Increased risk for cardiotoxicity

Xanthine Derivative Bronchodilators

Xanthine derivatives (also called *methylxanthines*) are a different class of drugs from the adrenergics and also have bronchodilating activity. Examples are theophylline and aminophylline. Additional information concerning the xanthine derivatives is found in the Summary Drug Table: Lower Respiratory System Drugs.

Actions

The xanthine derivatives are drugs that stimulate the central nervous system (CNS) to promote bronchodilation. They cause direct relaxation of the smooth muscles of the bronchi.

Uses

The xanthine derivatives are used for the following:

- Symptomatic relief or prevention of bronchial asthma
- Treatment of reversible bronchospasm associated with chronic bronchitis and emphysema

Adverse Reactions

Central Nervous System Reactions

- Restlessness, irritability, headache
- Nervousness, tremors

Cardiac and Respiratory System Reactions

- Tachycardia
- Palpitations

- Electrocardiographic changes
- Increased respirations

Other Reactions

- Nausea, vomiting, fever
- Hyperglycemia, flushing, alopecia

Contraindications

The xanthine derivatives are contraindicated in those with known hypersensitivity to the drugs, peptic ulcers, seizure disorders (unless well controlled with appropriate anticonvulsant medication), and serious uncontrolled arrhythmias.

Precautions

The xanthine derivatives are used cautiously in patients with cardiac disease, hypoxemia, hypertension, congestive heart failure, and liver disease. They are also used cautiously in older adult patients and those who use alcohol habitually. Aminophylline, dyphylline, oxtriphylline, and theophylline are pregnancy category C drugs and are used cautiously during pregnancy and lactation.

Interactions

When taken with theophylline, the following agents have an effect on theophylline levels:

Interacting Drug	Common Use	Effect of Interaction
barbiturates	Sedation	**Decreased** theophylline levels result when the drug is taken with the interacting drug noted to the left.
charcoal (in large amounts)	Neutralize poisoning	
hydantoins	Anticonvulsant	
ketoconazole	Antifungal agent	
rifampin	Antitubercular agent	
nicotine (tobacco, nicotine gum, and patches)	Effect from smoking tobacco or to aid smoking cessation	
adrenergic agents	Treatment of hypotension and shock	
isoniazid	Antitubercular agent	
loop diuretics	Treatment of hypertension	
allopurinol	Antigout agent	**Increased** theophylline levels result when the drug is taken with the interacting drug noted to the left.
β-adrenergic blockers	Treatment of hypertension	
calcium channel blockers	Treatment of angina and hypertension	
cimetidine	Treatment of gastrointestinal (GI) problems	

Interacting Drug	Common Use	Effect of Interaction
oral contraceptives	Birth control	**Increased** theophylline levels result when the drug is taken with the interacting drug noted to the left.
corticosteroids	Anti-inflammatory agents	
influenza virus vaccine	Prevention of flu	
macrolide, quinolone antibiotics	Treatment of infections	
thyroid hormones	Treatment of hypothyroidism	
isoniazid	Antitubercular agent	
loop diuretics	Treatment of edema	

ANTIASTHMA DRUGS

Long-term control medications are used daily to achieve and maintain control of persistent asthma. The most effective are those that reduce the underlying inflammation of asthma.

Inhaled Corticosteroids

ICSs are the most consistently effective long-term control medication at all steps of care for persistent asthma. ICS and LABA drugs may be combined to ease administration of the medications and produce positive outcomes in the management of asthma; these ICS/LABA combinations can be found in the Summary Drug Table: Lower Respiratory System Drugs.

Actions

ICSs are anti-inflammatory medications that reduce airway hyperresponsiveness, reduce the number of mast cells in the airway, and block reaction to allergens. ICSs, such as beclomethasone (QVAR) or flunisolide (AeroBid), are given by inhalation and decrease the inflammatory process directly in the airways. In addition, the corticosteroids increase the sensitivity of the β_2 receptors, which in turn increases the effectiveness of the β_2 receptor agonist drugs.

Uses

The ICSs are used in the management and prophylactic treatment of the inflammation associated with chronic asthma. A number of these preparations may be used intranasally for the treatment of nasal polyps and **rhinitis** (see Chapter 31).

Adverse Reactions

When used to manage chronic asthma, the corticosteroids are most often given by inhalation. Adverse reactions to the corticosteroids are less likely to occur when the drugs are given by inhalation rather than taken orally. Occasionally, patients may experience reactions.

Respiratory System Reactions

• Throat irritation
• Hoarseness
• Upper respiratory tract infection
• Fungal infection of the mouth and throat

See Chapter 43 for adverse reactions after oral administration of the corticosteroids. A more complete listing of the adverse reactions associated with the ICSs is found in the Summary Drug Table: Lower Respiratory System Drugs.

Contraindications

The ICSs are contraindicated in patients with hypersensitivity to the corticosteroids, acute bronchospasm, status asthmaticus, or other acute episodes of asthma. Beclomethasone is contraindicated for the relief of symptoms that can be controlled by a bronchodilator and other nonsteroidal medications and in the treatment of nonasthmatic bronchitis.

Precautions

The ICSs are used cautiously in patients with compromised immune systems, glaucoma, kidney disease, liver disease, convulsive disorders, and diabetes. Combining ICSs with systemic corticosteroids can increase the risk of hypothalamic-pituitary-adrenal (HPA) suppression, resulting in adrenal insufficiency. These drugs are also used with caution during pregnancy (pregnancy category C) and lactation (pregnancy category B—budesonide).

> **NURSING ALERT**
>
> During periods of stress or a severe asthmatic attack, patients who have been withdrawn from systemic corticosteroids should be instructed to resume systemic steroids immediately and to contact the primary health care provider. Patient deaths can result from adrenal insufficiency that may occur during and after transfer from systemic corticosteroids to inhaled corticosteroids.

Interactions

Ketoconazole may increase plasma levels of budesonide and fluticasone.

Mast Cell Stabilizer

Cromolyn (Intal) is a mast cell stabilizer.

Actions

Although its action is not fully understood, this drug is thought to stabilize the mast cell membrane, possibly by preventing calcium ions from entering mast cells, thus preventing the release of inflammatory mediators such as histamine and **leukotrienes**.

Uses

The mast cell stabilizer is used in combination with other drugs in the treatment of asthma and allergic disorders, including allergic rhinitis (nasal solution). It is also used to prevent EIB. They are typically used in Step 2 care for chronic asthma (see Display 32.1).

Adverse Reactions
Respiratory System Reactions

• Throat irritation and dryness
• Unpleasant taste sensation
• Cough or wheeze

This drug may cause a nauseated feeling. A more complete listing of the adverse reactions associated with the mast cell stabilizer is found in the Summary Drug Table: Lower Respiratory System Drugs.

Contraindications and Precautions

The mast cell stabilizer is contraindicated in patients with known hypersensitivity to the drugs and during attacks of acute asthma, because they may worsen bronchospasm during the acute asthma attack.

A mast cell stabilizer is used cautiously during pregnancy (pregnancy category B) and lactation and in patients with impaired renal or hepatic function.

Interactions

No significant drug interactions have been reported.

Leukotriene Modifiers and Immunomodulators

Leukotriene receptor antagonists include montelukast (Singulair) and zafirlukast (Accolate). Zileuton (Zyflo) is classified as a leukotriene formation inhibitor. Omalizumab (Xolair) is a monoclonal antibody used in the treatment of asthma. Additional information concerning these drugs is found in the Summary Drug Table: Lower Respiratory System Drugs.

Actions

Asthma attacks are often triggered by allergens or exercise. Inflammatory substances called *leukotrienes* are one of several substances that are released by mast cells during an asthma attack. Leukotrienes are primarily responsible for bronchoconstriction. When leukotriene production is inhibited, bronchodilation is facilitated. Zileuton (an inhibitor) acts by decreasing the formation of leukotrienes. Although the result is the same, montelukast and zafirlukast work in a manner slightly different from that of zileuton. Montelukast and zafirlukast are considered leukotriene receptor antagonists because they inhibit

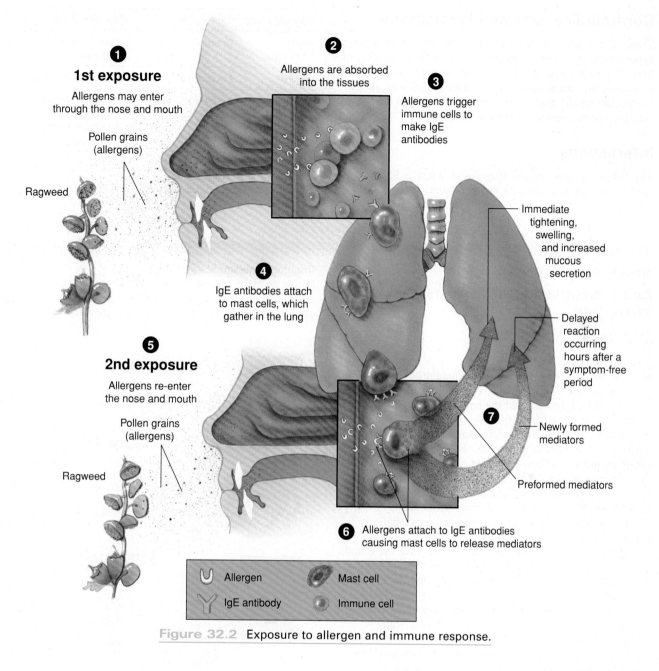

1 **1st exposure**
Allergens may enter through the nose and mouth

Pollen grains (allergens)

Ragweed

2 Allergens are absorbed into the tissues

3 Allergens trigger immune cells to make IgE antibodies

Immediate tightening, swelling, and increased mucous secretion

4 IgE antibodies attach to mast cells, which gather in the lung

Delayed reaction occurring hours after a symptom-free period

5 **2nd exposure**
Allergens re-enter the nose and mouth

Pollen grains (allergens)

Ragweed

7

Newly formed mediators

Preformed mediators

6 Allergens attach to IgE antibodies causing mast cells to release mediators

| Allergen | Mast cell |
| IgE antibody | Immune cell |

Figure 32.2 Exposure to allergen and immune response.

leukotriene receptor sites in the respiratory tract, preventing airway edema and facilitating bronchodilation. Omalizumab modulates the immune response by preventing the binding of immunoglobulin to the receptors on basophils and mast cells, thereby limiting the allergic reaction. The action of these drugs is illustrated in Figure 32.2, which shows how exposure to an allergen triggers the antibody response in the respiratory system.

Uses

Leukotriene modifiers are used in the prophylaxis and treatment of chronic asthma in adults and children older than 12 years. Omalizumab is used as adjunctive therapy for patients 12 years of age and older who are sensitive to allergens (e.g., dust mites, cockroaches, cat or dog dander) and who require Step 5 or 6 care (see Display 32.1).

Adverse Reactions

- CNS reaction includes headache.
- Generalized body system reactions include flu-like symptoms.
- Immunomodulators may cause anaphylactic reactions.
- Emergency equipment should be available when administering this medication.

Lower Respiratory System Drugs

Contraindications and Precautions

These drugs are contraindicated in patients with known hypersensitivity, bronchospasm in acute asthma attacks, or liver disease (zileuton). They should be used cautiously in pregnancy and not at all during lactation (zafirlukast, montelukast, and omalizumab are pregnancy category B drugs and zileuton is a pregnancy category C drug).

Interactions

The following interactions may occur when a leukotriene modifier is administered with another agent:

Interacting Drug	Common Use	Effect of Interaction
aspirin	Pain relief	Increased plasma levels of zafirlukast
warfarin	Anticoagulant	Increased anticoagulant effect
theophylline	Treatment of asthma and COPD	Decreased level of zafirlukast; increased serum theophylline levels with zileuton use
erythromycin	Treatment of bacterial infection	Decreased level of zafirlukast

NURSING PROCESS
PATIENT RECEIVING A LOWER RESPIRATORY SYSTEM DRUG

ASSESSMENT

Preadministration Assessment

Because the bronchodilators or antiasthma drugs may be given for asthma, emphysema, or chronic bronchitis, the preadministration assessment of the patient requires careful observation and documentation. Many respiratory problems are chronic conditions with acute exacerbations. Quick recognition and immediate action are essential in treating acute breathing problems. Long-term control of respiratory conditions consists of assessment and monitoring, patient education, environmental control, and medication management. Patients are encouraged to use asthma action plans for daily self-management and for acute respiratory exacerbations (see Fig. 32.4).

In situations of acute breathing distress, take the blood pressure, pulse, and respiratory rate before therapy with a bronchodilator or antiasthma drug. Respiratory rates below 12 breaths/min or above 24 breaths/min are considered abnormal. It is important to assess the lung fields and carefully document the sounds heard before therapy is begun. Note any dyspnea, cough, wheezing, "noisy" respirations, or use of accessory muscles when breathing. If the patient is raising sputum, document a description of the sputum. It is also important to record nonrespiratory signs of hypoxia, such as mental confusion, restlessness, anxiety, and cyanosis (bluish discoloration of the skin and mucous membranes). In some instances, the primary health care provider may order arterial blood gas analysis or pulmonary function tests.

If the patient is able to talk comfortably, ask about possible triggers of the asthma attack causing the inability to breathe. Figure 32.3 illustrates common triggers of asthma. Has the patient been around different environmental items, such as a new pet or changes in environmental temperature? Has the patient been under undue stress either physically or emotionally? Has the patient been monitoring lung function with a peak flow meter, and has a change been noted?

Ongoing Assessment

During an acute attack, assess the respiratory status about 30 minutes after a drug is administered or every 4 hours as the patient returns to a normal breathing pattern (or more often

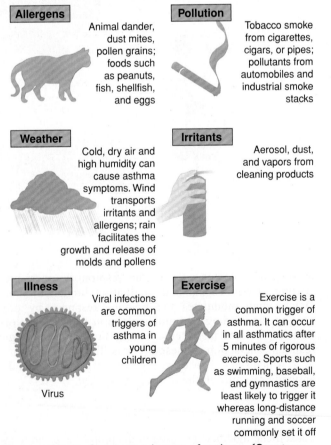

Common Triggers of Asthma

Triggers are those factors that set off asthma symptoms. They may vary among asthmatics, making it important to identify which factors bring on an attack.

Allergens
Animal dander, dust mites, pollen grains; foods such as peanuts, fish, shellfish, and eggs

Pollution
Tobacco smoke from cigarettes, cigars, or pipes; pollutants from automobiles and industrial smoke stacks

Weather
Cold, dry air and high humidity can cause asthma symptoms. Wind transports irritants and allergens; rain facilitates the growth and release of molds and pollens

Irritants
Aerosol, dust, and vapors from cleaning products

Illness
Viral infections are common triggers of asthma in young children

Virus

Exercise
Exercise is a common trigger of asthma. It can occur in all asthmatics after 5 minutes of rigorous exercise. Sports such as swimming, baseball, and gymnastics are least likely to trigger it whereas long-distance running and soccer commonly set it off

Figure 32.3 Common triggers of asthma. (Courtesy of Anatomical Chart Co.)

if needed). Note the respiratory rate, lung sounds, and use of accessory muscles in breathing. Additionally, keep a careful record of the intake and output and report any imbalance, which may indicate a fluid overload or excessive diuresis.

During stable chronic phases the patient assumes responsibility to monitor for changes. When an asthma action plan is used, the primary health care provider prescribes daily medications for the patient as well as quick-relief medications. The patient in turn monitors for symptoms such as wheezing and coughing, peak flow meter changes, and triggers that might be making the asthma worsen. During follow-up sessions ask the patient about changes seen on the asthma action plan.

Action plans use a "traffic signal" approach to monitoring breathing status (Fig. 32.4). Has the patient's condition stayed within the parameters of the green zone or has the patient's status moved to the yellow or red zones? It is important to monitor any patient with a history of cardiovascular problems for chest pain and changes in the electrocardiogram. The primary health care provider may order periodic pulmonary function tests, particularly for patients with emphysema or bronchitis, to help monitor respiratory status.

NURSING DIAGNOSES
Drug-specific nursing diagnoses include the following:

- **Anxiety** related to feelings of breathlessness
- **Ineffective Airway Clearance** related to bronchospasm
- **Impaired Oral Mucous Membranes** related to dryness or irritation
- **Imbalanced Nutrition: Less Than Body Requirements** related to decreased appetite caused by nausea, heartburn, or unpleasant taste

Nursing diagnoses related to drug administrations are discussed in Chapter 4.

PLANNING
The expected outcomes for the patient depend on the specific reason for administering the drug but may include an optimal response to therapy, support of patient needs related to managing adverse reactions, and confidence in an understanding of the medication regimen.

IMPLEMENTATION

Promoting an Optimal Response to Therapy
Nursing care of the patient receiving a bronchodilating drug or an antiasthma drug requires careful monitoring of the patient and instruction for proper administration of the various drugs. These drugs may be given orally, parenterally, or topically by inhalation or nebulization. Dosages are individualized for each patient, which allows the smallest effective dose to be given.

ACUTE SYMPTOM INTERVENTIONS. SABA bronchodilators are used to treat acute respiratory symptoms. Instruct the patient to administer 2 to 4 puffs of the inhaled medication when acute distress occurs. Depending on the severity of the exacerbation, up to three treatments at 20-minute intervals may be administered. A nebulizer may be ordered to deliver the medication rather than an inhaler device. These treatments are given less frequently.

Older adults taking the adrenergic bronchodilators are at increased risk for adverse reactions related to both the cardiovascular system (tachycardia, arrhythmias, palpitations, and hypertension) and the CNS (restlessness, agitation, and insomnia).

If the patient seeks care at an urgent or emergent facility, health care providers may administer epinephrine subcutaneously for an acute bronchospasm. Doses of drugs, such as epinephrine, are measured in tenths of a milliliter. Minimize distractions that may prevent you from reading the primary health care provider's order when preparing these drugs for administration to prevent error. Therapeutic effects occur within 5 minutes after administration and last as long as 4 hours. Anticholinergic medications or intravenous (IV) steroids may also be used when the situation is emergent.

Rapid theophyllinization using one of the xanthine derivatives may be required for acute respiratory symptoms. Patients are encouraged to use the Step Method to resolve acute respiratory symptoms, yet theophylline remains a low-cost effective alternative. Theophyllinization is accomplished by giving the patient a higher initial dose, called a *loading dose*, to bring blood levels to a therapeutic range more quickly than waiting several days for the drug to exert a therapeutic effect. Typically this is achieved in an inpatient setting and the primary health care provider may prescribe loading doses to be administered orally or IV over 12 to 24 hours. It is important to monitor the patient closely for signs of theophylline toxicity (Table 32.1). If a bronchodilator is given IV, it is administered through an infusion pump. Check the IV infusion site at frequent intervals, because these patients may be extremely restless and extravasation can occur.

LONG-TERM CONTROL OF SYMPTOMS. Controlling respiratory mucosal inflammation is the goal of long-term medications. The stepwise method of self-care (see Display 32.1) is a guideline for patients and is the basis for an individualized plan made by the primary health care provider. Using the Step Method, patients manage the first step without daily medications. ICSs

Table 32.1 Theophyllinization Process		
Drug administered (IV or orally) over 12 to 24 hours		
Serum blood level measured 1–2 hours after dose (5–9 hours with sustained-release drug)		
Therapeutic range: 10–20 mcg/L	Monitor for toxicity: 15–20 mcg/L	Toxicity: +20 mcg/L
	anorexia	abdominal cramping confusion
	nausea	restlessness
	vomiting	tachycardia
	diarrhea	arrhythmias
	headache	seizures
	insomnia	

My Asthma Plan ENGLISH

Patient Name: _____

Medical Record #: _____

Provider's Name: _____ DOB: _____

Provider's Phone #: _____ Completed by: _____ Date: _____

Controller Medicines	How Much to Take	How Often	Other Instructions
		_____ times per day **EVERY DAY!**	❑ Gargle or rinse mouth after use
		_____ times per day **EVERY DAY!**	
		_____ times per day **EVERY DAY!**	
		_____ times per day **EVERY DAY!**	

Quick-Relief Medicines	How Much to Take	How Often	Other Instructions
❑ Albuterol (ProAir, Ventolin, Proventil) ❑ Levalbuterol (Xopenex)	❑ 2 puffs ❑ 4 puffs ❑ 1 nebulizer treatment	Take ONLY as needed (see below — starting in Yellow Zone or before excercise)	NOTE: If you need this medicine more than two days a week, call physician to consider increasing controller medications and discuss your treatment plan.

Special instructions when I am ⬤ *doing well,* ◯ *getting worse,* ⬤ *having a medical alert.*

GREEN ZONE

Doing *well.*

- No cough, wheeze, chest tightness, or shortness of breath during the day or night.
- Can do usual activities.

Peak Flow (for ages 5 and up):
is _____ or more. (80% or more of personal best)
Personal Best Peak Flow (for ages 5 and up): _____

PREVENT asthma symptoms every day:

☐ Take my controller medicines (above) every day.

☐ Before exercise, take _____ puff(s) of _____

☐ Avoid things that make my asthma worse. (See back of form.)

YELLOW ZONE

Getting *worse.*

- Cough, wheeze, chest tightness, shortness of breath, or
- Waking at night due to asthma symptoms, or
- Can do some, but not all, usual activities.

Peak Flow (for ages 5 and up):
_____ to _____ (50 to 79% of personal best)

CAUTION. Continue taking every day controller medicines, AND:
☐ Take ____ puffs or ____ one nebulizer treatment of quick-relief medicine. If I am not back in the **Green Zone** within 20-30 minutes take ____ more puffs or nebulizer treatments. If I am not back in the **Green Zone** within one hour, then I should:
☐ Increase_____
☐ Add_____
☐ Call_____
☐ Continue using quick-relief medicine every 4 hours as needed. Call provider if not improving in _____ days.

RED ZONE

Medical Alert

- Very short of breath, or
- Quick-relief medicines have not helped, or
- Cannot do usual activities, or
- Symptoms are same or get worse after 24 hours in Yellow Zone.

Peak Flow (for ages 5 and up):
less than_____(50% of personal best)

MEDICAL ALERT! Get help!

☐ Take quick-relief medicine: _____ puffs every _____ minutes and get help immediately.

☐ Take _____

☐ Call _____

Danger! Get help immediately! Call 911 if trouble walking or talking due to shortness of breath or if lips or fingernails are gray or blue. For child, call 911 if skin is sucked in around neck and ribs during breaths or child doesn't respond normally.

Health Care Provider: My signature provides authorization for the above written orders. I understand that all procedures will be implemented in accordance with state laws and regulations. Student may self-carry asthma medications: ❑ Yes ❑ No self-administer asthma medications: ❑ Yes ❑ No (This authorization is for a maximum of one year from signature date.)

_____ _____
Healthcare Provider Signature   Date

ORIGINAL (Patient) / CANARY (School/Child Care/Work/Other Support Systems) / PINK (Chart)

©2008, Public Health Institute (RAMP)

Figure 32.4 Example of asthma action plan. (Reprinted with permission from *The Asthma Action Plan*, developed by a committee facilitated by the Regional Asthma Management and Prevention [RAMP] Initiative, a program of the Public Health Institute. Source: http://www.rampasthma.org/actionplan. This publication was supported by Cooperative Agreement Number 1U58DP001016-01 from the CDC. Its contents are solely the responsibility of the authors and do not necessarily represent the official views of the CDC.)

are used in the second step of the plan. It is important to remind the patient to refrain from swallowing the medication and to rinse the mouth thoroughly after using the inhaler.

LIFESPAN CONSIDERATIONS
Pediatric/Gerontology

When taking oral corticosteroids or higher doses of the inhalant form:

- Children are at risk for growth reduction. Document the patient's growth record consistently, particularly during growth periods such as puberty and adolescence.
- For older adults at risk for osteoporosis, a calcium or vitamin D supplement may be prescribed.

Instruct the patient to ensure confidence in understanding that the purpose of step care is a self-management program for worsening symptoms. Part of a step care program is to start the patient on the lowest number and dosage of drugs that will treat the respiratory condition. As the patient's breathing becomes distressed, doses are changed by the patient, and different medications are added at each step. As the symptoms lessen, the patient reduces medications, and the patient's medication routine moves down a step. Providing emotional support and encouragement as the patient makes adjustments in accordance with each step is a key factor to success.

The patient learns to adjust according to daily experiences of breathing distress or peak expiratory flow readings. LABA bronchodilators are not administered more frequently than twice daily (morning and evening). LABA drugs, such as salmeterol or formoterol, do not replace the fast-acting inhalers for sudden symptoms, nor are they used to treat acute asthma symptoms. The drugs may be administered by a metered-dose inhaler (Display 32.2). If a dry-powder inhaler is used for administration, you should teach the patient how to use it.

! NURSING ALERT

Formoterol (Foradil Aerolizer) comes in capsule form and is administered only by oral inhalation using the Aerolizer inhaler. Be sure to remind the patient that this capsule is not to be taken orally.

Display 32.2 Using a Metered-Dose Inhaler

How to Use an Inhaler
When a patient is first diagnosed with asthma and prescribed inhalation therapy, he or she may need to learn how to use the inhaler that will deliver drug therapy. You may be the health care provider who supplies instructions such as these:

Metered-Dose Inhaler (MDI)
1. When using a new inhaler, or one that has not been used in several days, point the inhaler away from you and prime the inhaler 1–2 times.
2. Hold the device upright and shake it.
3. Tilt the head back slightly.
4. Exhale and open mouth.
5. Position the inhaler in one of three ways:
   - Held 1–2 inches from the mouth (this is preferred)
   - Using a spacer
   - With the inhaler between the lips
6. Start to inhale slowly and press down on the inhaler to release the medication.
7. Breathe in for 3–5 seconds.
8. Hold your breath for 10 seconds to allow the drug to reach deep into the lungs.

9. Repeat for the ordered number of puffs, allowing 1 minute between each puff.

Spacers are recommended for children, older adults, and anyone who has difficulty using a nebulizer alone. Spacers are indicated when using inhaled steroids.

Dry-Powder Inhaler (DPI)
1. Prepare the medication for inhalation.
2. Place the mouthpiece to the lips.
3. Inhale quickly.
4. Hold your breath for 10 seconds to allow the drug to reach deep into the lungs.
5. Capsules for inhalation (such as those used in Foradil Aerolizer or Spiriva HaniHaler) must not be swallowed.
6. Do not place your device in water.

When the patient is prescribed more than one type of inhaler, instruct the patient to use the bronchodilator first to open the air passages, and then use other prescribed medications.

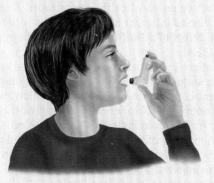

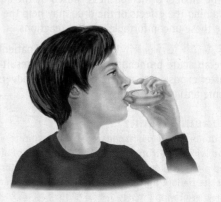

The mast cell stabilizer cromolyn (Intal) may be added to the patient's existing treatment regimen (e.g., ICSs). If use of the mast cell stabilizer must be discontinued for any reason, the dosage is gradually tapered. When administered orally, cromolyn is given one half hour before meals and at bedtime. The oral form of the drug comes in an ampule. The ampule is opened and its contents poured into a glass of water. The patient or care provider stirs the mixture thoroughly. The patient must drink all of the mixture. The drug may not be mixed with any other substance (e.g., fruit juice, milk, or foods).

Leukotriene receptor antagonists, leukotriene inhibitors, and immunomodulators are drugs used for managing asthma and are never administered during an acute asthma attack. If used during an acute attack, these drugs may worsen the attack. These drugs are administered orally.

Zileuton may cause liver damage. Because of the danger of liver toxicity, the primary health care provider may order hepatic aminotransferase levels at the beginning of treatment and during therapy. Patients are instructed to immediately report any symptoms of liver dysfunction, such as upper right quadrant pain, nausea, fatigue, lethargy, pruritus, and jaundice. Patients may be hypersensitive to monoclonal antibodies (e.g., omalizumab), which are used to modulate the immune response. It is administered subcutaneously every 2 to 4 weeks, typically in the clinic setting, where the patient can be monitored after the injection for an anaphylactic reaction. Be sure to tell the patient a reaction may occur up to 4 days following the injection and to have emergency contact information close at hand.

Monitoring and Managing Patient Needs

ANXIETY. Patients who have difficulty breathing and are receiving a bronchodilator or antiasthma drug may experience extreme anxiety, nervousness, and restlessness, which may be caused by their breathing difficulty or by the action of the drug. In these patients, it may be difficult for the primary health care provider to determine whether the patient is having an adverse drug reaction or the problem is related to the respiratory disorder. Reassure the patient that the drug being administered will most likely relieve the respiratory distress in a short time. Patients who are extremely apprehensive are observed more frequently until their respirations are near normal. Closely monitor the patient's blood pressure and pulse during therapy and report any significant changes. If you remember to speak and act in a calm manner, this will help to decrease the anxiety or nervousness caused by the adrenergic drug. Explaining the effects of the drug may help the patient to tolerate these uncomfortable adverse reactions.

INEFFECTIVE AIRWAY CLEARANCE. Occasionally the patient may experience an acute bronchospasm either as a result of the disease, after exposure to an allergen, or as an adverse reaction to some antiasthma drugs, such as ICSs.

⚠ NURSING ALERT

Acute bronchospasm causes severe respiratory distress and wheezing from the forceful expiration of air and is considered a medical emergency. Initiate medical intervention, or instruct the patient and family to call emergency services if this happens at home.

During an acute bronchospasm, check the blood pressure, pulse, respiratory rate, and response to the drug every 5 to 15 minutes until the patient's condition stabilizes and respiratory distress is relieved.

IMPAIRED ORAL MUCOUS MEMBRANES. Inhalers, particularly the corticosteroid or mast cell aerosols, may cause throat irritation and promote infection with *Candida albicans.* Instruct the patient to use strict oral hygiene, cleanse the inhaler as directed in the package directions, and use the proper technique when taking an inhalation. These interventions will decrease the incidence of candidiasis and help to soothe the throat. Occasionally an antifungal drug may be prescribed by the primary health care provider to manage the candidiasis.

IMBALANCED NUTRITION: LESS THAN BODY REQUIREMENTS. Some antiasthma drugs cause nausea. The patient with nausea should be offered frequent smaller meals rather than three large meals. Meals should be followed by good mouth care. Limiting fluids with meals can help lessen nausea. Teach the family ways to provide a pleasant, relaxed atmosphere for meals.

The patient taking theophylline may report heartburn, because the drug relaxes the lower esophageal sphincter, allowing gastroesophageal reflux. Heartburn is minimized if the patient remains in an upright position and sleeps with the head of the bed elevated. Some antiasthma drugs may cause an unpleasant taste in the mouth. Asking the patient to take frequent sips of water, suck on sugarless candy, or chew gum helps to alleviate the problem.

Educating the Patient and Family

Due to the chronic nature of respiratory illnesses, the nurse's role is to instruct the patient and family in methods to monitor the condition, control triggers in the environment, and manage medications properly for optimal breathing.

Asthma action plans in multiple languages can be found on the Internet. You can provide websites to the patient or demonstrate how to fill out the plans during a patient teaching session. These can be printed, or the individual can fill out the information and use it to monitor daily asthma management and acute episodes.

Teach the patient to monitor breathing status and regulate medications based on the asthma action plan. Demonstrate to the patient how to fill in the medications prescribed to maintain optimal breathing. Then instruct the patient to monitor his or her own breathing pattern based on zones defined by specific symptoms, peak flow meter readings, and corresponding adjusted medications as defined by the primary health care provider. A commonly used method to interpret breathing status is to relate it to the three colors of a traffic light: green, yellow, and red (see Fig. 32.4).

The patient uses a peak flow meter at home to monitor breathing status and the effectiveness of the drug regimen. The patient is taught how to use the peak flow meter and when to notify the primary health care provider (see Patient Teaching for Improved Patient Outcomes: Using a Peak Flow Meter). A majority of the medications prescribed will be delivered by inhalation. If the patient is to use an aerosol inhaler for administration of the medication, provide thorough explanation of its use (see Display 32.2). Do not assume

Patient Teaching for Improved Patient Outcomes

Using a Peak Flow Meter

Patients receiving bronchodilators or antiasthma drugs often need to monitor their lung function at home with a peak flow meter. Doing so provides the patient and the primary health care provider with valuable information about the status of the patient's condition and the effectiveness of therapy. Often, trends in the readings can detect changes in the patient's airway and airflow even before any signs and symptoms are experienced. This allows possible intervention before a major problem arises.

Because a variety of meters are commercially available, explain about the type of meter that will be used, how often the peak flow should be checked, and the ranges for the readings along with instructions on what to do for each range. Use the following steps to instruct the patient on the use of the peak flow meter:

✔ Check to make sure that the indicator is at the lowest level of the scale.
✔ Stand upright to allow the best inhalation possible. (Be sure to remove gum or food from your mouth.)
✔ Inhale as deeply as you can and then place your lips around the mouthpiece, making sure you have a tight seal.
✔ Exhale as forcibly and as quickly as possible in one large "huff."
✔ Watch the indicator rise on the scale, noting where it stops. The number below the indicator's position is your *peak flow reading.*
✔ Repeat the procedure two more times.
✔ Compare the three readings. Record the highest reading on your action plan. Do not calculate an average.
✔ Bring the action plan with peak flow meter readings to your follow-up visits.
✔ Measure the peak flow rate close to the same time each day. (Your physician may provide you with a suggested time. Some patients measure the peak flow rate twice daily between 7 and 9 a.m. and between 6 and 8 p.m. Others measure the peak flow rate before or after taking their medication.)
✔ Follow the medication instructions written on your action plan next to the zone color of your reading (see Fig. 32.4).
✔ Clean your meter with mild soap and hot water after use.

that the patient understands how to use an aerosol inhaler correctly. Many different devices are on the market; these are used with specific medications and do not all work the same. Review the written instructions and examine the device with the patient. Then have the patient demonstrate the use of the inhaler to evaluate whether he or she is using the proper technique. It is important to review instructions at each follow-up visit.

Display 32.3 Promoting Environmental Control for Asthma

You need to know what things bring on your asthma symptoms. Then do what you can to avoid or limit contact with these things.

* If animal dander is a problem for you, keep your pet out of the house or at least out of your bedroom, or find it a new home.
* Do not smoke or allow smoking in your home.
* If pollen is a problem for you, stay indoors with the air conditioner on, if possible, when the pollen count is high.
* To control dust mites, wash your sheets, blankets, pillows, and stuffed toys once a week in hot water. You can get special dust-proof covers for your mattress and pillows.
* If cold air bothers you, wear a scarf over your mouth and nose in the winter.
* If you have symptoms when you exercise or do routine physical activities like climbing stairs, work with your doctor to find ways to be active without having asthma symptoms. Physical activity is important.
* If you are allergic to sulfites, avoid foods (like dried fruit) or beverages (like wine) that contain them.

As the patient becomes more confident in managing the asthma medications, you can begin to help the patient assess the living environment. Display 32.3 describes ways to reduce or limit exposure to environmental triggers. Patients may be able to reduce asthma attacks if they feel they have control to modify exposure to the trigger elements.

As you develop a teaching plan for the patient or family member, include the following points:

■ Take the drug regularly as prescribed by the primary health care provider, even during symptom-free times. Long-acting medications are taken to prevent acute attacks and maintain a level of breathing—do not use to treat acute episodes of asthma.

■ If symptoms become worse, increase the dose or frequency of use as directed to do so by the primary health care provider or as established in the action plan.

■ Ask before using nonprescription drugs or herbal preparations. Some may contain similar drugs and may cause you to increase doses unknowingly.

■ Check medications weekly to be sure you can reorder prescriptions and avoid running out of medication when stores are closed. Do not chew or crush coated or sustained-release tablets.

■ Be sure you understand how the inhaler unit is assembled, used, and cleaned.

■ If LABAs are used for preventing EIB, the drug is administered at least 30 minutes before exercise. Additional doses are not to be given for at least 12 hours.

■ *For patients using adrenergic bronchodilators*—these drugs may cause nervousness, insomnia, and restlessness. Contact the primary health care provider if the symptoms become severe.

■ *For patients using xanthine derivatives*—follow your primary health care provider's instructions concerning monitoring of theophylline serum levels. Avoid foods that contain xanthine, such as colas, coffee, chocolate, and charcoal-prepared foods.

■ *For patients using ICSs*—wear a medical alert item (e.g., bracelet) indicating the need for supplemental systemic steroids in the event of stress or severe asthmatic attack that is unresponsive to bronchodilators. Do not stop therapy abruptly.

■ *For patients using immunomodulators*—be aware that an anaphylactic reaction can occur for up to a year after dosing. Contact the primary health care provider should you begin itching or get hives, and seek emergent care if you have trouble breathing.

EVALUATION

■ Therapeutic response is achieved and breathing is easier and more effective.

■ Adverse reactions are identified, reported to the primary health care provider, and managed successfully with appropriate nursing interventions:
  • Anxiety is managed successfully.
  • Patient has a clear patent airway.

• Mucous membranes are moist and intact.
• Nutrition is adequately maintained.

■ Patient and family express confidence and demonstrate an understanding of the drug regimen and use of both the peak flow meter and inhalator device.

PHARMACOLOGY IN PRACTICE
THINK CRITICALLY

Mrs. Chase has been diagnosed with asthma by her primary care provider, and the following plan is established:

  • Goal of peak flow meter should be 350.
• Asmanex Twisthaler 1 puff daily at bedtime.
• Albuterol inhaler, 2 puffs 30 minutes before exercise, or if peak flow reading is in yellow zone, or if feel short of breath.
• Call for medication changes if in red zone.

Mrs. Chase remarks that she does not want to use the inhaler because when her older mother used inhaled medication it smelled like rotten eggs.

KEY POINTS

• COPD includes asthma, chronic bronchitis, obstructive bronchitis, and emphysema, or any combination of these conditions. Asthma is a chronic lung condition causing spasmodic constriction of the bronchi and lung inflammation. Many Americans suffer from the ailment, and it is one of the most common childhood chronic conditions.

• Bronchodilators are used for patients with COPD who experience difficulty breathing (dyspnea) and an interference of gas exchange at the alveoli level in the lungs.

• Antiasthma drugs are used for both long-term management and short-term breathing relief. Guidelines for medication use are called the Step Method. Inhaled corticosteroids reduce inflammation, while bronchodilators relieve bronchospasm. Providers define parameters and help the patient make an asthma action plan to help the patient in self-management of the condition.

• Common adverse reactions to the medications include nervousness and restlessness, nausea, anorexia, vomiting, and tachycardia, or the feeling of heart palpitations.

Summary Drug Table LOWER RESPIRATORY SYSTEM DRUGS

Generic Name	Trade Name	Uses	Adverse Reactions	Dosage Ranges
Bronchodilators				
Short-Acting β₂ Agonists (SABAs—Adrenergics or Sympathomimetics Used for Acute Symptom Relief)				
albuterol *al-byoo'-ter-roll*	Proventil, Ventolin	Bronchospasm, prevention of EIB	Headache, palpitations, tachycardia, tremor, dizziness, shakiness, nervousness, hyperactivity	2–4 mg TID, QID orally; 1–2 inhalations q 4–6 hr; 2 inhalations before exercise; may also be given by nebulizer
ephedrine *eh-fed'-rin*		Asthma, bronchospasm	Precordial pain, urinary hesitancy	12.5–25 mg orally q 3–4 hr PRN; 25–50 mg IM, subcut, IV
epinephrine *ep-ih-nef'-rin*	Adrenalin, Epinephrine Mist, Primatene Mist	Asthma, bronchospasm	Palpitations, tremor, dizziness, drowsiness, vertigo, shakiness, nervousness, headache, nausea, vomiting, anxiety, fear, pallor	Inhalation aerosol: individualize dose Injection: Solution 1:1000, 0.3–0.5 mL subcut, IM Suspension (1:200), 0.1–0.3 mL subcut only
levalbuterol *lev-al-byoo'-ter-roll*	Xopenex	Treat and prevent bronchospasm	Tachycardia, nervousness, anxiety, pain, dizziness, rhinitis, cough, cardiac arrhythmias	0.63 mg TID, q 6–8 hr by nebulization; if no response, dose may be increased to 1.25 mg TID by nebulizer
metaproterenol *met-ah-proe-ter'-eh-noll*		Asthma, bronchospasm	Tachycardia, tremor, nervousness, shakiness, nausea, vomiting	20 mg TID orally, aerosol 2–3 inhalations q 3–4 hr; do not exceed 12 inhalations
pirbuterol *peer-byoo'-ter-roll*	Maxair Autohaler	Asthma, bronchospasm	Tremor, dizziness, shakiness, nervousness	2 inhalations q 4–6 hr; do not exceed 12 inhalations
terbutaline *ter-byoo'-tah-leen*		Treat and prevent bronchospasm	Palpitations, tremor, dizziness, vertigo, shakiness, nervousness, drowsiness, headache, nausea, vomiting, GI upset	2.5–5 mg q 6 hr orally TID during waking hours; 0.25 mg subcut (may repeat once if needed)
Long-Acting β₂ Agonists (LABAs—Adrenergics or Sympathomimetics Used for Long-Term Management)				
arformoterol *ar- for- moe'-ter-ol*	Brovana	Long-term treatment and prevention of bronchospasm in COPD	Nervousness, tremor, dizziness, headache, insomnia, nausea, vomiting, diarrhea, leg cramps, back pain	15 mcg inhalation BID morning and evening
formoterol *for-moh'-te-rol*	Foradil	Long-term treatment and prevention of bronchospasm	Palpations, tachycardia, dizziness, nervousness	One 12-mg capsule q 12 hr using inhalation device, not for oral use; EIB use 15 min before exercise
indacaterol *in'-da-ka'-ter-ol*	Arcapta Neohaler	Long-term treatment and prevention of bronchospasm	Palpations, tachycardia, weakness, cramping, thirst, increased urination	One 75-mcg capsule daily
salmeterol *sal-mee'-ter-ol*	Serevent Diskus	Long-term treatment and prevention of bronchospasm	Tremor, headache, cough	1 inhalation BID morning and evening; inhalation powder, do not use spacer
Xanthine Derivatives				
aminophylline *am-in-off'-lin*		Symptomatic relief or prevention of bronchial asthma and reversible bronchospasm of chronic bronchitis and emphysema	Nausea, vomiting, restlessness, nervousness, tachycardia, tremors, headache, palpitations, hyperglycemia, electrocardiographic changes, cardiac arrhythmias	Individualize dosage: base adjustments on clinical responses, monitor serum aminophylline levels, maintain therapeutic range of 10–20 mcg/mL; base dosage on lean body mass

(table continues on page 340)

Lower Respiratory System Drugs

Summary Drug Table LOWER RESPIRATORY SYSTEM DRUGS (continued)

Generic Name	Trade Name	Uses	Adverse Reactions	Dosage Ranges
dyphylline *dye'-fi-lin*	Lufyllin	Same as aminophylline	Same as aminophylline	Up to 15 mg/kg orally q 6 hr
oxtriphylline *ox-trye'-fi-lin*	Choledyl SA	Same as aminophylline	Same as aminophylline	4.7 mg/kg orally q 8 hr; sustained-action: 1 tablet orally q 12 hr
theophylline *thee-off'-i-lin*	Theolair,	Same as aminophylline	Same as aminophylline	Initial dosing: 16 mg/kg/day or 400 mg/day
Cholinergic Blocking Drug (Anticholinergics Used for Acute Symptom Relief)				
ipratropium *ih-prah-trow'-pea-um*	Atrovent	Bronchospasm associated with COPD, chronic bronchitis and emphysema, rhinorrhea	Dryness of the oropharynx, nervousness, irritation from aerosol, dizziness, headache, GI distress, dry mouth, exacerbation of symptoms, nausea, palpitations	Aerosol: 2 inhalations QID, not to exceed 12 inhalations Solution: 500 mg (1 unit dose vial) TID, QID by oral nebulization Nasal spray: 2 sprays per nostril BID, TID of 0.03%, or 2 sprays per nostril TID, QID of 0.06%
tiotropium *tee-oh-tro'-pee-um*	Spiriva	Same as ipratropium	Same as ipratropium, increased stroke potential	1 capsule per day using inhalation device, not for oral use
Antiasthma Drugs				
Inhaled Corticosteroids				
beclomethasone *beh-kloe-meth'-ah-soan*	QVAR	Maintenance treatment of asthma	Oral, laryngeal, pharyngeal irritation; fungal infections; suppression of HPA function	Starting dose used with bronchodilators alone: 40–80 mcg BID; when used with ICSs: 40–160 mcg BID; maximum 320 mcg BID Children 5–12 yr: 40 mcg BID when used with bronchodilators alone or with ICSs
budesonide *byoo-dess'-oh-nyde*	Pulmicort	Maintenance treatment of asthma	Same as beclomethasone	Individualized dosage by oral inhalation Adults: 200–800 mcg BID Children 6 yr and older: 200–400 mcg BID Children 12 mo to 8 yr: 0.5–1 mcg total daily dose administered once or twice daily in divided doses
flunisolide *floo-niss'-oh-lyde*	Aerospan, AeroBid,	Maintenance treatment of asthma, especially those on systemic corticosteroid therapy	Same as beclomethasone	Adults: 2 inhalations BID; maximum dose, 4 inhalations BID Children 6–15 yr: 2 inhalations BID
fluticasone *floo-tik'-ah-soan*	Flovent HFA, Flovent Diskus	Prophylactic maintenance and treatment of asthma	Same as beclomethasone	88–880 mcg BID
mometasone *moe-met'-ah-soan*	Asmanex Twisthaler	Maintenance treatment of asthma	Same as beclomethasone	1 inhalation (220 mcg) QD in the evening for patients previously maintained on bronchodilators alone or ICSs; 2 inhalations (440 mcg) BID for patients previously maintained on oral corticosteroids

Summary Drug Table LOWER RESPIRATORY SYSTEM DRUGS (continued)

Generic Name	Trade Name	Uses	Adverse Reactions	Dosage Ranges
ICS/LABA Combinations				
budesonide/ formoterol *byoo-dess'-oh-nyde/ for-moe'-ter-roll*	Symbicort	Long-term maintenance of asthma	See individual drugs	Low-medium dose (ICS) 80/4.5 mcg; medium-high dose (ICS) 160/4.5 mcg, 2 inhalations morning and evening
fluticasone/ salmeterol *floo-tik'-ah-soan/ sal-mee'-ter-roll*	Advair	Long-term maintenance of asthma, COPD	See individual drugs	2 inhalations twice daily
Mast Cell Stabilizer				
cromolyn *kroe'-moe-lin*	Gastrocrom	Bronchial asthma, prevention of bronchospasm, prevention of EIB Nasal preparations: prevention and treatment of allergic rhinitis	Cough, wheeze, unusual taste, dizziness, headache, nausea, dry and irritated throat, rash, joint swelling and pain	Inhalation solution: 20 mg (1 ampule/vial) administered by nebulizer QID Aerosol: adults and children 5 yr and older: 2 metered sprays QID EIB: 2 metered sprays shortly (10–15 min but not more than 60 min) before exposure to the precipitating factor Nasal solution: 1 spray each nostril 3–6 times/day Oral: adults and children 13 yr and older: 2 ampules QID 30 min before meals and at bedtime Children 2–12 yr: 1 ampule QID before meals and at bedtime; do not exceed 40 mg/kg/day
Leukotriene Modifiers and Immunomodulators				
montelukast *mon-teh-loo'-cast*	Singulair	Prophylaxis and treatment of chronic asthma in adults and pediatric patients 12 mo of age and older, seasonal allergic rhinitis in adults and pediatric patients 2 yr of age and older	Headache, influenza-like symptoms	Adults and children older than 15 yr: 10 mg orally in the evening Children 6–14 yr: one 5-mg chewable tablet daily, in the evening Children 1–5 yr: one 4-mg chewable tablet daily, in the evening, or one 4-mg oral granule packet daily
omalizumab *oh-mal-iz'-yoo-mab*	Xolair	Moderate to severe persistent asthma	Injection site reaction, anaphylaxis	150–375 mg subcut every 2–4 wk
roflumilast *roe-flue'-mi-last*	Daliresp	Severe COPD—phosphodiesterase inhibitor	Diarrhea	500 mcg orally daily
zafirlukast *zah-fur-loo'-cast*	Accolate	Prophylaxis and treatment of chronic asthma in adults and children 5 yr or older	Same as montelukast	Adults and children older than 12 yr: 20 mg orally BID Children 5–11 yr: 10 mg orally BID
zileuton *zye-loot'-on*	Zyflo	Prophylaxis and treatment of chronic asthma in adults and children 12 yr or older	Dyspepsia, nausea, headache	600 mg orally QID

Lower Respiratory System Drugs

● Chapter Review

Know Your Drugs

Clients sometimes know a medication by the brand (or trade) name and not the generic name. To help you recognize both names, match the brand name with the generic name of the same medication:

Generic Name	Brand Name
1. albuterol	A. Asmanex
2. mometasone	B. Proventil
3. montelukast	C. Singulair
4. tiotropium	D. Spiriva

Calculate Medication Dosages

1. A client is prescribed 0.25 mg of terbutaline subcutaneously. The drug is available for injection in a solution of 1 mg/mL. The nurse administers _____.

2. The client is prescribed zafirlukast 20 mg orally BID. The drug is available in 10-mg tablets. The nurse administers _____. How many milligrams of zafirlukast will the client receive each day?

● Prepare for the NCLEX®

Build Your Knowledge

1. COPD does not include which of the following conditions?

   1. acute asthma
   2. acute pneumonia
   3. chronic bronchitis
   4. emphysema

2. Which of the following actions are accomplished when using bronchodilators?

   1. reduce inflammatory response
   2. promote mucous removal
   3. reverse bronchoconstriction
   4. remove fluid from the lungs

3. When the SABA drugs are administered to older adults, there is a greater increased risk of _____.

   1. GI effects
   2. nephrotoxic effects
   3. neurotoxic effects
   4. cardiovascular effects

4. When administering aminophylline, a xanthine derivative bronchodilating drug, the nurse monitors the client for adverse reactions, which include _____.

   1. restlessness and nervousness
   2. hypoglycemia and hypothyroidism
   3. bradycardia and bronchospasm
   4. somnolence and lethargy

5. The nurse correctly administers montelukast (Singulair) _____.

   1. once daily in the evening
   2. twice daily in the morning and evening
   3. three times a day with meals
   4. once daily in the morning

Apply Your Knowledge

6. Which of the following laboratory tests would the nurse expect to be ordered for a client taking Theolair?

   1. thyroid hormone levels
   2. alanine aminotransferase
   3. sodium electrolytes
   4. serum theophylline levels

7. The body reacts to a trigger and stimulates the sympathetic branch of the nervous system causing bronchoconstriction and inflammation. Which neurotransmitter is stimulated?

   1. serotonin
   2. norepinephrine
   3. dopamine
   4. acetylcholine

8. The following statement indicates that the client understands the purpose of the peak flow meter.

   1. "I use the peak flow meter when I am short of breath."
   2. "I must wash the peak flow meter after every use."
   3. "I should measure my peak flow every day."
   4. "I put the medicine in the peak flow meter."

Alternate-Format Questions

9. The drug Advair is a combination of different medications. Which drugs are in this inhaler? **Select all that apply**.

   1. fluticasone
   2. omalizumab
   3. salmeterol
   4. zafirlukast

10. The drug Advair is a combination of which drug categories? **Select all that apply**.

    1. corticosteroids
    2. immunomodulators
    3. long-acting β agonists
    4. xanthine derivatives

To check your answers, see Appendix G.

thePoint *For more NCLEX-style questions, log on to* *http://thepoint.lww.com to access more than 1000 questions.*

Drugs That Affect the Cardiovascular System

Drugs used to treat disorders of the cardiovascular system are discussed in this unit. With nearly 2,500 deaths per day, coronary heart disease (CHD) is the single largest killer of both men and women in the United States. These seem like high numbers, yet the death rate from CHD and stroke decreased by 30% from 1998 to 2008 (American Heart Association, 2012). This is due in part to advances in diagnosis and treatment and changes in lifestyle, which result in reduced mortality. The drugs discussed in this unit range from those used early in heart disease (such as diuretics) to drugs used in critical care units when advanced disease is treated.

The first few chapters discuss drugs used to reduce risk of cardiovascular diseases. Individuals at risk for hypertension require health-promoting lifestyle modifications to prevent cardiovascular disease. Hypertension, if untreated, can lead to dysfunction not only in the cardiovascular system but also in other systems such as the renal and respiratory systems. In individuals between the ages of 40 and 70 years, every increase of 20 mm Hg in systolic pressure or every increase of 10 mm Hg in diastolic pressure doubles the risk of cardiovascular disease. Treating hypertension early reduces the risk for cardiovascular disease and death and protects against hypertension-related complications such as stroke, heart failure (HF), and renal disease.

Chapter 33 discusses the use of diuretics. These drugs make the kidneys filter more effectively and remove fluid as well as waste products from the body. Although the kidney is the target organ of these drugs, fluid removal is necessary for cardiac function. Sometimes reducing fluid, along with lifestyle changes, is all that is necessary.

Chapter 34 features the cholesterol-lowering drugs or antihyperlipidemic drugs. As blood cholesterol levels increase, so does the risk of CHD. In general, the higher the low-density lipoprotein (LDL) level and the more risk factors involved, the greater the risk for heart disease. Lowering blood cholesterol levels can arrest or reverse atherosclerosis in the vessels and can significantly decrease the incidence of heart disease.

In Chapter 35, specific drugs used to treat hypertension are discussed. Some of those include adrenergic blocking drugs, angiotensin-converting enzyme (ACE) inhibitors, calcium channel blockers, and other inhibitors or antagonists.

Chapter 36 discusses the antianginal drugs whose primary purpose is to increase blood supply to an area by dilating blood vessels. Sharp pains in the chest, jaw, or arm may be one of the first times a person will stop and consider his or her cardiac status. Diseases of the arteries—coronary artery disease, cerebral vascular disease, and peripheral vascular disease—are caused by narrowing

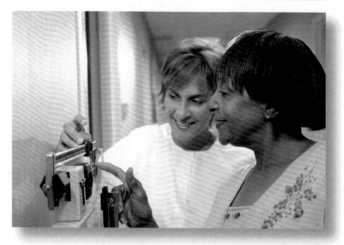

of the arteries and may result in pain when tissues are denied oxygen. Blockage of the vessels in the form of blood clots can occur in the cardiovascular system.

Chapter 37 discusses drugs used to prevent (anticoagulants or antiplatelets) and drugs used to remove (thrombolytics) blood clots from the blood vessels.

Almost 5 million Americans have HF (previously referred to as *congestive heart failure*). It is the most frequent cause of hospitalization for individuals older than 65 years. African Americans and obese individuals are at the highest risk for HF. With treatment, some patients may lead nearly normal lives, although more than 300,000 individuals with HF die each year. The ACE inhibitors are considered the first-choice treatment and are the cornerstones of HF drug therapy. These drugs are discussed in terms of their ability to reduce hypertension. Many older adults may continue to use a cardiotonic, for example, digoxin, discussed in Chapter 38. Digoxin is prescribed for patients with HF who do not respond to the ACE inhibitors and diuretics.

The last chapter in this unit (Chapter 39) discusses the antiarrhythmic drugs used to treat cardiac arrhythmia (a conduction disorder resulting in an abnormally slow or rapid regular heart rate, or a heart that beats with an irregular pace). Some arrhythmias do not require treatment, whereas others require immediate treatment because they are potentially fatal. Although these drugs are used to treat arrhythmia, they are also capable of causing or worsening an arrhythmia. The benefits of treatment must be carefully weighed by the primary health care provider against the risks of treatment with the antiarrhythmic drug.

Some of the drug classes may be repeated in multiple chapters because their use effectively reduces death from heart disease.

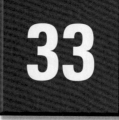

33

Diuretics

KEY TERMS

anuria • cessation of urine production
azotemia • absence of urine production
diuresis • production of urine
edema • accumulation of excess water in the body
gynecomastia • male breast enlargement
hyperkalemia • increase in potassium levels in the blood
hypokalemia • low blood potassium level

DRUG CLASSES

Loop diuretics
Thiazides and related diuretics
Potassium-sparing diuretics
Osmotic diuretics
Carbonic anhydrase inhibitors

Many conditions or diseases, such as heart failure (HF), endocrine disturbances, and kidney and liver diseases, can cause fluid overload or **edema** (retention of excess fluid). When the patient shows signs of excess fluid retention, the primary health care provider may order a diuretic to reduce the increased fluid. A diuretic is a drug that increases the excretion of urine (i.e., water, electrolytes, and waste products) by the kidneys. There are various types of diuretic drugs, and the primary health care provider selects the one that best suits the patient's needs and effectively reduces the amount of excess fluid in body tissues.

Hypertension is frequently treated with the administration of an antihypertensive drug and a diuretic. The diuretics used for this combination therapy include the loop diuretics and the thiazides. The specific uses of each type of diuretic drug are discussed in the following sections.

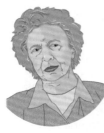

PHARMACOLOGY IN PRACTICE

You are concerned about Mrs. Moore because of the increase in calls from her out-of-town daughter. It is time to do a medication reconciliation. When she brings in a bag of pills you find that a prescription bottle for a daily diuretic filled 3 weeks ago is almost full. As you read on, see if you can determine what questions to ask Mrs. Moore.

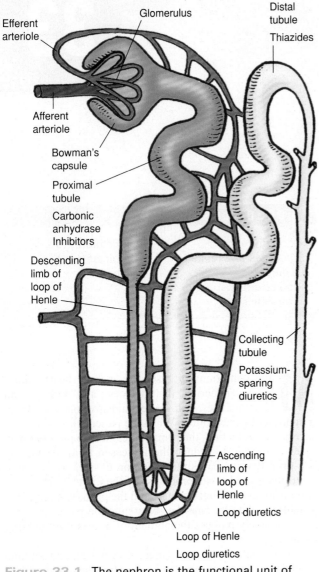

Figure 33.1 The nephron is the functional unit of the kidney. Note the various tubules, the site of most diuretic activity.

Actions

Diuretics work by altering the excretion or reabsorption of electrolytes (sodium and chloride) in the kidney. In turn, this determines the amount of water that becomes urine and is eliminated in the genitourinary system. Refer to the illustration of the kidney nephron (Fig. 33.1) for a better understanding of the actions as you read about the diuretics.

- *Loop diuretics* inhibit reabsorption of sodium and chloride in the distal and proximal tubules of the kidney and in the loop of Henle. Acting at three sites increases their effectiveness as diuretics.
- *Thiazide and related diuretics* inhibit the reabsorption of sodium and chloride ions in the ascending portion of the loop of Henle and the early distal tubule of the nephron. This action results in the excretion of sodium, chloride, and water.

Both of these types of diuretics will also cause the electrolyte potassium to be excreted in urine. If there is an issue of maintaining potassium in the body, another type of diuretic may be used.

- *Potassium-sparing diuretics* (or potassium saving) reduce the excretion of potassium from the kidney. Potassium-sparing diuretics work by blocking the reabsorption of sodium in the kidney tubules, thereby increasing sodium and water in the urine; this reduces the excretion of potassium. Spironolactone (Aldactone) works to antagonize the action of aldosterone. Aldosterone, a hormone produced by the adrenal cortex, enhances the reabsorption of sodium in the distal convoluted tubules of the kidney. When this is blocked by the drug, sodium (but not potassium) and water are excreted.
- *Osmotic diuretics* increase the density of the filtrate in the glomerulus. This prevents selective reabsorption of water, and it passes out as urine. Sodium and chloride excretion is also increased.
- *Carbonic anhydrase inhibitors* are sulfonamides, without bacteriostatic action, that inhibit the enzyme carbonic anhydrase. Carbonic anhydrase inhibition results in the excretion of sodium, potassium, bicarbonate, and water.

Uses

Diuretic drugs are used in the treatment of the following:

- Edema (fluid retention) associated with HF, corticosteroid/estrogen therapy, and cirrhosis of the liver
- Hypertension
- Renal disease (acute failure, renal insufficiency, and nephrotic syndrome)
- Cerebral edema
- Acute glaucoma (topically) and increased intraocular pressure (IOP; before and after eye surgery)
- Seizures and altitude sickness

Ethacrynic acid (a loop diuretic) is also used for the short-term management of ascites caused by a malignancy, idiopathic edema, or lymphedema. When patients are at risk for potassium loss, the potassium-sparing diuretics may be used with or in place of other categories of diuretics.

Adverse Reactions

Adverse reactions associated with any category of diuretics involve various body systems.

Neuromuscular System Reactions

- Dizziness, lightheadedness, headache
- Weakness, fatigue

Cardiovascular System Reactions

- Orthostatic hypotension
- Electrolyte imbalances, glycosuria

Gastrointestinal System Reactions

- Anorexia
- Nausea, vomiting

Other System Reactions

Dermatologic reactions include rash and photosensitivity. Extremity paresthesias (numbness or tingling) or flaccid muscles may indicate **hypokalemia** (low blood potassium). **Hyperkalemia** (an increase in potassium in the blood), a serious event, may occur with the administration of potassium-sparing diuretics. Hyperkalemia is most likely to occur in patients with an inadequate fluid intake and urine output, those with diabetes or renal disease, older adults, and those who are severely ill.

In male patients taking spironolactone, **gynecomastia** (breast enlargement) may occur. This reaction appears to be related to both dosage and duration of therapy. The gynecomastia is usually reversible when therapy is discontinued, but in rare instances some breast enlargement may remain.

Additional adverse reactions of these drugs are listed in the Summary Drug Table: Diuretics. When a potassium-sparing diuretic and another diuretic are given together, the adverse reactions associated with both drugs may be greater.

Contraindications

Diuretics are contraindicated in patients with known hypersensitivity to the drugs, electrolyte imbalances, severe kidney or liver dysfunction, and **anuria** (cessation of urine production). Mannitol (an osmotic diuretic) is contraindicated in patients with active intracranial bleeding (except during craniotomy). The potassium-sparing diuretics are contraindicated in patients with hyperkalemia and are not recommended for pediatric patients.

Precautions

Diuretics are used cautiously in patients with renal dysfunction. Most of the diuretics are pregnancy category C drugs (although ethacrynic acid, torsemide, isosorbide, amiloride, and triamterene are in pregnancy category B) and must be used cautiously during pregnancy and lactation. All of the thiazide diuretics are pregnancy category B drugs, with the exception of benzthiazide and methyclothiazide, which are pregnancy category C drugs. The safety of these drugs for use during pregnancy and lactation has not been established, so they should be used only when the drug is clearly needed and when the potential benefits to the patient outweigh the potential hazards to the fetus.

The thiazide and loop diuretics are used cautiously in patients with liver disease, diabetes, systemic lupus erythematosus (may exacerbate or activate the disease), or diarrhea. A cross-sensitivity reaction may occur with the thiazides and sulfonamides. Some of the thiazide diuretics contain tartrazine (a yellow food dye), which may cause allergic-type reactions or bronchial asthma in individuals sensitive to tartrazine. Patients with sensitivity to sulfonamides may show allergic reactions to loop diuretics (furosemide, torsemide, or bumetanide). The potassium-sparing diuretics should be used cautiously in patients with liver disease, diabetes, or gout.

Interactions

All the diuretics may cause an increased risk of hypotension when taken with antihypertensive drugs. The interactions for specific diuretic categories are listed here.

Interacting Drug	Common Use	Effect of Interaction
Carbonic Anhydrase Inhibitors		
primidone	Treatment of seizure activity	Decreased effectiveness
Loop Diuretics		
cisplatin, aminoglycosides	Cancer treatment, anti-infective, respectively	Increased risk of ototoxicity
anticoagulants or thrombolytics	Blood thinner	Increased risk of bleeding
digitalis	Cardiac problems	Increased risk of arrhythmias
lithium	Psychotic symptoms	Increased risk of lithium toxicity
hydantoins	Treatment of seizure activity	Decreased diuretic effectiveness
nonsteroidal anti-inflammatory drugs (NSAIDs) and salicylates	Pain relief	Decreased diuretic effectiveness
Potassium-Sparing Diuretics		
angiotensin-converting enzyme inhibitors or potassium supplements	Cardiovascular problems	Increased risk of hyperkalemia
NSAIDs and salicylates; anticoagulants	Pain relief and blood thinner, respectively	Decreased diuretic effectiveness
Thiazides and Related Diuretics		
allopurinol	Treatment of gout	Increased risk of hypersensitivity to allopurinol
anesthetics	Surgical anesthesia	Increased anesthetic effectiveness
antineoplastic drugs	Cancer treatment	Extended leukopenia
antidiabetic drugs	Control of diabetes	Hyperglycemia

HERBAL CONSIDERATIONS

Numerous herbal diuretics are available as over-the-counter (OTC) products. Most plant and herbal extracts available as OTC diuretics are nontoxic. The following herbals are believed to possess diuretic activity: celery, chicory, sassafras, juniper berries, St. John's wort, foxglove, horsetail, licorice, dandelion, digitalis purpurea, ephedra, hibiscus, parsley, and elderberry. However, most are either ineffective or no more effective than caffeine. There is very little scientific evidence to justify the use of these plants as diuretics. For example, dandelion root was once believed to be a strong diuretic. However, research has found dandelion root to be safe but ineffective as a diuretic. No herbal diuretic should be taken without discussing with your primary health care provider. Diuretic teas such as juniper berries and shave grass or horsetail are contraindicated. Juniper berries have been associated with renal damage, and horsetail contains severely toxic compounds. Teas with ephedrine should be avoided, especially by individuals with hypertension (DerMarderosian, 2003).

NURSING PROCESS
PATIENT RECEIVING A DIURETIC

ASSESSMENT

Preadministration Assessment
Before administering a diuretic, taking vital signs and measuring weight gives you baseline information to compare fluid loss. Laboratory results such as serum electrolytes are carefully reviewed. Patients with renal dysfunction should have blood urea nitrogen (BUN) and creatinine clearance levels monitored as well. If the patient has peripheral edema, inspect and measure the involved areas and document in the patient's chart the degree and extent of edema.

If the patient is to receive an osmotic diuretic, the focus of the assessment is on the patient's disease or disorder and the symptoms being treated. For example, if the patient has a low urinary output and the osmotic diuretic is given to increase urinary output, review the ratio between intake and output, and symptoms that the patient is experiencing.

Ongoing Assessment
The type of assessment depends on such factors as the reason for the administration of the diuretic, the type of diuretic administered, the route of administration, and the condition of the patient. When the patient is institutionalized, measure and record fluid intake and output and report to the primary health care provider any marked decrease in the output. Report fluid loss as measured by weighing the patient at the same time daily, making certain that the patient is wearing the same amount or type of clothing. Depending on the specific diuretic, frequent serum electrolyte, uric acid, and liver and kidney function tests may be performed during the first few months of therapy and periodically thereafter. When patients take diuretics on an outpatient basis, it is your responsibility to instruct patients or caregivers to do the same activities at home.

NURSING DIAGNOSES
Drug-specific nursing diagnoses include the following:

- **Impaired Urinary Elimination** related to action of the diuretics causing increased frequency
- **Risk for Deficient Fluid Volume** related to excessive diuresis secondary to administration of a diuretic
- **Risk for Injury** related to lightheadedness, dizziness, or cardiac arrhythmias

Nursing diagnoses related to drug administration are discussed in Chapter 4.

PLANNING
The expected outcomes for the patient depend on the reason for administration of the diuretic but may include an optimal response to drug therapy, support of patient needs related to adverse drug reactions, and confidence in an understanding of the medication regimen.

IMPLEMENTATION

Promoting an Optimal Response to Therapy
Diuretics are used to treat many different types of conditions. Therefore, promoting an optimal response to therapy for patients taking diuretics often depends on the specific diuretic and the patient's condition.

PATIENT WITH EDEMA. Patients with edema caused by HF or other causes are weighed daily or as ordered by the primary health care provider. Weight loss of about 2 lb daily is desirable to maintain fluid loss and prevent dehydration and electrolyte imbalances. Every 8 hours carefully measure and document the fluid intake and output. The critically ill patient or the patient with renal disease may require more frequent measurements of urinary output. The blood pressure, pulse, and respiratory rate are assessed every 4 hours or as ordered by the primary health care provider. An acutely ill patient may require more frequent monitoring of the vital signs.

Areas of edema are examined daily to evaluate the effectiveness of drug therapy. Note the patient's general appearance and condition daily or more often if the patient is acutely ill.

PATIENT WITH HYPERTENSION. Teach the hypertensive patient how to monitor the blood pressure and pulse rate when receiving a diuretic or a diuretic along with an antihypertensive drug. Vital signs, including respiratory rate, are more frequently monitored when the patient is critically ill or the blood pressure excessively high.

PATIENT WITH INCREASED INTRACRANIAL PRESSURE. Mannitol is administered only by the intravenous (IV) route. Because mannitol solution may crystallize when exposed to low temperatures, inspect the solution before administration. If this happens, return the solution to the pharmacy and request another dose. The rate of administration and concentration of the drug is individualized to maintain a urine flow of at least 30 to 50 mL/hour.

When a patient is receiving the osmotic diuretic mannitol or urea for treatment of increased intracranial pressure caused by cerebral edema, perform neurologic assessments (response of the pupils to light, level of consciousness, or response to a painful stimulus) in addition to vital signs at the time intervals ordered by the primary health care provider.

PATIENT WITH RENAL COMPROMISE. When thiazide diuretics are administered, renal function should be monitored periodically. These drugs may cause azotemia (accumulation of nitrogenous waste in the blood). If nonprotein nitrogen (NPN) or BUN increases, the primary health care provider may consider withholding the drug or discontinuing its use. In addition, serum uric acid concentrations are monitored periodically during treatment with thiazide diuretics, because these drugs may cause an acute attack of gout; therefore, be alert to patient complaints of joint pain or discomfort. Insulin or oral antidiabetic drug dosages may require alterations due to hyperglycemia; therefore, serum glucose concentrations are monitored periodically.

PATIENT AT RISK FOR ELECTROLYTE IMBALANCES. As fluids and electrolytes shift in the body, be alert for imbalances. Signs and symptoms of common imbalances are listed in Display 33.1. One of the primary imbalances to monitor is potassium. Patients who experience cardiac arrhythmias or who are being "digitalized" (initiating digoxin therapy) may be more susceptible to significant potassium loss when taking diuretics. The potassium-sparing diuretics are recommended for these patients.

Display 33.1 Signs and Symptoms of Common Fluid and Electrolyte Imbalances Associated With Diuretic Therapy

Dehydration (Excessive Water Loss)
- Thirst
- Poor skin turgor
- Dry mucous membranes
- Weakness
- Dizziness
- Fever
- Low urine output

Hyponatremia (Excessive Loss of Sodium)
Note: Sodium—normal laboratory values 132–145 mEq/L

- Cold, clammy skin
- Decreased skin turgor
- Confusion
- Hypotension
- Irritability
- Tachycardia

Hypomagnesemia (Low Levels of Magnesium)
Note: Magnesium—normal laboratory values 1.5–2.5 mEq/L or 1.8–3 mg/dL

- Leg and foot cramps
- Hypertension
- Tachycardia
- Neuromuscular irritability
- Tremor
- Hyperactive deep tendon reflexes
- Confusion
- Visual or auditory hallucinations
- Paresthesias

Hypokalemia (Low Blood Potassium)
Note: Potassium—normal laboratory values 3.5–5 mEq/L

- Anorexia
- Nausea
- Vomiting
- Depression
- Confusion
- Cardiac arrhythmias
- Impaired thought processes
- Drowsiness

Hyperkalemia (High Blood Potassium)
- Irritability
- Anxiety
- Confusion
- Nausea
- Diarrhea
- Cardiac arrhythmias
- Abdominal distress

NURSING ALERT

Symptoms of hyperkalemia include paresthesia (numbness, tingling, or prickling sensation), muscular weakness, fatigue, flaccid paralysis of the extremities, bradycardia, shock, and electrocardiographic abnormalities.

Monitor patients taking potassium-sparing diuretics, because they are at risk for *hyperkalemia*. If the serum potassium levels exceed 5.3 mEq/mL, the diuretic is stopped and the primary health care provider is notified immediately. Treatment to reduce the potassium can include administration of IV bicarbonate (if the patient is acidotic) or oral or parenteral glucose with rapid-acting insulin. Persistent hyperkalemia may require dialysis. Serum potassium levels are monitored frequently, particularly during initial treatment.

Monitoring and Managing Patient Needs
IMPAIRED URINARY ELIMINATION. Because many of the conditions treated are cardiac in nature, explain to the patient how eliminating fluids helps the heart and blood vessels work more efficiently. The patient should understand how quickly some of these drugs work and cause increased urination. Before a diuretic is given, explain to the patient when diuresis may be expected to occur, and how long diuresis will last (Table 33.1). These drugs are taken early in the day to prevent any nighttime sleep disturbance caused by increased urination.

Table 33.1 Examples of Onset and Duration of Activity of Diuretics

Drug	Onset	Duration of Activity
acetazolamide tablets	1–1.5 hr	8–12 hr
sustained-release capsules	2 hr	18–24 hr
IV route	2 min	4–5 hr
amiloride	2 hr	24 hr
bumetanide oral	30–60 min	4–6 hr
IV route	Within a few minutes	Less than 1 hr
ethacrynic acid oral	Within 30 min	6–8 hr
IV route	Within 5 min	2 hr
furosemide oral	Within 1 hr	6–8 hr
IV route	Within 5 min	2 hr
mannitol (IV route)	30–60 min	6–8 hr
spironolactone	24–48 hr	48–72 hr
thiazides and related diuretics	1–2 hr	Varies*
triamterene	2–4 hr	12–16 hr
urea (IV route)	30–45 min	5–6 hr

*Duration varies with drug used. Average duration is 12–24 hours. Indapamide has a duration of more than 24 hours.

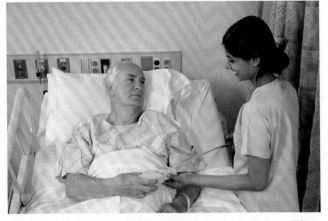

Figure 33.2 Reduce fear of incontinence by providing urinals or bedpans or answering call lights promptly for patients taking diuretics.

Some patients may become worried or anxious related to the fact that it will be necessary to urinate at frequent intervals and they may experience incontinence (Fig. 33.2). Reassure the patient on bed rest with prompt responses to a call light and, when necessary, have a bedpan or urinal within easy reach. Teach the patient using the drug at home to take it early in the day so nighttime sleep will not be interrupted. Although the duration of activity of most diuretics is about 8 hours or less, some diuretics have a longer activity, which may result in a need to urinate during nighttime hours. This is especially true early in therapy.

RISK FOR DEFICIENT FLUID VOLUME. The most common adverse reaction associated with the administration of a diuretic is the loss of fluid and electrolytes (see Display 33.1), especially during initial therapy with the drug. In some patients, the diuretic effect is moderate, whereas in others a large volume of fluid is lost. Regardless of the amount of fluid lost, there is always the possibility of excessive electrolyte loss, which is potentially serious.

The most common imbalances are a loss of potassium and water. Other electrolytes, particularly magnesium, sodium, and chloride, are also lost. When too much potassium is lost, hypokalemia occurs (see Patient Teaching for Improved Patient Outcomes: Preventing Potassium Imbalances). In certain patients, such as those also receiving a digitalis glycoside or those who currently have a cardiac arrhythmia, hypokalemia has the potential to create a more serious arrhythmia.

Hypokalemia is treated with potassium supplements or foods with high potassium content or by changing the diuretic to a potassium-sparing diuretic. In addition to hypokalemia, patients taking the loop diuretics are prone to magnesium deficiency (see Display 33.1). Whether a fluid or electrolyte imbalance occurs depends on the amount of fluid and electrolytes lost and the ability of the individual to replace them. For example, if a patient receiving a diuretic eats poorly and does not drink extra fluids, an electrolyte and water imbalance is likely to occur. However, preventive treatment is not always a guarantee; even when a patient drinks adequate amounts of fluid and eats a balanced diet, an electrolyte imbalance may still occur and require electrolyte

Patient Teaching for Improved Patient Outcomes

Preventing Potassium Imbalances

Diuretics increase the excretion of water and sodium. Some of these drugs also increase the excretion of potassium, which places the patient at risk for *hypokalemia,* a possibly life-threatening condition. Patients can reduce their risk of hypokalemia by eating foods rich in potassium, which will replace the loss caused by the diuretic.

When you teach, make sure your patient understands the following:

Potassium can be replenished by diet; take supplements only when instructed to do so by your primary health care provider. The following foods have higher levels of potassium than other foods:

✔ **Top 10 foods** with the highest amount of potassium per serving: white beans, dark leafy greens, baked potatoes with skin on, dried apricots, acorn squash, plain low-fat yogurt, salmon, avocado, mushrooms, bananas
✔ **Fruits (10 highest):** Apricots, prunes, dried currants/raisins, dates, figs, dried coconut, avocado, bananas, oranges, nectarines and peaches
✔ **Vegetables (10 highest):** Sun-dried tomatoes, spinach, Swiss chard, mushrooms, sweet potato, kale, brussels sprouts, zucchini, green beans, asparagus
✔ **Other sources:** Chocolate, molasses, nuts and nut butters
(http://www.healthaliciousness.com)

replacement (see Chapter 54 for additional discussion of fluid and electrolyte imbalances).

 LIFESPAN CONSIDERATIONS
Gerontology
Older adults are particularly prone to fluid volume deficit and electrolyte imbalances while taking diuretics. Dehydration can occur if the patient reduces fluid intake because of fear of incontinence.

Encourage oral fluids at frequent intervals during waking hours to prevent a fluid volume deficit. A balanced diet may help prevent electrolyte imbalances. Encourage potassium-rich snacks between meals and in the evening (when allowed). Monitor the fluid intake and output and notify the primary health care provider if the patient fails to drink an adequate amount of fluid, if the urinary output is low, if the urine appears concentrated, if the patient appears dehydrated, or if signs and symptoms of an electrolyte imbalance are apparent.

NURSING ALERT
Warning signs of a fluid and electrolyte imbalance include dry mouth, thirst, weakness, lethargy, drowsiness, restlessness, muscle pains or cramps, confusion, gastrointestinal (GI) disturbances, hypotension, oliguria, tachycardia, and seizures.

RISK FOR INJURY. Patients receiving a diuretic (particularly a loop or thiazide diuretic) and a digitalis glycoside concurrently require frequent monitoring of the pulse rate and rhythm because of the possibility of cardiac arrhythmias. Any significant changes in the pulse rate and rhythm are immediately reported to the primary health care provider.

Some patients experience dizziness or lightheadedness, especially during the first few days of therapy or when a rapid diuresis has occurred. Patients who are dizzy but who are allowed out of bed are assisted with ambulatory activities until these adverse drug effects disappear.

Educating the Patient and Family

The patient and the family may modify drug administration due to the excessive amount of urination or when the diuretic works at inappropriate times for patient activity. To ensure adherence to the prescribed drug regimen, be sure the patient is taking the drug correctly. Emphasize the importance of diuretic therapy in treating the patient's disorder. As you develop a teaching plan include the following information:

- Do not stop taking the drug or omit doses, except on the advice of a primary health care provider.

- If GI upset occurs, take the drug with food or milk.

- Take the drug early in the morning (once-a-day dosage) unless directed otherwise to minimize the effects on nighttime sleep. Twice-a-day dosing should be administered early in the morning (e.g., 7 a.m.) and early afternoon (e.g., 2 p.m.) or as directed by the primary health care provider.

- Do not reduce fluid intake to reduce the need to urinate. Be sure to continue the fluid intake recommended by the primary health care provider.

- Avoid alcohol and nonprescription drugs unless approved by the primary health care provider. Hypertensive patients should be careful to avoid medications that increase blood pressure, such as OTC drugs for appetite suppression and cold symptoms.

- Notify the primary health care provider if any of the following occur: muscle cramps or weakness, dizziness, nausea, vomiting, diarrhea, restlessness, excessive thirst, general weakness, rapid pulse, increased heart rate or pulse, or GI distress.

- If dizziness or weakness occurs, observe caution while driving or performing hazardous tasks, rise slowly from a sitting or lying position, and avoid standing in one place for an extended time.

- Weigh yourself weekly or as recommended by the primary health care provider. Keep a record of these weekly weights and contact the primary health care provider if weight loss exceeds 3 to 5 lb a week.

- If foods or fluids high in potassium are recommended by the primary health care provider, eat the amount recommended. Do not exceed this amount or eliminate these foods from the diet for more than 1 day, except when told to do so by the primary health care provider (see Patient Teaching for Improved Patient Outcomes: Preventing Potassium Imbalances).

- After a time, the diuretic effect of the drug may be minimal because most of the body's excess fluid has been removed. Continue therapy to prevent further accumulation of fluid.

- If taking thiazide or related diuretics, loop diuretics, potassium-sparing diuretics, carbonic anhydrase inhibitors, or triamterene, avoid exposure to sunlight or ultraviolet light (sunlamps, tanning beds), because exposure may cause exaggerated sunburn (a photosensitivity reaction). Wear sunscreen and protective clothing until tolerance is determined.

- For patients who have diabetes mellitus and who take loop or thiazide diuretics: Know that blood glucometer test results for glucose may be elevated. Contact the primary health care provider if home-tested blood glucose levels increase.

- For patients who take potassium-sparing diuretics: Avoid eating foods high in potassium and avoid the use of salt substitutes containing potassium. Read food labels carefully. Do not use a salt substitute unless a particular brand has been approved by the primary health care provider. Also avoid the use of potassium supplements. Male patients who take spironolactone may experience gynecomastia. This is usually reversible when therapy is discontinued.

- For patients who take thiazide diuretics: These agents may cause gout attacks. Contact the primary health care provider if significant, sudden joint pain occurs.

- For patients who take carbonic anhydrase inhibitors: During treatment for glaucoma, contact the primary health care provider immediately if eye pain is not relieved or if it increases. When a patient with epilepsy is being treated for seizures, a family member of the patient should keep a record of all seizures witnessed and bring this to the primary health care provider at the time of the next visit. Contact the primary health care provider immediately if the number of seizures increases.

EVALUATION

- Therapeutic effect is achieved and diuresis occurs.

- Adverse reactions are identified, reported to the primary health care provider, and managed successfully through appropriate nursing interventions.
  - Urinary elimination occurs without incident.
  - Fluid volume problems are corrected.
  - No injury is evident.

- Patient and family express confidence and demonstrate an understanding of the drug regimen.

PHARMACOLOGY IN PRACTICE
THINK CRITICALLY

 When you question Mrs. Moore, she tells you the water pills just don't do the job, and she needs to go out of the house too frequently to take them on a regular basis. Based on your understanding of diuretic medications, why do you think Mrs. Moore has decided not to take the medications as prescribed?

KEY POINTS

- Excessive fluid is involved in many conditions such as HF, endocrine disturbances, and kidney and liver diseases. Pressure of fluid in the blood vessels contributes to hypertension. Diuretics are drugs that reduce body fluid by increasing production of urine by altering the excretion or reabsorption of electrolytes in the kidney.

- Loop, thiazide, and potassium-sparing diuretics are used to treat the HF, endocrine disturbances, and kidney and liver diseases. Osmotic and carbonic anhydrase inhibitors are used in the treatment of cerebral edema and seizures, intraocular pressure, and altitude sickness.

- Fluid loss is monitored by vital signs and weight reduction as well as measured intake and output. Some people may be reluctant to take diuretics for fear of incontinence. Others may reduce fluid intake for the same reason. Dehydration and electrolyte imbalances are more likely to occur when patients engage in these behaviors.

- Common adverse reactions to the medications include dizziness, headache, weakness, anorexia, nausea, and vomiting. Rashes and photosensitivity may occur with sun exposure. Again, patients should be monitored for electrolyte imbalances to reduce these adverse reactions.

Summary Drug Table DIURETICS

Generic Name	Trade Name	Uses	Adverse Reactions	Dosage Ranges
Loop Diuretics				
bumetanide *byoo-met'-ah-nyde*		Edema due to HF, cirrhosis of the liver, renal disease, acute pulmonary edema	Electrolyte and hemato-logic imbalances, anorexia, nausea, vomiting, dizziness, rash, photo-sensitivity, orthostatic hypotension, glycosuria	0.5–10 mg/day orally, IV, IM
ethacrynic acid *eth-ah-krye'-nik*	Edecrin	Same as bumetanide plus ascites due to malignancy, idiopathic edema, lymphedema	Same as bumetanide, plus diarrhea	50–200 mg/day orally, IV
furosemide *fur-oh-seh-myde*	Lasix	Same as bumetanide plus hypertension	Same as bumetanide	Edema: 20–80 mg/day, may go up to 600 mg/day for severe edema; Hypertension: 40 mg orally BID HF/renal failure: up to 2.5 g/day
torsemide *tor-she-myde*	Demadex	Same as bumetanide plus hypertension	Same as bumetanide plus headache	HF/renal failure: 10–20 mg/day orally, IV Cirrhosis/hypertension: 5–10 mg/day orally, IV
Potassium-Sparing Diuretics				
amiloride *ah-mill'-oh-ryde*		HF, hypertension, preven-tion of hypokalemia in at-risk patients, polyuria prevention with lithium use	Headache, dizziness, nausea, anorexia, diar-rhea, vomiting, weakness, fatigue, rash, hypotension	5–20 mg/day orally
spironolactone *speer-on-oh-lak-tone*	Aldactone	Hypertension, edema due to HF, cirrhosis, renal disease; hypokalemia, prophylaxis of hypokale-mia in at-risk patients, hyperaldosteronism	Headache, diarrhea, drowsiness, lethargy, hyperkalemia, cramping, gastritis, erectile dysfunc-tion, gynecomastia	Up to 400 mg/day orally in single dose or divided doses
triamterene *trye-am'-ter-een*	Dyrenium	Prevention of hypokale-mia, edema due to HF, cirrhosis, renal disease, hyperaldosteronism	Diarrhea, nausea, vomiting, hyperkalemia, photosensitivity	Up to 300 mg/day orally in divided doses

Summary Drug Table DIURETICS (continued)

Generic Name	Trade Name	Uses	Adverse Reactions	Dosage Ranges
Thiazides and Related Diuretics				
chlorothiazide *klor-oh-thye'-ah-zyde*	Diuril	Hypertension, edema due to HF, cirrhosis, corticosteroid and estrogen therapy	Orthostatic hypotension, dizziness, vertigo, lightheadedness, weakness, anorexia, gastric distress, nausea, diarrhea, constipation, hematologic changes, rash, photosensitivity reactions, hyperglycemia, fluid and electrolyte imbalances, reduced libido	0.5–2 g orally or IV, QID or BID
chlorthalidone *klor-thal'-ih-doan*	Thalitone	Same as chlorothiazide	Same as chlorothiazide	Edema: 50–120 mg/day orally Hypertension: 25–100 mg/day orally
hydrochlorothiazide *hye-droe-klor-oh-thye'-ah-zyde*	Microzide, Oretic	Same as chlorothiazide	Same as chlorothiazide	Edema: 25–200 mg/day orally Hypertension: 12.5–50 mg/day orally
indapamide *in-dap'-ah-myde*		Hypertension, edema due to HF	Same as chlorothiazide	Edema: 2.5–5 mg/day orally Hypertension: 1.25–5 mg/day orally
metolazone *meh-toll'-ah-zoan*	Zaroxolyn	Edema in HF, cirrhosis, corticosteroids, estrogen therapy, renal dysfunction	Same as chlorothiazide	2.5–20 mg/day orally
methyclothiazide *meth-ih-kloe-thye'-ah-zyde*		Same as chlorothiazide	Same as chlorothiazide	Edema: 2.5–10 mg/day orally Hypertension: 2.5–5 mg/day orally
Carbonic Anhydrase Inhibitors				
acetazolamide *ah-set-ah-zoll'-ah-myde*	Diamox	Open-angle glaucoma, secondary glaucoma, preoperatively to lower IOP, edema due to HF, drug-induced edema, centrencephalic epilepsy	Weakness, fatigue, anorexia, nausea, vomiting, rash, paresthesias, photosensitivity	Glaucoma: up to 1 g/day orally in divided doses Acute glaucoma: 500 mg initially then 125–250 mg orally q 4 hr Epilepsy: 8–30 mg/kg/day in divided doses HF and edema: 250–375 mg/day orally
methazolamide *meth-ah-zoll'-ah-myde*		Glaucoma	Same as acetazolamide	50–100 mg orally BID, TID
Osmotic Diuretics				
glycerin (glycerol) *glíh-ser-in*		Glaucoma, before and after surgery	Headache, nausea, vomiting	1–2 g/kg orally in solution
isosorbide *eye-soe-sor-byde*		Same as glycerin	Same as glycerin	1–3 mg/kg orally, BID–QID
mannitol *man-ih-toll*	Osmitrol	To promote diuresis in acute renal failure, reduction of IOP, treatment of cerebral edema, irrigation solution in prostate surgical procedures	Edema, fluid and electrolyte imbalance, headache, blurred vision, nausea, vomiting, diarrhea, urinary retention	Diuresis: 50–200 g/24 hr IV IOP: 1.5–2 g/kg IV
urea *yoor-ee'-ah*		Reduction of IOP, reduction of intracranial pressure	Headache, nausea, vomiting, fluid and electrolyte imbalance, syncope	Up to 120 g/day IV

● Chapter Review

Know Your Drugs

Clients sometimes know a medication by the brand (or trade) name and not the generic name. To help you recognize both names, match the brand name with the generic name of the same medication.

Generic Name	Brand Name
1. acetazolamide	A. Aldactone
2. furosemide	B. Diamox
3. metolazone	C. Lasix
4. spironolactone	D. Zaroxolyn

Calculate Medication Dosages

1. The primary health care provider prescribes spironolactone (Aldactone) 100 mg orally. The drug is available in 50-mg tablets. The nurse administers _____.

2. Furosemide (Lasix) 20 mg oral solution is prescribed. The oral solution is available in a concentration of 40 mg/5 mL. The nurse administers into the nasogastric tube _____.

● Prepare for the NCLEX®

Build Your Knowledge

1. The best description of how diuretic medications work is that they:
   1. promote retention of fluid in the kidney
   2. achieve acid balance in the lungs
   3. increase the removal of potassium from the blood
   4. inhibit reabsorption of sodium in the nephron

2. When ordered two times daily, the best schedule for taking furosemide would be _____.
   1. 9 a.m. and 9 p.m.
   2. 7 a.m. and 9 a.m.
   3. 6 a.m. and 7 p.m.
   4. 8 a.m. and 2 p.m.

3. When evaluating the effectiveness of chlorothiazide, the nurse questions the client about _____.
   1. number of times voiding
   2. relief of eye pain
   3. amount of fluids drank
   4. daily weight

4. When administering spironolactone (Aldactone), the nurse monitors the client for which of the following electrolyte imbalances?
   1. hypernatremia
   2. hyponatremia
   3. hyperkalemia
   4. hypokalemia

5. Which electrolyte imbalance would the patient receiving a loop or thiazide diuretic most likely develop?
   1. hypernatremia
   2. hyponatremia
   3. hyperkalemia
   4. hypokalemia

Apply Your Knowledge

6. The nurse is seeing a client in the clinic 1 week after the client began taking a diuretic. Which finding would make you suspect that the client is not taking the diuretic?
   1. serum potassium of 3.0 mEq/mL
   2. urine output of 200 mL for the last 2 hours
   3. blood pressure of 130/90 mm Hg
   4. weight gain of 4 lb since last week

7. When a client is given mannitol for increased intracranial pressure, which of the following findings would be most important for the nurse to report?
   1. serum potassium of 3.5 mEq/mL
   2. urine output of 20 mL for the last 2 hours
   3. blood pressure of 140/80 mm Hg
   4. heart rate of 72 bpm

8. When a diuretic is being administered for HF, which of the following would be most indicative of an effective response to diuretic therapy?
   1. output of 30 mL/hour
   2. daily weight loss of 2 lb
   3. increase in blood pressure
   4. increasing edema of the lower extremities

Alternate-Format Questions

9. Which of the following foods would the nurse most likely recommend the client include in the daily diet to prevent hypokalemia? **Select all that apply**.
   1. potatoes
   2. apricots
   3. bananas
   4. corn

10. Match the diuretic with its use:

1. Reduce cerebral edema	A. acetazolamide
2. Reduce hypertension	B. Lasix
3. Remove fluid, spare potassium	C. mannitol
4. Treat altitude sickness	D. spironolactone
	E. Zaroxolyn

To check your answers, see Appendix G.

the**Point** *For more NCLEX-style questions, log on to http://thepoint.lww.com to access more than 1000 questions.*

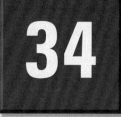

Antihyperlipidemic Drugs

LEARNING OBJECTIVES

On completion of this chapter, the student will:

1. Define cholesterol, high-density lipoprotein (HDL), low-density lipoprotein (LDL), and triglyceride levels and how they contribute to the development of heart disease.
2. Define therapeutic life changes and how they affect cholesterol levels.
3. Discuss the uses, general drug actions, general adverse reactions, contraindications, precautions, and interactions of antihyperlipidemic drugs.
4. Discuss important preadministration and ongoing assessment activities the nurse should perform on the patient taking an antihyperlipidemic drug.
5. List nursing diagnoses particular to a patient taking an antihyperlipidemic drug.
6. Discuss ways to promote an optimal response to therapy, how to manage common adverse reactions, and important points to keep in mind when educating patients about the use of antihyperlipidemic drugs.

KEY TERMS

atherosclerosis • disease characterized by deposits of fatty plaques on the inner walls of arteries

catalyst • substance that accelerates a chemical reaction without itself undergoing a change

cholecystitis • inflammation of the gallbladder

cholelithiasis • stones in the gallbladder

cholesterol • fat-like substance produced mostly in the liver of animals

high-density lipoproteins (HDLs) • macro (big) molecules that carry cholesterol from the body cells to the liver to be excreted

hyperlipidemia • increase in the lipids in the blood

lipids • group of fats or fat-like substances

lipoprotein • macromolecule consisting of lipid (fat) and protein; how fats are transported in the blood

low-density lipoproteins (LDLs) • macromolecules that carry cholesterol from the liver to the body cells

rhabdomyolysis • condition in which muscle damage results in the release of muscle cell contents into the bloodstream.

statins (HMG-CoA reductase inhibitors) • common name for drugs that inhibit the manufacture or promote breakdown of cholesterol

triglycerides • types of lipids that circulate in the blood

xanthomas • yellow deposits of cholesterol in tendons and soft tissues

DRUG CLASSES

HMG-CoA reductase inhibitors (statins)	Fibric acid derivatives
	Niacin
Bile acid resins	

PHARMACOLOGY IN PRACTICE

Lillian Chase is taking cholestyramine for hyperlipidemia. The primary health care provider has prescribed therapeutic life changes for the patient, who is on a low-fat diet and walks short distances daily for exercise. Her major complaint at this visit is constipation, which is very bothersome to her. She feels depressed and has started smoking again. She tells you the medicine isn't working and wants to stop taking it. As you read about medications in this chapter, think about Lillian's concerns.

Atherosclerosis is a disorder in which **lipid** (fat or fat-like substance) deposits accumulate on the lining of the blood vessels, eventually producing degenerative changes and obstructing blood flow. Atherosclerosis is considered to be a major contributor in the development of heart disease. **Cholesterol** and the **triglycerides** are the two lipids in our blood. Elevation of one or both of these lipids occurs in hyperlipidemia. **Hyperlipidemia** is an increase (*hyper*) in the lipids in the blood (*emia*). Serum cholesterol levels above 240 mg/dL and triglyceride levels above 150 mg/dL are associated with atherosclerosis.

Triglycerides and cholesterol are insoluble in water and must be bound to a lipid-containing protein (**lipoprotein**) for transportation throughout the body (Fig. 34.1). Although several lipoproteins are found in the blood, this chapter focuses on the low-density lipoproteins, the high-density lipoproteins (HDLs), and cholesterol.

Lipoproteins

Low-density lipoproteins (LDLs) transport cholesterol to the peripheral cells. When the cells have all the cholesterol they need, the excess cholesterol is discarded into the blood (see Fig. 34.1). This excess penetrates the walls of the arteries,

resulting in atherosclerotic plaque formation. Elevation of the LDL level increases the risk for heart disease. On the other hand, **high-density lipoproteins (HDLs)** take cholesterol from the peripheral cells and transport it to the liver, where it is metabolized and excreted; the higher the HDL level, the lower the risk for development of atherosclerosis. Therefore, it is desirable to see an increase in the HDL (the "good" lipoprotein) level, because of the protective nature of its properties against the development of atherosclerosis, and a decrease in the LDL level. A laboratory examination of blood lipids, called a *lipoprotein profile,* provides valuable information on the important cholesterol levels, such as:

- Total cholesterol
- LDL (the harmful lipoprotein)
- HDL (the protective lipoprotein)
- Triglycerides

Table 34.1 provides an analysis of cholesterol levels.

Cholesterol Levels

High-density lipoprotein cholesterol protects against heart disease, so the higher its numbers (i.e., blood level), the better. An HDL level less than 40 mg/dL is low and considered

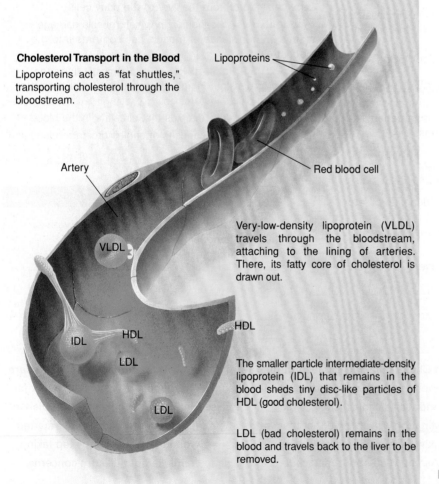

Cholesterol Transport in the Blood

Lipoproteins act as "fat shuttles," transporting cholesterol through the bloodstream.

Lipoproteins

Artery

Red blood cell

VLDL

Very-low-density lipoprotein (VLDL) travels through the bloodstream, attaching to the lining of arteries. There, its fatty core of cholesterol is drawn out.

HDL

IDL

HDL

LDL

The smaller particle intermediate-density lipoprotein (IDL) that remains in the blood sheds tiny disc-like particles of HDL (good cholesterol).

LDL

LDL (bad cholesterol) remains in the blood and travels back to the liver to be removed.

Figure 34.1 Cholesterol transport in the blood. (Courtesy of Anatomical Chart Co.)

Table 34.1 Cholesterol Level Analysis

Level	Category
Total Cholesterol*	
Less than 200 mg/dL	Desirable
200–239 mg/dL	Borderline
240 mg/dL and above	High
LDL Cholesterol*	
Less than 100 mg/dL	Optimal
100–129 mg/dL	Near optimal/above optimal
130–159 mg/dL	Borderline
160–189 mg/dL	High
190 mg/dL and above	Very high
HDL Cholesterol*	
Less than 40 mg/dL	Low
60 mg/dL and above	High

*Cholesterol levels are measured in milligrams (mg) of cholesterol per deciliter (dL) of blood.

a major risk factor for heart disease. Triglyceride levels that are borderline (150 to 190 mg/dL) or high (above 190 mg/dL) may need treatment in some individuals.

In general, the higher the LDL level and the more risk factors involved, the greater the risk for heart disease. Other risk factors, besides elevated cholesterol levels, that play a role in the development of *hyperlipidemia* are listed here. Uncontrollable risk factors include:

- Age (men older than 45 years and women older than 55 years)
- Gender (in women after menopause, LDL cholesterol levels increase)
- Family history of early heart disease (father/brother before age 55 years and mother/sister before age 65 years)

Those factors a person *can* control or modify include:

- Diet (saturated fat and cholesterol in food raise total and LDL cholesterol levels)
- Weight (overweight can make LDL cholesterol level go up and HDL level go down)
- Physical inactivity (increased physical activity helps to lower LDL cholesterol and raise HDL cholesterol levels)

The main goal of treatment in patients with hyperlipidemia is to lower the LDLs to a level that will reduce the risk of heart disease.

The primary health care provider may initially seek to control the cholesterol level by encouraging *therapeutic life changes* (TLCs). This includes a cholesterol-lowering diet (the TLC diet), physical activity, smoking cessation (if applicable), and weight management. The TLC diet is a low–saturated fat and low-cholesterol eating plan that includes less than 200 mg of dietary cholesterol per day. In addition, 30 minutes of physical activity each day is recommended for the TLC diet. Walking at a brisk pace for 30 minutes a day 5 to 7 days a week can help raise the HDL and lower the LDL levels.

Added benefits of a healthy diet and exercise program include a reduction of body weight. If TLCs do not result in bringing blood lipids to therapeutic levels, the primary health care provider may add one of the antihyperlipidemic drugs to the treatment plan. TLCs are continued along with the drug regimen.

In addition to control of the dietary intake of fat, particularly saturated fatty acids, antihyperlipidemic drug therapy is used to lower serum levels of cholesterol and triglycerides. The primary health care provider may use one drug or, in some instances, more than one antihyperlipidemic drug for those with poor response to therapy with a single drug. Three classes of antihyperlipidemic drugs are currently in use, as well as miscellaneous antihyperlipidemic drugs (see Summary Drug Table: Antihyperlipidemic Drugs for a complete listing of the drugs).

The target LDL level for treatment is less than 130 mg/dL. If the response to drug treatment is adequate, lipid levels are monitored every 4 months. If the response is inadequate, another drug or a combination of two drugs is used. Antihyperlipidemic drugs decrease cholesterol and triglyceride levels in several ways. Although the end result is a lower lipid blood level, each has a slightly different action.

HMG-COA REDUCTASE INHIBITORS

Actions

The antihyperlipidemic drugs, HMG-CoA reductase inhibitors, are typically referred to as **statins**. HMG-CoA (3-hydroxy-3-methylglutaryl coenzyme A) reductase is an enzyme that is a **catalyst** (a substance that accelerates a chemical reaction without itself undergoing a change) in the manufacture of cholesterol. These drugs appear to have one of two activities, namely, inhibiting the manufacture of cholesterol or promoting the breakdown of cholesterol. Either drug activity lowers the blood levels of cholesterol, LDLs, and serum triglycerides. Examples of these drugs can be found in the Summary Drug Table: Antihyperlipidemic Drugs.

Uses

Statin drugs, along with a diet restricted in saturated fat and cholesterol, are used for the following:

- Treatment of hyperlipidemia
- Primary prevention of coronary events (in patients with hyperlipidemia without clinically evident coronary heart disease to reduce the risk of myocardial infarction and death from other cardiovascular events, including strokes, transient ischemic attacks, and cardiac revascularization procedures)
- Secondary prevention of cardiovascular events (in patients with hyperlipidemia with evident coronary heart disease to reduce the risk of coronary death, slow the progression of coronary atherosclerosis, and reduce risk of death from stroke/transient ischemic attack; and in those undergoing myocardial revascularization procedures)

Adverse Reactions

The statins are usually well tolerated. Adverse reactions, when they do occur, are often mild and transient and do not require discontinuing therapy. These reactions may include the following.

Central Nervous System Reactions

• Headache
• Dizziness
• Insomnia
• Memory and cognitive impairment

Gastrointestinal System Reactions

• Flatulence, abdominal pain, cramping
• Constipation, nausea
• Hyperglycemia in nondiabetic patients

Contraindications and Precautions

The statins are contraindicated in individuals with hypersensitivity to the drugs or serious liver disorders, and during pregnancy (pregnancy category X) and lactation.

These drugs are used cautiously in patients with a history of alcoholism, non-alcohol-related liver disease, acute infection, hypotension, trauma, endocrine disorders, visual disturbances, and myopathy.

NURSING ALERT

The drug rosuvastatin in higher doses is linked to risks for serious muscle toxicity (myopathy/rhabdomyolysis) in certain populations. These include patients taking cyclosporine, Asian patients, and patients with severe renal insufficiency. A 5-mg dose is available as a starting dose for those individuals who do not require aggressive cholesterol reductions or who have predisposing factors for myopathy.

Interactions

The following interactions may occur when the statin drugs are administered with another agent:

Interacting Drug	Common Use	Effect of Interaction
macrolides, erythromycin, clarithromycin	Treatment of infections	Increased risk of severe myopathy or rhabdomyolysis
amiodarone	Cardiovascular problems	Increased risk of myopathy
niacin	Used to lower elevated cholesterol	Increased risk of severe myopathy or rhabdomyolysis
protease inhibitors	Treatment of human immunodeficiency virus (HIV) infection and acquired immunodeficiency syndrome (AIDS)	Elevated plasma levels of statins
verapamil	Treatment of cardiovascular problems and hypertension	Increased risk of myopathy
warfarin	Blood thinner (anticoagulant)	Increased anticoagulant effect

The statin drugs have an additive effect when used with the bile acid resins, which may provide an added benefit in treating

hypercholesterolemia that does not respond to a single-drug regimen. Due to a specific enzyme reaction, grapefruit or its juice should not be taken if the patient is on the following drugs: lovastatin or simvastatin.

HERBAL CONSIDERATIONS

Red yeast is a traditional Chinese medicine, currently sold as a supplement to lower cholesterol. It comes from an extract of fermented yeast (*Monascus purpureus*) grown on rice. Its use as an aid for gastric (indigestion, diarrhea, stomach, and spleen) ailments and blood circulation enhancement date back to 800 A.D. in China. It is also used as the red food coloring additive seen in Chinese meats and poultry dishes.

The red yeast naturally contains ingredients that help to control cholesterol levels; these include "healthy fats" and monacolin—the ingredient used in the drug lovastatin. Therefore, the supplement would have all the adverse reactions and drug interactions of the statin drugs. Taking this supplement with antihyperlipidemic drugs can cause serious reactions, notably liver or muscle damage (http://nccam.nih.gov/health/redyeastrice).

Patients may not volunteer information regarding their use of alternative or complementary remedies. You should always inquire about use of herbal products, especially niacin or red yeast purchased as a supplement. Be aware that a possible interaction with St. John's wort, used to relieve depression, causes a decrease in statin effectiveness.

BILE ACID RESINS

Actions

Bile, which is manufactured and secreted by the liver and stored in the gallbladder, emulsifies fat and lipids as these products pass through the intestine. Once emulsified, fats and lipids are readily absorbed in the intestine. The bile acid resins bind to bile acids to form an insoluble substance that cannot be absorbed by the intestine, so it is excreted in the feces. With increased loss of bile acids, the liver uses cholesterol to manufacture more bile. This is followed by a decrease in cholesterol levels.

Uses

The bile acid resins are used to treat the following:

• Hyperlipidemia (in patients who do not have an adequate response to a diet and exercise program)
• Pruritus associated with partial biliary obstruction (cholestyramine only)

Adverse Reactions

• Constipation (may be severe and occasionally result in fecal impaction), aggravation of hemorrhoids, abdominal cramps, flatulence, nausea
• Increased bleeding tendencies related to vitamin K malabsorption, and vitamin A and D deficiencies

Contraindications and Precautions

The bile acid resins are contraindicated in patients with known hypersensitivity to the drugs. Bile acid resins are also contraindicated in those with complete biliary obstruction.

These drugs are used cautiously in patients with liver and kidney disease; they are also used cautiously during pregnancy (pregnancy category C) and lactation (decreased absorption of vitamins may affect the infant).

Interactions

The following interactions may occur when the bile acid resins are administered with another agent:

Interacting Drug	Common Use	Effect of Interaction
anticoagulants	Blood thinners	Decreased effect of the anticoagulant (cholestyramine)
thyroid hormone	Treatment of hypothyroidism	Loss of efficacy of thyroid; also hypothyroidism (particularly with cholestyramine)
fat-soluble vitamins (A, D, E, K) and folic acid	Nutritional supplements	Reduced absorption of vitamins

When administered with the bile acid resins, a decreased serum level or decreased gastrointestinal (GI) absorption of the following drugs may occur:

- nonsteroidal anti-inflammatory drugs (NSAIDs; used to treat pain)
- penicillin G and tetracycline (used to treat infection)
- niacin (used to treat elevated cholesterol levels)
- digitalis glycosides (used to treat heart failure)
- furosemide and thiazide diuretics (used to treat edema)
- glipizide (used to treat diabetes)
- hydrocortisone (used to treat inflammation)
- methyldopa and propranolol (used to treat hypertension and cardiovascular problems, respectively)

Because the bile acids resins, particularly cholestyramine, can decrease the absorption of numerous drugs, the bile acid resins should be administered alone and other drugs given at least 1 hour before or 4 hours after administration of the bile acid resins.

FIBRIC ACID DERIVATIVES

Actions

Fibric acid derivatives, also known as fibrates, are the third group of antihyperlipidemic drugs and work in a variety of ways. Fenofibrate acts by reducing very-low-density lipoproteins (VLDLs) and stimulating the catabolism of triglyceride-rich lipoproteins, resulting in a decrease in plasma triglycerides and cholesterol. Gemfibrozil increases the excretion of cholesterol in the feces and reduces the production of triglycerides by the liver, thus lowering serum lipid levels.

Uses

Although the fibric acid derivatives have antihyperlipidemic effects, their use varies depending on the drug. For example, gemfibrozil is used to treat individuals with very high serum triglyceride levels who are at risk for abdominal pain and pancreatitis and who do not experience a response to dietary modifications. Fenofibrate is used as adjunctive treatment for reducing LDLs, total cholesterol, and triglycerides in patients with hyperlipidemia.

Adverse Reactions

The adverse reactions associated with fibric acid derivatives include the following:

- Nausea, vomiting, and GI upset
- Diarrhea
- **Cholelithiasis** (stones in the gallbladder) or **cholecystitis** (inflammation of the gallbladder)

If cholelithiasis is found, the primary health care provider may discontinue the drug. See the Summary Drug Table: Antihyperlipidemic Drugs for additional adverse reactions.

Contraindications and Precautions

The fibric acid derivatives are contraindicated in patients with hypersensitivity to the drugs and in those with significant hepatic or renal dysfunction or primary biliary cirrhosis because these drugs may increase the already elevated cholesterol. The drugs are used cautiously during pregnancy (pregnancy category C) and not during lactation or in patients with peptic ulcer disease or diabetes.

Interactions

The following interactions may occur when the fibric acid derivatives are administered with another agent:

Interacting Drug	Common Use	Effect of Interaction
anticoagulants	Blood thinners	Enhanced effects of the anticoagulants
cyclosporine	Immunosuppression after organ transplantation	Decreased effects of cyclosporine (particularly with gemfibrozil)
HMG-CoA reductase inhibitors (statins)	Treatment of elevated blood cholesterol levels	Increased risk of rhabdomyolysis
sulfonylureas	Treatment of diabetes	Increased hypoglycemic effects (particularly with gemfibrozil)

MISCELLANEOUS ANTIHYPERLIPIDEMIC DRUGS

Miscellaneous antihyperlipidemic drugs include niacin and ezetimibe. Refer to the Summary Drug Table: Antihyperlipidemic Drugs for information on combinations of more than one class of antihyperlipidemic drugs in one tablet.

Actions

The mechanism by which niacin (nicotinic acid) lowers blood lipid levels is not fully understood. Ezetimibe inhibits the absorption of cholesterol in the small intestine, leading to a decrease in cholesterol in the liver.

Uses

Niacin is used as adjunctive therapy for lowering very high serum triglyceride levels in patients who are at risk for pancreatitis (inflammation of the pancreas) and whose response to dietary control is inadequate. Ezetimibe is typically used in combinations with other antihyperlipidemics in lipid-lowering treatments.

Adverse Reactions

Gastrointestinal System Reactions

• Nausea, vomiting, abdominal pain
• Diarrhea

Other Reactions

• Severe, generalized flushing of the skin; sensation of warmth
• Severe itching or tingling

Contraindications, Precautions, and Interactions

Niacin is contraindicated in patients with known hypersensitivity to niacin, active peptic ulcer, hepatic dysfunction, and arterial bleeding. The drug is used cautiously in patients with renal dysfunction, high alcohol consumption, unstable angina, gout, and pregnancy (pregnancy category C). Pregnant and lactating women should not use ezetimibe.

HERBAL CONSIDERATIONS

Garlic has been used for many years throughout the world. The benefits of garlic on cardiovascular health are the best-known and most extensively researched benefits of the herb. Its benefits include lowering serum cholesterol and triglyceride levels, improving the ratio of HDL to LDL cholesterol, lowering blood pressure, and helping to prevent the development of atherosclerosis. The recommended dosages of garlic are 600 to 900 mg/day of the garlic powder tablets, 10 mg of garlic oil "perles," or one moderate-sized fresh clove of garlic a day. Adverse reactions include mild stomach upset or irritation that can usually be alleviated by taking garlic supplements with food. There is an increased risk of bleeding when garlic is taken with warfarin. Although no serious reactions have occurred in pregnant women taking garlic, its use is not recommended. Garlic is excreted in breast milk and may cause colic in some infants. As with all herbal therapy, when garlic is used for therapeutic purposes, the primary health care provider should be aware of its use (DerMarderosian, 2003).

NURSING PROCESS

PATIENT RECEIVING AN ANTIHYPERLIPIDEMIC DRUG

ASSESSMENT

Preadministration Assessment

Many individuals with hyperlipidemia have no symptoms, and the disorder is not discovered until laboratory tests reveal elevated cholesterol and triglyceride levels, elevated LDL levels, and decreased HDL levels. Often, these drugs are initially prescribed on an outpatient basis, but initial administration may occur in the hospitalized patient. Serum cholesterol levels (i.e., a lipid profile) and liver functions tests (LFTs) are obtained before the drugs are administered.

During the initial assessment, record a dietary history, focusing on the types of foods normally included in the diet. Vital signs and weight are recorded. The skin and eyelids are inspected for evidence of xanthomas (flat or elevated yellowish deposits) that may be seen in the more severe forms of hyperlipidemia.

Ongoing Assessment

Patients usually take antihyperlipidemic drugs on an outpatient basis and come to the clinic or the primary health care provider's office for periodic monitoring. The primary health care provider usually prescribes frequent monitoring of blood cholesterol and triglyceride levels as a part of the ongoing assessment. Liver monitoring should occur when doses are changed or if the patient shows signs or symptoms of liver disease (jaundice, nausea, or abdominal pain). One of the

best measurements for statin-caused liver compromise is fractionated (indirect) bilirubin levels. Your responsibility is to monitor these levels and report any increase to the primary health care provider. If aspartate aminotransferase (AST) levels increase to three times normal, the primary health care provider may discontinue drug therapy. Because the maximum effects of these drugs are usually evident within 4 weeks, periodic lipid profiles are ordered to determine the therapeutic effect of the drug regimen. The dose may be increased, another antihyperlipidemic drug added, or drug therapy discontinued, depending on the patient's response.

NURSING ALERT

Sometimes a paradoxical elevation of blood lipid levels occurs. Should this happen, bring this to the attention of the primary health care provider because he or she may prescribe a different antihyperlipidemic drug.

During the ongoing assessment, check vital signs and assess bowel functioning because an adverse reaction to these drugs is constipation. Constipation may become serious if not treated early in the medication regimen.

NURSING DIAGNOSES

Drug-specific nursing diagnoses include the following:

■ **Constipation** related to antihyperlipidemic drugs

■ **Risk for Imbalanced Nutrition: Less Than Body Requirements** related to malabsorption of vitamins

■ **Risk for Impaired Skin Integrity** related to rash and flushing

- Nausea related to antihyperlipidemic drugs
- Risk for Injury related to dizziness

Nursing diagnoses related to drug administration are discussed in depth in Chapter 4.

PLANNING

The expected outcomes of the patient depend on the specific reason for administering the drug but may include an optimal response to therapy, support of patient needs related to the management of adverse reactions, and confidence in an understanding of the medication regimen.

IMPLEMENTATION

Promoting an Optimal Response to Therapy

Because hyperlipidemia is often treated on an outpatient basis, it is your responsibility to explain the drug regimen and possible adverse reactions. If printed dietary guidelines are given to the patient, utilize language-appropriate printed materials to emphasize the importance of following these recommendations. Drug therapy usually is discontinued if the antihyperlipidemic drug is not effective after 3 months of treatment.

Monitoring and Managing Patient Needs

CONSTIPATION. Patients taking the antihyperlipidemic drugs, particularly the bile acid resins, may experience constipation. The drugs can produce or severely worsen pre-existing constipation. Instruct the patient to increase fluid intake, eat foods high in dietary fiber, and exercise daily to help prevent constipation. If the problem persists or becomes severe, a stool softener or laxative may be required. Some patients require decreased dosage or discontinuation of the drug therapy.

LIFESPAN CONSIDERATIONS
Gerontology

Older adults are particularly prone to constipation when taking the bile acid resins. Question older adults about hard, dry stools; difficulty passing stools; and any complaints of constipation. Early intervention with stool softeners or laxatives may improve adherence.

RISK FOR IMBALANCED NUTRITION: LESS THAN BODY REQUIREMENTS. Bile acid resins may interfere with the digestion of fats and prevent the absorption of the fat-soluble vitamins (vitamins A, D, E, and K) and folic acid. When the bile acid resins are used for long-term therapy, vitamins A and D may be given in a water-soluble form or administered parenterally.

RISK FOR IMPAIRED SKIN INTEGRITY. Patients taking nicotinic acid (niacin) may experience moderate to severe, generalized flushing of the skin; a sensation of warmth; and severe itching or tingling. They may also complain of ringing in the ears. Although these reactions are most often seen at higher dose levels, some patients may experience them even when small doses of nicotinic acid are administered. The sudden appearance of these reactions may frighten the patient.

NURSING ALERT

Advise the patient taking niacin to contact the primary health care provider if the skin reactions are severe or cause extreme discomfort. Aspirin may be recommended before taking niacin preparations to reduce adverse reactions.

NAUSEA. Some antihyperlipidemic drugs cause nausea. If nausea occurs, the drug should be taken with meals or with food. Other measures to help alleviate the nausea include providing a relaxed atmosphere for eating with no unpleasant odors or sights. Teach the patient to eat several small meals rather than three large meals. If nausea is severe or vomiting occurs, the primary health care provider is notified.

RISK FOR INJURY. Injury can occur when the patient falls as the result of dizziness as an adverse reaction from the fibrates or statins. Monitor the hospitalized patient starting this medication carefully, placing the call light within easy reach. The patient may require assistance with ambulation until the effects of the medication are known, especially with the initial doses of the antihyperlipidemic.

POTENTIAL MEDICAL COMPLICATION: VITAMIN K DEFICIENCY. To prevent deficiency, the patient is encouraged to include foods high in vitamin K in the diet, such as asparagus, broccoli, green beans, lettuce, turnip greens, beef liver, collard greens, green tea, and spinach. Teach the patient to check for bruises over the body as an indication of vitamin K deficiency. If bruising is observed or if bleeding tendencies occur, instruct the patient to contact the primary health care provider immediately. Parenteral vitamin K may be prescribed by the primary health care provider for immediate treatment, and oral vitamin K for preventing a deficiency in the future.

POTENTIAL MEDICAL COMPLICATION: RHABDOMYOLYSIS. Antihyperlipidemic drugs, particularly the statin drugs, have been associated with skeletal muscle effects leading to rhabdomyolysis. Rhabdomyolysis is a rare condition in which muscle damage results in the release of muscle cell contents into the bloodstream. Rhabdomyolysis may precipitate renal dysfunction or acute renal failure. Be alert for complaints of unexplained muscle pain, muscle tenderness, or weakness, especially if accompanied by malaise or fever. This reaction is more likely in Asian patients; therefore, a lower starting dose of the statin rosuvastatin is recommended. These symptoms should be reported to the primary health care provider because the drug may need to be discontinued.

Educating the Patient and Family

Many of the circulatory-related ailments require lifestyle changes. Diet is an important aspect of cholesterol management for the patient. Emphasize the importance of following the diet recommended by the primary health care provider because drug therapy alone will not significantly lower cholesterol and triglyceride levels. Contact the patient periodically to see how he or she is handling a new eating plan; in addition, provide a copy of the recommended diet. Learn about your resources and refer the patient or family member to a clinical dietitian, a cardiovascular dietary health workshop, Internet websites, or a lecture/workshop provided by a hospital or community agency (see Patient Teaching for Improved Patient Outcomes: Using Self-Management Skills to Control Blood Cholesterol Levels). As you develop a teaching plan include the following information:

STATINS (HMG-CoA REDUCTASE INHIBITORS)

- Usually statins are taken in the evening or at bedtime.
- Choose juices other than grapefruit juice due to an enzyme reaction.

Patient Teaching for Improved Patient Outcomes

Using Self-Management Skills to Control Blood Cholesterol Levels

Adherence to long-term medical management of chronic conditions such as hyperlipidemia or hypertension is more successful when patients feel they have an element of control. As the nurse, you can empower patients by supporting efforts rather than telling them to participate in strategies for self-care.

Encourage patients to participate in managing their abilities to reduce cardiovascular risk by accessing interactive tools on the Internet. Various sites use information from the Framingham Heart Study to predict heart attack risk (see example at National Cholesterol Education Program site). To use the interactive site, enter the following:

✔ Age
✔ Gender
✔ Cholesterol laboratory value
✔ Blood pressure reading

A prediction for heart attack risk in the next 10 years is calculated. By reviewing these notations periodically, adherence to treatment recommendations will be re-enforced as the patient sees risk reduced over time.

- Antacids should be taken at least 2 hours after rosuvastatin.
- When fluvastatin or pravastatin is prescribed with a bile acid resin, the statin should be taken 2 hours after the bile acid resin or at least 4 hours afterward.
- These drugs may cause photosensitivity; avoid exposure to the sun and wear both sunscreen and protective clothing.
- These drugs cannot be used during pregnancy (pregnancy category X). Use a barrier contraceptive while taking these drugs. If the patient wishes to become pregnant while taking these drugs, the primary health care provider should be consulted before efforts at conception.
- Advise the patient to contact the primary health care provider as soon as possible if muscle pain, tenderness, or weakness occurs.

BILE ACID RESINS

- Take the drug before meals unless the primary health care provider directs otherwise.
- Cholestyramine powder: The prescribed dose must be mixed in 2 to 6 fluid ounces of water or noncarbonated beverage and shaken vigorously. The powder can also be mixed with highly fluid soups or pulpy fruits (e.g., applesauce, crushed pineapple). The powder should not be ingested in the dry form. Other drugs are taken 1 hour

before or 4 to 6 hours after cholestyramine. Cholestyramine is available combined with the artificial sweetener aspartame for patients with diabetes or those who are concerned about weight gain.
- Colestipol granules: The prescribed dose must be mixed in liquids, soup, cereals, carbonated beverages, or pulpy fruits. Use approximately 90 mL of liquid and, when mixing with a liquid, slowly stir the preparation until ready to drink. The granules will not dissolve. Take the entire drug, rinse the glass with a small amount of water, and drink to ensure that all the medication is taken.
- Colestipol tablets: Tablets should be swallowed whole, one at a time, with a full glass of water or other fluid—not chewed, cut, or crushed.
- Sipping or holding the liquid preparations in the mouth can cause tooth discoloration or enamel decay.
- Constipation, nausea, abdominal pain, and distention may occur and may subside with continued therapy. Contact the primary health care provider if these effects become bothersome or if unusual bleeding or bruising occurs.

FIBRIC ACID DERIVATIVES

- Gemfibrozil may cause dizziness or blurred vision. Observe caution when driving or performing hazardous tasks. Notify the primary health care provider if epigastric pain, diarrhea, nausea, or vomiting occurs.

MISCELLANEOUS PREPARATIONS

- Nicotinic acid (niacin): Take this drug with meals. This drug may cause mild to severe facial flushing, a sensation of warmth, severe itching, or headache. These symptoms usually subside with continued therapy, but contact the primary health care provider as soon as possible if symptoms are severe. The primary health care provider may prescribe aspirin (325 mg) to be taken about 30 minutes before nicotinic acid to decrease the flushing reaction. If dizziness occurs, avoid sudden changes in posture.
- Ezetimibe: this drug should be taken at least 2 hours before or 4 hours after a bile acid sequestrant. Report unusual muscle pain, weakness or tenderness, severe diarrhea, or respiratory infections.

EVALUATION

- Therapeutic response is achieved and serum lipid levels are decreased.
- Adverse reactions are identified, reported to the primary health care provider, and managed successfully with appropriate nursing interventions:
  • Patient reports adequate bowel movements.
  • Patient maintains an adequate nutritional status.
  • Skin remains intact.
  • Nausea is controlled.
  • No evidence of injury is seen.
- Patient and family express confidence and demonstrate an understanding of the drug regimen.

PHARMACOLOGY IN PRACTICE
THINK CRITICALLY

 Lillian's first visit to the clinic was a year ago. Her blood pressure was 156/98 and lab work drawn that day was cholesterol = 320, LDL = 178, HDL = 20.

The following information from her medical record today shows that T = 98.6°F, P = 104, R = 18, and BP = 136/92. Lab work drawn had the following values: cholesterol = 256, LDL = 160, HDL = 36.

How can you use this information to help encourage Mrs. Chase to continue her medication? What information would you give the patient concerning her constipation?

KEY POINTS

- Atherosclerosis is a disorder in which lipid deposits accumulate on the lining of blood vessels. Cholesterol and triglycerides are two lipids in our blood; elevation of one or both is termed hyperlipidemia.

- Antihyperlipidemic drugs decrease cholesterol and triglycerides in the blood. When included with lifestyle changes such as diet modifications, physical activity, smoking cessation, and weight management, the risk of coronary heart disease is lessened.

- HMG-CoA reductase inhibitors are frequently called "statin" drugs. These drugs lower the blood level of LDL cholesterol and triglycerides. Bile acid resins and fibric acid derivatives act in a similar manner to reduce cholesterol by binding with bile so the liver will use more, putting less in the system.

- Common adverse reactions include headache, dizziness, insomnia, and GI complaints such as increased flatulence and constipation. Patients taking bile acid resins need to be alert for bleeding tendencies. Those taking niacin have experienced a sensation of warmth, flushing, and itching; a reduction in dose diminishes the reactions.

Summary Drug Table ANTIHYPERLIPIDEMIC DRUGS

Generic Name	Trade Name	Uses	Adverse Reactions	Dosage Ranges
HMG-CoA Reductase Inhibitors (Statins)				
atorvastatin *ah-tore'-vah-stah-tin*	Lipitor	Reduce risk of coronary heart disease (CHD) events, hyperlipidemia, familial hypercholesterolemia	Headache, diarrhea, sinusitis	10–80 mg/day orally
fluvastatin *floo-vah-stah'-tin*	Lescol	Atherosclerosis, hyperlipidemia, familial hypercholesterolemia	Headache, back pain, upper respiratory infection, flu-like syndrome	20–80 mg/day orally
lovastatin *loe-vah-stah'-tin*	Mevacor, Altoprev	Reduce risk of CHD events, atherosclerosis, hyperlipidemia, familial hypercholesterolemia	Headache, flatulence, infection	10–80 mg/day orally in single or divided doses Adolescents: 10–40 mg/day orally

(table continues on page 364)

Antihyperlipidemic Drugs

Summary Drug Table ANTIHYPERLIPIDEMIC DRUGS (continued)

Generic Name	Trade Name	Uses	Adverse Reactions	Dosage Ranges
pitavastatin pit-a'-va-stah'-tin	Livalo	Hyperlipidemia	Constipation, diarrhea, confusion, back pain	2–4 mg/day orally
pravastatin prah-vah-stah'-tin	Pravachol	Reduce risk of CHD events, atherosclerosis, hyperlipidemia, familial hypercholesterolemia	Headache, nausea, vomiting, diarrhea, localized pain, cold symptoms	40–80 mg/day orally Children 8–13 yr: 20 mg/day orally Adolescents 14–18 yr: 40 mg/day orally
rosuvastatin roe-soo'-vah-stah-tin	Crestor	Hyperlipidemia	Headache	5–40 mg/day orally
simvastatin sim-vah-stah'-tin	Zocor	Reduce risk of CHD events, hyperlipidemia, familial hypercholesterolemia	Constipation	5–80 mg/day orally
Bile Acid Resins				
cholestyramine koe-less'-teer-ah-meen	Prevalite	Hyperlipidemia, relief of pruritus associated with partial biliary obstruction	Constipation (may lead to fecal impaction), exacerbation of hemorrhoids, abdominal pain, distention and cramping, nausea, increased bleeding related to vitamin K malabsorption, vitamin A and D deficiencies	4 g orally 1–6 times/day; individualize dosage based on response
colestipol koe-less'-tih-poll	Colestid	Hyperlipidemia	Same as cholestyramine	Granules: 5–30 g/day orally in divided doses Tablets: 2–16 g/day
colesevelam koe-leh-sev'-eh-lam	WelChol	Hyperlipidemia	Same as cholestyramine	3–7 tablets/day orally
Fibric Acid Derivatives (Fibrates)				
fenofibrate fen-oh-fye'-brate	TriCor, Triglide, Antara, Lipofen	Hyperlipidemia, hypertriglyceridemia	Abnormal liver function test results, respiratory problems, abdominal pain	Tablet: 48–145 mg/day orally
gemfibrozil jem-fye'-broe-zill	Lopid	Reduce risk of CHD events, hypertriglyceridemia	Dyspepsia, abdominal pain, diarrhea, nausea, vomiting, fatigue	1200 mg/day orally in two divided doses 30 min before morning and evening meals
Miscellaneous Preparations				
ezetimibe ee-zet'-ah-mibe	Zetia	Primary hypercholesterolemia	Diarrhea, back pain, sinusitis, dizziness, abdominal pain, arthralgia, coughing, fatigue	10 mg/day orally
niacin (nicotinic acid) nye'-ah-sin	Niaspan, Niacor	Adjunctive treatment for hyperlipidemia	Generalized flushing sensation of warmth, severe itching and tingling, nausea, vomiting, abdominal pain	Immediate release: 1–2 g orally BID, TID Extended release: 500–2000 mg/day orally
Combination Drugs				
amlodipine/ atorvastatin	Caduet	Treat hypertension and hypercholesterolemia	See individual drugs	Titrate dose to no more than 10/80 mg/day combination orally
niacin/lovastatin	Advicor	Primary hypercholesterolemia	See individual drugs	Titrate dose between 500/20 mg/day combination orally, to maximum of 2000 mg of niacin
niacin/ simvastatin	Simcor	Hyperlipidemia, hypertriglyceridemia	See individual drugs	Titrate dose between 500/20 mg/day combination orally, to maximum of 2000 mg of niacin
ezetimibe/ simvastatin	Vytorin	Primary/familial hypercholesterolemia	See individual drugs	Titrate dose between 10/10 mg/day and 10/80 mg/day

Chapter Review

Know Your Drugs

Clients sometimes know a medication by the brand (or trade) name and not the generic name. To help you recognize both names, match the brand name with the generic name of the same medication.

Generic Name	Brand Name
1. atorvastatin	A. Crestor
2. lovastatin	B. Lipitor
3. rosuvastatin	C. Mevacor
4. simvastatin	D. Zocor

Calculate Medication Dosages

1. A client is prescribed 10-mg simvastatin orally daily for high cholesterol. The drug is available in 5-mg tablets. The nurse administers _____.

2. Lipitor comes in both 20-mg and 40-mg tablets. To use the least number of pills, what strength of tablet should be used for a client prescribed 80-mg orally daily?

Prepare for the NCLEX®

Build Your Knowledge

1. Which of the following blood elements has a protective property for heart disease?

   1. cholesterol
   2. low-density lipoproteins
   3. high-density lipoproteins
   4. triglycerides

2. Antihyperlipidemia drugs work to:

   1. reduce fat in dietary intake
   2. decrease cholesterol and triglycerides
   3. remove plaque from arterioles
   4. lessen gallbladder stones

3. Select the most common adverse reaction in a client taking a bile acid resin:

   1. anorexia
   2. vomiting
   3. constipation
   4. headache

4. Lovastatin is best taken _____.

   1. once daily, preferably with the evening meal
   2. three times daily with meals
   3. at least 1 hour before or 2 hours after meals
   4. twice daily without regard to meals

5. A client taking niacin reports flushing after each dose of the niacin. Which of the following drugs would the nurse expect to be prescribed to help alleviate the flushing?

   1. meperidine (Demerol)
   2. aspirin
   3. vitamin K
   4. diphenhydramine (Benadryl)

Apply Your Knowledge

6. When assessing a client taking cholestyramine for vitamin K deficiency, the nurse would _____.

   1. check the client for bruising
   2. keep a record of the client's intake and output
   3. monitor the client for myalgia
   4. keep a dietary record of foods eaten

7. Which of the following points is important for the nurse to tell the client when teaching about drug and diet therapy for hyperlipidemia?

   1. Fluids are taken in limited amounts when eating a low-fat diet
   2. The medication should be taken at least 1 hour before meals
   3. Medication alone will not lower cholesterol
   4. Meat is not allowed on a low-fat diet

8. As the client makes breakfast selections for tomorrow, which of the following items should the nurse recognize as a potential problem food?

   1. scrambled eggs
   2. oatmeal with cream and sugar
   3. stewed prunes
   4. grapefruit juice

Alternate-Format Questions

9. A client taking bile acid resins can become vitamin deficient in which of the following? **Select all that apply**.

   1. vitamin A
   2. vitamin B
   3. vitamin C
   4. vitamin D
   5. vitamin E

10. The primary health care provider prescribes fenofibrate for the treatment of hypertriglyceridemia. The client is now taking 200 mg/day orally. Is this an appropriate dosage? If not, what action would you take? If the dose is appropriate, how many capsules would you administer if the drug is available in 67-mg capsules?

   _____

To check your answers, see Appendix G.

the**Point** *For more NCLEX-style questions, log on to http://thepoint.lww.com to access more than 1000 questions.*

35

Antihypertensive Drugs

LEARNING OBJECTIVES

On completion of this chapter, the student will:

1. Discuss the various types of hypertension and risk factors involved.
2. Identify normal and abnormal blood pressure levels for adults.
3. List the various types of drugs used to treat hypertension.
4. Discuss the general drug actions, uses, adverse reactions, contraindications, precautions, and interactions of the antihypertensive drugs.
5. Discuss important preadministration and ongoing assessment activities the nurse should perform for the patient taking an antihypertensive drug.
6. Explain why blood pressure determinations are important during therapy with an antihypertensive drug.
7. List nursing diagnoses particular to a patient taking an antihypertensive drug.
8. Discuss ways to promote an optimal response to therapy, how to manage adverse reactions, and important points to keep in mind when educating patients about the use of an antihypertensive drug.

KEY TERMS

angioedema • localized wheals or swellings in subcutaneous tissues or mucous membranes, which may be due to an allergic response; also called angioneurotic edema

blood pressure • force of blood against artery walls

endogenous • pertaining to something that normally occurs or is produced within the organism

hyperkalemia • increase in potassium levels in the blood

hypertension • high blood pressure that stays elevated over time

hypertensive emergency • extremely high blood pressure that must be lowered immediately to prevent damage to target organs (i.e., heart, kidneys, eyes)

hypokalemia • low blood potassium level

hyponatremia • low blood sodium level

isolated systolic hypertension • systolic blood pressure over 140 mm Hg with diastolic blood pressure under 90 mm Hg

lumen • inner diameter of a tube; the space or opening within an artery

orthostatic hypotension • decrease in blood pressure occurring after standing in one place for an extended period

prehypertension • systolic blood pressure between 120 and 139 mm Hg or diastolic pressure between 80 and 89 mm Hg

primary hypertension • hypertension that has no known cause; also known as essential or idiopathic hypertension

secondary hypertension • hypertension with a known cause, such as kidney disease

vasodilation • increase in the diameter of the blood vessels that, when widespread, results in a drop in blood pressure

DRUG CLASSES

Beta (β)-adrenergic blocking drugs	Calcium channel blocking drugs
Alpha (α)/β and antiadrenergic drugs (centrally and peripherally acting)	Angiotensin-converting enzyme inhibitors (ACEIs)
	Angiotensin II receptor antagonists

PHARMACOLOGY IN PRACTICE

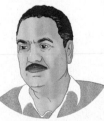

Mr. Alfredo Garcia was in a month ago for a respiratory infection. At that time his blood pressure was 210/120 mm Hg. He was prescribed a beta (β) blocking drug. When he returns today, his weight is down 15 lb and his blood pressure is 170/95 mm Hg. Read about the different drugs in this chapter to see if any changes should be made.

In the United States, about 72 million people have high blood pressure; this is about 1 in 3 adults. African Americans are twice as likely as whites to experience hypertension. After age 65, African American women have the highest incidence of hypertension. **Hypertension** as defined as a blood pressure of 140/90 mm Hg or higher.

What is meant by **blood pressure**? It is simply the force of the blood against the walls of the arteries. Blood pressure increases and decreases throughout the day. The condition in which blood pressure stays elevated over time is known as hypertension. A systolic blood pressure less than 120 mm Hg and a diastolic blood pressure less than 80 mm Hg (120/80) are considered normal. **Prehypertension** is defined as a systolic pressure between 120 and 139 mm Hg or a diastolic pressure between 80 and 89 mm Hg. Individuals with prehypertensive blood pressures are at risk for developing hypertension and should begin health-promoting lifestyle modifications.

Risks Factors for Hypertension

Hypertension is serious, because it causes the heart to work too hard and contributes to atherosclerosis. It also increases the risk of heart disease, heart failure (HF), kidney disease, blindness, and stroke. Yet, most cases of hypertension have no known cause and this is called **primary hypertension**. Although the cause may be unknown, certain risk factors, such as diet and lifestyle, can influence primary hypertension. Display 35.1 identifies the risk factors associated with hypertension.

Primary hypertension cannot be cured but it can be controlled. Although hypertension is not a part of healthy aging, many individuals experience hypertension as they grow older. For many older individuals, the *systolic* pressure gives the most accurate diagnosis of hypertension. Display 35.2 discusses the importance of the systolic pressure.

Nonpharmacologic Management for Hypertension

Once primary hypertension develops, management of the disorder becomes a lifetime task. When a direct cause of the hypertension can be identified, the condition is described as

---

Display 35.1 Risk Factors for Hypertension

- Age and sex (women older than 55 years and men older than 45 years of age)
- African American race (higher rates than Asian, Caucasian, or Hispanic individuals)
- Obesity
- Excessive dietary intake of salt and too little intake of potassium
- Chronic alcohol consumption
- Lack of physical activity
- Cigarette smoking
- Family history of high blood pressure and/or cardiovascular disease, diabetes, persistent stress
- Overweight in youth younger than 18 years has become a risk factor for prehypertension in teens

---

Display 35.2 Importance of the Systolic Blood Pressure

Individuals with only an elevated systolic pressure have a condition known as **isolated systolic hypertension** (ISH). In ISH, systolic blood pressure is 140 mm Hg or greater with diastolic blood pressure less than 90 mm Hg. When the systolic pressure is high, blood vessels become less flexible and stiffen, leading to cardiovascular disease and kidney damage. Research indicates that treating ISH saves lives and reduces illness. The treatment is the same for ISH as for other forms of hypertension. Diastolic pressure should not be reduced lower than 70 mm Hg. Therefore, caution is advised in treating those with ISH and existing heart disease (JNC 7, 2009).

---

secondary hypertension. Among the known causes of secondary hypertension kidney disease ranks first, with tumors or other abnormalities of the adrenal glands following. Most primary health care providers prescribe lifestyle changes to reduce risk factors before prescribing drugs. The primary health care provider may recommend measures such as:

- Weight loss (if the patient is overweight)
- Stress reduction (e.g., relaxation techniques, meditation, and yoga)
- Regular aerobic exercise
- Smoking cessation (if applicable)
- Moderation of alcohol consumption
- Dietary changes, such as a decrease in sodium (salt) intake

Many people with hypertension are "salt sensitive," in that any salt or sodium more than the minimum need is too much for them and leads to an increase in blood pressure. Dietitians usually recommend the Dietary Approaches to Stop Hypertension (DASH) diet. Studies indicate that blood pressure can be reduced by eating a diet low in saturated fat, total fat, and cholesterol and rich in fruits, vegetables, and low-fat dairy foods. The DASH diet includes whole grains, poultry, fish, and nuts and has reduced amounts of fats, red meats, sweets, and sugared beverages. Table 35.1 identifies current blood pressure classifications and management strategies for adults.

Drug Therapy for Hypertension

When nonpharmacologic measures do not control high blood pressure, drug therapy usually begins, and the primary health care provider may first prescribe a diuretic (see Chapter 33) or beta (β)-adrenergic blocker (see Chapter 25), because these drugs typically are highly effective. However, as in many other diseases and conditions, there is no "best" single drug, drug combination, or medical regimen for treatment of hypertension. After examination and evaluation of the patient, the primary health care provider selects the antihypertensive drug and therapeutic regimen that will probably be most effective. Figure 35.1 illustrates the recommendations of the National Heart, Lung and Blood Institute's seventh report on hypertension displayed as an algorithm for the treatment of hypertension.

Table 35.1 Classification and Management of Blood Pressure for Adults

Blood Pressure Classification	Systolic Blood Pressure* (mm Hg)	Diastolic Blood Pressure* (mm Hg)	Lifestyle Modification	Without Compelling Indications	With Compelling Indications
Normal	<120	and <80	Encourage	n/a	n/a
Prehypertension	120–139	or 80–89	Yes	No antihypertensive drug indicated	Drug(s) for compelling indications‡
Stage 1 hypertension	140–159	or 90–99	Yes	Thiazide-type diuretics for most.† May consider ACEI, ARB, BB, CCB, or combination	Drug(s) for the compelling indications.‡ Other antihypertensive drugs (diuretics, ACEI, ARB, BB, CCB) as needed
Stage 2 hypertension	≥160	or ≥100	Yes	Two-drug combination for most (usually thiazide-type diuretic and ACEI or ARB or BB or CCB)	

Drug abbreviations: ACEI, angiotensin-converting enzyme inhibitor; ARB, angiotensin receptor blocker; BB, β blocker; CCB, calcium channel blocker.

*Treatment determined by highest BP category.

†Initial combined therapy should be used cautiously in those at risk for orthostatic hypotension.

‡Treat patients with chronic kidney disease or diabetes to BP goal of <130/80 mm Hg.

Adapted from National Heart, Lung and Blood Institute. (2003). *The seventh report of the Joint National Committee on Prevention, Detection, Evaluation, and Treatment of High Blood Pressure*. Bethesda, MD: National Institutes of Health. Retrieved May 7, 2009, from http://www.nhlbi.nih.gov/guidelines/hypertension/.

When the patient does not experience a response to therapy, it may be necessary to change to another antihypertensive drug or add a second antihypertensive drug. The primary health care provider also recommends that the patient continue with stress reduction, dietary modifications, and other lifestyle modifications needed for controlling hypertension. The types of drugs used for the treatment of hypertension include the following:

- Diuretics—for example, furosemide and hydrochlorothiazide
- β-Adrenergic blocking drugs—for example, atenolol and propranolol
- Antiadrenergic drugs (centrally acting)—for example, clonidine and methyldopa
- Antiadrenergic drugs (peripherally acting)—for example, doxazosin and prazosin
- Calcium channel blocking drugs—for example, amlodipine and diltiazem
- Angiotensin-converting enzyme inhibitors—for example, captopril and enalapril
- Angiotensin II receptor antagonists—for example, irbesartan and losartan
- Vasodilating drugs—for example, hydralazine and minoxidil

Two drug types are relatively new—direct renin inhibitors (aliskiren) and selective aldosterone receptor antagonists (SARAs; eplerenone). Aliskiren inhibits renin and subsequently prevents the angiotensin conversion process. Eplerenone also blocks the angiotensin process by binding with aldosterone.

For additional information concerning the antiadrenergic drugs (both centrally and peripherally acting), and the alpha (α)- and β-adrenergic blocking drugs, see Chapter 25. Information on the vasodilating drugs and the diuretics can be found in Chapters 36 and 33, respectively. In addition to these antihypertensive drugs, many antihypertensive combinations are available, such as Capozide, Timolide, Aldoril, and Lopressor HCT (Table 35.2). Most combination antihypertensive drugs combine antihypertensive and diuretic agents.

Actions

Many antihypertensive drugs lower the blood pressure by dilating or increasing the size of the arterial blood vessels (**vasodilation**). Vasodilation creates an increase in the **lumen** (the space or opening within a blood vessel) of the arterial blood vessels, which in turn increases the amount of space available for the blood to circulate. Because blood volume (the amount of blood) remains relatively constant, an increase in the space in which the blood circulates (i.e., the blood vessels) lowers the pressure of the fluid (measured as blood pressure) in the blood vessels. Although the method by which antihypertensive drugs dilate blood vessels varies, the result remains basically the same. Figure 35.2 shows the organs affected by the different classes of antihypertensive drugs.

Antihypertensive drugs with vasodilating activity include the adrenergic blocking and calcium channel blocking drugs. Diuretics (Chapter 33) are also considered antihypertensive drugs. The mechanism by which the diuretics reduce elevated blood pressure is not completely understood, but it is thought to be based, in part, on their ability to increase the excretion of sodium from the body.

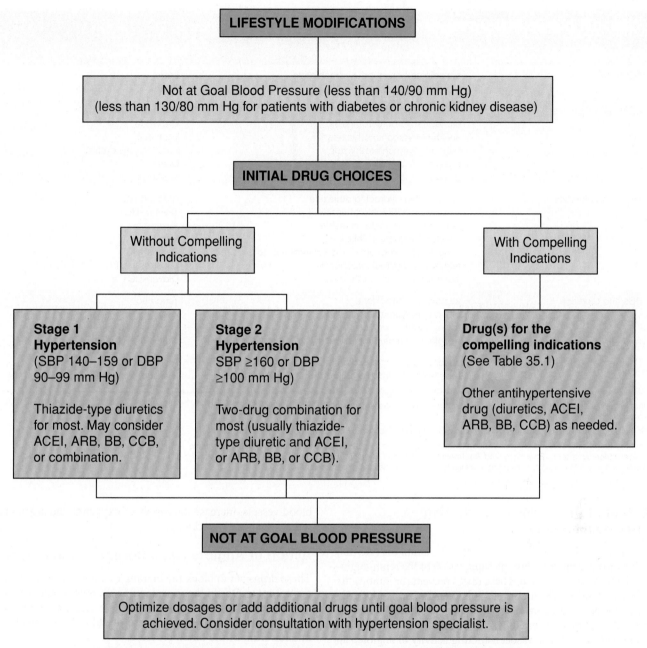

Figure 35.1 Algorithm for treatment of hypertension. Compelling indicators include HF, high risk for cardiovascular disease, post–myocardial infarction (MI), diabetes, stroke prevention, and chronic kidney disease. Key: DBP, diastolic blood pressure; SBP, systolic blood pressure; ACEI, angiotensin-converting enzyme inhibitor; ARB, angiotensin receptor blocker; BB, β blocker; CCB, calcium channel blocker; DBP, diastolic blood pressure; SBP, systolic blood pressure. (Adapted from National Heart, Lung and Blood Institute. [2003]. *The seventh report of the Joint National Committee on Prevention, Detection, Evaluation, and Treatment of High Blood Pressure.* Bethesda, MD: National Institutes of Health. Retrieved May 7, 2009, from http://www.nhlbi.nih.gov/guidelines/ hypertension/.)

Antihypertensive Drugs

Table 35.2 Examples of Antihypertensive Combinations

Combination Type	Generic Drug Combinations*	Trade Name
ACEIs and CCBs	amlodipine-benazepril hydrochloride	Lotrel
	trandolapril-verapamil	Tarka
ACEIs and diuretics	benazepril-hydrochlorothiazide	Lotensin HCT
	captopril-hydrochlorothiazide	Capozide
	enalapril-hydrochlorothiazide	Vaseretic
	lisinopril-hydrochlorothiazide	Prinzide, Zestoretic
	moexipril-hydrochlorothiazide	Uniretic
	quinapril-hydrochlorothiazide	Accuretic
ARBs and diuretics	candesartan-hydrochlorothiazide	Atacand HCT
	eprosartan-hydrochlorothiazide	Teveten-HCT
	irbesartan-hydrochlorothiazide	Avalide
	losartan-hydrochlorothiazide	Hyzaar
	olmesartan medoxomil- hydrochlorothiazide	Benicar HCT
	telmisartan-hydrochlorothiazide	Micardis-HCT
	valsartan-hydrochlorothiazide	Diovan-HCT
BBs and diuretics	atenolol-chlorthalidone	Tenoretic
	bisoprolol-hydrochlorothiazide	Ziac
	metoprolol-hydrochlorothiazide	Lopressor HCT
	nadolol-bendroflumethiazide	Corzide
Diuretic and diuretic	spironolactone-hydrochlorothiazide	Aldactazide
	triamterene-hydrochlorothiazide	Dyazide, Maxzide

Drug abbreviations: BB, β blocker; ACEI, angiotensin-converting enzyme inhibitor; ARB, angiotensin receptor blocker; CCB, calcium channel blocker.

*Some drug combinations are available in multiple fixed doses. Each drug dose is reported in milligrams.

Adapted from National Heart Lung and Blood Institute. (2003). *The seventh report of the Joint National Committee on Prevention, Detection, Evaluation, and Treatment of High Blood Pressure.* Bethesda, MD: National Institutes of Health. Retrieved May 7, 2009, from http://www.nhlbi.nih.gov/guidelines/hypertension/.

Action of Angiotensin-Converting Enzyme Inhibitors

The angiotensin-converting enzyme (ACE) inhibitors (ACEIs) appear to act primarily through suppression of the renin-angio-tensin-aldosterone system. These drugs prevent (or inhibit) the activity of ACE, which converts angiotensin I to angiotensin II, a powerful vasoconstrictor. Both angiotensin I and ACE normally are manufactured by the body and are called **endogenous** substances. The vasoconstricting activity of angiotensin II stimulates the secretion of the endogenous hormone aldosterone by the adrenal cortex. Aldosterone promotes the retention of sodium and water, which may contribute to a rise in blood pressure. By preventing the conversion of angiotensin I to angiotensin II, this chain of events is interrupted, sodium and water are not retained, and blood pressure decreases.

Action of Calcium Channel Blockers

Systemic and coronary arteries are influenced by movement of calcium across cell membranes of vascular smooth muscle. The contractions of cardiac and vascular smooth muscle depend on movement of extracellular calcium ions into these walls through specific ion channels.

Calcium channel blockers act by inhibiting the movement of calcium ions across cell membranes of cardiac and arterial muscle cells. This results in less calcium available for the transmission of nerve impulses. As a result, these drugs relax blood vessels, increase the supply of oxygen to the heart, and reduce the heart's workload.

Action of Angiotensin II Receptor Antagonists

These drugs act to block the binding of angiotensin II at various receptor sites in the vascular smooth muscle and adrenal gland, which blocks the vasoconstrictive effect of the renin-angiotensin system and the release of aldosterone, resulting in a lowering of the blood pressure.

Uses

Antihypertensive drugs are used in the treatment of hypertension. Although many antihypertensive drugs are available, not all drugs work equally well for a given patient. In some instances, the primary health care provider may find it necessary to prescribe a different antihypertensive drug when the patient does not experience a response to therapy. Some antihypertensive drugs are used only in severe cases of hypertension and when other, less potent drugs fail to lower the blood pressure. At times, two antihypertensive drugs may be given together to achieve a better response (see Fig. 35.1).

Nitroprusside (Nitropress) is an example of an intravenous (IV) drug that may be used to treat hypertensive emergencies. A **hypertensive emergency** is a case of extremely high blood pressure in which blood pressure must be lowered immediately to prevent damage to the target organs. Target organs

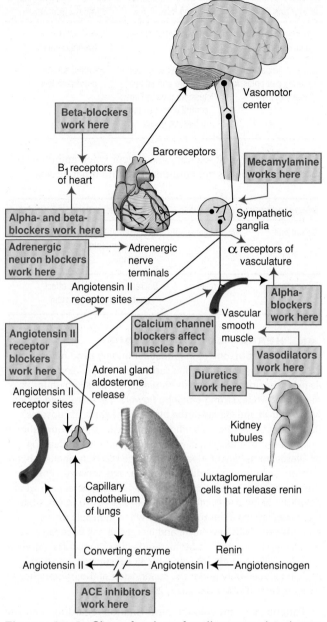

Figure 35.2 Sites of action of antihypertensive drugs.

of hypertension include the heart, kidney, and eyes (retinopathy). Additional uses of the antihypertensive drugs are given in the Summary Drug Table: Antihypertensive Drugs.

Adverse Reactions

When any antihypertensive drug is given, orthostatic (or postural) hypotension may result in some patients, especially early in therapy. **Orthostatic hypotension** occurs when the individual has a significant drop in blood pressure (usually 10 mm Hg systolic or more) when assuming an upright position. The patient can become dizzy and may fall, resulting in an injury. Butt (2012) reported that the risk of hip fracture is increased by almost 50% for those older than 66 when they are started on antihypertensives. This is

thought to be from fainting and falling related to orthostatic hypotension.

Central Nervous System Reactions

• Fatigue, depression, dizziness, headache, and syncope

Respiratory System Reactions

• Upper respiratory infections and cough

Gastrointestinal System Reactions

• Abdominal pain, nausea, diarrhea, constipation, gastric irritation, and anorexia

Other Reactions

• Rash, pruritus, dry mouth, tachycardia, hypotension, proteinuria, and neutropenia

Additional adverse reactions that may occur when an antihypertensive drug is administered are listed in the Summary Drug Table: Antihypertensive Drugs. For the adverse reactions that may result when a diuretic is used as an antihypertensive drug, see the Summary Drug Table: Diuretics in Chapter 33.

Contraindications

Antihypertensive drugs are contraindicated in patients with known hypersensitivity to the individual drugs.

The ACEIs and angiotensin II receptor blockers are contraindicated if the patient has impaired renal function, HF, salt or volume depletion, bilateral stenosis, or angioedema. They are also contraindicated during pregnancy (pregnancy category C during first trimester and pregnancy category D in the second and third trimesters) or during lactation. Use of the ACEIs and the angiotensin II receptor blockers during the second and third trimesters of pregnancy is contraindicated, because use may cause fetal and neonatal injury or death.

Calcium channel blockers are contraindicated in patients who are hypersensitive to the drugs and those with sick sinus syndrome, second- or third-degree atrioventricular (AV) block (except with a functioning pacemaker), hypotension (systolic pressure less than 90 mm Hg), ventricular dysfunction, or cardiogenic shock.

Precautions

Antihypertensive drugs are used cautiously in patients with renal or hepatic impairment or electrolyte imbalances, during lactation and pregnancy, and in older patients. The calcium channel blockers are used cautiously in patients with HF or renal or hepatic impairment. The calcium channel blockers are used cautiously during pregnancy (pregnancy category C) and lactation. ACEIs are used cautiously in patients with sodium depletion, hypovolemia, or coronary or cerebrovascular insufficiency and in those receiving diuretic therapy or dialysis. The angiotensin II receptor agonists are used cautiously in patients with renal or hepatic dysfunction, hypovolemia, or volume or salt depletion, and in patients receiving high doses of diuretics.

Interactions

The hypotensive effects of most antihypertensive drugs are increased when administered with diuretics and other antihypertensives. Many drugs can interact with the antihypertensive drugs and decrease their effectiveness (e.g., monoamine oxidase inhibitor antidepressants, antihistamines, and sympathomimetic bronchodilators).

The following interactions may occur when the calcium channel blockers are used with another agent:

Interacting Drug	Common Use	Effect of Interaction
cimetidine or ranitidine	Gastrointestinal (GI) disorders	Increased effects of calcium channel blockers
theophylline	Control of asthma and chronic obstructive pulmonary disease	Increased pharmacologic and toxic effects of theophylline
digoxin	HF	Increased risk for digitalis toxicity
rifampin	Antitubercular agent	Decreased effect of calcium channel blocker

The following interactions may occur when ACEI drugs are administered with another agent:

Interacting Drug	Common Use	Effect of Interaction
nonsteroidal anti-inflammatory drugs (NSAIDs)	Relief of pain and inflammation	Reduced hypotensive effects of the ACEIs
rifampin	Antitubercular agent	Decreased pharmacologic effect of ACEIs (particularly of enalapril)
allopurinol	Antigout agent	Higher risk of hypersensitivity reaction
digoxin	Management of HF	Increased or decreased plasma digoxin levels
loop diuretics	Reduce/eliminate edema	Decreased diuretic effects
lithium	Management of bipolar disorder	Increased serum lithium levels, possible lithium toxicity

Interacting Drug	Common Use	Effect of Interaction
hypoglycemic agents and insulin	Management of diabetes	Increased risk of hypoglycemia
potassium-sparing diuretics or potassium preparations	Diuretics: reduce blood pressure and edema Potassium preparations: control of low serum potassium levels	Elevated serum potassium level

The following interactions may occur when angiotensin II receptor antagonists are administered with other agents:

Interacting Drug	Common Use	Effect of Interaction
fluconazole	Antifungal agent	Increased antihypertensive and adverse effects (particularly with losartan)
indomethacin	Pain relief	Decreased hypotensive effect (particularly with losartan)

HERBAL CONSIDERATIONS

Hawthorn, one of the most commonly used natural agents to treat various cardiovascular problems such as hypertension, angina, arrhythmias, and HF, is known for its masses of white, strong-smelling flowers. They are used, along with the fruit and leaves of the plant, in the form of capsules, fluid extract, tea, tinctures, and topical creams. Hawthorn should not be taken by individuals who are pregnant, breastfeeding, or allergic to the agent. Possible adverse reactions include hypotension, arrhythmias, sedation, nausea, and anorexia. Possible drug–hawthorn interactions include a risk of hypotension when hawthorn is used with other antihypertensive drugs, possible increased effects of inotropic drugs when inotropic drugs are administered with hawthorn, and increased risk of sedative effects when hawthorn is administered with other central nervous system (CNS) depressants. As with all substances, hawthorn should be used only under the supervision of the primary health care provider (DerMarderosian, 2003).

Patients may not volunteer information regarding their use of complementary and alternative remedies. Always inquire about use of herbal products. Medical reports indicate a possible interaction with St. John's wort, used to relieve depression, causing a decrease in serum levels of calcium channel blockers. Due to a specific enzyme reaction, grapefruit or its juice should not be taken if a patient is prescribed a calcium channel blocker.

NURSING PROCESS
PATIENT RECEIVING AN ANTIHYPERTENSIVE DRUG

ASSESSMENT

Preadministration Assessment
Before therapy with an antihypertensive drug starts, assess the blood pressure and pulse rate on both arms with the patient in standing, sitting, and lying positions. Correctly label the readings for each extremity and position (e.g., the pressure readings on each arm and the three positions used to obtain the readings) as you document these on the patient's chart. Obtain the patient's weight, especially if a diuretic is part of therapy or if the primary health care provider prescribes a weight loss regimen.

When ACE inhibitors, angiotensin antagonists, or renin inhibitors are prescribed for female patients of childbearing age, it is important to ensure that the patient is not pregnant before beginning therapy. Teach the patient how to use a reliable birth control method such as barrier birth control while taking these drugs.

LIFESPAN CONSIDERATIONS
Menopause
Women experiencing the start of menopause may have irregular ovulation and periods. Some women are reluctant to use birth control as they age, because they feel they are not capable of becoming pregnant. Because the ACEIs and angiotensin II receptor antagonists can cause injury and death to a developing fetus, it is important to teach the hypertensive woman who is entering menopause that pregnancy can still occur. Birth control measures should be discussed. Should a woman taking the aforementioned hypertensive medicines become pregnant, medications should be discontinued immediately.

Ongoing Assessment
Monitoring and recording the blood pressure is an important part of the ongoing assessment, especially early in therapy. The primary health care provider may need to adjust the dose of the drug upward or downward, try a different drug, or add another drug to the therapeutic regimen if the patient's response to drug therapy is inadequate.

Each time the blood pressure is measured, use the same arm with the patient in the same position (e.g., standing, sitting, or lying down). In some instances, the primary health care provider may order the blood pressure taken in one or more positions, such as standing and lying down. When the patient has severe hypertension, does not have the expected response to drug therapy, or is critically ill, continuous monitoring is performed (Fig. 35.3).

NURSING ALERT
The blood pressure is taken before each administration of an antihypertensive drug when therapy is started in the inpatient setting. If the blood pressure is significantly decreased from baseline values, do not give the drug but notify the primary health care provider. In addition, the primary health care provider is notified if there is a significant increase in the blood pressure.

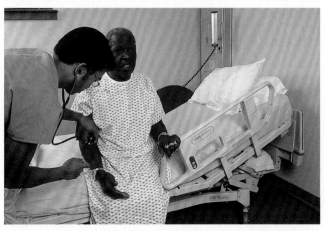

Figure 35.3 Nurse takes the patient's blood pressure before administering an antihypertensive drug.

Patients taking an antihypertensive drug occasionally retain sodium and water, resulting in edema and weight gain. Assess the patient's weight and examine the extremities for edema daily when the patient is an inpatient. Report a weight gain of 2 lb or more per day and any evidence of edema in the hands, fingers, feet, legs, or sacral area. The patient is also weighed at regular intervals if a weight reduction diet is used to lower the blood pressure or if the patient is receiving a thiazide or related diuretic as part of antihypertensive therapy.

In the ambulatory setting, help the patient to plan a schedule of regular self-monitoring of weight and blood pressure. Teach the patient to record weight and blood pressure readings, and to find local resources for taking blood pressures in the community. The patient is instructed to bring these records in to the primary care provider at each appointment.

NURSING DIAGNOSES
Drug-specific nursing diagnoses include the following:

■ **Risk for Deficient Fluid Volume** related to excessive diuresis secondary to administration of a diuretic

■ **Risk for Injury** related to dizziness or lightheadedness secondary to postural or orthostatic hypotensive episodes

■ **Risk for Ineffective Sexuality Patterns** related to impotence secondary to effects of antihypertensive drugs

■ **Risk for Activity Intolerance** related to fatigue and weakness

■ **Pain** (acute headache) related to antihypertensive drugs

Nursing diagnoses related to drug administration are discussed in Chapter 4.

PLANNING
The expected outcomes for the patient may include an optimal response to therapy (blood pressure maintained in an acceptable range), support of patient needs related to managing adverse reactions, and confidence in an understanding of the medication regimen.

IMPLEMENTATION

Promoting an Optimal Response to Therapy
Most of the antihypertensive drugs can be taken without regard to meals. If GI upset occurs, the drug should be taken with meals. The ACEIs inhibitors, captopril and moexipril, should be taken 1 hour before or 2 hours after meals to enhance absorption. The drugs are sustained-release capsules that should not be crushed, opened, or chewed. Increased serum potassium, or hyperkalemia, can occur with direct renin inhibitor medications; therefore, teach the patient to refrain from using potassium-based salt substitutes in the preparation of foods.

Some patients taking an ACEI experience a dry cough that does not subside until the drug therapy is discontinued. This reaction may need to be tolerated. If the cough becomes too bothersome, the primary health care provider may discontinue use of the drug. The ACEIs may cause a significant drop in blood pressure after the first dose. This effect can be minimized if the primary health care provider discontinues the diuretic therapy (if the patient is taking a diuretic) or begins treatment with small doses.

Clonidine is available as an oral tablet (Catapres) and transdermal patch (Catapres-TTS). If using the transdermal patch, apply it to a hairless area of intact skin on the upper arm or torso; the patch is kept in place for 7 days. The adhesive overlay is applied directly over the system to ensure the patch remains in place for the required time. A different body area is selected for each application. If the patch loosens before 7 days, the edges can be reinforced with nonallergenic tape. The date the patch was placed and the date the patch is to be removed can be written on the surface of the patch with a fiber-tipped pen.

⚠ NURSING ALERT

Advise patients that **angioedema** may occur at any time when taking aliskiren. If the patient experiences swelling of the face, throat, or extremities, he or she should hold the next dose of medication and call the primary health care provider immediately to report symptoms and get instruction regarding antihypertensive treatment.

Nitroprusside, a vasodilator, is used to treat patients with a hypertensive emergency. When vasodilators are used, hemodynamic monitoring of the patient's blood pressure and cardiovascular status is required throughout the course of therapy.

LIFESPAN CONSIDERATIONS
Gerontology

Older adults are particularly sensitive to the hypotensive effects of nitroprusside. To minimize hypotensive effects, the drug is initially given in lower dosages. Older adults require more frequent monitoring during the administration of nitroprusside.

Monitoring and Managing Patient Needs

Observe the patient for adverse drug reactions, because their occurrence may require a change in the dose of the drug. In some instances, the patient may have to tolerate mild adverse reactions, such as dry mouth or mild anorexia. Contact the primary health care provider to determine if the medication should be changed or the reactions tolerated.

⚠ NURSING ALERT

If it becomes necessary to discontinue antihypertensive therapy, never discontinue use of the drug abruptly. The primary health care provider will prescribe the parameters by which the dosage is to be discontinued. The dosage is usually gradually reduced over 2 to 4 days to avoid rebound hypertension (a rapid rise in blood pressure).

DEFICIENT FLUID VOLUME. The patient receiving a diuretic is observed for dehydration and electrolyte imbalances. A fluid volume deficit is most likely to occur if the patient fails to drink a sufficient amount of fluid. This is especially true in the older or confused patient. To prevent a fluid volume deficit, encourage patients to drink adequate oral fluids (up to 2000 mL/day, unless contraindicated because of a medical condition). This is especially important when a person excessively perspires or has episodes of vomiting or diarrhea.

Electrolyte imbalances that may occur during therapy with a diuretic include hyponatremia (low blood sodium level) and hypokalemia (low blood potassium level), although other imbalances may also be seen. (See Chapter 54 for the signs and symptoms of electrolyte imbalances.) When administering aliskiren or eplerenone, monitor for hyperkalemia. The primary health care provider is notified if any signs or symptoms of an electrolyte imbalance occur.

RISK FOR INJURY. Dizziness or weakness along with orthostatic hypotension can occur with the administration of antihypertensive drugs. If orthostatic hypotension occurs, instruct the patient to rise slowly from a sitting or lying position. Explain how to rise from a lying position, by sitting on the edge of the bed for 1 or 2 minutes, which often minimizes these symptoms. In addition, rising slowly from a chair and then standing for 1 to 2 minutes also minimizes the symptoms of orthostatic hypotension. When symptoms of orthostatic hypotension, dizziness, or weakness do occur, teach the patient to call for assistance in getting out of bed or a chair and with ambulatory activities.

INEFFECTIVE SEXUALITY PATTERNS. Antihypertensive drugs can cause sexual dysfunction ranging from impotence to inhibition of ejaculation. Provide an open and understanding atmosphere when discussing sexuality. You can get literature in different languages that explains potential problems with sexual patterns that can occur with these drugs. If sexual patterns are affected negatively, suggest that the partners use other means of expressing caring, such as touching, massage, and personal closeness. Allow the patient time to express feelings and concerns and encourage the patient and partner to discuss ways to satisfy intimacy needs. You may suggest that the patient discuss the use of drugs for erectile dysfunction (ED) with the primary care provider. Many ED medications are safe to take with antihypertensives when the dose is modified.

ACTIVITY INTOLERANCE. Some patients on the antihypertensive drugs have decreased exercise tolerance and feel fatigued, weak, and lethargic. In addition, patients with hypertension may have other health problems (either cardiovascular or respiratory problems) that may affect their ability to perform activities. The patient is encouraged to walk and ambulate as he or she can tolerate. Assistive devices may be used if needed. Gradually increase tolerance by increasing the daily amount of activity. Plan rest periods according to the individual's tolerance. Rest can take many forms, such as sitting in a chair, napping, watching television, or sitting with legs elevated. Reassure the patient that often the fatigue diminishes after 4 to 6 weeks of therapy.

ACUTE PAIN. Patients taking the antihypertensive drugs may complain of a headache that could be an adverse reaction to the drugs, particularly antiadrenergics or the angiotensin II receptor blocking drugs. If the headache is acute, the patient may need to remain in bed with a cool cloth on the forehead, or offer the patient a back and neck rub. Relaxation techniques such as guided imagery or progressive body relaxation may prove helpful. If nursing measures are not successful, the primary health care provider is notified, because an analgesic may be required.

Educating the Patient and Family

Educate all patients on the importance of having their blood pressure checked at periodic intervals. This includes people of all ages, because hypertension is not a disease that affects only older individuals. Once hypertension is detected, patient teaching becomes an important factor in successfully returning the blood pressure to normal or near-normal levels.

To ensure lifetime adherence to the prescribed therapeutic regimen, emphasize the importance of drug therapy, as well as other treatments recommended by the primary health care provider. Educate the patient by describing the adverse reactions from a particular antihypertensive drug and advise the patient to contact the primary health care provider if any should occur.

The primary health care provider will want the patient or family to monitor blood pressure during therapy. If the patient purchases equipment, have him or her bring it in and teach the technique of taking blood pressure and pulse rate to the patient or family member, allowing sufficient time for supervised practice. If the patient or family is unable to do this, provide information on community resources where blood pressures are checked, such as local pharmacies or fire stations. Show the patient how to keep a record of the blood pressure and to bring this record to each visit to the primary health care provider's office or clinic. A wallet-size card can be obtained for use from the National Institutes of Health. As you develop a teaching plan include the following information:

- Never discontinue use of this drug except on the advice of the primary health care provider. These drugs control but do not cure hypertension. Skipping doses of the drug or voluntarily discontinuing the drug may cause severe rebound hypertension.

- Avoid the use of any nonprescription drugs (some may contain drugs that can increase the blood pressure) unless approved by the primary health care provider.

- ! Avoid alcohol unless its use has been approved by the primary health care provider.

- This drug may produce dizziness or lightheadedness when rising suddenly from a sitting or lying position. To avoid these effects, rise slowly from a sitting or lying position (see Patient Teaching for Improved Patient Outcomes: Preventing Injury From Orthostatic Hypotension).

- If the drug causes drowsiness, avoid hazardous tasks such as driving or performing tasks that require alertness. Drowsiness may disappear with time.

- If unexplained weakness or fatigue occurs, contact the primary health care provider.

- Follow the diet restrictions recommended by the primary health care provider. Do not use salt substitutes unless a particular brand of salt substitute is approved by the primary health care provider.

- Notify the primary health care provider if the diastolic pressure suddenly increases to 130 mm Hg or higher; this may signal a hypertensive emergency.

EVALUATION

- Therapeutic response is achieved and blood pressure is controlled.

Patient Teaching for Improved Patient Outcomes

Preventing Injury From Orthostatic Hypotension

Many patients receiving antihypertensive therapy commonly receive more than one drug, placing them at risk for orthostatic hypotension. If it occurs, the patient may fall and be injured. Teach the following measures to follow while in the acute care facility and at home:

- ✔ Place items close to the bed at night such as the cell phone to reduce need to sit up suddenly.
- ✔ Change your position slowly, and sleep with the head of the bed slightly elevated.
- ✔ Exercise calf muscles before getting out of bed or going from a sitting to standing position.
- ✔ Sit at the edge of the bed or chair for a few minutes before standing up.
- ✔ Stand for a few minutes before starting to walk.
- ✔ Avoid bending at the waist; use implements to reach items on the floor.
- ✔ Ask for assistance when necessary.
- ✔ If you feel dizzy or lightheaded, sit or lie down immediately.
- ✔ Make sure to drink adequate amounts of fluid throughout the day.

- Adverse reactions are identified, reported to the primary health care provider, and managed successfully with appropriate nursing interventions:
  - Proper fluid volume is maintained.
  - No evidence of injury is seen.
  - Patient is satisfied with sexual activity.
  - Patient engages in activity as able.
  - Patient is free of headache pain.

- Patient and family express confidence and demonstrate an understanding of the drug regimen.

PHARMACOLOGY IN PRACTICE
THINK CRITICALLY

 The primary health care provider asks you to explain to Mr. Alfredo Garcia how and where to monitor blood pressure readings on a weekly basis. As you compliment Mr. Garcia on his weight loss, he tells you nothing tastes good anymore. How will you educate a person with limited English proficiency about both diet and blood pressure measurement?

KEY POINTS

- Hypertension is defined by a blood pressure of 140/90 mm Hg or greater. Unchecked, it can lead to heart and kidney disease, heart failure, or stroke.

- Prehypertension exists when the blood pressure is 121/81 to 139/89 mm Hg, and the patient should engage in lifestyle modifications to reduce risk factors for the diseases mentioned.

- Primary hypertension is the term used when a direct cause is not established. When lifestyle changes do not reduce the pressures measured, then antihypertensive drugs are used to lower the blood pressure.

- Various drugs are used alone or in combinations to cause vasodilation and reduce the pressure in the circulatory system. This may be done through a direct effect on blood vessels or the various hormonal/glandular processes that impact blood pressure in the body.

- Common adverse reactions include headache, dizziness, and GI complaints. Many of the drug classes used can injure a developing fetus, so it is important to check for pregnancy in women and discuss birth control. Also, those older than 66 years are at a greater risk of hip fracture due to orthostatic hypotension.

Summary Drug Table ANTIHYPERTENSIVE DRUGS

Generic Name	Trade Name	Uses	Adverse Reactions	Dosage Ranges
β-Adrenergic Blocking Drugs				
acebutolol *ah-seh-byoo'-toe-loll*	Sectral	Hypertension, ventricular arrhythmias	Bradycardia, dizziness, weakness, hypotension, nausea, vomiting, diarrhea, nervousness	Hypertension: 400 mg orally in 1–2 doses
atenolol *ah-ten'-oh-loll*	Tenormin, Tenoretic	Hypertension, angina, acute myocardial infarction (MI)	Bradycardia, dizziness, fatigue, weakness, hypotension, nausea, vomiting, diarrhea, nervousness	Hypertension/angina: 50–200 mg/day orally
bisoprolol *bye-soe'-proe-loll*	Zebeta	Hypertension	Same as acebutolol	2.5–10 mg orally daily; maximum dose, 20 mg orally daily
metoprolol *meh-toe'-proe-loll*	Lopressor, Toprol-XL	Hypertension, angina, MI, HF	Dizziness, hypotension, HF, cardiac arrhythmia, nausea, vomiting, diarrhea	Hypertension/angina: 100–450 mg/day orally Extended release: 50–100 mg/day orally
nadolol *nay-doe'-loll*	Corgard	Hypertension, angina	Dizziness, hypotension, nausea, vomiting, diarrhea, HF, cardiac arrhythmia	Hypertension: 40–80 mg/day orally
nebivolol *neh-biv'-oh-loll*	Bystolic	Hypertension	Dizziness, headache, nausea, diarrhea, tingling extremities	5–40 mg/daily
penbutolol *pen-byoo'-toe-loll*	Levatol	Hypertension	Bradycardia, dizziness, hypotension, nausea, vomiting, diarrhea	20 mg orally daily
pindolol *pin'-doe-loll*		Hypertension	Bradycardia, dizziness, hypotension, nausea, vomiting, diarrhea	5–60 mg/day orally BID
propranolol *pro-pran'-oh-loll*	Inderal	Cardiac arrhythmias, MI, angina, hypertension, migraine prophylaxis, hypertrophic subaortic stenosis, pheochromocytoma, primary tremor	Bradycardia, dizziness, hypotension, nausea, vomiting, diarrhea, bronchospasm, hyperglycemia, pulmonary edema	Hypertension: 120–240 mg/day orally in divided doses
timolol *tih'-moe-loll*		Hypertension, MI, migraine prophylaxis	Dizziness, hypotension, nausea, vomiting, diarrhea, pulmonary edema	Hypertension: 10–40 mg/day orally in divided doses MI: 10 mg orally BID

Summary Drug Table ANTIHYPERTENSIVE DRUGS (continued)

Generic Name	Trade Name	Uses	Adverse Reactions	Dosage Ranges
Antiadrenergic Drugs: Centrally Acting				
clonidine *kloe'-nih-deen*	Catapres, Catapres-TTS (transdermal)	Hypertension, severe pain in patients with cancer	Drowsiness, dizziness, sedation, dry mouth, constipation, syncope, dreams, rash	100–600 mcg/day orally Transdermal: release rate 0.1–0.3 mg/24 hr
guanabenz *gwan'-ah-benz*		Hypertension	Dry mouth, sedation, dizziness, headache, weakness, arrhythmias	4–32 mg orally BID
guanfacine *gwan'-fah-seen*	Tenex	Hypertension	Dry mouth, somnolence, asthenia, dizziness, headache, constipation, fatigue	1–3 mg/day orally at bedtime
methyldopa or methyldopate *meth'-ill-doe-pah,* *meth'-ill-doe-pate*		Hypertension, hypertensive crisis	Bradycardia, aggravation of angina pectoris, HF, sedation, headache, rash, nausea, vomiting, nasal congestion	250 mg orally BID or TID; maintenance dose, 2 g/day; 250–500 mg q 6 hr IV
Antiadrenergic Drugs: Peripherally Acting				
doxazosin *dok-say-zoe'-sin*	Cardura	Hypertension, benign prostatic hyperplasia (BPH)	Headache, dizziness, fatigue	Hypertension: 1–8 mg orally daily BPH: 1–16 mg orally daily
prazosin *pray-zoe'-sin*	Minipress	Hypertension	Dizziness, postural hypotension, drowsiness, headache, loss of strength, palpitation, nausea	1–20 mg orally daily in divided doses
reserpine *reh-ser'-pyne*	Serpalan	Hypertension, psychosis	Bradycardia, dizziness, nausea, vomiting, diarrhea, nasal congestion	Hypertension: 0.1–0.5 mg orally daily Psychosis: 0.1–1 mg orally daily
terazosin *tare-ah'-zoe-sin*	Hytrin	Hypertension, BPH	Dizziness, postural hypotension, headache, dyspnea, nasal congestion	Hypertension: 1–20 mg orally daily BPH: 1–10 mg orally daily
α/β-Adrenergic Blocking Drugs				
carvedilol *car-veh'-dih-loll*	Coreg	Hypertension, HF, left ventricular dysfunction (LVD)	Bradycardia, hypotension, cardiac insufficiency, fatigue, dizziness, diarrhea	6.25–25 mg orally BID
labetalol *lah-beh'-tah-loll*	Trandate	Hypertension	Fatigue, drowsiness, insomnia, hypotension, impotence, diarrhea	200–400 mg/day orally in divided doses IV: 20 mg over 2 min with blood pressure monitoring, may repeat
Calcium Channel Blockers				
amlodipine *am-loe'-dih-peen*	Norvasc	Hypertension, chronic stable angina, vasospastic angina (Prinzmetal's angina)	Headache	Individualize dosage; 5–10 mg/day orally
clevidipine *kle-vid'-a-peen*	Cleviprex	Hypertension	Rebound hypertension	IV only when unable to provide oral therapy
diltiazem *dil-tye'-ah-zem*	Cardizem, Cardizem CD, Dilacor XR	Hypertension, chronic stable angina, atrial fibrillation/flutter, paroxysmal supraventricular tachycardia	Headache, dizziness, atrioventricular block, bradycardia, edema, dyspnea, rhinitis	Extended-release tablets/capsules—hypertension: 120–540 mg/day

(table continues on page 378)

Antihypertensive Drugs

Summary Drug Table ANTIHYPERTENSIVE DRUGS (continued)

Generic Name	Trade Name	Uses	Adverse Reactions	Dosage Ranges
felodipine *fell-oh'-dih-peen*	Plendil	Hypertension	Headache, dizziness	2.5–10 mg/day orally
isradipine *iz-rah'-dih-peen*	DynaCirc CR	Hypertension	Headache, edema	5–10 mg/day orally
nicardipine *nye-kar'-dih-peen*	Cardene, Cardene IV, Cardene SR	Hypertension, chronic stable angina	Headache	Hypertension: immediate release 20–40 mg/TID; extended release 30–60 mg/BID
nifedipine *nye-fed'-ih-peen*	Procardia, Procardia XL	Hypertension (sustained release only), vasospastic angina, chronic stable angina	Headache, dizziness, weakness, edema, nausea, muscle cramps, cough, nasal congestion, wheezing	10–20 mg TID orally; may increase to 120 mg/day Sustained release: 30–60 mg/day orally; may increase to 120 mg/day
nisoldipine *nye-sole'-dih-peen*	Sular	Hypertension	Headache, edema	20–40 mg/day orally
verapamil *ver-app'-ah-mill*	Calan, Calan SR, Verelan	Hypertension, chronic stable angina, vaso-spastic angina, chronic atrial flutter, paroxysmal superventricular tachycardia	Headache, constipation	Individualize dosage; do not exceed 480 mg/day orally in divided doses Sustained release: 120–180 mg/day orally; maximum dose, 480 mg Extended release: 120– 180 mg/day orally, maximum dose, 480 mg/day
Angiotensin-Converting Enzyme Inhibitors				
benazepril *ben-ah'-zeh-prill*	Lotensin	Hypertension	Headache, dizziness, fatigue	10–40 mg/day orally in single dose or two divided doses, maximum dose 80 mg
Ⓡ captopril *kap'-toe-prill*	Capoten	Hypertension, HF, LVD after MI, diabetic nephropathy	Rash	Hypertension: 25–100 mg/day orally in divided doses, not to exceed 450 mg/day
enalapril *eh-nal'-ah-prill*	Vasotec, Enalaprilat	Hypertension, HF, asymptomatic LVD	Headache, dizziness	Hypertension: 5–40 mg/day orally as a single dose or in two divided doses CHF: 2.5–20 mg BID
fosinopril *foh-sin'-oh-prill*		Hypertension, HF	Dizziness, cough	10–40 mg/day orally in a single dose or two divided doses
lisinopril *lye-sin'-oh-prill*	Prinivil, Zestril	Hypertension, HF, post-MI	Headache, dizziness, diarrhea, orthostatic hypotension, cough	Hypertension: 10–40 mg/day orally as a single dose
Ⓡ moexipril *moe-ex'-ah-prill*	Univasc	Hypertension	Dizziness, cough, bronchospasm	7.5–30 mg orally as a single dose or two divided doses
perindopril *per-in'-doh-prill*	Aceon	Hypertension	Dizziness, headache, cough, upper respiratory infection (URI) symptoms, asthenia	4–8 mg/day orally, maximum dose 16 mg
quinapril *kwin'-ah-prill*	Accupril	Hypertension, HF	Dizziness	Hypertension: 10–80 mg/day orally as a single dose or two divided doses
ramipril *rah-mih'-prill*	Altace	Hypertension, HF, decrease risk of cardio-vascular disease, coro-nary artery disease	Dizziness, cough	Hypertension: 2.5–20 mg/day orally as a single dose or two divided doses
trandolapril *tran-dole'-ah-prill*	Mavik	Hypertension, patients post-MI with symptoms of HF and LVD	Dizziness, cough	Hypertension: 1–4 mg/day orally

Summary Drug Table ANTIHYPERTENSIVE DRUGS (continued)

Generic Name	Trade Name	Uses	Adverse Reactions	Dosage Ranges
Angiotensin II Receptor Antagonists				
azilsartan *ay'-zil-sar-tan*	Edarbi	Hypertension	Dizziness, fainting, diarrhea	80 mg orally daily
candesartan *can-dah-sar'-tan*	Atacand	Hypertension, HF	Dizziness, URI symptoms	8–32 mg/day orally in divided doses
eprosartan *ep-roe-sar'-tan*	Teveten	Hypertension	Cough, URI, and urinary tract infection symptoms	400–800 mg/day orally in two divided doses
irbesartan *er-beh-sar'-tan*	Avapro	Hypertension, nephropathy in type 2 diabetes	Headache, URI symptoms	150–300 mg/day orally as one dose
losartan *loe-sar'-tan*	Cozaar	Hypertension, hypertension in patients with LVD, diabetic nephropathy in type 2 diabetes	Dizziness, URI symptoms	Hypertension: 25–100 mg/day orally in one or two doses
olmesartan *ol-mah-sar'-tan*	Benicar	Hypertension	Dizziness	20–40 mg/day orally
telmisartan *tell-mah-sar'-tan*	Micardis	Hypertension	Diarrhea, URI symptoms, sinusitis	40–80 mg/day orally
valsartan *val-sar'-tan*	Diovan	Hypertension, HF, post-MI	Viral infections	Hypertension: 80–320 mg/day orally
Direct Renin Inhibitors				
aliskiren *ah-liss-kye'-ren*	Tekturna	Hypertension	Diarrhea, URI symptoms	150 mg/day orally, may increase to 300 mg/day
Selective Aldosterone Receptor Antagonists				
eplerenone *eh-pler'-eh-noan*	Inspra	Hypertension, HF	Hyperkalemia	50 mg/day orally, may increase to 100 mg/day

Ⓡ This drug should be administered at least 1 hour before or 2 hours after a meal.

● Chapter Review

Know Your Drugs

Clients sometimes know a medication by the brand (or trade) name and not the generic name. To help you recognize both names, match the brand name with the generic name of the same medication.

Generic Name	Brand Name
1. lisinopril	A. Altace
2. moexipril	B. Mavik
3. ramipril	C. Prinivil
4. trandolapril	D. Univasc

Calculate Medication Dosages

1. Oral nadolol 80 mg is prescribed. The drug is available in 40-mg tablets. The nurse administers _____.

2. Nifedipine 10-mg capsules are available. How many capsules will the client be instructed to take when the dose is 30 mg?

● Prepare for the NCLEX®

Build Your Knowledge

1. The best description of how antihypertensives work is that they:
   1. promote workload of the heart
   2. vasodilate vessels to reduce pressure
   3. increase angiotensin production
   4. increase reabsorption of sodium in the nephron

2. Which of the following pressures is considered prehypertension?
   1. 110/80
   2. 122/70
   3. 136/84
   4. 145/92

3. The nurse instructs the client using the transdermal system Catapres-TTS to _____.
   1. place the patch on the torso and keep it in place for 24 hours
   2. change placement of the patch every day after bathing
   3. place the patch on the upper arm or torso and keep it in place for 7 days
   4. avoid getting the patch wet because it might detach from the skin

4. To avoid symptoms associated with orthostatic hypotension, the nurse advises the client to _____.
   1. sleep in a side-lying position
   2. avoid sitting for prolong periods
   3. change position slowly
   4. get up from a sitting position quickly

5. During the preadministration assessment of a client prescribed an antihypertensive drug, the nurse _____.
   1. places the client in a high Fowler's position
   2. places the client in a supine position
   3. darkens the room to decrease stimuli
   4. takes the client's blood pressure

Apply Your Knowledge

6. Before the first dose of an ACEI, the nurse monitors a female client for _____.
   1. elevated cardiac enzymes
   2. positive pregnancy test
   3. low serum sodium
   4. complete blood count

7. The nurse gives the following instruction to the client when discontinuing use of an antihypertensive drug:
   1. Monitor the blood pressure every hour for 8 hours after the drug therapy is discontinued
   2. Gradually decrease the medication over a period of 2 to 4 days to avoid rebound hypertension
   3. Check the blood pressure and pulse every 30 minutes after discontinuing the drug therapy
   4. Expect to taper the dosage of the drug over a period of 2 weeks to avoid a return of hypertension

8. Nifedipine extended-release tablets are prescribed. A nasogastric (NG) tube has recently been placed in the client. The nurse should:
   1. give the drug as ordered orally
   2. crush the tablet and give via the NG tube
   3. contact the primary health care provider for a new order
   4. return the medication unused to the pharmacy

Alternate-Format Questions

9. Which of the following drugs should not be taken with food? **Select all that apply**.
   1. captopril
   2. fosinopril
   3. moexipril
   4. ramipril

10. Diltiazem 180 mg is prescribed. The drug is available in 60-mg, 90-mg, and 120-mg tablets. Which tablet should you select as it is least likely to cause drug errors? How many tablets would you administer? _____

To check your answers, see Appendix G.

the**Point** *For more NCLEX-style questions, log on to http://thepoint.lww.com to access more than 1000 questions.*

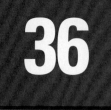

36

Antianginal and Vasodilating Drugs

LEARNING OBJECTIVES

On completion of this chapter, the student will:

1. Describe the two types of antianginal drugs.
2. Discuss the general actions, uses, adverse reactions, contraindications, precautions, and interactions of antianginal and vasodilating drugs.
3. Discuss important preadministration and ongoing assessment activities the nurse should perform on the patient taking an antianginal or vasodilating drug.
4. List nursing diagnoses particular to a patient taking an antianginal or vasodilating drug.
5. Discuss ways to promote an optimal response to therapy, how to manage common adverse reactions, and important points to keep in mind when educating patients about the use of antianginal or vasodilating drugs.

KEY TERMS

angina • acute pain in the chest resulting from decreased blood supply to the heart muscle

atherosclerosis • disease characterized by deposits of fatty plaques on the inner walls of arteries

buccal • space in the mouth between the gum and the cheek in either the upper or lower jaw

prophylaxis • prevention

sublingual • under the tongue

topical • pertaining to a substance applied directly to the skin by patch, ointment, gel, or other formulation

transdermal system • drug delivery system by which the drug is applied to and absorbed through the skin

DRUG CLASSES

Nitrates
Calcium channel blockers

Atherosclerosis is a disease characterized by deposits of fatty plaques on the inner walls of arteries. These deposits result in a narrowing of the lumen (inside diameter) of the artery and a decrease in blood supply to the area served by the artery. Diseases of the arteries can cause serious problems: coronary artery disease, cerebral vascular disease, and peripheral vascular disease. Drug therapy for vascular diseases may include drugs that dilate blood vessels and thereby increase blood supply to an area.

This chapter discusses drugs whose primary purpose is to increase blood supply to an area by dilating blood vessels. Vasodilating drugs relax the smooth muscle layer of arterial blood vessels, which results in vasodilation, an increase in the size of blood vessels, primarily small arteries and arterioles. Because peripheral, cerebral, or coronary artery disease usually results in decreased blood flow to an area, drugs that dilate narrowed arterial vessels permit the vessels to carry more blood, resulting in an increase in blood flow to the affected area. Increasing the blood flow to an area may result in complete or partial relief of symptoms. In some cases, however, drug therapy provides only minimal and temporary relief. Many of the calcium channel blockers and vasodilating drugs are also used to treat hypertension. Their use as antihypertensives is discussed in Chapter 35.

Angina is a disorder characterized by atherosclerotic plaque formation in the coronary arteries, which causes decreased

PHARMACOLOGY IN PRACTICE

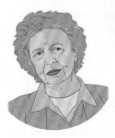

Mrs. Moore was hospitalized with severe chest pain and a possible myocardial infarction. After tests were completed, her primary health care provider prescribed sublingual nitroglycerin for her angina. Her daughter is calling about severe pain. As you assess the situation you find out it is not her heart but what the daughter calls "severe migraine headaches." As you read this chapter determine if this pain is related to cardiac function or medications.

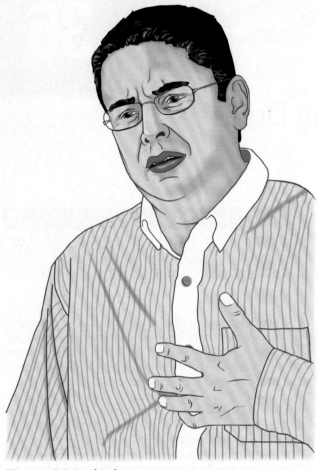

Figure 36.1 Angina can present as pressure or discomfort as well as a sharp pain.

oxygen supply to the heart muscle and results in chest pain or pressure (Fig. 36.1). Any activity that increases the workload of the heart, such as exercise or simply climbing stairs, can precipitate a painful angina attack. Antianginal drugs relieve chest pain or pressure by dilating coronary arteries, increasing the blood supply to the myocardium.

The antianginal drugs include the nitrates and the calcium channel blockers. Chapter 25 and its Summary Drug Table: Adrenergic Blocking Drugs discuss the adrenergic blocking drugs that also are used to treat angina and other disorders.

Actions

The *nitrates* act by relaxing the smooth muscle layer of blood vessels, increasing the lumen of the artery or arteriole, and increasing the amount of blood flowing through the vessels.

Calcium channel blockers have several effects on the heart:

- Slowing the conduction velocity of the cardiac impulse
- Depressing myocardial contractility
- Dilating coronary arteries and arterioles, which in turn deliver more oxygen to cardiac muscle

Dilation of peripheral arteries reduces the workload of the heart. The end effect of these drugs is the same as that of the

nitrates. An increased blood flow results in an increase in the oxygen supply to surrounding tissues.

Uses

The antianginal drugs are used in the treatment of cardiac disease to:

- Relieve pain of acute anginal attacks
- Prevent angina attacks (**prophylaxis**)
- Treat chronic stable angina pectoris

Typically the nitrate group of drugs is used to relieve symptoms when an anginal attack happens, as opposed to the use of the "blocking" drugs to prevent angina from occurring by taking the drug on a regular basis.

Intravenous (IV) nitroglycerin is used to control perioperative hypertension associated with surgical procedures. Calcium channel blocking drugs are also used to treat hypertension (see Chapter 35) and other cardiac conditions. For example, verapamil affects the conduction system of the heart and is used to treat cardiac arrhythmias. See the Summary Drug Table: Antianginal and Vasodilating Drugs for additional uses of the nitrates and calcium channel blockers.

Adverse Reactions

Adverse reactions to the calcium channel blocking drugs usually are not serious and rarely require discontinuation of the drug therapy (see Chapter 35 for specifics). Adverse reactions associated with the nitrates include the following:

- Central nervous system (CNS) reactions, such as headache (may be severe and persistent), dizziness, weakness, and restlessness
- Other body system reactions, such as hypotension, flushing (caused by dilation of small capillaries near the surface of the skin), and rash

The nitrates are available in various forms (e.g., **sublingual**, translingual spray, transdermal, and parenteral). Some adverse reactions are a result of the method of administration. For example, sublingual nitroglycerin may cause a local burning or tingling in the oral cavity. However, the patient must be aware that an absence of this effect does not indicate a decrease in the drug's potency. Contact dermatitis may occur from use of the transdermal delivery system.

In many instances, the adverse reactions associated with the nitrates lessen and often disappear with prolonged use of the drug. However, for some patients, these adverse reactions become severe, and the primary health care provider may lower the dose until symptoms subside. The dose may then be slowly increased if the lower dosage does not provide relief from the symptoms of angina. See the Summary Drug Table: Antianginal and Vasodilating Drugs for more information.

Contraindications and Precautions

Nitrates are contraindicated in patients with known hypersensitivity to the drugs, severe anemia, closed-angle glaucoma, postural hypertension, early myocardial infarction (sublingual form), head trauma, cerebral hemorrhage (may increase intracranial hemorrhage), allergy to adhesive (transdermal system), or constrictive pericarditis. Patients taking phosphodiesterase inhibitors (drugs for erectile dysfunction) should not use nitrates.

Nitrates are used cautiously in patients with the following:

• Severe hepatic or renal disease
• Severe head trauma
• Hypothyroidism

These drugs are used cautiously during pregnancy and lactation (pregnancy category C).

Interactions

The following interactions may occur when the nitrates are used with another agent:

Interacting Drug	Common Use	Effect of Interaction
aspirin	Pain reliever	Increased nitrate plasma concentrations and action may occur
calcium channel blockers	Treatment of angina	Increased symptomatic orthostatic hypotension
dihydroergotamine	Migraine headache treatment	Increased risk of hypertension and decreased antianginal effect
heparin	Anticoagulant	Decreased effect of heparin
phosphodiesterase inhibitors	Erectile dysfunction (ED)	Severe hypotension and cardiovascular collapse may occur
alcohol	Relaxation and enjoyment of social situations	Severe hypotension and cardiovascular collapse may occur

NURSING PROCESS
PATIENT RECEIVING AN ANTIANGINAL DRUG

ASSESSMENT

Preadministration Assessment
The person using an antianginal drug for episodic pain is typically an outpatient; therefore, instruction about use is an essential intervention. When you engage in a teaching session, first conduct and document a thorough pain assessment (see Chapter 14) as well as a history of allergy to the nitrates or calcium channel blockers and of other disease processes that would contraindicate administration of the drug. Display 36.1 lists angina-specific example questions. Remember to assess the patient's health literacy by asking about what he or she may think causes the pain. Also, ask what remedies the patient has used to relieve the pain and whether he or she is able to read and understand directions that you will prepare for the patient.

Be sure to assess the physical appearance of the patient (e.g., skin color, lesions) and auscultate the lungs for adventitious sounds. Tests frequently include a baseline electrocardiogram, stress test, chest x-ray, and laboratory panels. Include weighing the patient when you perform vital signs and note any problem with orthostatic hypotension.

Ongoing Assessment
As a part of the ongoing assessment, monitor the patient for the frequency and severity of any episodes of anginal pain. This assessment may be conducted by telephone for the patient at home. With treatment, the patient may expect that episodes of angina should be eliminated or decrease in frequency and severity. Instruct the patient to call for emergency assistance if the chest pain does not respond to three doses of nitroglycerin given every 5 minutes for 15 minutes.

Teach the patient or caregiver to monitor vital signs frequently during administration of the antianginals. If the patient's heart rate falls below 50 bpm or the systolic blood pressure drops below 90 mm Hg, hold the drug and notify the primary health care provider. A dosage adjustment may be necessary. For the patient at home, instruct the patient or the caregiver to also call the primary health care provider and ask if the drug should be given for the next episode of heart-related pain.

Assess patients receiving the calcium channel blockers for signs of heart failure (HF): dyspnea, weight gain, peripheral edema, abnormal lung sounds (crackles/rales), and jugular vein distention. Any symptoms of HF are reported promptly to the primary health care provider. The dosage may be increased more rapidly in hospitalized patients under close supervision. When the drug is being titrated to a therapeutic dose, the patient is typically monitored by telemetry.

Display 36.1 Angina-Specific Pain Assessment

History
• Describe the pain (e.g., tightness, pressure, sharp, stabbing).
• Location—is it in a specific place or generalized?
• Does the pain spread and where does it spread?
• Does it start suddenly or is it gradual? How long does it last?
• What events tend to cause anginal pain (e.g., exercise, emotion, other triggers)?
• What makes it feel worse (e.g., movement, breathing, activity)?
• What seems to relieve the pain (e.g., resting, position change)?

NURSING DIAGNOSES

Drug-specific nursing diagnoses include the following:

- **Risk for Injury** related to hypotension, dizziness, light-headedness
- **Pain** related to narrowing of peripheral arteries, decreased blood supply to the extremities

Nursing diagnoses related to drug administration are discussed in Chapter 4.

PLANNING

The expected outcomes of the patient depend on the specific reason for administering the drug but may include an optimal response to therapy, support of patient needs related to the management of adverse reactions, and confidence in an understanding of the medication regimen.

IMPLEMENTATION

Promoting an Optimal Response to Therapy

NITRATES—STOPPING AN ATTACK. Nitrates may be administered by the sublingual (under the tongue), buccal (between the cheek and gum), oral, IV, or transdermal route. If the buccal form of nitroglycerin has been prescribed, you may want to show the patient how and where to place the tablet in the mouth by using a small sugarless candy. Be sure the patient understands that absorption of sublingual and buccal forms depends on salivary secretion and a dry mouth may decrease the effect.

Nitroglycerin may also be administered by a metered spray canister that is used to stop an acute anginal attack. Be sure the patient understands that the spray is directed from the canister onto or under the tongue. Each dose is metered so that when the canister top is depressed, the same dose is delivered each time. Instruct the patient not to shake the canister or inhale the spray. For some individuals, this is more convenient than placing small tablets under the tongue.

> **NURSING ALERT**
>
> The dose of sublingual nitroglycerin may be repeated every 5 minutes until pain is relieved or until the patient has received three doses in a 15-minute period. One to two sprays of translingual nitroglycerin may be used to relieve angina, but no more than three metered doses are recommended within a 15-minute period.

When the pain is not relieved or worsens or the frequency of attacks increases in the inpatient setting, the primary health care provider is notified, because a change in the dosage of the drug or morphine may be ordered for pain relief.

Administering Oral Nitrates. Nitrates are also available as oral tablets that are swallowed. The sustained-released preparation may not be crushed or chewed.

Administering Nitroglycerin Ointment. The dose of topical (ointment) nitroglycerin is measured in inches or millimeters. Check the vital signs frequently, and if the blood pressure is appreciably lower or the pulse rate higher than the patient's baseline, contact the primary health care provider before applying the drug. The first step in application is to remove the paper from the previous application, fold the paper so no one can touch the drug, and cleanse the area. Applicator paper is supplied with the drug; one paper is used for each application. Wear disposable gloves to prevent contact with the ointment. While holding the paper, express the prescribed amount of ointment from the tube onto the paper. Use the applicator or dose-measured paper to gently spread a thin uniform layer over at least a $2^1/_4$- by $3^1/_2$-inch area. The ointment is usually applied to the chest or back. Application sites are rotated to prevent inflammation of the skin. Areas that may be used for application include the chest (front and back), abdomen, and upper arms and legs. After application of the ointment, you may secure the paper with nonallergenic tape.

> **NURSING ALERT**
>
> Do not rub the nitroglycerin ointment into the patient's skin, because this will immediately deliver a large amount of the drug through the skin. Exercise care in applying topical nitroglycerin and do not allow the ointment to come in contact with your fingers or hands while measuring or applying the ointment, because the drug will be absorbed through your skin, causing a severe headache.

Administering Transdermal Nitroglycerin. For most people, nitroglycerin transdermal systems are more convenient and easier to use because the drug is absorbed through the skin. A transdermal system has the drug imbedded in a pad. The primary health care provider may prescribe the system to be applied to the skin once a day for 10 to 12 hours. Tolerance to the vascular and antianginal effects of the nitrates may develop, particularly in patients taking higher dosages, those who are prescribed longer-acting products, or those who are on more frequent dosing schedules. Patients using the transdermal nitroglycerin patches are particularly prone to tolerance, because the nitroglycerin is released at a constant rate, and steady plasma concentrations are maintained. Applying the patch in the morning and leaving it in place for 10 to 12 hours, followed by leaving the patch off for 10 to 12 hours, typically yields better results and delays tolerance to the drug.

When applying the transdermal system, inspect the skin site to be sure it is dry, free of hair, and not subject to excessive rubbing or movement. If needed, shave the application site. The transdermal system should be applied at the same time each day and the placement sites should be rotated. Optimal sites include the chest, abdomen, and thighs. The system is not applied to distal extremities. The best time to apply the transdermal system is after daily care (bed bath, shower, tub bath), because it is important that the skin be clean and thoroughly dry before applying the system. When removing the system, fold the adhesive side onto itself to prevent adhesion to another person or pet. To avoid errors in applying and removing the patch, the person applying the patch uses a fiber-tipped pen to write his or her name (or initials), date, and time of application on the top side of the patch; also document location in the record. Patches should be removed before cardioversion or defibrillation to prevent patient burns.

Administering IV Nitroglycerin. IV nitroglycerin is diluted in normal saline solution or 5% dextrose in water (D₅W) for continuous infusion using an infusion pump to ensure an accurate rate. Because nitroglycerin can be absorbed by plastic, the drug comes in glass IV bottles and special infusion sets provided by the manufacturer. Nurses regulate the dosage according to the patient's response and the primary health care provider's instructions. Nitroglycerin solutions should not be mixed with any other drugs or blood products.

CALCIUM CHANNEL BLOCKERS—PREVENTING AN ATTACK. With a few exceptions, the calcium channel blockers may be taken without regard to meals. If gastrointestinal upset occurs, the drug may be taken with meals. Verapamil frequently causes gastric upset and should routinely be given with meals. Verapamil tablets may be opened and sprinkled on foods or mixed in liquids. Sometimes the tablet coverings of verapamil are expelled in the stool. This causes no change in the effect of the drug and need not cause the patient concern.

For patients who have difficulty swallowing diltiazem (except Dilacor XR), tablets can be crushed and mixed with food or liquids. However, the patient should swallow the sustained-released tablets whole and not chew or divide them.

ADMINISTERING VASODILATING DRUGS. Carefully monitor the patient receiving minoxidil, because the drug increases the heart rate. The primary health care provider is notified if any of the following occur:

■ Heart rate of 20 bpm or more above the normal rate
■ Rapid weight gain of 5 lb or more
■ Unusual swelling of the extremities, face, or abdomen
■ Dyspnea, angina, severe indigestion, or fainting

Monitoring and Managing Patient Needs
Carefully monitor patients receiving these drugs for adverse reactions. Hypotension may be accompanied by paradoxical bradycardia and increased angina. Adverse reactions such as headache, flushing, and postural hypotension that are seen with the administration of the antianginal drugs often become less severe or even disappear after a period of time.

 LIFESPAN CONSIDERATIONS
Men
Quality of life has been enhanced for some patients with the advent of drugs for erectile dysfunction (phosphodiesterase inhibitors). When taken with nitrates, severe hypotension can occur; their use is contraindicated. Always assess for and discuss the use of erectile dysfunction drugs when a male patient is prescribed a nitrate preparation.

RISK FOR INJURY. When postural hypotension is suspected, be sure to offer assistance with all ambulatory activities. Instruct those with episodes of postural hypotension to take the drug in a sitting or supine position and to remain in that position until symptoms disappear. The blood pressure should be frequently monitored in the patient with dizziness or lightheadedness.

 LIFESPAN CONSIDERATIONS
Adolescents and Young Adults
"Rush poppers" (amyl nitrite, butyl nitrite, and isobutyl nitrite) are popular among the gay community and young people at clubs and raves. The head rush, euphoria, uncontrollable laughter or giggling, and other sensations that result from the blood pressure drop are often felt to increase sexual arousal and desire. Historically, amyl nitrite was used to treat angina. Amyl nitrite and several other alkyl nitrites used in over-the-counter products such as air fresheners and video head cleaners are also inhaled to enhance sexual pleasure. The reduction in blood pressure can result in loss of balance and fainting, especially if people are involved in physical activity like dancing. The likelihood of accidents can increase, and people with heart conditions or high blood pressure are at greater risk. Inquire about popper use when injury and low blood pressure are presenting symptoms in the urgent care or emergency department.

PAIN. In some patients, the anginal pain may be entirely relieved, whereas in others it may be less intense or less frequent or may occur only with prolonged exercise. Document all information in the patient's record, because this helps the primary health care provider plan future therapy as well as make dosage adjustments if required.

Educating the Patient and Family
The patient and family should have a thorough understanding of the treatment of chest pain with an antianginal drug. These drugs are used either to prevent angina from occurring or to relieve the pain of angina. Explain the therapeutic regimen (dose, time of day the drug is taken, how often to take the drug, how to take or apply the drug) to the patient. Include the following general areas, as well as those points relevant to specific routes of administration of the drug, in a teaching plan:

■ ♥ Avoid the use of alcohol unless use has been permitted by the primary health care provider.
■ Notify your emergency response providers if the drug does not relieve pain or if pain becomes more intense despite use of this drug.
■ Follow the recommendations of the primary health care provider regarding frequency of use.
■ Keep an adequate supply of the drug on hand for events, such as vacations, bad weather conditions, and holidays.
■ Keep a record of the frequency of acute anginal attacks (date, time of the attack, drug, and dose used to relieve the acute pain), and bring this record to each primary health care provider or clinic visit.

For more teaching points related specifically to administration routes of nitrates, see the Patient Teaching for Improved Patient Outcomes: Directions for Administering Nitrates.

Patient Teaching for Improved Patient Outcomes

Directions for Administering Nitrates

General Instructions

✔ Headaches result from vasodilation and are an uncomfortable adverse reaction. If headache persists or becomes severe, notify the primary health care provider, because a change in dosage may be needed. Do not try to avoid headaches by altering the treatment schedule or dose. Ask about aspirin or acetaminophen for headache relief.

✔ Sit or lie down when you take your nitroglycerin. To relieve severe lightheadedness or dizziness, lie down, elevate the extremities, move the extremities, and breathe deeply.

✔ Store capsules and tablets in their original containers, because nitroglycerin must be kept in a dark container and protected from exposure to light. Never mix this drug with any other drug in a container. Nitroglycerin will lose its potency if stored in containers made of plastic or if mixed with other drugs.

✔ Always replace the cover or cap of the container as soon as the oral drug or ointment is removed from the container or tube. Replace caps or covers tightly, because the drug deteriorates on contact with air.

✔ Seek prompt medical attention if chest pain persists, changes character, increases in severity, or is not relieved by following the recommended dosing regimen.

✔ Do not use erectile dysfunction drugs while taking nitrates.

Oral Nitrates

✔ The drug works best on an empty stomach; if nausea occurs take the preparation with food.

Sublingual or Buccal Nitrates

✔ Do not handle the tablets any more than necessary. Perform thorough hand hygiene after use.

✔ Place the buccal tablet between the cheek and gum or between the upper lip and gum above the incisors.

✔ Do not swallow or chew sublingual or transmucosal tablets; allow them to dissolve slowly. The tablet may cause a burning or tingling in the mouth. Absence of this effect does not indicate a decrease in potency. A dry mouth lessens absorption; you may want to rinse with water *before* placing the tablet in your cheek.

Translingual (Aerosol Spray) Nitrates

✔ Directions for use of translingual nitroglycerin are supplied with the product. Follow the instructions regarding using and cleaning the canister.
  ■ This drug may be used prophylactically 5 to 10 minutes before engaging in activities that precipitate an anginal attack.
  ■ Do not shake the canister before use.

✔ At the onset of an anginal attack, spray 1 to 2 metered doses onto or under the tongue. Do not exceed 3 metered doses within 15 minutes.

Topical Ointment or Transdermal System

✔ Instructions for application of the topical ointment or transdermal system are available with the product. Read these instructions carefully.
  ■ Apply the topical ointment or topical transdermal system at approximately the same time each day.
  ■ Remove the old system and inspect the body to be sure no other papers or systems have been missed.

✔ Be sure the area is clean and thoroughly dry before applying the topical ointment or transdermal system, and rotate the application sites. Apply the transdermal system to the chest (front and back), abdomen, and upper legs. Firmly press the patch to ensure contact with the skin. If the transdermal system comes off or becomes loose, apply a new system. Apply the topical ointment to the front or the back of the chest. If applying to the back, another person should apply the ointment.

✔ When using the topical ointment form or transdermal system, cleanse old application sites with soap and warm water as soon as the ointment or transdermal system is removed. Fold the old patch in half to prevent adherence to others.

✔ To use the topical ointment, apply a thin layer on the skin using the paper applicator (the patient or family member may need practice regarding this technique). Avoid finger contact with the ointment.

✔ Wear disposable gloves when applying the ointment.

✔ Notify the primary health care provider if any of the following occurs: increased severity of chest pain or discomfort, irregular heartbeat, palpitations, nausea, shortness of breath, swelling of the hands or feet, or severe and prolonged episodes of lightheadedness and dizziness.

✔ Make position changes slowly to minimize hypotensive effects.

✔ Because these drugs can cause dizziness or drowsiness, do not drive or engage in hazardous activities until response to the drug is known.

EVALUATION

■ Therapeutic response is achieved.

■ Adverse reactions are identified, reported to the primary health care provider, and managed successfully with appropriate nursing interventions:
  • No evidence of injury is seen.
  • Pain is relieved.

■ Patient and family express confidence and demonstrate an understanding of the drug regimen.

PHARMACOLOGY IN PRACTICE
THINK CRITICALLY

 What you have discovered in your phone conversation is that Mrs. Moore is actually chewing the sublingual tablets, which is causing the vasodilation of cerebral arteries and headache. After reading this chapter, what do you think would be a better alternative?

KEY POINTS

• When the fatty deposits of atherosclerosis involve the coronary vessels supplying the heart, anginal pain can occur. Other diseases of the arteries can cause serious problems: coronary artery disease, cerebral vascular disease, and peripheral vascular disease.

• Antianginal drugs vasodilate and relax the smooth muscle of arterioles around the heart; this promotes blood flow and reduces pain. Some drugs are used for immediate relief of pain; others are used routinely to prevent

painful episodes. These drugs are administered in multiple ways, from different oral to topical preparations.

• Because the purpose of these drugs is to vasodilate, that is also a concern with the adverse reactions. Headache, from rapid vasodilation of cerebral arteries, is a very unpleasant reaction. Also, men taking antianginals need to be assessed and cautioned for use of erectile dysfunction medications because these drugs also cause vasodilation.

Summary Drug Table ANTIANGINAL AND VASODILATING DRUGS

Generic Name	Trade Name	Uses	Adverse Reactions	Dosage Ranges
Nitrates				
isosorbide *eye-soe-sor'-byde*	Isordil, Dilatate SR, Monoket	Treatment and prevention of angina	Headache, hypotension, dizziness, weakness, flushing, restlessness, rash	Initial dose 5–20 mg orally; maintenance dose 10–40 mg BID, TID orally Sublingually: 2.5–5 mg Prevention: 5–10 mg sublingually, 5 mg chewable
nitroglycerin, parenteral form *nye-troe-glih'-ser-in*		Angina, HF, perioperative hypertension, induce intraoperative hypotension	Same as isosorbide	Initially 5 mcg/min by IV infusion pump; may increase to 20 mcg/min postoperative period
nitroglycerin, oral	Nitrostat (sublingual) Nitrolingual Pump Spray, NitroMist (aerosol used sublingually)	Acute relief of an attack or prophylaxis of angina	Same as isosorbide dinitrate	1 tablet under tongue or in buccal pouch at first sign of an acute anginal attack—may repeat every 5 min until relief or 3 tablets have been taken Pump spray: 1–2 metered doses onto or under the tongue; maximum of 3 metered doses in 15 min
nitroglycerin, ointment		Prevention and treatment of angina	Same as isosorbide dinitrate	Used supplied ruled papers to give ½–2 inches twice daily
nitroglycerin transdermal systems	Minitran, Nitro-Dur	Prevention of angina	Same as isosorbide dinitrate	One system daily, 0.2–0.8 mg/hr

(table continues on page 388)

Antianginal and Vasodilating Drugs

Summary Drug Table ANTIANGINAL AND VASODILATING DRUGS (continued)

Generic Name	Trade Name	Uses	Adverse Reactions	Dosage Ranges
Calcium Channel Blockers				
amlodipine *am-low'-dih-peen*	Norvasc	Hypertension, chronic stable angina, vasospastic angina (Prinzmetal's angina)	Headache	Individualize dosage; 5–10 mg/day orally
diltiazem *dill-tye'-ah-zem*	Cardizem, Cardizem CD, Dilacor XR	Hypertension, chronic stable angina, atrial fibrillation/flutter, paroxysmal superventricular tachycardia	Headache, dizziness, atrioventricular block, bradycardia, edema, dyspnea, rhinitis	Extended-release tablets/capsules: Angina: 120–580 mg/day Exertional angina—immediate-release tablets: 30 mg/QID Heart arrhythmias—injection: 0.25 mg/kg over 2 min, then titrated continuous infusion
nicardipine *nye-kar'-deh-peen*	Cardene, Cardene IV, Cardene SR	Hypertension, chronic stable angina	Headache	Angina: individualize dosage; immediate-release only, 20–40 mg TID orally
nifedipine *nye-fed'-ih-peen*	Procardia, Procardia XL	Vasospastic angina (Prinzmetal's variant angina), chronic stable angina, hypertension (sustained release only)	Headache, dizziness, weakness, edema, nausea, muscle cramps, cough, nasal congestion, wheezing	10–20 mg TID orally; may increase to 120 mg/day Sustained release: 30–60 mg/day orally; may increase to 120 mg/day
nimodipine *nye-moe'-dih-peen*		Subarachnoid hemorrhage	Headache, hypotension, diarrhea	60 mg every 4 hr orally
ranolazine *ra-noe'-la-zeen*	Ranexa	Chronic angina	Dizziness, headache, nausea, constipation	500–1000 mg orally, twice daily
verapamil *ver-ap'-ah-mill*	Calan, Calan SR, Verelan	Hypertension, chronic stable angina, vasospastic angina (Prinzmetal's variant angina), chronic atrial flutter, paroxysmal superventricular tachycardia	Headache, constipation	Individualize dosage; do not exceed 480 mg/day orally in divided doses Sustained release: 120–180 mg/day orally; maximum dose, 480 mg Extended release: 120–180 mg/day orally, maximum dose, 480 mg/day Parenteral: 5–10 mg IV over 2 min
Peripheral Vasodilators				
hydralazine *hye-drah'-lah-zeen*		Primary hypertension (oral); when need to lower blood pressure is urgent (parenteral)	Dizziness, palpitations, tachycardia, numbness/tingling in legs, nasal congestion	10–50 mg QID orally, up to 300 mg/day; 20–40 mg IM or IV
minoxidil *mih-nok'-sih-dill*		Severe hypertension	Dizziness, hypotension, electrocardiogram changes, tachycardia, sodium and water retention, gynecomastia, hair growth	5–100 mg/day orally; dose greater than 5 mg given in divided doses
nitroprusside *nye-troe-pruss'-syde*	Nitropress	Hypertensive crisis	Apprehension, headache, restlessness, nausea, vomiting, palpitations, diaphoresis	3 mcg/kg/min, not to exceed infusion rate of 10 mcg/min (if blood pressure is not reduced within 10 min, discontinue administration)

● Chapter Review

Know Your Drugs

Clients sometimes know a medication by the brand (or trade) name and not the generic name. To help you recognize both names, match the brand name with the generic name of the same medication.

Generic Name	Brand Name
1. amlodipine	A. Isordil
2. isosorbide	B. Norvasc
3. nifedipine	C. Procardia
4. ranolazine	D. Ranexa

Calculate Medication Dosages

1. The primary care provider prescribed verapamil (Calan) 120 mg TID orally. The drug is available in 40-mg tablets. The nurse administers _____.

2. The client is prescribed isosorbide (Isordil) 40 mg orally BID. The drug form available is 20-mg tablets. The nurse administers _____.

● Prepare for the NCLEX®

Build Your Knowledge

1. The nitrates for anginal pain are used to dilate which of the following vessels?

   1. cerebral arteries
   2. coronary arteries
   3. peripheral veins
   4. coronary veins

2. Which class of drug is used for the *prevention* of anginal pain?

   1. calcium channel blockers
   2. nitrates
   3. Beta-adrenergics
   4. phosphodiesterase inhibitors

3. When administering the nitrates for angina, the nurse monitors the client for which common adverse reaction?

   1. hyperglycemia
   2. headache
   3. fever
   4. anorexia

4. When teaching a client about prescribed sublingual nitroglycerin, the nurse informs the client that if pain is not relieved, the dose can be repeated in ____ minute(s).

   1. 1
   2. 5
   3. 15
   4. 30

5. When administering nitroglycerin ointment, the nurse _____.

   1. rubs the ointment into the skin
   2. applies the ointment every hour or until the angina is relieved
   3. applies the ointment to a clean, dry area
   4. rubs the ointment between his or her palms and then spreads it evenly onto the client's chest

Apply Your Knowledge

6. A client taking a calcium channel blocker experiences orthostatic hypotension. The nurse instructs the client with orthostatic hypotension to _____.

   1. remain in a supine position until the effects subside
   2. make position changes slowly to minimize hypotensive effects
   3. increase the dosage of the calcium channel blocker
   4. discontinue use of the calcium channel blocker until the hypotensive effects diminish

7. A client has seen his primary health care provider for his heart condition. The provider gives you the prescription for sublingual nitrate to fax to the pharmacy. The client hands you more prescriptions from another provider to refill. Which one should you review with the primary health care provider first?

   1. cimetidine
   2. ibuprofen
   3. lisinopril
   4. sildenafil

8. Which of the following statements if made by the client taking a nitrate would indicate that he needs to be seen immediately by an urgent response team?

   1. "I had some chest pressure a week ago."
   2. "My wife had chest pain so I gave her one of my pills."
   3. "I woke this morning with swollen legs."
   4. "My heart feels worse after putting three of those little heart pills under my tongue."

Alternate-Format Questions

9. Best placement of a nitroglycerin transdermal system would be _____. **Select all that apply**.

   1. abdomen
   2. thigh
   3. chest
   4. forearm

10. The client has just been discharged with sublingual nitrate. He is experiencing chest tightness and has taken one tablet 4 minutes ago with minimal relief. He is calling confused about taking two more doses. When can he take those two additional doses? _____

To check your answers, see Appendix G.

the**Point** *For more NCLEX-style questions, log on to http://thepoint.lww.com to access more than 1000 questions.*

37

Anticoagulant and Thrombolytic Drugs

LEARNING OBJECTIVES

On completion of this chapter, the student will:

1. Describe hemostasis and thrombosis.
2. Discuss the uses, general drug actions, adverse reactions, contraindications, precautions, and interactions of anticoagulant, antiplatelet, and thrombolytic drugs.
3. Discuss important preadministration and ongoing assessment activities the nurse should perform on the patient taking an anticoagulant, antiplatelet, or thrombolytic drug.
4. List nursing diagnoses particular to a patient taking an anticoagulant, antiplatelet, or thrombolytic drug.
5. Discuss ways to promote an optimal response to therapy, how to manage common adverse reactions, and important points to keep in mind when educating patients about the use of anticoagulant, antiplatelet, and thrombolytic drugs.

KEY TERMS

aggregate • clumping of blood elements

embolus • thrombus that detaches from a blood vessel wall and travels through the bloodstream

fibrolytic • drug that dissolves clots already formed within blood vessel walls

hemostasis • complex process by which fibrin forms and blood clots

lysis • dissolution or destruction of cells

petechiae • pinpoint-sized red hemorrhagic spots on the skin

prothrombin • substance that is essential for the clotting of blood; clotting factor II

thrombolytic • drug that helps to eliminate blood clots

thrombosis • formation of a blood clot

thrombus • blood clot (pl. thrombi)

DRUG CLASSES

Anticoagulants
Antiplatelets
Thrombolytics

Clotting is an essential body mechanism. When a blood vessel is injured, a series of events occurs to form a clot and stop the bleeding. This process is called **hemostasis**. It involves a complex process also called the *coagulation cascade*. Figure 37.1 shows the blood clotting pathway and the extrinsic and intrinsic factors involved. The blood clotting or coagulation cascade is so named because as each factor is activated, it acts as a catalyst that enhances the next reaction, with the net result being a large collection of fibrin (the clot) that forms a plug in the vessel, thus stopping the bleeding. This is a normal event, taking a few minutes, that happens daily in response to tears and leaks in blood vessels throughout the body.

Clotting can also cause damage to both blood vessels and the tissues nourished by those vessels. **Thrombosis** is the formation of a blood clot, or **thrombus**. A thrombus may form in any vessel (artery or vein), impeding blood flow. For example,

---

PHARMACOLOGY IN PRACTICE

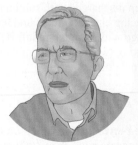

Mr. Phillip is a widower and lives alone. He had not been seen in a number of years, and his physical exam shows that he has atrial fibrillation, for which he was prescribed Coumadin to take at home. The clinical pharmacist asks you about Mr. Phillip's mental status. It seems that the weekly lab work for Mr. Phillip fluctuates considerably despite weekly teaching. After you read about these drugs, think about what action could be taken.

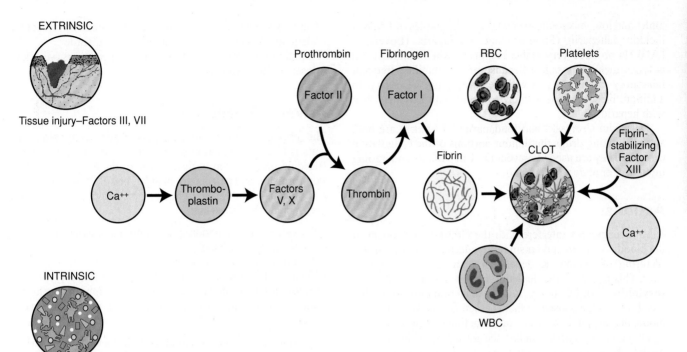

EXTRINSIC

Tissue injury–Factors III, VII

INTRINSIC

Platelets Thromboplastin Precursors
Factors VIII, IX, XI, XII

Figure 37.1 Blood clotting pathway. Blood coagulation results in the formation of a stable fibrin clot. Formation of this clot involves a cascade of interactions of clotting factors, platelets, and other substances. Clotting factors exist in the blood in inactive form and must be converted to an active form before the next step in the clotting pathway can occur. Each factor is stimulated in turn until the process is complete and a fibrin clot is formed. In the intrinsic pathway, all of the components necessary for clot formation are in the circulating blood. Clot formation in the intrinsic pathway is initiated by factor XII. In the extrinsic pathway, coagulation is initiated by release of tissue thromboplastin, a factor not found in circulating blood. RBC, red blood cell; WBC, white blood cell.

a venous thrombus can develop as the result of venous stasis (decreased blood flow), injury to the vessel wall, or altered blood coagulation. Venous thrombosis most often occurs in the lower extremities and is associated with venous stasis. Deep vein thrombosis (DVT) occurs in the lower extremities and is the most common type of venous thrombosis.

Arterial thrombosis can occur because of atherosclerosis or arrhythmias, such as atrial fibrillation. The thrombus may begin small, but fibrin, platelets, and red blood cells attach to the thrombus, increasing its size. When a thrombus detaches itself from the wall of the vessel and is carried along through the bloodstream, it becomes an **embolus**. The embolus travels until it reaches a vessel that is too small to permit its passage. If the embolus goes to the lung and obstructs a pulmonary vessel, it is called a *pulmonary embolism* (PE). Similarly, if the embolus detaches and occludes a vessel supplying blood to the heart, it can cause a myocardial infarction (MI).

The type of drugs discussed in this chapter include drugs that prevent the formation of blood clots (anticoagulants), drugs that suppress platelet aggregation (antiplatelets), and drugs that help to eliminate the clot (thrombolytics). For more information about specific drugs, see the Drug Summary Table: Anticoagulant, Antiplatelet, and Thrombolytic Agents.

ORAL AND PARENTERAL ANTICOAGULANTS

Anticoagulants are used to prevent the formation and extension of a thrombus. Anticoagulants have no direct effect on an existing thrombus and do not reverse any damage from the thrombus. However, once the presence of a thrombus has been established, anticoagulant therapy can prevent additional clots from forming. Although they do not thin the blood, they are commonly called *blood thinners* by patients. The anticoagulant group of drugs includes warfarin (Coumadin; a coumarin derivative) and fractionated and unfractionated heparin. The anticoagulant drugs are used prophylactically in patients who are at high risk for clot formation.

Warfarin is the oral anticoagulant most commonly prescribed. Although primarily given by the oral route, warfarin is also available for parenteral administration. Because it can be given orally, it is the drug of choice for patients requiring long-term therapy with an anticoagulant. Peak activity is reached 1.5 to 3 days after therapy is initiated.

Heparin preparations are available as heparin sodium and the low–molecular-weight heparins (LMWHs; fractionated heparins). Heparin is not a single drug, but rather a mixture of high– and low–molecular-weight drugs. Examples of LMWH include dalteparin (Fragmin) and enoxaparin (Lovenox). LMWHs produce very stable responses when administered at recommended dosages. Because of this stability, frequent laboratory monitoring, as with heparin, is not necessary. In addition, bleeding is less likely to occur with LMWHs than with heparin.

Desirudin (Iprivask) and fondaparinux (Arixtra) are both anticoagulating drugs that inhibit portions of the coagulation cascade. They are used to prevent DVT in patients undergoing hip, knee, or abdominal surgeries.

Actions

All anticoagulants interfere with the clotting mechanism of the blood. Warfarin and anisindione interfere with the manufacturing of vitamin K–dependent clotting factors by the liver. This results in the depletion of clotting factors II (**prothrombin**), VII, IX, and X. It is the depletion of prothrombin (see Fig. 37.1), a substance that is essential for the clotting of blood, that accounts for most of the action of warfarin.

By contrast, heparin inhibits the formation of fibrin clots, inhibits the conversion of fibrinogen to fibrin, and inactivates several of the factors necessary for the clotting of blood. Heparin cannot be taken orally, because it is inactivated by gastric acid in the stomach; therefore, it must be given by injection. The LMWHs act to inhibit clotting reactions by binding to antithrombin III, which inhibits the synthesis of factor X and the formation of thrombin. These drugs have no effect on clots that have already formed and aid only in preventing the formation of new blood clots.

Desirudin and fondaparinux produce strong anticoagulant effects with a different mechanism of action than heparin. Additionally, their therapeutic index is narrower than heparin and can be associated with hemorrhagic complications.

Uses

Anticoagulants are used for the following:

- Prevention (prophylaxis) and treatment of DVT
- Prevention and treatment of atrial fibrillation with embolization
- Prevention and treatment of PE
- Adjuvant treatment of MI
- Prevention of thrombus formation after valve replacement surgery

Parenteral anticoagulants are used specifically for the following:

- Prevention of postoperative DVT and PE in certain patients undergoing surgical procedures, such as major abdominal surgery
- Prevention of clotting in arterial and heart surgery, in the equipment used for extracorporeal (occurring outside the body) circulation (e.g., in dialysis procedures), in blood transfusions, and in blood samples for laboratory purposes
- Prevention of a repeat cerebral thrombosis in some patients who have experienced a stroke
- Treatment of coronary occlusion, acute MI, and peripheral arterial embolism

- Diagnosis and treatment of disseminated intravascular coagulation (DIC), a severe hemorrhagic disorder
- Maintaining patency of intravenous (IV) catheters (very low doses of 10 to 100 units)

Adverse Reactions

The principal adverse reaction associated with anticoagulants is bleeding, which may range from very mild to severe. Bleeding may be seen in many areas of the body, such as the skin (bruising and petechiae), bladder, bowel, stomach, uterus, and mucous membranes. Other adverse reactions are rare but may include the following:

- Nausea, vomiting, abdominal cramping, diarrhea
- Alopecia (loss of hair)
- Rash or urticaria (hives)
- Hepatitis (inflammation of the liver), jaundice (yellowish discoloration of the skin and mucous membranes), thrombocytopenia (low platelet count), and blood dyscrasias (disorders)

Additional adverse reactions include local irritation when heparin is given by the subcutaneous (subcut) route. Hypersensitivity reactions may also occur with any route of administration and include fever and chills. More serious hypersensitivity reactions include an asthma-like reaction and an anaphylactic reaction. See the Summary Drug Table: Anticoagulant, Antiplatelet, and Thrombolytic Agents for additional adverse reactions.

Contraindications

Anticoagulants are contraindicated in patients with known hypersensitivity to the drugs, active bleeding (except when caused by DIC), hemorrhagic disease, tuberculosis, leukemia, uncontrolled hypertension, gastrointestinal (GI) ulcers, recent surgery of the eye or central nervous system, aneurysms, or severe renal or hepatic disease, and during lactation. Use during pregnancy can cause fetal death (oral agents are in pregnancy category X and parenteral agents are in pregnancy category C). The LMWHs are also contraindicated in patients with a hypersensitivity to pork products.

 LIFESPAN CONSIDERATIONS
Jewish/Muslim Cultural Practices
Use of pork or porcine products is prohibited by some religious groups. Alert the primary health care provider if the patient notes a Jewish or Muslim religious preference and is likely to undergo anticoagulant therapy. The drug fondaparinux (Arixtra) is artificially produced and does not contain pork products; this may be used as a substitute for one of the pork derivative heparin products.

Precautions

Anticoagulants are used cautiously in patients with fever, heart failure, diarrhea, diabetes, malignancy, hypertension, renal or hepatic disease, psychoses, or depression. Precaution is taken with patients undergoing spinal procedures (anesthesia or diagnostic) to be aware of the potential of spinal or epidural hematoma formation when parenteral anticoagulants are used. Women of childbearing age must use a reliable contraceptive to prevent pregnancy. These drugs are used with caution in all patients with a potential site for bleeding or hemorrhage.

Interactions

The following interactions may occur when an anticoagulant is administered with another agent:

Interacting Drug	Common Use	Effect of Interaction
aspirin, acetaminophen, nonsteroidal anti-inflammatory drugs (NSAIDs), and chloral hydrate	Pain relief and sedation	Increased risk for bleeding
penicillin, aminoglycosides, isoniazid, tetracyclines, and cephalosporins	Anti-infective agents	Increased risk for bleeding
beta (β) blockers and loop diuretics	Treatment of cardiac problems	Increased risk for bleeding
disulfiram and cimetidine	Management of GI distress	Increased risk for bleeding
oral contraceptives, barbiturates, diuretics, and vitamin K	Birth control, sedation, treatment of cardiac problems, and treatment of bleeding disorders, respectively	Decreased effectiveness of the anticoagulant

HERBAL CONSIDERATIONS

Any herbal remedy should be used with caution in patients taking warfarin. Warfarin, a drug with a narrow therapeutic index, has the potential to interact with many herbal remedies. For example, warfarin should not be combined with any of the following substances, because they may have additive or synergistic activity and increase the risk for bleeding: celery, chamomile, clove, dong quai, feverfew, garlic, ginger, ginkgo biloba, ginseng, green tea, onion, passion flower, red clover, St. John's wort, and turmeric.

ANTIPLATELET DRUGS

Thrombi forming in the venous system are composed primarily of fibrin and red blood cells. In contrast, it is believed that arterial thrombosis formation is due to clumping of platelet aggregates. Therefore, anticoagulant drugs prevent thrombosis in the venous system, and the antiplatelet drugs prevent thrombus formation in the arterial system. In addition to aspirin therapy, the antiplatelet drugs include adenosine diphosphate (ADP) receptor blockers and glycoprotein receptor blockers.

Actions and Uses

These drugs work by decreasing the platelets' ability to stick together (**aggregate**) in the blood, thus forming a clot. Aspirin works by prohibiting the aggregation of the platelets

for the lifetime of the platelet. The ADP blockers alter the platelet cell membrane, preventing aggregation. Glycoprotein receptor blockers work to prevent enzyme production, again inhibiting platelet aggregation. Antiplatelet drug therapy is designed primarily to treat patients at risk for acute coronary syndrome, MI, stroke, and intermittent claudication.

Adverse Reactions

Some of the more common adverse reactions include the following:

• Heart palpitations
• Bleeding
• Dizziness and headache
• Nausea, diarrhea, constipation, dyspepsia

Contraindications and Precautions

Antiplatelet drugs are contraindicated in pregnant or lactating patients and those with known hypersensitivity to the drugs, congestive heart failure, active bleeding, or thrombotic thrombocytopenic purpura (TTP). These drugs are to be used cautiously in older adult patients, pancytopenic patients, or those with renal or hepatic impairment. If TTP is diagnosed, the antiplatelet treatment should be stopped immediately. Clopidogrel is a pregnancy category B and the others are pregnancy category C; none of these drugs have been well studied in humans. Antiplatelet drugs should be discontinued 1 week before any surgical procedure.

Interactions

The following interactions may occur when an antiplatelet is administered with another agent:

Interacting Drug	Common Use	Effect of Interaction
aspirin and NSAIDs	Pain relief	Increased risk of bleeding
macrolide antibiotics	Anti-infective agents	Increased effectiveness of anti-infective
digoxin	Management of cardiac problems	Decreased digoxin serum levels
phenytoin	Control of seizure activity	Increased phenytoin serum levels

Although these agents produce strong anticoagulant effects, their mechanism of action is distinct from that of heparins; thus, these agents should be used carefully using specific guidelines provided for each product. Thrombin inhibitors are effective anticoagulants; however, their therapeutic index is narrower than heparin and as such their nonoptimized use is potentially associated with hemorrhagic complications.

THROMBOLYTIC DRUGS

Whereas the anticoagulant agents prevent thrombus formation, the **thrombolytic** class of drugs dissolves blood clots that have already formed within the walls of a blood vessel. These drugs reopen blood vessels after they become occluded. Another term used to describe the thrombolytic drugs is **fibrolytic**. Examples of the thrombolytics include alteplase recombinant (Activase), streptokinase (Streptase), and tenecteplase (TNKase).

Actions

Although the exact action of each of the thrombolytic drugs is slightly different, these drugs break down fibrin clots by converting plasminogen to plasmin. Plasmin is an enzyme that breaks down the fibrin of a blood clot. This reopens blood vessels after their occlusion and prevents tissue necrosis. Because thrombolytic drugs dissolve all clots encountered (both occlusive and those repairing vessel leaks), bleeding is a great concern when using these agents. Before these drugs are used, their potential benefits must be weighed carefully against the potential dangers of bleeding.

Uses

These drugs are used to treat the following:

• Acute stroke or MI by **lysis** (breaking up) of blood clots in the coronary arteries
• Blood clots causing pulmonary emboli and DVT
• Suspected occlusions in central venous catheters

See the Summary Drug Table: Anticoagulant, Antiplatelet, and Thrombolytic Agents for a more complete listing of the use of these drugs.

Adverse Reactions

Bleeding is the most common adverse reaction seen with the use of these drugs. Bleeding may be internal and involve areas such as the GI tract, genitourinary tract, and brain. Bleeding may also be external (superficial) and seen at areas of broken skin, such as venipuncture sites and recent surgical wounds. Allergic reactions may also be seen.

Contraindications and Precautions

Thrombolytic drugs are contraindicated in a patient with known hypersensitivity to the drugs, active bleeding, and history of stroke, aneurysm, and recent intracranial surgery.

These drugs are used cautiously in patients who have recently undergone major surgery (within 10 days), such as coronary artery bypass grafting; who experienced stroke, trauma, vaginal or cesarean section delivery, GI bleeding, or trauma within the last 10 days; who have hypertension, diabetic retinopathy, or any condition in which bleeding is a significant possibility; or who are currently receiving oral anticoagulants. All of the thrombolytic drugs discussed in this chapter are classified in pregnancy category C, with the exception of urokinase, which is a pregnancy category B drug.

Interactions

When a thrombolytic is administered with medications that prevent blood clots, such as aspirin, dipyridamole, or an anticoagulant, the patient is at increased risk for bleeding.

NURSING PROCESS

PATIENT RECEIVING AN ANTICOAGULANT, ANTIPLATELET, OR THROMBOLYTIC DRUG

ASSESSMENT

Preadministration Assessment
When immobilization is anticipated, patients are often started on preventative anticoagulant therapy. Routinely examine the extremities for color and skin temperature. In addition to vital signs, check immobile patients for a pedal pulse, noting the rate and strength of the pulse. Should a patient have a DVT, it usually occurs in a lower extremity. It is important to record any difference between the affected extremity and the unaffected extremity. Document areas of redness or tenderness and asks the patient to describe current symptoms. The affected extremity may appear edematous and a positive Homans' sign (pain in the calf when the foot is dorsiflexed) may be elicited. A positive Homans' sign suggests DVT.

Before administering the first dose of an anticoagulant or thrombolytic, ask the patient about all drugs taken during the previous 2 to 3 weeks (if the patient was recently admitted to the hospital). If the patient was taking any drugs before admission, review the drugs with the primary health care provider before starting an anticoagulant. The first dose of warfarin is not given until blood is drawn for a baseline

prothrombin time (PT) and the international normalized ratio (INR). The dosage is individualized based on the results of the PT or the INR.

The most commonly used test to monitor heparin is the activated partial thromboplastin time (aPTT).

A complete blood count is usually drawn before the administration of the thrombolytic agents. Radiologic testing such as a computed tomography (CT) scan will be performed. Most patients receiving a thrombolytic agent are admitted or transferred to an intensive care unit, because close monitoring is necessary for 48 hours or more after therapy. If the patient is experiencing pain because of the blood clot, include a thorough pain assessment.

Ongoing Assessment
In the ongoing assessment, a patient receiving an anticoagulant, antiplatelet, or thrombolytic drug requires close observation and careful monitoring. During the course of therapy for both oral and parenteral drugs, continually assess the patient for any signs of bleeding and hemorrhage. Areas of assessment include the gums, nose, stools, urine, or nasogastric drainage. Level of consciousness should be assessed on a routine basis to monitor for intracranial bleeding.

Patients receiving warfarin for the first time often require daily adjustment of the dose, which is based on the daily PT/INR results. In settings such as long-term care or rehabilitation, this may be done with an INR monitor, similar to the

Display 37.1 Understanding Prothrombin Time and International Normalized Ratio

Prothrombin time (also called pro-time or abbreviated as "PT") and the *international normalized ratio* (INR) are used to monitor the patient's response to warfarin therapy. The daily dose of the oral anticoagulant is based on the patient's daily PT/INR. The therapeutic range of the PT is 1.2 to 1.5 times the control value. Studies indicate that levels greater than 2 times the control value do not provide additional therapeutic effects in most patients and are associated with a higher incidence of bleeding.

Laboratories report results for the INR along with the patient's PT and the control value. The INR "corrects" the routine PT results from different laboratories. By measuring against a known standard, the INR gives a more consistent value. The INR is maintained between 2 and 3. Values above 5 can be dangerous, and values below 1 are ineffective.

glucometers used for monitoring blood glucose. If the PT exceeds 1.2 to 1.5 times the control value or the INR ratio exceeds 3, the primary health care provider is notified before the drug is given. A daily PT/INR is performed until it stabilizes and when any other drug is added to or removed from the patient's drug regimen. After the INR has stabilized, it is monitored every 4 to 6 weeks. See Display 37.1 for more information on the laboratory tests for monitoring warfarin.

The dosage of heparin is adjusted according to daily aPTT monitoring. A therapeutic dosage is attained when the aPTT is 1.5 to 2.5 times the normal. The LMWHs have little or no effect on the aPTT values. Special monitoring of clotting times is not necessary when administering the drugs. Periodic platelet counts, hematocrit, and tests for occult blood in the stool should be performed throughout the course of heparin therapy.

! NURSING ALERT

Blood coagulation tests for those receiving heparin by continuous IV infusion are taken at periodic intervals (usually every 4 hours) determined by the primary health care provider. If the patient is receiving long-term heparin therapy, blood coagulation tests may be performed at less frequent intervals.

Remember to monitor for any indication of hypersensitivity reaction. Report reactions such as chills, fever, or hives to the primary health care provider. Examine the skin temperature and color in the patient with a DVT for signs of improvement. Check and document vital signs every 4 hours or more frequently, if needed. When heparin is given to prevent the formation of a thrombus, observe the patient for signs of thrombus formation every 2 to 4 hours. Because the signs and symptoms of thrombus formation vary and depend on the area or organ involved, evaluate and report any complaint the patient may have or any change in the patient's condition to the primary health care provider.

NURSING DIAGNOSES

Drug-specific nursing diagnoses include the following:

■ **Risk for Injury** related to excessive bleeding due to drug therapy

■ **Individual Effective Self-Health Management** related to inability to communicate drug use if incapacitated

■ **Anxiety** related to fear of atypical bleeding during thrombolytic drug therapy

Nursing diagnoses related to drug administration are discussed in depth in Chapter 4.

PLANNING

The expected outcomes for the patient may include an optimal response to therapy, support of patient needs related to the management of adverse reactions, and confidence in an understanding of the medication regimen.

IMPLEMENTATION

Promoting an Optimal Response to Therapy

ORAL ADMINISTRATION OF ANTICOAGULANTS. To hasten the onset of the therapeutic effect, a higher dosage (loading dose) may be prescribed for 2 to 4 days, followed by a maintenance dosage adjusted according to the daily PT/INR. Otherwise, the drug takes 3 to 5 days to reach therapeutic levels. When rapid anticoagulation is required, heparin is preferred as a loading dose, followed by maintenance dose of warfarin based on the PT or INR. The dose is typically given in the evening at a specified time. This prevents errors in administration of doses too high or too low by providing ample time to allow time for adjustments based on lab results.

Optimal therapeutic results are obtained when the patient's PT is 1.2 to 1.5 times the control value. In certain instances, such as in recurrent systemic embolism, a PT of 1.5 to 2 may be prescribed. Studies indicate that diet can influence the PT/INR values. A study at the Massachusetts General Hospital in Boston looked at the effect of varying dietary vitamin K intake on the INR in patients receiving anticoagulation therapy with warfarin. As vitamin K intake increased, INR became more consistent and stable. By contrast, as vitamin K intake decreased, INR became more variable and fluctuated to a greater extent. The key to vitamin K management for patients receiving warfarin is maintaining a consistent daily intake of vitamin K.

PARENTERAL ADMINISTRATION OF ANTICOAGULANTS. Heparin preparations, unlike warfarin, must be given by the parenteral route, preferably subcut or IV. The onset of anticoagulation is almost immediate after a single dose. Maximum effects occur within 10 minutes of administration. Clotting time returns to normal within 4 hours unless subsequent doses are given. Although warfarin is most often administered orally, an injectable form may be used as an alternative route for patients who are unable to receive oral drugs.

Heparin may be given by intermittent IV administration, continuous IV infusion, and the subcut route. Intramuscular (IM) administration is avoided because of the possibility of the development of local irritation, pain, or hematoma (a collection of blood in the tissue). The dosage of heparin is measured in units and is available in various dosage strengths as units per milliliter (e.g., 10,000 units/mL). When selecting the strength used for administration, choose the strength closest to the prescribed dose. For example, if 5000 units are ordered, and the available strengths are 1000, 5000, 7500, 20,000, and 40,000 units/mL, use 1 mL of the 5000 units/mL for administration.

NURSING ALERT

Errors have been made by misreading the numbers on the bottles of heparin. Doses of 10,000 units have been misread as 100 units; as a result, patients have been put at risk for hemorrhage when receiving these higher doses. It is important for the nurse to prepare medications without distraction to minimize risk to patients.

An infusion pump must be used for the safe administration of heparin by continuous IV infusion. The infusion pump is checked every 1 to 2 hours to ensure that it is working properly. The needle site is inspected for signs of inflammation, pain, and tenderness along the pathway of the vein. If these occur, the infusion is discontinued and restarted in another vein.

When heparin or other anticoagulants are given by the subcutaneous route, administration sites are rotated and the site used is documented on the patient's chart. The recommended sites of administration are those on the abdomen, but areas within 2 inches of the umbilicus are avoided because of the increased vascularity of that area. Other areas of administration of heparin are the buttocks, lateral thighs, and upper arms (Fig. 37.2). No fluctuation in absorption has been found by using the arms and legs. Drugs for DVT prevention are available in prefilled syringes; do not expel the air bubble.

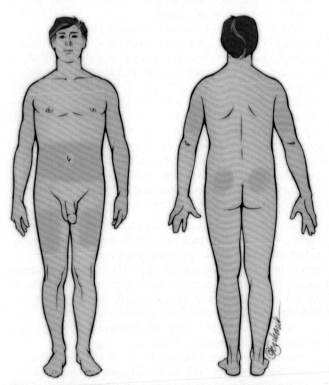

Figure 37.2 Sites for subcutaneous anticoagulant parenteral injection. (From Smeltzer, S. C., & Bare, B. G. [2000]. *Textbook of medical-surgical nursing* [9th ed.]. Philadelphia: Lippincott Williams & Wilkins.)

They are administered deep in subcutaneous tissue by pinching a fold of skin. Insert the needle into the tissue at a 90-degree angle so the air bubble is injected last. It is not necessary to aspirate before injecting the drug; this may activate the needle guard. Be careful not to let go of the plunger until the syringe is empty and pulled out of the skin; letting go causes the needle to withdraw into the barrel of the syringe, thus preventing injury from a needle stick following the injection. The application of firm pressure after the injection helps to prevent hematoma formation. Each time heparin is given by this route, inspect all recent injection sites for signs of inflammation (redness, swelling, tenderness) and hematoma formation.

Blood coagulation tests are usually ordered before and during heparin therapy, and the dose of heparin is adjusted to the test results. Coagulation tests are usually performed 30 minutes before the scheduled dose and from the extremity opposite the infusion site. When administering heparin by the subcutaneous route, an aPTT test is performed 4 to 6 hours after the injection. Optimal results of therapy are obtained when the aPTT is 1.5 to 2.5 times the control value. The LMWHs do not require close monitoring of blood coagulation tests.

A complete blood count, platelet count, and stool analysis for occult blood may be ordered periodically throughout therapy. Thrombocytopenia may occur during heparin or antiplatelet administration. A mild, transient thrombocytopenia may occur 2 to 3 days after heparin therapy is begun. This early development of thrombocytopenia tends to resolve itself despite continued therapy. As you check periodic lab reports, a platelet count of less than 100,000 mm^3 should be brought to the attention of the primary health care provider, who may choose to discontinue the heparin therapy. Overdose of antiplatelet drugs is typically managed by withholding treatment or by infusion of platelets.

NURSING ALERT

Withhold the drug and immediately contact the primary health care provider for any of the following:

The PT exceeds 1.5 times the control value.
There is evidence of bleeding.
The INR is greater than 3.

Administration of Thrombolytics. For optimal therapeutic effect, the thrombolytic drugs are used as soon as possible after the formation of a thrombus, preferably within 4 to 6 hours or as soon as possible after the symptoms are identified. The greatest benefit follows drug administration within 4 hours, but significant benefits occur when the agents are used within the first 24 hours. The patient is brought to a facility where a CT scan is performed and blood will be taken for testing. Timing of the onset of symptoms is important. Here you can help the family or person coming with the patient to remember the situation and get estimates of the timing of symptoms.

Assess the patient for bleeding every 15 minutes during the first 60 minutes of therapy, every 15 to 30 minutes for the next 8 hours, and at least every 4 hours until therapy is completed. Vital signs are monitored continuously. If pain is present, the primary health care provider may order an opioid analgesic. Once the clot dissolves and blood flows freely through the obstructed blood vessel, severe pain usually decreases.

Monitoring and Managing Patient Needs

Risk For Injury. Bleeding can occur any time during therapy with warfarin or the heparin preparations, even when the INR appears to be within a safe limit (e.g., 2 to 3). All nursing personnel and medical team members should be made aware of any patient receiving warfarin and the observations necessary with administration. If bleeding should occur, the primary health care provider may decrease the dose, discontinue the heparin therapy for a time, or order the administration of protamine sulfate. *Be alert to the following indicators of bleeding:*

- If a decided drop in blood pressure or rise in the pulse rate occurs, notify the primary health care provider, because this may indicate internal bleeding. Hemorrhage can begin as a slight bleeding or bruising tendency; frequently observe the patient for these occurrences. Sometimes, hemorrhage occurs without warning.

- Urinal, bedpan, catheter drainage unit—Inspect the urine for a pink to red color and the stool for signs of GI bleeding (bright red to black stools). Visually check the catheter drainage every 2 to 4 hours and when the unit is emptied. Oral anticoagulants may impart a red-orange color to alkaline urine, making hematuria difficult to detect visually. A urinalysis may be necessary to determine if blood is in the urine.

- Emesis basin, nasogastric suction units—Visually check the nasogastric suction unit every 2 to 4 hours and when the unit is emptied. Check the emesis basin each time it is emptied.

- Skin, mucous membranes—Inspect the patient's skin daily for evidence of easy bruising or bleeding. Be alert for bleeding from minor cuts and scratches, nosebleeds, or excessive bleeding after IM, subcut, or IV injections or after a venipuncture. After oral care, check the toothbrush and gums for signs of bleeding.

NURSING ALERT

When patients using anticoagulants have spinal anesthesia or undergo spinal punctures, they are at risk for potential spinal or epidural hematoma formation, which can lead to long-term or permanent paralysis. These patients should be frequently monitored for signs and symptoms of neurologic impairment.

Individual Effective Self–Health Management. The patient needs to be aware of the many food and drug interactions that can cause a higher risk for bleeding when taking anticoagulants, or make the drugs less effective. A medical alert bracelet and list of drugs being taken should be on the patient at all times in case the patient becomes incapacitated by accident or illness, because other care providers need to know that anticoagulant or antiplatelet drugs are being taken.

The patient is instructed to notify all health care providers of the anticoagulant or antiplatelet therapy when diagnostic tests or other treatments are performed. When the skin is pierced during procedures, explain why you must apply prolonged pressure to needle or catheter sites after venipuncture, removal of central or peripheral IV lines, and IM and subcut injections. Laboratory personnel or those responsible for drawing blood for laboratory tests are made aware of anticoagulant therapy, because prolonged pressure on the venipuncture

site is necessary. All laboratory requests should be flagged that the patient is receiving anticoagulant therapy.

Anxiety. Bleeding is the most common adverse reaction when thrombolytic drugs are administered. Conditions requiring thrombolytic treatment are typically of an urgent nature, and treatment occurs in special care units of the hospital such as the intensive care unit or operating room. Combined with the potential for bleeding, all this can be frightening and cause anxiety to the patient and any family members present. As you monitor the patient's status, it is important to reassure the patient and communicate with family members that measures are being taken to diagnose and intervene early for any adverse reactions.

Throughout administration of the thrombolytic drug, assess for signs of bleeding and hemorrhage. Internal bleeding may involve the GI tract, genitourinary tract, intracranial sites, or respiratory tract. Signs and symptoms of internal bleeding may include abdominal pain; coffee-ground emesis; black, tarry stools; hematuria; joint pain; and spitting or coughing up blood.

Superficial bleeding may occur at venous or arterial puncture sites or recent surgical incision sites. Again, this can be disturbing to the patient and family, and they may become anxious. Because fibrin is lysed during therapy, bleeding from recent injection sites may occur. Carefully monitor all potential bleeding sites (including catheter insertion sites, arterial and venous puncture sites, cutdown sites, and needle puncture sites). Reassure the patient that bleeding will be reported to the primary health care provider and steps taken to minimize the bleeding. Minor bleeding at a puncture site can usually be controlled by applying pressure for at least 30 minutes at the site, followed by the application of a pressure dressing. The puncture site is checked frequently for evidence of further bleeding. IM injections and nonessential handling of the patient are avoided during treatment. Venipunctures are done only when absolutely necessary.

NURSING ALERT

Heparin may be given along with or after administration of a thrombolytic drug to prevent another thrombus from forming. However, administration of an anticoagulant increases the risk for bleeding. The patient must be monitored closely for internal and external bleeding.

If uncontrolled bleeding is noted or the bleeding appears to be internal, stop the drug and immediately contact the primary health care provider, because whole blood, packed red cells, or fresh frozen plasma may be required. Vital signs are monitored every hour (or more frequently) for at least 48 hours after the drug is discontinued. Contact the primary health care provider if there is a marked change in one or more of the vital signs. Any signs of an allergic (hypersensitivity) reaction, such as difficulty breathing, wheezing, hives, skin rash, and hypotension, are reported immediately to the primary health care provider.

Managing Anticoagulant Overdosage

Oral Anticoagulants. Symptoms of warfarin overdosage include blood in the stool (melena); petechiae (pinpoint-sized red hemorrhagic spots on the skin); oozing from superficial injuries, such as cuts from shaving or bleeding from the gums after brushing the teeth; or excessive menstrual bleeding.

Immediately report any of these adverse reactions or evidence of bleeding to the primary health care provider.

If bleeding occurs, the PT exceeds 1.5 times the control value, or the INR exceeds 3, the primary health care provider may either discontinue the anticoagulant therapy for a few days or order vitamin K (phytonadione), an oral anticoagulant antagonist, which should be readily available when a patient is receiving warfarin. Because warfarin interferes with the synthesis of vitamin K–dependent clotting factors, the administration of vitamin K reverses the effects of warfarin by providing the necessary ingredient to enhance clot formation and stop bleeding. However, withholding one or two doses of warfarin may quickly bring the PT to an acceptable level.

Assess the patient for additional evidence of bleeding until the PT is below 1.5 times the control value or until the bleeding episodes cease. The PT usually returns to a safe level within 6 hours of administration of vitamin K. Administration of whole blood or plasma may be necessary if severe bleeding occurs because of the delayed onset of action of vitamin K.

Parenteral Anticoagulants. In most instances, discontinuation of the drug is sufficient to correct overdosage, because the duration of action of heparin is brief. However, if hemorrhaging is severe, the primary health care provider may order protamine, the specific heparin antagonist or antidote. Protamine is also used to treat overdosage of the LMWHs. Protamine has an immediate onset of action and a duration of 2 hours. It counteracts the effects of heparin and brings blood coagulation test results to within normal limits. The drug is given slowly by the IV route over a period of 10 minutes.

If administration of this drug is necessary, monitor the patient's blood pressure and pulse rate every 15 to 30 minutes for 2 hours or more after administration of the heparin antagonist. Immediately report to the primary health care provider any sudden decrease in blood pressure or increase in the pulse rate. Observe the patient for new evidence of bleeding until blood coagulation test results are within normal limits. To replace blood loss, the primary health care provider may order blood transfusions or fresh frozen plasma.

Educating the Patient and Family
In many facilities the clinical pharmacist is responsible for anticoagulant teaching. A thorough review of the dosage regimen, possible adverse drug reactions, and early signs of bleeding dencies help the patient cooperate with the prescribed ther You can provide further explanation or validate learning on part of the patient and family. Validate understanding of th following points in a patient and family teaching plan:

- Follow the dosage schedule prescribed by the primary health care provider, and report any signs of active bleeding immediately.
- The INR will be monitored periodically. Keep all primary health care provider and laboratory appointments, because dosage changes may be necessary during therapy.
- Do not take or stop taking other drugs except on the advice of the primary health care provider. This includes nonprescription drugs, as well as those prescribed by a primary health care provider or dentist.
- Inform the dentist or other primary health care providers of therapy with this drug before any treatment or procedure is started or drugs are prescribed.

- Take the drug at the same time each day.
- Do not change brands of anticoagulants without consulting a physician or pharmacist.
- ⚠ Avoid alcohol unless use has been approved by the primary health care provider.
- Be aware of foods high in vitamin K, such as leafy green vegetables, beans, broccoli, cabbage, cauliflower, cheese, fish, and yogurt. Maintaining a healthy diet including these foods may help maintain a consistent INR value.
- Keep in mind that antiplatelet drugs can lower all blood counts, including the white cell count. Patients may be at greater risk of infection during the first 3 months of treatment.
- If evidence of bleeding occurs, such as unusual bleeding or bruising, bleeding gums, blood in the urine or stool, black stool, or diarrhea, omit the next dose of the drug and contact the primary health care provider immediately (anisindione may cause a red-orange discoloration of alkaline urine).
- Use a soft toothbrush and consult a dentist regarding routine oral hygiene, including the use of dental floss. Use an electric razor when possible to avoid small skin cuts.
- Women of childbearing age should use a reliable contraceptive to prevent pregnancy.
- Wear or carry medical identification, such as a MedicAlert bracelet, to inform medical personnel and others of therapy with this drug.

EVALUATION

- Therapeutic response is achieved and blood coagulation is controlled.
- Adverse reactions are identified, reported to the primary health care provider, and managed successfully with appropriate nursing interventions:
  - No evidence of injury is seen.
  - Patient manages the therapeutic regimen effectively.
  - Anxiety is managed successfully.
- Patient and family express confidence and demonstrate an understanding of the drug regimen.

PHARMACOLOGY IN PRACTICE
THINK CRITICALLY

 Mr. Phillip's last INR was 2.9; the week before it was 1.5. You ask him to bring in his medication and find seven different bottles and four different strengths of Coumadin. When asked he tells you he has a weekly calendar and takes as many tablets as it says on the sheet. You know that Coumadin pills come in strengths from 1 to 10 mg. When you ask about the bottles, he states, "They are all green, so they must be the same." What action would you take next?

KEY POINTS

- Hemostasis is the process of clotting; this is beneficial when injury tears a vessel. A thrombus is a clot that forms in a vessel and impedes blood flow.

- Anticoagulants are used to prevent the formation or extension of a thrombus (or blood clot). These drugs do not affect existing clots, nor do they reverse damage already done by a clot. These drugs are used to prevent further clot development. Although they do not thin the blood, they are commonly called blood thinners.

- Antiplatelet drugs decrease the platelets' ability to aggregate (or stick together). This reduces the chance of

thrombus formation in the arterial circulation for conditions such as acute coronary syndrome, MI, and stroke.

- Thrombolytic drugs are used to dissolve blood clots that have already formed within the walls of a blood vessel.

- Many of these drugs are monitored with frequent lab tests because bleeding is an adverse reaction of all these drugs. The GI system, mental status, and pain should be monitored for signs of internal bleeding. Precautions with lab draws and previous skin punctures and monitoring of the skin can detect superficial bleeding.

Summary Drug Table ANTICOAGULANT, ANTIPLATELET, AND THROMBOLYTIC AGENTS

Generic Name	Trade Name	Uses	Adverse Reactions	Dosage Ranges
Oral Anticoagulants				
warfarin *war'-fah-rin*	Coumadin, Jantoven	Prophylaxis/treatment of venous thrombosis	Bleeding, fatigue, dizziness, abdominal cramping	2–10 mg/day orally, individualized dose based on PT or INR: IV form for injection
Parenteral Anticoagulants				
heparin *hep'-ah-rin*		Thrombosis/embolism, diagnosis and treatment of disseminated intravascular coagulation, prophylaxis of DVT, clotting prevention	Bleeding, chills, fever, urticaria, local irritation, erythema, mild pain, hematoma or bruising at the injection site (subcut)	10,000–20,000 units subcut in divided doses q 8–12 hr; 5000–10,000 units q 4–6 hr intermittent IV; 5000–40,000 units/day IV infusion
heparin sodium lock flush solution		Clearing intermittent infusion lines (heparin lock) to prevent clot formation at site	None significant	10–100 units/mL heparin solution
Parenteral Anticoagulants: Low–Molecular-Weight Heparins				
dalteparin *dal-tep'-ah-rin*	Fragmin	Unstable angina/non–Q-wave MI, DVT prophylaxis	Bleeding, bruising, rash, fever, erythema and irritation at site of injection	Angina/MI: 120 units/kg subcut q 12 hr with concurrent oral aspirin; DVT: 2500 units/day subcut
enoxaparin *en-ox'-ah-par-in*	Lovenox	DVT and presurgical prophylaxis, PE treatment, unstable angina/non–Q-wave MI	Same as dalteparin	DVT prophylaxis: 30–40 mg subcut q 12 hr Treatment: 1 mg/kg subcut q 12 hr
Miscellaneous Anticoagulant Agents				
dabigatran *da'-bi-gat-ran*	Pradaxa	Stroke and embolism prevention	Bleeding, nausea, diarrhea	150 mg orally BID
desirudin *deh-sih'-rue-din*	Iprivask	DVT prophylaxis	Bleeding (at injection site)	15 mg subcut every 12 hr for 9–12 days postoperatively
fondaparinux *fon-dah-par'-ih-nux*	Arixtra	DVT prophylaxis	Bleeding (at injection site)	2.5 mg subcut 6–8 hr following surgery, then daily for 5–9 days postoperatively
rivaroxaban *riv'-a-rox'-a-ban*	Xarelto	DVT prophylaxis and stroke prevention	Bleeding	10–10 mg orally daily

(table continues on page 400)

Summary Drug Table ANTICOAGULANT, ANTIPLATELET, AND THROMBOLYTIC AGENTS (continued)

Generic Name	Trade Name	Uses	Adverse Reactions	Dosage Ranges
Antiplatelet Agents				
abciximab *ab-six'-ih-mab*	ReoPro	Adjunct in coronary angioplasty	Bleeding, pain	0.125 mcg/kg/min IV during procedure
anagrelide *an-ag'-greh-lyde*	Agrylin	Thrombocythemia	Heart palpitations, dizziness, headache, nausea, abdominal pain, diarrhea, edema	1 mg orally BID
cilostazol *sill-ah'-stah-zoll*	Pletal	Intermittent claudication	Heart palpitations, dizziness, diarrhea, headache, rhinitis	100 mg orally BID
clopidogrel *kloe-pid'-oh-grel*	Plavix	Recent MI, stroke, and acute coronary syndrome	Dizziness, skin rash, chest pain, constipation	Single loading dose: 300 mg; 75 mg/day orally
dipyridamole *dye-peer-id'-ah-mole*	Persantine	Postoperative thromboembolic prevention in valve replacement	Dizziness, abdominal distress	75–100 mg orally QID
eptifibatide *ep-tiff-ib'-ah-tyde*	Integrilin	Adjunct in coronary angioplasty, acute coronary syndrome	Bleeding, pain	1 mcg/kg/min IV infusion
prasugrel *pra'-soo-grel*	Effient	Acute coronary syndrome	Bleeding, anemia	5–10 mg orally daily
ticagrelor *tye'-ka-grel*	Brilinta	Acute coronary syndrome	Bleeding	90–180 mg orally daily
ticlopidine *tye-kloe'-pih-deen*		Thrombotic stroke	Nausea, dyspepsia, diarrhea	250 mg orally BID
tirofiban *tye-roe'-fih-ban*	Aggrastat	Acute coronary syndrome	Bleeding, pain	0.4–0.1 mcg/kg/min IV infusion
Thrombolytics				
alteplase *al'-teh-plaze*	Activase, Cathflo Activase (for IV catheter occlusions only)	Acute MI, acute ischemic stroke, PE, IV catheter clearance	Bleeding (genitourinary [GU], gingival, intracranial) and epistaxis, ecchymosis	Total dose of 90–100 mg IV, given as a 2- to 3-hr infusion
reteplase *ret'-ah-plaze*	Retavase	Acute MI	Bleeding (GI, GU, or at injection site), intracranial hemorrhage, anemia	Prepackaged: 2- to 10-unit IV bolus injections
streptokinase *strep-toe-kye'-nase*	Streptase	Acute MI, DVT, PE, embolism	Minor bleeding (superficial and surface) and major bleeding (internal and severe)	250,000 units IV loading dose, followed by 100,000 units for 24–72 hr
tenecteplase *teh-nek'-tih-plaze*	TNKase	Acute MI	Bleeding (GI, GU, or at injection site), intracranial hemorrhage, anemia	Dosage based on weight, not to exceed 50 mg IV
Anticoagulant Antagonists				
phytonadione (vitamin K) *fye-toe-nah-dye'-own*	Mephyton	Treatment of warfarin overdosage	Gastric upset, unusual taste, flushing, rash, urticaria, erythema, pain and/or swelling at injection site	2.5–10 mg orally, IM, may repeat orally in 12–48 hr or in 6–8 hr after parenteral dose
protamine *proe'-tah-meen*		Treatment of heparin overdose	Flushing and warm feeling, dyspnea, bradycardia, hypotension	Dose is determined by amount of heparin to be neutralized; generally, 1 mg IV neutralizes 100 units of heparin

● Chapter Review

Know Your Drugs

Clients sometimes know a medication by the brand (or trade) name and not the generic name. To help you recognize both names, match the brand name with the generic name of the same medication.

Generic Name	Brand Name
1. clopidogrel	A. Brilinta
2. dalteparin	B. Coumadin
3. ticagrelor	C. Fragmin
4. warfarin	D. Plavix

Calculate Medication Dosages

1. The client is prescribed 5000 units of heparin. The drug is available as a solution of 2500 units/mL. The nurse administers _____.

2. Oral warfarin 5 mg is prescribed. On hand are 2.5-mg tablets. The nurse administers _____.

● Prepare for the NCLEX®

Build Your Knowledge

1. Hemostasis is best defined as _____.

   1. thinning the blood for better flow in the vessels
   2. stopping all evidence of bleeding
   3. events forming a clot, stopping bleeding
   4. formation of a thrombus in the venous circulation

2. When a clot detaches from the vessel wall and begins to travel, this is termed _____.

   1. thrombus
   2. aggregation
   3. hemostasis
   4. embolus

3. Optimal INR during therapy is _____.

   1. more than 5
   2. less than 1
   3. between 1.8 and 2
   4. between 2 and 3

4. There is an increased risk for bleeding when the client receiving heparin is also taking _____.

   1. allopurinol
   2. NSAIDs
   3. digoxin
   4. furosemide

5. In which of the following situations would the nurse expect dalteparin to be prescribed?

   1. to prevent a DVT
   2. for a client with DIC
   3. to prevent hemorrhage
   4. for a client with atrial fibrillation

Apply Your Knowledge

6. The patient is receiving oral anticoagulant drug therapy. Before administering the drug, the nurse _____.

   1. administers a loading dose of heparin
   2. has the laboratory draw blood for a serum potassium level
   3. takes the apical pulse
   4. sees that blood has been drawn for a baseline PT evaluation

7. If bleeding is noted while a client is receiving a thrombolytic drug, the client may receive _____.

   1. heparin
   2. whole blood or fresh frozen plasma
   3. a diuretic
   4. protamine sulfate

8. The clinic nurse prepares teaching materials to give a client using Coumadin. Which statement would cause her to contact the primary health care provider?

   1. "I noticed my bowel movements were black yesterday."
   2. "I ordered a medical alert bracelet."
   3. "My mother died of a stroke."
   4. "A nutritious meal will make my blood better."

Alternate-Format Questions

9. Clients on blood-thinning medications should be monitored for bleeding. Which of the following may indicate internal bleeding? **Select all that apply**.

   1. sudden decrease in blood pressure
   2. INR of 1.5
   3. cloudy, amber urine
   4. multiple red spots on skin
   5. black, tarry stool

10. Match the drug class with its function.

1. anticoagulant	A. prevents cell aggregation
2. antiplatelet	B. dissolves existing thrombi
3. thrombolytic	C. prevents formation of new thrombi

To check your answers, see Appendix G.

thePoint *For more NCLEX-style questions, log on to http://thepoint.lww.com to access more than 1000 questions.*

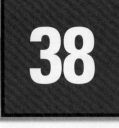

38

Cardiotonic and Inotropic Drugs

LEARNING OBJECTIVES

On completion of this chapter, the student will:

1. Discuss heart failure in relationship to left ventricular failure, right ventricular failure, neurohormonal activity, and treatment options.
2. Discuss the uses, general drug actions, general adverse reactions, contraindications, precautions, and interactions of the cardiotonic and inotropic drugs.
3. Discuss the use of other drugs with positive inotropic action.
4. Discuss important preadministration and ongoing assessment activities the nurse should perform on the patient taking a cardiotonic or inotropic drug.
5. List nursing diagnoses particular to a patient taking a cardiotonic or inotropic drug.
6. Identify the symptoms of digitalis toxicity.
7. Discuss ways to promote an optimal response to therapy, how to manage common adverse reactions, and important points to keep in mind when administering cardiotonic drugs.

KEY TERMS

atrial fibrillation • quivering of the atria of the heart
cardiac output • volume of blood discharged from the left or right ventricle per minute
digitalis toxicity • toxic drug effects from administration of digoxin
heart failure • condition in which the heart cannot pump enough blood to meet the tissue needs of the body; commonly called congestive heart failure

left ventricular dysfunction • condition in which fluids back up previous to the left ventricle of the heart and is characterized by shortness of breath and moist cough in heart failure
neurohormonal activity • in heart failure, increased secretions of epinephrine and norepinephrine, resulting in arteriolar vasoconstriction, tachycardia, and myocardial contractility, resulting in a worsening of heart failure and reduced ability of the heart to contract effectively
positive inotropic activity • increase in the force of cardiac contraction
right ventricular dysfunction • condition in which fluid backs up previous to the right ventricle of the heart and is characterized by peripheral edema and venous congestion in heart failure

DRUG CLASSES

Cardiotonic
Inotropic

The cardiotonics are drugs used to increase the efficiency and improve the contraction of the heart muscle, which leads to improved blood flow to all tissues of the body. These drugs have long been used to treat **heart failure**, a condition in which the heart cannot pump enough blood to meet the tissue needs of the body. Although the term *congestive heart failure* is commonly used, a more accurate term is simply *heart failure*.

Heart failure is a complex clinical syndrome that can result from any number of cardiac or metabolic disorders, such as ischemic heart disease, hypertension, or hyperthyroidism.

PHARMACOLOGY IN PRACTICE

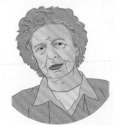

Mrs. Moore's daughter calls the clinic after her hospital discharge. She is concerned because her mother lives alone and that her mother will not be able to recognize toxicity symptoms and have to return to the hospital. Read about the drugs and their toxic effects and then think about what your approach to Mrs. Moore's daughter would be.

Display 38.1 Neurohormonal Responses Affecting Heart Failure

The body activates the neurohormonal compensatory mechanisms, which result in:

- Increased secretion of the neurohormones by the sympathetic nervous system
- Activation of the renin-angiotensin-aldosterone (RAA) system
- Remodeling of the cardiac tissue

Any condition that impairs the ability of the ventricle to pump blood can lead to heart failure. In heart failure, the heart fails in its ability to pump enough blood to meet the needs of the body or can do so only with an elevated filling pressure. Heart failure causes a number of neurohormonal changes as the body tries to compensate for the increased workload of the heart. Display 38.1 discusses this neurohormonal response.

The sympathetic nervous system increases the secretion of the catecholamines (the neurohormones epinephrine and norepinephrine), which results in increased heart rate and vasoconstriction. The activation of the renin-angiotensin-aldosterone (RAA) system occurs because of decreased perfusion to the kidneys. As the RAA system is activated, angiotensin II and aldosterone levels increase, which increases the blood pressure, adding to the workload of the heart. These increases in **neurohormonal activity** cause a remodeling (restructuring) of the cardiac muscle cells, leading to hypertrophy (enlargement) of the heart, increased need for oxygen, and cardiac necrosis, which worsens the heart failure. The tissue of the heart is changed such that there is an increase in the cellular mass of cardiac tissue, the shape of the ventricle(s) is changed, and the heart's ability to contract effectively is reduced.

Heart failure is best described by denoting the area of initial ventricular dysfunction: left-sided (left ventricular) dysfunction or right-sided (right ventricular) dysfunction. **Left ventricular dysfunction** leads to pulmonary symptoms, such as dyspnea and moist cough with the production of frothy, pink (blood-tinged) sputum. **Right ventricular dysfunction** leads to neck vein distention, peripheral edema, weight gain, and hepatic engorgement. Because both sides of the heart work together, ultimately both sides are affected in heart failure. Typically the left side of the heart is affected first, followed by right ventricular involvement. The most common symptoms associated with heart failure include the following:

- Left ventricular dysfunction
- Shortness of breath with exercise
- Dry, hacking cough or wheezing
- Orthopnea (difficulty breathing while lying flat)
- Restlessness and anxiety
- Right ventricular dysfunction
- Swollen ankles, legs, or abdomen, leading to pitting edema
- Anorexia
- Nausea
- Nocturia (the need to urinate frequently at night)
- Weakness
- Weight gain as the result of fluid retention

Other symptoms include:

- Palpitations, fatigue, or pain when performing normal activities
- Tachycardia or irregular heart rate
- Dizziness or confusion

Left ventricular dysfunction, also called left ventricular systolic dysfunction, is the most common form of heart failure and results in decreased **cardiac output** and decreased ejection fraction (the amount of blood that the ventricle ejects per beat in relationship to the amount of blood available to eject). Typically, the ejection fraction should be greater than 60%. With left ventricular systolic dysfunction, the ejection fraction is less than 40%, and the heart is enlarged and dilated.

In the past, the cardiotonics were the mainstay in heart failure treatment; currently, however, they are used in the treatment of patients who continue to experience symptoms *after* using the angiotensin-converting enzyme (ACE) inhibitors, diuretics, and beta (β) blockers. Although their use is diminished, they remain a low-cost option for therapy.

CARDIOTONICS

Cardiotonic drugs are used for patients with persistent symptoms or recurrent hospitalizations or as indicated in conjunction with ACE inhibitors, loop diuretics, and β blockers.

Digoxin (Lanoxin) is the most commonly used cardiotonic drug. Other terms used to identify the cardiotonics are cardiac glycosides or digitalis glycosides. The digitalis or cardiac glycosides are obtained from the leaves of the foxglove plant (*Digitalis purpurea* and *Digitalis lanata*).

Another drug with positive inotropic action is milrinone, a nonglycoside used in the short-term management of heart failure. See the Summary Drug Table: Cardiotonic and Inotropic Drugs for information concerning these drugs.

Actions

Cardiotonics increase cardiac output through **positive inotropic activity** (an increase in the force of the contraction). They slow the conduction velocity through the atrioventricular (AV) node in the heart and decrease the heart rate through a negative chronotropic effect. Milrinone has inotropic action and is used in the short-term management of severe heart failure that is not controlled by the digitalis preparation.

Uses

The cardiotonics are used to treat the following:

- Heart failure
- **Atrial fibrillation**

Atrial fibrillation is a cardiac arrhythmia characterized by rapid contractions and quivering of the atrial myocardium, resulting in an irregular and often rapid ventricular rate. See Chapter 39 for more information on arrhythmias and their treatment. These drugs do not cure heart failure; rather, they control its signs and symptoms.

Adverse Reactions

Central Nervous System Reactions

- Headache
- Weakness, drowsiness
- Visual disturbances (blurring or yellow halo)

Cardiovascular and Gastrointestinal System Reactions

- Arrhythmias
- Nausea and anorexia

Because some patients are more sensitive to side effects of digoxin, dosage is calculated carefully and adjusted as the clinical condition indicates. There is a narrow margin of safety between the full therapeutic effects and the toxic effects of cardiotonic drugs. Even normal doses of a cardiotonic drug can cause toxic drug effects. Because substantial individual variations may occur, it is important to individualize the dosage. The term **digitalis toxicity** (or *digitalis intoxication*) is used to describe toxic drug effects that occur when digoxin is administered.

Contraindications and Precautions

The cardiotonics are contraindicated in the presence of digitalis toxicity and in patients with known hypersensitivity, ventricular failure, ventricular tachycardia, cardiac tamponade, restrictive cardiomyopathy, or AV block.

The cardiotonics are given cautiously to patients with electrolyte imbalance (especially hypokalemia, hypocalcemia, and hypomagnesemia), thyroid disorders, severe carditis, heart block, myocardial infarction, severe pulmonary disease, acute glomerulonephritis, and impaired renal or hepatic function.

Digoxin is classified as a pregnancy category C drug and is used cautiously during pregnancy and lactation. Exposure to digoxin in a nursing infant is typically below an infant maintenance dose, yet caution should be exercised when digoxin is taken by a nursing woman.

Interactions

When the cardiotonics are taken with food, absorption is slowed, but the amount absorbed is the same. However, if taken with high-fiber meals, absorption of the cardiotonics may be decreased. The following interactions may occur with the cardiac glycosides:

Interacting Drug	Common Use	Effect of Interaction
thyroid hormones	Treatment of hypothyroidism	Decreased effectiveness of digitalis glycosides, requiring a larger dosage of digoxin
thiazide and loop diuretics	Management of edema and hypertension	Increased diuretic-induced electrolyte disturbances, predisposing the patient to digitalis-induced arrhythmias

Patients may not always volunteer information regarding their use of complementary and alternative remedies. Be sure to inquire about use of herbal products. St. John's wort (used to relieve depression) causes a decrease in serum digitalis levels. Certain drugs may increase or decrease serum digitalis levels as follows:

Interacting Drug	Common Use	Effect of Interaction
amiodarone	Cardiac problems	**Increased** serum digitalis levels leading to toxicity
benzodiazepines (alprazolam, diazepam)	Treatment of seizures and anxiety	
indomethacin	Pain relief	
itraconazole	Fungal infections	
macrolides (erythromycin, clarithromycin)	Infections	
propafenone	Cardiac problems	
quinidine	Cardiac problems	
spironolactone	Edema	
tetracyclines, macrolides	Infections	
verapamil	Cardiac problems	
oral aminoglycoside	Infections	
antacids	Gastrointestinal (GI) problems	**Decreased** serum digitalis levels
antineoplastics (bleomycin, carmustine, cyclophosphamide, methotrexate, and vincristine)	Anticancer agents	
activated charcoal	Antidote to poisoning with certain toxic substances	
cholestyramine	Agent to lower high blood cholesterol levels	
colestipol	Agent to lower high blood cholesterol levels	
neomycin	Agent to suppress GI bacteria before surgery	
rifampin	Antitubercular agent	

NURSING PROCESS
PATIENT RECEIVING A CARDIOTONIC DRUG

ASSESSMENT

Preadministration Assessment
The cardiotonics are potentially toxic drugs. Therefore, patients are observed closely, especially during initial therapy. The physical assessment of a person in heart failure should include information to establish a database for comparison during therapy. The physical assessment should include the following:

- Taking blood pressure, apical-radial pulse rate, respiratory rate
- Auscultating the lungs, noting any unusual sounds during inspiration and expiration
- Examining the extremities for edema
- Checking the jugular veins for distention
- Measuring weight
- Inspecting sputum raised (if any) and noting the appearance (e.g., frothy, pink tinged, clear, yellow)
- Looking for evidence of other problems such as cyanosis, shortness of breath on exertion (if the patient is allowed out of bed) or when lying flat, and mental changes

The primary health care provider also may order laboratory and diagnostic tests, such as an electrocardiogram, renal and hepatic function tests, complete blood count, and serum enzyme and electrolyte levels. Renal function is particularly important because diminished renal function could affect the prescribed dosage of digoxin. Because digoxin interacts with many medications, take a careful drug history.

Ongoing Assessment
Before administering each dose of a cardiotonic, take the apical pulse rate for 60 seconds (Fig. 38.1). Document the apical pulse rate in the designated area on the chart or the medication administration record. If the pulse rate is below 60 bpm in adults or greater than 100 bpm, withhold the drug and notify the primary health care provider, unless there is a written order giving different guidelines for withholding the drug.

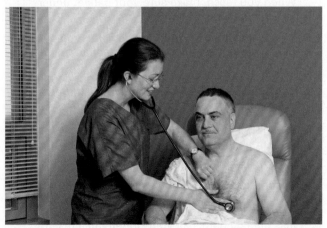

Figure 38.1 Nurse counts the apical pulse for 1 minute before administering the cardiotonic.

LIFESPAN CONSIDERATIONS
Pediatric
The drug is withheld and the primary health care provider notified before administration of the drug if the apical pulse rate in a child is below 70 bpm, or below 90 bpm in an infant.

Weigh patients receiving a cardiotonic drug daily or as ordered. Intake and output are measured, especially if the patient has edema or heart failure or is also receiving a diuretic. Throughout therapy, assess the patient for peripheral edema and auscultate the lungs for crackles (formerly called *rales*). Serum electrolyte levels should be assessed periodically. Hypokalemia, hypomagnesemia, or hypercalcemia may increase the risk for toxicity. Any electrolyte imbalance is reported to the primary health care provider.

NURSING DIAGNOSES
Drug-specific nursing diagnoses include the following:

- **Imbalanced Nutrition: Less Than Body Requirements** related to anorexia, nausea, vomiting
- **Activity Intolerance** related to weakness and drowsiness

Nursing diagnoses related to drug administration are discussed in Chapter 4.

PLANNING
The expected outcomes of the patient depend on the specific reason for administering the drug but may include an optimal response to therapy, support of patient needs related to the management of adverse reactions, and confidence in an understanding of the medication regimen.

IMPLEMENTATION

Promoting an Optimal Response to Therapy
Because other drugs are typically chosen to treat heart failure, it is the patient who has been on this drug for a long time, often in a long-term care facility, who will be treated with digoxin. Great care must be taken when administering a cardiotonic drug because patients can become toxic.

> **NURSING ALERT**
> Plasma digoxin levels are monitored closely. Blood for plasma level measurements should be drawn immediately before the next dose or 6 to 8 hours after the last dose regardless of route. Therapeutic drug levels are between 0.8 and 2 nanograms/mL. Plasma digoxin levels greater than 2 nanograms/mL are considered toxic and are reported to the primary health care provider.

Periodic electrocardiograms, serum electrolytes, hepatic and renal function tests, and other laboratory studies also may be ordered. Diuretics (see Chapter 33) may be ordered for some patients receiving a cardiotonic drug. Diuretics, along with other conditions or factors, such as GI suction, diarrhea, and old age, may produce low serum potassium levels (hypokalemia). The primary health care provider may order a potassium salt to be given orally or intravenously (IV).

> **NURSING ALERT**
> Hypokalemia makes the heart muscle more sensitive to digitalis, thereby increasing the possibility of developing digitalis toxicity. At frequent intervals, observe patients with hypokalemia closely for signs of digitalis toxicity.

Patients with hypomagnesemia (low plasma magnesium levels) are at increased risk for digitalis toxicity. If low magnesium levels are detected, the primary health care provider may prescribe magnesium replacement therapy.

A cardiotonic can be given orally, IV, or intramuscularly (IM). When a cardiotonic drug is given IV, it is administered slowly (over at least 5 minutes), and the administration site is assessed for redness or infiltration. IM injection is not recommended for these drugs yet; it may be given through this route when needed urgently and IV access is not available. When giving a cardiotonic drug IM, give the injection deep in the muscle and follow with massage to the site. No more than 2 mL should be injected IM. Oral preparations can be given without regard to meals. Tablets can be crushed and mixed with food or fluids if the patient has difficulty swallowing. Do not alternate between the dosage forms (i.e., tablets and capsules); these dosages are not the same. Owing to better absorption, the recommended dosage of the capsules is 80% of the dosage for tablets and elixir.

Monitoring and Managing Patient Needs

IMBALANCED NUTRITION: LESS THAN BODY REQUIREMENTS. If toxicity is suspected, closely observe the patient for adverse drug reactions such as anorexia, nausea, and vomiting. Carefully consider any patient complaint or comment, document it on the patient's chart, and bring it to the attention of the primary health care provider. Other signs of digitalis toxicity include abdominal pain, visual disturbances (blurred, yellow, or green vision and white halos, borders around dark objects), and arrhythmias (any type).

If the nausea or anorexia is not a result of toxicity but an adverse reaction to the drug, use nursing measures to help control the reactions. Offer frequent small meals rather than three large meals. Restricting fluids at meals and avoiding fluids 1 hour before and after meals helps to control nausea. Helping the patient to maintain good oral hygiene by brushing teeth or rinsing the mouth after ingesting food will also help with nausea.

ACTIVITY INTOLERANCE. The patient may experience weakness or drowsiness as adverse reactions associated with digoxin, which may lead to activity intolerance. The patient is encouraged to increase daily activities gradually as tolerance increases and to plan adequate rest periods during the day.

Digitalis toxicity can occur even when normal doses are being administered or when the patient has been receiving a maintenance dose. Many symptoms of toxicity are similar to the symptoms of the heart conditions for which the patient is receiving the cardiotonic. The signs of digitalis toxicity are listed in Display 38.2. When digitalis toxicity develops, the primary health care provider may discontinue digitalis use until all signs of toxicity are gone. If severe bradycardia occurs, atropine may be ordered. If digoxin has been given, the primary health care provider may order blood tests to determine serum drug levels. A digoxin serum level greater than 2.0 nanograms/mL indicates toxicity.

Digoxin has a rapid onset and a short duration of action. Once the drug is withheld, the toxic effects of digoxin subside rapidly. Most often, digoxin toxicity can be treated successfully by simply withdrawing the drug.

Display 38.2 Signs of Digitalis Toxicity

- Gastrointestinal—anorexia (usually the first sign), nausea, vomiting, diarrhea
- Muscular—weakness, lethargy
- Central nervous system—headache, drowsiness, visual disturbances (blurred vision, disturbance in yellow or green vision, halo effect around dark objects), confusion, disorientation, delirium
- Cardiac—changes in pulse rate or rhythm: electrocardiographic changes, such as bradycardia, tachycardia, premature ventricular contractions

---

LIFESPAN CONSIDERATIONS
Gerontology

Older adults are particularly prone to digitalis toxicity. Some conditions such as dementia may have similar signs, such as confusion, as those of digitalis toxicity.

Educating the Patient and Family

In some instances, a cardiotonic drug may be prescribed for a prolonged period. If the primary health care provider wants the patient to monitor the pulse rate daily during cardiotonic therapy, show the patient or a family member the correct technique for taking the pulse (see Patient Teaching for Improved Patient Outcomes: Monitoring Pulse Rate).

The primary health care provider may also want the patient to omit the next dose of the drug and call him or her

---

Patient Teaching for Improved Patient Outcomes

Monitoring Pulse Rate

Monitoring a patient's pulse rate is second nature when the patient is in an acute care facility. However, when the patient goes home with digoxin, he or she will need to monitor the pulse rate to prevent possible adverse reactions.

When you teach, make sure your patient understands the following:

- ✔ Have a watch with a second hand with you.
- ✔ Sit down and rest your nondominant arm on a table or chair armrest.
- ✔ Place the index and third fingers of your dominant hand just below the wrist bone on the thumb side of your nondominant arm.
- ✔ Feel lightly for a beating or pulsing sensation. This is your pulse.
- ✔ Count the number of beats for 30 seconds (if the pulse is regular) and multiply by 2. If the pulse is irregular, count the number of beats for 60 seconds.
- ✔ Record the number of beats of your pulse and keep a log of your reading.
- ✔ If you notice the pulse is greater than 100 bpm or less than 60 bpm, call your primary health care provider immediately.

if the pulse rate falls below a certain level (usually 60 bpm in an adult, 70 bpm in a child, and 90 bpm in an infant). These instructions are emphasized at the time of patient teaching.

As you develop a teaching plan include the following information:

- Do not discontinue use of this drug without first checking with the primary health care provider (unless instructed to do otherwise). Do not miss a dose or take an extra dose.
- Take this drug at the same time each day; a compartmentalized pill container may be helpful.
- Take your pulse before taking the drug, and withhold the drug and notify the primary health care provider if your pulse rate is less than 60 bpm or greater than 100 bpm.
- Avoid antacids and nonprescription cough, cold, allergy, antidiarrheal, and diet (weight-reducing) drugs unless their use has been approved by the primary health care provider. Some of these drugs interfere with the action of the cardiotonic drug or cause other, potentially serious problems (see Interactions, earlier).
- Contact the primary health care provider if nausea, vomiting, diarrhea, unusual fatigue, weakness, vision change (such as blurred vision, changes in colors of objects, or halos around dark objects), or mental depression occurs.
- Carry medical identification describing the disease process and your medication regimen.
- Do not substitute tablets for capsules or vice versa.
- Follow the dietary recommendations (if any) made by the primary health care provider.

- The primary health care provider will closely monitor therapy. Keep all appointments for primary health care provider visits or laboratory or diagnostic tests.

EVALUATION

- Therapeutic response is achieved, and the heart beats more efficiently.
- Adverse reactions are identified, reported to the primary health care provider, and managed successfully with appropriate nursing interventions:
  - Patient maintains an adequate nutritional status.
  - Patient carries out activities of daily living.
- Patient and family express confidence and demonstrate an understanding of the drug regimen.

PHARMACOLOGY IN PRACTICE
THINK CRITICALLY

 In talking with the primary health care provider you learn that Mrs. Moore is now on an ACE inhibitor. What are the different teaching points you will emphasize when you return her daughter's phone call?

KEY POINTS

- Heart failure, also called congestive heart failure, is a condition in which the heart cannot pump enough blood to meet the tissue needs of the body. Left-sided failure (left ventricular dysfunction) leads to pulmonary symptoms such as dyspnea and moist cough. Right-sided failure (right ventricular dysfunction) can be seen with fluid backup in the body such as distended neck veins, peripheral edema, and hepatic engorgement.
- Cardiotonics increase the efficiency and improve the contraction of the heart muscle. Due to their toxic effects

and use of other drugs such as ACE inhibitors, they are not used as frequently.

- When a cardiotonic is used, the pulse rate is monitored and the drug held if the patient's heart rate is less than 60 bpm. Adverse reactions are typically GI in nature, and patients need to be monitored for toxicity to the drug, which can appear as GI distress, changes in vision, or muscle weakness.

Summary Drug Table CARDIOTONIC AND INOTROPIC DRUGS

Generic Name	Trade Name	Uses	Adverse Reactions	Dosage Ranges
Cardiotonics				
digoxin *dih-jox'-in*	Lanoxin	Heart failure, atrial fibrillation	Headache, weakness, drowsiness, visual disturbances, nausea, vomiting, anorexia, arrhythmias	Loading dose:* 0.75–1.25 mg orally or 0.6–1 mg IV Maintenance: 0.125–0.25 mg/day orally Lanoxicaps: 0.1–0.3 mg/day orally
Miscellaneous Inotropic Drugs				
milrinone *mill'-rih-noan*		Short-term management of heart failure	Ventricular arrhythmias, hypotension, angina/chest pain, headaches, hypokalemia	Loading dose: 50 mcg/kg IV IV: Up to 1.13 mg/kg/day

*Based on patient lean body weight of 70 kg.

● Chapter Review

Calculate Medication Dosages

1. Digoxin 0.5 mg IV is prescribed. The drug is available in a solution of 0.25 mg/mL. How many milliliters will the nurse prepare?

● Prepare for the NCLEX®

Build Your Knowledge

1. Which of the following is commonly associated with left ventricular systolic dysfunction?

   1. ejection fraction of 60% or more
   2. ejection fraction below 40%
   3. increased cardiac output
   4. normal cardiac output

2. Which of the following serum digoxin levels in an adult would be most indicative that the client may be experiencing digoxin toxicity?

   1. 0.5 nanograms/mL
   2. 0.8 nanograms/mL
   3. 1.0 nanograms/mL
   4. 2.0 nanograms/mL

3. In which of the following situations would the nurse withhold a dose of digoxin and notify the primary health care provider?

   1. pulse rate of 50 bpm
   2. pulse rate of 87 bpm
   3. pulse rate of 92 bpm
   4. pulse rate of 62 bpm

Apply Your Knowledge

4. The nurse suspects a client is experiencing digoxin toxicity. Which of the following symptoms did the client report to make the nurse suspicious of a toxic reaction?

   1. insatiable hunger
   2. constipation
   3. halo in vision field
   4. muscle cramping

Alternate-Format Questions

5. Digoxin (Lanoxin) is prescribed for a client with heart failure. The primary health care provider prescribes digoxin (Lanoxin) 0.75 mg orally as the initial dose. Available are digoxin tablets of 0.5 and 0.25 mg. The nurse administers _____.

To check your answers, see Appendix G.

the**Point** *For more NCLEX-style questions, log on to http://thepoint.lww.com to access more than 1000 questions.*

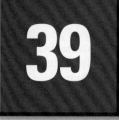

Antiarrhythmic Drugs

39

LEARNING OBJECTIVES

On completion of this chapter, the student will:

1. Describe the different types of cardiac arrhythmias.
2. Discuss the uses, general drug actions, general adverse reactions, contraindications, precautions, and interactions of the antiarrhythmic drugs.
3. Discuss important preadministration and ongoing assessments the nurse should perform on a patient taking an antiarrhythmic drug.
4. List nursing diagnoses particular to a patient taking an antiarrhythmic drug.
5. Discuss ways to promote an optimal response to therapy, how to manage common adverse reactions, and important points to keep in mind when educating patients about the use of antiarrhythmic drugs.

KEY TERMS

action potential • electrical impulse that passes from cell to cell in the myocardium of the heart and stimulates the fibers to shorten, causing the heart muscle to contract

agranulocytosis • decrease or lack of granulocytes (a type of white blood cell)

arrhythmia • abnormal heart rate or rhythm; also called *dysrhythmia*

bradycardia • slow heart rate, usually below 60 bpm

cinchonism • quinidine toxicity or poisoning

depolarization • movement of ions in a nerve cell from inside to outside and vice versa

myocardium • the striated, muscle tissue of the heart

polarization • status of a nerve cell at rest, with positive ions on the outside of the cell membrane and negative ions on the inside

proarrhythmic effect • creation of new arrhythmia or worsening of existing arrhythmia, resulting from administration of an antiarrhythmic drug

refractory period • quiet period between the transmission of nerve impulses along a nerve fiber

repolarization • return of positive and negative ions to their original place on the nerve cell after an impulse has passed along the nerve fiber (*see polarization*)

tachycardia • heart rate above 100 bpm

threshold • term applied to any stimulus of the lowest intensity that will give rise to a response in a nerve fiber

DRUG CLASSES

Class I sodium channel blockers	Class III potassium channel blockers
Class II beta (β)-adrenergic blockers	Class IV calcium channel blockers

A number of the drugs in this section are used to treat chronic heart conditions and have been discussed in previous chapters. In this chapter familiar drug names and classes, along with some new ones, will be studied as the category of antiarrhythmic drugs used to treat cardiac arrhythmias. A cardiac **arrhythmia** (also referred to as a dysrhythmia or irregular heart beat) is an electrical disturbance or irregularity in the rate or rhythm of the heart. This electrical disturbance makes

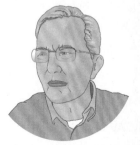

PHARMACOLOGY IN PRACTICE

Mr. Phillip was recently diagnosed with atrial fibrillation and prescribed both propranolol and Coumadin to take at home. When he comes in for weekly lab work, the phlebotomist tells you that Mr. Phillip is very dizzy and she is concerned about his safety. Read about the antiarrhythmic drugs and determine what should happen next.

the blood pumping action inefficient because the heart beats too fast (**tachycardia**) or too slow (**bradycardia**). Table 39.1 describes some examples of conduction problems known as arrhythmias.

Problems occur as a result of heart disease or from a disorder that affects cardiovascular function. Conditions such as emotional stress, hypoxia, and electrolyte imbalance also may trigger an arrhythmia. The goal of antiarrhythmic drug therapy is to restore normal cardiac function and prevent life-threatening conduction problems.

Actions

The cardiac muscle (**myocardium**) has both nerve and muscle tissues and therefore has the properties of both. Figure 39.1 illustrates how the electrical impulse is generated throughout the heart. Typically, the electrical impulse signals the heart muscle to contract (the heartbeat) in a regular, steady pattern. Some cardiac arrhythmias are caused by the generation of an abnormal number of electrical impulses (stimuli). These abnormal impulses may come from the sinoatrial (SA) node or may be generated in other areas of the myocardium. The antiarrhythmic drugs are classified according to their effects on what is termed the **action potential** (see Display 39.1 for a description). The pathophysiology of the cardiac condition guides the use of drugs to treat these conduction problems. The drugs used include four basic classes and several subclasses. Drugs in

Table 39.1 Types of Arrhythmias	
Arrhythmia	**Description**
Atrial flutter	Rapid contraction of the atria (up to 300 bpm) at a rate too rapid for the ventricles to pump efficiently
Atrial fibrillation	Irregular and rapid atrial contraction, resulting in a quivering of the atria and causing an irregular and inefficient ventricular contraction
Premature ventricular contractions	Beats originating in the ventricles instead of the sinoatrial node in the atria, causing the ventricles to contract before the atria and resulting in a decrease in the amount of blood pumped to the body
Ventricular tachycardia	A rapid heart beat with a rate of more than 100 bpm, usually originating in the ventricles
Ventricular fibrillation	Rapid, disorganized contractions of the ventricles resulting in the inability of the heart to pump any blood to the body, which will result in death unless treated immediately

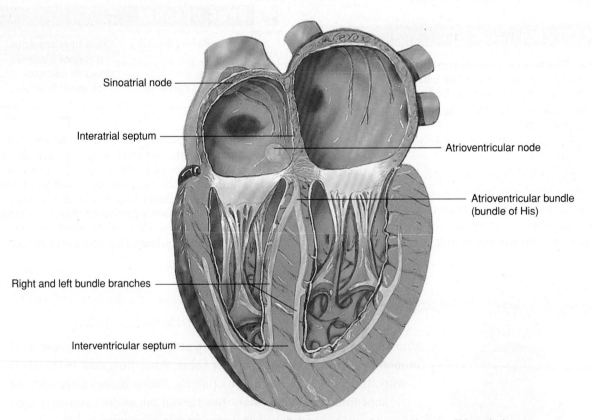

Figure 39.1 Conduction of the heart. SA node is the blue pathway; AV node is the yellow pathway. (Courtesy of Anatomical Chart Co.)

each group, or class, have certain similarities, yet each drug has subtle differences that make it unique.

Class I Sodium Channel Blockers

Class I antiarrhythmic drugs have a membrane-stabilizing or anesthetic effect on the cells of the myocardium. Class I contains the largest number of drugs of the four antiarrhythmic drug classifications. Because their actions differ slightly, the drugs are subdivided into classes IA, IB, and IC.

Class IA Drugs

In general, class IA drugs act to:

• Prolong the action potential
• Produce moderate slowing of cardiac conduction

For example, disopyramide (Norpace) decreases depolarization of myocardial fibers, prolongs the **refractory period**, and increases the action potential duration of cardiac cells (Display 39.1).

Quinidine depresses myocardial excitability or the ability of the myocardium to respond to an electrical stimulus. By depressing the myocardium and its ability to respond to some, but not all, electrical stimuli, the pulse rate decreases and the heartbeat is corrected.

Class IB Drugs

Class IB drugs generally act to:

• Shorten the action potential duration
• Selectively depress cardiac conduction

Lidocaine (Xylocaine) decreases diastolic depolarization, decreases automaticity of ventricular cells, and raises the **threshold** of the ventricular myocardium. *Threshold* is a term applied to any stimulus of the lowest intensity that will give rise to a response in a nerve fiber. A stimulus must be of a specific intensity (strength, amplitude) to pass along a given nerve fiber.

Some cardiac arrhythmias result from many stimuli present in the myocardium. Some of these are weak or of low intensity but are still able to excite myocardial tissue. Lidocaine raises the threshold of myocardial fibers, which in turn reduces the number of stimuli that will pass along these fibers and therefore decreases the pulse rate and corrects the arrhythmia.

Class IC Drugs

The general action of class IC drugs includes:

• Slight effect on **repolarization**
• Profound slowing of conduction

Specifically, flecainide (Tambocor) depresses fast sodium channels, decreases the height and rate of rise of action potentials, and slows conduction of all areas of the heart. Propafenone (Rythmol), which has a direct membrane-stabilizing effect on the myocardial membrane, prolongs the refractory period.

Class II Beta-Adrenergic Blockers

The general action of drugs in class II is to indirectly block calcium channels and block catecholamine-caused arrhythmias.

Display 39.1 Understanding Cardiac Conduction Terminology

Action Potential

All cells are electrically polarized, with the inside of the cell more negatively charged than the outside. The difference in the electrical charge is called the *resting membrane potential*. Nerve and muscle cells are excitable and can change the resting membrane potential in response to electrochemical stimuli. The *action potential* is an electrical impulse that passes from cell to cell in the myocardium, stimulating the fibers to shorten, and causing muscular contraction (systole). An action potential generated in one part of the myocardium passes almost simultaneously through all of the myocardial fibers, causing rapid contraction.

Refractory Period

Only one impulse can pass along a nerve fiber at any given time. After the passage of an impulse, there is a brief pause, or interval, before the next impulse can pass along the nerve fiber. This pause is called the *refractory period,* which is the period between the transmission of nerve impulses along a nerve fiber. Lengthening the refractory period decreases the number of impulses traveling along a nerve fiber within a given time.

Polarization

Nerve cells have positive ions on the outside and negative ions on the inside of the cell membrane when they are at rest. This is called **polarization**.

Depolarization

When a stimulus passes along the nerve, the positive ions move from outside the cell into the cell, and the negative ions move from inside the cell to outside the cell. This movement of ions is called **depolarization**. Unless positive ions move into and negative ions move out of a nerve cell, a stimulus (or impulse) cannot pass along the nerve fiber.

Repolarization

Once the stimulus has passed along the nerve fiber, the positive and negative ions move back to their original place, that is, the positive ions on the outside and the negative ions on the inside of the nerve cell. This movement back to the original place is called **repolarization**.

Acebutolol (Sectral) and propranolol (Inderal) act by blocking beta (β)-adrenergic receptors of the heart and kidney, reducing the influence of the sympathetic nervous system on these areas, decreasing the excitability of the heart and the release of renin (lowering heart rate and blood pressure). These drugs have membrane-stabilizing effects that contribute to their antiarrhythmic activity.

Class III Potassium Channel Blockers

The general action of class III antiarrhythmic drugs is prolongation of repolarization. Amiodarone (Cordarone) appears to act directly on the cardiac cell membrane, prolonging the refractory period and repolarization and increasing the ventricular fibrillation threshold. Ibutilide acts by prolonging the action potential, producing a mild slowing of the sinus rate and atrioventricular (AV) conduction.

Class IV Calcium Channel Blockers

In general, the class IV antiarrhythmic drugs act by:

• Depressing depolarization (phase 4)
• Lengthening phase 1 and 2 of repolarization

Verapamil (Calan) is a calcium channel blocker. These drugs inhibit the movement of calcium through channels across the myocardial cell membranes and vascular smooth muscle. Cardiac and vascular smooth muscle depends on the movement of calcium ions into the muscle cells through specific ion channels. When this movement is inhibited, the coronary and peripheral arteries dilate, thereby decreasing the force of cardiac contraction. This drug also reduces heart rate by slowing conduction through the SA and AV nodes. Additional information about the calcium channel blockers can be found in the chapter about antihypertensives (Chapter 35).

Uses

In general, the antiarrhythmic drugs are used to treat:

• Premature ventricular contractions (PVCs)
• Ventricular tachycardia
• Premature atrial contractions
• Paroxysmal atrial tachycardia
• Other atrial arrhythmias, such as atrial fibrillation or flutter
• Tachycardia when rapid but short-term control of ventricular rate is desirable

Some of the antiarrhythmic drugs are used for other conditions. For example, propranolol is also used for patients with myocardial infarction. This drug has reduced the risk of death and repeated myocardial infarctions in those surviving the acute phase of a myocardial infarction. See the Summary Drug Table: Antiarrhythmic Drugs for more uses.

Adverse Reactions

Adverse reactions associated with the administration of specific antiarrhythmic drugs are given in the Summary Drug Table: Antiarrhythmic Drugs. General adverse reactions common to most antiarrhythmic drugs include the following:

Central Nervous System Reactions

• Lightheadedness
• Weakness
• Somnolence

Cardiovascular System Reactions

• Hypotension
• Arrhythmias
• Bradycardia

Other Reactions

• Urinary retention
• Local inflammation

All antiarrhythmic drugs may cause new arrhythmias or worsen existing arrhythmias, even though they are administered to resolve an existing arrhythmia. This phenomenon is called the **proarrhythmic effect**. This effect ranges from an increase in frequency of PVCs to the development of more severe ventricular tachycardia to ventricular fibrillation, and the effect may lead to death. Proarrhythmic effects may occur at any time, but they occur more often when excessive dosages are given, when the pre-existing arrhythmia is life-threatening, or when the drug is given intravenously (IV).

Contraindications

The antiarrhythmic drugs are contraindicated in patients with known hypersensitivity to these drugs. They are contraindicated during pregnancy and lactation. The antiarrhythmic drug amiodarone is a pregnancy category D drug, indicating that fetal harm can occur when the agent is administered to a pregnant woman. It is used only if the potential benefits outweigh the potential hazards to the fetus. Antiarrhythmic drugs are contraindicated in patients with second- or third-degree AV block (if the patient has no artificial pacemaker), severe heart failure (HF), aortic stenosis, hypotension, and cardiogenic shock. Quinidine is contraindicated in patients with myasthenia gravis or systemic lupus erythematosus.

Precautions

Antiarrhythmic drugs are used cautiously in patients with hepatic disease, electrolyte disturbances, HF (quinidine, flecainide, and disopyramide), and renal impairment. Most antiarrhythmics are pregnancy category B or C drugs, indicating that safe use of these drugs during pregnancy or lactation, or in children, has not been established. Disopyramide is used cautiously in patients with myasthenia gravis, urinary retention, or glaucoma, and in men with prostate enlargement.

Interactions

Because of a specific enzyme reaction, grapefruit or its juice should not be taken if on the following drugs: amiodarone or the calcium channel blockers. When antiarrhythmics are used with other medications, various interactions may occur. See Table 39.2 for more interactions.

Table 39.2 Interactions of Antiarrhythmics With Other Agents

Interacting Drug	Common Uses	Effect of Interaction
Disopyramide		
clarithromycin, erythromycin	Bacterial infections	Increased serum disopyramide levels
fluoroquinolones	Infections	Risk of life-threatening arrhythmias
quinidine	Cardiac problems	Increased serum levels of disopyramide
rifampin	Antitubercular agent	Decreased disopyramide serum levels
thioridazine, ziprasidone	Management of mental illness	Increased risk of life-threatening arrhythmias
Quinidine		
cholinergic drugs	Treatment of glaucoma	Failure to terminate paroxysmal supraventricular tachycardia
cimetidine	GI problems	Increased serum quinidine level
hydantoins	Seizure control	Decreased therapeutic effect of quinidine
nifedipine	Treatment of angina	Decreased action and serum level of quinidine
cholinergic blocking drugs	GI problems	Additive vagolytic effect
Lidocaine		
β blockers	Hypertension and angina	Increased lidocaine levels
cimetidine	GI problems	Decreased lidocaine clearance with possible toxicity
Flecainide		
amiodarone	Cardiac problems	Increased serum flecainide levels
cimetidine	GI problems	Increased serum flecainide levels
disopyramide, verapamil	Cardiovascular problems	May increase negative inotropic properties. Avoid using either of these drugs with flecainide
propranolol and other β blockers	Cardiovascular problems	Increased serum levels of propranolol and flecainide, and additive negative inotropic effects
local anesthetics	Anesthesia	Concurrent use (e.g., during pacemaker implantation, surgery, or dental use) may increase the risk of central nervous system (CNS) side effects
quinidine	Cardiac problems	Increased serum propafenone levels
selective serotonin reuptake inhibitors (SSRIs)	Relief of depression	Increased serum propafenone levels
anticoagulants (e.g., warfarin)	Blood thinners	Increased prothrombin time and increased plasma warfarin levels
digoxin	Heart failure	Increased serum digoxin level
theophylline	Management of asthma and chronic obstructive pulmonary disease (COPD)	Increased serum theophylline level

NURSING PROCESS

PATIENT RECEIVING AN ANTIARRHYTHMIC DRUG

ASSESSMENT

Preadministration Assessment

Antiarrhythmic drugs are used to treat various types of cardiac arrhythmias. Cardiovascular assessment is performed before starting therapy and should include the following:

- Take and document the blood pressure, apical and radial pulses, and respiratory rate. This provides a database for comparison during therapy.
- Perform or arrange for an electrocardiogram (ECG), which provides a picture of the electrical activity of the heart.

Interpretation of the ECG along with a thorough physical assessment is necessary to determine the cause and type of arrhythmia.

■ Assess the patient's general condition and include observations such as skin color (pale, cyanotic, flushed), orientation, level of consciousness, and the patient's general status (e.g., appears acutely ill or appears somewhat ill). All observations must be documented to provide a means of evaluating the response to drug therapy.

■ Record any symptoms (subjective data) described by the patient.

Because all antiarrhythmic drugs may produce proarrhythmic effects, baseline information is important to distinguish a proarrhythmic effect from the patient's underlying rhythm disorder.

The primary health care provider may also order laboratory and diagnostic tests, renal and hepatic function tests, complete blood count, and serum enzymes and electrolyte analyses. Review these test results before an antiarrhythmic drug is given and report any abnormalities to the primary health care provider. The patient is usually placed on cardiac monitoring before antiarrhythmic drug therapy is initiated.

Ongoing Assessment

When the patient is hospitalized, his or her blood pressure, apical and radial pulses, and respiratory rate are continually monitored. Continual cardiac monitoring assists you in assessing the patient for adverse drug reactions. Be sure to closely observe the patient for a response to drug therapy, signs of HF, the development of a new cardiac arrhythmia, or worsening of the arrhythmia being treated. Immediately report to the primary health care provider any significant changes in the blood pressure, pulse rate or rhythm, respiratory rate or rhythm, or the patient's general condition.

> **NURSING ALERT**
>
> When giving an oral antiarrhythmic drug, withhold the drug and immediately notify the primary health care provider when the pulse rate is above 120 bpm or below 60 bpm. In some instances, the primary health care provider may establish additional or different guidelines for withholding the drug.

If the patient is acutely ill or is receiving one of the antiarrhythmics parenterally, the fluid intake and output should be measured and documented. The primary health care provider may order subsequent laboratory tests to monitor the patient's progress for comparison with tests performed in the preadministration assessment. Review and report any abnormalities.

NURSING DIAGNOSES

Drug-specific nursing diagnoses include the following:

■ **Nausea** related to antiarrhythmic drugs
■ **Urinary Retention** related to cholinergic blocking effects of drugs
■ **Impaired Oral Mucous Membranes** related to dry mouth
■ **Risk for Injury** related to dizziness, lightheadedness
■ **Risk for Infection** related to agranulocytosis

Nursing diagnoses related to drug administration are discussed in Chapter 4.

PLANNING

The expected outcomes for the patient depend on the reason for administration of the antiarrhythmic drug but may include obtaining an optimal therapeutic response to drug therapy, support of patient needs related to managing adverse reactions, and confidence in an understanding of the medication regimen.

IMPLEMENTATION

Promoting an Optimal Response to Therapy

Cardiac monitoring is recommended when drugs are given IV and allows for observation of ECG activity, because severe bradycardia and hypotension may occur. Written instructions from the primary health care provider for titrating administration may be provided. The drug is titrated to the patient's response and in accord with institutional protocols. For example, the primary health care provider may want the drug to be withheld for a systolic blood pressure less than 90 mm Hg or a pulse rate less than 50 bpm.

Be familiar with the location of life support equipment and vasopressors in case of adverse reaction. Any sudden change in mental state should be reported to the primary health care provider immediately, because a decrease in the dosage may be necessary.

Monitoring and Managing Patient Needs

NAUSEA. Many of the antiarrhythmic drugs cause nausea and should not be crushed or chewed, especially the sustained-release tablets. Taking the drugs with food aids in reducing gastrointestinal (GI) upset. Help the patient to select small, frequent meals, which may be better tolerated than three full meals daily. Help the patient to avoid lying flat for approximately 2 hours after meals. When the patient rests or reclines, the head should be at least 4 inches higher than the feet. Some GI distress may be due to blood levels of the drugs, so scan labs frequently and report abnormal findings.

URINARY RETENTION. Because of the cholinergic blocking effects of disopyramide (see Chapter 27), urinary retention may occur. Monitor the urinary output closely, especially during the initial period of therapy. If the patient's intake is sufficient but the output is low, the lower abdomen is palpated and scanned for bladder distention. If urinary retention occurs, and noninvasive nursing measures do not produce results, notify the primary health care provider, because catheterization may be necessary.

IMPAIRED ORAL MUCOUS MEMBRANES. Dryness of the mouth and throat caused by the cholinergic blocking action of disopyramide may occur. Provide an adequate amount of fluid and instruct the patient to take frequent sips of water to relieve this problem. If the patient is able to take oral foods, offer hard candy (preferably sugarless) to keep the mouth moist.

RISK FOR INJURY. Hypotension and bradycardia caused by the antiarrhythmic drugs may cause dizziness and lightheadedness, especially during early therapy. This places the patient at risk for injury from falling. Postural hypotension also may occur during the first few weeks of therapy. Assist patients who are not on complete bed rest to ambulate until these symptoms subside. The patient is advised to make position changes slowly.

RISK FOR INFECTION. Some antiarrhythmic drugs, such as quinidine, mexiletine, or verapamil, may cause agranulocytosis. A complete blood count is usually ordered every 2 to 3 weeks during the first 3 months of therapy. Report any signs of agranulocytosis, such as fever, chills, sore throat, or unusual bleeding or bruising. If a decrease in the blood levels of leukocytes or platelets occurs or the hematocrit falls, report this to the primary health care provider immediately, because the drug may be discontinued. Blood levels usually return to normal within 1 month after discontinuing the antiarrhythmic drug.

POTENTIAL MEDICAL COMPLICATION: PROARRHYTHMIC EFFECTS. Proarrhythmic effects may occur, such as ventricular tachycardia or ventricular fibrillation. It is often difficult to distinguish proarrhythmic effects from the patient's pre-existing arrhythmia. Report any new arrhythmia or exacerbation of an existing arrhythmia to the primary health care provider immediately.

LIFESPAN CONSIDERATIONS
Gerontology

Older adults are at greater risk for adverse reactions such as additional arrhythmias or aggravation of existing arrhythmias, hypotension, and HF. Careful monitoring is necessary for early identification and management of adverse reactions. Monitor the intake and output and report any signs of HF, such as an increase in weight, a decrease in urinary output, or shortness of breath. A dosage reduction may be indicated.

POTENTIAL MEDICAL COMPLICATION: QUINIDINE TOXICITY. Monitor the patient for the most common adverse reactions associated with quinidine (nausea, vomiting, abdominal pain, diarrhea, or anorexia). Cinchonism is the term used to describe quinidine toxicity. Cinchonism occurs with high blood levels of quinidine (greater than 6 mcg/mL). Report any quinidine levels greater than 6 mcg/mL and the occurrence of any of the following signs or symptoms of cinchonism: ringing in the ears (tinnitus), hearing loss, headache, nausea, dizziness, vertigo, and lightheadedness. These symptoms may be experienced after a single dose.

Educating the Patient and Family

These medications do not cure heart disease. Used with lifestyle changes they can improve the quality of life, yet adherence to the prescribed drug regimen is important. As you develop a teaching plan include the following information:

■ Take the drug at the prescribed intervals. Do not omit a dose or increase or decrease the dose unless advised to do so by the primary health care provider. Do not stop taking the drug unless advised to do so by the primary health care provider.

■ Always check with your primary health care provider before taking any nonprescription drug, supplement, or herbal preparation.

■ ⚠ Avoid drinking alcoholic beverages or smoking unless these have been approved by the primary health care provider.

■ Follow the directions on the drug label, such as taking the drug with food.

■ Do not chew tablets or capsules; instead, swallow them whole. Contact the pharmacy if this is a problem for you to take the drug in the form provided.

■ Do not attempt to drive or perform hazardous tasks if lightheaded or dizzy.

■ Notify the primary health care provider as soon as possible if any adverse effects occur.

■ To relieve dry mouth, take frequent sips of water; allow ice chips to dissolve in the mouth, or chew (sugar-free) gum.

■ Keep all appointments with the primary health care provider, clinic, or laboratory, because therapy will be closely monitored.

■ If you have diabetes and are taking propranolol, adhere to the prescribed diet and check the blood glucose levels one to two times a day (or as recommended by the primary health care provider). Report elevated glucose levels to the primary health care provider as soon as possible, because an adjustment in the dosage of insulin or oral hypoglycemic drugs may be necessary.

EVALUATION

■ Therapeutic response is achieved and the arrhythmia is controlled.

■ Adverse reactions are identified, reported to the primary health care provider, and managed successfully with appropriate nursing interventions:
  • Patient is free of nausea.
  • Patient urinates adequately.
  • Oral mucous membranes are intact and moist.
  • No evidence of infection is seen.
  • No evidence of injury is seen.

■ Patient and family express confidence and demonstrate an understanding of the drug regimen.

PHARMACOLOGY IN PRACTICE
THINK CRITICALLY

You asked Mr. Phillip to bring in his medications. Here is what he brought:

• seven bottles of various Coumadin strengths
• two bottles Zoloft 100 mg strength
• Ambien
• two bottles atenolol 50 mg strength
• propranolol 60 mg strength

He does not use a medication container because he "knows what to take out of each bottle." What action would you take next?

KEY POINTS

- The heart has cardiac and nerve tissue; the nerves transmit an electrical impulse through the heart, which makes the muscles contract (a heartbeat). When there is an electrical conduction problem it can affect the rate or the rhythm of the heartbeat. This irregularity is called a cardiac arrhythmia or dysrhythmia, which ranges from causing fatigue to being life-threatening.

- Antiarrhythmic drugs include drugs that block impulses and are classified as class I—sodium channel blockers, class II—β-adrenergic blockers, class III—potassium channel blockers, and class IV—calcium channel blockers.

- These drugs are also used for treating hypertension and heart failure.

- Cardiac monitoring is important when therapy is started. Although the drugs are designed to correct an electrical conduction problem, they can also create new ones or extenuate existing problems—a proarrhythmic effect.

- As with many of the drugs that affect the cardiovascular system, hypotension, lightheadedness, dizziness, and weakness are all adverse reactions that can lead to injury.

Summary Drug Table ANTIARRHYTHMIC DRUGS

Generic Name	Trade Name	Uses	Adverse Reactions	Dosage Ranges
Class I Sodium Channel Blockers				
disopyramide *dye-soe-pee'-ah-myde*	Norpace, Norpace CR	Life-threatening ventricular arrhythmias	Dry mouth, constipation, urinary hesitancy, blurred vision, nausea, fatigue, dizziness, headache, rash, hypotension, HF, proarrhythmic effect	Ventricular arrhythmias: dosage individualized, 400–800 mg/day orally in divided doses
flecainide *fleh-kaye'-nyde*	Tambocor	Paroxysmal atrial fibrillation/flutter and supraventricular tachycardia	Dizziness, headache, faintness, unsteadiness, blurred vision, headache, nausea, dyspnea, HF, fatigue, palpitations, chest pain, proarrhythmic effect	Initial dose: 100 mg orally q 12 hr; maximum dosage, 390 mg/day
lidocaine *lye'-doe-kane*	Xylocaine	Ventricular arrhythmias	Lightheadedness, nervousness, bradycardia, hypotension, drowsiness, apprehension, proarrhythmic effect	50–100 mg IV bolus; 1–4 mg/min IV infusion, 20–50 mg/kg/min; 300 mg IM
mexiletine *max-ill'-ih-teen*		Life-threatening ventricular arrhythmias	Palpitations, nausea, vomiting, chest pain, heartburn, dizziness, lightheadedness, rash, agranulocytosis, proarrhythmic effect	Initial dose: 200 mg orally q 8 hr; maximum dosage, 1200 mg/day orally
propafenone *proe-paff'-ah-non*	Rythmol	Atrial fibrillation, ventricular arrhythmias, paroxysmal supraventricular tachycardia	Dizziness, nausea, vomiting, constipation, unusual taste, first-degree atrioventricular block, agranulocytosis, proarrhythmic effect	Initial dose: 150 mg orally q 8 hr; may be increased to 300 mg orally q 8 hr
quinidine *kwin'-ih-deen*		Premature atrial and ventricular contractions, atrial tachycardia, chronic atrial fibrillation	Ringing in the ears, hearing loss, nausea, vomiting, dizziness	Administer test dose of 1 tablet orally or 200 mg IM to test for idiosyncratic reaction
Class II β-Adrenergic Blockers				
acebutolol *ah-see-byoo'-toe-loll*	Sectral	Ventricular arrhythmias, hypertension	Hypotension, nausea, dizziness, bradycardia, vomiting, diarrhea, nervousness	Arrhythmias: 400–1200 mg/day orally in divided doses
propranolol *proe-pran'-oh-loll*	Inderal	Cardiac arrhythmias, angina pectoris, hypertension, essential tremor, myocardial infarction, migraine headache, pheochromocytoma	Nausea, vomiting, bradycardia, dizziness, hypotension, hyperglycemia, diarrhea, bronchospasm, pulmonary edema	Cardiac arrhythmias: 10–30 mg orally TID or QID Life-threatening arrhythmias: 1–3 mg IV, may repeat once in 2 min Angina pectoris: 80–320 mg/day orally in 2–4 divided doses

Summary Drug Table ANTIARRHYTHMIC DRUGS (continued)

Generic Name	Trade Name	Uses	Adverse Reactions	Dosage Ranges
Class III Potassium Channel Blockers				
amiodarone *ah-mee'-oh-dah-rone*	Cordarone, Pacerone	Life-threatening ventricular arrhythmias	Malaise, fatigue, tremor, proarrhythmic effect, nausea, vomiting, constipation, ataxia, anorexia, bradycardia, photosensitivity	Loading dose: 800–1600 mg/day orally in divided doses Maintenance dose, 390 mg/day orally; up to 1000 mg/day over 24 hr IV
dofetilide *doe-feh'-tih-lyde*	Tikosyn	Conversion of atrial fibrillation/flutter to normal sinus rhythm, maintenance of normal sinus rhythm	Headache, chest pain, dizziness, respiratory tract infection, dyspnea, nausea, flu-like syndrome, insomnia, proarrhythmic effect	Dosage based on electrocardiogram response and creatinine clearance; range, 125–500 mg BID
ibutilide *eye-byoo'-tih-lyde*		Atrial fibrillation/flutter	Headache, nausea, hypotension or hypertension, ventricular arrhythmias, proarrhythmic effect	Adults 60 kg and more: 1 mg infused over 10 in min; may repeat 10 min Adults under 60 kg: 0.1 mL/kg infused over 10 min; may repeat in 10 min
sotalol *soe'-tah-loll*	Betapace, Betapace AF	Treatment of life-threatening ventricular arrhythmias, reduction and delay of atrial fibrillation and flutter for ventricular arrhythmias (Betapace AF)	Drowsiness, difficulty sleeping, unusual tiredness or weakness, depression, decreased libido, bradycardia, HF, cold hands and feet, nausea, vomiting, nasal congestion, anxiety, life-threatening arrhythmias, proarrhythmic effect	Initially: 80 mg BID orally; may increase up to 239–320 mg/day (Betapace); up to 120 mg BID (Betapace AF)
Class IV Calcium Channel Blockers				
verapamil *ver-ap'-ah-mill*	Calan, Covera HS, Verelan, Verelan PM	Supraventricular tachyarrhythmias, temporary control of rapid ventricular rate in atrial flutter/fibrillation, angina, unstable angina, hypertension	Constipation, dizziness, lightheadedness, headache, asthenia, nausea, vomiting, peripheral edema, hypotension, mental depression, agranulocytosis, proarrhythmic effect	Adults: oral—initial dose 80–120 mg TID; maintenance, 320–480 mg/day Hypertension: 239 mg/day orally; sustained release, in a.m. 80 mg TID; extended-release capsules, 100–300 mg orally at bedtime Parenteral: IV use only; initial dose 5–10 mg over 2 min; may repeat 10 mg 30 min later

● Chapter Review

Know Your Drugs

Clients sometimes know a medication by the brand (or trade) name and not the generic name. To help you recognize both names, match the brand name with the generic name of the same medication.

Generic Name	Brand Name
1. lidocaine	A. Betapace
2. propranolol	B. Calan
3. sotalol	C. Inderal
4. verapamil	D. Xylocaine

Calculate Medication Dosages

1. The primary health care provider prescribes verapamil 80 mg orally. The drug is available in 40-mg tablets. The nurse prepares _____.

2. Disopyramide 200 mg orally is prescribed. The pharmacy sends disopyramide (Norpace) 100-mg tablets to the nursing facility. The nurse administers _____.

● Prepare for the NCLEX®

Build Your Knowledge

1. An irregular, rapid atrial contraction resulting in quivering atria is best described as which of the following arrhythmias?

   1. atrial fibrillation
   2. premature ventricular contraction
   3. ventricular tachycardia
   4. ventricular fibrillation

2. Which of the following antiarrhythmic drugs are also used as antihypertensives?

   1. sodium and calcium channel blockers
   2. β-adrenergic and calcium channel blockers
   3. potassium and sodium channel blockers
   4. β-adrenergic and potassium channel blockers

3. Which of the following adverse reactions of lidocaine (Xylocaine) should be reported immediately to the primary health care provider?

   1. sudden change in mental status
   2. dry mouth
   3. occipital headache
   4. lightheadedness

4. Which of the following drugs, when given with disopyramide (Norpace), would possibly increase the serum disopyramide levels?

   1. verapamil (Calan)
   2. propranolol (Inderal)
   3. flecainide (Tambocor)
   4. quinidine

5. Common adverse reactions of the antiarrhythmic drugs include _____.

   1. lightheadedness, hypotension, and weakness
   2. headache, hypertension, and lethargy
   3. weakness, lethargy, and hyperglycemia
   4. anorexia, GI upset, and hypertension

Apply Your Knowledge

6. When administering quinidine, the nurse reports a blood level greater than _____.

   1. 2 mcg/mL
   2. 3 mcg/mL
   3. 4 mcg/mL
   4. 6 mcg/mL

7. Which of the following statements would the nurse include in a teaching plan for the client taking an antiarrhythmic drug on an outpatient basis?

   1. Take the drug without regard to meals.
   2. Limit fluid intake during the evening hours.
   3. Avoid drinking alcoholic beverages unless approved by the primary health care provider.
   4. Eat a diet high in potassium.

8. Which of the following adverse reactions, if observed in a client prescribed propafenone, would indicate that the patient may be developing agranulocytosis?

   1. fever
   2. ataxia
   3. hyperactivity
   4. dizziness

Alternate-Format Questions

9. The client's ventricular fibrillation has stabilized and the client is scheduled to see the nurse for medication review. The prescribed dose is amiodarone 400 mg daily. Look at the medication brought from home: how many tablets should the client be taking?

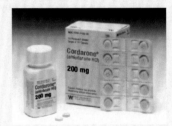

10. Match the specific drug with the correct class of drug.

Antiarrhythmia Drug Class	Brand Name
1. Class I	A. Betapace
2. Class II	B. Calan
3. Class III	C. Inderal
4. Class IV	D. Xylocaine

To check your answers, see Appendix G.

the**Point** *For more NCLEX-style questions, log on to http://thepoint.lww.com to access more than 1000 questions.*

Drugs That Affect the Gastrointestinal System

The gastrointestinal (GI) system is responsible for the ingestion and exchange of body nutrients. The process of digestion in the GI system begins with the breakdown of food and fluids in the mouth (oral cavity). In the stomach, foodstuffs are broken down by gastric acids and enzymes to prepare for absorption in the small intestine. After nutrients are absorbed in the small intestine, the large intestine is responsible for the reabsorption of water and the elimination of waste materials in the form of feces.

As people age, the personal focus of health often centers on this body system. As aging occurs, individuals experience wear and tear on their teeth and the ability to produce saliva decreases; this changes the taste of foods. Also, as the body ages, motility and absorption in the GI system slow. Drugs are used to assist in the absorption of nutrients, either by altering the gastric acids for purposes of protection or by controlling the transit of food through the system by speeding up or slowing down the process. Chapter 40 describes drugs used for protecting the structures of the upper GI system—mouth, esophagus, and stomach—from the effects of gastric acid. Drugs used to speed up or prevent emesis are also covered in this chapter.

Chronic illness, such as inflammatory bowel diseases, can affect how water and nutrients are absorbed. Drugs used to slow down or facilitate transit in the lower GI system—the small and large intestines—are covered in Chapter 41. The drugs used in the treatment of chronic GI diseases are also presented in Chapter 41.

An area of concern to you as the nurse caring for patients is the availability of nonprescription drugs for the GI system, thereby creating the potential for problems of misuse and overuse of the drugs, which may, in turn, disguise or delay diagnosis of more serious medical problems. This issue is addressed in Chapter 41 as well.

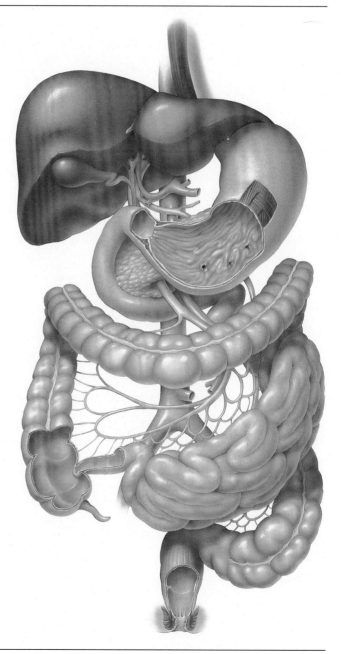

Drugs That Affect the Gastrointestinal System

Upper Gastrointestinal System Drugs

The upper GI system consists of the mouth, esophagus, and stomach (Fig. 40.1). The GI system is essentially a long tube in the body where ingested food and fluids are processed for absorption of nutrients. The mouth is responsible for breaking down food parts and mixing them with saliva to begin the digestion process. The tubular esophagus connects the mouth to the stomach,

PHARMACOLOGY IN PRACTICE

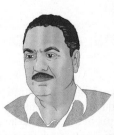

Alfredo Garcia is being seen in the clinic for an upper respiratory infection. During the intake assessment, you find that his blood pressure is high and he complains of "heartburn." You ask him what helps relieve the heartburn. Mr. Garcia is attempting to use home remedies to decrease acid production in his stomach, and he tells you that he thinks he might have an ulcer, so he has been drinking cream and half-and-half to coat the ulcer. At one time, antiulcer diets included the use of dairy products with the intent of coating the mucosal lining of the stomach, protecting it from acid secretion. While reading this chapter, you will learn about the current method to treat peptic ulcers in the stomach.

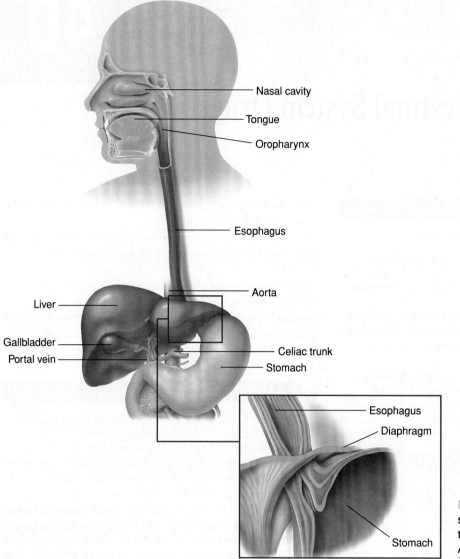

Figure 40.1 The upper GI system with esophagogastric junction featured. (Courtesy of the Anatomical Chart Co.)

where food is mixed with acids and enzymes to become a solution for absorption. Some of the cells of the stomach secrete **hydrochloric acid (HCl)**, a substance that aids in the initial digestive process. Problems occur when acids or stomach contents reverse direction and come back up into the esophagus or stomach, which can create tissue damage and ulcers.

Drugs are presented in this chapter according to their function, whether they treat gastric acid production or prevent vomiting. Drugs that neutralize HCl and protect the mucosal lining are called *antacids*. Drugs that reduce the production and release of HCl include histamine type 2 receptor (H_2) antagonists, proton pump inhibitors, and miscellaneous acid-reducing agents. The proton pump inhibitors are particularly important in the treatment of *Helicobacter pylori* infection in patients with active duodenal ulcers. *H. pylori* are believed to cause a type of chronic gastritis and some peptic and duodenal ulcers as well. GI stimulants facilitate emptying of stomach contents into the small intestine and are used both as ulcer treatments and as antiemetics. Antiemetics are used to treat and prevent nausea and vomiting. Some of the more common drugs are listed in the Summary Drug Table: Upper Gastrointestinal System Drugs.

ACID NEUTRALIZERS: ANTACIDS

Actions

Antacids ("against acids") are drugs that neutralize or reduce the acidity of stomach and duodenal contents by combining with HCl and increasing the pH of the stomach acid. Antacids do not "coat" the stomach lining, although they may increase the sphincter tone of the lower esophagus. Examples of antacids include aluminum (Amphojel), magaldrate (Riopan), and magnesium (Milk of Magnesia).

Uses

Antacids are used in the treatment of hyperacidity caused by the following:

- Heartburn, acid indigestion, or sour stomach
- **Gastroesophageal reflux disease (GERD**; a reflux or backup of gastric contents into the esophagus)
- Peptic ulcer

Antacids may be used to treat conditions that are not associated with the GI system. For example, aluminum carbonate is a phosphate-binding agent and is used in treating hyperphosphatemia (often associated with chronic renal failure) or as an adjunct to a low-phosphate diet to prevent formation of phosphate-based urinary stones. Calcium may be used in treating calcium deficiency states such as menopausal osteoporosis. Magnesium may be used for treating magnesium deficiencies or magnesium depletion from malnutrition, restricted diet, or alcoholism.

Adverse Reactions

The magnesium- and sodium-containing antacids may have a laxative effect and may produce diarrhea. Aluminum- and calcium-containing products tend to produce constipation. Although the antacids have the potential for serious adverse reactions, they have a wide margin of safety, especially when used as prescribed. Adverse reactions of concern include:

- *Aluminum-containing antacids*—constipation, intestinal impaction, anorexia, weakness, tremors, and bone pain
- *Magnesium-containing antacids*—severe diarrhea, dehydration, and hypermagnesemia (nausea, vomiting, hypotension, decreased respirations)
- *Calcium-containing antacids*—rebound hyperacidity, metabolic alkalosis, hypercalcemia, vomiting, confusion, headache, renal calculi, and neurologic impairment
- *Sodium bicarbonate*—systemic alkalosis and rebound hyperacidity

Contraindications and Precautions

The antacids are contraindicated in patients with severe abdominal pain of unknown cause and during lactation. Sodium-containing antacids are contraindicated in patients with cardiovascular problems, such as hypertension or heart failure, and those on sodium-restricted diets. Calcium-containing antacids are contraindicated in patients with renal calculi or hypercalcemia.

Aluminum-containing antacids are used cautiously in patients with gastric outlet obstruction or those with upper GI bleeding. Magnesium- and aluminum-containing antacids are used cautiously in patients with decreased kidney function. The calcium-containing antacids are used cautiously in patients with respiratory insufficiency, renal impairment, or cardiac disease. Antacids are classified as pregnancy category C drugs and should be used with caution during pregnancy.

Interactions

The following interactions may occur when an antacid is administered with another agent:

Interacting Drug	Common Use	Effect of Interaction
digoxin, isoniazid, phenytoin, and chlorpromazine	Treatment of cardiac problems, infection, seizures, and nausea and vomiting, respectively	Decreased absorption of the interacting drugs results in a decreased effect of those drugs
tetracycline	Anti-infective agent	Decreased effectiveness of anti-infective
corticosteroids	Treatment of inflammation and respiratory problems	Decreased anti-inflammatory properties
salicylates	Pain relief	Pain reliever is excreted more rapidly in the urine

ACID-REDUCING AGENTS

Drugs that reduce the production of HCl include histamine H_2 antagonists, proton pump inhibitors, and miscellaneous drugs such as pepsin inhibitors, prostaglandins, and cholinergic blockers.

Histamine H_2 Antagonists

Actions

These drugs inhibit the action of histamine at H_2 receptor cells of the stomach, which then reduces the secretion of gastric acid. Because cholinergic blocking drugs typically block the action of histamine throughout the entire body, they are used less frequently. Histamine H_2 antagonists do not cause the effects of the cholinergic blockers, because they are selective only for the H_2 receptors in the stomach and not the general body H_2 receptors. When ulcers are present, the decrease in acid allows the ulcerated areas to heal. Examples of histamine H_2 antagonists include cimetidine (Tagamet), famotidine (Pepcid), and ranitidine (Zantac).

Uses

These drugs are used prophylactically to treat stress-related ulcers and acute upper GI bleeding in critically ill patients. They are also used for the treatment of the following:

- Heartburn, acid indigestion, and sour stomach (frequently sold as over-the-counter remedies)
- GERD
- Gastric or duodenal ulcer
- Gastric **hypersecretory** conditions (excessive gastric secretion of HCl)

Adverse Reactions

Histamine H_2 antagonist adverse reactions are usually mild and transient as well as rare (affecting less than 2% of users), and include:

• Dizziness, somnolence, headache
• Confusion, hallucinations, diarrhea, and reversible impotence

Contraindications and Precautions

The histamine H_2 antagonists are contraindicated in patients with a known hypersensitivity to the drugs. These drugs are used cautiously in patients with renal or hepatic impairment and in severely ill, older, or debilitated patients. Cimetidine is used cautiously in patients with diabetes. Histamine H_2 antagonists are pregnancy category B (cimetidine, famotidine, and ranitidine) and C (nizatidine) drugs and should be used with caution during pregnancy and lactation.

Interactions

The following interactions may occur when a histamine H_2 antagonist is administered with another agent:

Interacting Drug	Common Use	Effect of Interaction
antacids and metoclopramide	GI distress	Decreased absorption of the H_2 antagonists
carmustine	Anticancer therapy	Decreased white blood cell count
opioid analgesics	Pain relief	Increased risk of respiratory depression
oral anticoagulants	Blood thinners	Increased risk of bleeding
digoxin	Cardiac problems	May decrease serum digoxin levels

Proton Pump Inhibitors

Actions

Proton pump inhibitors, such as lansoprazole, omeprazole, pantoprazole, and rabeprazole, are a group of drugs with antisecretory properties. These drugs suppress gastric acid secretion by inhibition of the hydrogen-potassium adenosine triphosphatase (ATPase) enzyme system of the gastric parietal cells. The ATPase enzyme system is also called the acid (proton) pump system. The proton pump inhibitors suppress gastric acid secretion by blocking the final step in the production of gastric acid by the gastric mucosa. Examples of proton pump inhibitors include esomeprazole (Nexium) and omeprazole (Prilosec).

Uses

Proton pump inhibitors are used for treatment or symptomatic relief of various gastric disorders, including:

• Gastric and duodenal ulcers (specifically associated with *H. pylori* infections)
• GERD and erosive esophagitis
• Pathologic hypersecretory conditions
• Prevention of bleeding in high-risk patients using antiplatelet drugs

An important use of these drugs is combination therapy for the treatment of *H. pylori* infection in patients with duodenal ulcers.

One treatment regimen used to treat infection with *H. pylori* is a triple-drug therapy, such as one of the proton pump inhibitors (e.g., omeprazole or lansoprazole) and two anti-infectives (e.g., amoxicillin and clarithromycin). Another triple-drug treatment regimen consists of bismuth plus two anti-infective drugs. Helidac, a triple-drug treatment regimen (bismuth, metronidazole, and tetracycline), may be given along with a histamine H_2 antagonist to treat disorders of the GI tract infected with *H. pylori*. Table 40.1 lists various drug combinations used in the treatment of *H. pylori* infection. Additional information concerning anti-infective agents is found in Chapters 6 through 9. The Summary Drug Table: Upper Gastrointestinal System Drugs provides additional information on the proton pump inhibitor drugs used in treating *H. pylori* infection.

Adverse Reactions

The most common adverse reactions seen with the proton pump inhibitors include headache, nausea, diarrhea, and abdominal pain.

Contraindications and Precautions

Proton pump inhibitors are contraindicated in patients who are hypersensitive to any of the drugs. Proton pump inhibitors are used cautiously in older adults and in patients with hepatic impairment. Prolonged treatment may decrease the body's ability to absorb vitamin B_{12}, resulting in anemia. Omeprazole (pregnancy category C) and lansoprazole, rabeprazole, and pantoprazole (pregnancy category B) are contraindicated during pregnancy and lactation.

 LIFESPAN CONSIDERATIONS
Menopausal Women
An increase in fractures of the hip, wrist, and spine have been seen in those taking high doses of proton pump inhibitors and undergoing treatment of osteoporosis with bisphosphonates.

Interactions

The following interactions may occur when a proton pump inhibitor is administered with another agent:

Interacting Drug	Common Use	Effect of Interaction
sucralfate	Management of GI distress	Decreased absorption of the proton pump inhibitor
ketoconazole and ampicillin	Anti-infective agent	Decreased absorption of the anti-infective
oral anticoagulants	Blood thinners	Increased risk of bleeding
digoxin	Cardiac problems	Increased absorption of digoxin
benzodiazepines, phenytoin	Management of anxiety and seizure disorders	Risk for toxic level of antiseizure drugs
clarithromycin (with omeprazole, specifically)	Anti-infective agent	Risk for an increase in plasma levels of both drugs
bisphosphonates	Bone strengthening	Increased risk of fracture

Table 40.1 Agents Used to Eradicate *Helicobacter pylori* in Patients With Duodenal Ulcers

Drug	Recommended Usage	Dosage Range
amoxicillin	In combination with lansoprazole and clarithromycin or lansoprazole alone	1 g BID for 14 days (triple therapy) or 1 g TID (double therapy)
bismuth (Bismatrol)	In combination with other products	525 mg QID
clarithromycin (Biaxin)	In combination with amoxicillin	500 mg TID
lansoprazole (Prevacid)	In combination with clarithromycin or amoxicillin	30 mg BID for 14 days (triple therapy) or 30 mg TID for 14 days (double therapy)
metronidazole (Flagyl)	In combination with other products	250 mg QID
omeprazole (Prilosec)	In combination with clarithromycin	40 mg BID for 4 wk and 20 mg/day for 15–28 days
tetracycline	In combination with other products	500 mg QID
Combination Drug Packs		
bismuth, metronidazole, tetracycline (Helidac, Pylera)	*H. pylori* eradication in patients with duodenal ulcer	Each drug provided separately in daily administration pack for QID dosing
lansoprazole, amoxicillin, clarithromycin (Prevpac)	*H. pylori* eradication in patients with duodenal ulcer	Each drug provided separately in daily administration pack for BID dosing

Miscellaneous Acid Reducers

Three other types of acid-reducing drugs that are less frequently used are the cholinergic blocking drugs (also called *anticholinergic* drugs), a pepsin inhibitor, and a prostaglandin drug. Cholinergic blocking drugs reduce gastric motility and decrease the amount of acid secreted by the stomach. These drugs have been largely replaced by histamine H_2 antagonists, which appear to be more effective and have fewer adverse effects. Examples of cholinergic blocking drugs used for GI disorders include propantheline and glycopyrrolate (Robinul). For information about specific cholinergic blocking drugs, see Chapter 27.

Sucralfate (Carafate) is known as a pepsin inhibitor or mucosal protective drug. The drug binds with protein molecules to form a viscous substance that buffers acid and protects the mucosal lining. Sucralfate is used in the short-term treatment of duodenal ulcers. The most common adverse reaction is constipation. Drug interactions of sucralfate are similar to those of the proton pump inhibitors.

A prostaglandin drug, misoprostol (Cytotec), has been used to reduce the risk of nonsteroidal anti-inflammatory drug (NSAID)–induced gastric ulcers in high-risk patients, such as older adults or the critically ill. Misoprostol both inhibits the production of gastric acid and has mucosal protective properties. Because this drug can cause abortion or birth defects, it is not recommended for use in ulcer reduction in women who are pregnant or may become pregnant or who are lactating. Adverse reactions include headache, nausea, diarrhea, and abdominal pain. The drug effects are decreased when it is taken with antacids.

Gastrointestinal Stimulants

Actions

Metoclopramide (Reglan) is used to treat delayed gastric emptying and emesis—that is, it increases the motility of the upper GI tract without increasing the production of secretions. By sensitizing tissue to the effects of acetylcholine, the tone and amplitude of gastric contractions are increased, resulting in faster emptying of gastric contents into the small intestine. It also inhibits stimulation of the vomiting center in the brain.

Uses

The GI stimulants are used in the treatment of the following:

• GERD
• **Gastric stasis** (failure to move food normally out of the stomach) in diabetic patients, in patients with nausea and vomiting associated with cancer chemotherapy, and in patients in the immediate postoperative period

Adverse Reactions

Adverse reactions associated with metoclopramide are usually mild. Higher doses or prolonged administration may produce central nervous system (CNS) symptoms, such as restlessness, drowsiness, dizziness, extrapyramidal effects (tremor, involuntary movements of the limbs, muscle rigidity), facial grimacing, and depression.

Contraindications and Precautions

The GI stimulant is contraindicated in patients with known hypersensitivity to the drug, GI obstruction, gastric perforation or hemorrhage, or pheochromocytoma. Patients with Parkinson's disease or a seizure disorder who are taking drugs likely to cause extrapyramidal symptoms should not take these drugs.

This drug is used cautiously in patients with diabetes and cardiovascular disease. Metoclopramide is a pregnancy category B drug. The drug is secreted in breast milk and should be used with caution during pregnancy and lactation.

Interactions

The following interactions may occur when a GI stimulant is administered with another agent:

Interacting Drug	Common Use	Effect of Interaction
cholinergic blocking drugs or opioid analgesics	Management of GI distress or pain relief	Decreased effectiveness of metoclopramide
cimetidine	Management of GI distress	Decreased absorption of cimetidine
digoxin	Management of cardiac problems	Decreased absorption of digoxin
monoamine oxidase inhibitor antidepressants	Management of depression	Increased risk of hypertensive episode
levodopa	Management of disease	Decreased metoclopramide and levodopa

ANTIEMETICS

An antiemetic drug is used to treat or prevent **nausea** (unpleasant gastric sensation usually preceding vomiting) or **vomiting** (forceful expulsion of gastric contents through the mouth). The drugs discussed in this section are used to treat severe nausea and vomiting. Individuals may experience nausea due to motion sickness or a condition called **vertigo** (a sensation of spinning or a rotation-type motion). Many of the drugs used to treat motion sickness can be purchased over the counter. Table 40.2 lists examples of drugs used in the treatment of motion sickness or vertigo.

Actions

The brain is involved in the sensation of nausea. The medulla has an area called the vomiting center. The process of vomiting happens when the area is stimulated directly by GI irritation, motion sickness, and vestibular neuritis (inflammation of the vestibular nerve). An adjacent area, the **chemoreceptor trigger zone (CTZ)**, is a group of nerve fibers that sends signals to the vomiting center in the medulla when the metabolism is unbalanced. When these nerves are stimulated by chemicals, such as drugs or toxic substances, impulses are sent to the vomiting center located in the medulla. Vomiting caused by drugs, radiation, and metabolic disorders often occurs because of stimulation of the CTZ. These drugs appear to act primarily by inhibiting the CTZ and the brain's primary neurotransmitters dopamine and acetylcholine.

The 5-hydroxytryptamine type 3 (5-HT3) receptor antagonists target serotonin receptors both at the CTZ and peripherally at the nerve endings in the stomach. This action reduces the non-GI adverse effects that are often evident when nonspecific cholinergic blocking drugs are used. Because of their localized action in the GI system, these drugs are being tested for use in irritable bowel syndrome as well.

Uses

An antiemetic is used to treat nausea and vomiting, typically by preventive administration (prophylaxis):

- Before surgery to prevent vomiting during surgery
- Immediately after surgery when the patient is recovering from anesthesia
- Before, during, and after administration of antineoplastic drugs that induce a high degree of nausea and vomiting
- During radiation therapy when the GI tract is in the treatment field
- During pregnancy for hyperemesis

Other causes of nausea and vomiting that may be treated with an antiemetic include bacterial and viral infections and adverse drug reactions. Some antiemetics also are used for motion sickness and vertigo. Dronabinol (Marinol) is the only medically available cannabinoid (marijuana derivative) prescribed for antiemetic use. Approximately 20 states allow marijuana use for medical purposes such as nausea.

Adverse Reactions

The most common adverse reactions resulting from these drugs are varying degrees of drowsiness. Additional adverse reactions for each drug are listed in the Summary Drug Table: Upper Gastrointestinal System Drugs.

Contraindications

Antiemetic drugs are contraindicated in patients with known hypersensitivity to these drugs or with severe CNS depression. The 5-HT3 receptor antagonists should not be used by patients with heart block or prolonged QT intervals. In general, these drugs are not recommended during pregnancy and lactation, or for uncomplicated vomiting in young children. Prochlorperazine is contraindicated in patients with bone marrow depression, blood dyscrasia, Parkinson's disease, or severe liver or cardiovascular disease.

Precautions

Severe nausea and vomiting should not be treated with antiemetic drugs alone. The cause of the vomiting must be investigated. Antiemetic drugs may hamper the diagnosis of disorders such as brain tumor or injury, appendicitis, intestinal obstruction, and drug toxicity (e.g., digitalis toxicity). Delayed diagnosis of any of these disorders could have serious consequences for the patient.

Cholinergic blocking antiemetics are used cautiously in patients with glaucoma or obstructive disease of the GI or genitourinary system, in those with renal or hepatic dysfunction,

Table 40.2 **Motion Sickness Drugs**	
Generic Name	**Trade Name**
dimenhydrinate	Dramamine
diphenhydramine	Benadryl
meclizine	Antivert
scopolamine	Transderm-Scop (transdermal system)

and in older men with possible prostatic hypertrophy. Promethazine is used cautiously in patients with hypertension, sleep apnea, or epilepsy. The 5-HT3 receptor antagonists should be used cautiously in patients with cardiac conduction problems or electrolyte imbalances.

Perphenazine, prochlorperazine, promethazine, scopolamine, and chlorpromazine are pregnancy category C drugs. Other antiemetics are classified as pregnancy category B.

Interactions

The following interactions may occur when an antiemetic is administered with another agent:

Interacting Drug	Common Use	Effect of Interaction
CNS depressants	Analgesia, sedation, or pain relief	Increased risk of sedation
antihistamines	Management of allergy and respiratory distress	Increased adverse cholinergic blocking effects
antacids	Management of gastric distress	Decreased absorption of antiemetic
rifampin with 5-HT3 receptor antagonist	Tuberculosis/human immunodeficiency virus infection management	Decreased effectiveness of 5-HT3 receptor antagonist
lithium with prochlorperazine	Management of bipolar disorder	Increased risk of extrapyramidal effects

EMETICS

An emetic is a drug that *induces* vomiting. This is caused by local irritation of the stomach and by stimulation of the vomiting center in the medulla. Emetics are used to empty the stomach rapidly when an individual has accidentally or intentionally ingested a poison or drug overdose. Not all poison ingestions or drug overdoses are treated with emetics. This is because more harm can occur from the vomiting of many substances. As a result, guidelines were established for the use of syrup of ipecac (see Patient Teaching for Improved Patient Outcomes: Using Emetics Properly).

HERBAL CONSIDERATIONS

Ginger, a pungent root, has been used medicinally for GI problems such as motion sickness, nausea, vomiting, and indigestion. In addition, it is recommended for the pain and inflammation of arthritis, and it may help lower cholesterol. The dosage of the dried form of ginger is 1 g (1000 mg) per day. Adverse reactions are rare, although heartburn has been reported by some individuals. Ginger should be used cautiously in patients with hypertension or gallstones and during pregnancy or lactation. As with any substance, a primary health care provider should be consulted before any ginger remedy is taken, although ginger has been consumed safely as a food by millions of individuals for centuries (DerMarderosian, 2003).

NURSING PROCESS
PATIENT RECEIVING A DRUG FOR AN UPPER GASTROINTESTINAL CONDITION

ASSESSMENT

Preadministration Assessment
When a patient is nauseated, ask about the type and intensity of symptoms (e.g., pain, discomfort, nausea, vomiting) to provide a baseline for evaluating the effectiveness of drug therapy. As part of the preadministration assessment for a patient receiving a drug for nausea and vomiting, document the number of times the patient has vomited and the approximate amount of fluid lost. Before starting therapy, take vital signs and assess for signs of fluid and electrolyte imbalances.

In the case of preventative administration of an antiemetic, explain the rationale for preventing an episode of nausea rather than waiting for symptoms to occur when the primary health care provider knows the drugs or treatments being given will cause this problem. Ask the patient about any episodes of nausea or vomiting in anticipation of the therapy.

Ongoing Assessment
Monitor the patient frequently for continued complaints of pain, sour taste, or the production of bloody or coffee-ground emesis. If vomiting is severe, observe the patient for signs and symptoms of electrolyte imbalance and monitor the blood pressure, pulse, and respiratory rate every 2 to 4 hours or as

ordered by the primary health care provider. Measure intake and output (urine, emesis) carefully until vomiting ceases and the patient can take oral fluids in sufficient quantity.

Document in the patient's chart each time the patient vomits, and notify the primary health care provider if there is blood in the emesis or if vomiting suddenly becomes more severe. If vomiting is severe you may anticipate a nasogastric (NG) tube being inserted for suctioning to prevent aspiration of emesis (Fig. 40.2). You may need to measure the patient's

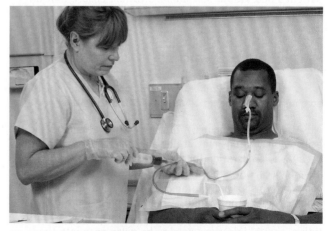

Figure 40.2 Placement of a nasogastric tube may be indicated with nausea and vomiting.

weight daily to weekly in patients with prolonged and repeated episodes of vomiting (e.g., those receiving chemotherapy for cancer). Assess the patient at frequent intervals for the effectiveness of the drug in relieving symptoms (e.g., nausea, vomiting, or vertigo) and notify the primary health care provider if the drug fails to relieve or diminish symptoms.

NURSING DIAGNOSES

Drug-specific nursing diagnoses include the following:

- **Risk for Deficient Fluid Volume** related to diarrhea, nausea, and vomiting
- **Imbalanced Nutrition: Less Than Body Requirements** related to impaired ability to ingest and retain food and fluids, or offensive tastes and smells
- **Individual Effective Self-Health Management** related to inability to take oral form of medication
- **Risk for Injury** related to adverse drug effects of drowsiness

Nursing diagnoses related to drug administration are discussed in Chapter 4.

PLANNING

The expected outcomes for the patient depend on the reason the upper GI drug is administered but may include an optimal response to drug therapy, support of patient needs related to the management of adverse reactions, and confidence in an understanding of the medication regimen.

IMPLEMENTATION

Promoting an Optimal Response to Therapy

ANTACIDS. The antacid may be administered hourly for the first 2 weeks when used to treat acute peptic ulcer. After the first 2 weeks, the drug is administered 1 to 2 hours after meals and at bedtime. It is important for the patient to understand that acid will be reduced, but with reduction comes less absorption of food and drugs from the stomach. Therefore, the antacids need to be taken later so that medicines have the opportunity to enter the circulation, before the acid is reduced. The primary health care provider may order that the antacid be left at the patient's bedside for self-administration. Ensure that an adequate supply of water and cups for measuring the dose is available.

> **! NURSING ALERT**
> Because of the possibility of an antacid interfering with the activity of other oral drugs, no oral drug should be administered within 1 to 2 hours of an antacid.

NON-ORAL METHODS OF DRUG ADMINISTRATION. Patients taking acid-reducing drugs may not be able to take oral medications because of preparation for an operative procedure, postoperative nausea, or physical condition. Many of these drugs come in forms for both intramuscular (IM) and intravenous (IV) administration. The IV route is typically preferred if the patient has an existing IV line, because these drugs are irritating, and IM injections need to be given deep into the muscular tissue to minimize harm.

> **! NURSING ALERT**
> When one of these drugs is given IV, monitor the rate of infusion at frequent intervals. Too rapid an infusion may induce cardiac arrhythmias.

Patients who are debilitated and require feeding from an NG tube are at risk for gastric ulcer development and may be prescribed acid-reducing drugs. Always check the medication label to see if the pill can be crushed or the capsule opened before doing so. These can be mixed with 40 mL of apple juice and administered through the NG tube. The tube is flushed with fluid afterward. Many of these drugs come in a liquid form as well as tablet or capsule. Request the liquid form when administration is in a tube to decrease the chance of a clogged NG tube due to improper flushing.

PREVENTION OF NAUSEA IN PATIENTS UNDERGOING CANCER THERAPY. Different protocols for prechemotherapy nausea depend on the type of cancer treatment. Some cancer (antineoplastic) drugs rarely cause nausea, and others are highly emetogenic. Granisetron (Kytril), ondansetron (Zofran), and dolasetron (Anzemet) are examples of antiemetics used when cancer chemotherapy drugs are very likely to cause nausea and vomiting. These drugs are administered regardless of emesis history before the chemotherapy is given. The first dose is typically given IV during therapy, and then the patient is asked to take it orally at home for a specified period. It is important to explain to the patient that the drug prevents nausea and vomiting and to be sure to take the entire dose prescribed, even when the patient feels fine at home. You may be asked to assist in the preadministration of antiemetics, yet the antineoplastics should always be given by a nurse trained in the administration of cancer chemotherapy.

Monitoring and Managing Patient Needs

RISK FOR DEFICIENT FLUID VOLUME. When antacids are given, keep a record of the patient's bowel movements, because these drugs may cause constipation or diarrhea. If the patient experiences diarrhea, accurately record fluid intake and output along with a description of the diarrhea stool. Uncontrolled diarrhea can lead to fluid loss and dehydration. Changing to a different antacid usually alleviates the problem. Diarrhea may be controlled by combining a magnesium antacid with an antacid containing aluminum or calcium.

Dehydration is a serious concern in the patient experiencing nausea and vomiting. It is important to observe the patient for signs of dehydration, which include poor skin turgor, dry mucous membranes, decrease in or absence of urinary output, concentrated urine, restlessness, irritability, increased respiratory rate, and confusion. Monitor the input and output (urine and emesis) and document findings every 8 hours. If the patient is able to take and retain small amounts of oral fluids, offer sips of water at frequent intervals. In addition, it is important to observe the patient for signs of electrolyte imbalance, particularly sodium and potassium deficit (see Chapter 54). If signs of dehydration or electrolyte imbalance are noted, contact the primary health care provider, because parenteral administration of fluids or fluids with electrolytes may be necessary.

LIFESPAN CONSIDERATIONS
Chronic Care

Observations for fluid and electrolyte disturbances are particularly important in the older adult or chronically ill patients in whom severe dehydration may develop quickly. Immediately report symptoms of dehydration, such as dry mucous membranes, decreased urinary output, concentrated urine, restlessness, or confusion. Dehydration can lead to confusion and dizziness. Dizziness increases the risk for falls in the older adult. Assistance is needed for ambulatory activities. The environment is made safe by removing throw rugs, small pieces of furniture, and the like. Report any change in orientation to the primary health care provider.

IMBALANCED NUTRITION: LESS THAN BODY REQUIREMENTS. Nausea, vomiting, vertigo, and dizziness are disagreeable sensations. Provide the patient with an emesis basin and check the patient at frequent intervals. If vomiting occurs, empty the emesis basin, and measure and document the volume in the patient's record. Offer comfort measures such as giving the patient a damp washcloth and a towel to wipe the hands and face as needed. It also is a good idea to give the patient mouthwash or frequent oral rinses to remove the disagreeable taste that accompanies vomiting (Fig. 40.3).

Nausea may make the patient lose his or her appetite and decrease nutritional intake. It is important to make the environment as pleasant as possible to enhance the patient's appetite. Remove items with strong smells and odors. Change the patient's bedding and clothing or gown as needed, because the odor of vomit may intensify the sensations of nausea and further decrease appetite. Ask visitors to refrain from wearing strong perfumes and colognes.

INDIVIDUAL EFFECTIVE SELF-HEALTH MANAGEMENT. When antacids are given, instruct the patient to chew the tablets thoroughly before swallowing and then drink a full glass of water or milk. If the patient expresses a dislike for the taste of the antacid or has difficulty chewing the tablet form, contact the primary health care provider. A flavored antacid may be ordered if the patient finds the taste unpleasant. A liquid form may be ordered if the patient has difficulty chewing a tablet. Liquid antacid preparations must be shaken thoroughly

immediately before administration. Liquid antacids are followed by a small amount of water.

If the patient cannot retain the oral form of the drug (other than the antacids), it may be given parenterally or as a rectal suppository (if the prescribed drug is available in these forms). If only the oral form has been ordered and the patient cannot retain the drug, contact the primary health care provider regarding an order for a parenteral or suppository form of this or another antiemetic drug. Should you send a patient home with instructions to use a suppository, be sure to include disposable gloves or finger cots (medical supplies used to cover one or more fingers when a full glove is unnecessary) for administration.

When administering scopolamine for motion sickness, one transdermal system is applied behind the ear approximately 4 hours before the antiemetic effect is needed. Approximately 1 g of scopolamine is administered every 24 hours for 3 days. Advise the individual to discard any disk that becomes detached and to replace it with a fresh disk applied behind the opposite ear.

RISK FOR INJURY. Administration of these drugs may result in varying degrees of drowsiness. To prevent accidental falls and other injuries, assist the patient who is allowed out of bed with ambulatory activities. If extreme drowsiness is noted, instruct the patient to remain in bed and provide a call light for assistance.

! NURSING ALERT

Tardive dyskinesia (nonreversible, involuntary muscle spasms), which is typically associated with conventional antipsychotics, is known to occur with long-term use (12 weeks or more) of metoclopramide. Immediately report extrapyramidal symptoms to prevent tardive dyskinesia from occurring.

Educating the Patient and Family

When a drug to treat the upper GI system is prescribed for outpatient use, and as you develop a teaching plan, include the following information:

■ If drowsy, avoid driving or performing other hazardous tasks when taking these drugs.

■ Do not use antacids indiscriminately. Check with a primary health care provider before using an antacid if other medical problems, such as a cardiac condition, exist (some antacids contain sodium).

■ Do not increase the frequency of use or the dose if your symptoms become worse; instead, see the primary health care provider as soon as possible.

■ Because antacids impair the absorption of some drugs, do not take other drugs within 2 hours before or after taking the antacid unless use of an antacid with a drug is recommended by the primary health care provider.

■ If pain or discomfort remains the same or becomes worse, if the stools turn black, or if vomitus resembles coffee grounds, contact the primary health care provider as soon as possible.

■ Magnesium-containing products may produce a *laxative* effect and may cause diarrhea; aluminum- or calcium-containing antacids may cause *constipation.*

■ Taking too much antacid may cause the stomach to secrete excess stomach acid. Consult the primary health

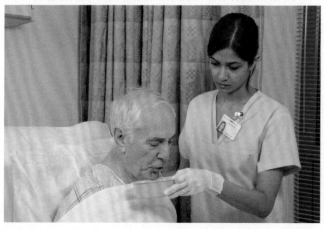

Figure 40.3 Provide comfort measures for the nauseated patient.

care provider or pharmacist about appropriate dose. Do not use the maximum dose for more than 2 weeks, except under the supervision of a primary health care provider.

- When taking proton pump inhibitors, swallow the tablet whole at least 1 hour before eating. Do not chew, open, or crush.

- When taking metoclopramide, immediately report any of the following signs: difficulty speaking or swallowing; mask-like face; shuffling gait; rigidity; tremors; uncontrolled movements of the mouth, face, or extremities; and uncontrolled chewing or unusual movements of the tongue.

- ❢ Avoid the use of alcohol and other sedative-type drugs unless use has been approved by the primary health care provider.

- Take antiemetics for cancer chemotherapy as prescribed. Do not omit a dose. Consult the primary health care provider if you have forgotten a dose of the medication.

- When using rectal suppositories, remove foil wrapper and immediately insert the pointed end into the rectum without using force.

- Take the drug for motion sickness about 1 hour before travel.

- Misoprostol: Because this drug may cause spontaneous abortion, women of childbearing age need to use a reliable contraceptive. If pregnancy is suspected, discontinue use of the drug and notify the primary health care provider. Report severe menstrual pain, bleeding, or spotting as well.

EVALUATION

- Therapeutic effect is achieved and nausea or pain is controlled.
- Adverse reactions are identified, reported to the primary health care provider, and managed successfully through appropriate nursing interventions:
  - Fluid volume balance is maintained.
  - Patient maintains an adequate nutritional status.
  - Patient manages the therapeutic regimen effectively.
  - No evidence of injury is seen.
- Patient or family express confidence and demonstrate an understanding of the drug regimen.

PHARMACOLOGY IN PRACTICE
THINK CRITICALLY

 Alfredo Garcia was found to have GERD, not a peptic ulcer. During your patient teaching, how would you explain to Mr. Garcia that using dairy products to coat the stomach lining is not helpful in reducing acid secretions? Instead, he is instructed to buy the antacid of his choice for the heartburn. He can't understand why he should coat his stomach with medicine instead of cream. Explain how antacids work.

Patient Teaching for Improved Patient Outcomes
Using Emetics Properly

Before an emetic is given, it is extremely important to know the chemicals or substances that have been ingested, the time they were ingested, and what symptoms were noted before seeking medical treatment. This information will probably be obtained from a family member or friend, but the adult patient may also contribute to the history. You should inform patients there are times when syrup of ipecac is contraindicated.

The U.S. Food and Drug Administration approved the following warnings for the labeling of syrup of ipecac:

- ✔ Do not use in persons who are not fully conscious.
- ✔ Do not use this product unless directed by a health care professional. Do not use if turpentine; corrosives, such as alkalis (lye) or strong acids; or petroleum distillates, such as kerosene, paint thinner, cleaning fluid, or furniture polish, have been ingested.

Clinicians (Manoguerra, 2005) have expanded the contraindications for ipecac syrup to include situations in which:

- ✔ The patient is comatose or has altered mental status, and the risk of aspiration of stomach contents is high.
- ✔ The patient is having convulsions.
- ✔ The substance ingested is capable of causing altered mental status or convulsions.
- ✔ The substance ingested is a caustic or corrosive agent.
- ✔ The substance ingested is a low-viscosity petroleum distillate (e.g., gas or kerosene) with the potential for pulmonary aspiration and the development of chemical pneumonitis.
- ✔ The patient has a medical condition that may be exacerbated by vomiting (e.g., severe hypertension, bradycardia, hemorrhagic diathesis).

Remember: The primary health care provider or nurse should also contact the local poison control center to obtain information regarding treatment.

KEY POINTS

- The upper GI system includes the mouth, esophagus, and stomach. We take in food and fluids that are processed and absorbed for use by our cells. Hydrochloric acid is secreted in the stomach to help in the digestion process.

- Problems occur when the digestive juices reverse and go into the esophagus or backflow into the stomach from the small intestine. Drugs discussed in this chapter focus on acid reduction or neutralization and increasing motility to move contents through the system. Antiemetics used to reduce or prevent nausea and vomiting are also discussed.

- Antacids do not actually coat the stomach; instead, they neutralize the acid in the stomach. Because acid is needed for proper absorption, these drugs should not be taken within 2 hours of other drugs. Acid-reducing drugs such as the histamine antagonists and proton pump inhibitors

reduce the gastric acid secretion. The decrease in acid aids in the healing process when an ulcer is present. Stimulants are used to promote GI motility, which, in turn, will reduce nausea. Antiemetics currently used inhibit neuronal transmission of sensation from the gut or the signal to vomit.

- Common adverse reactions include headache, nausea, diarrhea, or abdominal pain. Metoclopramide, when used long term, can cause extrapyramidal effects, which can lead to the irreversible condition of tardive dyskinesia.

- Multiple over-the-counter products exist to treat GI symptoms. Patients need confidence in understanding how to purchase and take these products because the majority of users do so without health care provider supervision.

Summary Drug Table UPPER GASTROINTESTINAL SYSTEM DRUGS

Generic Name	Trade Name	Uses	Adverse Reactions	Dosage Ranges
Acid Neutralizers				
aluminum carbonate *ah-loo-mih-num*	Basaljel	Symptomatic relief of peptic ulcer and stomach hyperacidity, hyperphosphatemia	Constipation, bone softening, neurotoxicity	2 tablets or capsules (10 mL of regular oral suspension) as often as q 2 hr, up to 12 times daily
aluminum hydroxide	ALternaGEL, Alu-Tab, Amphojel, Dialume	Same as aluminum carbonate	Same as aluminum carbonate	500–1500 mg (5–30 mL in oral suspension) 3–6 times daily orally between meals and at bedtime
calcium carbonate *kal'-see um car'-boe-nate*	Tums, Mylanta (multiple trade names)	Symptomatic relief of peptic ulcer and stomach hyperacidity, calcium deficiencies (osteoporosis)	Acid rebound	0.5–1.5 g orally
magnesia (magnesium hydroxide) *mag-nee'-zee-ah*	Milk of Magnesia, Phillips MOM	Symptomatic relief of peptic ulcer and stomach hyperacidity, constipation	Diarrhea, bone loss in patients with chronic renal failure	Antacid: 622–1244 mg (5–15 mL in suspension) orally QID Laxative: 15–60 mL orally
magnesium oxide *mag-nee'-zee-um*	Mag-Ox 400, Maox 420, Uro-Mag	Same as magnesia	Same as magnesia	140–800 mg/day orally
sodium bicarbonate *soe'-dee-um*	Bell/ans	Symptomatic relief of peptic ulcer and stomach hyperacidity	Electrolyte imbalance and metabolic alkalosis	0.3–2 g orally 1–4 times daily
Combined-Product Acid Neutralizer				
magaldrate (magnesium/aluminate) *mag-al-drate*	Iosopan, Riopan	Symptomatic relief of peptic ulcer and stomach hyperacidity	Constipation, diarrhea	5–10 mL orally between meals and at bedtime
Acid Reducers				
Histamine H₂ Antagonists				
cimetidine* *sye-meh'-tih-deen*	Tagamet	Gastric/duodenal ulcers, GERD, gastric hypersecretory conditions, GI bleeding, heartburn	Headache, somnolence, diarrhea	800–1600 mg/day orally; 300 mg q 6 hr IM or IV

(table continues on page 432)

Summary Drug Table UPPER GASTROINTESTINAL SYSTEM DRUGS (continued)

Generic Name	Trade Name	Uses	Adverse Reactions	Dosage Ranges
famotidine* *fah-moe-tih-deen*	Pepcid	Same as cimetidine	Same as cimetidine	20–40 mg orally; IV if unable to take orally
nizatidine* *nih-zah'-tih-deen*	Axid	Same as cimetidine	Same as cimetidine	150–300 mg/day orally in one dose or divided doses
ranitidine* *rah-nye'-tih-deen*	Zantac	Same as cimetidine, erosive esophagitis	Same as cimetidine	150–600 mg orally in one dose or divided doses orally; 50 mg q 6–8 hr IM, IV (do not exceed 400 mg/day)
Proton Pump Inhibitors				
dexlansoprazole *deks-lan-soe'-prah-zoll*	Dexilant	Erosive esophagitis, reflux disease	Headache, nausea, diarrhea	30–60 mg/day orally
esomeprazole *ess-oh-meh'-prah-zoll*	Nexium	Erosive esophagitis, GERD, *H. pylori* eradication, NSAID-associated gastric ulcers	Headache, nausea, diarrhea	20–40 mg/day orally
lansoprazole *lan-soe'-prah-zoll*	Prevacid	Same as esomeprazole, hypersecretory conditions, cystic fibrosis (intestinal malabsorption)	Same as esomeprazole	15–30 mg/day orally
omeprazole *oh-meh'-prah-zoll*	Prilosec, (Zegerid—combined with sodium bicarbonate)	Same as esomeprazole, hypersecretory conditions, heartburn, reduce risk of upper GI bleeding	Same as esomeprazole	20–60 mg/day orally
pantoprazole *pan-toe-prah-zoll*	Protonix	GERD, erosive esophagitis and hypersecretory conditions	Same as esomeprazole	40 mg/day orally or IV Hypersecretion: 80 mg IV q 12 hr
rabeprazole *rah-beh-prah-zoll*	AcipHex	Same as esomeprazole	Same as esomeprazole	20 mg/day orally
Miscellaneous Acid Reducers				
sucralfate *soo-kral-fate*	Carafate	Short-term duodenal ulcer treatment	Constipation	1 g/day orally in divided doses
misoprostol *mye-soe-prah'-stoll*	Cytotec	Prevention of gastric ulcers in patients taking NSAIDs	Headache, nausea, diarrhea, abdominal pain	100–200 mcg orally QID
GI Stimulant				
Ⓡ metoclopramide *meh-toe-kloe'-prah-mide*	Reglan	Diabetic gastroparesis, GERD, prevention of nausea and vomiting	Restlessness, dizziness, fatigue, extrapyramidal effects	10–15 mg orally; 10–20 mg IM, IV
Antiemetics				
Antidopaminergics				
chlorpromazine *klor-proe'-mah-zeen*		Control of nausea and vomiting, intractable hiccoughs	Drowsiness, hypotension, dry mouth, nasal congestion	Nausea and vomiting: 10–25 mg orally q 4–6 hr; 50–100 mg rectal suppository q 6–8 hr; 25–50 mg IM q 3–4 hr Hiccoughs: 25–50 mg orally, IM, slow IV infusion
perphenazine *per-fen-ah-zeen*		Same as chlorpromazine	Same as chlorpromazine	8–16 mg/day orally in divided doses, 5–10 mg IM, IV q 6 hr

Summary Drug Table UPPER GASTROINTESTINAL SYSTEM DRUGS (continued)

Generic Name	Trade Name	Uses	Adverse Reactions	Dosage Ranges
prochlorperazine *proe-klor-per'-ah-zeen*		Control of nausea and vomiting	Same as chlorpromazine	Orally: 5–10 mg TID or QID IM, IV: 5–10 mg Rectal suppository: 25 mg BID Sustained release: 10–15 mg
promethazine *proe-meth'-ah-zeen*		Control of nausea and vomiting associated with anesthesia and surgery, motion sickness	Same as diphenhydramine (Benadryl)	Nausea and vomiting: 12.5–25 mg orally, IM, IV, rectally Motion sickness: 25 mg orally 1–2 hr before travel, repeat 8–12 hr
Cholinergic Blocking Drug				
trimethobenzamide *trye-meth-oh-ben'-zah-myde*	Tigan	Control of nausea and vomiting	Hypotension (IM use), Parkinson-like symptoms, blurred vision, drowsiness, dizziness	250 mg orally or 200 mg IM, rectal suppository TID or QID
5-HT3 Receptor Antagonists				
dolasetron[†] *doe-laz-ee-tron*	Anzemet	Prevention of chemotherapy-induced and postoperative nausea, vomiting	Headache, fatigue, fever, abdominal pain	100 mg orally or 1.8 mg/kg IV
granisetron[†] *gran-iz-ee-tron*	Kytril, Sancuso (transdermal)	Same as dolasetron	Headache, asthenia, diarrhea, constipation	1–2 mg orally or 10 mcg/kg IV; transdermal patch applied 2 days before to 5 days after chemotherapy treatment
ondansetron[†] *on-dan-see-tron*	Zofran	Same as dolasetron, hyperemesis in pregnancy, bulimia, spinal analgesia– or gallbladder-induced pruritus	Headache, fatigue, drowsiness, sedation, constipation, hypoxia	8 mg orally BID or TID; 32 mg IV
palonosetron[†] *pal-oe-noh-see-tron*	Aloxi	Same as dolasetron	Same as dolasetron	0.25–0.5 mg in a single dose
Miscellaneous Antiemetic				
aprepitant[†] *ap-re'-pih-tant*	Emend	Prevention of chemotherapy-induced and postoperative nausea, vomiting	Headache, fatigue, stomatitis, constipation	125 mg 1 hr before chemotherapy and 80 mg daily for 3 days
dronabinol[†] *droe-nab-ih-nol*	Marinol	Prevention of chemotherapy-induced nausea and vomiting, appetite stimulant for patients with human immunodeficiency virus infection	Drowsiness, somnolence, euphoria, dizziness, vomiting	5 mg/m^2 1–3 hr before chemotherapy Appetite stimulant: 2.5 mg orally BID
nabilone[†] *nab'-ih-loan*	Cesamet	Prevention of chemotherapy-induced nausea and vomiting	Drowsiness, vertigo, euphoria, dry mouth	1–2 mg BID up to 48 hr following chemotherapy dose

® These drugs are taken at least 30 minutes before meals and at bedtime.

*These drugs are sold over the counter in smaller doses than those listed for therapeutic interventions.

[†]These drugs are administered according to specific protocols; consult the order before administration.

● Chapter Review

Know Your Drugs

Clients sometimes know a medication by the brand (or trade) name and not the generic name. To help you recognize both names, match the brand name with the generic name of the same medication.

Generic Name	Brand Name
1. cimetidine	A. Nexium
2. esomeprazole	B. Pepcid
3. famotidine	C. Tagamet
4. ranitidine	D. Zantac

Calculate Medication Dosages

1. Esomeprazole 40 mg once daily is prescribed. The drug is available in 20-mg capsules. How many will the nurse administer? _____

2. Sucralfate 2 g twice daily is prescribed. The drug comes in an oral suspension sucralfate 1 g/10 mL. How many milliliters will the nurse administer in each dose? _____

● Prepare for the NCLEX®

Build Your Knowledge

1. How would the nurse correctly administer an antacid to a client taking other oral medications?

    1. with the other drugs
    2. 30 minutes before or after administration of other drugs
    3. 2 hours before or after administration of other drugs
    4. in early morning and at bedtime

2. When a histamine H₂ antagonist drug is prescribed for the treatment of a peptic ulcer, the nurse observes the client for which of the following adverse effects?

    1. dry mouth, urinary retention
    2. edema, tachycardia
    3. constipation, anorexia
    4. headache, somnolence

3. What is the most common adverse reaction the nurse would expect in a client receiving an antiemetic?

    1. occipital headache
    2. drowsiness
    3. edema
    4. nausea

4. When explaining how to use transdermal scopolamine, the nurse tells the client to apply the system to _____.

    1. a nonhairy region of the chest
    2. the upper back
    3. behind the ear
    4. the forearm

Apply Your Knowledge

5. Select the most helpful resource for the nurse assisting the client to determine the best antacid to purchase.

    1. scan magazines and newspaper ads
    2. discuss with the clinical pharmacist
    3. search the Internet for drug ads
    4. contact the drug company

6. Which of the following statements made by the client would be of concern to the nurse?

    1. "Take this pill if I feel nauseated."
    2. "I will take this antacid right before I eat."
    3. "I should avoid drinking alcoholic beverages for a while."
    4. "Eating a diet high in protein will help me feel better."

7. If a client is taking metoclopramide, which of the following behaviors indicates an irreversible condition that should be reported immediately to the primary health care provider?

    1. muscle rigidity, dry mouth, insomnia
    2. rhythmic, involuntary movements of the tongue, face, mouth, or jaw
    3. muscle weakness, paralysis of the eyelids, diarrhea
    4. dyspnea, somnolence, muscle spasms

Alternate-Format Questions

8. Match the antacid with the adverse reaction it causes:

1. constipation	A. Milk of Magnesia
2. diarrhea	B. Amphojel
	C. Mylanta
	D. Bell/ans

9. Prochlorperazine (Compazine) 10 mg orally is prescribed. Use the drug label below to prepare the correct dosage. The nurse would administer _____.

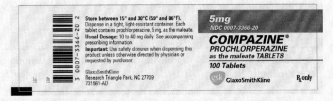

10. The client is to receive 400 mg cimetidine (Tagamet) orally. Available for use is the cimetidine shown below. The nurse administers _____.

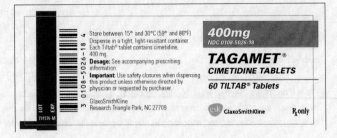

To check your answers, see Appendix G.

the**Point** *For more NCLEX-style questions, log on to http://thepoint.lww.com to access more than 1000 questions.*

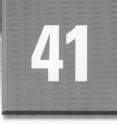

Lower Gastrointestinal System Drugs

LEARNING OBJECTIVES

On completion of this chapter, the student will:

1. Describe how inflammatory bowel disease alters function of the lower gastrointestinal (GI) system.
2. List the types of drugs prescribed or recommended for lower GI disorders.
3. Discuss the uses, general drug actions, general adverse reactions, contraindications, precautions, and interactions associated with lower GI drugs.
4. Discuss important preadministration and ongoing assessment activities the nurse should perform on the patient taking a lower GI drug.
5. List nursing diagnoses particular to a patient taking a lower GI drug.
6. Discuss ways to promote an optimal response to therapy, how to manage common adverse reactions, and important points to keep in mind when educating patients about the use of lower GI drugs.

KEY TERMS

antiflatulents • drugs that work against flatus (gas)

constipation • hardened fecal material that is difficult to pass

diarrhea • loose, watery stool

dyspepsia • fullness or epigastric discomfort

inflammatory bowel disease • inflammation of the bowel (e.g., Crohn's disease and ulcerative colitis)

obstipation • watery stool leakage around a hard fecal impaction

DRUG CLASSES

Aminosalicylates	Antiflatulents
Antidiarrheals	Laxatives

The large intestine is responsible for the absorption of water and some of the nutrients from the food and fluids we eat. The speed of transit determines what will be absorbed. Transit of contents rapidly through the bowel is called **diarrhea**. When contents move sluggishly, more water is absorbed, and the fecal material gets harder, resulting in **constipation**. Transit can be triggered by many things. Illness, such as irritable bowel syndrome or ulcerative colitis; bacterial infection; or drugs such as anti-infectives can make transit faster, resulting in diarrhea. Conditions such as Parkinson's disease can slow the bowel, causing constipation. Treatment with opioid drugs and the aftereffects of abdominal surgery can also cause constipation.

Conditions that affect the function of the lower GI system can have a significant impact on activities of daily living; if proper absorption does not occur, people may not have the energy to engage in activities. One such condition that affects function is **inflammatory bowel disease** (IBD; Fig. 41.1). Another condition, irritable bowel syndrome (IBS), also affects the lower GI system. The pain and bloating of a sluggish bowel or fear of stool incontinence may prevent people from socializing, again affecting daily life. The drugs described in this chapter affect the function of the bowel. Antidiarrheals and laxatives, as well as drugs to treat IBD and IBS, are presented. Some of the more common drugs are listed in the Summary Drug Table: Lower Gastrointestinal System Drugs.

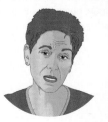

PHARMACOLOGY IN PRACTICE

Betty Peterson comes into the clinic and states, "Things just aren't right." During your assessment you learn she has become constipated after taking a cold preparation recently. After reading this chapter, determine why Betty has constipation and what should be recommended to help her.

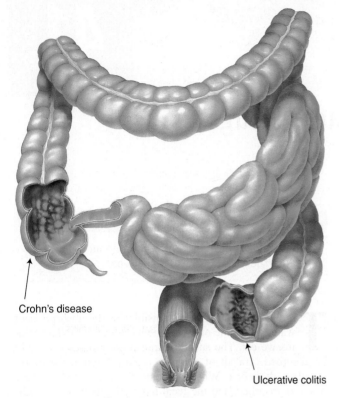

Crohn's disease

Ulcerative colitis

Figure 41.1 Examples of inflammatory bowel diseases. (Courtesy of Anatomical Chart Co.)

Inflammatory Bowel Disease

According to the Crohn's and Colitis Foundation of America (2012), as many as 1.4 million Americans have IBD. The term IBD is used collectively for Crohn's disease and ulcerative colitis, diseases that cause inflammation in the intestines. The cause of these diseases is unknown, although it is thought that a virus or bacterial organism interacting with the body's immune system may be the cause. Clinical manifestations of Crohn's disease include abdominal pain and distention. As the disease progresses, other GI symptoms present, such as anorexia, diarrhea, weight loss, dehydration, and nutritional deficiencies. Ulcerative colitis has a more abrupt onset; patients experience the sudden need to defecate, resulting in severe, blood- and mucus-filled diarrhea or no stool at all. Pain and fatigue accompany this disorder as well. No evidence has been found to support the theory that IBD is caused by tension, anxiety, or any other psychological factor or disorder (NIH, 2012). Drugs used to treat IBD include antibiotics, corticosteroids, biologic agents, and aminosalicylates. Aminosalicylates are described in this chapter; other drugs used in the treatment of IBD are included in their respective chapters.

AMINOSALICYLATES

Actions and Uses

Aminosalicylates are aspirin-like compounds with anti-inflammatory action. The drugs exert a topical anti-inflammatory effect in the bowel. The exact mechanism of action

of these drugs is unknown. The aminosalicylates are used to treat Crohn's disease and ulcerative colitis as well as other inflammatory diseases.

Adverse Reactions

Because these drugs are topical anti-inflammatory drugs, the most common adverse reactions happen in the GI system and include abdominal pain, nausea, and diarrhea. Other general adverse reactions include headache, dizziness, fever, and weakness.

Contraindications and Precautions

Aminosalicylates are contraindicated in patients with a known hypersensitivity to the drugs or salicylate-containing drugs. In addition, these drugs are contraindicated in patients who have hypersensitivity to sulfonamides and sulfites or intestinal obstruction, and in children younger than 2 years. Aminosalicylates are pregnancy category B drugs (except olsalazine, which is in pregnancy category C); all are used with caution during pregnancy and lactation (safety has not been established).

Interactions

The following interactions may occur when an aminosalicylate is administered with another agent:

Interacting Drug	Common Use	Effect of Interaction
digoxin	Cardiac problems	Reduced absorption of digoxin
methotrexate	Cancer and autoimmune conditions	Increased risk of immunosuppression
oral hypoglycemic drugs	Diabetes mellitus management	Increased blood glucose level
warfarin	Blood thinner	Increased risk of bleeding

HERBAL CONSIDERATIONS

Chamomile has several uses in traditional herbal therapy, including as a mild sedative and for treatment of digestive upsets, menstrual cramps, and stomach ulcers. It has been used topically for skin irritation and inflammation. Chamomile is on the U.S. Food and Drug Administration (FDA) list of herbs generally recognized as safe. It is one of the most popular teas in Europe. When used as an infusion, it appears to produce an antispasmodic effect on the smooth muscle of the GI tract and to protect against the development of stomach ulcers. Although the herb is generally safe and nontoxic, the infusion is prepared from the pollen-filled flower heads and has resulted in mild symptoms of contact dermatitis to severe anaphylactic reactions in individuals hypersensitive to ragweed, asters, and chrysanthemums (DerMarderosian, 2003).

ANTIDIARRHEALS

Actions and Uses

Antidiarrheals are used in the treatment of diarrhea. Difenoxin (Motofen) and diphenoxylate (Lomotil) are chemically related to opioid drugs; therefore, they decrease intestinal peristalsis, which often is increased when the patient has diarrhea. Because these drugs are opioid related, they may have sedative and euphoric effects, but no analgesic activity. A drug dependence potential exists; therefore, the drugs are combined with atropine (a cholinergic blocking drug), which causes dry mouth and other mild adverse effects. Abuse potential is reduced because of these unpleasant adverse effects.

Loperamide (Imodium) acts directly on the muscle wall of the bowel to slow motility and is not related to the opioids. It therefore is also used in treating chronic diarrhea associated with IBD.

Adverse Reactions

Gastrointestinal System Reactions

• Anorexia, nausea, vomiting, and constipation
• Abdominal discomfort, pain, and distention

Other System Reactions

• Dizziness, drowsiness, and headache
• Sedation and euphoria
• Rash

Contraindications and Precautions

These drugs are contraindicated in patients whose diarrhea is associated with organisms that can harm the intestinal mucosa (*Escherichia coli*, *Salmonella* and *Shigella* spp.). Patients with pseudomembranous colitis, abdominal pain of unknown origin, and obstructive jaundice also should not take antidiarrheals. Antidiarrheal drugs are contraindicated in children younger than 2 years of age.

 NURSING ALERT

If diarrhea persists for more than 2 days when over-the-counter (OTC) antidiarrheal drugs are being used, the patient should discontinue use and seek treatment from the primary health care provider.

The antidiarrheal drugs are used cautiously in patients with severe hepatic impairment. Antidiarrheals are classified as pregnancy category C drugs and should be used cautiously during pregnancy and lactation. Loperamide is a pregnancy category B drug but is not recommended for use during pregnancy and lactation.

Interactions

The following interactions may occur when an antidiarrheal drug is administered with another agent:

Interacting Drug	Common Use	Effects of Interaction
antihistamines, opioids, sedatives, or hypnotics	Allergy treatment (antihistamines), sedation, or pain relief	Increased risk of central nervous system (CNS) depression
antihistamines and general antidepressants	Allergy relief and depression management	Increased cholinergic blocking adverse reactions

Interacting Drug	Common Use	Effects of Interaction
monoamine oxidase inhibitor (MAOI) antidepressants	Depression management	Increased risk of hypertensive crisis

ANTIFLATULENTS

Actions

Simethicone (Mylicon) and charcoal are used as **antiflatulents** (drugs that reduce flatus or gas in the intestinal tract). These drugs do not absorb or remove gas; rather, they act to help the body release the gas by belching or flatus (passing gas). Simethicone has a defoaming action that disperses and prevents the formation of gas pockets in the intestine. Charcoal helps bind gas for expulsion.

Uses

Antiflatulents are used to relieve painful symptoms of excess gas in the digestive tract that may be caused by the following:

• Postoperative gaseous distention and air swallowing
• **Dyspepsia** (fullness or epigastric discomfort)
• Peptic ulcer
• Irritable bowel syndrome or diverticulosis

In addition to its use for the relief of intestinal gas, charcoal may be used in the prevention of nonspecific pruritus associated with kidney dialysis treatment and as an antidote in poisoning. Simethicone is in some antacid products, such as Mylanta Liquid and Di-Gel Liquid.

Adverse Reactions

No adverse reactions have been reported with the use of antiflatulents.

Contraindications and Precautions

Antiflatulents are contraindicated in patients with known hypersensitivity to any components of the drug. The pregnancy category of simethicone has not been determined; because it is not absorbed, it may be safe for use during pregnancy, although the primary health care provider should be consulted whenever any drug is to be taken. Charcoal is a pregnancy category C drug.

Interactions

There may be a decreased effectiveness of other drugs because of adsorption by charcoal, which can also adsorb other drugs in the GI tract. There are no known interactions with simethicone.

LAXATIVES

Actions

There are various types of laxatives (see the Summary Drug Table: Lower Gastrointestinal System Drugs). The action of

---

Display 41.1 **Actions of Different Types of Laxatives**

- *Bulk-producing laxatives* are not digested by the body and therefore add bulk and water to the contents of the intestines. The added bulk in the intestines stimulates peristalsis, moves the products of digestion through the intestine, and encourages evacuation of the stool. Examples of bulk-forming laxatives are psyllium (Metamucil) and polycarbophil (FiberCon). Sometimes these laxatives are used with severe diarrhea to add bulk to the watery bowel contents and slow transit through the bowel.
- *Emollient laxatives* lubricate the intestinal walls and soften the stool, thereby enhancing passage of fecal material. Mineral oil is an emollient laxative.
- *Stool softeners* promote water retention in the fecal mass and soften the stool. One difference between emollient laxatives and stool softeners is that the emollient laxatives do not promote the retention of water in the stool. Examples of stool softeners include docusate (Colace).
- *Hyperosmolar drugs* dehydrate local tissues, which causes irritation and increased peristalsis, with consequent evacuation of the fecal mass. Glycerin is a hyperosmolar drug.
- *Irritant or stimulant laxatives* increase peristalsis by direct action on the intestine. An example of an irritant laxative is senna (Senokot) or bisacodyl.
- *Saline laxatives* attract or pull water into the intestine, thereby increasing pressure in the intestine, followed by an increase in peristalsis. Magnesium (Milk of Magnesia) is a saline laxative.

Display 41.2 **Drugs That Cause Constipation**

- Anticholinergic (cholinergic blocking drugs)
- Antihistamines
- Phenothiazines
- Tricyclic antidepressants
- Opioids
- Non–potassium-sparing diuretics
- Iron preparations
- Barium
- Clonidine
- Antacids containing calcium or aluminum

---

each laxative is somewhat different, yet they all produce the same result—relief of constipation. The manner of action of the various laxative groups is explained in Display 41.1.

Uses

A laxative is most often prescribed for the short-term relief or prevention of constipation. Specific uses of laxatives include:

- *Stimulant, emollient, and saline laxatives*—evacuate the colon for rectal and bowel examinations
- *Stool softeners or mineral oil*—prevention of strain during defecation (after anorectal surgery or a myocardial infarction)
- *Psyllium and polycarbophil*—irritable bowel syndrome and diverticular disease
- *Hyperosmotic (lactulose) agents*—reduction of blood ammonia levels in hepatic encephalopathy

Adverse Reactions

Constipation may occur as an adverse drug reaction. When the patient has constipation as an adverse reaction to another drug, the primary health care provider may prescribe a stool

softener or another laxative to prevent constipation during the drug therapy. Display 41.2 lists some of the drug classifications known to cause constipation.

Laxatives may cause diarrhea and a loss of water and electrolytes, abdominal pain or discomfort, nausea, vomiting, perianal irritation, fainting, bloating, flatulence, cramps, and weakness.

Prolonged use of a laxative can result in serious electrolyte imbalances, as well as the "laxative habit," that is, dependence on a laxative to have a bowel movement. Some of these products contain tartrazine (a yellow food dye), which may cause allergic-type reactions (including bronchial asthma) in susceptible individuals. Obstruction of the esophagus, stomach, small intestine, and colon has occurred when bulk-forming laxatives are administered without adequate fluid intake or in patients with intestinal stenosis.

 LIFESPAN CONSIDERATIONS
Chronic Care
The very young, the very old, and debilitated patients are at greatest risk for aspiration of mineral oil into the lungs when it is taken orally for constipation. Aspiration of mineral oil can lead to a lipid pneumonitis.

Contraindications and Precautions

Laxatives are contraindicated in patients with known hypersensitivity and those with persistent abdominal pain, nausea, vomiting of unknown cause, or signs of acute appendicitis, fecal impaction, intestinal obstruction, or acute hepatitis. These drugs are used only as directed because excessive or prolonged use may cause physical dependence on them for normal bowel movements.

Magnesium is used cautiously in patients with any degree of renal impairment. Laxatives are used cautiously in patients with rectal bleeding, in pregnant women, and during lactation. The following laxatives are pregnancy category C drugs: cascara sagrada, docusate, glycerin, phenolphthalein, magnesium, and senna. These drugs are used during pregnancy only when the benefits clearly outweigh the risks to the fetus.

Interactions

- Mineral oil may impair the GI absorption of fat-soluble vitamins (A, D, E, and K).

- Laxatives may reduce absorption of other drugs present in the GI tract by combining with them chemically or hastening their passage through the intestinal tract.
- When surfactants are administered with mineral oil, they may increase mineral oil absorption.

- Milk, antacids, histamine H₂ antagonists, and proton pump inhibitors should not be administered 1 to 2 hours before bisacodyl tablets because the enteric coating may dissolve early (before reaching the intestinal tract), resulting in gastric lining irritation or dyspepsia and decreasing the laxative effect of the drug.

NURSING PROCESS
PATIENT RECEIVING A DRUG FOR A LOWER GASTROINTESTINAL CONDITION

ASSESSMENT

Preadministration Assessment
Often when dealing with lower GI complaints you should review the patient's chart for the course of treatment and find the reason for administration of the prescribed drug. Question the patient regarding the type and intensity of symptoms (e.g., pain, discomfort, diarrhea, or constipation) to provide a baseline for evaluation of the effectiveness of drug therapy. Listen first to bowel sounds and then palpate the abdomen, monitoring the patient for signs of guarding or discomfort. Loose stool may indicate diarrhea; however, hypoactive bowel sounds in severe cases of obstipation (liquid stool leaked around the fecal mass, presenting as loose stool) are evidence that the patient is constipated, which would indicate very different drug therapy.

Ongoing Assessment
Assess the patient receiving one of these drugs for relief of symptoms (e.g., diarrhea, pain, or constipation). Instruct the patient regarding loose, frequent stools and diarrhea. The patient may report multiple trips to the bathroom with formed stool as diarrhea. For the best treatment you need to know the difference so you can report relief or continued symptoms to the primary health care provider. Monitoring vital signs if the patient has severe diarrhea may help you to discover issues such as dehydration in addition to the bowel problem. Observe the patient for adverse drug reactions associated with the specific GI drug being administered and report any adverse reactions to the primary health care provider before the next dose is due (Fig. 41.2).

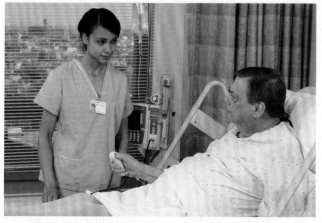

Figure 41.2 Disruption in bowel routine can have an impact on the activities of daily living for the patient.

NURSING DIAGNOSES
A drug-specific nursing diagnosis is the following:

- **Risk for Imbalanced Fluid Volume** related to diarrhea

Nursing diagnoses related to drug administration are discussed in Chapter 4.

PLANNING
The expected outcomes for the patient depend on the reason for administration of the drug but may include an optimal response to drug therapy, support of patient needs related to the management of adverse reactions, and confidence in an understanding of the medication regimen.

IMPLEMENTATION

Promoting an Optimal Response to Therapy
Ways in which you can help promote an optimal response to therapy when administering lower GI drugs follow.

ANTIDIARRHEALS. When diarrhea is severe, these drugs may be ordered to be given after each loose bowel movement. This may concern the patient that the opposite will happen, that is, becoming constipated. Ask the patient to describe or check each bowel movement before making a decision to administer the drug.

LAXATIVES. Give bulk-producing or stool-softening laxatives with a full glass of water or juice. The administration of a bulk-producing laxative is followed by an additional full glass of water. Mineral oil preferably is given to the patient with an empty stomach in the evening. Immediately before administration, thoroughly mix and stir laxatives that are in powder, flake, or granule form. If the laxative has an unpleasant or salty taste, explain this to the patient. The taste of some of these preparations may be disguised by chilling, adding to juice, or pouring over cracked ice.

> **! NURSING ALERT**
> Because activated charcoal can absorb other drugs in the GI tract, when used as an antiflatulent it should not be taken 2 hours before or 1 hour after the administration of other drugs.

Monitoring and Managing Patient Needs
RISK FOR IMBALANCED FLUID VOLUME. Notify the primary health care provider if the patient experiences an elevation in body temperature, severe abdominal pain, or abdominal rigidity or distention because this may indicate a complication of the disorder, such as infection or intestinal perforation. If diarrhea is severe, additional treatment measures, such as intravenous fluids and electrolyte replacement, may be necessary.

If diarrhea is chronic, encourage the patient to drink extra fluids. Weak tea, water, bouillon, or a commercial electrolyte preparation may be used.

Monitor fluid intake and output closely. In some instances, the primary health care provider may prescribe an oral electrolyte supplement to replace electrolytes lost by frequent loose stools. Patients with fluid volume losses taking drugs that cause drowsiness or dizziness are at greater risk for injury. The patient may require assistance with ambulatory activities. For perianal irritation caused by loose stools, instruct the patient or caregiver to cleanse the area with mild soap and water after each bowel movement, dry the area with a soft cloth, and apply an emollient, such as petrolatum.

When a laxative is administered, document the bowel movement results on the patient's chart. If excessive bowel movements or severe, prolonged diarrhea occurs, or if the laxative is ineffective, notify the primary health care provider. If a laxative is ordered for constipation, encourage a liberal fluid intake and an increase in foods high in fiber to prevent a repeat of this problem.

Educating the Patient and Family

Because patients frequently will begin use of OTC products for lower GI conditions before discussing with health care providers, develop teaching plans to include the following general points about these medications at any teaching session:

ANTIDIARRHEALS

- Do not exceed the recommended dosage.
- Observe caution when driving or performing other hazardous tasks because the drug may cause drowsiness.
- ⚠ Avoid the use of alcohol or other central nervous system (CNS) depressants (e.g., tranquilizers, sleeping pills) and other nonprescription drugs unless use has been approved by the primary health care provider.
- Notify the primary health care provider if diarrhea persists or becomes more severe.

ANTIFLATULENTS

- Take simethicone after each meal and at bedtime. Thoroughly chew tablets because complete particle dispersion enhances antiflatulent action.
- Notify the health care provider if symptoms are not relieved within several days.

LAXATIVES

- Avoid long-term use of these products unless use of the product has been recommended by the primary health care

provider. Long-term use may result in the "laxative habit," which is dependence on a laxative to have a normal bowel movement. Constipation may also occur with overuse of these drugs. Laxatives are not to be used for weight loss. Read and follow the directions on the label.

- Do not use these products in the presence of abdominal pain, nausea, or vomiting.
- Notify the primary health care provider if constipation is not relieved or if rectal bleeding or other symptoms occur.
- To avoid constipation, drink plenty of fluids, get exercise, and eat foods high in bulk or roughage.
- Cascara sagrada or senna—Pink-red, red-violet, red-brown, yellow-brown, or black discoloration of urine may occur.

EVALUATION

- Therapeutic drug effect is achieved, and bowel movements are appropriate for the patient's normal routine.
- Adverse reactions are identified, reported to the primary health care provider, and managed successfully through appropriate nursing interventions:
  - Patient maintains an adequate fluid volume.
- Patient and family express confidence and demonstrate an understanding of the drug regimen.

PHARMACOLOGY IN PRACTICE
THINK CRITICALLY

 Betty shares the medications she is currently taking:

amitriptyline
acetaminophen
diphenhydramine cold preparation

Based on this list of medications being taken, what type of laxative preparation would be best for Betty's constipation problem?

KEY POINTS

- The lower GI system includes the small and large intestines. Other organs secrete into the system but are not mentioned in this chapter. Absorption of both nutrients and fluids occurs in the intestines, as does the exchange of waste products.
- Drugs that slow down transit or speed up the process also are used for chronic conditions such as inflammatory bowel disease. Adverse reactions include abdominal

pain or perianal irritation associated with moving or slowing content transit in the bowel, or issues associated with fluid imbalances such as dizziness, drowsiness, or headache.
- Multiple OTC products exist to treat GI symptoms. Patients need confidence in understanding how to purchase and take these products because the majority of users do so without health care provider supervision.

Chapter 41 Lower Gastrointestinal System Drugs 441

Summary Drug Table LOWER GASTROINTESTINAL SYSTEM DRUGS

Generic Name	Trade Name	Uses	Adverse Reactions	Dosage Ranges
Drugs Used to Treat Inflammatory Bowel Disease				
Aminosalicylates				
balsalazide *bal-sal'-ah-zyde*	Colazal	Active ulcerative colitis	Headache, abdominal pain	2250 mg orally TID for 8 wk
mesalamine *meh-sal'-ah-meen*	Asacol, Pentasa, Rowasa (rectal form)	Active ulcerative colitis, proctosigmoiditis or proctitis	Headache, abdominal pain, nausea	800–1000 mg orally TID or QID Suspension enema: 4 g daily
olsalazine *ohl-sal'-ah-zeen*	Dipentum	Maintenance of remission of ulcerative colitis	Diarrhea, abdominal pain and cramping	1 g/day orally in two divided doses
sulfasalazine *sul-fah-sal'-ah-zeen*	Azulfidine	Ulcerative colitis, rheumatoid arthritis	Headache, nausea, anorexia, vomiting, gastric distress, reduced sperm count	Initial: 3–4 g/day orally in divided doses Maintenance: 2 g orally QID
Miscellaneous Drugs for Bowel Disorders				
alosetron *ah-loe'-seh-tron*	Lotronex	Second-line treatment of female irritable bowel syndrome with severe diarrhea	Gastric distress, hemorrhoids, constipation	Special permission must be obtained for therapy
alvimopan *al'-vi-moe'-pan*	Entereg	Accelerate upper/lower GI recovery following surgery	Indigestion, hypokalemia, fatigue	12 mg orally twice daily for no more than 15 doses
infliximab *in-flik'-sih-mab*	Remicade	Crohn's disease, ulcerative colitis, rheumatoid arthritis	Sore throat, cough, sinus infection, gastric distress	5 mg/kg IV every 2–8 wk
Antidiarrheals				
bismuth *biz'-muth*	Bismatrol Pepto-Bismol, Pink Bismuth	Nausea, diarrhea, abdominal cramps, *Helicobacter pylori* infection with duodenal ulcer	Same as difenoxin	2 tablets or 30 mL orally every 30 min to 1 hr, up to 8 doses in 24 hr
difenoxin with atropine *dye-fen-ok'-sin, ah'-troe-peen*	Motofen	Symptomatic relief of acute diarrhea	Dry skin and mucous membranes, nausea, constipation, lightheadedness	Initial dose: 2 tablets orally, then 1 tablet after each loose stool (not to exceed 8 tablets/day)
diphenoxylate with atropine *dye-fen-ok'-sih-late*	Lomotil, Lonox	Same as difenoxin	Same as difenoxin	5 mg orally QID
loperamide *loe-pare'-ah-myde*	Imodium, Kaopectate, Maalox Anti-Diarrheal Caplets	Same as difenoxin	Same as difenoxin	Initial dose 4 mg orally; then 2 mg after each loose stool (not to exceed 16 mg/day)
tincture of opium	Paregoric	Severe diarrhea	Somnolence, constipation	0.6 mL orally QID
Antiflatulents				
charcoal	CharcoCaps, Flatulex (combined with simethicone)	Intestinal gas, diarrhea, poisoning antidote	Vomiting, constipation, diarrhea, black stools	520 mg orally after meals (not to exceed 4–16 g/day)
simethicone *sye-meth'-ih-kone*	Gas-X, Mylicon, Maalox Anti-Gas, Mylanta Gas	Postoperative distention, dyspepsia, irritable bowel syndrome, peptic ulcer	Bloating, constipation, diarrhea, heartburn	40–125 mg orally QID after meals and at bedtime
Laxatives				
Bulk-Producing Laxatives				
methylcellulose *meth-ill-sell'-yoo-loas*	Citrucel, Unifiber	Relief of constipation, irritable bowel syndrome, severe watery diarrhea	Diarrhea, nausea, vomiting, bloating, flatulence, cramping, perianal irritation, fainting	Follow directions given on the container

(table continues on page 442)

Summary Drug Table LOWER GASTROINTESTINAL SYSTEM DRUGS (continued)

Generic Name	Trade Name	Uses	Adverse Reactions	Dosage Ranges
psyllium *sill'-ee-um*	Fiberall, Genfiber, Hydrocil, Konsyl, Metamucil, Perdiem	Same as methylcellulose	Same as methylcellulose	Powder, granules, or wafers taken as directed on package
polycarbophil *pol-ee-kar'-boe-fill*	Equalactin, FiberCon, Mitrolan	Same as methylcellulose	Same as methylcellulose	1 g daily to QID or as needed (do not exceed 4 g in 24 hr)
Emollients				
mineral oil	Kondremul Plain, Milkinol	Relief of constipation, fecal impaction	Perianal discomfort and itching due to anal seepage	15–45 mL orally at bedtime
Stool Softeners/Surfactants				
docusate (dioctyl; DDS) *dok'-yoo-sate*	Colace, Ex-Lax Stool Softener, Modane Soft, Surfak Liquigels	Relief of constipation, prevention of straining during bowel movement	Diarrhea, nausea, vomiting, bloating, flatulence, cramping, perianal irritation, fainting	Follow directions given on the container; comes in enema form
Hyperosmotic Agents				
glycerine *glih'-ser-in*	Colace Suppositories, Sani-Supp, Fleet Babylax	Relief of constipation	Same as docusate sodium	Rectal suppository, use as directed
lactulose *lak'-tyoo-loas*	Constilac	Relief of constipation, hepatic encephalopathy	Same as docusate sodium	Constipation: 15–30 mL/day orally Hepatic encephalopathy: 30–45 mL orally QID, may give enema form
lubiprostone *loo-bih-pros'-tone*	Amitiza	Chronic idiopathic constipation	Headache, nausea, diarrhea	24 mcg orally BID
Irritant or Stimulant Laxatives				
cascara sagrada *kas-kar'-ah sah-grah'-dah*	Aromatic Cascara	Relief of constipation	Same as docusate sodium, darkening of colon mucosa, brownish color to urine	Follow directions given on the container
sennosides *sen'-oh-sydes*	Agoral, Ex-Lax, Senokot	Same as cascara	Same as cascara	Follow directions given on the container
bisacodyl *bis-ah-koe'-dill*	Dulcolax, Modane, Correctol	Same as cascara	Diarrhea, nausea, vomiting, bloating, flatulence, cramping, perianal irritation	Tablets: 10–15 mg daily orally Rectal suppositories: 10 mg daily; comes in enema form
Saline Laxatives				
magnesium preparations *mag-nee'-zee-um*	Milk of Magnesia, Magnesium Citrate, Fleets (enema preparation)	Evacuate colon for endoscopy, relieve constipation	Same as docusate sodium	Follow directions given on the container
Bowel Evacuants				
polyethylene glycol (PEG) solution *pol-ee-eth'-ih-leen*	MiraLAX	Relieve constipation	Same as sodium docusate	Follow directions given on the container
polyethylene glycol-electrolyte solution (PEG-ES) *pol-ee-eth'-ih-leen*	Colyte, GoLYTELY, NuLYTELY, OCL	Evacuate colon for endoscopy, relieve constipation	Same as sodium docusate	4 L oral solution to be drunk in 3 hr
sodium picosulfate/magnesium oxide/citric acid	Prepopik	Evacuate colon for endoscopy	Same as sodium docusate	Follow directions given on the container

Chapter Review

Know Your Drugs

Clients sometimes know a medication by the brand (or trade) name and not the generic name. To help you recognize both names, match the brand name with the generic name of the same medication.

Generic Name	Brand Name
1. diphenoxylate	A. Colace
2. docusate	B. Lomotil
3. polyethylene glycol	C. Metamucil
4. psyllium	D. MiraLAX

Calculate Medication Dosages

1. Balsalazide (Colazal) 2250 mg orally TID is prescribed. If the drug comes in 750-mg capsules, the nurse administers _____ capsules with each dose.

2. Diphenoxylate (Lomotil) 1 tablet BID is prescribed. If the drug comes in 2.5-mg tablets, how much diphenoxylate will the client take in 24 hours?

Prepare for the NCLEX®

Build Your Knowledge

1. In which area of the GI tract is water primarily reabsorbed?
   1. stomach
   2. small intestine
   3. large intestine (colon)
   4. pancreas

2. Which of the following is the best description of the cause of Crohn's disease?
   1. somatic response to psychological stress
   2. infection due to bacteria or parasites
   3. inflammatory response in the colon
   4. precancerous stage in the bowel

3. The client asks how stool softeners relieve constipation. Which of the following would be the best response by the nurse? Stool softeners relieve constipation by _____.
   1. stimulating the walls of the intestine
   2. promoting the retention of sodium in the fecal mass
   3. promoting water retention in the fecal mass
   4. lubricating the intestinal walls

4. The nurse administers antidiarrheal drugs _____.
   1. after each loose bowel movement
   2. hourly until diarrhea ceases
   3. with food
   4. twice a day, in the morning and at bedtime

5. The pregnancy category for the antiflatulent drug simethicone is _____.
   1. pregnancy category A
   2. pregnancy category C
   3. pregnancy category X
   4. pregnancy category unknown

Apply Your Knowledge

6. When recording the administration of diphenoxylate for multiple loose stools:
   1. document the daily number of drugs given
   2. record all stools once each shift
   3. indicate all stools on the medication administration record (MAR) next to the drug
   4. document each dose on the MAR

7. Which of the following points should be included in a teaching plan for a client taking a laxative?
   1. They may be used for minor weight loss
   2. Drink more fluid and eat more high-fiber foods
   3. The abdominal pain is probably gas buildup
   4. Using daily promotes good bowel health

8. Why is atropine put in an antidiarrheal?
   1. to neutralize acid
   2. to kill bacteria in the bowel
   3. to reduce addictive property
   4. to promote bowel health

Alternate-Format Questions

9. Harmful drug interactions exist when aminosalicylates are taken with the following drugs. **Select all that apply**.
   1. cardiotonics
   2. beta-adrenergic blockers
   3. oral hypoglycemics
   4. anticoagulants

10. A client is to drink 4 liters of polyethylene glycol-electrolyte solution (GoLYTELY) the night before an outpatient colonoscopy. If the directions state, "Drink 240 mL every 10 minutes," the nurse tells the client the solution must be completely drunk in _____ hours.

To check your answers, see Appendix G.

thePoint *For more NCLEX-style questions, log on to http://thepoint.lww.com to access more than 1000 questions.*

Drugs That Affect the Endocrine System

The endocrine system consists of a group of glands throughout the body. The work of the endocrine system is to provide hormones (chemicals that assist in function) to various organs in the body. Hormones are produced and circulated through the blood to target receptors on certain cells in specific organs to assist in function. Glands that make up the endocrine system and are discussed in this unit include the pituitary, thyroid, pancreas, adrenal glands, and sex organs.

The pancreas is part of the gastrointestinal (GI) system. This organ provides enzymes to assist in the digestion of food and provides the body with the hormone insulin to help cells use the glucose from food sources. The American Diabetes Association (ADA) estimates that, since 2008, there has been an increase from 7.8% to 8.3% of the people in the United States who now have diabetes (25.8 million people; ADA, 2012). Diabetes mellitus is a chronic condition characterized by problems with the body's production or use of insulin. Chapter 42 discusses both insulin and the oral antidiabetic drugs used in treating diabetes mellitus.

The pituitary gland sits at the base of the brain and helps with the function of many different organs in the body. Its hormones are secreted and sent to a variety of organs to promote and regulate growth and maturation, fluid and electrolyte balance, and metabolism. These hormones and the drugs that affect them are covered in Chapter 43. The adrenal glands are crucial in the secretion of corticosteroids, which are also covered in that chapter.

Located in the lower anterior portion of the neck, the thyroid's purpose is to help control metabolism. Chapter 44 covers the function of the thyroid and its hormones as well as drugs used to supplement function of the thyroid gland.

Hormones play a major role in the development of the reproductive system as people go through puberty. The ovaries in the female and the testes in the male produce hormones that aid in the development of secondary sexual characteristics such as hair, voice, and musculature. Reproduction is controlled by the secretion of hormones. Chapters 45 and 46 describe the function of these hormones and the drugs used to promote optimal reproductive health.

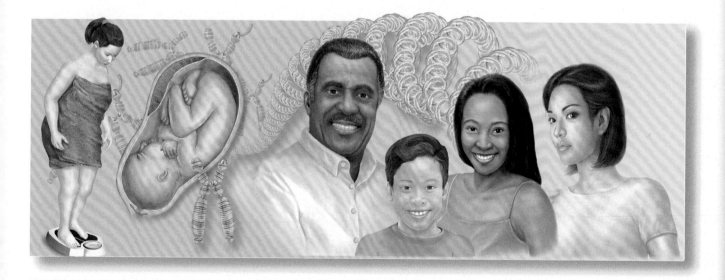

Antidiabetic Drugs

42

LEARNING OBJECTIVES

On completion of this chapter, the student will:

1. Describe the two types of diabetes mellitus.
2. Discuss the types, uses, general drug actions, adverse reactions, contraindications, precautions, and interactions of the antidiabetic drugs.
3. Discuss important preadministration and ongoing assessment activities the nurse should perform with the patient taking an antidiabetic drug.
4. List nursing diagnoses particular to a patient taking an antidiabetic drug.
5. Discuss ways to promote an optimal response to therapy, how to manage common adverse reactions, and important points to keep in mind when educating patients about the use of antidiabetic drugs.

KEY TERMS

diabetes mellitus • disease in which insulin does not help glucose enter the cell

diabetic ketoacidosis (DKA) • life-threatening deficiency of insulin resulting in severe hyperglycemia and excessively high levels of ketones in the blood

glucagon • hormone secreted by the alpha cells of the pancreas that increases the concentration of glucose in the blood

glucometer • device to monitor blood glucose level

glycosylated hemoglobin • blood test that monitors average blood glucose level over a 3- to 4-month period

hyperglycemia • high blood glucose (sugar) level

hypoglycemia • low blood glucose (sugar) level

lipodystrophy • atrophy of subcutaneous fat

polydipsia • excessive thirst

polyphagia • eating large amounts of food

polyuria • increased urination

secondary failure • in diabetes mellitus, loss of the effectiveness of sulfonylurea, an oral antidiabetic drug

DRUG CLASSES

Insulins	Nonsulfonylureas
Sulfonylureas	Incretin mimetics

PHARMACOLOGY IN PRACTICE

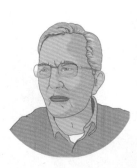

When Mr. Phillip was seen for atrial fibrillation, it was discovered that he had not been seen by a health care provider in more than 5 years. The first priority was to stabilize his heart and coagulation status. He was then given an appointment to come to the clinic for a complete physical examination. During the clinic visit, Mr. Phillip was found to be in relatively good physical condition, yet his blood chemistries showed an elevation in his blood glucose level (153 mg/dL) and his HbA$_{1c}$ reading was 9%. When his wife was alive, he remembers she started fixing food in a different way because of the doctor's concerns about eating too much sugar. When you finish this chapter, you should better understand the meaning of these laboratory values and know what patient interventions and instruction should follow.

Insulin is essential for cells to utilize glucose for energy and for the proper metabolism of protein and fat in our bodies. A hormone produced by the pancreas, insulin is required for the proper use of glucose (carbohydrate). This is accomplished by the release of small amounts of insulin into the bloodstream throughout the day in response to changes in blood glucose levels. Insulin lowers blood glucose levels by inhibiting glucose production by the liver. Insulin also controls the storage and utilization of amino acids and fatty acids.

Diabetes mellitus (often referred to as simply *diabetes*) is a complicated, chronic disorder characterized either by insufficient insulin production by the beta (β) cells of the pancreas or by cellular resistance to insulin. Insulin insufficiency results in elevated blood glucose levels, or **hyperglycemia**. As a result of the disease, individuals with diabetes are at greater risk for a number of disorders, including myocardial infarction,

cerebrovascular accident (stroke), blindness, kidney disease, and lower limb amputations.

Insulin and antidiabetic drugs, along with diet and exercise, are the cornerstones of treatment for diabetes. They are used to prevent episodes of **hypoglycemia** and normalize carbohydrate metabolism.

There are two major types of diabetes mellitus:

- Type 1—formerly known as insulin-dependent diabetes mellitus or IDDM
- Type 2—formerly known as non–insulin-dependent diabetes mellitus or NIDDM

Those with type 1 diabetes produce insulin in insufficient amounts and therefore must have insulin supplementation to survive (Fig. 42.1). Type 1 diabetes usually has a rapid onset, occurs before age 20 years, produces more severe symptoms

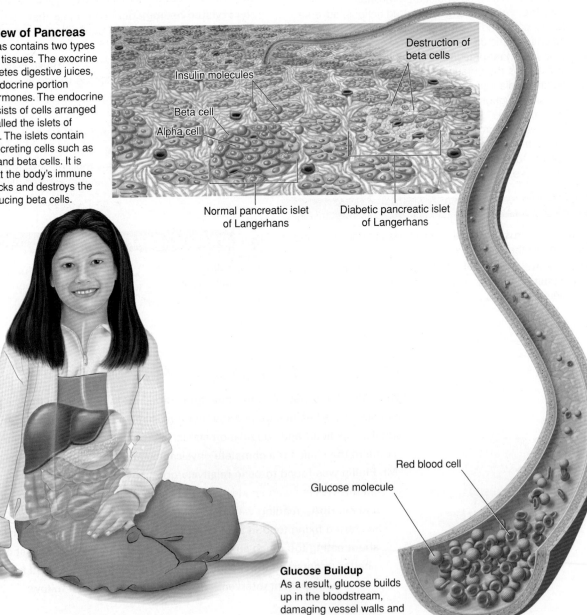

Cellular View of Pancreas
The pancreas contains two types of secretory tissues. The exocrine portion secretes digestive juices, while the endocrine portion releases hormones. The endocrine portion consists of cells arranged in groups called the islets of Langerhans. The islets contain hormone-secreting cells such as alpha cells and beta cells. It is believed that the body's immune system attacks and destroys the insulin-producing beta cells.

Insulin molecules

Beta cell

Alpha cell

Destruction of beta cells

Normal pancreatic islet of Langerhans

Diabetic pancreatic islet of Langerhans

Red blood cell

Glucose molecule

Glucose Buildup
As a result, glucose builds up in the bloodstream, damaging vessel walls and hurting vital processes.

Figure 42.1 Cellular view of type 1 diabetes. (Courtesy of Anatomical Chart Co.)

than type 2 diabetes, and is more difficult to control. Major symptoms of type 1 diabetes include hyperglycemia, **polydipsia** (increased thirst), **polyphagia** (increased appetite), **polyuria** (increased urination), and weight loss. Control of type 1 diabetes is particularly difficult because of the lack of insulin production by the pancreas. Treatment requires a strict regimen that typically includes a carefully calculated diet,

planned physical activity, home glucose testing several times a day, and daily supplement of insulin by injections or pump.

Type 2 diabetes mellitus affects about 90% to 95% of individuals with diabetes. Those with type 2 diabetes are affected either by decreased production of insulin by the β cells of the pancreas or by decreased sensitivity of the body cells to insulin, making the cells insulin resistant (Fig. 42.2). Although

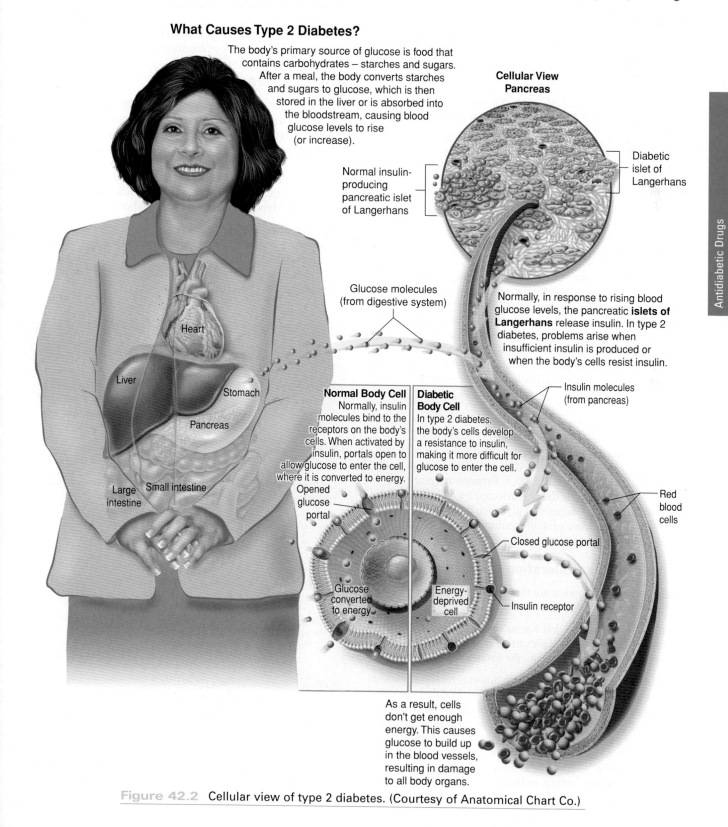

What Causes Type 2 Diabetes?

The body's primary source of glucose is food that contains carbohydrates – starches and sugars. After a meal, the body converts starches and sugars to glucose, which is then stored in the liver or is absorbed into the bloodstream, causing blood glucose levels to rise (or increase).

Cellular View Pancreas

Normal insulin-producing pancreatic islet of Langerhans

Diabetic islet of Langerhans

Glucose molecules (from digestive system)

Normally, in response to rising blood glucose levels, the pancreatic **islets of Langerhans** release insulin. In type 2 diabetes, problems arise when insufficient insulin is produced or when the body's cells resist insulin.

Insulin molecules (from pancreas)

Heart

Liver

Stomach

Pancreas

Normal Body Cell
Normally, insulin molecules bind to the receptors on the body's cells. When activated by insulin, portals open to allow glucose to enter the cell, where it is converted to energy.

Diabetic Body Cell
In type 2 diabetes, the body's cells develop a resistance to insulin, making it more difficult for glucose to enter the cell.

Opened glucose portal

Large intestine

Small intestine

Glucose converted to energy

Energy-deprived cell

Closed glucose portal

Insulin receptor

Red blood cells

As a result, cells don't get enough energy. This causes glucose to build up in the blood vessels, resulting in damage to all body organs.

Figure 42.2 Cellular view of type 2 diabetes. (Courtesy of Anatomical Chart Co.)

type 2 diabetes may occur at any age, the disorder occurs most often after age 40 years. The onset of type 2 diabetes is usually insidious. Symptoms are less severe than in type 1 diabetes, and because it tends to be more stable, type 2 diabetes is easier to control than type 1. Risk factors for type 2 diabetes include:

• Obesity
• Older age
• Family history of diabetes
• History of gestational diabetes (diabetes that develops during pregnancy but disappears when pregnancy is over)
• Impaired glucose tolerance
• Minimal or no physical activity
• Race/ethnicity (African Americans, Hispanic/Latino Americans, Native Americans, and some Asian Americans)

In many individuals with type 2 diabetes, the disorder can be controlled with diet, exercise, and oral antidiabetic drugs. However, about 40% of those with type 2 diabetes respond poorly to the oral antidiabetic drugs and require insulin to control the disorder.

INSULIN

Insulin is a hormone manufactured by the β cells of the pancreas. Pharmaceutical human insulin is derived from a biosynthetic process (recombinant DNA or rDNA). Animal-source insulins are used less frequently today than in the past. They have been replaced by synthetic insulins, such as human insulin or insulin analogs. Insulin analogs, insulin lispro, and insulin aspart are newer forms of insulin made using recombinant DNA technology and are structurally similar to human insulin.

Actions

Insulin appears to activate a process that helps glucose molecules enter the cells of striated muscle and adipose tissue. Figure 42.2 depicts the difference between normal glucose metabolism and that of the cell affected by diabetes. Insulin also stimulates the synthesis of glycogen by the liver. In addition, insulin promotes protein synthesis and helps the body store fat by preventing its breakdown for energy.

Onset, Peak, and Duration of Action

Onset, peak, and duration are three clinically important properties of insulin:

• Onset—when insulin first begins to act in the body
• Peak—when the insulin is exerting maximum action
• Duration—the length of time the insulin remains in effect

To meet the needs of those with diabetes mellitus, various insulin preparations have been developed to delay the onset and prolong the duration of action of insulin. When insulin is combined with protamine (a protein), its absorption from the injection site is slowed and its duration of action is prolonged. The addition of zinc also modifies the onset and duration of action of insulin. Insulin preparations are classified as rapid acting, intermediate acting, or long acting. See the Summary

Drug Table: Insulin Preparations for information concerning the onset, peak, and duration of various insulins.

Uses

Insulin is used to:

• Control type 1 diabetes
• Control type 2 diabetes when uncontrolled by diet, exercise, or weight reduction
• Treat severe **diabetic ketoacidosis** (DKA) or diabetic coma
• Treat hypokalemia in combination with glucose

Adverse Reactions

The two major adverse reactions seen with insulin administration are hypoglycemia (low blood glucose, or sugar level) and hyperglycemia (elevated blood glucose, or sugar level). The symptoms of hypoglycemia and hyperglycemia are listed in Table 42.1.

Hypoglycemia may occur when there is too much insulin in the bloodstream in relation to the available glucose (hyperinsulinism). Hypoglycemia may occur when:

• The patient eats too little food.
• The insulin dose is incorrectly measured and is greater than that prescribed.
• The patient has drastically increased demands (activity or illness).

Table 42.1 Hypoglycemia Versus Hyperglycemia

Symptoms	Hypoglycemia (Insulin Reaction)	Hyperglycemia (Diabetic Coma, Ketoacidosis)
Onset	Sudden	Gradual (hours or days)
Blood glucose level	Less than 60 mg/dL	More than 200 mg/dL
Central nervous system	Fatigue, weakness, nervousness, agitation, confusion, headache, diplopia, convulsions, dizziness, unconsciousness	Drowsiness, dim vision
Respirations	Normal to rapid, shallow	Deep, rapid (air hunger)
Gastrointestinal	Hunger, nausea	Thirst, nausea, vomiting, abdominal pain, loss of appetite
Skin	Pale, moist, cool, diaphoretic	Dry, flushed, warm
Pulse	Normal or uncharacteristic	Rapid, weak
Miscellaneous	Numbness, tingling of the lips or tongue	Acetone breath, excessive urination

Display 42.1 Drugs That Alter Insulin Effectiveness

Selected Drugs That Decrease the Effect (More Insulin May Be Required)

acetazolamide
albuterol
antipsychotics (atypical or second generation)
asparaginase
calcitonin
contraceptives, oral
corticosteroids
cyclophosphamide
danazol
diltiazem
diuretics
dobutamine
epinephrine
estrogens
glucagon
human immunodeficiency virus (HIV) antivirals
isoniazid
lithium
morphine sulfate
niacin
nicotine
phenothiazines
phenytoin
progestogens
protease inhibitors
somatropin
terbutaline
thiazide diuretics
thyroid hormones

Drugs That Increase the Effect (Less Insulin May Be Required)

angiotensin-converting enzyme (ACE) inhibitors
alcohol
anabolic steroids
antidiabetic drugs, oral
β-blocking drugs
calcium
clonidine
disopyramide
fluoxetine
fibrates
lithium
MAOIs
mebendazole
pentamidine
pentoxifylline
pyridoxine
salicylates
somatostatin analog
sulfonamides
tetracycline

Hyperglycemia may occur if there is too little insulin in the bloodstream in relation to the available glucose (hypoinsulinism). Hyperglycemia may occur when:

- The patient eats too much food.
- Too little or no insulin is given.
- The patient experiences emotional stress, infection, surgery, pregnancy, or an acute illness.

An individual can also become insulin resistant because antibodies develop against insulin. These patients have impaired receptor function and become so unresponsive to insulin that the dose requirement may be in excess of 500 units/day, rather than the usual 40 to 60 units/day. High-potency insulin in a concentrated form (U500) is used for patients requiring more than 200 units/day.

Contraindications and Precautions

Specific insulin products are contraindicated when the patient is hypoglycemic. Insulin is used cautiously in patients with renal or hepatic impairment and during pregnancy and lactation. The insulins are grouped in pregnancy category B, except for insulin glargine and insulin aspart, which are in pregnancy category C. Insulin appears to inhibit

milk prowduction in lactating women and could interfere with breastfeeding. Lactating women may require adjustment in insulin dose and diet.

LIFESPAN CONSIDERATIONS
Pregnancy
Pregnancy makes diabetes more difficult to manage. Insulin requirements usually decrease in the first trimester, increase during the second and third trimesters, and decrease rapidly after delivery. The patient with diabetes or a history of gestational diabetes must be encouraged to maintain good metabolic control before conception and throughout pregnancy.

Interactions

When certain drugs are administered with insulin, a resultant decrease or increase in hypoglycemic effect can occur. Display 42.1 identifies selected drugs that decrease and increase the hypoglycemic effect of insulin.

Patients may not volunteer information regarding their use of complementary and alternative remedies. You should always inquire about use of herbal products. Although lab testing is not conclusive, medical reports indicate a possible interaction with eucalyptus products, causing decreased blood sugar.

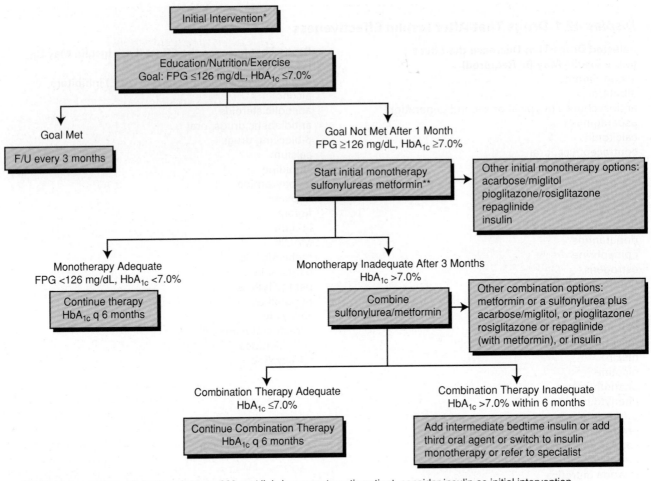

Figure 42.3 Pharmacologic algorithm for treating type 2 diabetes. FPG, fasting plasma glucose; HbA₁c, glycosylated hemoglobin; F/U, follow-up.

ORAL ANTIDIABETIC DRUGS AND OTHER AGENTS

Oral antidiabetic drugs are used to treat patients with type 2 diabetes that is not controlled by diet and exercise alone. These drugs are not effective for treating type 1 diabetes. These drugs may also be called oral hypoglycemics. A number of oral antidiabetic drugs are currently in use and can be categorized into two groups:

- Sulfonylureas
- Nonsulfonylureas

Newer agents include those that interact or mimic the action of incretin hormones. These additional drugs are listed in the Summary Drug Table: Antidiabetic Drugs.

Uses

Oral antidiabetic drugs are used in the treatment of patients with type 2 diabetes mellitus whose condition cannot be controlled by diet alone. These drugs may also be used with insulin in the management of some patients with diabetes. Use of an oral antidiabetic drug with insulin may help to decrease the insulin dosage in some individuals. Two oral antidiabetic drugs (e.g., a sulfonylurea and metformin) may also be used together when one antidiabetic drug and diet do not control blood glucose levels of those with type 2 diabetes. Figure 42.3 illustrates an example of a treatment protocol for type 2 diabetes.

Actions

Sulfonylureas

Sulfonylureas appear to lower blood glucose by stimulating the β cells of the pancreas to release insulin. Sulfonylureas are not effective if the β cells of the pancreas cannot release a sufficient amount of insulin to meet the individual's needs. The most commonly used sulfonylureas are the second- and third-generation drugs, such as glimepiride (Amaryl), glipizide (Glucotrol), and glyburide (DiaBeta). The first-generation sulfonylureas (e.g., chlorpropamide [Diabinese], tolazamide, and tolbutamide) are not commonly used today because they have a long duration of action and a higher incidence of adverse reactions and are more likely to react with other drugs.

Like the sulfonylureas, the meglitinides act to lower blood glucose levels by stimulating the release of insulin from the pancreas. This action depends on the ability of the β cells in the pancreas to produce some insulin. However, the action of the meglitinides is more rapid than that of the sulfonylureas and their duration of action much shorter. Because of this, they must be taken three times a day. Examples of the meglitinides include nateglinide (Starlix) and repaglinide (Prandin).

Nonsulfonylureas

The liver normally releases glucose by detecting the level of circulating insulin. When insulin levels are high, glucose is available in the blood, and the liver produces little or no glucose. When insulin levels are low, there is little circulating glucose, so the liver produces more glucose. In type 2 diabetes, the liver may not detect levels of glucose in the blood and, instead of regulating glucose production, releases glucose despite adequate blood glucose levels.

Metformin sensitizes the liver to circulating insulin levels and reduces hepatic glucose production. The alpha (α)-glucosidase inhibitors acarbose (Precose) and miglitol (Glyset) lower blood glucose levels by delaying the digestion of carbohydrates and absorption of carbohydrates in the intestine. The thiazolidinediones, also called glitazones, decrease insulin resistance and increase insulin sensitivity by modifying several processes, resulting in decreased hepatic glucogenesis (formation of glucose from glycogen) and increased insulin-dependent muscle glucose uptake. Examples of the thiazolidinediones are rosiglitazone (Avandia) and pioglitazone (Actos).

Adverse Reactions

Sulfonylureas

Adverse reactions associated with sulfonylureas include hypoglycemia, anorexia, nausea, vomiting, epigastric discomfort, weight gain, heartburn, and various vague neurologic symptoms, such as weakness and numbness of the extremities. Often, these can be eliminated by reducing the dosage or giving the drug in divided doses. If these reactions become severe, the primary health care provider may try another oral antidiabetic drug or discontinue the use of these drugs. If the drug therapy is discontinued, it may be necessary to control the diabetes with insulin. Adverse reactions associated with the administration of the meglitinides include upper respiratory tract infection, headache, rhinitis, bronchitis, headache, back pain, and hypoglycemia.

Nonsulfonylureas

Adverse reactions associated with nonsulfonylureas include GI upset (e.g., metallic taste, abdominal bloating, nausea, cramping, flatulence, and diarrhea). These adverse reactions are self-limiting and can be reduced if the patients are started on a low dose with dosage increased slowly, and if the drug is taken with meals. Hypoglycemia rarely occurs when a nonsulfonylurea is used alone. However, patients receiving these drugs in combination with insulin or other oral hypoglycemics (e.g., sulfonylureas) are at greater risk for hypoglycemia. A

reduction in the dosage of insulin or the sulfonylurea may be required to prevent episodes of hypoglycemia.

Adverse reactions associated with the administration of thiazolidinediones include upper respiratory infections, sinusitis, headache, pharyngitis, myalgia, diarrhea, and back pain. Lactic acidosis (buildup of lactic acid in the blood) may also occur with the administration of metformin. Although lactic acidosis is a rare adverse reaction, its occurrence is serious and can be fatal. Lactic acidosis occurs mainly in patients with kidney dysfunction. Symptoms of lactic acidosis include malaise (vague feeling of bodily discomfort), abdominal pain, rapid respirations, shortness of breath, and muscular pain. In some patients, vitamin B_{12} levels are decreased. This can be reversed with vitamin B_{12} supplements or with discontinuation of the drug therapy. Because weight loss can occur, metformin is sometimes recommended for obese patients or patients with insulin-resistant diabetes.

Contraindications, Precautions, and Interactions

Sulfonylureas

Oral antidiabetic drugs are contraindicated in patients with known hypersensitivity to the drugs, DKA, severe infection, or severe endocrine disease. The first-generation sulfonylureas (chlorpropamide, tolazamide, and tolbutamide) are contraindicated in patients with coronary artery disease or liver or renal dysfunction. Other sulfonylureas are used cautiously in patients with impaired liver function because liver dysfunction can prolong the drug's effect. In addition, sulfonylureas are used cautiously in patients with renal impairment and severe cardiovascular disease. There is a risk for cross-sensitivity with sulfonylureas and sulfonamides (sulfa anti-infectives).

Many drugs may affect the action of sulfonylureas; monitor blood glucose carefully when beginning therapy, when discontinuing therapy, and any time any change is made in the drug regimen with these drugs. Sulfonylureas may have an increased hypoglycemic effect when administered with anticoagulants, chloramphenicol, clofibrate, fluconazole, histamine H_2 antagonists, methyldopa, monoamine oxidase inhibitors (MAOIs), nonsteroidal anti-inflammatory drugs (NSAIDs), salicylates, sulfonamides, and tricyclic antidepressants. The hypoglycemic effect of sulfonylureas may be decreased when the agents are administered with β blockers, calcium channel blockers, cholestyramine, corticosteroids, estrogens, hydantoins, isoniazid, oral contraceptives, phenothiazines, rifampin, thiazide diuretics, and thyroid agents.

Nonsulfonylureas

Nonsulfonylureas are contraindicated in patients with heart failure (HF), renal disease, hypersensitivity to the individual drug, and acute or chronic metabolic acidosis, including ketoacidosis. The drug is also contraindicated in patients older than 80 years and during pregnancy (pregnancy category B, the thiazolidinediones are pregnancy category C) and lactation.

Metformin use is temporarily discontinued for surgical procedures. The drug therapy is restarted when the patient's oral intake has been resumed and renal function is normal. There is a risk of acute renal failure when iodinated contrast material used for radiologic studies is administered with metformin. Metformin therapy is stopped for 48 hours before and after radiologic studies using iodinated material. There is an increased risk of lactic acidosis when metformin is administered with the glucocorticoids.

Digestive enzymes may reduce the effect of miglitol. Acarbose and miglitol are used cautiously in patients with renal impairment or pre-existing GI problems, such as irritable bowel syndrome or Crohn's disease. Thiazolidinediones are used cautiously in patients with edema, cardiovascular disease, and liver or kidney disease. These drugs may alter the effects of oral contraceptives.

HORMONE MIMETIC AGENTS

These hormones are released in response to increases in glucose that occur after eating. Incretin hormones cause insulin to be made and reduce the amount of glucagon made by the pancreas. Hormone mimetic agents help control blood glucose levels by maintaining β cell function of the pancreas, enhancing insulin secretion, and suppressing glucagon, which signals the liver to decrease release of glucose. Gastric emptying is also delayed, which slows carbohydrate absorption.

Sitagliptin (Januvia) lowers the blood glucose level of those with type 2 diabetes by enhancing the secretion of the endogenous incretin hormone. Exenatide (Byetta) mimics the action of the incretin hormone. Pramlintide (Symlin) mimics the action of another secretion, amylin.

An incretin mimetic should be used cautiously in patients with chronic kidney disease or in older adults. This drug has not been studied in pregnant women but is believed to be a category B drug from animal studies, and it should be used cautiously in lactating women.

NURSING PROCESS

PATIENT RECEIVING INSULIN AND/OR AN ORAL ANTIDIABETIC DRUG

ASSESSMENT

Preadministration Assessment
When conducting a physical assessment, note that a general inspection of the skin is important for the patient with diabetes. Visualize the mucous membranes and extremities, with special attention given to any sores or cuts that appear to be infected or healing poorly, as well as any ulcerations or other skin or mucous membrane changes. Obtain the following information and include it in the patient's record:

- Dietary habits
- Family history of diabetes (if any)
- Type and duration of symptoms experienced

Scan the patient's record for recent laboratory and diagnostic tests. If the patient has diabetes and has been receiving insulin or an oral antidiabetic drug, include the type and dosage of drug used, dietary habits, and the frequency and methods used for glucose testing in the patient's record.

Ongoing Assessment
The most important aspect of the ongoing assessment is tracking and treatment of high or low blood sugars (see Table 42.1). Frequent observation of the patient for symptoms of hypoglycemia, particularly during initial therapy or after a change in dosage, is an important ongoing assessment. The patient is particularly prone to hypoglycemic reactions at the time of peak insulin action (see the Summary Drug Table: Insulin Preparations) or when he or she has not eaten for some time or has skipped a meal. In acute care settings, frequent blood glucose monitoring is routinely done to help detect abnormalities of blood glucose.

Patients in the acute care setting are also monitored closely for hyperglycemia. Insulin needs increase in times of stress or illness. For a person without diabetes, blood glucose levels are considered within normal limits when the measure is 60 to 100 mg/dL. For a person with diabetes, the health care provider may have higher levels as the parameters for the patient. When products such as insulin glargine (Lantus) are used, the insulin levels do not fluctuate as often.

When ready for discharge, patients will need to be taught to use a glucometer for self-monitoring of blood glucose levels (see Patient Teaching for Improved Patient Outcomes: Obtaining a Blood Glucose Reading Using a Glucometer). The best way to monitor long-term glycemic control and response to treatment is with HbA$_{1c}$ levels measured at 3-month intervals. If the first HbA$_{1c}$ indicates that glycemic control during the last 3 months was inadequate, the dosages may be increased for better control.

NURSING DIAGNOSES
Drug-specific nursing diagnoses include the following:

- **Acute Confusion** related to hypoglycemia effects on mentation
- **Deficient Fluid Volume** related to fluid loss during DKA
- **Anxiety** related to uncertainty of diagnosis, testing own glucose levels, self-injection, dietary restrictions, other factors (specify)
- **Ineffective Breathing Pattern** related to hyperventilation in lactic acidosis with metformin use

Nursing diagnoses related to drug administration are discussed in Chapter 4.

PLANNING
The expected outcomes of the patient may include an optimal response to therapy, support of patient needs related to the management of adverse reactions, a reduction in anxiety, improved ability to cope with the diagnosis, and confidence in an understanding of the medication regimen.

IMPLEMENTATION
Nursing management of a patient with diabetes requires diligent, skillful, and comprehensive nursing care.

Patient Teaching for Improved Patient Outcomes

Obtaining a Blood Glucose Reading Using a Glucometer

When you teach, make sure your patient understands the following:

✔ Before initial use, carefully read the manufacturer's instructions, because blood glucose monitoring devices vary greatly.
✔ Prepare the finger by cleansing the area with warm, soapy water. Rinse with warm water and dry well. (If the patient cannot prepare the area, the caregiver should wear gloves to comply with Standard Precautions, the guidelines of the Centers for Disease Control and Prevention.)
✔ Remove a test strip and close the container to prevent damage to the remaining strips. Insert the strip into the meter if the instructions call for this before obtaining the blood sample.
✔ Using the lancet (needle) device, perform a finger stick *on the side* of a finger (not the tip), where there are fewer nerve endings and more capillaries.
✔ Gently massage the finger to produce a large, hanging drop of blood. Using this technique to obtain a blood sample will help prevent inaccurate readings. *Note:* Do not smear the blood or try to obtain an extra drop.
✔ Drop the blood sample on the test strip and read the number on the meter. *Note:* Some glucometers, especially institutional devices, may have slightly different procedures.
✔ Record the time and test results in the record-keeping book recommended by your primary health care provider.
✔ Clean and calibrate the device according to the manufacturer's recommendations to maintain accurate readings.

Promoting an Optimal Response to Therapy

There are no fixed drug dosages in antidiabetic therapy. The drug regimen is individualized on the basis of the effectiveness and tolerance of the drug(s) used and the maximum recommended dose of the drug(s).

BLOOD GLUCOSE MONITORING. Blood glucose levels are monitored often in the patient with diabetes. The primary health care provider may order blood glucose levels to be tested before meals, after meals, and at bedtime. Less frequent monitoring may be performed if the patient's glucose levels are well controlled. The glucometer is a device used by the patient with diabetes or the nursing personnel to monitor blood glucose levels. Nursing or laboratory personnel are responsible for obtaining blood glucose levels during hospitalization, but the patient must be taught to monitor blood glucose levels after discharge from the acute care setting (see Patient Teaching for Improved Patient Outcomes: Obtaining a Blood Glucose Reading Using a Glucometer).

Urine testing was widely used to monitor glucose levels in the past, but this method has largely been replaced with blood glucose monitoring. Urine testing can play a role in identifying kidney involvement or ketone excretion in patients prone to ketoacidosis. If urine testing is done, it is usually recommended to use the second voided specimen (i.e., fresh urine collected 30 minutes after the initial voiding) to check glucose or acetone levels, rather than the first specimen obtained.

The glycosylated hemoglobin (HbA$_{1c}$) test is a blood test used to monitor the patient's average blood glucose level throughout a 3- to 4-month period. When blood glucose levels are high, glucose molecules attach to hemoglobin in the red blood cell. The longer the hyperglycemia lasts, the more glucose binds to the red blood cell and the higher the glycosylated hemoglobin. This binding lasts for the life of the red blood cell (about 4 months). When the patient's diabetes is well controlled with normal or near-normal blood glucose levels, the overall HbA$_{1c}$ level will not be greatly elevated. However, if blood glucose levels are consistently high, the HbA$_{1c}$ level will be elevated. The test result (expressed as a percentage) refers to the average amount of glucose that has been in the blood throughout the last 4 months. Results vary with the laboratory method used for analysis, but, in general, levels between 6.5% and 7% indicate good control of diabetes. Results of 10% or greater indicate poor blood glucose control for the last several months. The HbA$_{1c}$ is useful in evaluating the success of diabetes treatment, comparing new treatment regimens with past regimens, and individualizing treatment.

INSULIN ADMINISTRATION. Sometimes the health care provider finds that the patient achieves best control with one injection of insulin per day; sometimes the patient requires two or more injections per day. In addition, two different types of insulin may be combined, such as a rapid-acting and a long-acting preparation. The number of insulin injections, dosage, times of administration, and type of insulin are determined by the health care provider after careful evaluation of the patient's metabolic needs and response to therapy. The dosage prescribed for the patient may require changes until the dosage is found that best meets the patient's needs.

❗ NURSING ALERT

Insulin requirements may change when the patient experiences any form of stress and with any illness, particularly illnesses resulting in nausea and vomiting.

Insulin is ordered by the generic name (e.g., insulin zinc suspension, extended) or the trade (brand) name (e.g., Lantus; see the Summary Drug Table: Insulin Preparations). One brand of insulin must never be substituted for another unless the substitution is approved by the primary health care provider, because some patients may be sensitive to changes in brands of insulin. In addition, it is important never to substitute one type of insulin for another. For example, do not use insulin zinc suspension instead of the prescribed protamine zinc insulin.

When administering insulin, care must be taken to use the correct insulin. Names and packaging are similar and can easily be confused. Carefully read all drug labels before preparing any insulin preparation. For example, Humalog (insulin lispro) and Humulin R (regular human insulin) are easily confused because of the similar names.

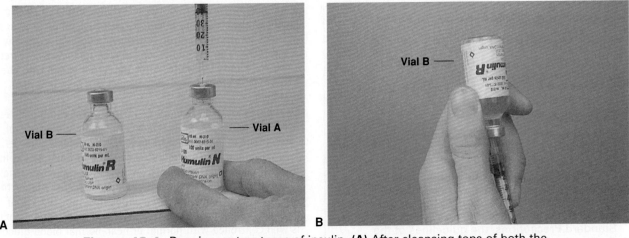

A   **B**

Figure 42.4 Drawing up two types of insulin. **(A)** After cleansing tops of both the Humulin R (regular) insulin and Humulin N (intermediate-acting) insulin, with the container upright, the nurse injects air into the Humulin N insulin equal to the pre-scribed dosage of Humulin N. The nurse removes the needle without touching any fluid, then injects the amount of air equal to the prescribed dosage of the regular insulin and withdraws the prescribed dosage of regular insulin into the syringe. **(B)** After removing any air bubbles and determining what the total combined volume of the two insulins would measure, the nurse inverts the vial with the NPH insulin and carefully withdraws the correct volume of medication. *Note:* The nurse should have a second nurse independently check medication and dosage again before adminis-tering the insulin.

Insulin cannot be administered orally, because it is a protein and readily destroyed in the GI tract. Insulin must be administered by the parenteral route, usually the subcu-taneous (subcut) route. Aspiration for blood return does not need to be done when given subcutaneously. Regular insulin is the only insulin preparation given intravenously (IV). Regular insulin is given 30 to 60 minutes before a meal to achieve optimal results.

Insulin aspart is given immediately before a meal (within 5 to 10 minutes of beginning a meal). Insulin lispro is given 15 minutes before a meal or immediately after a meal. Insulin aspart and lispro make insulin administration more convenient for many patients who find taking a drug 30 to 60 minutes before meals bothersome. In addition, insulin lispro (Humalog) appears to lower the blood glucose level 1 to 2 hours after meals better than does regular human insulin, because it more closely mimics the body's natural insulin. It also lowers the risk of low blood glucose reactions from midnight to 6 a.m. in patients with type I diabetes. The longer-acting insulins are given before breakfast or at bedtime (depending on the primary health care provider's instructions). Many patients are maintained on a single dose of intermediate-acting insulin administered subcutaneously in the morning.

Insulin glargine is given subcutaneously once daily at bedtime. This type of insulin maintains a steady blood level and is used in treating adults and children with type 1 diabetes and in adults with type 2 diabetes who need long-acting insulin for the control of hyperglycemia.

Insulin is available in concentrations of U100 and U500. You must read the label of the insulin bottle carefully for the name and the number of units per milliliter. The dose of insulin is measured in units. U100 insulin has 100 units in each mil-liliter; U500 has 500 units in each milliliter. Most people with diabetes use the U100 concentration. Patients who are resis-tant to insulin and require large insulin doses use the U500 concentration.

Mixing Insulins. If the patient is to receive regular insulin and NPH (isophane insulin suspension) insulin, or regular and Lente (insulin zinc suspension) insulin, clarify with the primary health care provider whether two separate injections are to be given or if the insulins may be mixed in the same syringe. If the two insulins are to be given in the same syringe, the short-acting insulin (regular or lispro) is drawn into the syringe first (Fig. 42.4). Even small amounts of intermediate- or long-acting insulin, if mixed with the short-acting insulin, can bind with the short-acting insulin and delay its onset.

! NURSING ALERT

Regular insulin is clear, whereas intermediate- and long-acting insulins are cloudy. The clear insulin should be drawn up first. When insulin lispro is mixed with a longer-acting insulin, the insulin lispro is drawn up first.

An unexpected response may be obtained when changing from mixed injections to separate injections or vice versa. If the patient had been using insulin mixtures before admission, ask whether the insulins were given separately or together.

Several types of premixed insulins are available. These insulins combine regular insulin with the longer-acting NPH insulin. The mixtures are available in ratios of 70/30 and 50/50 of NPH to regular. Although these premixed insulins are helpful for patients who have difficulty drawing up their insulin or seeing the markings on the syringe, they prohibit individualizing the dosage. For patients who have difficulty controlling their diabetes, these premixed insulins may not be effective.

> **! NURSING ALERT**
>
> Do not mix or dilute insulin glargine with any other insulin or solution, because glucose control will be lost and the insulin will not be effective.

Preparing Insulin for Administration. Always check the expiration date printed on the label of the insulin bottle before withdrawing the insulin. An insulin syringe that matches the concentration of insulin to be given is always used. For example, a syringe labeled as U100 is used only with insulin labeled U100. U500 insulin is given only by the subcut or intramuscular (IM) route. Never substitute a tuberculin syringe for an insulin syringe.

When insulin is in a suspension (this can be seen when looking at a vial that has been untouched for about 1 hour), gently rotate the vial between the palms of the hands and tilt it gently end to end immediately before withdrawing the insulin. This ensures even distribution of the suspended particles. Care is taken not to shake the insulin vigorously.

Carefully check the primary health care provider's order for the type and dosage of insulin immediately before withdrawing the insulin from the vial. All air bubbles must be eliminated from the syringe barrel and hub of the needle before withdrawing the syringe from the insulin vial.

> **! NURSING ALERT**
>
> Accuracy is of the utmost importance when measuring any insulin preparation because of the potential danger of administering an incorrect dosage. If possible, check and consult with another nurse for accuracy of the insulin dosage by comparing the insulin container, the syringe, and the primary health care provider's order before administration.

Rotating Injection Sites. Insulin may be injected into the arms, thighs, abdomen, or buttocks. Because absorption rates vary at the different sites, with the abdomen having the most rapid rate of absorption, followed by the upper arm, thigh, and buttocks, some health care providers recommend rotating the injection sites within one specific area, rather than rotating areas. For example, all available sites within the abdomen would be used before moving to the thigh.

Sites of insulin injection are rotated to prevent lipodystrophy (atrophy of subcutaneous fat), a problem that can interfere with the absorption of insulin from the injection site. Lipodystrophy appears as a slight dimpling or pitting of the subcutaneous fat.

With many tasks to learn in caring for diabetes, some manufactures provide numbered charts or templates to guide site rotation. Use these teaching tools as a method to instruct patients in self-management as well as providing care. Before each dose of insulin is given, check the patient's record for the site of the previous injection and use the next site (according to the rotation plan) for injection. Ask the patient to validate the site last used, too. If able, always ask the patient if he or she prefers to self-inject, rather than assuming the person is too sick to do the task. After giving the injection, document the site used. Every time insulin is given, previous injection sites are inspected for inflammation, which may indicate a localized allergic reaction.

Methods of Administering Insulin. Several methods can be used to administer insulin. The most common method is the use of a needle and syringe. Use of microfine needles has reduced the discomfort associated with an injection. Another method is the pen injection system, which uses a cartridge that is prefilled with a specific type of insulin (e.g., NPH insulin). The desired units are selected by turning a dial and the locking ring. The insulin dose is determined by the number of clicks heard. Although expensive, these are helpful for patients with trouble holding or seeing the syringe. The pens are meant for single patient use and should never be used with more than one patient.

> **! NURSING ALERT**
>
> Insulin pens are patient specific. They are designed for one patient to use multiple times. A needle is used in these devices, which will be contaminated by the patient's blood and should never be shared by more than one patient.

Another method of insulin delivery is the insulin pump. This system attempts to mimic the body's normal pancreatic function, uses only regular insulin, is battery powered, and requires insertion of a needle into subcutaneous tissue. The needle is changed every 1 to 3 days. The amount of insulin injected can be adjusted according to blood glucose levels, which are monitored four to eight times per day.

Depending on the patient's condition, an order for regular insulin as a supplement to the drug regimen to "cover" any episodes of hyperglycemia may be used. For example, blood glucose levels are monitored every 6 hours or before meals and at bedtime, with regular (short-acting) insulin prescribed to cover any hyperglycemia detected. This coverage is sometimes referred to by the health care providers as a sliding scale, or insulin coverage. The supplemental insulin is administered based on blood glucose readings and the amount of insulin prescribed by the primary health care provider in the regular insulin coverage protocol. Even when a protocol is in use, you should immediately notify the primary health care provider if the blood glucose level is greater than 400 mg/dL.

The insulin dosage pattern that most closely follows normal insulin production is a multiple-dose plan sometimes called *intensive insulin therapy*. Used for type 1 diabetes mainly, in this regimen, a single dose of intermediate- or long-acting insulin is taken in the morning or at bedtime. Small doses of regular insulin are taken before meals based on the patient's blood glucose levels and HbA$_{1c}$. This allows for greater flexibility in the patient's lifestyle, but can also be an inconvenience to the patient (e.g., the need always to carry supplies, the lack of privacy, inconvenient schedules).

Inhaled insulin delivery was considered at one time but was pulled from the market due to expense. It is now in the research process for use in patients with mild cognitive impairment and Alzheimer's disease (Craft, 2012).

ORAL HYPOGLYCEMICS. Glycemic control can often be improved when a second oral medication is added to the drug regimen. The choice of a second medication varies from patient to patient and is prescribed by the primary health care provider. Glucovance, which includes both glyburide and metformin, is one example of the use of combination drugs for glycemic control. The combination drugs are useful for individuals needing dual therapy and those who are forgetful (only once-daily dosing is required) or mildly confused.

CHRONIC CARE CONSIDERATIONS

Exposure to stress, such as infection, fever, surgery, or trauma, may cause a loss of control of blood glucose levels in patients who have been stabilized with oral antidiabetic drugs. Should this occur, the primary health care provider may discontinue use of the oral drug and administer insulin.

Oral antidiabetic drugs are given as a single daily dose or in divided doses. The following sections provide specific information for each group of oral antidiabetic drugs.

Sulfonylureas. Chlorpropamide, tolazamide, and tolbutamide are given with food to prevent GI upset. However, because food delays absorption, glipizide should be given 30 minutes before a meal. Glyburide and glimepiride are administered with breakfast or with the first main meal of the day. Repaglinide can be taken immediately or up to 30 minutes before meals. Nateglinide is taken up to 30 minutes before meals.

After the patient has been taking sulfonylureas for a period of time, a condition called secondary failure may occur, in which the sulfonylurea loses its effectiveness. When a normally adherent patient has a gradual increase in blood glucose levels, secondary failure may be the cause. This increase in blood glucose levels can be caused by an increase in the severity of the diabetes or a decreased response to the drug. When secondary failure occurs, the primary health care provider may prescribe another sulfonylurea or add an oral antidiabetic drug such as metformin to the drug regimen. See the Summary Drug Table: Antidiabetic Drugs for additional drugs that can be used in combination with sulfonylureas.

Nonsulfonylureas. Acarbose and miglitol are given three times a day with the first bite of the meal, because food increases absorption. Some patients begin therapy with a lower dose once daily to minimize GI effects such as abdominal discomfort, flatulence, and diarrhea. The dose is then gradually increased to three times daily. Response to these drugs is monitored by periodic testing. Dosage adjustments are made at 4- to 16-week intervals based on blood glucose levels.

The patient is instructed to take metformin two or three times a day with meals. If the patient has not experienced a response in 4 weeks using the maximum dose of metformin, the primary health care provider may add an oral sulfonylurea while continuing metformin at the maximum dose. Glucophage XR (metformin, extended release) is administered once daily with the evening meal.

The thiazolidinediones, pioglitazone and rosiglitazone, are given with or without meals. If the dose is missed at the usual meal, the drug is taken at the next meal. If the dose is missed on one day, it is not doubled the following day. If the drug is taken, the meal must not be delayed. Delay of a meal for as little as 30 minutes can cause hypoglycemia.

Monitoring and Managing Patient Needs

Acute Confusion. Mental confusion may be a sign that a patient has low blood sugar. Close observation of the patient with diabetes is important, especially when diabetes is newly diagnosed, the medication dosage changes, the patient is pregnant, the patient has a medical illness or surgery, or the patient fails to adhere to the prescribed diet. Older, debilitated, or malnourished patients are also more likely to experience hypoglycemia. Episodes of hypoglycemia are corrected as soon as the symptoms are recognized. A patient who has had this reaction before may be able to tell you that his or her blood sugar is low; check his or her blood sugar.

Methods of terminating a hypoglycemic reaction include the administration of one or more of the following:

- 4 ounces of orange juice or other fruit juice
- Hard candy or 1 tablespoon of honey
- Commercial glucose products such as glucose gel or glucose tablets
- Glucagon by the subcut, IM, or IV routes
- Glucose 10% or 50% IV

Selection of any one or more of these methods for terminating a hypoglycemic reaction, as well as other procedures to be followed, such as drawing blood for glucose levels, depends on the written order of the primary health care provider or hospital policy. Never give oral fluids or substances (such as candy) to a patient when the swallowing and gag reflexes are absent. Absence of these reflexes may result in aspiration of the oral fluid or substance into the lungs, which can result in extremely serious consequences and even death. If swallowing and gag reflexes are absent, or if the patient is unconscious, glucose or glucagon is given by the parenteral route.

NURSING ALERT

When a hypoglycemic patient is taking an α-glucosidase inhibitor (e.g., acarbose or miglitol), give the patient an oral form of glucose, such as glucose tablets or dextrose, rather than juice, honey, or candy (sucrose). Absorption of sugar is blocked by acarbose or miglitol.

Glucagon is a hormone produced by the α cells of the pancreas; it acts to increase blood glucose by stimulating the conversion of glycogen to glucose in the liver. A return of consciousness is observed within 5 to 20 minutes after parenteral administration of glucagon. Glucagon is effective in treating hypoglycemia only if glycogen is available from the liver.

Contact the primary health care provider when a hypoglycemic reaction occurs; note the substance and amount used to terminate the reaction, blood samples drawn (if any), the length of time required for the symptoms of hypoglycemia to disappear, and the current status of the patient. After termination of a hypoglycemic reaction, closely observe the patient for additional hypoglycemic reactions. The length of time that close observation is required depends on the peak and duration of the insulin administered.

Deficient Fluid Volume. Dehydration occurs with DKA. DKA is a potentially life-threatening deficiency of insulin (hypoinsulinism), resulting in severe hyperglycemia and requiring prompt diagnosis and treatment. Because insulin is unavailable to allow glucose to enter the cell, dangerously high levels of glucose build up in the blood (hyperglycemia). The body, needing energy, begins to break down fat for energy.

Summary Drug Table ANTIDIABETIC DRUGS (continued)

Generic Name	Trade Name	Uses	Adverse Reactions	Dosage Ranges
pioglitazone/ glimepiride	Duetact	Type 2 diabetes	See individual drugs	Individualized; maximum daily dose, 45 mg/8 mg
rosiglitazone/ glimepiride	Avandaryl	Type 2 diabetes	See individual drugs	Individualized; maximum daily dose, 8 mg/4 mg
sitagliptin/metformin	Janumet	Type 2 diabetes	See individual drugs	Individualized; maximum daily dose, 100 mg/2000 mg
Glucose-Elevating Agents				
diazoxide *dye-az-ok'-syde*	Proglycem	Hypoglycemia due to hyperinsulinism	Sodium and fluid retention, hyperglycemia, glycosuria, tachycardia, congestive heart failure	3–8 mg/kg/day orally in two or three equal doses q 8–12 hr
glucagon *gloo-kah'-gahn*	Glucagon Emergency Kit	Hypoglycemia	Nausea, vomiting, generalized allergic reactions	See instructions on the product

Antidiabetic Drugs

● Chapter Review

Know Your Drugs

Clients sometimes know a medication by the brand (or trade) name and not the generic name. To help you recognize both names, match the brand name with the generic name of the same medication.

Generic Name	Brand Name
1. glyburide	A. DiaBeta
2. metformin	B. Fortamet
3. nateglinide	C. Januvia
4. sitagliptin	D. Starlix

Calculate Medication Dosages

1. A client is prescribed rosiglitazone (Avandia) 8 mg orally daily. Available are 2-mg tablets. The nurse would administer _____.

2. A client is prescribed 40 units NPH insulin mixed with 5 units of regular insulin. What is the total insulin dosage?

● Prepare for the NCLEX®

Build Your Knowledge

1. Where is insulin produced in the body?

   1. Lining of the gut
   2. Pancreas
   3. Gallbladder
   4. Thyroid

2. Which of the following medications may be used for both type 1 and 2 diabetes?

   1. regular insulin
   2. Januvia injection
   3. metformin
   4. chlorpropamide

3. Which of the following would the nurse mostly likely choose to treat a hypoglycemic reaction?

   1. regular insulin
   2. NPH insulin
   3. orange juice
   4. crackers and soda

4. Which of the following would be the correct method of administering insulin glargine?

   1. within 10 minutes of meals
   2. immediately before meals
   3. any time within 30 minutes before or 30 minutes after a meal
   4. at bedtime

5. Which of the following symptoms would alert the nurse to a possible hyperglycemic reaction?

   1. fatigue, weakness, confusion
   2. pale skin, elevated temperature
   3. thirst, abdominal pain, nausea
   4. rapid, shallow respirations, headache, nervousness

Apply Your Knowledge

6. A client with diabetes received a glycosylated hemoglobin test result of 10%. This indicates _____.

   1. the diabetes is well controlled
   2. poor blood glucose control
   3. the need for an increase in the insulin dosage
   4. the client is at increased risk for hypoglycemia

7. The mental health center is writing new admission protocols. Which client population should be routinely tested for elevated blood sugars?

   1. obsessive-compulsive clients on antianxiety drugs
   2. clinically depressed patients
   3. schizophrenic clients on second-generation antipsychotics
   4. older clients on haloperidol

Alternate-Format Questions

8. List in order the following steps in drawing up two types of insulin.

   1. Remove air bubbles from syringe, and withdraw the Humulin N insulin prescribed.
   2. Remove the needle from the vial without getting fluid (insulin) on the needle.
   3. After cleansing both vials, inject air into the Humulin N insulin vial.
   4. Inject air into the regular insulin vial, and invert and withdraw the prescribed amount.

9. A client is prescribed 40 units NPH insulin mixed with 5 units of regular insulin. What is the total insulin dosage? Describe how you would prepare the insulins.

10. A client is prescribed metformin (Glucophage) 1000 mg orally BID. The drug is available in 500-mg tablets. The nurse administers _____. What is the total daily dosage of metformin? _____

To check your answers, see Appendix G.

the**Point** *For more NCLEX-style questions, log on to http://thepoint.lww.com to access more than 1000 questions.*

Pituitary and Adrenocortical Hormones

On completion of this chapter, the student will:

1. List the hormones produced by the pituitary gland and the adrenal cortex.
2. Discuss general actions, uses, adverse reactions, contraindications, precautions, and interactions of the pituitary and adrenocortical hormones.
3. Discuss important preadministration and ongoing assessment activities the nurse should perform with the patient taking a pituitary or adrenocortical hormone.
4. List nursing diagnoses particular to a patient taking a pituitary or adrenocortical hormone.
5. Discuss ways to promote an optimal response to therapy, how to manage common adverse reactions, and important points to keep in mind when educating patients about the use of pituitary and adrenocortical hormones.

KEY TERMS

adrenal insufficiency • diminished adrenal gland production resulting in a deficiency in corticosteroids

anovulatory • a menstrual cycle in which ovulation (release of egg) does not occur

cryptorchism • failure of the testes to descend into the scrotum

cushingoid • group of symptoms (including moon face, buffalo hump) due to the disease caused by the overproduction of endogenous glucocorticoids

diabetes insipidus • disease caused by failure of the pituitary gland to secrete vasopressin or by surgical removal of the pituitary

feedback mechanism • method used by glands to signal need for or cessation of hormonal production

gonads • glands responsible for sexual activity and characteristics

hirsutism • excess growth of facial and body hair in women

hyperstimulation syndrome • sudden ovarian enlargement caused by overstimulation

DRUG CLASSES

Posterior pituitary hormones
 • Vasopressin
Anterior pituitary hormones
 • Gonadotropins
• Somatropin
• Adrenocorticotropic hormone (ACTH)
Glucocorticoids
Mineralocorticoids

The pituitary gland is about the size of a green pea and lies deep within the cranial vault. The gland is not part of the brain; rather, it is suspended from the hypothalamus by the pituitary stalk and is protected by an indentation of the sphenoid bone called the *sella turcica*. The pituitary gland has two lobes:

• Anterior pituitary (adenohypophysis)
• Posterior pituitary (neurohypophysis)

The pituitary gland is often referred to as the "master gland" because it secretes many hormones that regulate numerous

PHARMACOLOGY IN PRACTICE

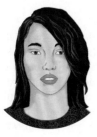

Janna Wong is at the clinic for a sports physical. As you measure her height and weight she tells you about a girl on the team who was sick and is now taking hormones and has grown 4 inches over the summer. Janna says that the coach favored this girl and let her use the bathroom whenever she felt like it. The classmate that Janna is describing had a pituitary tumor and needs to receive hormonal replacement for the rest of her life. Think about this situation as you read this chapter.

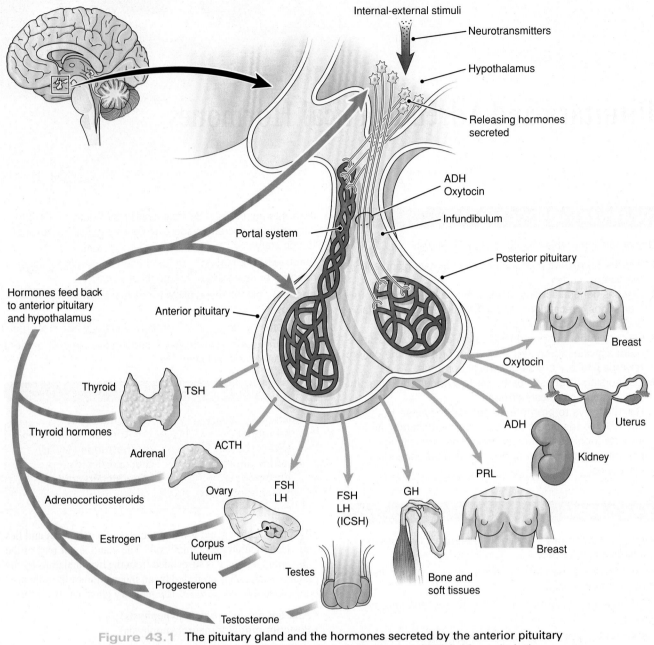

Figure 43.1   The pituitary gland and the hormones secreted by the anterior pituitary and the posterior pituitary. (From Cohen, B. J., & Taylor, J. J. [2005]. *Memmler's the human body in health and disease* [10th ed.]. Baltimore: Lippincott Williams & Wilkins.)

vital processes. The pituitary regulates growth, metabolism, the reproductive cycle, electrolyte balance, and water retention or loss. The hormones secreted by the anterior and posterior pituitary and the organs influenced by these hormones are shown in Figure 43.1.

POSTERIOR PITUITARY HORMONES

The posterior pituitary gland produces two hormones: vasopressin (antidiuretic hormone) and oxytocin (uterine stimulant). Vasopressin is discussed in this chapter and oxytocin is presented in Chapter 46.

VASOPRESSIN

Actions and Uses

Vasopressin and its derivative, desmopressin (DDAVP), regulate the reabsorption of water by the kidneys. Vasopressin is secreted by the pituitary when body fluids must be conserved. This mechanism may be activated when, for example, an individual has severe vomiting and diarrhea with little or no fluid intake. When this and similar conditions are present, the posterior pituitary releases the hormone vasopressin, water in the kidneys is reabsorbed into the blood (i.e., conserved), and the urine becomes concentrated. Vasopressin exhibits its greatest activity on the renal tubular epithelium, where it promotes water resorption and smooth muscle contraction throughout the vascular bed. Vasopressin also has some vasopressor activity.

Vasopressin and its derivative are used in treating **diabetes insipidus**, a disease resulting from the failure of the pituitary to secrete vasopressin or from surgical removal of the pituitary. Diabetes insipidus is characterized by a marked increase in urination (as much as 10 L in 24 hours) and excessive thirst by inadequate secretion of vasopressin (antidiuretic hormone). Treatment with vasopressin therapy replaces the hormone in the body and restores normal urination and thirst. Vasopressin may also be used for preventing and treating postoperative abdominal distention and for dispelling gas interfering with abdominal roentgenography (x-ray studies).

Adverse Reactions

Local or systemic hypersensitivity reactions may occur in some patients receiving vasopressin, and the following may also be seen:

- Tremor, sweating, vertigo
- Nasal congestion
- Nausea, vomiting, abdominal cramps
- Water intoxication (overdosage, toxicity)

Contraindications and Precautions

Vasopressin is contraindicated in patients hypersensitive to the drug or its components. Vasopressin is used cautiously in patients with a history of seizures, migraine headaches, asthma, congestive heart failure (HF), or vascular disease (because the substance may precipitate angina or myocardial infarction) and in those with perioperative polyuria. Vasopressin is classified as a pregnancy category C drug. Desmopressin acetate (a pregnancy category B drug) is typically used when diabetes insipidus occurs during pregnancy; however, it still must be used cautiously then and during lactation.

Interactions

The following interactions may occur when vasopressin is administered with another agent:

Interacting Drug	Common Use	Effect of Interaction
norepinephrine	Neurostimulant	Decreased antidiuretic effect
lithium	Management of psychological problems	Decreased antidiuretic effect
oral anticoagulants	Blood thinners	Decreased antidiuretic effect
carbamazepine	Anticonvulsant	Increased antidiuretic effect
chlorpropamide	Antidiabetic (diabetes mellitus) agent	Increased antidiuretic effect

NURSING PROCESS
PATIENT RECEIVING VASOPRESSIN

ASSESSMENT

Preadministration Assessment
Patients experiencing diabetes insipidus process large amounts of fluid in their bodies. To assess drug response the weight, vital signs, and a patient history of fluid intake and output are taken. Serum electrolyte levels and other laboratory tests may be ordered by the primary health care provider.

Before administering vasopressin to relieve abdominal distention, document the patient's blood pressure, pulse, and respiratory rate. Auscultate the abdomen and record the findings. Additionally, measure and document the patient's abdominal girth.

Ongoing Assessment
During the ongoing assessment of a hospitalized patient, monitor the blood pressure, pulse, and respiratory rate every 4 hours or as ordered by the primary health care provider. The patient's fluid intake and output are strictly measured. The primary health care provider is notified if there are any significant changes in these vital signs, because a dosage adjustment may be necessary.

The dosage of vasopressin or its derivatives may require periodic adjustments. After administration of the drug, observe the patient every 10 to 15 minutes for signs of an excessive dosage (e.g., blanching of the skin, abdominal cramps, and nausea). If these occur, reassure the patient that recovery from these effects will occur in a few minutes.

NURSING DIAGNOSES
Drug-specific nursing diagnoses include the following:

- **Deficient Fluid Volume** related to inability to replenish fluid intake secondary to diabetes insipidus
- **Acute Pain** related to abdominal distention

Nursing diagnoses related to drug administration are discussed in Chapter 4.

PLANNING
The expected outcomes for the patient may include an optimal response to therapy, support of patient needs related to the management of adverse reactions, and confidence in an understanding of the medication regimen.

IMPLEMENTATION

Promoting an Optimal Response to Therapy
Vasopressin may be given intramuscularly (IM) or subcutaneously (subcut) to an inpatient to treat diabetes insipidus. To prevent or relieve abdominal distention, the first dose is given 2 hours before x-ray examination and the second dose 30 minutes before the testing. An enema may be given before the first dose.

Desmopressin may be given orally, intranasally, subcut, or intravenously (IV). When the condition becomes chronic and the patient learns to self-administer the drug, adjustments are made according to the patient's response to therapy. Patients learn to regulate their dosage based on the frequency of urination and increase of thirst. A higher dose of the drug may be taken at night to reduce thirst and urination while sleeping.

Monitoring and Managing Patient Needs

The adverse reactions associated with vasopressin, such as skin blanching, abdominal cramps, and nausea, may be decreased by administering the agent with one or two glasses of water. If these adverse reactions occur, inform the patient that they are not serious and should subside within a few minutes.

NURSING ALERT

Excessive dosage is manifested as water intoxication (fluid overload). Symptoms of water intoxication include drowsiness, listlessness, confusion, and headache (which may precede convulsions and coma). If signs of excessive dosage occur, notify the primary health care provider before the next dose of the drug is due; a change in the dosage, the restriction of oral or IV fluids, and the administration of a diuretic may be necessary.

DEFICIENT FLUID VOLUME. The symptoms of diabetes insipidus include the voiding of a large volume of urine at frequent intervals during the day and throughout the night. Accompanying this frequent urination is the need to drink large volumes of fluid, because patients with diabetes insipidus are continually thirsty and need to be supplied with large amounts of drinking water. Take care to refill the water container at frequent intervals. This is especially important when the patient has limited ambulatory activities. Until controlled by a drug, the symptoms of frequent urination and excessive thirst may cause a great deal of anxiety. Reassure the patient that with the proper drug therapy, these symptoms will most likely be reduced or eliminated.

Fluid intake and output are accurately measured and the patient is observed for signs of dehydration (dry mucous membranes, concentrated urine, poor skin turgor, flushing, dry skin, confusion). This is especially important early in treatment and until such time as the optimum dosage is determined and symptoms have diminished. If the patient's output greatly exceeds intake, contact the primary health care provider. In some instances, the primary health care provider may order specific gravity and volume measurements of each voiding or at hourly intervals. Document these results in the chart to aid the primary health care provider in adjusting the dosage to the patient's needs.

CHRONIC CARE CONSIDERATIONS

If a person with diabetes insipidus is unable to take routine medication, a fluid deficit can rapidly occur. Therefore, individuals with diabetes insipidus should wear a medical alert bracelet so emergency personnel can be aware of this need for the medication and dosing can be continued if the patients are unable to take the drug themselves.

ACUTE PAIN. If the patient is receiving vasopressin for abdominal distention, explain the details of treating this problem and the necessity of monitoring drug effectiveness (e.g., auscultation of the abdomen for bowel sounds, insertion of a rectal tube, and measurement of the abdomen). If a rectal tube is ordered after administration of vasopressin for abdominal distention, the lubricated end of the tube is inserted past the anal sphincter and taped in place. The tube is left in place for 1 hour or as prescribed by the primary health care provider. Auscultate the abdomen every 15 to 30 minutes and measure abdominal girth hourly, or as ordered by the primary health care provider.

Educating the Patient and Family

If desmopressin is to be used nasally, ensure that the patient masters the technique of instillation. Provide illustrated patient instructions with the drug and review them with the patient. You should discuss the need to take the drug as directed by the primary health care provider. The patient should change the dosage (i.e., the prescribed number or frequency of sprays) only after consulting with the primary health care provider.

Emphasize the importance of adhering to the prescribed treatment program to control symptoms. In addition to instruction in administration, include the following in a patient and family teaching plan:

- Wear medical identification naming the disease and the drug regimen.
- Carry a sport drink bottle to be sure to have liquids available at all times.
- Monitor the amount of fluids taken each day.
- Monitor the amount and frequency of urine for each 24-hour period, reporting changes to daily patterns to your nurse.
- Carry extra doses of the drug in case you do not make it home in time for your next dose.
- ❗ Avoid the use of alcohol while taking these drugs.
- Rotate injection sites for parenteral administration.
- Contact the primary health care provider immediately if any of the following occurs: a significant increase or decrease in urine output, abdominal cramps, blanching of the skin, nausea, signs of inflammation or infection at the injection sites, confusion, headache, or drowsiness.

EVALUATION

- Therapeutic effect is achieved.
- Adverse reactions are identified, reported to the primary health care provider, and managed successfully through appropriate nursing interventions:
  - Fluid volume balance is maintained.
  - Acute pain is relieved.
- Patient and family express confidence and demonstrate an understanding of the drug regimen.

ANTERIOR PITUITARY HORMONES

The hormones of the anterior pituitary include:

- Thyroid-stimulating hormone (TSH)
- Adrenocorticotropic hormone (ACTH)
- Luteinizing hormone (LH)
- Follicle-stimulating hormone (FSH)
- Growth hormone (GH)
- Prolactin

The anterior pituitary hormone TSH is discussed in Chapter 44. The remaining hormones are covered in this chapter and can be classified as follows:

- ACTH is produced by the anterior pituitary and stimulates the adrenal cortex to secrete the corticosteroids in response to biological stress.
- FSH and LH are called gonadotropins because they influence the **gonads** (the organs of reproduction).
- GH, also called somatropin, contributes to the growth of the body during childhood, especially the growth of muscles and bones.
- Prolactin, which is also secreted by the anterior pituitary, stimulates the production of breast milk in the postpartum patient. Additional functions of prolactin are not well understood. Prolactin is the only anterior pituitary hormone that is not used medically.

GONADOTROPINS: FOLLICLE-STIMULATING HORMONE AND LUTEINIZING HORMONE

The gonadotropins (FSH and LH) influence the secretion of sex hormones, the development of secondary sex characteristics, and the reproductive cycle in both men and women.

Action and Uses

These drugs are purified preparations of the gonadotropins (FSH and LH) extracted from the urine of postmenopausal women or produced by a recombinant form of DNA. Gonadotropins are used to induce ovulation and pregnancy in **anovulatory** women (women whose bodies fail to produce an ovum or fail to ovulate). Menopur is also used in assisted reproductive technology (ART) programs to stimulate multiple follicles for in vitro fertilization. Besides their use in treating female infertility, some of these drugs are used in men. Human chorionic gonadotropin (HCG) is extracted from human placentas. The actions of HCG are identical to those of the pituitary LH. This drug is

also used in boys to treat prepubertal **cryptorchism** (failure of the testes to descend into the scrotum) and in men to treat selected cases of hypogonadotropic hypogonadism. Follistim AQ is used to induce sperm production (spermatogenesis). For additional information on the gonadotropins, see the Summary Drug Table: Pituitary and Adrenocortical Hormones.

Clomiphene and ganirelix are synthetic nonsteroidal compounds that bind to estrogen receptors, decreasing the amount of available estrogen receptors and causing the anterior pituitary to increase secretion of FSH and LH. These drugs are used to induce ovulation in anovulatory (nonovulating) women.

Adverse Reactions

Hormone-Associated Reactions

- Vasomotor flushes (which are like the hot flashes of menopause)
- Breast tenderness
- Abdominal discomfort, ovarian enlargement
- Hemoperitoneum (blood in the peritoneal cavity)

Generalized Reactions

- Nausea, vomiting
- Headache, irritability, restlessness, fatigue
- Edema and irritation at the injection site

LIFESPAN CONSIDERATIONS
Childbearing Women
Fetal effects have been demonstrated in animal studies when gonadotropins have been administered. Birth defects have been reported in human studies; therefore, gonadotropins should not be administered to women known to be pregnant.

Contraindications, Precautions, and Interactions

These drugs are contraindicated in patients who are hypersensitive to the drug or any component of the drug. The gonadotropins are contraindicated in patients with high gonadotropin levels, thyroid dysfunction, adrenal dysfunction, liver disease, abnormal bleeding, ovarian cysts, or sex hormone–dependent tumors, or those with an organic intracranial lesion (pituitary tumor). Gonadotropins are contraindicated during pregnancy (pregnancy category X).

These drugs are used cautiously in patients with epilepsy, migraine headaches, asthma, or cardiac or renal dysfunction, and during lactation. There are no known clinically significant interactions with the gonadotropins.

NURSING PROCESS
PATIENT RECEIVING A GONADOTROPIN

ASSESSMENT

Preadministration Assessment
These drugs are almost always administered on an outpatient basis and may be self-administered by the patient. Before

prescribing any of these drugs, the primary health care provider takes a thorough medical history and performs a physical examination. Additional laboratory and diagnostic tests for ovarian function and tubal patency may also be performed. A pelvic examination may be performed by the primary health care provider to rule out ovarian enlargement, pregnancy, or uterine problems.

Ongoing Assessment

At the time of each office or clinic visit, ask the patient about the occurrence of adverse reactions and document the patient's vital signs and weight.

NURSING DIAGNOSES

Drug-specific nursing diagnoses include the following:

- **Acute Pain** related to adverse reactions (ovarian enlargement, irritation at the injection site)
- **Anxiety** related to inability to conceive, treatment outcome, other factors

Nursing diagnoses related to drug administration are discussed in Chapter 4.

PLANNING

The expected outcomes of the patient may include an optimal response to drug therapy, support of patient needs related to the management of adverse reactions, reduction in anxiety, and confidence in an understanding of the medication regimen.

IMPLEMENTATION

Promoting an Optimal Response to Therapy

Gonadotropin injections are given in the primary health care provider's office or the clinic or may be self-administered. These drugs must be administered IM or subcut because they are destroyed in the gastrointestinal (GI) tract; therefore, they cannot be taken orally. Injection sites are rotated and previous sites are checked for redness and irritation.

NURSING ALERT

If the patient complains of visual disturbances, the drug therapy is discontinued and the primary health care provider notified. An examination by an ophthalmologist is usually indicated.

Monitoring and Managing Patient Needs

ACUTE PAIN. Female patients taking these drugs are usually examined by the primary health care provider frequently to detect excessive ovarian stimulation, called hyperstimulation syndrome (sudden ovarian enlargement with ascites). The patient may or may not report pain. This syndrome usually develops quickly, within 3 to 4 days.

NURSING ALERT

The patient is checked for signs of excessive ovarian enlargement (abdominal distention, pain, ascites [with serious cases]). The drug is discontinued at the first sign of ovarian stimulation or enlargement. The patient is usually admitted to the hospital for supportive measures.

ANXIETY. Patients seeking treatment to become pregnant often experience a great deal of anxiety due to past failed attempts. In addition, when taking these drugs, the patient faces the possibility of multiple births. The success rate of these drugs varies and depends on many factors. The primary health care provider usually discusses the value of this, as well as other approaches, with the patient and her sexual partner. Allow the patient time to talk about her concerns about the proposed treatment program.

Educating the Patient and Family

Patients are instructed by the primary health care provider about the frequency of sexual intercourse. You can assess whether the patient understands the directions given by the primary health care provider. When a gonadotropin is prescribed, you may instruct the patient how to use the device to inject the hormone and to keep all primary health care provider appointments and to report adverse reactions to the nurse or primary health care provider. Include the following information when a gonadotropin is prescribed:

HORMONAL OVARIAN STIMULANTS

- Before beginning therapy, be aware of the possibility of multiple births and birth defects.
- It is a good idea to use a calendar to track the treatment schedule and ovulation.
- Report bloating, abdominal pain, flushing, breast tenderness, and pain at the injection site.

NONHORMONAL OVARIAN STIMULANTS

- Take the drug as prescribed (5 days) and do not stop taking the drug before the course of therapy is finished unless told to do so by the primary health care provider.
- Notify the primary health care provider if bloating, stomach or pelvic pain, jaundice, blurred vision, hot flashes, breast discomfort, headache, nausea, or vomiting occurs.
- Keep in mind that if ovulation does not occur after the first course of therapy, a second or third course may be used. If therapy does not succeed after three courses, the drug is considered unsuccessful and is discontinued.

EVALUATION

- Therapeutic effect is achieved.
- Adverse reactions are identified, reported to the primary health care provider, and managed successfully through appropriate nursing interventions:
  - Patient is free of pain.
  - Anxiety is managed successfully.
- Patient expresses confidence and demonstrates an understanding of the drug regimen.

GROWTH HORMONE

GH, also called *somatotropic hormone,* is secreted by the anterior pituitary. This hormone regulates the growth of the individual until approximately early adulthood or the time when the person no longer gains height.

Action and Uses

GH is available as the synthetic product somatropin. Of recombinant DNA origin, somatropin is identical to human GH and produces skeletal growth in children. This drug is administered to children who have not grown because of a deficiency of pituitary GH; it must be used before closure of the child's bone epiphyses. Bone epiphyses are the ends of bones. They are separated from the main bone but joined to it by cartilage, which allows for growth or lengthening of the bone. GH is ineffective in patients with closed epiphyses, because when the epiphyses close, growth (in length) can no longer occur.

Growth hormone is used in adults to supplement the lack of endogenous (naturally occurring) hormone. This may occur in conditions such as chronic renal failure or pituitary disease. The drug Serostim is also used in patients with human immunodeficiency virus to stop severe muscle wasting.

Adverse Reactions

Somatropin causes few adverse reactions when administered as directed. Antibodies to somatropin may develop in a small number of patients, resulting in a failure to experience response to therapy, namely, failure of the drug to produce growth in the child. Some patients may experience hypothyroidism or insulin resistance. Swelling, joint pain, and muscle pain may also occur.

Contraindications, Precautions, and Interactions

Somatropin is contraindicated in patients with known hypersensitivity to somatropin or sensitivity to benzyl alcohol and those with epiphyseal closure or underlying cranial lesions (e.g., pituitary tumor). The drug is used cautiously in patients with thyroid disease or diabetes and during pregnancy (pregnancy category C) and lactation. Excessive amounts of glucocorticoids may decrease the response to somatropin.

NURSING PROCESS
PATIENT RECEIVING GROWTH HORMONE

ASSESSMENT

Preadministration Assessment
A thorough physical examination and laboratory and diagnostic tests are performed before a child is accepted into a GH program. Assessments include the patient's vital signs, height, and weight.

Ongoing Assessment
Children may increase their growth rate from 3.5 to 4 cm/year before treatment to 8 to 10 cm/year during the first year of treatment. Each time the child visits the primary health care provider's office or clinic (usually every 3 to 6 months), measure and document the child's height and weight to evaluate the response to therapy. Bone age is monitored periodically for growth and to detect epiphyseal closure, at which time therapy must stop.

NURSING DIAGNOSES
A key nursing diagnosis for patients receiving GH therapy is:

- **Disturbed Body Image** related to changes in appearance, physical size, or failure to grow

    Nursing diagnoses related to drug administration are discussed in Chapter 4.

PLANNING
The expected outcomes of the patient may include an optimal response to drug therapy, support of patient needs related to the management of adverse reactions, reduction in anxiety, and confidence in an understanding of the medication regimen.

IMPLEMENTATION

Promoting an Optimal Response to Therapy
GH is administered subcutaneously. The vial containing the hormone is not shaken but swirled to mix. The solution is clear; do not administer it if it is cloudy. The weekly dosage is divided and given in three to seven doses throughout the week. The drug may (if possible) be given at bedtime to adhere most closely to the body's natural release of the hormone. Periodic testing of GH levels, glucose tolerance, and thyroid function may be done during treatment.

Monitoring and Managing Patient Needs
DISTURBED BODY IMAGE. Children requiring treatment are usually of short stature. The parents, and sometimes the children, may be concerned about the success or possible failure of treatment with GH. The child is provided with the opportunity to share fears, concerns, or anger. Acknowledge these feelings as normal and discuss any misconceptions the child or parents may have concerning treatment. Families may be surprised by the growth changes once treatment is started. Children may experience stretch marks or sizable changes in body structure and appearance. A child may become shy, reserved, or uncomfortable with his or her new body image. Time is allowed for the parents and children to ask questions not only before therapy is started but also during the months of treatment.

Educating the Patient and Family
When the patient is receiving GH, the primary health care provider discusses in detail the therapeutic regimen for increasing growth (height) with the child's parents or guardians. If the drug is to be given at bedtime and not in the outpatient clinic, instruct the parents on the proper injection technique. The parents are encouraged to keep all clinic or office visits with the child. You will want to explain that the child may experience sudden growth and increase in appetite and instruct the parents to report lack of growth, symptoms of diabetes (e.g., increased hunger, increased thirst, or frequent voiding), or symptoms of hypothyroidism (e.g., fatigue, dry skin, intolerance to cold).

EVALUATION

- Therapeutic effect is achieved and the child grows in height.
- Adverse reactions are identified, reported to the primary health care provider, and managed successfully through appropriate nursing interventions:
    - Positive body image is maintained.
- Patient and family express confidence and demonstrate an understanding of the drug regimen.

Pituitary and Adrenocortical Hormones

ADRENOCORTICAL HORMONES AND CORTICOTROPIN

This section discusses the hormones produced by the adrenal cortex or the adrenocortical hormones, which are the glucocorticoids and mineralocorticoids. These hormones are essential to life and influence many organs and structures of the body. The glucocorticoids and mineralocorticoids are collectively called *corticosteroids*.

Corticotropin (ACTH) is an anterior pituitary hormone that stimulates the adrenal cortex to produce and secrete adrenocortical hormones, primarily the glucocorticoids. Corticotropin is used for diagnostic testing of adrenocortical function.

The adrenal gland lies on the superior surface of each kidney. It is a double organ composed of an outer cortex and an inner medulla (Fig. 43.2). In response to ACTH secreted by the anterior pituitary, the adrenal cortex secretes several hormones (glucocorticoids, mineralocorticoids, and small amounts of sex hormones).

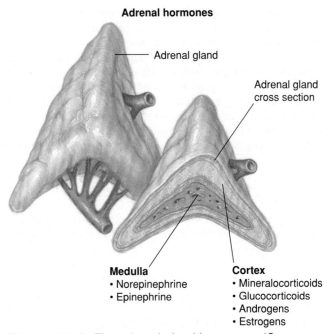

Adrenal hormones

— Adrenal gland

Adrenal gland cross section

Medulla
• Norepinephrine
• Epinephrine

Cortex
• Mineralocorticoids
• Glucocorticoids
• Androgens
• Estrogens

Figure 43.2 The adrenal gland hormones. (Courtesy of Anatomical Chart Co).

GLUCOCORTICOIDS

Glucocorticoids influence or regulate functions such as the immune response; glucose, fat, and protein metabolism; and the anti-inflammatory response. Table 43.1 describes the activity of glucocorticoids in the body.

Actions

Glucocorticoids enter target cells and bind to receptors, initiating many complex reactions in the body. Some of the actions are considered undesirable, depending on the indication for which these drugs are used. Examples of the glucocorticoids include cortisone, hydrocortisone, prednisone, prednisolone, and triamcinolone. The Summary Drug Table: Pituitary and Adrenocortical Hormones provides information concerning these hormones.

Table 43.1 Activity of Glucocorticoids in the Body	
Function Within the Body	**Description of Bodily Activity**
Anti-inflammatory	Stabilizes lysosomal membrane and prevents the release of proteolytic enzymes during the inflammatory process.
Regulation of blood pressure	Potentiates vasoconstrictor action of norepinephrine. Without glucocorticoids the vasoconstricting action is decreased, and blood pressure decreases.
Metabolism of carbohydrates and protein	Facilitates the breakdown of protein in the muscle, leading to increased plasma amino acid levels. Increases activity of enzymes necessary for glucogenesis, producing hyperglycemia, which can aggravate diabetes, precipitate latent diabetes, and cause insulin resistance.
Metabolism of fat	A complex phenomenon that promotes the use of fat for energy (a positive effect) and permits fat stores to accumulate in the body, causing buffalo hump and moon-shaped or round face (a negative effect).
Interference with the immune response	Decreases the production of lymphocytes and eosinophils in the blood by causing atrophy of the thymus gland; blocks the release of cytokines, resulting in a decreased performance of T and B monocytes in the immune response. (This action, coupled with the anti-inflammatory action, makes the corticosteroids useful in delaying organ rejection in patients with transplants.)
Protection during stress	As a protective mechanism, the corticosteroids are released during periods of stress (e.g., injury or surgery). The release of epinephrine or norepinephrine by the adrenal medulla during stress has a synergistic effect along with the corticosteroids.
Central nervous system responses	Affects mood and possibly causes neuronal or brain excitability, causing euphoria, anxiety, depression, psychosis, and an increase in motor activity in some individuals.

Uses

Glucocorticoids are used to treat the following:

- Adrenocortical insufficiency (replacement therapy)
- Allergic reactions
- Collagen diseases (e.g., systemic lupus erythematosus)
- Dermatologic conditions
- Rheumatic disorders
- Shock
- Multiple other conditions (see Display 43.1)

The anti-inflammatory activity of these hormones makes them valuable for suppressing inflammation and modifying the immune response.

Display 43.1 Uses of Glucocorticoids

- **Endocrine disorders:** Primary or secondary adrenal cortical insufficiency, congenital adrenal hyperplasia, nonsuppurative thyroiditis, hypercalcemia associated with cancer
- **Rheumatic disorders:** Short-term management of acute ankylosing spondylitis, acute and subacute bursitis, acute nonspecific tenosynovitis, acute gouty arthritis, psoriatic arthritis, rheumatoid arthritis, posttraumatic osteoarthritis, synovitis of osteoarthritis, epicondylitis
- **Collagen diseases:** Systemic lupus erythematosus, acute rheumatic carditis, systemic dermatomyositis
- **Dermatologic disorders:** Pemphigus, bullous dermatitis herpetiformis, severe erythema multiforme (Stevens-Johnson syndrome), exfoliative dermatitis, mycosis fungoides, severe psoriasis, severe seborrheic dermatitis, angioedema, urticaria, various skin disorders (e.g., lichen planus or keloids)
- **Allergic states:** Control of severe or incapacitating allergic conditions not controlled by other methods, bronchial asthma (including status asthmaticus), contact dermatitis, atopic dermatitis, serum sickness, drug hypersensitivity reactions
- **Ophthalmic diseases:** Severe acute and chronic allergic and inflammatory processes, keratitis, allergic corneal marginal ulcers, herpes zoster of the eye, iritis, iridocyclitis, chorioretinitis, diffuse posterior uveitis, optic neuritis, sympathetic ophthalmia, anterior segment inflammation
- **Respiratory diseases:** Seasonal allergic rhinitis, berylliosis, fulminating or disseminating pulmonary tuberculosis, aspiration pneumonia
- **Hematologic disorders:** Idiopathic or secondary thrombocytopenic purpura, hemolytic anemia, red blood cell anemia, congenital hypoplastic anemia
- **Neoplastic diseases:** Leukemia, lymphomas
- **Edematous states:** Induction of diuresis or remission of proteinuria in nephrotic syndrome
- **GI diseases:** During critical period of ulcerative colitis, regional enteritis, intractable sprue
- **Nervous system disorders:** Acute exacerbations of multiple sclerosis

---

Adverse Reactions

The adverse reactions that may result from the administration of the glucocorticoids are given in Display 43.2. Long- or short-term high-dose therapy may also produce many of the signs and symptoms seen with Cushing's syndrome, a disease caused by the overproduction of endogenous glucocorticoids. Some of the signs and symptoms of this Cushing-like (**cushingoid**) state include a buffalo hump (a hump on the back of

---

Display 43.2 Adverse Reactions Associated With Glucocorticoids

- **Fluid and electrolyte disturbances:** Sodium and fluid retention, potassium loss, hypokalemic alkalosis, hypertension, hypocalcemia, hypotension or shock-like reactions
- **Musculoskeletal disturbances:** Muscle weakness, loss of muscle mass, tendon rupture, osteoporosis, aseptic necrosis of femoral and humeral heads, spontaneous fractures
- **Cardiovascular disturbances:** Thromboembolism or fat embolism; thrombophlebitis; necrotizing angiitis; syncopal episodes; cardiac arrhythmias; aggravation of hypertension; fatal cardiac arrhythmias with rapid, high-dose IV methylprednisolone administration; HF in susceptible patients
- **GI disturbances:** Pancreatitis, abdominal distention, ulcerative esophagitis, nausea, vomiting, increased appetite and weight gain, possible peptic ulcer or bowel perforation, hemorrhage
- **Dermatologic disturbances:** Impaired wound healing; thin, fragile skin; petechiae; ecchymoses; erythema; increased sweating; suppression of skin test reactions; subcutaneous fat atrophy; purpura; striae; hirsutism; acneiform eruptions; urticaria; angioneurotic edema; perineal itch
- **Neurologic disturbances:** Convulsions, increased intracranial pressure with papilledema (usually after treatment is discontinued), vertigo, headache, neuritis or paresthesia, steroid psychosis, insomnia
- **Endocrine disturbances:** Amenorrhea, other menstrual irregularities, development of cushingoid state, suppression of growth in children, secondary adrenocortical and pituitary unresponsive (particularly in times of stress), decreased carbohydrate tolerance, manifestation of latent diabetes mellitus, increased requirements for insulin or oral hypoglycemic agents (in diabetic patients)
- **Ophthalmic disturbances:** Posterior subcapsular cataracts, increased intraocular pressure, glaucoma, exophthalmos
- **Metabolic disturbances:** Negative nitrogen balance (due to protein catabolism)
- **Other disturbances:** Anaphylactoid or hypersensitivity reactions, aggravation of existing infections, malaise, increase or decrease in sperm motility and number

the neck), moon face, oily skin and acne, osteoporosis, purple striae on the abdomen and hips, altered skin pigmentation, and weight gain. When a serious disease or disorder is treated, it is often necessary to allow these effects to occur, because therapy with these drugs is absolutely necessary.

Contraindications, Precautions, and Interactions

Glucocorticoids are contraindicated in patients with serious infections, such as tuberculosis and fungal and antibiotic-resistant infections. Glucocorticoids are administered with caution to patients with renal or hepatic disease, hypothyroidism, ulcerative colitis, diverticulitis, peptic ulcer disease, inflammatory bowel disease, hypertension, osteoporosis, convulsive disorders, or diabetes. Glucocorticoids are classified as pregnancy category C drugs and should be used with caution during pregnancy and lactation. Patients taking ACTH should avoid any vaccinations with live virus. The live virus vaccines can potentiate virus replication with ACTH, increase any adverse reaction to the vaccine, and decrease the patient's antibody response to the vaccine.

Multiple drug interactions may occur with the glucocorticoids. Table 43.2 identifies selected clinically significant interactions.

MINERALOCORTICOIDS

Actions and Uses

The natural mineralocorticoids consist of aldosterone and desoxycorticosterone and play an important role in conserving sodium and increasing potassium excretion. Because of these activities, mineralocorticoids are important in controlling salt and water balance. Aldosterone is the more potent of these two hormones. Deficiencies of mineralocorticoids result in a loss of sodium and water and a retention of potassium. Fludrocortisone is a drug that has both glucocorticoid and mineralocorticoid activity and is the only currently available mineralocorticoid drug. Fludrocortisone is used for replacement therapy for primary and secondary adrenocortical deficiency. Even though this drug has both mineralocorticoid and glucocorticoid activity, it is used only for its mineralocorticoid effects.

Adverse Reactions

Adverse reactions may occur if the dosage is too high or prolonged or if withdrawal is too rapid. Administration of fludrocortisone may cause:

- Edema, hypertension, HF, enlargement of the heart
- Increased sweating, allergic skin rash
- Hypokalemia, muscular weakness, headache, hypersensitivity reactions

Because this drug has glucocorticoid and mineralocorticoid activity and is often given with glucocorticoids, adverse reactions of glucocorticoids must be closely monitored as well (see Display 43.2).

Contraindications, Precautions, and Interactions

Fludrocortisone is contraindicated in patients with hypersensitivity to fludrocortisone and those with systemic fungal

Table 43.2 Selected Drug Interactions of Glucocorticoids		
Precipitant Drug	**Object Drug**	**Description**
cholestyramine	hydrocortisone	Effects of hydrocortisone may be decreased.
oral contraceptives	corticosteroids	Effects of corticosteroid may be increased.
estrogens	corticosteroids	Effects of corticosteroid may be increased.
hydantoins	corticosteroids	Effects of corticosteroid may be decreased.
ketoconazole	corticosteroids	Effects of corticosteroid may be increased.
rifampin	corticosteroids	Effects of corticosteroid may be decreased.
corticosteroids	anticholinesterases	Anticholinesterase effects may be antagonized in myasthenia gravis.
corticosteroids	oral anticoagulants	Anticoagulant dose requirements may be reduced. Corticosteroids may decrease the anticoagulant action.
corticosteroids	digitalis glycosides	Coadministration may enhance the possibility of digitalis toxicity associated with hypokalemia.
corticosteroids	isoniazid	Isoniazid serum concentrations may be decreased.
corticosteroids	potassium-depleting diuretics	Hypokalemia may occur.
corticosteroids	salicylates	Corticosteroids will reduce serum salicylate levels and may decrease their effectiveness.
corticosteroids	theophyllines	Alterations in the pharmacologic activity of either agent may occur.

infections. Fludrocortisone is used cautiously in patients with Addison's disease or infection and during pregnancy (pregnancy category C) and lactation. Fludrocortisone decreases the effects of hydantoins and rifampin. There is a decrease in serum levels of salicylates when those agents are administered with fludrocortisone.

NURSING PROCESS
PATIENT RECEIVING A GLUCOCORTICOID OR MINERALOCORTICOID

ASSESSMENT

Preadministration Assessment
Assessments depend on the patient's condition and diagnosis. The primary health care provider may order baseline diagnostic tests, such as chest or upper GI x-ray studies and serum electrolytes, urinalysis, or complete blood count. When feasible, perform a physical assessment of the area of disease involvement, such as the respiratory tract or skin, and document the findings in the patient's record. These findings provide baseline data for evaluating the patient's response to drug therapy. Weigh patients who are acutely ill and those with a serious systemic disease before starting therapy.

Ongoing Assessment
Ongoing assessments of the patient receiving a glucocorticoid, and the frequency of these assessments, depend largely on the disease being treated. Take and record vital signs every 4 to 8 hours if the patient is not continuously monitored. Weigh the patient daily to weekly, depending on the diagnosis and the primary health care provider's orders. More frequent assessment may be necessary if a glucocorticoid is used for emergency situations.

Assess for signs of adverse effects of the mineralocorticoid or glucocorticoid, particularly signs of electrolyte imbalance, such as hypocalcemia, hypokalemia, and hypernatremia (see Chapter 54). Be alert for changes in the patient's mental status, especially if there is a history of depression or other psychiatric problems or if high doses of the drug are prescribed. Monitor for signs of an infection, which may be masked by glucocorticoid therapy. The blood of the patient without diabetes is checked weekly for elevated glucose levels because glucocorticoids may aggravate latent diabetes. Those with diabetes must be checked more frequently.

When administering fludrocortisone, check the patient's blood pressure at frequent intervals. Hypotension may indicate insufficient dosage. Weigh the patient daily and assess for edema, particularly swelling of the feet and hands. The lungs are auscultated for adventitious sounds (e.g., crackles).

NURSING DIAGNOSES
Drug-specific nursing diagnoses include the following:

- **Risk for Infection** related to immune suppression or impaired wound healing
- **Acute Confusion** related to adverse drug reactions
- **Risk for Injury** related to muscle atrophy, osteoporosis, or spontaneous fractures
- **Acute Pain** related to epigastric distress of gastric ulcer formation

- **Excess Fluid Volume** related to adverse reactions (sodium and water retention)
- **Disturbed Body Image** related to adverse reactions (cushingoid appearance)

Nursing diagnoses related to drug administration are discussed in Chapter 4.

PLANNING
The expected outcomes of the patient include an optimal response to therapy, support of patient needs related to the management of adverse reactions, and confidence in an understanding of the medication regimen.

IMPLEMENTATION

Promoting an Optimal Response to Therapy
Glucocorticoids may be administered orally, IM, subcut, IV, topically, or as an inhalant. The primary health care provider may also inject the drug into a joint (intra-articular), a lesion (intralesional), soft tissue, or bursa. The drug dosage is individualized and based on the severity of the condition and the patient's response.

> **! NURSING ALERT**
> Never omit a dose of a glucocorticoid. If the patient cannot take the drug orally because of nausea or vomiting, contact the primary health care provider immediately, because the drug needs to be ordered given by the parenteral route. Patients who can receive nothing by mouth for any reason must have the glucocorticoid given by the parenteral route.

Daily oral doses are usually given before 9 a.m. to minimize adrenal suppression and to coincide with normal adrenal function. However, alternate-day therapy may be prescribed for patients receiving long-term therapy. Fludrocortisone is given orally and is well tolerated in the GI tract.

 LIFESPAN CONSIDERATIONS
Gerontology
Corticosteroids are administered with caution in older adults, because they are more likely to have pre-existing conditions, such as HF, hypertension, osteoporosis, and arthritis, which may be worsened by use of such agents. Monitor older adults for exacerbation of existing conditions during corticosteroid therapy. In addition, lower dosages may be needed because of the effects of aging, such as decreases in muscle mass, renal function, and plasma volume.

ALTERNATE-DAY THERAPY. The alternate-day therapy approach to glucocorticoid administration is used in treating diseases and disorders requiring long-term therapy, especially arthritic disorders. This regimen involves giving twice the daily dose of the glucocorticoid every other day. The drug is given only once on the alternate day, before 9 a.m. The purpose of alternate-day administration is to provide the patient requiring long-term glucocorticoid therapy with the beneficial effects of the drug while minimizing certain undesirable reactions (see Display 43.2).

Plasma levels of the endogenous adrenocortical hormones vary throughout the daytime and nighttime hours. They are normally higher between 2 a.m. and 8 a.m. and lower between 4 p.m. and midnight. When plasma levels are lower, the anterior pituitary releases ACTH, which in turn stimulates the adrenal cortex to manufacture and release glucocorticoids. When plasma levels are high, the pituitary gland does not release ACTH. The response of the pituitary to high or low plasma levels of glucocorticoids and the resulting release or nonrelease of ACTH is an example of the feedback mechanism, which may also be seen in other glands of the body, such as the thyroid gland.

The feedback mechanism (also called the *feedback control*) is the method by which the body maintains most hormones at relatively constant levels in the bloodstream. When the hormone concentration falls, the rate of production of that hormone increases. Likewise, when the hormone level becomes too high, the body decreases production of that hormone.

Administration of a short-acting glucocorticoid on alternate days and before 9 a.m., when glucocorticoid plasma levels are still relatively high, does not affect the release of ACTH later in the day yet gives the patient the benefit of exogenous glucocorticoid therapy.

PATIENT WITH DIABETES. Patients with diabetes who are receiving a glucocorticoid may require frequent adjustment of their insulin or oral antidiabetic drug dosage. Blood glucose levels may be monitored more frequently than when the patient is at home. If the blood glucose levels increase or urine is positive for ketones, notify the primary health care provider. Some patients may have latent (hidden) diabetes. In these cases, the corticosteroid may precipitate hyperglycemia. Therefore, all patients, those with diabetes and those without, should have blood glucose levels checked frequently.

ADRENAL INSUFFICIENCY. Administration of the glucocorticoids poses the threat of adrenal gland insufficiency (particularly if the alternate-day therapy is not prescribed). Administration of glucocorticoids several times a day and during a short time (as little as 5 to 10 days) results in shutting off the pituitary release of ACTH, because there are always high levels of glucocorticoids in the plasma (caused by the body's own glucocorticoid production plus the administration of a glucocorticoid drug). Eventually, the pituitary atrophies and ceases to release ACTH. Without ACTH, the adrenals fail to manufacture and release (endogenous) glucocorticoids. When this happens, the patient has acute adrenal insufficiency, which is a life-threatening situation until corrected with the administration of an exogenous glucocorticoid.

Adrenal insufficiency is a critical deficiency of mineralocorticoids and glucocorticoids; the disorder requires immediate treatment. Symptoms of adrenal insufficiency include fever, myalgia, arthralgia, malaise, anorexia, nausea, orthostatic hypotension, dizziness, fainting, dyspnea, and hypoglycemia. Death due to circulatory collapse will result unless the condition is treated promptly. Situations producing stress (e.g., trauma, surgery, severe illness) may precipitate the need for an increase in dosage of corticosteroids until the crisis or stressful situation is resolved.

❗ NURSING ALERT

Glucocorticoid therapy should never be discontinued suddenly. When administration of a glucocorticoid extends beyond 5 days and the drug therapy is to be discontinued, the dosage must be reduced gradually (tapered) over several days. In some instances, it may be necessary to taper the dose over 7 to 10 or more days. Tapering the dosage allows normal adrenal function to return gradually, thereby preventing adrenal insufficiency.

Monitoring and Managing Patient Needs

RISK FOR INFECTION. Report any slight rise in temperature, sore throat, or other signs of infection to the primary health care provider as soon as possible, because decreased resistance to infection may occur during glucocorticoid therapy. Nursing personnel and visitors with any type of infection or recent exposure to an infectious disease should avoid patient contact.

ACUTE CONFUSION. Glucocorticoid drugs can also cause disturbances in mental processing. Monitor and report any evidence of behavior change, such as depression, insomnia, euphoria, mood swings, or nervousness. If disturbances occur provide a quiet, nonthreatening environment, and spend time actively listening as the patient talks. It is important to encourage verbalization of fears and concerns. Anxiety usually decreases with understanding of the therapeutic regimen. Allow time for a thorough explanation of the drug regimen and answering of questions.

RISK FOR INJURY. Patients receiving long-term glucocorticoid therapy, especially those with limited activity, should be monitored for signs of compression fractures of the vertebrae and pathologic fractures of the long bones. If the patient reports back or bone pain, contact the primary health care provider. Extra care is also necessary to prevent falls and other injuries when the patient is confused or is allowed out of bed. If the patient is weak, provide assistance to the patient to the bathroom or when ambulating. Edematous extremities are handled with care to prevent skin tears and trauma.

ACUTE PAIN. Peptic ulcer has been associated with glucocorticoid therapy. Encourage the patient to report complaints of epigastric burning or pain, bloody or coffee-ground emesis, or the passing of tarry stools. Giving oral corticosteroids with food or a full glass of water may minimize gastric irritation.

EXCESS FLUID VOLUME. Fluid and electrolyte imbalances, particularly excess fluid volume, are common with corticosteroid therapy. Scan the patient for visible edema, keep an accurate fluid intake and output record, obtain daily weights, and restrict sodium if indicated by the primary health care provider. Edematous extremities are elevated and the patient's position is changed frequently. Inform the primary health care provider if signs of electrolyte imbalance or glucocorticoid drug effects are noted. Dietary adjustments are made for the increased potassium loss and sodium retention if necessary. Consultation with a dietitian may be indicated.

DISTURBED BODY IMAGE. A body image disturbance may occur, especially if the patient experiences cushingoid effects (e.g., buffalo hump, moon face), acne, or hirsutism. If continuation of drug therapy is necessary, explain the reason for the cushingoid appearance and emphasize the necessity of continuing the drug regimen. Assess the patient's emotional state and help the patient express feelings and concerns. Offer positive reinforcement, when possible. Instruct the patient experiencing acne to keep the affected areas clean and in the use of over-the-counter acne drugs and water-based cosmetics or creams.

Educating the Patient and Family
To support adherence, provide the patient and family with thorough instructions and educational materials about the drug regimen:

- These drugs may cause GI upset. To decrease GI effects, take the oral drug with meals or snacks.
- Take antacids between meals to help prevent peptic ulcer.
- Carry patient identification, such as a MedicAlert tag, so that drug therapy will be known to medical personnel during an emergency situation.
- Keep follow-up appointments to determine if a dosage adjustment is necessary.

SHORT-TERM GLUCOCORTICOID THERAPY

- Take the drug exactly as directed in the prescription container. Do not increase, decrease, or omit a dose unless advised to do so by the primary health care provider.
- Take single daily doses before 9:00 a.m.
- Follow the instructions for tapering the dose, because they are extremely important.
- If the problem does not improve, contact the primary health care provider.

ALTERNATE-DAY ORAL GLUCOCORTICOID THERAPY

- Take this drug before 9 a.m. once every other day. Use a calendar or some other method to identify the days of each week to take the drug.
- Do not stop taking the drug unless advised to do so by the primary health care provider.
- If the problem becomes worse, especially on the days the drug is not taken, contact the primary health care provider.

Most of the following teaching points may also apply to alternate-day therapy, especially when higher doses are used and therapy extends over many months.

LONG-TERM OR HIGH-DOSE GLUCOCORTICOID THERAPY

- Do not omit this drug or increase or decrease the dosage except on the advice of the primary health care provider.
- Inform other primary health care providers, dentists, and all medical personnel of therapy with this drug. Wear medical identification or another form of identification to alert medical personnel of long-term therapy with a glucocorticoid.
- Do not take any nonprescription drug unless its use has been approved by the primary health care provider.

- If you go to get a vaccine, ask if it is a "live virus." Do not receive the vaccine if it is a live preparation because of the risk for a lack of antibody response. (This does not include patients receiving corticosteroids as replacement therapy.)
- Whenever possible, avoid exposure to infections. Contact the primary health care provider if minor cuts or abrasions fail to heal, persistent joint swelling or tenderness is noted, or fever, sore throat, upper respiratory infection, or other signs of infection occur.
- If the drug cannot be taken orally for any reason or if diarrhea occurs, contact the primary health care provider immediately. If you are unable to contact the primary health care provider before the next dose is due, go to the nearest urgent care or hospital emergency department (preferably where the original treatment was started or where the primary health care provider is on the hospital staff), because the drug must be given by injection.
- Weigh yourself weekly. If significant weight gain or swelling of the extremities is noted, contact the primary health care provider.
- Remember that dietary recommendations made by the primary health care provider are an important part of therapy and must be followed.
- Follow the primary health care provider's recommendations regarding periodic eye examinations and laboratory tests.

INTRA-ARTICULAR OR INTRALESIONAL ADMINISTRATION

- Do not overuse the injected joint, even if the pain is gone.
- Follow the primary health care provider's instructions concerning rest and exercise.

MINERALOCORTICOID (FLUDROCORTISONE) THERAPY

- Take the drug as directed. Do not increase or decrease the dosage except as instructed to do so by the primary health care provider.
- Do not discontinue use of the drug abruptly.
- Inform the primary health care provider if the following adverse reactions occur: edema, muscle weakness, weight gain, anorexia, swelling of the extremities, dizziness, severe headache, or shortness of breath.

EVALUATION

- Therapeutic effect is achieved.
- Adverse reactions are identified, reported to the primary health care provider, and managed successfully through appropriate nursing interventions:
  - No evidence of infection is seen.
  - Orientation and mentation remain intact.
  - No evidence of injury is seen.
  - Patient is free of pain.
  - Fluid volume balance is maintained.
  - Positive body image is maintained.
- Patient expresses confidence and demonstrates an understanding of the drug regimen.

PHARMACOLOGY IN PRACTICE
THINK CRITICALLY

Janna's classmate was showing her the numerous medications she has to take on a daily basis. She wonders why her friend has to take two tablets of desmopressin during the day and three in the evening. Explain the reasoning for this schedule for the drug desmopressin.

KEY POINTS

- The pituitary is a small gland suspended from the hypothalamus in the brain. Called the "master gland," the pituitary controls many of the body processes. The gland has two lobes, the anterior and posterior pituitary.

- The posterior pituitary secretes two hormones, oxytocin and vasopressin. Vasopressin regulates the reabsorption of fluid by the kidney. Diabetes insipidus occurs when vasopressin is not secreted properly. This results in unquenchable thirst and copious urination.

- Patients taking vasopressin replacement can easily become dehydrated if unable to take the medication; therefore, a medical alert identification should always be worn.

- The anterior pituitary secretes many hormones, including prolactin, luteinizing hormone, follicle-stimulating hormone, thyroid-stimulating hormone, adrenocorticotropic hormone, and growth hormone. These all help in the regulation of growth, metabolism, reproduction, and stress.

- Hormones to stimulate ovulation are given as an injection because the hormones are destroyed by GI fluids. Pain may be an indicator of hyperstimulation syndrome and the medication is then stopped. Injection of growth hormones can lead to sudden growth spurts and leave the patient with body image issues. ACTH influences the adrenal glands to secrete glucocorticoids; often this is triggered by biological stress.

- Corticosteroids influence metabolism, the immune response, and electrolyte and fluid balance. When replacement or supplementation is indicated, the drugs should be tapered off rather than stopped abruptly, as adrenal insufficiency can result.

Summary Drug Table PITUITARY AND ADRENOCORTICAL HORMONES

Generic Name	Trade Name	Uses	Adverse Reactions	Dosage Ranges
Posterior Pituitary Hormones				
desmopressin *des-moe-press'-in*	DDAVP, Stimate	Diabetes insipidus, hemophilia A, von Willebrand's disease, nocturnal enuresis	Headache, nausea, nasal congestion, abdominal cramps	Doses are individualized, administered orally, intranasally, or subcut
vasopressin *vay-soe-press'-in*		Diabetes insipidus, prevention and treatment of postoperative abdominal distention, to dispel gas interfering with abdominal x-ray examination	Tremor, sweating, vertigo, nausea, vomiting, abdominal cramps, headache	Diabetes insipidus: 5–10 units IM, subcut q 3–4 hr, parenteral solution may be used intranasally

Summary Drug Table PITUITARY AND ADRENOCORTICAL HORMONES (continued)

Generic Name	Trade Name	Uses	Adverse Reactions	Dosage Ranges
Anterior Pituitary Hormones and Hormone Inhibitors				
Gonadotropins: Ovarian Stimulants				
choriogonadotropin alfa *kore-ee-oh-goe-nad'-oh-troe-pin*	Ovidrel	Ovulation induction, follicular maturation	Vasomotor flushes, breast tenderness, abdominal pain, ovarian overstimulation, nausea, vomiting	Injection following follicle stimulation drugs
gonadotropin *goe-nad'-oh-troe-pin*	Bravelle, Follistim AQ, Gonal-f, Gonal-f RFF, Menopur, Repronex	Ovulation induction, multifollicular development, male infertility	Same as choriogonadotropin	Individualized dosing dependent on patient outcome
Gonadotropin-Releasing Hormones/Synthetics				
nafarelin *naf'-ah-rell-in*	Synarel	Endometriosis, precocious puberty	Hot flashes, decreased libido, vaginal dryness, headache, emotional lability	400 mcg/day intranasally in 2 doses
Gonadotropin-Releasing Hormone Antagonists				
cetrorelix *seh-tro'-rell-iks*	Cetrotide	Infertility	Ovarian overstimulation, nausea, vomiting	Dose individualized during cycle
ganirelix *gan-ih-rell'-iks*		Infertility	Abdominal pain, fetal death, headache	250 mcg/day subcut during cycle
Nonsteroidal Ovarian Stimulant				
clomiphene *kloe'-mih-feen*	Clomid, Serophene	Ovulatory failure	Vasomotor flushes, breast tenderness, abdominal discomfort, ovarian enlargement, nausea, vomiting	50 mg/day orally for 5 days, may be repeated
Growth Hormone and Hormone Inhibitors				
somatropin *soe-mah-troe'-pin*	Genotropin, Humatrope, Norditropin, Nutropin, Serostim	Growth failure due to deficiency of pituitary GH in children, replacement of endogenous GH in adults	With injection: diarrhea, arthralgia Long term: growth problems—bone, ear, edema	Doses are individualized, administered by subcut injection weekly
octreotide *ok-tree'-oh-tyde*	Sandostatin	Reduction of GH in acromegaly and treatment of certain tumors	Nausea, diarrhea, abdominal pain, sinus bradycardia, hypoglycemia, injection site pain	50 mcg subcut or IV BID or TID
Adrenocorticotropic Hormone				
adrenocorticotropic hormone *ah-dreen-oh-core-tih-koe-troe'-pik*	ACTH	Diagnose adrenocortical function, nonsuppurative thyroiditis, hypercalcemia, multiple sclerosis	See Display 43.2	20 units IM, subcut QID
cosyntropin	Cortrosyn	Screening for adrenal insufficiency	Dizziness, nausea, vomiting	See package insert

(table continues on page 480)

Summary Drug Table   PITUITARY AND ADRENOCORTICAL HORMONES (continued)

Generic Name	Trade Name	Uses	Adverse Reactions	Dosage Ranges
Glucocorticoids				
betamethasone *bay-tah-meth'-ah-zoan*	Celestone Soluspan	See Display 43.1	See Display 43.2	Individualize dosage; syrup or injectable, see package insert
budesonide *byoo-dess'-oh-nyde*	Entocort EC	Crohn's disease	See Display 43.2	9 mg QD in a.m. for 8 wk
cortisone *kore'-tih-zoan*		See Display 43.1	See Display 43.2	25–300 mg/day orally
dexamethasone *dex-ah-meth'-ah-zoan*		Cerebral edema, other conditions listed in Display 43.1	See Display 43.2	Individualize dosage based on severity of condition and response
hydrocortisone (cortisol) *hye-droe-kore'-tih-zoan*	Cortef, Solu-Cortef, A-Hydrocort	See Display 43.1	See Display 43.2	Individualize dosage based on severity of condition and response
methylprednisolone *meh-thill-pred-niss'-oh-loan*	Medrol, Depo-Medrol, Solu-Medrol	See Display 43.1	See Display 43.2	Individualize dosage based on severity of condition and response
prednisolone *pred-niss'-oh-loan*	Prelone	See Display 43.1	See Display 43.2	200 mg/day for 1 wk, then 80 mg every other day
prednisone *pred'-nih-zoan*		See Display 43.1	See Display 43.2	Individualize dosage: initial dose usually between 5 and 60 mg/day orally
triamcinolone *trye-am-sin'-oh-loan*	Aristospan, Kenalog	See Display 43.1	See Display 43.2	Joint and soft tissue injection: 2–80 mg
Mineralocorticoid				
fludrocortisone *floo-droe-kore'-tih-zoan*		Partial replacement therapy for Addison's disease, salt-losing adrenogenital syndrome	See Display 43.2	0.1 mg 3 times a week to 0.2 mg/day orally
Miscellaneous Hormones and Hormone Inhibitors				
bromocriptine *broe-moe-krip'-tin*	Parlodel	Hyperprolactinemia, acromegaly, Parkinson's disease	Headache, dizziness, fatigue, nausea	5–7.5 mg/day orally
cabergoline *cah-ber'-goe-leen*		Same as bromocriptine	Same as bromocriptine	1 mg twice weekly orally
gonadotropin, chorionic (HCG)	Pregnyl	Testicular descent induction, hypogonadism, ovulation induction	Headache, irritability, fluid retention, fatigue, gynecomastia, aggressive behavior	500–5000 units IM up to 3 times weekly depending on results

● Chapter Review

Know Your Drugs

Clients sometimes know a medication by the brand (or trade) name and not the generic name. To help you recognize both names, match the brand name with the generic name of the same medication.

Generic Name	Brand Name
1. betamethasone	A. Prelone
2. hydrocortisone	B. Medrol
3. methylprednisolone	C. Cortef
4. prednisolone	D. Celestone

Calculate Medication Dosages

1. Hydrocortisone 5 mg twice daily is prescribed. The drug is available in 2.5-mg tablets. The nurse prepares to administer _____.

2. Desmopressin 0.2 mg orally is prescribed. The drug is available in 0.1-mg tablets. The nurse administers _____.

● Prepare for the NCLEX®

Build Your Knowledge

1. Where is the pituitary gland located?
   1. inside the brain
   2. on top of the kidney
   3. suspended from the hypothalamus
   4. directly in front of the trachea

2. The pituitary gland secretes hormones. Which one is secreted by the posterior lobe?
   1. growth hormone
   2. luteinizing hormone
   3. prolactin
   4. vasopressin

3. Which of the following adverse reactions would the nurse expect with the administration of clomiphene?
   1. edema
   2. vasomotor flushes
   3. sedation
   4. hypertension

4. Which of the following signs would lead the nurse to suspect a cushingoid appearance adverse reaction in a client taking a corticosteroid?
   1. moon face, hirsutism
   2. kyphosis, periorbital edema
   3. pallor of the skin, acne
   4. exophthalmos

5. Adverse reactions to the administration of fludrocortisone include _____.
   1. hyperactivity, headache
   2. sedation, lethargy
   3. edema, hypertension
   4. dyspnea, confusion

Apply Your Knowledge

6. Which of the following assessments would be most important for the nurse to make when a child receiving GH comes to the primary health care provider's office?
   1. blood pressure, pulse, and respiration
   2. diet history
   3. height and weight
   4. measurement of abdominal girth

7. Which of the following statements, if made by the client, would indicate a possible adverse reaction to the administration of vasopressin?
   1. "I am unable to see well at night."
   2. "My stomach is cramping."
   3. "I have a sore throat."
   4. "I am hungry all the time."

8. The client makes the following statement: "This is our last try to have a baby." Select the most appropriate nursing diagnosis.
   1. Body Image Disturbance
   2. Anxiety
   3. Acute Confusion
   4. Deficient Fluid Volume

Alternate-Format Questions

9. Harmful drug interactions exist when glucocorticoids are taken with selected drugs. Which drugs increase the effect of the glucocorticoids when taken together? **Select all that apply**.
   1. cholestyramine
   2. oral contraceptives
   3. hydantoins
   4. rifampin

10. Match the lobe of the pituitary gland with the hormone it secretes:

1. anterior	A. ACTH
2. posterior	B. FSH
	C. Oxytocin
	D. TSH

To check your answers, see Appendix G.

the**Point** *For more NCLEX-style questions, log on to http://thepoint.lww.com to access more than 1000 questions.*

44

Thyroid and Antithyroid Drugs

LEARNING OBJECTIVES

On completion of this chapter, the student will:

1. Identify the hormones produced by the thyroid gland.
2. Discuss the uses, general drug actions, adverse reactions, contraindications, precautions, and interactions of thyroid and antithyroid drugs.
3. Discuss important preadministration and ongoing assessment activities the nurse should perform with the patient taking a thyroid or antithyroid drug.
4. Discuss ways to promote an optimal response to therapy, how to manage adverse reactions, and important points to keep in mind when educating patients about the use of thyroid and antithyroid drugs.

KEY TERMS

euthyroid • normal thyroid function

goiter • enlargement of the thyroid gland causing a swelling in the front part of the neck, usually caused by hyperthyroidism

Grave's disease • autoimmune disorder leading to overactivity of the thyroid gland

Hashimoto's thyroiditis • autoimmune disease attacking the thyroid typically resulting in hypothyroid function

hyperthyroidism • overactive thyroid function

hypothyroidism • underactive thyroid function

thyrotoxicosis • severe hyperthyroidism characterized by high fever, extreme tachycardia, and altered mental status (also called *thyroid storm*)

DRUG CLASSES

Antithyroid drugs
Thyroid hormones

The thyroid gland is located in the neck in front of the trachea (Fig. 44.1). This highly vascular gland manufactures and secretes two hormones: thyroxine (T_4) and tri-iodothyronine (T_3). These hormones help to control body metabolism. When the thyroid functions properly this is known as a **euthyroid** (normal thyroid) state. When the thyroid does not work correctly one of two conditions related to the hormone-producing activity of the thyroid gland may occur:

• **Hypothyroidism**—a decrease in the amount of thyroid hormones manufactured and secreted
• **Hyperthyroidism**—an increase in the amount of thyroid hormones manufactured and secreted

In a normal functioning thyroid, when the level of circulating thyroid hormone decreases, the anterior pituitary secretes thyroid-stimulating hormone (TSH), which then activates the cells of the thyroid to release stored thyroid hormones. This process is an example of the feedback mechanism described in Chapter 43.

When a disease such as **Hashimoto's thyroiditis** causes hypothyroidism, thyroid hormones are taken for supplement until the condition can be corrected. When the patient has a condition such as **Grave's disease** (autoimmune disorder), the thyroid gland works harder to produce hormone and individuals may develop a **goiter**. Hyperthyroidism is also caused by inflammation and is called **thyrotoxicosis**. If the condition,

---

PHARMACOLOGY IN PRACTICE

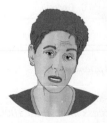

Betty Peterson's neighbor will receive a dose of radioactive iodine for a hyperthyroid illness. Betty is concerned about bringing her daughter's new baby home, thinking that her neighbor may be radioactive after the procedure. Learn in this chapter how to respond to Betty's concerns.

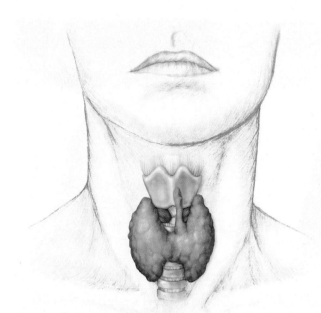

Figure 44.1 Normal thyroid gland. (Courtesy of Anatomical Chart Co.)

such as hyperthyroidism, is due to pregnancy and is correctable, it may be treated with one of the antithyroid drugs. If the condition is not correctable, then radioactive iodine is swallowed to destroy the thyroid so it stops overproducing the hormones. In some cases the thyroid is removed surgically; however, it is more difficult to remove the entire gland.

Unfortunately, when the thyroid is surgically or radiologically removed, the patient becomes *hypothyroid,* and without a functioning thyroid the individual must take thyroid supplements for the remainder of his or her life. The symptoms of hypothyroidism and hyperthyroidism are described in Table 44.1.

THYROID HORMONES

Thyroid hormones used as supplements include both the natural and synthetic hormones. The synthetic hormones are generally preferred because they are more uniform in potency than are the natural hormones obtained from animals. Thyroid hormones are listed in the Summary Drug Table: Thyroid and Antithyroid Drugs.

Actions

The thyroid hormones influence every organ and tissue of the body. These hormones increase the metabolic rate of tissues, which results in increases in the heart and respiratory rate, body temperature, cardiac output, oxygen consumption, and the metabolism of fats, proteins, and carbohydrates. The exact mechanisms by which the thyroid hormones exert their influence on body organs and tissues are not well understood.

Uses

Thyroid hormones are used in the treatment or prevention of *hypothyroidism* caused by the following:

- Subacute or chronic thyroiditis (Hashimoto's disease or viral thyroiditis)

- Hormone supplement after hyperthyroid treatment
- Euthyroid goiter (enlargement of a normal thyroid gland)
- Thyroid nodules and multinodular goiter
- Some types of depression
- Thyroid cancer

Levothyroxine (Synthroid) is the drug of choice for hypothyroidism, because it is relatively inexpensive, requires once-a-day dosage, and has a more uniform potency than do other thyroid hormone replacement drugs. Thyroid hormones also may be used as a diagnostic measure to differentiate suspected hyperthyroidism from euthyroidism.

> **! NURSING ALERT**
>
> Thyroid hormone replacement drugs are not equivalent to each other. Patients should not change brands or types of thyroid hormone without first checking with the primary health care provider. The primary health care provider needs to determine the equivalent dosages when changing medication brands.

Adverse Reactions

Treatment of hypothyroidism is based on individualized doses of the hormone. During initial therapy, the most common adverse reactions are signs of overdose and hyperthyroidism as titration of the drug is being attempted (see Table 44.1). Adverse reactions other than symptoms of hyperthyroidism are rare.

Contraindications and Precautions

These drugs are contraindicated in patients with known hypersensitivity to the drug, an uncorrected adrenal cortical insufficiency, or thyrotoxicosis. These drugs should not be used as a treatment for obesity or infertility. Thyroid hormone should not be used after a recent myocardial infarction. When hypothyroidism is a cause or contributing factor to a myocardial infarction or heart disease, the physician may prescribe small doses of thyroid hormone.

These drugs are used cautiously in patients with cardiac disease and during lactation. Thyroid hormones are classified as pregnancy category A and should be continued by hypothyroid women during pregnancy.

Interactions

The following interactions may occur with thyroid hormones:

Interacting Drug	Common Use	Effect of Interaction
digoxin, beta (β) blockers	Management of cardiac problems	Decreased effectiveness of cardiac drug
oral antidiabetics and insulin	Treatment of diabetes	Increased risk of hypoglycemia
oral anticoagulants	Blood thinners	Prolonged bleeding
Selective serotonin reuptake inhibitor (SSRI) antidepressants	Treatment of depression	Decreased effectiveness of thyroid drug
All other antidepressant drug categories	Treatment of depression	Increased effectiveness of thyroid drug

Table 44.1 Signs and Symptoms of Thyroid Dysfunction

Bodily System or Function	Hypothyroidism	Hyperthyroidism
Metabolism	Decreased, with anorexia, intolerance to cold, low body temperature, weight gain despite anorexia	Increased, with increased appetite, intolerance to heat, elevated body temperature, weight loss despite increased appetite
Cardiovascular	Bradycardia, moderate hypotension	Tachycardia, moderate hypertension
Central nervous system	Lethargy, sleepiness	Nervousness, anxiety, insomnia, tremors, exophthalmos
Skin, skin structures	Pale, cool, dry skin; face appears puffy; coarse hair; nails thick and hard	Flushed, warm, moist skin; thinning hair; goiter
Ovarian function	Heavy menses, may be unable to conceive, loss of fetus possible	Irregular or scant menses
Testicular function	Low sperm count	

ANTITHYROID DRUGS

Antithyroid drugs or thyroid antagonists are used to treat *hyperthyroidism.* In addition to the antithyroid drugs, hyperthyroidism may be treated by the use of radioactive iodine (^{131}I), or by surgical removal of some or almost all of the thyroid gland (subtotal thyroidectomy).

Actions

Antithyroid drugs inhibit the manufacture of thyroid hormones. They do not affect existing thyroid hormones circulating in the blood or stored in the thyroid gland. For this reason, therapeutic effects of the antithyroid drugs may not be observed for 3 to 4 weeks. Antithyroid drugs are listed in the Summary Drug Table: Thyroid and Antithyroid Drugs.

Radioactive iodine (^{131}I) is used because the thyroid has an affinity for iodine. The radioactive isotope accumulates in the cells of the thyroid gland, where destruction of thyroid cells occurs without damaging other cells throughout the body.

Although using isotopes is preferable, it may not be recommended for all patients; therefore, a thyroidectomy may be necessary. Antithyroid drugs may be administered before surgery to return the patient temporarily to a euthyroid state. When used for this reason, the vascularity of the thyroid gland is reduced typically using potassium iodide, and the tendency to bleed excessively during and immediately after surgery is decreased.

Uses

Methimazole (Tapazole) and propylthiouracil (PTU) are used for the medical management of hyperthyroidism. Potassium iodide may be given orally with methimazole or propylthiouracil to prepare for thyroid surgery. Radioactive iodine (^{131}I) is used for treatment of hyperthyroidism and cancer of the thyroid. The drug is given orally either as a solution or in a gelatin capsule.

Adverse Reactions

Generalized System Reactions

- Hay fever, sore throat, skin rash, fever, headache
- Nausea, vomiting, paresthesias

Severe System Reactions

- Agranulocytosis (decrease in the number of white blood cells)
- Exfoliative dermatitis, granulocytopenia, hypoprothrombinemia
- Drug-induced hepatitis

Contraindications, Precautions, and Interactions

The antithyroid drugs are contraindicated in patients with hypersensitivity to the drug or any constituent of the drug.

Mothers taking methimazole or propylthiouracil should not breastfeed their children. Radioactive iodine (pregnancy category X) is contraindicated during pregnancy and lactation.

Methimazole and propylthiouracil are used with extreme caution during pregnancy (pregnancy category D) because they can cause hypothyroidism in the fetus. However, if an antithyroid drug is necessary during pregnancy, propylthiouracil is the preferred drug, because it does not cross the placenta. The potential for bleeding increases when these products are taken with oral anticoagulants.

NURSING PROCESS

PATIENT RECEIVING AN ANTITHYROID DRUG, FOLLOWED BY THYROID HORMONE SUPPLEMENT

ASSESSMENT

Preadministration Assessment

Often a patient is diagnosed with hyperthyroidism, is treated and becomes hypothyroid, and subsequently requires supplementation. Nursing care described here covers the entire continuum of that care. Before a patient starts therapy with either an antithyroid drug or a thyroid hormone, document the history of thyroid-related symptoms (see Table 44.1). It is important to include vital signs, weight, and a notation regarding the subjective symptoms felt by the patient. Lab work will include measuring the TSH as well as T_3 and T_4 levels. When thyroid dysfunction is suspected, serum thyroid antibodies and the TSH level are the best indicators for treatment. If the patient is prescribed an iodine procedure, it is essential to ask about the allergy history, particularly to iodine or seafood (which contains iodine).

 LIFESPAN CONSIDERATIONS
Gerontology
Hypothyroidism may be confused with other conditions associated with aging, such as depression, cold intolerance, weight gain, confusion, or unsteady gait. These symptoms should be thoroughly evaluated before thyroid treatment is started.

Ongoing Assessment

During the ongoing assessment, observe the patient for adverse drug effects.

ANTITHYROID TREATMENT. During the short-term therapy of radioactive treatment, adverse drug reactions are usually minimal. Long-term therapy is usually on an outpatient basis. Ask the patient about relief of symptoms, as well as signs or symptoms indicating agranulocytosis, a possible adverse reaction related to a decrease in blood cells. Inquire about symptoms such as fatigue, fever, sore throat, easy bruising or bleeding, fever, cough, or any other signs of infection. Also monitor the patient for signs of thyrotoxicosis (high fever, extreme tachycardia, and altered mental status), which can occur in patients whose hyperthyroidism increases rather than decreases during therapy.

THYROID SUPPLEMENT. The full effects of thyroid hormone replacement therapy may not be apparent for several weeks or more, but early effects may be apparent in as little as 48 hours. Signs of a therapeutic response include weight loss, mild diuresis, increased appetite, an increased pulse rate, and decreased puffiness of the face, hands, and feet. The patient may also report an increased sense of well-being and increased mental activity.

NURSING DIAGNOSES

Drug-specific nursing diagnoses include the following:

- **Ineffective Protection** related to urinary elimination of radioactive isotopes
- **Risk for Ineffective Self-Health Management** related to consistent dosing or titrating doses
- **Risk for Infection** related to adverse reactions
- **Risk for Impaired Skin Integrity** related to adverse reactions

Nursing diagnoses related to drug administration are discussed in Chapter 4.

PLANNING

The expected outcomes of the patient may include an optimal response to therapy, support of patient needs related to the management of adverse reactions, and confidence in an understanding of the medication regimen.

IMPLEMENTATION

Promoting an Optimal Response to Therapy

ANTITHYROID TREATMENT. The patient with hyperthyroidism may also have cardiac symptoms such as tachycardia or palpitations. Propranolol, an adrenergic blocking drug (see Chapter 25), may be prescribed by the primary health care provider as adjunctive treatment for several weeks until the therapeutic effects of the antithyroid drug are obtained.

Prior home arrangements are made for isolated activities when the patient with an enlarged thyroid gland is given radioactive iodine. The patient stops taking antithyroid drugs about 3 days before the procedure. After midnight, no food or drink is taken; the patient comes to the nuclear medicine department of a facility, swallows the preparation, and returns home. The effects of iodides are evident within 24 hours, with maximum effects attained after 10 to 15 days. If the patient is hospitalized, radiation safety precautions identified by the hospital's department of nuclear medicine are followed.

THYROID SUPPLEMENT. Once a euthyroid state is achieved, the primary health care provider may begin a thyroid hormone supplement to prevent or treat hypothyroidism, which may develop slowly during long-term antithyroid drug therapy or after administration of ^{131}I. Thyroid hormones are administered once a day, early in the morning and preferably before breakfast. An empty stomach increases the absorption of the drug. Thyroid hormone replacement therapy in patients with diabetes may increase the intensity of the symptoms or the diabetes. Closely monitor the patient with diabetes during thyroid hormone replacement therapy for signs of hyperglycemia (see Chapter 42), and notify the primary health care provider if this problem occurs.

Carefully monitor patients with cardiovascular disease who take thyroid hormones. The development of chest pain or worsening of cardiovascular disease should be reported to the primary health care provider immediately, because the patient may require a reduction in the dosage of the thyroid hormone.

LIFESPAN CONSIDERATIONS
Gerontology

The older adult is at increased risk for adverse cardiovascular reactions when taking thyroid drugs. The initial dosage is smaller for an older adult, and increases, if they are necessary, are made in smaller increments during a period of about 8 weeks.

Monitoring and Managing Patient Needs

INEFFECTIVE PROTECTION. When the patient returns home after taking the radioactive preparation, a place in the home where other individuals can be avoided should have been arranged. Avoiding contact with small children and pregnant women is especially important. Private toilet facilities should be provided and the patient flushes twice each time. Eating utensils and laundry should be cleaned separately and the patient should sleep alone. Instructions will be given as to how long the patient should do activities by himself or herself and away from others; typically this lasts for 2 to 4 days.

RISK FOR INEFFECTIVE SELF-HEALTH MANAGEMENT. The patient with hyperthyroidism may be concerned with the results of medical treatment and with the problem of taking the drug at regular intervals around the clock (usually every 8 hours). Whereas some patients may be awake early in the morning and retire late at night, others may experience difficulty with an 8-hour dosage schedule. Another concern may be a tendency to forget the first dose early in the morning, thus causing a problem with the two following doses.

If the patient expresses a concern about the dosage schedule, suggest other options such as an 8-hour interval schedule: 7 a.m., 3 p.m., and 11 p.m. Medication dispensers with alarms are available as well as simply posting a notice on a bathroom mirror to remind the individual that the first dose is due immediately after rising. After a week or more of therapy, most patients remember to take their morning dose on time.

For the hypothyroid patient, once thyroid supplement is started, dosing is individualized to the needs of the patient. If the dosage is inadequate, the patient will continue to experience signs of hypothyroidism. If the dosage is excessive, the patient will exhibit signs of hyperthyroidism. It is important to teach the patient how to monitor reactions and document them well to provide information for correct dosing. This may be a frustrating process for the patient as the primary health care provider makes dose adjustments based on the patient's hormone responses.

RISK FOR INFECTION. Monitor the patient throughout therapy for adverse drug reactions. Teach the patient about signs of agranulocytosis. It is important that the patient learn these signs because reduced white blood cells will put the patient at greater risk for infections, particularly upper respiratory tract infections.

RISK FOR IMPAIRED SKIN INTEGRITY. If the patient experiences a rash while taking methimazole or propylthiouracil, soothing creams or lubricants may be applied, and soap is used sparingly, if at all, until the rash subsides. Drug dosing may need to be changed; report any indication of rash immediately.

Educating the Patient and Family

Thyroid hormones and antithyroid drugs are usually taken on an outpatient basis. Patient instruction should include the importance of taking the drug exactly as directed and not stopping the drug even though symptoms have improved. The drugs absorb better on an empty stomach, so meal timing should be taken into consideration. As you develop a teaching plan for the patient, include the following points:

METHIMAZOLE AND PROPYLTHIOURACIL

- Take these drugs at regular intervals around the clock (e.g., every 8 hours) unless directed otherwise by the primary health care provider.
- Do not take these drugs in larger doses or more frequently than as directed on the prescription container.
- Notify the primary health care provider promptly if any of the following occur: sore throat, fever, cough, easy bleeding or bruising, headache, or a general feeling of malaise.
- Record weight twice a week and notify the primary health care provider if there is any sudden weight gain or loss. (Note: the primary health care provider may also want the patient to monitor pulse rate. If this is recommended, the patient needs instruction in the proper technique and a recommendation to record the pulse rate and bring the record to the primary health care provider's office or clinic.)
- Avoid the use of nonprescription drugs unless the primary health care provider has approved the use of a specific drug.

RADIOACTIVE IODINE

- Follow the directions of the department of nuclear medicine regarding precautions to be taken.
- Keep in mind that tenderness and swelling of the neck, sore throat, and cough may occur in 2 to 3 days after the procedure

THYROID HORMONE

- Replacement therapy is for life, with the exception of transient hypothyroidism seen in those with thyroiditis.
- Do not increase, decrease, or skip a dose unless advised to do so by the primary health care provider.

■ Take this drug in the morning, preferably before breakfast, unless advised by the primary health care provider to take it at a different time of day.

■ Notify the primary health care provider if any of the following occur: headache, nervousness, palpitations, diarrhea, excessive sweating, heat intolerance, chest pain, increased pulse rate, or any unusual physical change or event.

■ Do not change from one brand of this drug to another without consulting the primary health care provider.

EVALUATION

■ Therapeutic effect is achieved.

■ Adverse reactions are identified, reported to the primary health care provider, and managed successfully through appropriate nursing interventions:
  • Patient protects others effectively.
  • Patient manages the therapeutic regimen effectively.

• No evidence of infection is seen.
• Skin remains intact.

■ Patient and family express confidence and demonstrate an understanding of the drug regimen.

PHARMACOLOGY IN PRACTICE
THINK CRITICALLY

 Does Betty have cause for concern about her neighbor being able to contaminate the baby? Discuss how you would present information to Betty to help deal with her fear.

KEY POINTS

• The thyroid gland secretes the hormones thyroxine and tri-iodothyronine, which help to control metabolism. This process is controlled by the pituitary gland when it secretes thyroid-stimulating hormone.

• Hashimoto's thyroiditis is an example of a condition that causes hypothyroidism. When a person has hypothyroidism, presenting problems include decreased metabolism, weight gain, low body temperature, lethargy, and pale, cool, dry skin, along with other symptoms. Grave's disease is an example of a condition that causes hyperthyroidism. When a person has hyperthyroidism, presenting

problems include increased metabolism; weight loss; intolerance to heat; tachycardia; nervousness; anxiety; exophthalmos; flushed, warm skin; and possible goiter, along with other symptoms.

• Hyperthyroid conditions are treated with antithyroid drugs or radioactive iodine to slow or completely eliminate function. Hypothyroidism is treated with thyroid hormone supplementation.

• Common adverse reactions include the opposite action, such as symptoms of hyperthyroidism resulting from too much thyroid hormone replacement.

Summary Drug Table THYROID AND ANTITHYROID DRUGS

Generic Name	Trade Name	Uses	Adverse Reactions	Dosage Ranges
Thyroid Hormones				
levothyroxine (T_4) *lee-voe-thye-rox'-een*	Levothroid, Levoxyl, Synthroid, Unithroid	Hypothyroidism, thyroid- stimulating hormone suppression, thyrotoxicosis, thyroid diagnostic testing	Palpitations, tachycardia, headache, nervousness, insomnia, diarrhea, vomiting, weight loss, fatigue, sweating, flushing	100–125 mcg/day orally
liothyronine (T_3) *lye'-oh-thye'-roe-neen*	Cytomel, Trio stat	Same as levothyroxine	Same as levothyroxine	25–75 mcg/day orally
liotrix (T_3, T_4) *lye'-oh-trix*	Thyrolar	Same as levothyroxine	Same as levothyroxine	Initial: 1 Thyrolar half-grain tablet/day orally Maintenance: 1 Thyrolar, 1-grain or 2-grain tablet/day orally Initial: 30 mg/day orally
thyroid, desiccated	Armour	Same as levothyroxine	Same as levothyroxine	Maintenance: 60–120 mg/day orally
Antithyroid Preparations				
methimazole *meh-thim'-ah-zoll*	Tapazole	Hyperthyroidism	Numbness, headache, loss of hair, skin rash, nausea, vomiting, agranulocytosis	5–40 mg/day orally, divided doses at 8-hr intervals
propylthiouracil (PTU) *proe-pill-thye-oh-yoor'-ah-sill*		Same as methimazole	Same as methimazole	300–900 mg/day orally, divided doses at 8-hr intervals
Iodine Products				
sodium iodide (^{131}I) *eye'-oh-dyde*	Iosotope	Eradicate hyperthyroidism, selected cases of thyroid cancer	Bone marrow depression, nausea, vomiting, tachycardia, itching, rash, hives	Measured by a radioactivity calibration system before administering orally 4–10 microcuries Thyroid cancer: 50–150 mCi

● Chapter Review

Know Your Drugs

Clients sometimes know a medication by the brand (or trade) name and not the generic name. To help you recognize both names, match the brand name with the generic name of the same medication.

Generic Name	Brand Name
1. levothyroxine	A. Armour
2. methimazole	B. PTU (a more commonly used abbreviation)
3. propylthiouracil	C. Synthroid
4. thyroid, desiccated	D. Tapazole

Calculate Medication Dosages

1. Methimazole 40 mg is prescribed. The drug is available in 10-mg tablets. The client is taught to take _____.

2. Levothyroxine 0.2 mg orally is prescribed. Available are 0.1-mg tablets. The client is taught to take _____.

● Prepare for the NCLEX®

Build Your Knowledge

1. What is the function of the thyroid gland?
   1. secrete hormones produced in the pituitary gland
   2. aid in digestion
   3. control metabolism
   4. facilitate breathing

2. Grave's disease is an autoimmune disorder that causes which of the following symptoms?
   1. tachycardia
   2. low body temperature
   3. thick, hard fingernails
   4. low sperm count

3. Hypothyroidism is treated with which of the following interventions?
   1. surgery
   2. hormone replacement
   3. radioactive iodine
   4. Tapazole

4. What adverse reaction is most likely to occur in a client taking a thyroid hormone?
   1. congestive heart failure
   2. hyperthyroidism
   3. hypothyroidism
   4. euthyroidism

5. The nurse informs the client that therapy with a thyroid hormone may not produce a therapeutic response for _____.
   1. 24 to 48 days
   2. 1 to 3 days
   3. several weeks or more
   4. 8 to 12 months

Apply Your Knowledge

6. Which of the following symptoms best indicates a rare but serious adverse reaction is developing in a client receiving methimazole (Tapazole)?
   1. fever, sore throat, bleeding from an injection site
   2. cough, periorbital edema, constipation
   3. constipation, anorexia, blurred vision
   4. unsteady gait, blurred vision, insomnia

7. Which of the following statements made by a client would indicate to the nurse that the client is experiencing an adverse reaction to radioactive iodine?
   1. "I am sleepy most of the day."
   2. "I am unable to sleep at night."
   3. "My throat hurts when I swallow."
   4. "My body aches all over."

8. Which of the following food allergies is of highest concern to the client about to take radioactive iodine?
   1. peanut or other tree nuts
   2. seafood
   3. wheat products
   4. lactose intolerance

Alternate-Format Questions

9. Which drugs are used to treat hypothyroidism? **Select all that apply**.
   1. T_4
   2. Synthroid
   3. thyroid-stimulating hormone
   4. PTU

10. Which hormones are produced by the thyroid gland? **Select all that apply**.
    1. T_3
    2. T_4
    3. thyroid-stimulating hormone
    4. thyroxine

To check your answers, see Appendix G.

thePoint *For more NCLEX-style questions, log on to* http://thepoint.lww.com *to access more than 1000 questions.*

45

Male and Female Hormones

LEARNING OBJECTIVES

On completion of this chapter, the student will:

1. Discuss the medical uses, actions, adverse reactions, contraindications, precautions, and interactions of the male and female hormones.
2. Discuss important preadministration and ongoing assessment activities the nurse should perform with the patient taking male or female hormones.
3. List nursing diagnoses particular to a patient taking male or female hormones.
4. Discuss ways to promote an optimal response to therapy, how to manage adverse reactions, and important points to keep in mind when educating the patient about the use of male or female hormones.

KEY TERMS

anabolism • tissue-building process

androgens • male hormones, responsible for sexual maturity and characteristics

catabolism • tissue-depleting process

endogenous • pertaining to something that normally occurs or is produced within the organism

estrogen • female hormones, responsible for sexual maturity and characteristics

gynecomastia • male breast enlargement

menarche • age of onset of first menstruation

progesterone • female hormone produced by the corpus luteum that works in the uterus (along with estrogen) to prepare the uterus for possible conception

testosterone • primary male sex hormone; acts to stimulate development of the male reproductive organs and secondary sex characteristics

virilization • acquisition of male sexual characteristics by a woman

DRUG CLASSES

Androgens
Estrogens
Progestins

Male and female hormones play a vital role in the development and maintenance of secondary sex characteristics; they are necessary for human reproduction. Although hormones are naturally produced by the body, administration of a male or female hormone may be indicated in the treatment of certain disorders, such as an advanced-stage cancer, male hypogonadism, and male or female hormone deficiency. Hormones also are used as contraceptives and for treating the symptoms of menopause (Chapter 47).

MALE HORMONES

Male hormones—**testosterone** and its derivatives—are collectively called **androgens**. Androgen secretion is influenced by the anterior pituitary gland. Small amounts of male and female hormones are also produced by the adrenal cortex (see Chapter 43). The anabolic steroids are closely related to the

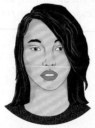

PHARMACOLOGY IN PRACTICE

Janna Wong is at the clinic for a sports physical. After the physical, Janna lingers in the examination room. You knock and ask if everything is okay. She asks you to come in and says she would like to get birth control. After reading the chapter, determine how you would respond to Janna's request.

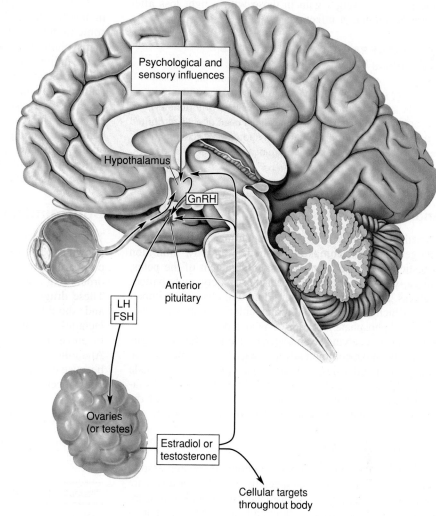

Figure 45.1 The sex hormone relationship to the pituitary and hypothalamus. (From Bear, M. F., Connors, B. W., & Parasido, M. A. [2001]. *Neuroscience–exploring the brain* [2nd ed.]. Philadelphia: Lippincott Williams & Wilkins.)

androgen testosterone and have both androgenic and anabolic (stimulate cellular growth and repair) activity. Androgen hormone inhibitors reduce the conversion of testosterone into a potent androgen (Fig. 45.1).

Actions

Androgens

The male hormone testosterone and its derivatives cause the reproductive maturation in the adolescent boy. From puberty onward, androgens continue to aid in the development and maintenance of secondary sex characteristics: facial hair, deep voice, body hair, body fat distribution, and muscle development. Testosterone also stimulates the growth in size of the sex organs (penis, testes, vas deferens, prostate) at the time of puberty. The androgens also promote tissue-building processes (**anabolism**) and reverse tissue-depleting processes (**catabolism**).

Anabolic Steroids

Anabolic steroids are synthetic drugs chemically related to the androgens. Like the androgens, they promote tissue-building

processes. Given in normal doses, they have a minimal effect on the accessory sex organs and secondary sex characteristics.

Uses

Androgen therapy may be given as replacement therapy for the following:

- Testosterone deficiency
- Hypogonadism (failure of the testes to develop)
- Delayed puberty
- Development of testosterone deficiency after puberty

In the female patient, androgen therapy may be used for:

- Postmenopausal, metastatic breast carcinoma
- Premenopausal, hormone-dependent metastatic breast carcinoma

The transdermal testosterone system is used as replacement therapy when **endogenous** (produced by the body) testosterone is deficient or absent.

Anabolic steroid use includes the following:

- Management of anemia of renal insufficiency
- Control of metastatic breast cancer in women

• Promotion of weight gain in those with weight loss after surgery, trauma, or infections

LIFESPAN CONSIDERATIONS
Young Males
The use of anabolic steroids to promote an increase in muscle mass and strength has become a serious problem. Anabolic steroids are not intended for this use. Unfortunately, deaths in young, healthy individuals have been directly attributed to the use of these drugs. Young men should be discouraged from the illegal use of anabolic steroids to increase muscle mass.

Adverse Reactions

Androgens

In men, administration of an androgen may result in breast enlargement (**gynecomastia**), testicular atrophy, inhibition of testicular function, impotence, enlargement of the penis, nausea, vomiting, jaundice, headache, anxiety, male-pattern baldness, acne, and depression. Fluid and electrolyte imbalances, which include sodium, water, chloride, potassium, calcium, and phosphate retention, may also occur.

In women receiving an androgen preparation for breast carcinoma, the most common adverse reactions are amenorrhea, menstrual irregularities, and **virilization** (acquisition of male sexual characteristics by a woman). Virilization produces facial hair, a deepening of the voice, and enlargement of the clitoris. Male-pattern baldness and acne may also result.

Anabolic Steroids

Virilization in a woman is the most common reaction associated with anabolic steroids, especially when higher doses are used. Acne occurs frequently in all age groups and both sexes. Nausea, vomiting, diarrhea, fluid and electrolyte imbalances (the same as for the androgens, discussed previously), testicular atrophy, jaundice, anorexia, and muscle cramps may also be seen. Blood-filled cysts of the liver and sometimes the spleen, malignant and benign liver tumors, an increased risk of atherosclerosis, and mental changes are the most serious adverse reactions that may occur during prolonged use.

Many serious adverse drug reactions are being reported in healthy individuals using anabolic steroids. There is some indication that prolonged high-dose use has resulted in psychological and possibly physical dependence, and some individuals have required treatment in drug rehab centers. Severe mental changes, such as uncontrolled rage (called "roid rage"), severe depression, and suicidal tendencies; malignant and benign liver tumors; aggressive behavior; increased risk of atherosclerosis; inability to concentrate; and personality changes are not uncommon. In addition, the incidence of the severe adverse reactions cited earlier appears to be increased in those using anabolic steroids for this purpose.

Contraindications and Precautions

The male hormones are contraindicated in patients with known hypersensitivity to the drugs, liver disorders, or serious cardiac disease, and in men with prostate gland disorders (e.g., prostate carcinoma and prostate enlargement). These drugs are classified as pregnancy category X drugs and should not be administered during pregnancy and lactation. Anabolic steroids are contraindicated for use to enhance physical appearance or athletic performance. Anabolic steroids should be used cautiously in older men because of increased risk of prostate enlargement and prostate cancer.

Interactions

The following interactions may occur with the male hormones:

Interacting Drug	Common Use	Effect of Interaction
oral anticoagulants	Blood thinners	Increased antidiuretic effect
imipramine and androgen	Treatment of depression	Increased risk of paranoid behavior
sulfonylureas and anabolic steroids	Diabetes	Increased risk of hypoglycemia

---

NURSING PROCESS
PATIENT RECEIVING A MALE HORMONE

ASSESSMENT

Preadministration Assessment
Assessment of the patient receiving an androgen or anabolic steroid depends on the drug, the patient, and the reason for administration.

ANDROGENS. In most instances, androgens are administered to the man on an outpatient basis. Before and during therapy, the primary health care provider may order electrolyte studies, because use of these drugs can result in fluid and electrolyte imbalances.

When these drugs are given to the female patient with advanced breast carcinoma, evaluate the patient's current status (physical, emotional, and nutritional) carefully and record the findings in the patient's chart. Problem areas such as pain, any limitation of motion, and the ability to participate in the activities of daily living are carefully evaluated and recorded in the patient's record. You should take and document vital signs and weight. Baseline laboratory tests may include a complete blood count, hepatic function tests, serum electrolytes, and serum and urinary calcium levels. Review these tests and note any abnormalities.

ANABOLIC STEROIDS. Evaluate and document the patient's physical and nutritional status before starting therapy with anabolic steroids. Note the patient's weight, blood pressure, pulse, and respiratory rate. Baseline laboratory studies may include a complete blood count, hepatic function tests, and serum electrolytes and serum lipid levels. Review these studies and note any abnormalities.

Ongoing Assessment

The ongoing assessment depends on the reason the drug was prescribed and the condition of the patient. Men receiving an androgen or anabolic steroid are questioned regarding the effectiveness of drug therapy.

Track the weight of the patient with advanced breast carcinoma daily or as ordered by the primary health care provider. Contact the primary health care provider if there is a significant (5-lb) increase or decrease in the weight. Check the lower extremities frequently for signs of edema.

Teach the patient or caregiver to observe for adverse drug reactions, especially signs of fluid and electrolyte imbalance, jaundice (which may indicate hepatotoxicity), and virilization. The primary health care provider must be alerted to any signs of fluid and electrolyte imbalance or jaundice.

When the patient is hospitalized, review vital signs every 4 to 8 hours, depending on the patient's condition, and then evaluate the patient's response to drug therapy based on original assessment findings. Possible responses include a decrease in pain, an increase in appetite, and a feeling of well-being.

LIFESPAN CONSIDERATIONS
Chronic Care

When the androgens are administered to a patient with diabetes, blood glucose levels should be measured frequently because glucose tolerance may be altered. Adjustments may need to be made in insulin dosage, oral antidiabetic drugs, or diet.

When anabolic steroids are used for weight gain, the patient is weighed at intervals ranging from daily to weekly. A good dietary regimen is necessary to promote weight gain. Consult the dietitian if the patient eats poorly.

NURSING DIAGNOSES

Drug-specific nursing diagnoses include the following:

- **Excess Fluid Volume** related to adverse reactions (sodium and water retention)
- **Disturbed Body Image** (in the female) related to adverse reactions (virilization)

Nursing diagnoses related to drug administration are discussed in Chapter 4.

PLANNING

The expected outcomes of the patient may include an optimal response to therapy, support of patient needs related to the management of adverse reactions, and confidence in an understanding of the medication regimen.

IMPLEMENTATION

Promoting an Optimal Response to Therapy

If the androgen is to be administered as a buccal tablet, show the patient how to place the tablet and warn the patient not to swallow the tablet but to allow it to dissolve in the mouth. Remind the patient not to smoke or drink water until the tablet is dissolved. Oral and parenteral androgens are often

taken or given by injection on an outpatient basis. When given by injection, the injection is administered deep intramuscularly (IM) into the gluteal muscle. Alternatively, a pellet dose is placed under the skin and repeated every 3 to 6 months. Oral testosterone is given with or before meals to decrease gastrointestinal (GI) upset.

Androderm is a transdermal system that is applied nightly to clean, dry skin on the abdomen, thigh, back, or upper arm. This system is not applied to the scrotum. Sites are rotated, with 7 days between applications to any specific site. The system is applied immediately after opening the pouch and removing the protective covering. If the patient has not exhibited a therapeutic response after 8 weeks of therapy, another form of testosterone replacement therapy should be considered. When the system is removed it should be folded in half on itself to prevent accidental dosing if touched.

Testosterone gel (AndroGel) is applied once daily (preferably in the morning) to clean, dry, intact skin of the shoulders and upper arms or abdomen. After the packet is opened, the contents are squeezed into the palm of the hand and immediately applied to the application sites. The application sites are allowed to dry before the patient gets dressed. The gel is not applied to the genitals. Wear gloves if applying to another person; wash hands well with soap and water for self-applications.

Axiron is a liquid preparation that is sprayed into the axillae daily. It is a fast-drying liquid being tested for ease of use.

Monitoring and Managing Patient Needs

Observe the patient receiving an androgen or anabolic steroid for signs of adverse drug reactions.

EXCESS FLUID VOLUME. Sodium and water retention may also occur with androgen or anabolic steroid administration, causing the patient to become edematous. In addition, other electrolyte imbalances, such as hypercalcemia, may occur. Monitor the patient for fluid and electrolyte disturbances.

LIFESPAN CONSIDERATIONS
Gerontology

Older adults with cardiac problems or kidney disease are at increased risk for sodium and water retention when taking androgens or anabolic steroids.

To monitor for fluid retention, make a daily comparison of the patient's preadministration weight with current weights and make sure to note the appearance of puffy eyelids and dependent swelling of the hands or feet (if the patient is ambulatory) or the sacral area (if the patient is nonambulatory), and report any findings to the primary health care provider. Daily fluid intake and output should be used to calculate fluid balance, too.

DISTURBED BODY IMAGE. With long-term administration of a male hormone, the female patient may experience mild to moderate masculine changes (virilization), namely, facial hair, a deepening of the voice, and enlargement of the clitoris. Male-pattern baldness, patchy hair loss, skin pigmentation, and acne may also result. Although these adverse effects are not life-threatening, they often are distressing and only add to the patient's discomfort and anxiety. These problems may be easy to identify, but they are not always easy to solve. If hair loss occurs, suggest wearing head coverings such as hats, scarves, or a wig; mild skin pigmentation may be covered with makeup, but severe and widespread pigmented areas and acne are often difficult to conceal. Each patient is different, and the emotional responses to these outward changes may range from severe depression to a positive attitude and acceptance. Work with the patient as an individual, first identifying the problems, and then helping the patient, when possible, to deal with these changes.

Educating the Patient and the Family

Explain the dosage regimen and possible adverse drug reactions to the patient and family and develop a teaching plan to include the following points:

ANDROGENS

- *Notify the primary health care provider if any of the following occurs:* nausea, vomiting, swelling of the legs, or jaundice. Women should report any signs of virilization to the primary health care provider.
- *Oral tablets*—Take with food or a snack to avoid GI upset.
- *Buccal tablets*—Place the tablet between the cheek and molars and allow it to dissolve in the mouth. Do not smoke or drink water until the tablet is dissolved.
- *Testosterone transdermal system*—Apply according to the directions supplied with the product. Be sure the skin is clean and dry and the placement area is free of hair. Do not store outside the pouch or use damaged systems. Discard systems in household trash in a safe manner to prevent ingestion by children or pets.

ANABOLIC STEROIDS

- Anabolic steroids may cause nausea and GI upset. Take this drug with food or meals.
- Keep all primary health care provider or clinic visits, because close monitoring of therapy is essential.
- Female patients: Notify the primary health care provider if signs of virilization occur.

EVALUATION

- Therapeutic response is achieved.
- Adverse reactions are identified, reported to the primary health care provider, and managed successfully with appropriate nursing interventions:
  - Adequate fluid volume is maintained.
  - Perceptions of body changes are managed successfully.
- Patient and family express confidence and demonstrate an understanding of the drug regimen.

FEMALE HORMONES

The two endogenous (produced by the body) female hormones are **estrogen** and **progesterone**. Like the androgens, their production is under the influence of the anterior pituitary gland. The endogenous estrogens are estradiol, estrone, and estriol. The most potent of these three estrogens is estradiol. Examples of estrogens used as drugs include estropipate (Ortho-Est) and estradiol (Estrace).

There are natural and synthetic progesterones, which are collectively called progestins. Examples of progestins used as drugs include medroxyprogesterone (Provera) and norethindrone (Aygestin).

Actions

Estrogens

Estrogens are secreted by the ovarian follicle and in smaller amounts by the adrenal cortex. Estrogens are important in the development and maintenance of the female reproductive system and the primary and secondary sex characteristics. At puberty, they promote growth and development of the vagina, uterus, fallopian tubes, and breasts. They also affect the release of pituitary gonadotropins (see Chapter 43).

Other actions of estrogen include fluid retention, protein anabolism, thinning of the cervical mucus, and inhibition or facilitation of ovulation. Estrogens contribute to the conservation of calcium and phosphorus, the growth of pubic and axillary hair, and pigmentation of the breast areolae and genitals. Estrogens also stimulate contraction of the fallopian tubes (which promotes movement of the ovum). They modify the physical and chemical properties of the cervical mucus and restore the endometrium after menstruation.

Progestins

Progesterone is secreted by the corpus luteum, placenta, and (in small amounts) adrenal cortex. Progesterone and its derivatives (the progestins) transform the proliferative endometrium into a secretory endometrium. Progestins are necessary for the development of the placenta and inhibit the secretion of pituitary gonadotropins, which in turn prevents maturation of the ovarian follicle and ovulation. The synthetic progestins are usually preferred for medical use because of the decreased effectiveness of progesterone when administered orally.

Uses

Estrogens

Estrogen is most commonly used in combination with progesterones as a contraceptive agent (Table 45.1) or as estrogen replacement therapy (ERT) in postmenopausal women. ERT and other uses of postmenopausal estrogen are discussed in Chapter 47.

Progestins

Progestins are used in the treatment of amenorrhea, endometriosis, and functional uterine bleeding. Progestins are also used as oral contraceptives, either alone or in combination with an estrogen (see the Summary Drug Table: Male and Female Hormones; see also Table 45.1).

Contraceptive Hormones

Combination estrogens and progestins are used as oral contraceptives. There are three types of estrogen and progestin combination oral contraceptives: monophasic, biphasic,

Table 45.1 Examples of Oral Contraceptives

Generic Name	Trade Name
Monophasic Oral Contraceptives	
20 mcg ethinyl estradiol, 0.1 mg levonorgestrel	Alesse, Aviane, Lessina, Levlite
35 mcg ethinyl estradiol, 0.25 mg norgestimate	Ortho-Cyclen, Sprintec
35 mcg ethinyl estradiol, 0.5 mg norethindrone	Brevicon, Modicon
30 mcg ethinyl estradiol, 0.15 mg levonorgestrel	Jolessa, Levlen, Levora, Nordette, Portia, Quasense, Seasonale
30 mcg ethinyl estradiol, 0.3 mg norgestrel	Lo/Ovral, Low-Ogestrel, Cryselle
35 mcg ethinyl estradiol, 1 mg norethindrone	Norinyl 1 + 35, Ortho-Novum 1/35
50 mcg ethinyl estradiol, 1 mg norethindrone	Norinyl 1 + 50, Ortho-Novum 1/50
30 mcg ethinyl estradiol, 1.5 mg norethindrone	Junel 21 1.5/30, Junel Fe, Loestrin 21 1.5/30, Loestrin Fe 1.5/30, Microgestin Fe 1.5/30
20 mcg ethinyl estradiol, 1 mg norethindrone	Junel 21 1/20, Junel Fe 1/20, Loestrin 21 1/20, Loestrin Fe 1/20, Microgestin Fe 1/20
50 mcg ethinyl estradiol, 1 mg ethynodiol	Demulen 1/50, Zovia 1/50E
35 mcg ethinyl estradiol, 0.5 mg norethindrone	Brevicon, Modicon
35 mcg ethinyl estradiol, 0.4 mg norethindrone	Ovcon-35
20/10 mcg ethinyl estradiol, 0.15 mg desogestrel	Kariva, Mircette
30 mcg ethinyl estradiol, 0.15 mg desogestrel	Apri, Desogen, Ortho-Cept, Reclipsen
35 mcg ethinyl estradiol, 1 mg ethynodiol	Demulen 1/35, Zovia 1/35E
30 mcg ethinyl estradiol, 3 mg drospirenone	Yasmin
20 mcg ethinyl estradiol, 3 mg drospirenone	YAZ
Biphasic Oral Contraceptives	
Phase one: 35 mcg ethinyl estradiol, 0.5 mg norethindrone	Necon 10/11, Ortho-Novum 10/11
Phase one: 30 mcg ethinyl estradiol, 0.15 mg levonorgestrel	Seasonique
Triphasic Oral Contraceptives	
Phase one: 25 mcg ethinyl estradiol, 0.18 mg norgestimate	Ortho Tri-Cyclen Lo
Phase one: 30 mcg ethinyl estradiol, 0.05 mg levonorgestrel	Triphasil, Tri-Levlen, Trivora, Enpresse
Phase one: 35 mcg ethinyl estradiol, 0.18 mg norgestimate	Ortho Tri-Cyclen, Tri-Sprintec, Tri-Previfem, TriNessa
Phase one: 35 mcg ethinyl estradiol, 0.5 mg norethindrone	Aranelle, Leena, Tri-Norinyl
Phase one: 35 mcg ethinyl estradiol, 0.5 mg norethindrone	Necon 7/7/7, Ortho-Novum 7/7/7
Phase one: 1 mg norethindrone acetate, 20 mcg ethinyl estradiol	Estrostep Fe, Estrostep 21
Phase one: 25 mcg ethinyl estradiol, 0.1 mg desogestrel	Cesia, Cyclessa
Progestin-Only Contraceptive	
0.35 mg norethindrone	Camila, Errin

and triphasic. Monophasic oral contraceptives provide a fixed dose of estrogen and progestin throughout the cycle. The biphasic and triphasic oral contraceptives deliver hormones similar to the levels naturally produced by the body (see Table 45.1). Oral contraceptives have changed a great deal since their introduction in the 1960s. Today, lower hormone dosages provide reduced levels of hormones compared with the older formulations, while retaining the same degree of effectiveness (more than 99% when used as prescribed).

Taking contraceptive hormones provides health benefits not related to contraception, such as regulating the menstrual cycle and decreasing menstrual blood loss, the incidence of iron deficiency anemia, and dysmenorrhea. Health benefits related to the inhibition of ovulation include a decrease in ovarian cysts and ectopic pregnancies. In addition, there is a decrease in fibrocystic breast disease, acute pelvic inflammatory disease, endometrial cancer, and ovarian cancer; improved maintenance of bone density; and a decrease in symptoms related to endometriosis in women taking contraceptive hormones. Newer combination contraceptives such as drospirenone and ethinyl estradiol combinations (YAZ) have been shown to help reduce moderate acne and maintain clear skin in women 15 years of age or older (who menstruate, want contraception, and have no response to topical antiacne medications).

Adverse Reactions: Estrogens

Administration of estrogens by any route may result in many adverse reactions, although the incidence and intensity of these reactions vary. Some of the adverse reactions seen with the administration of estrogens follow.

Central Nervous System Reactions

• Headache, migraine
• Dizziness, mental depression

Dermatologic Reactions

• Dermatitis, pruritus
• Chloasma (pigmentation of the skin) or melasma (discoloration of the skin), which may continue when use of the drug is discontinued

Gastrointestinal Reactions

• Nausea, vomiting
• Abdominal bloating and cramps

Genitourinary Reactions

• Breakthrough bleeding, withdrawal bleeding, spotting, change in menstrual flow
• Dysmenorrhea, premenstrual-like syndrome, amenorrhea
• Vaginal candidiasis, cervical erosion, vaginitis

Local Reactions

• Pain at injection site or sterile abscess with parenteral form of the drug
• Redness and irritation at the application site with transdermal system

Ophthalmic Reactions

• Steepening of corneal curvature
• Intolerance to contact lenses

Miscellaneous Reactions

• Edema, rhinitis, changes in libido
• Breast pain, enlargement, and tenderness
• Reduced carbohydrate tolerance
• Venous thromboembolism, pulmonary embolism
• Weight gain or loss
• Generalized and skeletal pain

Warnings associated with the administration of estrogen include an increased risk of endometrial cancer, gallbladder disease, hypertension, hepatic adenoma (a benign tumor of the liver), cardiovascular disease, and thromboembolic disease, and hypercalcemia in those with breast cancer and bone metastases.

Adverse Reactions: Progestins

Administration of progestins by any route may result in many adverse reactions, although the incidence and intensity of these reactions vary. Progestin administration may result in the following:

• Breakthrough bleeding, spotting, change in menstrual flow, amenorrhea
• Breast tenderness, edema, weight increase or decrease
• Acne, chloasma or melasma, insomnia, mental depression

In addition to the adverse reactions seen with progestins, the use of a levonorgestrel implant system may result in bruising after insertion, scar tissue formation at the site of insertion, and hyperpigmentation at the implant site. The use of medroxyprogesterone contraceptive injection may result in the same adverse reactions as those associated with administration of any progestin.

Adverse Reactions: Contraceptive Hormones

When estrogen–progestin combinations are used as oral contraceptives, these drugs may exhibit adverse reactions that vary depending on their estrogen or progestin content, so the adverse reactions of each must be considered. Table 45.2 identifies the symptoms of estrogen and progestin excess or

Table 45.2 Estrogen and Progestin: Excess and Deficiency		
Hormone*	**Signs of Excess**	**Signs of Deficiency**
estrogen	Nausea, bloating, cervical mucorrhea (increased cervical discharge), polyposis (numerous polyps), hypertension, migraine headache, breast fullness or tenderness, edema	Early or midcycle breakthrough bleeding, increased spotting, hypomenorrhea, melasma (discoloration of the skin)
progestin	Increased appetite, weight gain, tiredness, fatigue, hypomenorrhea, acne, oily scalp, hair loss, hirsutism (excessive growth of hair), depression, monilial vaginitis, breast regression	Late breakthrough bleeding, amenorrhea, hypermenorrhea

*Hormonal balance is achieved by adjusting the estrogen/progestin dosage. Oral contraceptives have different amounts of progestin and estrogen, varying the estrogenic and progestational activity in each product.

deficiency. The adverse effects are minimized by adjusting the estrogen–progestin balance or dosage.

Contraindications and Precautions

Estrogen and progestin therapy is contraindicated in patients with known hypersensitivity to the drugs, breast cancer (except for metastatic disease), estrogen-dependent neoplasms, undiagnosed abnormal genital bleeding, and thromboembolic disorders. The progestins also are contraindicated in patients with cerebral hemorrhage or impaired liver function. Both the estrogens and progestins are classified as pregnancy category X drugs and are contraindicated during pregnancy.

Estrogens are used cautiously in patients with gallbladder disease, hypercalcemia (may lead to severe hypercalcemia in patients with breast cancer and bone metastasis), cardiovascular disease, and liver impairment. Cardiovascular complications are greater in women who smoke and use estrogen. Progestins are used cautiously in patients with a history of migraine headaches, epilepsy, asthma, and cardiac or renal impairment.

The warnings associated with the use of oral contraceptives, notably the combined drug contraceptives, are the same as those for the estrogens and progestins and include cigarette smoking (especially those older than 35 years of age), which increases the risk of cardiovascular side effects, such as venous and arterial thromboembolism, myocardial infarction, and thrombotic and hemorrhagic stroke. Also reported with oral contraceptive use are hepatic adenomas and other tumors, visual disturbances, gallbladder disease, hypertension, and fetal abnormalities.

Interactions

The following interactions may occur with female hormones:

Interacting Drug	Common Use	Effect of Interaction
Estrogens		
oral anticoagulants	Blood thinners	Decreased anticoagulant effect
tricyclic antidepressants	Treatment of depression	Increased effectiveness of antidepressant
rifampin	anti-infective	Increased risk of breakthrough bleeding
hydantoins	Seizure control	Increased risk of breakthrough bleeding and pregnancy
Progestins		
anticonvulsants or rifampin	Seizure control or anti-infective, respectively	Decreased effectiveness of progestin
penicillins or tetracyclines	Anti-infective agents	Decreased effectiveness of oral contraceptives

NURSING PROCESS
PATIENT RECEIVING A FEMALE HORMONE

ASSESSMENT

Preadministration Assessment
Before administering an estrogen or progestin, obtain a complete patient health history, including a menstrual history, which includes the menarche (age of onset of first menstruation), menstrual pattern, and any changes in the menstrual pattern (including a menopause history when applicable). Document the patient's sexual history and reason for contraception. Evaluate the patient's understanding of safe sexual practices and understanding that hormonal contraceptives do not protect against sexually transmitted infections (STIs). Inquire about a history of thrombophlebitis or other vascular disorders, a smoking history, and a history of liver diseases. Blood pressure, pulse, and respiratory rate are taken and documented. The primary health care provider usually performs a breast and pelvic examination and a Papanicolaou (Pap) test before starting therapy.

If the female patient is being treated for cancer, enter in the patient's record a general evaluation of the patient's physical and mental status. The primary health care provider may also order laboratory tests, such as serum electrolytes and liver function tests.

Ongoing Assessment
At the time of each office or clinic visit, the blood pressure, pulse, respiratory rate, and weight are checked. Ask the patient about any adverse drug effects as well as the result of drug therapy. Weigh the patient and report a steady weight gain or loss. A periodic (usually annual) physical examination is performed by the primary health care provider and may include a pelvic examination, breast examination, Pap test, and laboratory tests.

NURSING DIAGNOSES
Drug-specific nursing diagnoses include the following:

- **Effective Self-Health Management** related to administration of medications routinely despite adverse reactions
- **Excess Fluid Volume** related to sodium and water retention
- **Ineffective Tissue Perfusion** related to thromboembolic effects
- **Imbalanced Nutrition: More or Less Than Body Requirements** related to weight gain or loss

Nursing diagnoses related to drug administration are discussed in Chapter 4.

PLANNING
The expected outcomes of the patient may include an optimal response to therapy, support of patient needs related to the management of adverse reactions, and confidence in an understanding of the medication regimen.

IMPLEMENTATION

Promoting an Optimal Response to Therapy

ESTROGENS. Estrogens may be administered orally, IM, intravenously (IV), transdermally, or intravaginally. Outpatient use as a contraceptive is typically self-administered by the oral route. The transdermal delivery route has been found to be safer, especially for women with elevated triglycerides, type 2 diabetes, hypertension, or migraine headaches, or those who smoke.

CONTRACEPTIVE HORMONES. Monophasic oral contraceptives are administered on a 21-day regimen, with the first tablet taken on the first Sunday after the menses begin or on the day the menses begin if the menses begin on Sunday. After the 21-day regimen, the next 7 days are skipped, and then the cycle is begun again. With the biphasic oral contraceptives, the first phase is 10 days of a smaller dosage of progestin, and the second phase is a larger amount of progestin. The estrogen dosage remains constant for 21 days, followed by no estrogen for 7 days. Some regimens contain seven placebo tablets for easier management of the therapeutic regimen. With the triphasic oral contraceptives, the estrogen amount stays the same or may vary, and the progestin amount varies throughout the 21-day cycle. Progestin-only oral contraceptives are taken daily and continuously.

CONTRACEPTIVE IMPLANT SYSTEM. Levonorgestrel, a progestin, is available as an implant contraceptive system (Norplant System). Six capsules, each containing levonorgestrel, are implanted using local anesthesia in the subdermal (below the skin) tissues of the midportion of the upper arm. The capsules provide contraceptive protection for 5 years but may be removed at any time at the request of the patient. See Display 45.1 for more information on ways to promote an optimal response when taking the contraceptive hormones.

MEDROXYPROGESTERONE CONTRACEPTIVE INJECTION. Medroxyprogesterone (Depo-Provera), a synthetic progestin used in the treatment of abnormal uterine bleeding and secondary amenorrhea, is also used as a contraceptive. This drug is given IM every 3 months, and the initial dosage is given within the first 5 days of menstruation or within 5 days postpartum. When this drug is given IM, the solution must be shaken vigorously before use to ensure uniform suspension, and the drug is given deep IM into the gluteal or deltoid muscle.

! NURSING ALERT

If the interval is greater than 14 weeks between the IM injections of medroxyprogesterone, be certain that the patient is not pregnant before administering the next injection.

Monitoring and Managing Patient Needs

EFFECTIVE SELF-HEALTH MANAGEMENT. The patient prescribed female hormones usually takes them for several months or years. Throughout that time, the patient must be monitored for adverse reactions. These drugs are self-administered at home. Patients may decide to regulate their own drug doses to alleviate adverse reactions; this can lead to ineffective dosing and more unwanted reactions such as pregnancy. Therefore, patient education is an important avenue for detecting and managing adverse reactions.

With estrogens, it is important to monitor for breakthrough bleeding. If breakthrough bleeding occurs with either estrogen or progestin, the patient notifies the primary health care provider. A dosage change may be necessary.

GI upsets such as nausea, vomiting, abdominal cramps, and bloating may also occur. Nausea usually decreases or subsides within 1 to 2 months of therapy. However, until then the discomfort may be decreased if the drug is taken with food. If nausea is continual, frequent small meals may help. If nausea and vomiting persist, an antiemetic may be prescribed. Bloating may be alleviated with light to moderate exercise or by limiting fluid intake with meals.

Carefully monitor the patient with diabetes who is taking female hormones. The primary health care provider is notified if blood glucose levels are elevated or the urine is positive for ketone bodies, because a change in the dosage of insulin or the oral antidiabetic drug may be required. See Chapter 42 for the management of hypoglycemic and hyperglycemic episodes.

EXCESS FLUID VOLUME. Sodium and water retention may occur during female hormone therapy. In addition to reporting any swelling of the hands, ankles, or feet to the primary health care provider, weigh the hospitalized patient daily, keep an accurate record of the intake and output, encourage ambulation (if not on bed rest), and help the patient to eat a diet low in sodium (if prescribed by the primary health care provider).

INEFFECTIVE TISSUE PERFUSION. Teach the patient how to monitor for signs of thromboembolic effects, such as pain, swelling, and tenderness in the extremities, headache, chest pain, and blurred vision. These adverse effects are reported immediately to the primary health care provider. Patients with previous venous insufficiency, who are on bed rest for other medical reasons, taking combined drug contraceptives, or who smoke are at increased risk for thromboembolic effects. Encourage the patient to elevate the lower extremities when sitting, if possible, and to exercise the lower extremities by walking.

! NURSING ALERT

There is an increased risk of postoperative thromboembolic complications in women taking oral contraceptives. If possible, use of the drug is discontinued at least 4 weeks before a surgical procedure associated with thromboembolism or during prolonged immobilization.

IMBALANCED NUTRITION: MORE OR LESS THAN BODY REQUIREMENTS. Alterations in nutrition can occur, resulting in significant weight gain or loss. Weight gain occurs more frequently than weight loss. Encourage a daily diet that includes adequate amounts of protein and carbohydrates and is low in fats. A variety of nutritious foods (fruits, vegetables, grains, cereals, meats, and poultry) should be included in the daily diet, with portion sizes decreased to meet individual needs. A dietitian may be consulted if necessary. An exercise program is helpful in both losing weight and maintaining weight loss.

Weight loss is often as difficult to manage as weight gain. When a patient taking the female hormones has a decrease in appetite and loses weight, encourage the individual to increase protein, carbohydrates, and calories in the diet. Small feedings with several daily snacks are usually better tolerated in those with a loss of appetite than are three larger

Display 45.1 Alternatives to Oral Contraceptive Hormones

Patients who choose to use contraceptive hormone preparations need to be fully informed of their benefits and drawbacks. You can be instrumental in educating patients about these drugs. Included here are contraceptive methods used by women in place of the traditional oral contraceptive pills.

Emergency Contraceptives (Plan B)
These preparations are used for emergency contraception after unprotected intercourse or known contraceptive failure. They prevent pregnancy; they do not work if the patient is already pregnant.

• When using high-dose levonorgestrel (Plan B), take one tablet within 72 hours after unprotected intercourse. Take the second dose of Plan B 12 hours later.
• This drug can be used any time during the menstrual cycle.
• If vomiting occurs within 1 hour after taking either dose, notify the primary health care provider.
• Emergency contraceptives are not effective in terminating an existing pregnancy.
• Emergency contraceptives should not be used as a routine form of contraception.

Etonogestrel/Ethinyl Estradiol Vaginal Ring (NuvaRing)
• The woman inserts the vaginal ring into the vagina, where it remains continuously for 3 weeks. It is removed for 1 week, during which bleeding usually occurs (usually 2 to 3 days after removal).
• Insert a new ring 1 week after the last ring was removed, on the same day of the week as it was inserted in the previous cycle. Do this even if bleeding is not finished.
• *Insertion:* Position for insertion by the woman may be standing with one leg up, squatting, or lying down. Compress the ring and insert into the vagina. (The exact position of the vaginal ring inside the vagina is not critical to its effectiveness.)
• The vaginal ring is removed after 3 weeks on the same day of the week as it was started. Removal is accomplished by hooking the index finger under the forward rim or by grasping the rim between the thumb and index finger and pulling it out. Discard the used ring in the foil pouch in a waste receptacle out of the reach of children or pets. (Do not flush the ring down the toilet.)
• Consider the menstrual cycle, timing of ovulation, and possibility of pregnancy before beginning treatment.
• The vaginal ring may be accidentally expelled (e.g., when it was not inserted properly, during straining for defecation, while removing a tampon, or with severe constipation). If this occurs, rinse the vaginal ring with lukewarm water and reinsert promptly. (If the ring has been out of the vagina

for more than 3 hours, contraceptive effectiveness may be reduced and an alternative contraceptive must be used for the next 7 days.)
• The most common adverse effects leading to discontinuation of contraceptive use involve device-related problems, such as foreign body sensations, coital problems, and device expulsion.
• Other adverse effects include vaginitis, headache, upper respiratory tract infection, leukorrhea, sinusitis, weight gain, and nausea.

Levonorgestrel Implants (Norplant System)
This is a long-term (5-year) reversible contraceptive system, and an informed consent may be required in some institutions before implementing this procedure. The patient needs to know that a surgical incision is required to insert six capsules and that removal also requires surgical intervention.

Levonorgestrel-Releasing Intrauterine System (Mirena)
The capsules of the levonorgestrel-releasing intrauterine system (LRIS) are inserted during the first 7 days of the menstrual cycle or immediately after a first-trimester abortion. LRIS is an intrauterine contraception device for use for not more than 5 years. Before insertion, provide the patient with the patient package insert. Also before insertion, a complete medical and social history, including that of the partner, is obtained to determine conditions that might influence the use of an intrauterine device (IUD). Several patient teaching points follow:

• Irregular menstrual bleeding, spotting, prolonged episodes of bleeding, and amenorrhea may occur. These symptoms diminish with continued use. The patient should check after each menstrual period to ensure that the thread attached to the LRIS still protrudes from the cervix. Caution her not to pull the thread.
• If pregnancy occurs with the LRIS in place, the LRIS should be removed. If the LRIS is not removed there is an increased risk of miscarriage/abortion, sepsis, premature labor, and premature delivery.
• The patient should self-monitor for flu-like symptoms, fever, chills, cramping, pain, bleeding, vaginal discharge, or leakage of fluid.
• Re-examination and evaluation are done shortly after the first menses or within the first 3 months after insertion.
• Menstrual flow usually decreases after the first 3 to 6 months of LRIS use; therefore, an increase of menstrual flow may indicate expulsion of the device.
• Symptoms of partial or complete expulsion include pain and bleeding. However, the LRIS also can be expelled without any noticeable effects.

(display continues on page 500)

Display 45.1 Alternatives to Oral Contraceptive Hormones (continued)

Medroxyprogesterone Contraceptive Injection (Depo-Provera)

Medroxyprogesterone is available as a long-term injectable contraceptive administered IM every 3 months. The injection is given only during the first 5 days after the onset of a normal menstrual period, within 5 days postpartum if the woman is not breast-feeding, or at 6 weeks postpartum. Patient teaching points include the following:

- Bleeding irregularities may occur (i.e., irregular or unpredictable bleeding or spotting, or heavy continuous bleeding). Bleeding usually decreases to amenorrhea as treatment continues.
- Women tend to gain weight while using this form of contraception.
- The drug is not readministered if there is a sudden partial or complete loss of vision or if the patient experiences ptosis, diplopia, depression, or migraine.

Norelgestromin/Ethinyl Estradiol Transdermal System (Ortho Evra)

- The system is designed around a 28-day cycle, with a new patch applied each week for 3 weeks. Week 4 is patch free.
- Apply the new patch on the same day each week (note patch change day on the calendar).
- Discard used patch (only wear one patch at a time).
- Use no creams or lotions on area where patch is to be applied. Apply patch to clean, dry, intact, healthy skin

on the buttock, abdomen, upper outer arm, or upper torso in a place where the patch will not be rubbed by clothing. Patch should not be placed on the breast or on areas that are red or irritated.

- *Beginning treatment:* First day start (apply first patch on the first day of the menstrual cycle) or Sunday start (apply first patch on the first Sunday after the menstrual period begins).
- A backup contraceptive should be used for the first week of the *first* treatment cycle.
- If the patch partially or completely detaches for less than 24 hours, reapply to the same place or replace with a new patch immediately (no backup contraception needed).
- If the patch detaches for more than 24 hours, apply a new patch immediately (new patch change day). Backup contraception is needed for the first week (7 days) of the new cycle.
- If the patch change is forgotten, begin again immediately, making this day the new patch change day. (Backup contraception is needed for the first 7 days.)
- If breakthrough bleeding continues longer than a few cycles, a cause other than the patch should be considered. Do not stop patch if bleeding occurs.
- Bleeding should occur during the patch-free week. If no bleeding occurs, consider the possibility of pregnancy.
- If pregnancy is confirmed, discontinue treatment.

---

meals. Patients are encouraged to eat foods they like. Dietary supplements may be necessary if a significant weight loss occurs. A dietitian may be consulted if necessary. Weights are usually taken on a weekly, rather than daily, basis.

Educating the Patient and Family

The instructions for starting oral contraceptive therapy vary with the product used. Each product has detailed patient instruction sheets regarding starting oral contraceptive therapy. The instructions for missed doses also are included in the package insert and are reviewed with the patient. Advise those taking oral contraceptives that skipping a dose could result in pregnancy. See Display 45.1 for more information to include in a teaching plan for a woman taking contraceptive hormones. Be sure the patient is confident in understanding the directions provided for contraception.

In most instances, the primary health care provider performs periodic examinations, such as laboratory analyses, a pelvic examination, or a Pap test. The patient is encouraged to keep all appointments for follow-up evaluation of therapy. Include the following points in your teaching plan:

ESTROGENS AND PROGESTINS

- Carefully read the patient package insert available with the drug. If there are any questions about this information, discuss them with the primary health care provider.

- If GI upset occurs, take the drug with food.
- Notify the primary health care provider if any of the following occurs: pain in the legs or groin area; sharp chest pain or sudden shortness of breath; lumps in the breast; sudden severe headache; dizziness or fainting; vision or speech disturbances; weakness or numbness in the arms, face, or legs; severe abdominal pain; depression; or yellowing of the skin or eyes.
- If pregnancy is suspected or abnormal vaginal bleeding occurs, stop taking the drug and contact the primary health care provider immediately.
- Patient with diabetes: Check the blood glucose daily, or more often. Contact the primary health care provider if the blood glucose is elevated. An elevated blood glucose level may require a change in diabetic therapy (insulin, oral antidiabetic drug) or diet; these changes must be made by the primary health care provider.

ORAL CONTRACEPTIVES

- A package insert is available with the drug. Read the information carefully. Begin the first dose as directed in the package insert or as directed by the primary health care provider. If there are any questions about this information, discuss them with the primary health care provider.

■ To obtain a maximum effect, take this drug as prescribed and at intervals not exceeding once every 24 hours. An oral contraceptive is best taken with a routine daily behavior, such as with the evening meal or at bedtime. The effectiveness of this drug depends on following the prescribed dosage schedule. Failure to comply with the dosage schedule may result in a pregnancy.

■ Use an additional method of birth control (as recommended by the primary health care provider) until after the first week in the next cycle.

■ If one day's dose is missed, take the missed dose as soon as remembered or take two tablets the next day. If 2 days are missed, take two tablets for the next 2 days and continue on with the normal dosing schedule. However, another form of birth control must be used until the cycle is completed and a new cycle is begun. If 3 days in a row or more are missed, discontinue use of the drug and use another form of birth control until a new cycle can begin. Before restarting the dosage regimen, make sure a pregnancy did not result from the break in the dosage regimen.

■ If there are any questions regarding what to do about a missed dose, discuss the procedure with the primary health care provider.

■ Avoid smoking or excessive exposure to second-hand smoke while taking these drugs; cigarette smoking during estrogen therapy may increase the risk of cardiovascular effects.

■ Report adverse reactions such as fluid retention or edema to the extremities; weight gain; pain, swelling, or tenderness in the legs; blurred vision; chest pain; yellowed skin or eyes; dark urine; or abnormal vaginal bleeding.

■ Remember that while taking these drugs, patients need periodic examinations by the primary health care provider and laboratory tests.

EVALUATION

■ Therapeutic effect is achieved.

■ Adverse reactions are identified, reported to the primary health care provider, and managed using appropriate nursing interventions.
  • Patient manages the therapeutic regimen effectively.
  • Adequate fluid volume is maintained.
  • Tissue perfusion is maintained.
  • Patient maintains an adequate nutritional status.

■ Patient expresses confidence and verbalizes the importance of adhering to the prescribed therapeutic regimen.

PHARMACOLOGY IN PRACTICE
THINK CRITICALLY

 What are some assessment questions you will ask Janna about her request for birth control? Can she make this request without her mother's permission at age 16 in your community? How might you help Janna discuss the question of using birth control with her mother?

KEY POINTS

• Secondary sex characteristics as well as human reproduction are directed by male and female hormones. Supplement of naturally occurring hormones is necessary for some conditions, in treating certain cancers, and when a deficiency occurs.

• Testosterone and its derivatives are called androgens—or the male hormones—and are secreted by the anterior pituitary gland. These hormones promote reproductive maturation and the development of secondary sex characteristics (e.g., facial hair and deeper voice). They also promote tissue and muscle building. Anabolic steroids are synthetic drugs chemically similar to androgens.

• Adverse reactions include gynecomastia, testicular atrophy, impotence, nausea, vomiting, and male-pattern baldness. When used to reduce female hormone production in women, menstrual issues and virilization are adverse reactions.

• Estrogen and progesterone are the two hormones produced in the female body. Estrogen is secreted by the anterior pituitary gland and progesterone by the corpus luteum of the ovary. These hormones promote reproductive maturation and the development of secondary sex characteristics (e.g., breast development and pigmentation of areolae and genitals). Estrogen is used for contraception and replacement therapy following menopause, and progestin is used for both contraception and menstrual issues.

• Adverse reactions include headache, depressive mood, nausea, vomiting, skin discoloration, and menstrual irregularities.

Summary Drug Table MALE AND FEMALE HORMONES

Generic Name	Trade Name	Uses	Adverse Reactions	Dosage Ranges
Androgens				
fluoxymesterone *floo-oxi-mes'-ter-own*		Males: hypogonadism, delayed puberty Females: inoperable advanced breast cancer	Nausea, vomiting, acne, hair thinning, headache, libido changes, anxiety, mood changes, hematopoietic and electrolyte imbalances Males: gynecomastia, testicular atrophy, erectile dysfunction Females: amenorrhea, virilization	Males: 5–20 mg/day orally Females: 10–40 mg/day orally
methyltestosterone *meth-ill-tess-toss'-ter-own*	Testred	Same as fluoxymesterone	Same as fluoxymesterone	Males: 10–50 mg/day orally Females: 50–200 mg/day orally
testosterone *tess-toss'-ter-own*	AndroGel, Androderm & Testim (Transdermal) Delatestryl, Depo-Testosterone (injectable), Striant (oral, buccal) Testopel (pellet insert), Axiron (axilla spray)	Primary or hypogonadotropic hypogonadism, delayed puberty	Same as fluoxymesterone	Buccal: 30 mg BID Gel: apply daily Injectable: 50–400 mg every 2–4 wk Pellet: 150–450 mg subcut every 3–6 mo Transdermal: 6 mg/day, apply patch daily Spray: 30–120 mg daily
Anabolic Steroids				
nandrolone *nan'-droe-loan*		Anemia of renal insufficiency, human immunodeficiency virus (HIV) wasting syndrome	Nausea, vomiting, diarrhea, acne, hair thinning, libido changes, anxiety, mood changes, edema, anemia, electrolyte imbalances Males: gynecomastia, testicular atrophy, sexual dysfunction Females: amenorrhea, virilization	50–200 mg/wk IM
oxymetholone *ox-e-meth'-o-loan*	Anadrol-50	Anemia	Same as nandrolone	1–5 mg/kg/day orally
oxandrolone *ox-an'-droe-loan*	Oxandrin	Bone pain, weight gain, protein catabolism	Acne, hair thinning, libido changes, anxiety, mood changes, edema, electrolyte imbalances Males: gynecomastia, testicular atrophy, sexual dysfunction Females: amenorrhea, virilization	2.5–20 mg/day orally in divided doses
Estrogens				
estrogens, conjugated *ess'-troe-jens*	Premarin	Oral: hypogonadism, primary ovarian failure Parenteral: abnormal uterine bleeding from hormonal imbalance	Headache, dizziness, melasma, venous thromboembolism, nausea, vomiting, abdominal bloating and cramps, breakthrough bleeding/spotting, vaginal changes, rhinitis, changes in libido, breast enlargement and tenderness, weight changes, generalized pain	0.3–2.5 mg/day orally IM: 25 mg/injection

Summary Drug Table MALE AND FEMALE HORMONES (continued)

Generic Name	Trade Name	Uses	Adverse Reactions	Dosage Ranges
estrogens, esterified	Menest	Same as conjugated estrogens	Same as conjugated estrogens	0.3–1.25 mg/day orally
estradiol cypionate *ess-trah-dye'-ole 'sip-ee-oh-nate*	Depo-Estradiol	Female hypogonadism	Same as conjugated estrogens; pain at injection site	1–5 mg IM every 3–4 wk
estradiol transdermal system	Alora, Climara, Estraderm, Menostar, Vivelle	Same as conjugated estrogens	Same as conjugated estrogens	Variable doses, applied to skin weekly
estropipate *ess-troe-pye'-pate*	Ogen (cream), Ortho-Est (tablet)	Female hypogonadism, ovarian failure	Same as conjugated estrogens	0.625–9 mg/day orally
Progestins				
progesterone *pro-jess'-ter-own*	Crinone, Prometrium	Endometrial hyperplasia (oral), amenorrhea, abnormal uterine bleeding (injection), infertility (gel)	Breakthrough bleeding, spotting, change in menstrual flow, amenorrhea, breast tenderness, weight gain or loss, melasma, insomnia	Orally: 200 mg for 12 days of cycle IM: 5–10 mg/day for 6–8 days Gel: 90 mg/day
medroxyprogesterone *meh-drox'-ee-proe-jess'-ter-own*	Provera	Amenorrhea, abnormal uterine bleeding, endometrial hypoplasia	Same as progesterone	5–10 mg/day orally
norethindrone *nor-eth-in'-drone*	Aygestin	Amenorrhea, abnormal uterine bleeding, endometriosis	Same as hydroxyprogesterone caproate	2.5–10 mg/day for 5–10 days of cycle

● Chapter Review

Know Your Drugs

Clients sometimes know a medication by the brand (or trade) name and not the generic name. To help you recognize both names, match the brand name with the generic name of the same medication.

Generic Name	Brand Name
1. conjugated estrogen	A. Climara
2. medroxyprogesterone	B. Premarin
3. methyltestosterone	C. Provera
4. transdermal estradiol	D. Testred

Calculate Medication Dosages

1. Medroxyprogesterone 650 mg IM is prescribed. The drug is available in a solution of 400 mg/mL. The nurse administers _____.

2. Nandrolone 100 mg IM is prescribed. The drug is available in a solution of 100 mg/mL. The nurse administers _____.

● Prepare for the NCLEX®

Build Your Knowledge

1. Which hormone is secreted by the anterior pituitary gland?
   1. estrogen
   2. oxytocin
   3. progesterone
   4. testosterone

2. The nurse monitors the client taking an anabolic steroid for the more severe adverse reactions, which include _____.
   1. anorexia
   2. nausea and vomiting
   3. severe mental changes
   4. acne

3. The nurse must be aware that older men taking androgens are _____.
   1. prone to urinary problems
   2. at greater risk for hypertension
   3. at increased risk for confusion
   4. at increased risk for prostate cancer

4. When monitoring a client taking an oral contraceptive, the nurse would observe the client for signs of excess progestin. Which of the following reactions would indicate to the nurse that a client has an excess of progestin?
   1. increased appetite, hair loss
   2. virilization, constipation
   3. nausea, early breakthrough bleeding
   4. deepening of the voice, lightheadedness

5. When teaching the client taking an oral contraceptive for the first time, the nurse emphasizes the importance of taking _____.
   1. two tablets per day at the first sign of ovulation
   2. the drug at the same time each day
   3. the drug early in the morning before arising
   4. the drug each day for 20 days beginning on the first of the month

6. Which hormone when given to women can cause virilization?
   1. androgen
   2. estrogen
   3. progesterone
   4. thyroid

Apply Your Knowledge

7. A client calls the outpatient clinic and says that she missed 1 day's dose of her "birth control pills." Which of the following statements would be most appropriate for the nurse to make to the client?
   1. Do not take an additional tablet but resume the regular schedule today.
   2. Discontinue use of the drug and use another type of contraceptive until after your next menstrual period.
   3. Take two tablets today; then resume the regular daily schedule.
   4. Come into the office immediately for a pregnancy test.

8. The following statement indicates that the client understands the purpose of birth control pills:
   1. "These will protect me from STIs."
   2. "I must take one each time I have sex to prevent pregnancy."
   3. "If I miss a couple of days, I should use an additional birth control method."
   4. "I put the medicine in water and it works better."

Alternate-Format Questions

9. The drug YAZ is a combination of different medications. Which drugs are in this pill? **Select all that apply**.
   1. estradiol
   2. drospirenone
   3. levonorgestrel
   4. norethindrone

10. The anabolic steroids can cause which of the following unpleasant adverse reactions? **Select all that apply**.
    1. gynecomastia
    2. jaundice
    3. testicular atrophy
    4. virilization

To check your answers, see Appendix G.

thePoint *For more NCLEX-style questions, log on to http://thepoint.lww.com to access more than 1000 questions.*

Uterine Drugs

KEY TERMS

albuminuria • excessive protein in the urine

antepartum • the time during pregnancy before childbirth

eclampsia • a condition where seizures and possible coma happen in pregnancy after 20 weeks in a woman who has become hypertensive, with excess protein found in the urine

placenta previa • during pregnancy the placenta implants in the lower part of the uterus, possibly over the cervix

preeclampsia • a condition in pregnancy after 20 weeks in a woman when she becomes hypertensive, with excess protein found in the urine

tocolysis • to prevent preterm labor

uterine atony • marked relaxation of the uterine muscle

water intoxication • fluid overload in the body when electrolytes are imbalanced

DRUG CLASSES

Oxytocic drugs
Tocolytics

D rug therapy is beneficial for use in labor and delivery to promote the well-being of a woman and her fetus. Depending on the patient's need, drugs may be used to stimulate, intensify, or inhibit uterine contractions. The two types of drugs discussed in this chapter for their effect on the uterus are the oxytocics and the tocolytics. Drugs acting on the uterus are listed in the Summary Drug Table: Uterine Drugs.

OXYTOCIC DRUGS

Oxytocic drugs are used **antepartum** (before birth of the neonate) to induce uterine contractions similar to those of normal labor. These drugs are desirable when vaginal delivery has not begun and when it is in the best interest of the woman and the fetus to initiate it. An oxytocic drug is one that stimulates the uterus.

Action and Uses

Oxytocin

Oxytocin is an endogenous hormone produced by the posterior pituitary gland (Fig. 46.1). This hormone has uterus-stimulating properties, acting on the smooth muscle

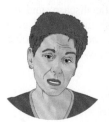

PHARMACOLOGY IN PRACTICE

Betty Peterson's daughter has been admitted to the obstetric unit and is being induced. This is her daughter's first child, and Betty is extremely anxious. After reading this chapter, think about the information that would be helpful to the family.

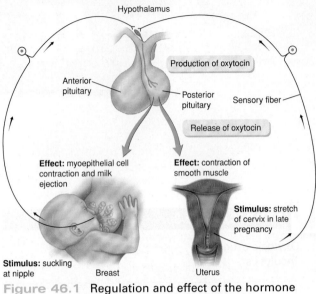

Figure 46.1 Regulation and effect of the hormone oxytocin. (From Premkumar, K. [2004]. *The massage connection: Anatomy and physiology.* Baltimore: Lippincott Williams & Wilkins.)

of the uterus, especially on the pregnant uterus. As pregnancy progresses, the sensitivity of the uterus to oxytocin increases, reaching a peak immediately before the birth of the infant. This sensitivity enables oxytocic drugs to exert their full therapeutic effect on the uterus and produce the desired results. Oxytocin also has antidiuretic and vasopressor effects.

Oxytocin is administered intravenously (IV) for starting or improving labor contractions. Drugs may be used to induce an early vaginal delivery when there are fetal or maternal problems, such as a woman with diabetes and a large fetus, Rh problems, premature rupture of the membranes, uterine inertia, and **preeclampsia** (also called pregnancy-induced hypertension). Preeclampsia is a condition of pregnancy characterized by hypertension, headache, **albuminuria**, and edema of the lower extremities occurring at, or near, term. The condition may progressively worsen until **eclampsia** (a serious condition occurring between the 20th week of pregnancy and the end of the first week postpartum and characterized by convulsive seizures and coma) occurs. Oxytocin may also be used in managing inevitable or incomplete abortion. Oxytocin can be given intramuscularly (IM) during the third stage of labor (period from the time the neonate is expelled until the placenta is expelled) to produce uterine contractions and control postpartum bleeding and hemorrhage. Some women find that when taken intranasally to stimulate the milk ejection (milk letdown) reflex they can breastfeed successfully. Although intranasal preparations are not commercially available, compounding pharmacies have made them for women.

Other Uterine Stimulants

Uterine stimulants increase the strength, duration, and frequency of uterine contractions and decrease the incidence of uterine bleeding. They are given after the delivery of the placenta and are used to prevent postpartum and postabortal hemorrhage caused by **uterine atony** (marked relaxation of the uterine muscle). These drugs include carboprost, methylergonovine, and misoprostol.

Adverse Reactions

Oxytocin

Administration of oxytocin may result in the following:

- Fetal bradycardia, uterine rupture, uterine hypertonicity
- Nausea, vomiting, cardiac arrhythmias, anaphylactic reactions

Oxytocin is similar to the hormone vasopressin and because of its antidiuretic effect, serious **water intoxication** (fluid overload, fluid volume excess) may occur, particularly when the drug is administered by continuous infusion and the patient is receiving fluids by mouth.

Other Uterine Stimulants

Adverse reactions associated with other uterine stimulants include the following:

- Nausea, vomiting, diarrhea
- Elevated blood pressure, temporary chest pain
- Dizziness, water intoxication, headache

Allergic reactions may also occur. In some instances hypertension associated with seizure or headache may occur.

Contraindications, Precautions, and Interactions

Oxytocin is contraindicated in patients with known hypersensitivity to the drug, cephalopelvic disproportion, and unfavorable fetal position or presentation. It is also contraindicated in obstetric emergencies, situations of fetal distress when delivery is not imminent, severe preeclampsia, eclampsia, and hypertonic uterus, as well as during pregnancy when there is total **placenta previa**. It is contraindicated as an agent to induce labor when vaginal delivery is contraindicated. Oxytocin is not expected to be a risk to the fetus when administered as indicated. When oxytocin is administered with vasopressors, however, severe maternal hypertension may occur.

Methylergonovine is not used before delivery of the placenta. It is contraindicated in those with known hypersensitivity to the drug or hypertension. This drug is used cautiously in patients with heart disease, vascular disease with narrowed vessels, and renal or hepatic disease, and during lactation. When methylergonovine is administered concurrently with vasopressors or to patients who are heavy cigarette smokers, excessive vasoconstriction may occur.

NURSING PROCESS

PATIENT RECEIVING AN OXYTOCIC DRUG

ASSESSMENT

Preadministration Assessment

Before starting an IV infusion of oxytocin to induce labor, obtain an obstetric history (e.g., parity, gravidity, previous obstetric problems, type of labor, stillbirths, abortions, live-birth infant abnormalities) and a general health history.

Keep a record of the activity of the uterus (strength, duration, and frequency of contractions, if any). Monitoring uterine contractions for strength and length of the contractions can be done with an external monitor or by an internal uterine catheter with an electronic monitor. A fetal monitor is placed to assess the fetal heart rate (FHR). Immediately before starting the IV infusion of oxytocin, assess and document the FHR and the patient's blood pressure, pulse, and respiratory rate.

The other uterine stimulants may be given orally or IM during the postpartum period to reduce the possibility of postpartum hemorrhage and to prevent relaxation of the uterus. When the patient is to receive any of these drugs after delivery, it is important to take the blood pressure, pulse, and respiratory rate before administration.

Ongoing Assessment

After injecting an oxytocic drug, both the mother's contractions and the fetal heart rate are monitored continuously. Three to four firm uterine contractions should occur every 10 minutes, followed by a palpable relaxation of the uterus. Hyperstimulation of the uterus during labor may lead to uterine tetany with marked impairment of the uteroplacental blood flow, uterine rupture, cervical rupture, amniotic fluid embolism, and trauma to the infant. Overstimulation of the uterus is dangerous to both the fetus and the mother and may occur even when the drug is administered properly in a uterus that is hypersensitive to oxytocin.

> **NURSING ALERT**
>
> All patients receiving IV oxytocin must be under constant observation to identify complications. In addition, the health care provider attending the delivery should be immediately available at all times.

When monitoring uterine contractions, notify the health care provider attending the delivery immediately if any of the following occurs:

- A significant change in the FHR or rhythm
- A marked change in the frequency, rate, or rhythm of uterine contractions; uterine contractions lasting more than 60 seconds; or contractions occurring more frequently than every 2 to 3 minutes, or no palpable relaxation of the uterus
- A marked increase or decrease in the patient's blood pressure or pulse or any significant change in the patient's general condition (vital signs are typically obtained every 15 to 30 minutes in active labor)

If any of these conditions are noted, immediately discontinue the oxytocin infusion and run the primary IV line at the rate prescribed by the health care provider attending the delivery until the patient is examined.

Report any signs of water intoxication or fluid overload (e.g., drowsiness, confusion, headache, listlessness, and wheezing, coughing, or rapid breathing) to the health care provider attending the delivery.

Oxytocin may be given IM after delivery of the placenta. After administering the drug, continue to take vital signs every 5 to 10 minutes. Palpate the patient's uterine fundus for firmness and position. Report immediately any excess bleeding to the health care provider attending the delivery.

When administering methylergonovine after delivery, monitor vital signs every 4 hours and also note the character and amount of vaginal bleeding. The patient may report abdominal cramping with the administration of these drugs. If cramping is moderately severe to severe, contact the health care provider attending the delivery because it may be necessary to discontinue use of the drug.

NURSING DIAGNOSES

Drug-specific nursing diagnoses include the following:

- **Anxiety** related to fears associated with the process of labor and delivery
- **Risk for Injury** (fetal) related to adverse drug effects of oxytocin on the fetus (fetal bradycardia)
- **Excess Fluid Volume** related to administration of IV fluids and the antidiuretic effects associated with oxytocin
- **Acute Pain** related to adverse reactions (abdominal cramping, nausea, headache)

Nursing diagnoses related to drug administration are discussed in Chapter 4.

PLANNING

The expected patient outcomes may include an optimal response to drug therapy (e.g., initiation of the normal labor process), adverse reactions (e.g., absence of a fluid volume excess with oxytocin administration) identified and reported to the health care provider attending the delivery, and confidence in an understanding of the medication regimen.

IMPLEMENTATION

Promoting an Optimal Response to Therapy

OXYTOCIN. When oxytocin is prescribed, the drug may come in a premixed solution such as 10 units in 1,000 mL of solution (0.01 units/1 mL). By using premixed solutions, errors are prevented because all patients are using the same dilution in a solution. An electronic infusion device is used to control the infusion rate. Frequently, health care providers attending deliveries establish protocol guidelines for administering the oxytocin solution and for increasing or decreasing the flow rate or discontinuing the administration of oxytocin. The flow rate is usually increased every 20 to 30 minutes, but this may vary according to the patient's response. The strength, frequency, and duration of contractions and the FHR are monitored closely.

METHYLERGONOVINE. Administer methylergonovine at the direction of the health care provider attending the delivery. Methylergonovine is usually given IM at the time of the delivery of the anterior shoulder or after the delivery of the placenta. The drug is not given routinely IV because it may produce sudden hypertension and stroke. If the drug is ordered IV, administer it slowly over a period of 1 minute or more with close monitoring of the patient's blood pressure. Although you may try to explain the purpose of the drug, which is to improve the tone of the uterus and help the uterus to return to its (near) normal size, the excitement of a new baby may interfere with the mother's understanding. You may need to repeat this should she wonder about the uterine sensations.

Misoprostol tablets are administered vaginally to induce or augment uterine contractions. Care should be taken that hyperstimulation of the uterus causing uterine tetany does not occur.

Monitoring and Managing Patient Needs

ANXIETY. When given to induce or stimulate contractions, oxytocin is given IV. The patient receiving oxytocin may have concern over the use of the drug to produce contractions. This may be contrary to the birth plan of the mother. By explaining the purpose of the IV infusion and the expected results to the patient, you can be supportive of her desires for a successful birth. Because the patient receiving oxytocin must be closely supervised, use the time with the patient to offer encouragement and reassurance to help reduce anxiety.

RISK FOR INJURY (FETAL). When oxytocin is administered, some adverse reactions must be tolerated or treated symptomatically until therapy is discontinued. For example, if the patient is nauseated, provide an emesis basin and perhaps a cool towel for the forehead. If vomiting occurs, provide rinsing solutions to freshen the mouth.

If contractions are frequent, prolonged, or excessive, the infusion is stopped to prevent fetal anoxia or trauma to the uterus. Excessive stimulation of the uterus can cause uterine hypertonicity and possible uterine rupture. Place the patient on her left side and provide supplemental oxygen. The effects of the drug diminish rapidly, because oxytocin is a short-acting drug.

EXCESS FLUID VOLUME. Track fluid intake and output; when oxytocin is administered IV, there is a danger of an excessive fluid volume (water intoxication), because oxytocin has an antidiuretic effect. In some instances, hourly measurements of output are necessary. Observe the patient for signs of fluid overload (see Chapter 54). If any of these signs or symptoms is noted, immediately discontinue the oxytocin infusion but let the primary IV line run at the rate ordered until the patient is examined.

ACUTE PAIN. When methylergonovine is administered for uterine atony and hemorrhage, abdominal cramping can occur and is usually an indication of drug effectiveness. The uterus is palpated in the lower abdomen as small, firm, and round. However, report persistent or severe cramping to the primary health care provider.

Educating the Patient and Family

The treatment regimen is explained to the patient and family (when appropriate). Answer any questions the patient may have regarding treatment and instruct the patient to report any adverse reactions. Also inform the patient and family about the therapeutic response during administration of the drug, and if nasal spray is to be used, teach the patient the proper technique.

EVALUATION

- Therapeutic effect is achieved and normal labor is initiated.
- Adverse reactions are identified, reported to the primary health care provider, and managed successfully through appropriate nursing interventions:
  - Anxiety is managed successfully.
  - No evidence of injury is seen.
  - Fluid volume balance is maintained.
  - Patient is free of pain.
- Patient expresses confidence and demonstrates an understanding of the drug regimen.

TOCOLYTICS

Premature births make up 11% of all the births in the United States. When a baby is born early the organs are not mature, especially the lungs. This leads to significant problems and even death. In some of the developing countries, the rate of premature birth is as high as 25%. Minority groups also have more premature births with the highest rate seen in black women. Preterm labor (PTL) is one of the leading causes of premature births. **Tocolysis** is a term meaning to prevent PTL. Therefore, tocolytic drugs are used to stop labor (Fig. 46.2). Although a number of studies have been done, the conclusions do not strongly support using drugs to stop PTL. Researchers do agree that gaining a few days for the fetus to stay in the uterus is beneficial (Valdes, 2012).

Actions and Uses

Tocolytics are generally used during a pregnancy of between 24 and 33 weeks' gestation. Indomethacin is a nonsteroidal anti-inflammatory drug that blocks the production of substances called *prostaglandins* (see Chapter 14), which contribute to uterine contractions. Beta (β)-2-adrenergic and calcium channel blockers are used to delay the delivery process for 24 to 48 hours. These drugs block the contractions of the smooth muscle of the uterus. This amount of time is often sufficient to allow the pregnant woman to be transferred to an acute care facility that deals with preterm deliveries or gives time to administer corticosteroids to the fetus in utero to enhance organ maturity. Magnesium at one time was one of the most commonly used drugs to decrease uterine muscle contractions, and is used for seizure control with eclampsia.

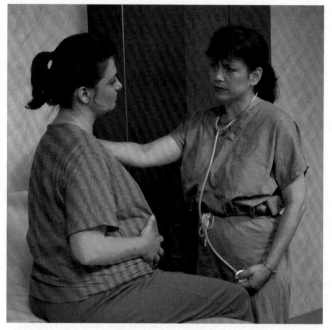

Figure 46.2 Tocolytic agents help gain time for fetal organ maturity.

Magnesium is a calcium antagonist that works to decrease the force of uterine contractions. Because of the risk of serious adverse reactions, the use of terbutaline for more than 48 hours or in the home setting is not advised.

Adverse Reactions

Adverse reactions include the following:

- Fatigue, flushing, headache, dizziness, diplopia
- Nausea, vomiting, stomach upset, heartburn
- Prolonged vaginal bleeding
- Sweating, hypotension, depressed reflexes, and flaccid paralysis are other adverse reactions associated with IV administration. They are related to hypocalcemia induced by the therapy.

Contraindications, Precautions, and Interactions

Magnesium and calcium channel blockers are contraindicated in patients with known hypersensitivity to these drugs, in patients with heart block or myocardial damage, and when the woman is within 2 hours of delivery. Magnesium is classified as a pregnancy category A drug, calcium channel blockers are pregnancy category C, and indomethacin is a pregnancy category B drug. Although these drugs are given for preterm labor, they still should be given cautiously during pregnancy.

There is an increased effectiveness of central nervous system depressants (e.g., opioids, analgesics, and sedatives) when magnesium is administered. The effectiveness of neuromuscular blocking agents is enhanced as well. See Chapters 14 and 35, respectively, for drug interactions with indomethacin and calcium channel blockers.

Uterine Drugs

NURSING PROCESS
PATIENT RECEIVING A TOCOLYTIC AGENT

ASSESSMENT

Preadministration Assessment
A patient history is taken of previous pregnancy experiences (such as PTL or preeclampsia) as well as other risk factors (such as infections or cigarette smoking). Ask the patient about symptoms such as back pain or cramping, discharge, or fluid from the vagina. A fetal fibronectin test (protein) to gauge PTL will be done. Once PTL is established, vital signs are taken and a respiratory system assessment is made before starting an IV infusion containing a tocolytic drug. The patient has a monitoring device in place to determine uterine contractions and the FHR before and during administration.

Before magnesium is initiated, baseline blood tests (e.g., complete blood count and creatinine level) are performed. Because magnesium affects the neuromuscular system, a neurologic examination is performed as well. Mentation, cranial nerve function, and deep tendon reflexes are assessed. When indomethacin is used as the tocolytic drug, additional tests include liver function tests and amniotic fluid index.

Ongoing Assessment
During the ongoing assessment of a patient receiving a tocolytic drug, nursing activities include the following at 15- to 30-minute intervals:

- Obtaining blood pressure, pulse, and respiratory rate
- Monitoring FHR
- Checking the IV infusion rate
- Examining the area around the IV needle insertion site for signs of infiltration
- Monitoring uterine contractions (frequency, intensity, length)
- Measuring maternal intake and output
- Maternal reflexes (if using magnesium)

NURSING DIAGNOSES
Drug-specific nursing diagnoses include the following:

- **Anxiety** related to fears concerning preterm labor
- **Impaired Gas Exchange** related to pulmonary edema from drug therapy and IV fluids

Nursing diagnoses related to drug administration are discussed in Chapter 4.

PLANNING

The expected outcomes of the patient may include an optimal response to therapy, a reduction in anxiety, and confidence in an understanding of the treatment of preterm labor.

IMPLEMENTATION

Promoting an Optimal Response to Therapy

For IV administration, the solution is prepared according to the primary health care provider's instructions. An infusion pump is used to control the flow rate. The medication will be piggy-backed to the primary line, allowing the patient to maintain IV access should it become necessary temporarily to discontinue infusion of the drug. In some cases, the primary health care provider may prescribe indomethacin for administration by the rectal or oral route throughout the treatment, rather than by the IV route. Terbutaline may be given orally or by subcutaneous (subcut) injection. In any case, the patient is continuously monitored to recognize hypotension should it occur, at which time the patient is placed in a left lateral position unless the primary health care provider orders a different position.

The primary health care provider is kept informed of the patient's response to the drug, because a dosage change may be necessary. The primary health care provider establishes guidelines for the regulation of the IV infusion rate, as well as the blood pressure and pulse ranges that require stopping the IV infusion.

Monitoring and Managing Patient Needs

During administration of the drug, monitor maternal and fetal vital signs every 15 minutes and uterine contractions frequently throughout the infusion.

ANXIETY. The patient in preterm labor may have many concerns about her pregnancy as well as the effectiveness of drug therapy. The woman is encouraged to verbalize any fears or concerns. Actively listen to the patient's concerns and carefully and accurately answer any questions she may have concerning drug therapy. In addition, offer emotional support and encouragement while the drug is being administered. The presence of family members may decrease anxiety in the woman experiencing preterm labor; learn your institutional policy for the number of visitors that can be at the bedside.

IMPAIRED GAS EXCHANGE. If the pulse rate increases to 140 bpm or there is persistent elevation of pulse rate, irregular pulse, or increase in respiratory rate of more than 20 respirations per minute, notify the primary health care provider. Assess the respiratory status for symptoms of pulmonary edema (e.g., dyspnea, tachycardia, increased respiratory rate, crackles, and frothy sputum). If

these reactions occur, the primary health care provider is notified immediately, because use of the drug may be discontinued or the dosage may be decreased. After contractions cease, taper the dosage to the lowest effective dose by decreasing the drug infusion rate at regular intervals prescribed by the primary health care provider. The infusion continues for at least 12 hours after uterine contractions cease. Because treatment duration is brief, mild adverse reactions may be tolerated. If adverse reactions are severe, use of the drug is discontinued or the dosage decreased.

Educating the Patient and Family

Carefully and gently explain the treatment regimen to the patient. Remember that anxiety about the condition of the fetus may hamper her ability to focus on your words. The primary health care provider usually discusses the expected outcome of treatment with the patient and answers any questions regarding therapy. Although the patient is monitored closely during therapy, the patient is instructed to immediately use the call light if any of the following occur: nausea, vomiting, palpitations, or shortness of breath.

EVALUATION

- Therapeutic drug effect is achieved and labor is stopped.
- Adverse reactions are identified, reported to the primary health care provider, and managed successfully through appropriate nursing interventions:
  - Anxiety is managed successfully.
  - Gas exchange is maintained.
- Patient expresses confidence and demonstrates an understanding of the drug regimen.

PHARMACOLOGY IN PRACTICE
THINK CRITICALLY

As the clinic nurse you know that Betty has some mental health issues and gets anxious about issues easily. What role might anxiety play in the birthing process? How can you explain induction while being supportive to Betty and her daughter?

KEY POINTS

- Oxytocin is a hormone produced in the posterior pituitary gland. The hormone stimulates the smooth muscle of the uterus. In a pregnant woman, oxytocin stimulation causes uterine contractions. The hormone is used to start or induce labor in pregnant women and may be used to expel the placenta after the baby is delivered.
- The oxytocin hormone also has antidiuretic and vasopressor effects. Adverse reactions to be aware of include water intoxication (holding water in the body due to the hormone) or high blood pressure. Use of the hormone is contraindicated when the fetus is not in proper position

- or when placenta previa or other conditions exist as described.
- If premature labor threatens a pregnancy, tocolytic drugs may be used to diminish contractions to allow for maturity of fetal organs before delivery. These drugs affect the mother in the opposite manner of the hormone oxytocin, reducing uterine contractions and possibly lowering the mother's blood pressure.
- Both maternal and fetal vital signs should be monitored when these drugs are used.

Summary Drug Table UTERINE DRUGS

Generic Name	Trade Name	Uses	Adverse Reactions	Dosage Ranges
Oxytocics				
carboprost *kar'-boe-prosst*	Hemabate	Postpartum uterine hemorrhage	Nausea, flushing	250 mcg IM may repeat in 15–90 minutes, not to exceed 2 mg total dose
methylergonovine *meh-thill-er-goe-noe'-veen*	Methergine	Control of postpartum bleeding and hemorrhage, uterine atony	Dizziness, headache, nausea, vomiting, elevated blood pressure	0.2 mg IM, IV after delivery of the placenta; 0.2 mg orally TID, QID
misoprostol *mye-soe-prosst-ole*	Cytotec	Postpartum hemorrhage, cervical ripening	Headache, nausea, diarrhea, abdominal pain	100-mcg tablet vaginally administered
oxytocin *ox-ih-toe'-sin*	Pitocin	Antepartum: to initiate or improve uterine contractions Postpartum: control of postpartum bleeding and hemorrhage	Nausea, vomiting, pelvic hematoma, postpartum bleeding, cardiac arrhythmias, anaphylactic reactions	Induction of labor: individualize dose not to exceed 10 units/min Postpartum bleeding: IV infusion of 10–40 units in 1000-mL IV solution or 10 units IM after placenta delivery
Agents for Cervical Ripening				
dinoprostone *dye-noe-prost'-one*	Cervidil, Prepidil	Prepare near/term cervix for labor induction	Uterine contraction, GI effect	As directed on package insert
Tocolytics				
nifedipine *nye-fed'-ih-peen*	Procardia	Preterm labor	Headache, dizziness, weakness, edema, nausea, muscle cramps, cough, nasal congestion, wheezing	20 mg orally q 3–8 hr
indomethacin *in-doe-meth'-ah-sin*	Indocin	Preterm labor before 31 weeks' gestation	Headache, dizziness, nausea, vomiting, stomach upset or heartburn, prolonged vaginal bleeding	100 mg rectally, then 50 mg orally q 6 hr for a total of 8 doses
magnesium *mag-nee'-zee-um*		Preterm labor, seizure control	Fatigue, headaches, flushing, diplopia	4–6 g IV over 2 min, then infuse 1–4 g/hr
terbutaline *ter-byoo'-tah-leen*	Brethine	Preterm labor	Nervousness, restlessness, tremor, headache, anxiety, hypertension, palpitations, arrhythmias, hypokalemia, pulmonary edema	Subcut: 250 mcg hourly until contractions stop Orally: 2.5 mg q 4–6 hr until delivery

Uterine Drugs

● Chapter Review

Know Your Drugs

Clients sometimes know a medication by the brand (or trade) name and not the generic name. To help you recognize both names, match the brand name with the generic name of the same medication.

Generic Name	Brand Name
1. dinoprostone	A. Indocin
2. indomethacin	B. Pitocin
3. nifedipine	C. Prepidil
4. oxytocin	D. Procardia

Calculate Medication Dosages

1. Terbutaline 2.5 mg is prescribed. The drug is available in 5-mg tablets. The nurse administers _____.

2. Methylergonovine 0.2 mg IM is prescribed. The drug is available as 0.2 mg/mL. The nurse administers _____.

● Prepare for the NCLEX®

Build Your Knowledge

1. The function of the hormone oxytocin is to stimulate_____
   1. blood pressure
   2. cardiac muscle
   3. kidney processing
   4. uterine smooth muscle

2. Which gland produces oxytocin?
   1. adrenal
   2. pituitary
   3. thyroid
   4. uterus

3. When oxytocin is administered over a prolonged time, which of the following adverse reactions would be most likely to occur?
   1. hyperglycemia
   2. renal impairment
   3. increased intracranial pressure
   4. water intoxication

4. What percentage of births in the United States is considered preterm?
   1. less than 2%
   2. 11%
   3. 45%
   4. 89%

5. Which nursing diagnosis would the nurse anticipate when administering either a uterine stimulant or tocolytic?
   1. Anxiety
   2. Impaired Gas Exchange
   3. Excess Fluid Volume
   4. Impaired Tissue Perfusion

6. Magnesium is used as a tocolytic drug. What other condition is treated with this drug?
   1. uterine atony
   2. preeclampsia
   3. placenta previa
   4. eclampsia

Apply Your Knowledge

7. Intravenous oxytocic and tocolytic drugs should be administered:
   1. as immediate push drugs in a syringe
   2. in a syringe pump into a heparin lock device
   3. directly in a primary IV line
   4. secondary or piggybacked into a primary line

8. When the client is receiving oxytocin, the nurse would notify the health care provider attending the delivery of which of the following situations?
   1. uterine contractions occurring every 5 to 10 minutes
   2. uterine contractions lasting more than 60 seconds or contractions occurring more frequently than every 2 to 3 minutes
   3. client experiencing pain during a uterine contraction
   4. client experiencing increased thirst

Alternate-Format Questions

9. Oxytocin is prepared in a solution of 10 units in 1,000 mL (0.01 units/1 mL). If the nurse is ordered to give 0.05 units of oxytocin per minute, how many mL would that be? _____

10. Name the drug and class of the nonobstetric drugs that have tocolytic properties.
    1. a class of drugs used for pain relief
    2. a class of drugs used for lowering blood pressure
    3. a class of drugs used for bronchial dilation

To check your answers, see Appendix G .

the**Point** *For more NCLEX-style questions, log on to http://thepoint.lww.com to access more than 1000 questions.*

Drugs That Affect the Urinary System

The urinary system includes the kidneys, ureters, bladder, and urethra and is responsible for the regulation and elimination of body fluids. Each kidney contains about one million nephrons, which filter the bloodstream to remove waste products. During this process, water and electrolytes are also selectively removed. It is an important body system to consider when discussing drug therapy because it is one of the primary systems used to eliminate drugs from the body. If the system does not work properly, drugs continue to circulate in the body. This can lead to drug buildup, increased adverse reactions, or toxicity from the drug.

Another body system that works directly with the urinary system is the reproductive system (male and female reproductive organs). Although this system is not covered in detail in this unit, it plays a key role in the aging process. On January 1, 2011 (1–1–11), the first baby boomer turned 65 years of age. It is estimated that for 20 years after that date, 10,000 individuals will turn 65 *on a daily basis*. As people age, their concerns about staying active and healthy increase. Issues that have an impact on both the urinary and reproductive systems as individuals age are the focus of Chapter 47. Issues arise as female hormones diminish and the reduction in estrogen affects many body systems. Because the uterus and vagina are interconnected structures, estrogen reduction also affects the function of the urinary system. In men, the urinary system is affected when there is enlargement of the prostate. This leads to concerns for both function and quality of relationships.

The bladder is the storage area for urine before it is excreted from the body and is the focus of Chapter 48. The nature of the bladder and its contents make it susceptible to infection. In this chapter discussion pertains to the drugs used specifically for treating urinary tract infections (UTIs) and the discomfort associated with those infections.

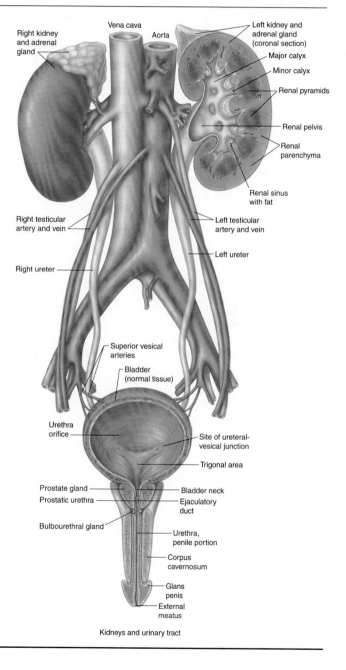

Right kidney and adrenal gland
Vena cava
Aorta
Left kidney and adrenal gland (coronal section)
Major calyx
Minor calyx
Renal pyramids
Renal pelvis
Renal parenchyma
Renal sinus with fat
Right testicular artery and vein
Left testicular artery and vein
Left ureter
Right ureter
Superior vesical arteries
Bladder (normal tissue)
Urethra orifice
Site of ureteral-vesical junction
Trigonal area
Prostate gland
Bladder neck
Prostatic urethra
Ejaculatory duct
Bulbourethral gland
Urethra, penile portion
Corpus cavernosum
Glans penis
External meatus

Kidneys and urinary tract

Menopause and Andropause Drugs

LEARNING OBJECTIVES

On completion of this chapter, the student will:

1. Describe changes occurring in the urinary and reproductive systems because of aging.
2. Discuss the uses, general drug actions, adverse reactions, contraindications, precautions, and interactions of the drugs used to treat symptoms associated with menopause and andropause.
3. Discuss important preadministration and ongoing assessment activities the nurse should perform with the patient taking a drug for a change resulting from menopause or andropause.
4. List nursing diagnoses for a patient taking a drug for a change resulting from menopause or andropause.
5. Discuss ways to promote an optimal response to therapy, how to manage adverse reactions, and important points to keep in mind when educating patients about the use of drugs to treat a change resulting from menopause or andropause.

KEY TERMS

andropause • male menopause

dysuria • painful urination

menarche • age of onset of first menstruation

menopause • the end of monthly cycles, referring to the fertility cycle of women

neurogenic bladder • impaired bladder function caused by a nervous system abnormality, typically an injury to the spinal cord

nocturia • voiding at night

overactive bladder syndrome (OBS) • conditions of urgency, frequency, and nocturia, with or without incontinence

priapism • prolonged, painful penile erection

stress incontinence • losing urine without meaning to during physical activity

urge incontinence • strong, sudden need to void due to bladder spasm or contraction

uroselective • antiadrenergic drug that is selective for alpha (α) receptors in the urinary system and not generalized

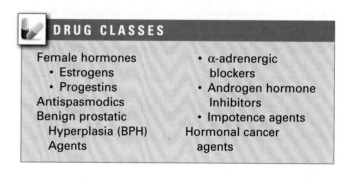

DRUG CLASSES

Female hormones
- Estrogens
- Progestins

Antispasmodics

Benign prostatic Hyperplasia (BPH) Agents

- α-adrenergic blockers
- Androgen hormone Inhibitors
- Impotence agents

Hormonal cancer agents

In both men and women, aging reproductive system changes are closely related to changes in the urinary system. **Menopause** makes changes for women very pronounced because fertility stops. For men change is not as overt. Hormonal and urinary changes may be more subtle and are referred to as **andropause**. Changes to a woman's reproductive system, the shared changes to the genitourinary

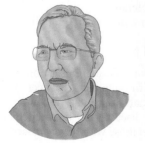

PHARMACOLOGY IN PRACTICE

Mr. Phillip, a 72-year-old widower who lives alone, was diagnosed with a UTI 8 weeks ago. Having failed to come in for a follow-up urine sample 2 weeks after completing the course of drug therapy, he is at the clinic to see a primary health care provider because the UTI symptoms are now worse.

system, and changes to the male are described in this chapter. The goal of drug treatment is to reduce symptoms related to the changes of aging reproductive and urinary systems.

Menopause

The female fertility cycle, which is under the influence of estrogen and progesterone, is described in Chapter 45. As women age there is a complex change in these and other hormones. Estrogen diminishes and the menstrual cycle can become irregular until it stops altogether. As the hormonal influence lessens women are said to be in the *female climacteric* or menopause.

The purpose of this section is to provide you with information to support the woman who has opted for hormone replacement therapy (HRT). Estrogen replacement therapy has been studied extensively. When a woman is premenopausal, this is a good time to discuss options with her primary health care provider. She should discuss the benefit of relief of symptoms (e.g., hot flashes) with negative impact on her body (e.g., blood pressure and lipid changes). Many of the physical changes throughout the body associated with loss of estrogen are illustrated in Figure 47.1. Information about medications used to deal with heart disease or bone changes of older women are discussed in Unit VIII and Chapter 30, respectively.

Aging of the female genitourinary system includes fat atrophy and hormonal changes, which are responsible for the following:

- Vaginal walls become thinner, shorten, and lose some of their elasticity.
- The vagina produces less lubrication and at a slower rate during sexual arousal.
- The pH environment changes, making the vagina more susceptible to yeast infections.
- Pelvic floor muscles weaken and lead to stress incontinence.

Symptoms related to these changes can be reduced by replacing the lost hormones.

ESTROGENS

Actions and Uses

In addition to contraception, estrogen is most commonly used in HRT (or estrogen replacement therapy [ERT]) in postmenopausal women. Changes to aging tissues can be lessened when estrogens are used for the following:

- Relief of moderate to severe vasomotor symptoms of menopause (flushing, sweating)
- Treatment of atrophic vaginitis
- Treatment of osteoporosis in women past menopause
- Palliative treatment of advanced prostatic carcinoma (in men)
- Selected cases of advanced breast carcinoma

The estradiol transdermal system is also used after removal of the ovaries in premenopausal women (female castration) and primary ovarian failure. Estrogen is given intramuscularly (IM) or intravenously (IV) to treat uterine bleeding caused by

hormonal imbalance. When estrogen is used to treat menopausal symptoms in a woman with an intact uterus, concurrent use of progestin is recommended to decrease the risk of endometrial cancer. After a hysterectomy, estrogen alone may be used for ERT.

Adverse Reactions

Administration of estrogens by any route may result in many adverse reactions, although the incidence and intensity of these reactions vary. Some of the adverse reactions seen with the administration of estrogens are as follows.

Central Nervous System Reactions

- Headache, migraine
- Dizziness, mental depression

Dermatologic Reactions

- Dermatitis, pruritus
- Chloasma (pigmentation of the skin) or melasma (discoloration of the skin), which may continue when use of the drug is discontinued

Gastrointestinal Reactions

- Nausea, vomiting
- Abdominal bloating and cramps

Genitourinary Reactions

- Breakthrough bleeding, withdrawal bleeding, spotting, changes in menstrual flow
- Dysmenorrhea, premenstrual-like syndrome, amenorrhea
- Vaginal candidiasis, cervical erosion, vaginitis

Local Reactions

- Pain at injection site or sterile abscess with parenteral form of the drug
- Redness and irritation at the application site with transdermal system

Ophthalmic Reactions

- Steepening of corneal curvature
- Intolerance to contact lenses

Miscellaneous Reactions

- Edema, rhinitis, changes in libido
- Breast pain, enlargement, and tenderness
- Reduced carbohydrate tolerance
- Venous thromboembolism, pulmonary embolism
- Weight gain or loss
- Generalized and skeletal pain

Warnings associated with the administration of estrogen include an increased risk of endometrial cancer, gallbladder disease, hypertension, hepatic adenoma (a benign tumor of the liver), cardiovascular disease, and thromboembolic disease, and hypercalcemia in those with breast cancer and bone metastases.

Changes Due to Menopause

Hair Growth
- Thinning of scalp hair.
- Darkening or thickening of other body hair, such as facial hair.

Skin
- Loss of firmness, tension, and fluid.
- Decrease in melanocytes, which give skin pigment.
- Increased sensitivity to sun exposure.

Bone
- Becomes progressively more porous and brittle.
- Increased risk of osteoporosis.
- More subject to fractures.

Circulatory System
- Increased heart disease risk.
- Increased high blood pressure risk.
- Increased high cholesterol risk.

Breasts
- Less firm breasts. Glandular tissue is replaced with fat.

Reproductive System
- Few remaining follicles (egg cells) in ovaries.
- Reproductive organs decrease in size.
- Vaginal mucosa become thinner, less lubricated.
- Vaginal pH changes, increasing susceptibility to infection.
- Endometriosis disappears.

Urinary System
- Thinning of tissues in bladder and urethra.
- Increased risk of urinary tract infections.

Another health concern associated with menopause is weight gain.

Suspensory ligaments

Fat

Gland lobules

Ureter

Ovary

Uterus

Bladder

Vagina

Urethra

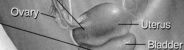

Figure 47.1 Menopausal changes in the female body.

Menopause and Andropause Drugs

Contraindications and Precautions

Estrogen and progestin therapy is contraindicated in patients with known hypersensitivity to the drugs, breast cancer (except for metastatic disease), estrogen-dependent neoplasms, undiagnosed abnormal genital bleeding, and thromboembolic disorders. The progestins also are contraindicated in patients with cerebral hemorrhage or impaired liver function. Both the estrogens and progestins are classified as pregnancy category X drugs and are contraindicated during pregnancy.

Estrogens are used cautiously in patients with gallbladder disease, hypercalcemia (may lead to severe hypercalcemia in patients with breast cancer and bone metastasis), cardiovascular disease, and liver impairment. Cardiovascular complications are greater in women who smoke and use estrogen. Progestins are used cautiously in patients with a history of migraine headaches, epilepsy, asthma, and cardiac or renal impairment.

Interactions

The following interactions may occur with female hormones:

Interacting Drug	Common Use	Effect of Interaction
oral anticoagulants	Blood thinners	Decreased anticoagulant effect
tricyclic antidepressants	Treatment of depression	Increased effectiveness of antidepressant
rifampin	Anti-infective	Increased risk of breakthrough bleeding
hydantoins	Seizure control	Increased risk of breakthrough bleeding and pregnancy

Urinary Aging

As a person's age increases, so do the number of urinary system disorders. All parts of the urinary system are affected by aging. Changes in kidney size and blood flow to the kidney reduce renal function by almost 50% in older individuals. These changes decrease the filtration and the urine becomes more dilute. Diuretics (Chapter 33) are used to maintain function in the kidney as well as to reduce fluid in the body for hypertension control.

The urinary bladder diminishes in strength, flexibility, and capacity resulting in frequent urination, especially at night (**nocturia**). The urethra shortens and its lining becomes thinner, increasing susceptibility to infection. In addition to the effects of childbirth and loss of muscle tone in pelvic structures, the urinary sphincter becomes less flexible and is less able to close tightly, resulting in urine leakage (**stress incontinence**). This type of incontinence is typically treated with surgical or behavior interventions.

Another continence issue can occur when the sensation of having to urinate is not as strong and may not be felt until the bladder is completely full. Then the need to void is sudden and urgent and there may be a loss of urine (**urge incontinence**). This type of incontinence can be treated with drugs called antispasmodics. **Overactive bladder syndrome** (OBS, or involuntary contractions of the detrusor or bladder muscle) also presents with urinary urgency. OBS is estimated to affect more than 16 million individuals in the United States. This problem sometimes results from such disorders as cystitis or prostatitis or from abnormalities related to affected structures, such as the kidney or the urethra. Symptoms of an overactive bladder include urinary urgency (a strong and sudden desire to urinate), frequent urination throughout the day and night, and urge incontinence. Another urinary issue in men involves an enlarged prostate, which can eventually interfere with urination. The enlarged prostate compresses the urethra, reducing the flow of urine from the bladder. This also makes men more susceptible to urinary tract infections.

ANTISPASMODICS

Actions and Uses

Antispasmodics are cholinergic blocking drugs that inhibit bladder contractions and delay the urge to void. These drugs counteract the smooth muscle spasm of the urinary tract by relaxing the detrusor and other muscles through action at the parasympathetic nerve receptors (see Chapter 27). Flavoxate (Urispas) is used to relieve symptoms of **dysuria** (painful or difficult urination), urinary urgency, nocturia (excessive urination during the night), suprapubic pain and frequency, and urge incontinence. The other antispasmodic drugs are also used to treat bladder instability (i.e., urgency, frequency, leakage, incontinence, and painful or difficult urination) caused by a **neurogenic bladder** (impaired bladder function caused by a nervous system abnormality, typically an injury to the spinal cord).

Adverse Reactions

Adverse reactions to these drugs are similar to those with other cholinergic blocking drugs. They include the following:

• Dry mouth, drowsiness, constipation or diarrhea, decreased production of tears, decreased sweating, gastrointestinal (GI) disturbances, dim vision, and urinary hesitancy
• Nausea and vomiting, nervousness, vertigo, headache, rash, and mental confusion (particularly in older adults)

Patients should be told that antispasmodic drugs can discolor the urine (dark orange to brown) and stain undergarments that come in contact with the urine.

Contraindications and Precautions

Antispasmodic drugs are contraindicated in those patients with known hypersensitivity to the drugs or with glaucoma. Other patients for whom antispasmodics are contraindicated are those with intestinal or gastric blockage, abdominal bleeding, myasthenia gravis, or urinary tract blockage.

These drugs should be used with caution in patients with GI infections, benign prostatic hypertrophy, urinary retention, hyperthyroidism, hepatic or renal disease, and hypertension. Antispasmodic drugs are classified as pregnancy category C drugs and are used only when the benefit to the woman outweighs the risk to the fetus.

Interactions

The following interactions may occur when an antispasmodic drug is administered with another agent:

Interacting Drug	Common Use	Effect of Interaction
antibiotics/antifungals	Fight infection	Decreased effectiveness of anti-infective drug
meperidine, flurazepam, phenothiazines	Preoperative sedation	Increased effect of the antispasmodic
tricyclic antidepressants	Management of depression	Increased effect of the antispasmodic
haloperidol (Haldol)	Antianxiety/antipsychotic agent	Decreased effectiveness of the antipsychotic drug
digoxin	Management of cardiac problems	Increased serum levels of digoxin

Andropause

Unlike women, men do not go through a major change in fertility like women experience (menopause). Instead, changes occur gradually and are called andropause or the *male climacteric.* Aging changes in the male reproductive system occur primarily in the testes. Like the ovary, testicular tissue diminishes; what is different is that the male sex hormone levels (of testosterone) remain relatively constant.

The change men often notice is prostate enlargement. The prostate gland is about the size of a walnut, sits below the bladder, and wraps around the urethra. Scar tissue replaces prostate cells and causes the enlargement. Fifty percent of men will experience benign prostatic hypertrophy (BPH) as they age (Fig. 47.2). BPH may cause difficulty in urination, retention of urine, and incontinence. Prostate gland infections or inflammation (prostatitis) may also occur. The risk of prostate cancer is no greater in men with BPH, although symptoms may be similar, prostate cancer is due to a change in the prostate cells (see Chapter 50). Treatment for BPH is aimed at relieving symptoms and improving urinary flow.

> **NURSING ALERT**
> Early-stage prostate cancer may not have signs or symptoms. When men present with issues such as difficulty with urination, reduced flow, or blood in the urine, prostate cancer should always be ruled out before treatment is started for BPH.

DRUGS TO TREAT BENIGN PROSTATIC HYPERTROPHY

Treatment for BPH includes monitoring, medications, or invasive procedures. Drugs are used for mild to moderate symptoms of BPH (e.g., frequency, reduced flow, nocturia, and dysuria) and include androgen inhibitors and adrenergic blockers.

Actions and Uses

The most widely used drugs to treat BPH are the alpha (α)-adrenergic blockers. As discussed in Chapter 25, adrenergic blockers prevent the neurotransmission of norepinephrine. The drugs used for BPH are peripherally acting, α_{1a}-adrenergic blockers that exert their action primarily on the smooth muscle of the prostate and the bladder neck. By blocking norepinephrine, the muscles relax and this allows urine to flow from the bladder. Adrenergic blockers can be **uroselective**; therefore, the α_{1a}-adrenergic blockers exert their action on the bladder with minimal action on the vascular system.

Androgen hormone inhibitors (AHIs) have been used for many years to deal with symptoms of BPH. The biggest drawback has been the adverse effects of erectile dysfunction (ED) and decreased libido. The androgen hormone inhibitors prevent the conversion of testosterone into the androgen 5-α-dihydrotestosterone (DHT). The growth of the prostate gland depends on DHT. The lowering of serum levels of DHT reduces the effect of this hormone on the prostate gland, resulting in a decrease in the size of the gland and the symptoms associated with prostatic gland enlargement.

Currently the use of both types of drugs is being studied (Dhingra, 2011) and is proving successful based on the different sites of action of the drugs. There is one drug on the market

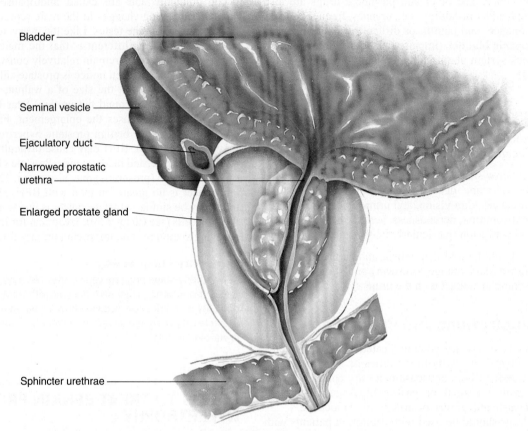

Bladder

Seminal vesicle

Ejaculatory duct

Narrowed prostatic
urethra

Enlarged prostate gland

Sphincter urethrae

Figure 47.2 Enlarged prostate and narrowing of urethra results in reduced urinary flow. (Asset provided by Anatomical Chart Co.)

that combines an α_{1a}-adrenergic blocker with an AHI—Jalyn, a combination of dutasteride and tamsulosin.

Adverse Reactions

Adverse reactions usually are mild and do not require discontinuing use of the drug. Some of the adverse reactions seen with the administration of α-adrenergic blockers are as follows: weight gain, fatigue, dizziness, and transient orthostatic hypotension. Adverse reactions of the AHI drugs, when they occur, are related to the sexual drive and include impotence, decreased libido, and a decreased volume of ejaculate. Changes to breast tissue—pain or tenderness, nipple discharge, or enlargement—can occur while taking AHIs.

Contraindications and Precautions

Both α-adrenergic blockers and AHI drugs should be used with caution in patients with hepatic or renal disease. Caution the patient with hypertension when using both beta (β) and α blockers that hypotensive symptoms may be increased. These drugs should be discontinued and the primary health care provider called if angina or a heart-like pain occurs. Although not typically taken by women, AHIs are pregnancy category X. Therefore, women of childbearing age should not handle the drug.

Interactions

The following interactions may occur when an α-adrenergic blocking drug is administered with another agent:

Interacting Drug	Common Use	Effect of Interaction
antibiotics/antifungals	Fight infection	Decreased effectiveness of anti-infective drug
β blockers	Hypertension	Increased hypotension
Phosphodiesterase type 5 inhibitors	Erectile dysfunction	Increased hypotension

HERBAL CONSIDERATIONS

Saw palmetto is used to relieve the symptoms of BPH (urinary frequency, decreased flow of urine, and nocturia). The herb is believed to reduce inflammation and the hormone DHT (responsible for prostate enlargement). Saw palmetto does not cause impotence, yet it can aggravate GI disorders such as peptic ulcer disease. Men report reduction in urinary symptoms in 1 to 3 months when 160 mg twice daily is taken. It is not recommended as a tea, because the active constituents are not water soluble. It is usually recommended that the herb be taken for 6 months, followed by evaluation by a primary health care provider (Bent, 2006).

DRUGS TO TREAT ERECTILE DYSFUNCTION

In addition to slowed urination, BPH causes problems with ejaculation or the ability to have an erection. ED may be a concern for aging men. It is normal for erections to occur less frequently as men age. The ability to experience repeated ejaculation is reduced. However, ED is most often the result of a medical (90%) or psychological (10%) problem rather than simple aging. Medications (especially antihypertensive and antidepressants) can cause the inability to develop or maintain an erection. Disorders such as diabetes can also cause ED. Erectile dysfunction that is caused by medications or illness is oftentimes successfully treated.

Actions and Uses

Sexual stimulation causes a series of steps where chemicals are released and the smooth muscles of the penis (corpus cavernosum) become engorged with blood. Erectile dysfunction results from a failure of the penis to become engorged, preventing sexual intercourse. Phosphodiesterase type 5 inhibitors are oral drugs that facilitate the enzyme that allows blood flow into the penis, resulting in an erection.

Adverse Reactions, Contraindications, and Precautions

The most common adverse reactions include headache, flushing, GI upset, nausea, and runny nose or congestion. Drugs for ED should not be taken by men who use nitrates (e.g., for anginal pain). Because these drugs affect smooth muscle, patients with pre-existing cardiac problems, especially those using drugs to lower blood pressure, should discuss use with their primary health care provider before using the drug. Doses should be reduced in men with renal or hepatic impairment. Medical attention should be sought for erections sustained for more than 4 hours. Ocular problems may occur when using these drugs; again, the primary health care provider should be consulted before use.

Interactions

The following interactions may occur when a phosphodiesterase type 5 inhibitor is administered with another agent:

Interacting Drug	Common Use	Effect of Interaction
antiretrovirals	Viral infection	Increased effectiveness of ED drug
antihypertensives	Reduce blood pressure	Increased effectiveness of antihypertensive

HORMONES FOR CANCER TREATMENT

Another issue with an aging urinary system is the ability for the kidneys to handle aggressive cancer treatment (see Chapter 50). Hormones may be used in cancer therapy especially for advanced disease. Receptors for specific hormones needed for cell growth are found on the surface of some tumor cells. By stopping the production of a hormone, blocking hormone receptors, or substituting a drug for the actual hormone, cancer cells can be killed or their growth slowed. These drugs also appear to counteract the effect of male or female hormones in hormone-dependent tumors. Hormones are not used as curative drugs in cancer treatment; rather, they have an adjuvant role because of their ability to slow or reverse tumor growth.

Examples of hormones used as antineoplastic drugs include the androgen testolactone (Teslac), conjugate estrogen, and the progestin megestrol (Megace). Gonadotropin-releasing hormone analogs, such as goserelin (Zoladex), appear to act by inhibiting the anterior pituitary secretion of gonadotropins, thus suppressing the release of pituitary gonadotropins. One drug on the market, sipuleucel-T (Provenge), uses a man's own cells to sensitize the drug to target the prostate cancer cells. This requires taking white blood cells from the patient, preparing the drug, then infusing the drug solution back into the patient. For a listing of names, categories, and typical adverse reactions, see the Summary Drug Table: Aging Urinary and Reproductive Drugs, Hormonal Therapy for Cancer.

Menopause and Andropause Drugs

NURSING PROCESS

Patient Receiving an Aging Urinary or Reproductive Drug

ASSESSMENT

Preadministration Assessment

Many patients seeking treatment for urinary or reproductive issues related to aging will be seen as an outpatient or as a resident in a long-term care facility. For some providers it may be embarrassing to ask questions about urinary problems or sexual history. Because these are topics infrequently discussed, the provider should remember that it is also probably difficult for the patient to bring these issues to his or her attention.

Obtain a complete patient health history, including a menstrual history, which includes the menarche (age of onset of first menstruation), menstrual pattern, and any changes in the menstrual pattern (including a menopause history when applicable). Ask about symptoms of BPH, such as frequency of voiding during the day and night and difficulty starting the urinary stream. Document any issues with overactive bladder syndrome or incontinence and if the patient wears protection, such as pads or disposable undergarments, including how many are used in a day. The primary health care provider may order laboratory tests such as urinalysis or blood work. If the patient is being treated hormonally for a cancer, ask about and document previous treatments.

Include questions to obtain a history of thrombophlebitis or other vascular disorders, a smoking history, and a history of liver diseases, especially if hormone replacement is being offered. Blood pressure, pulse, and respiratory rate are taken and recorded. The primary health care provider may perform breast and pelvic examinations and a Papanicolaou (Pap) test for women or a rectal exam (uterine/ovary exam for women or prostate exam for men) before starting therapy.

Ongoing Assessment

At the time of each office or clinic visit, the blood pressure, pulse, respiratory rate, and weight are checked. Ask the patient about any adverse drug effects, as well as the result of drug therapy. For example, if the patient is receiving an estrogen for the symptoms of menopause, ask her to compare her original symptoms with the symptoms she is currently experiencing, if any. You may want to ask about any breakthrough bleeding or adverse reactions such as weight gain or leg pain (thromboembolism). When antispasmodics are prescribed, monitor the patient for a reduction in the symptoms identified in the preadministration assessment, such as dysuria, urinary frequency, urgency, or nocturia. Ask about the relief of any pain associated with irritation of the lower genitourinary tract. For men being treated for BPH, inquire about changes in urinary flow patterns or if an ED medication has provided satisfactory results.

NURSING DIAGNOSES

Drug-specific nursing diagnoses include the following:

- **Deficient Knowledge** related to diagnosis, use of ERT, or other factors
- **Impaired Oral Mucous Membranes** related to dry mouth from anticholinergic
- **Risk for Injury** related to drowsiness, dizziness, or hypotension
- **Acute Pain** related to priapism

Nursing diagnoses related to drug administration are discussed in Chapter 4.

PLANNING

The expected outcomes for the patient may include an optimal response to drug therapy, support of patient needs related to the management of adverse reactions, and confidence in an understanding of the medication regimen.

IMPLEMENTATION

Promoting an Optimal Response to Therapy

Estrogens may be administered orally, IM, IV, transdermally, or intravaginally. Outpatient use as a contraceptive is typically self-administered orally. The transdermal delivery route has been found to be safer, especially for women with elevated triglycerides, type 2 diabetes, hypertension, or migraine headaches, or those who smoke. When estrogens are given vaginally for atrophic vaginitis, the nurse gives the patient instructions on proper use.

! **NURSING ALERT**

Women who are pregnant or may become pregnant should not handle crushed or broken finasteride (Propecia, Proscar) or dutasteride (Avodart) tablets or capsules. Absorption of the drug poses substantial risk for abnormal growth to a male fetus.

Monitoring and Managing Patient Needs

DEFICIENT KNOWLEDGE. The woman taking female hormones may have many concerns about therapy with these drugs. Some concerns may be based on inaccurate knowledge, such as incorrect facts about certain dangers associated with female hormones. Although there are dangers associated with long-term use of female hormones, these adverse reactions occur in a small number of patients. When the patient is closely monitored by the primary health care provider, the dangers associated with long-term use are often minimized.

Some women may be anxious because of a fear of experiencing uterine cancer as the result of HRT. You may explain that taking progestin, which counteracts the negative effect of estrogen, can prevent estrogen-induced cancer of the uterus. Other women may fear the development of breast cancer or heart disease. Most research studies find that there is little risk for breast cancer developing and that the benefits of HRT often outweigh the risk of breast cancer. Studies questioned the effectiveness of HRT for postmenopausal women and the increased risk of cardiovascular disease. Newer studies demonstrate that lower doses orally or transdermally help reduce bone fractures in postmenopausal women. Encourage the patient to ask questions about her therapy. Inaccurate information is clarified before starting therapy. Refer questions that cannot or should not be answered by a nurse to the primary health care provider.

The male patient with advanced prostatic carcinoma also may have concerns about taking a female hormone. Assure the patient that the dosage is carefully regulated and that feminizing effects, if they occur, are usually minimal.

IMPAIRED MUCOUS MEMBRANES. A common adverse reaction to antispasmodics (cholinergic blocking drugs) includes dry mouth. You may suggest that the patient not only suck on hard candy, sugarless lozenges, or small pieces of ice but also perform frequent mouth care. Sometimes patients may think if they reduce fluid intake that will reduce urination and urinary issues. Be sure to instruct patients in ways to maintain fluid intake and that reducing fluids will actually make urinary problems worse. Tell patients that by increasing oral fluids this will minimize the chance of also becoming constipated. Should the patient become constipated, again encourage fluids, a high-fiber diet, and fruits and vegetables with a high water content, such as watermelon, strawberries, or spinach.

RISK FOR INJURY. Should a patient be prescribed adrenergic blocking drugs for BPH, instruct the patient on his risk for injury due to a hypotensive reaction. A patient may experience immediate lowering of his blood pressure, termed "first-dose orthostatic hypotension," when first starting these drugs. When starting the medication, the patient may become dizzy during the first 60 to 90 minutes after taking the drug. Instruct the patient to take the drug at bedtime or when less activity is anticipated. The important issue is to take the medication at about the same time each day. This reaction can also happen if the drug is stopped and started a week or more later.

ACUTE PAIN. An uncommon but potentially serious adverse reaction of the ED drugs is priapism (an erection lasting more than 4 to 6 hours). This can be very painful and if not treated within a few hours, priapism can result in tissue damage and possible permanent impotence. Those more prone to priapism include patients with sickle cell anemia, multiple myeloma, leukemia, or an anatomic deformity of the penis. Because this can be an embarrassing adverse reaction, the patient may be reluctant to seek medical attention. The drug is discontinued immediately and the primary care provider notified. When a patient with priapism seeks care, injection of α-adrenergic stimulants (e.g., phenylephrine or norepinephrine) may be helpful in treating priapism once the engorgement is drained. In some cases, surgical intervention may be required.

Educating the Patient and Family

When educating the patient and family about drugs to relieve symptoms of aging genitourinary and reproductive systems, remember that your patient is typically older and may need repeated instruction to understand how to self-manage his or her issues and medications. The patient and family should feel confident in understanding that the drug is to help reduce symptoms experienced that may be hard to discuss with others. As you develop a teaching plan be sure to include one or more of the following items of information:

ESTROGENS AND PROGESTINS

- Carefully read the patient package insert available with the drug. If there are any questions about this information, discuss them with the primary health care provider.
- If GI upset occurs, take the drug with food.
- Notify the primary health care provider if any of the following occurs: pain in the legs or groin area; sharp chest pain or sudden shortness of breath; lumps in the breast; sudden severe headache; dizziness or fainting; vision or speech disturbances; weakness or numbness in the arms, face, or legs; severe abdominal pain; depression; or yellowing of the skin or eyes.
- If pregnancy is suspected or abnormal vaginal bleeding occurs, stop taking the drug and contact the primary health care provider immediately.
- Patient with diabetes: Check the blood glucose daily, or more often. Contact the primary health care provider if the blood glucose is elevated. An elevated blood glucose level may require a change in diabetic therapy (insulin, oral antidiabetic drug) or diet; these changes must be made by the primary health care provider.

ESTRADIOL TRANSDERMAL SYSTEM

- Be sure to read the package insert carefully. Some systems are applied twice weekly; others are applied every 7 days.
- Apply the system immediately after opening the pouch, with the adhesive side down. Apply to clean, dry skin of the trunk, buttocks, abdomen, upper inner thigh, or upper arm. Do not apply to breasts, waistline, or a site exposed to sunlight. The area should not be oily or irritated. Be careful with heat sources such as an electric blanket that can increase the rate of absorption.
- Press the system firmly in place with the palm of the hand for about 10 seconds. The application site is rotated, with at least 1-week intervals between applications to a particular site.
- Avoid areas that may be exposed to rubbing or where clothing may rub the system off or loosen the edges.
- Remove the old system before applying a new system. Rotate application sites to prevent skin irritation.
- Follow the directions of the primary health care provider regarding application of the system (e.g., continuous, 3 weeks of use followed by 1 week off, changed weekly, or applied twice weekly).
- If the system falls off, reapply it or apply a new system. Continue the original treatment schedule.

INTRAVAGINAL APPLICATION

- Use the applicator correctly. Refer to the package insert for correct procedure. The applicator is marked with the correct dosage and accompanies the drug when purchased.
- Wash the applicator after each use in warm water with a mild soap and rinse well.
- Maintain a recumbent position for at least 30 minutes after instillation.
- Use a panty liner to protect clothing if necessary.
- Do not double the dosage if a dose is missed. Instead, skip the dose and resume treatment the next day.

ANDROGEN HORMONE INHIBITOR

- Inform the primary health care provider immediately if sexual partner is or may become pregnant, because additional measures, such as discontinuing the drug or use of a condom, may be necessary.
- Women who are or may become pregnant should not handle this medication.
- Do not donate blood for at least 6 months after stopping medication due to potential effects on pregnant women who may receive the blood product.

ANTISPASMODIC DRUGS

- Flavoxate: Take this drug three to four times daily as prescribed. This drug is used to treat symptoms; other drugs are given to treat the cause.
- Oxybutynin: Take this drug with or without food. Oxybutynin (Ditropan XL) contains an outer coating that may not disintegrate and sometimes may be observed in the stool. This is not a cause for concern. If using the transdermal form (patch) of the drug, be sure to apply to a clean, dry area of the hip, abdomen, or buttocks. Remove the old patch and rotate sites of new application every 7 days.
- Antispasmodic drugs can cause heat prostration (fever and heat stroke caused by decreased sweating) in high temperatures. If you live in hot climates or will be exposed to high temperatures, take appropriate precautions.

Menopause and Andropause Drugs

EVALUATION

- Therapeutic effect is achieved and urinary or reproductive symptoms are relieved.
- Adverse reactions are identified, reported to the primary health care provider, and managed successfully through appropriate nursing interventions.
  - Knowledge level is enhanced.
  - Mucous membranes are moist and intact.
  - No injury is evident.
  - Patient is free of pain.
- Patient and family express confidence and demonstrate an understanding of the drug regimen.

PHARMACOLOGY IN PRACTICE
THINK CRITICALLY

 Mr. Phillip has returned to the clinic with continued UTI symptoms. The primary health care provider suspects that Mr. Phillip may have BPH and is reducing his fluid intake to prevent Mr. Phillip from having to get up at night to urinate. Analyze the situation to determine what points you would stress in a teaching plan for this patient.

KEY POINTS

- During menopause, the hormone estrogen diminishes and the menstrual cycle can become irregular until it stops. This period is also called the female climacteric. Changes related to the cardiovascular, skeletal, urinary, and reproductive systems can cause uncomfortable symptoms. The hormone estrogen can be replaced, which helps to relieve flushing, sweating, and atrophy of vaginal and urinary tissues, and improves bones.

- The number of urinary system disorders increases as people age. Renal function can be reduced to 50% and the urine becomes more dilute. Strength, flexibility, and the capacity of the bladder decreases. This can lead to

pain, frequency, or incontinence. Antispasmodic agents reduce urinary smooth muscle spasms and improves urinary flow.

- Urinary issues can also be a sign of prostate enlargement. BPH symptoms such as frequency, reduced flow, nocturia, and dysuria are treated with antiadrenergic or male hormone inhibitors. Erectile dysfunction may result from use of certain medications or a medical condition such as diabetes or BPH. Medications used to treat ED are similar to others used to dilate circulatory vessels. Similar adverse reactions can present such as hypotension.

Summary Drug Table — AGING URINARY AND REPRODUCTIVE DRUGS

Generic Name	Trade Name	Uses	Adverse Reactions	Dosage Ranges
Female Hormone: Estrogens				
estrogens, conjugated *ess'-troe-jens*	Premarin	Oral: vasomotor symptoms associated with menopause, atrophic vaginitis, osteoporosis, hypogonadism, primary ovarian failure, breast and prostate cancer palliation Parenteral: abnormal uterine bleeding from hormonal imbalance	Headache, dizziness, melasma, venous thromboembolism, nausea, vomiting, abdominal bloating and cramps, breakthrough bleeding/spotting, vaginal changes, rhinitis, changes in libido, breast enlargement and tenderness, weight changes, generalized pain	0.3–2.5 mg/day orally; IM: 25 mg/injection
estrogens, esterified	Menest	Same as conjugated estrogens	Same as conjugated estrogens	0.3–1.25 mg/day orally
estrogens, topical	Divigel, EstroGel (transdermal)	Vaginal atrophy and vasomotor symptoms associated with menopause	Rare: minor vaginal irritation or itching	Metered dose for daily application
estrogens, vaginal	Estring, Femring; Estrace, Ogen, and Premarin Vaginal Creams	Vaginal atrophy and vasomotor symptoms associated with menopause	Rare: minor vaginal irritation or itching	See package insert; used weekly or monthly

Summary Drug Table AGING URINARY AND REPRODUCTIVE DRUGS (continued)

Generic Name	Trade Name	Uses	Adverse Reactions	Dosage Ranges
estradiol, oral *ess-trah-dye'-ole*	Femtrace	Vasomotor symptoms associated with menopause, osteoporosis prevention, hypoestrogenism palliative therapy for breast and prostate cancer	Same as conjugated estrogens	0.5–10 mg/day orally
estradiol cypionate *ess-trah-dye'-ole 'sip-ee-oh-nate*	Depo-Estradiol	Moderate to severe vasomotor symptoms associated with menopause, female hypogonadism	Same as conjugated estrogens; pain at injection site	1–5 mg IM, every 3–4 wk
estradiol hemihydrate	Vagifem	Atrophic vaginitis	Same as conjugated estrogens	1 tablet vaginally daily
estradiol transdermal system	Alora, Climara, Estraderm, Menostar, Vivelle	Same as conjugated estrogens	Same as conjugated estrogens	Variable doses, applied to skin weekly
estradiol topical emulsion	Estrasorb	Vasomotor symptoms of menopause		Two prepackaged pouches/day
estradiol valerate *ess-trah-dye'-ole val'-eh-rate*	Delestrogen	Same as estradiol cypionate	Same as conjugated estrogens; pain at injection site	10–20 mg IM monthly
estropipate *ess-troe-pye'-pate*	Ogen (cream), Ortho-Est (tablet)	Moderate to severe vasomotor symptoms associated with menopause, female hypogonadism, ovarian failure, osteoporosis	Same as conjugated estrogens	0.625–9 mg/day orally
synthetic conjugated estrogens, A	Cenestin	Moderate to severe vasomotor symptoms associated with menopause, vaginal atrophy	Same as conjugated estrogens	0.45 mg/day orally, then adjust according to symptoms
synthetic conjugated estrogens, B	Enjuvia	Moderate to severe vasomotor symptoms associated with menopause	Same as conjugated estrogens	0.3 mg/day orally, then adjust according to symptoms
Progestins				
estrogens and progestins combined	Activella, Angeliq, Climara Pro, CombiPatch, Femhrt, Prefest, Prempro, YAZ	Treatment of moderate to severe vasomotor symptoms associated with menopause, treatment of vulval and vaginal atrophy, osteoporosis	Adverse reactions of both hormones; same as synthetic conjugated estrogens and progesterone	Oral or transdermal, variable dosing, used daily or weekly. See package insert
Miscellaneous Drug				
raloxifene *ral-ox'-i-feen*	Evista	Osteoporosis prevention and treatment	Hot flashes, flu-like symptoms, arthralgia, rhinitis, increased cough	60 mg/day orally

(table continues on page 526)

Menopause and Andropause Drugs

Summary Drug Table AGING URINARY AND REPRODUCTIVE DRUGS (continued)

Generic Name	Trade Name	Uses	Adverse Reactions	Dosage Ranges
Urinary Drugs (Antispasmodics)				
darifenacin
da-ree-fen'-ah-sin	Enablex	Overactive bladder	Dry mouth, constipation	7.5 mg/day orally
fesoterodine
fes-oh-ter'-oh-deen	Toviaz	Overactive bladder	Dry mouth	4–8 mg orally daily
flavoxate
fla-vox'-ate	Urispas	Urinary symptoms caused by cystitis, prostatitis, and other urinary problems	Dry mouth, drowsiness, blurred vision, headache, urinary retention	100–200 mg orally TID or QID
oxybutynin
ox-ee-byoo-tye'-nin	Ditropan	Overactive bladder, neurogenic bladder	Dry mouth, nausea, headache, drowsiness, constipation, urinary retention	5 mg orally BID or TID
solifenacin
soe-lih-fen'-ah-sin	Vesicare	Overactive bladder	Dry mouth, constipation, blurred vision, dry eyes	5 mg/day orally
tolterodine
toll-tare'-oh-dyne	Detrol, Detrol LA (long acting, extended release)	Overactive bladder	Dry mouth, constipation, headache, dizziness	2 mg orally TID; extended release: 4 mg/day
Ⓡ trospium
troz'-pee-um	Sanctura	Overactive bladder	Dry mouth, constipation, headache	20 mg orally TID
Benign Prostate Hyperplasia Drugs				
Androgen Hormone Inhibitors				
dutasteride
doo-tas'-teer-ryde	Avodart	BPH	Impotence, decreased libido	0.5 mg/day orally
finasteride
fin-as'-teh-ryde	Propecia, Proscar	Male-pattern baldness, BPH	Impotence, decreased libido, asthenia, dizziness, postural hypotension	1–5 mg/day orally
Antiadrenergic Drugs: Peripherally Acting				
alfuzosin
al-foo-zoe'-sin	Uroxatral	BPH	Headache, dizziness	10 mg orally daily
doxazosin
dok-say-zoe'-sin	Cardura	Hypertension, BPH	Headache, dizziness, fatigue	Hypertension: 1–8 mg orally daily; BPH: 1–16 mg orally daily
silodosin
sye'-lo-doe'-sin	Rapaflo	BPH	Headache, dizziness, ejaculatory dysfunction, diarrhea, rhinitis	8 mg orally daily
tamsulosin
tam-soo-loe' sin	Flomax	BPH	Headache, ejaculatory dysfunction, dizziness, rhinitis	0.4 mg orally daily
terazosin
tare-ah'-zoe-sin	Hytrin	Hypertension, BPH	Dizziness, postural hypotension, headache, dyspnea, nasal congestion	Hypertension: 1–20 mg orally daily; BPH: 1–10 mg orally daily
dutasteride/ tamsulosin combination	Jalyn	BPH	See each separate drug	1 capsule orally at the same time daily

Summary Drug Table AGING URINARY AND REPRODUCTIVE DRUGS (continued)

Generic Name	Trade Name	Uses	Adverse Reactions	Dosage Ranges
Impotence Agents				
avanafil *a-van'-a-fil*	Stendra	Erectile dysfunction	Headache, dyspepsia, nasal congestion, back pain	100–200 mg orally 30–60 min before sexual activity
sildenafil *sil-den'-a-fil*	Viagra	Erectile dysfunction	Headache, flushing, dyspepsia, nasal congestion	25–50 mg orally 30–60 min before sexual activity
tadalafil *ta-da'-a-fil*	Cialis	Erectile dysfunction, BPH	Headache, dyspepsia, nasal congestion, back pain	5–20 mg orally, take daily for BPH, as needed for sexual activity Up to 36 hours before sexual activity
vardenafil *var-den'-a-fil*	Levitra, Staxyn	Erectile dysfunction	Headache, flushing, dyspepsia, runny nose, back pain	5–20 mg orally 60 min before sexual activity 4 hours before sexual activity
Hormonal Therapy for Cancer				
Adrenal Steroid Inhibitors				
aminoglutethimide *ah-meen'-oh-glootih-thye-myde*	Cytadren	Metastatic breast, prostate cancers	Drowsiness, skin rash, nausea, vomiting	1–2 g/day orally
Gonadotropin-Releasing Hormone Analogs				
degarelix *deg-a-rel'-ix*	Firmagon	Advanced prostate cancer	Hot flashes, injection site pain, weight gain	80–240 mg subcut
goserelin *goe'-seh-rell-in*	Zoladex	Prostate and breast cancer, endometriosis, endometrial thinning	Headache, emotional lability, depression, sweating, acne, breast atrophy, sexual dysfunction, vaginitis, hot flashes, pain, edema	3.6-mg monthly implant, 10.8-mg q 3 mo implant
histrelin *hiss'-trell-in*	Vantas	Prostate cancer	Hot flashes, fatigue, implant site irritation	50–60 mcg/day delivered e.g., implant changed yearly
leuprolide *loo-proe'-lyde*	Eligard, Lupron	Prostate cancer, endometriosis, precocious puberty, uterine leiomyomata	Hot flashes, edema, bone pain, electrocardiographic changes, hypertension	1 mg/day subcut, provided in monthly injection form and implant
triptorelin *trip-toe-rell'-in*	Trelstar	Prostate cancer	Hot flashes, skeletal pain, headache, impotence	3.75 mg IM every 28 days
Antiandrogens				
abiraterone *a'-bir-a'-ter-one*	Zytiga	Prostate cancer	Hot flashes, nocturia, urinary frequency, peripheral edema, general pain, upper respiratory infection	1,000 g/day with prednisone
bicalutamide *bye-cal-loo'-tahmyde*	Casodex	Prostate cancer	Hot flashes, dizziness, constipation, nausea, diarrhea, nocturia, hematuria, peripheral edema, general pain, asthenia, infection	50 mg/day orally

(table continues on page 528)

Menopause and Andropause Drugs

Summary Drug Table AGING URINARY AND REPRODUCTIVE DRUGS (continued)

Generic Name	Trade Name	Uses	Adverse Reactions	Dosage Ranges
flutamide *floo'-tah-myde*	Eulexin	Prostate cancer	Hot flashes, loss of libido, impotence, diarrhea, nausea, vomiting, gynecomastia	250 mg/orally TID
nilutamide *nah-loo'-tah-myde*	Nilandron	Prostate cancer	Pain, headache, asthenia, flu-like symptoms, insomnia, nausea, constipation, testicular atrophy, dyspnea	300 mg/day for 1 mo, then 150 mg/day orally
Estrogen				
estramustine *es'-tra-mus-teen*	Emcyt	Prostate cancer	Breast tenderness and enlargement, nausea, diarrhea, edema	14 mg/kg/day orally in divided doses
Androgen				
testolactone *tess-toe-lak'-tone*	Teslac	Palliative treatment: breast cancer	Paresthesia, glossitis, anorexia, nausea, vomiting, maculopapular erythema, aches, alopecia, edema of the extremities, increase in blood pressure	250 mg orally QID
Aromatase Inhibitors				
anastrazole *an-ass'-troh-zoll*	Arimidex	Breast cancer	Vasodilation, mood disturbances, nausea, hot flashes, pharyngitis, asthenia, pain	1 mg/day orally
exemestane *ex-ah'-mess-tane*	Aromasin	Breast cancer	Same as anastrazole	25 mg/day orally
letrozole *leh'-troe-zoll*	Femara	Breast cancer	Same as anastrazole	2.5 mg/day orally
Progestins				
medroxyprogesterone *meh-drox'-ee-proe-jess'-ter-own*	Depo-Provera	Endometrial or renal cancer	Fatigue, nervousness, rash, pruritus, acne, edema	400–1000 mg/wk IM
megestrol *meh-jess'-troll*	Megace	Breast or endometrial cancer, appetite stimulant in human immunodeficiency virus (HIV) infection	Weight gain, nausea, vomiting, edema, breakthrough bleeding	40–320 mg/day orally in divided doses
Antiestrogens				
fulvestrant *full-vess'-trant*	Faslodex	Breast cancer	Nausea, vomiting, asthenia, pain, pharyngitis, headache	250 mg IM once monthly
tamoxifen *tah-mox'-ih-fen*		Breast cancer, prophylactic therapy for women at high risk for breast cancer	Hot flashes, rashes, headaches, vaginal bleeding and discharge	20–40 mg/day orally
toremifene *tore-em'-ih-feen*	Fareston	Breast cancer	Hot flashes, sweating, nausea, dizziness, edema, vaginal bleeding and discharge	60 mg/day orally

Ⓡ Take this drug at least 1 hour before or 2 hours after meals.

● Chapter Review

Know Your Drugs

Clients sometimes know a medication by the brand (or trade) name and not the generic name. To help you recognize both names, match the brand name with the generic name of the same medication.

Generic Name	Brand Name
1. avanafil	A. Ditropan
2. finasteride	B. Rapaflo
3. oxybutynin	C. Propecia
4. silodosin	D. Stendra

Calculate Medication Dosages

1. The primary health care provider prescribes fesoterodine 8 mg orally once a day for an overactive bladder problem. The pharmacy dispenses the drug in 4-mg tablets. The nurse instructs the client to take _____.

2. The primary health care provider prescribes sildenafil 50 mg orally as needed for sexual relations. If the maximum dose is 100 mg in 24 hours, how many pills can the client take in one day?

● Prepare for the NCLEX®

Build Your Knowledge

1. When a woman stops ovulating, this is referred to as _____.

   1. menarche
   2. andropause
   3. menopause
   4. HRT

2. Which of the following structures is in the upper urinary system?

   1. bladder
   2. prostate
   3. urethra
   4. kidney

3. What percentage of kidney function typically is reduced as people age?

   1. 10%
   2. 35%
   3. 50%
   4. 85%

4. The most common drugs used for BPH are _____.

   1. cholinergic blockers
   2. antiadrenergics
   3. hormones
   4. enzyme inhibitors

5. How many Americans suffer from OBS?

   1. 16 million
   2. 1.3 billion
   3. 46, 000
   4. 250,000

6. If a urinary drug has anticholinergic effects, the symptoms will be _____.

   1. slow heartbeat
   2. dry mouth
   3. wakefulness
   4. dry skin

Apply Your Knowledge

7. If the drug dutasteride is for BPH and used only for men, why is it rated pregnancy category X?

   1. To be sure it is not administered to women for menopausal symptoms
   2. It can harm a male fetus if absorbed by a pregnant woman
   3. To make it clear it is to be given to men only
   4. All drugs are ranked no matter if only for men or not

8. A client calls regarding taking vardenafil. Which of the following statements would be of concern and should be reported immediately?

   1. "Nurse, my cheeks look like I'm having a hot flash."
   2. "My penis is still poking out now after 4 hours."
   3. "I can't take those pills because they give me a headache!"
   4. "My nose is suddenly stuffy, wonder if I have a cold."

Alternate-Format Questions

9. A client says she is stopping the antispasmodic drug because of dry mouth and constipation. What are some teaching tips the nurse can offer to reduce these adverse reactions? **Select all that apply**.

   1. Add more fiber to your diet
   2. Limit fluid intake
   3. Eat a piece of watermelon daily
   4. Select meat cuts that are iron rich
   5. Brush and floss your teeth regularly

10. As the urinary bladder ages, which of the following cause nocturia? **Select all that apply**.

    1. capacity increases
    2. flexibility is reduced
    3. prostate tissue obstructs flow
    4. bladder strength diminishes

To check your answers, see Appendix G.

the**Point** *For more NCLEX-style questions, log on to http://thepoint.lww.com to access more than 1000 questions.*

Urinary Tract Anti-Infectives and Other Urinary Drugs

On completion of this chapter, the student will:

1. Discuss the uses, general drug actions, adverse reactions, contraindications, precautions, and interactions of the drugs used to treat infections and symptoms associated with urinary tract infections.
2. Discuss important preadministration and ongoing assessment activities the nurse should perform with the patient taking a drug for a urinary tract infection.
3. List nursing diagnoses particular to a patient taking a drug for a urinary tract infection.
4. Discuss ways to promote an optimal response to therapy, how to manage adverse reactions, and important points to keep in mind when educating patients about the use of drugs to treat urinary tract infections.

KEY TERMS

bactericidal • drug or agent that destroys or kills bacteria

bacteriostatic • drug or agent that slows or retards the multiplication of bacteria

cystitis • inflammation of the bladder

prostatitis • inflammation of the prostate gland

pyelonephritis • inflammation of the kidney nephron

urinary tract infection (UTI) • infection by pathogenic microorganisms of one or more structures of the urinary tract

DRUG CLASSES

Urinary anti-infectives
Urinary analgesics

This chapter discusses drugs used to treat **urinary tract infections** (UTIs). These types of infections are caused by pathogenic microorganisms of one or more structures of the urinary tract (Fig. 48.1). Because the female urethra is considerably shorter than the male urethra, women are affected by UTIs much more frequently than men. The most common structure affected is the bladder. Clinical manifestations of a UTI of the bladder (**cystitis**) include urgency, frequency, pressure, burning and pain on urination, and pain caused by spasm in the region of the bladder and the suprapubic area. With chronic UTIs, the urethra, prostate (**prostatitis**), and kidney (**pyelonephritis**) may also be affected.

The drugs discussed in this chapter are anti-infectives. They are used in the treatment of UTIs, and they have an effect on bacteria in the urinary tract. Although administered systemically, that is, by the oral or parenteral routes, they do not achieve significant levels in the bloodstream and are of no value in treating *systemic* infections. They are primarily excreted by the kidneys and exert their major antibacterial effects in the urine as it travels through the bladder.

Some drugs used in the treatment of UTIs, such as nitrofurantoin, do not belong to the antibiotic or sulfonamide groups of drugs. Examples of the most common drugs used in treating UTIs include amoxicillin (broad-spectrum penicillins; see Chapter 7), trimethoprim (sulfonamides; see Chapter 6), and nitrofurantoin. The anti-infective drugs known as fluoroquinolones (see Chapter 9) were initially approved for UTI treatment, but have become of greater use in systemic infection treatment. Combination drugs such as trimethoprim and sulfamethoxazole (Bactrim or Septra) are also used. The Summary Drug Table: Urinary Tract Anti-Infectives gives examples of the drugs used for UTIs.

Another drug frequently used to treat UTIs is phenazopyridine (Pyridium), a urinary analgesic, used to relieve discomfort associated with UTIs.

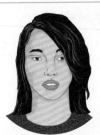

PHARMACOLOGY IN PRACTICE

Janna Wong is a 16-year-old high school gymnast. She is at the clinic for a routine physical. Vital signs show that Janna has a fever of 100.5°F. She says she feels tired, yet is fidgety. When asked if she would like some water, Janna says no because she does not want to urinate until she gets home. Think about her remarks as you read this chapter.

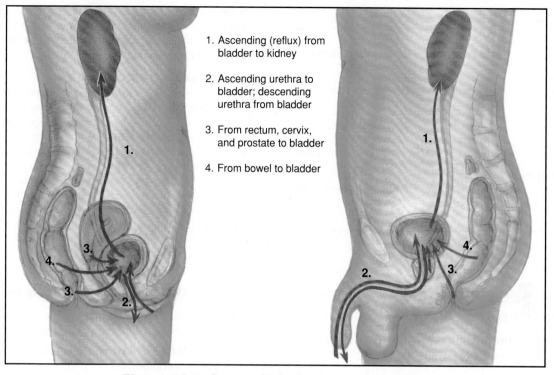

1. Ascending (reflux) from bladder to kidney

2. Ascending urethra to bladder; descending urethra from bladder

3. From rectum, cervix, and prostate to bladder

4. From bowel to bladder

Figure 48.1 Routes of infection in the urinary tract.

Actions and Uses

These drugs are used for UTIs that are caused by susceptible bacterial microorganisms. Many of the anti-infective drugs used for treating UTIs are chosen because of the rapid excretion rate of the drugs rather than the way they act inside the body. As a result, these anti-infectives have a high concentration in the urine and appear to act by interfering with bacterial multiplication in the urine. Nitrofurantoin (Macrodantin) may be **bacteriostatic** (slows or retards the multiplication of bacteria) or **bactericidal** (destroys bacteria), depending on the concentration of the drug in the urine. See the specific anti-infective chapters for the manner in which other anti-infective drugs work.

Phenazopyridine is a dye that exerts a topical analgesic effect on the lining of the urinary tract. It does not have anti-infective activity. Phenazopyridine is available as a separate drug but is also included in some urinary tract anti-infective combination drugs.

Adverse Reactions

Adverse reactions are primarily gastrointestinal (GI) disturbances and include the following:

- Anorexia, nausea, vomiting, and diarrhea
- Abdominal pain or stomatitis

Other generalized body system reactions include:

- Drowsiness, dizziness, headache, blurred vision, weakness, and peripheral neuropathy
- Rash, pruritus, photosensitivity reactions, and leg cramps

When these drugs are given in large doses, patients may experience burning on urination and bladder irritation; this should not be mistaken for a continued infection. Nitrofurantoin has been known to cause acute and chronic pulmonary reactions. Patients should be told that phenazopyridine will discolor the urine (dark orange to brown) and permanently stain undergarments that come in contact with the urine.

Contraindications and Precautions

Anti-infectives are contraindicated in patients with a hypersensitivity to the drugs and during pregnancy (pregnancy category C) and lactation. One exception is nitrofurantoin, which is classified as a pregnancy category B drug and is used with caution during pregnancy.

The anti-infectives should be used cautiously in those with renal or hepatic impairment. Patients who are allergic to tartrazine (a food dye) should not take methenamine (Hiprex). This drug is used cautiously in patients with gout, because it may cause crystals to form in the urine. Nitrofurantoin is used cautiously in patients with cerebral arteriosclerosis, diabetes, or a glucose-6-phosphate dehydrogenase (G6PD) deficiency.

Interactions

Anti-Infectives

The following interactions may occur when a specific urinary anti-infective is administered with another agent:

Interacting Drug	Common Use	Effect of Interaction
Sulfamethoxazole oral anticoagulants	Blood thinner	Increased risk for bleeding
Nitrofurantoin magnesium trisilicate or magaldrate	Relieve gastric upset	Decreased absorption of anti-infective
anticholinergics	Relieve bladder spasm/discomfort	Delay in gastric emptying, thereby increasing the absorption of nitrofurantoin
Fosfomycin (Monurol) metoclopramide (Reglan)	Relieve gastric upset	Lowers plasma concentration and urinary tract excretion of fosfomycin

An increased urinary pH (alkaline urine) decreases the effectiveness of methenamine. Therefore, to avoid raising the urine pH when taking methenamine, the patient should not use antacids containing sodium bicarbonate or sodium carbonate.

HERBAL CONSIDERATIONS

Cranberry juice has long been recommended for use in treating and preventing UTIs. Clinical studies have confirmed that cranberry juice is beneficial to individuals with frequent UTIs. Cranberry juice inhibits bacteria from attaching to the walls of the urinary tract and prevents certain bacteria from forming dental plaque in the mouth. Cranberry juice is safe for use as a food and for urinary tract health. Cranberry juice and capsules have no contraindications, no known adverse reactions, and no drug interactions. The recommended dosage is 9 to 15 capsules a day (400 to 500 mg/day) or 4 to 8 ounces of juice daily (Brown, 2012).

NURSING PROCESS
PATIENT RECEIVING A URINARY TRACT ANTI-INFECTIVE OR OTHER URINARY TRACT DRUG

ASSESSMENT

Preadministration Assessment
When a UTI has been diagnosed, urine culture and sensitivity tests are performed to determine bacterial sensitivity to the drugs (antibiotics and urinary tract anti-infectives) that will control the infection. Ask the patient about symptoms of the infection before instituting therapy. Document a description of the urine including the color (clear, straw, or amber) and the appearance (clear or cloudy). Typically you will check for fever by taking the vital signs and may perform a urine check for blood or protein.

Document the subjective symptoms the patient is experiencing to provide a baseline for future assessment. Record the patient's complaints of pain, urinary frequency, bladder distension, and other symptoms associated with the urinary system.

Ongoing Assessment
Many UTIs are treated on an outpatient basis because hospitalization is seldom required. UTIs may affect the hospitalized patient or nursing home resident with an indwelling urethral catheter or a disorder such as a stone in the urinary tract. The primary nursing intervention to prevent UTIs in the hospitalized patient is good hand hygiene (handwashing).

When caring for a hospitalized patient with a UTI, monitor the vital signs every 4 hours or as ordered by the primary health care provider. Any significant rise in body temperature is reported to the primary health care provider, because intervention to reduce the fever or culture and sensitivity tests may need to be repeated.

If after several days the symptoms of the UTI do not improve or they become worse, contact the primary health care provider as soon as possible. Periodic urinalysis and urine culture and sensitivity tests may be ordered to monitor the effects of drug therapy.

NURSING DIAGNOSES
Drug-specific nursing diagnoses include the following:

- **Impaired Urinary Elimination** related to discomfort of urinary tract infection
- **Ineffective Breathing Pattern** related to adverse reaction to drug

Nursing diagnoses related to drug administration are discussed in Chapter 4.

PLANNING
The expected outcomes for the patient may include an optimal response to drug therapy, support of patient needs related to the management of adverse reactions, and confidence in an understanding of the medication regimen.

IMPLEMENTATION

Promoting an Optimal Response to Therapy
To promote an optimal response to therapy, give urinary tract anti-infectives with food to prevent GI upset. Nitrofurantoin especially should be given with food, meals, or milk, because this drug is particularly irritating to the stomach. Fosfomycin (Monurol) has special administration requirements; it comes in a 3-gram, one-dose packet that must be dissolved in 90 to 120 mL of water (not hot water). Administer the drug immediately after dissolving it in water. Phenazopyridine is administered after meals to prevent GI upset.

NURSING ALERT
Phenazopyridine is not administered for more than 2 days when used in combination with an antibacterial drug to treat a UTI. When used for more than 2 days, the drug may mask the symptoms of a more serious disorder.

Monitoring and Managing Patient Needs
Observe the patient for adverse drug reactions. If an adverse reaction occurs, contact the primary health care provider before the next dose of the drug is due. However, serious drug reactions, such as a pulmonary reaction, are reported immediately.

Patient Teaching for Improved Patient Outcomes

Preventing and Treating UTIs

When you teach, make sure your patient understands the following:

✔ Describes UTIs and their causes, and identifies what may be their cause.
✔ Able to review the drug therapy regimen, including prescribed drug, dose, and frequency of administration.
✔ Knows the importance of taking the entire drug even if the patient feels better after a few doses.
✔ Describes ways to reduce UTIs, such as how to wipe front to back after going to the bathroom.
✔ Avoid tight clothing, prolonged wearing of pantyhose, tight pants, or wet bathing suits.
✔ Shower instead of bathing, rinsing well; avoid "overcleaning" and irritating the skin.
✔ Use tampons for menstrual periods instead of pads; make a habit of voiding every 4 hours and changing the tampon.
✔ After sexual contact, void and drink 2 to 8 ounces of water.
✔ Increase fluid intake, gauging the amount you drink to the color of your urine (it should be pale yellow during the day).
✔ ⚑ Avoid eating foods or drinking liquids that irritate the bladder, such as coffee, tea, alcohol, artificial sweeteners, chocolate, and pepper.
✔ Vitamin C supplements and cranberry juice help maintain an acid environment in the bladder.
✔ Be sure to drink fluids and void regularly when cycling or horseback riding.

IMPAIRED URINARY ELIMINATION. The patient is encouraged to drink at least 2000 mL of fluid daily (if condition permits) to dilute urine and decrease pain on voiding. Drinking extra fluids aids in the physical removal of bacteria from the genitourinary tract and is an important part of UTI treatment (see Patient Teaching for Improved Patient Outcomes: Preventing and Treating UTIs). Offer fluids, preferably water, to the patient at hourly intervals. Cranberry or prune juice is usually given rather than orange juice or other citrus or vegetable juices. Contact the primary health care provider if the patient fails to drink extra fluids, if the urine output is low, or if the urine appears concentrated during daytime hours. The urine of those drinking 2000 mL or more daily appears dilute and light in color.

Older patients often have a decreased thirst sensation and must be encouraged to increase fluid intake. This is especially true if the individual is not able to obtain or reach the fluid container. Develop a schedule to offer fluids at regular intervals to older adult patients or those who seem unable to increase their fluid intake without supervision.

When administering these drugs, monitor the fluid intake and urinary output for volume and frequency. Measure and record the fluid intake and output every 8 hours, especially when the primary health care provider orders an increase in fluid intake or when a kidney infection is being treated. The

primary health care provider may also order daily urinary pH levels when methenamine or nitrofurantoin is administered. These drugs work best in acid urine; failure of the urine to remain acidic may require administration of a urinary acidifier, such as ascorbic acid.

INEFFECTIVE BREATHING PATTERN. Pulmonary reactions have been reported with the use of nitrofurantoin and may occur within hours and up to 3 weeks after drug therapy is initiated. Signs and symptoms of an acute pulmonary reaction include dyspnea, chest pain, cough, fever, and chills. If these reactions occur, immediately notify the primary health care provider and withhold the next dose of the drug until the patient is seen by a primary health care provider. In addition to the aforementioned signs and symptoms, a nonproductive cough or malaise may indicate a chronic pulmonary reaction, which may occur during prolonged therapy.

Educating the Patient and Family

Educate regarding the importance for everyone to increase fluid intake to at least 2000 mL/day (unless contraindicated) to help remove bacteria from the genitourinary tract (see Patient Teaching for Improving Patient Outcomes: Preventing and Treating UTIs). Be sure the patient understands that phenazopyridine will cause a reddish-orange discoloration of the urine that stains clothing. In addition, the fluid that lubricates the eyes may change color, causing permanent discoloration of contact lenses. Reassure the patient that this discoloration is normal and will subside when use of the drug is discontinued.

To ensure adherence to the prescribed drug regimen, educate about the importance of completing the full course of drug therapy even though symptoms have been relieved. A full course of therapy is necessary to ensure that all bacteria have been eliminated from the urinary tract. Include the following drug teaching points in a patient and family teaching plan:

■ Take the drug with food or meals (nitrofurantoin must be taken with food or milk). If GI upset occurs despite taking the drug with food, contact the primary health care provider.

■ Take the drug at the prescribed intervals and complete the full course of therapy. Do not discontinue taking the drug even though the symptoms have disappeared, unless directed to do so by the primary health care provider.

■ If drowsiness or dizziness occurs, avoid driving and performing tasks that require alertness.

■ ⚑ Avoid alcoholic beverages and do not take any nonprescription drug unless its use has been approved by the primary health care provider.

■ Notify the primary health care provider immediately if symptoms do not improve after 3 or 4 days.

■ *Nitrofurantoin:* Take this drug with food or milk to improve absorption. Continue therapy for at least 1 week or for 3 days after the urine shows no signs of infection. Notify the primary health care provider immediately if any of the following occur: fever, chills, cough, shortness of breath, chest pain, or difficulty breathing. Do not take the next dose of the drug until the primary health care provider has been contacted. The urine may appear brown during therapy with this drug; this is not abnormal.

- *Methenamine:* Avoid excessive intake of citrus products, milk, and milk products.
- Fosfomycin comes in dry form as a one-dose packet to be dissolved in 90 to 120 mL of water (not hot water). Drink immediately after mixing and take with food to prevent gastric upset.
- *Phenazopyridine:* This drug may cause a reddish-orange discoloration of the urine and tears and may stain fabrics or contact lenses. This is normal. Take the drug after meals. Do not take this drug for more than 2 days if you are also taking an antibiotic for the treatment of a UTI.

EVALUATION

- Therapeutic effect is achieved and bladder symptoms are relieved.
- Adverse reactions are identified, reported to the primary health care provider, and managed successfully through appropriate nursing interventions.
  - Urinary elimination occurs without incident.
  - Adequate breathing pattern is maintained.
- Patient and family express confidence and demonstrate an understanding of the drug regimen.

PHARMACOLOGY IN PRACTICE
THINK CRITICALLY

 During your intake you find that Janna drinks minimal amounts of water at school, waiting to get home to void instead of using the school facilities. Urinalysis shows cloudy, dark amber urine with white cells when you test it using a dipstick. In addition to antibiotic treatment, what are some important teaching points to review with Janna?

KEY POINTS

- Urinary tract infections are caused by pathogenic microorganisms of one or more structures of the urinary tract. Because the female urethra is considerably shorter than the male urethra, women are affected by UTIs much more frequently than men. The most common structure affected is the bladder.
- The anti-infectives used are the same as for other bacterial infections although taken orally they do not achieve significant levels in the bloodstream. The purpose of use is that they are rapidly excreted by the kidneys and exert their major antibacterial effects in the urine as it travels through the bladder.
- Adverse reactions are GI such as nausea, diarrhea, and abdominal pain. If burning on urination occurs it should be determined if it is due to the medication or the infection.

Summary Drug Table URINARY TRACT ANTI-INFECTIVES

Generic Name	Trade Name	Uses	Adverse Reactions	Dosage Ranges
amoxicillin *ah-mox-ih-sill'-in*	Amoxil	Acute bacterial UTIs, other bacterial infections	Glossitis, stomatitis, gastritis, furry tongue, nausea, vomiting, diarrhea, rash, fever, pain at injection site, hypersensitivity reactions, hematopoietic changes	250–500 mg orally q 8 hr or 875 mg orally BID
fosfomycin *foss-foh-mye'-sin*	Monurol	Acute bacterial UTIs	Nausea, diarrhea, vaginitis, rhinitis, headache, back pain	3-g packet orally, provided in powder that must be mixed with fluid
methenamine *meth-en'-ah-meen*	Hiprex, Urex	Chronic bacterial UTIs	Nausea, vomiting, abdominal cramps, bladder irritation	1 g orally BID
nitrofurantoin *nye-troe-fyoor-an'-toyn*	Furadantin, Macrobid, Macrodantin	Acute bacterial UTIs	Nausea, anorexia, peripheral neuropathy, headache, bacterial superinfection	50–100 mg orally QID
trimethoprim (TMP) *trye-meth'-oh-prim*		Acute bacterial UTIs	Rash, pruritus, nausea, vomiting	200 mg/day orally
Urinary Anti-Infective Combinations				
trimethoprim and sulfamethoxazole (TMP-SMZ) *trye-meth'-oh-prim* *sul-fah-meth-ox'-ah-zoll*	Bactrim, Septra	Acute bacterial UTIs, shigellosis, and acute otitis media	GI disturbances, allergic skin reactions, headache, anorexia, glossitis, hypersensitivity	160 mg TMP/800 SMZ orally q 12 hr; 8–10 mg/kg/day (based on TMP) IV in 2–4 divided doses
Other Urinary Drug (Analgesic)				
phenazopyridine *fen-az-oh-peer'-ih-deen*	Pyridium	Relief of pain associated with irritation of the lower genitourinary tract	Headache, rash, pruritus, GI disturbances, red-orange discoloration of the urine, yellowish discoloration of the skin or sclera	200 mg orally TID

Ⓡ Take this drug at least 1 hour before or 2 hours after meals.

● Chapter Review

Know Your Drugs

Clients sometimes know a medication by the brand (or trade) name and not the generic name. To help you recognize both names, match the brand name with the generic name of the same medication.

Generic Name	Brand Name
1. trimethoprim/sulfamethoxazole	A. Amoxil
2. phenazopyridine	B. Bactrim
3. nitrofurantoin	C. Macrodantin
4. amoxicillin	D. Pyridium

Calculate Medication Dosages

1. Amoxicillin 500 mg is prescribed. The drug is available in 250-mg tablets. The nurse administers _____.

2. Nitrofurantoin oral suspension 50 mg is prescribed. The oral suspension contains 25 mg/5 mL. The nurse administers _____.

● Prepare for the NCLEX®

Build Your Knowledge

1. The nurse correctly administers nitrofurantoin (Macrodantin) _____.

   1. with food
   2. for no longer than 7 days
   3. without regard to food
   4. for no longer than 2 days

2. To avoid raising the pH when taking methenamine (Hiprex), the nurse advises the client to _____.

   1. use an antacid before taking the drug
   2. take an antacid immediately after taking the drug
   3. avoid antacids containing sodium bicarbonate or sodium carbonate
   4. avoid the use of antacids 1 hour before or 2 hours after taking the drug

3. What instruction would be most important to give a client prescribed fosfomycin (Monurol)?

   1. Drink one to two glasses of cranberry juice daily to promote healing of the urinary tract.
   2. You may take the drug without regard to meals.
   3. This drug comes in a one-dose packet that must be dissolved in 90 mL or more of fluids.
   4. This drug may cause mental confusion.

Apply Your Knowledge

4. What statement(s) would be included in a teaching plan for a client prescribed phenazopyridine (Pyridium)?

   1. There is a danger of heat prostration or heat stroke when taking phenazopyridine in a hot climate.
   2. This drug may turn the urine dark brown. This is an indication of a serious condition and should be reported immediately.
   3. This drug may cause photosensitivity. Take precautions when out in the sun by wearing sunscreen, a hat, and a long-sleeved shirt for protection.
   4. This drug may turn the urine reddish-orange. This is a normal occurrence that will disappear when use of the drug is discontinued.

Alternate-Format Questions

5. Match the inflammation to the organ effected.

1. Cystitis	A. Bladder
2. Prostatitis	B. Kidney
3. Pyelonephritis	C. Prostate
4. Urethritis	D. Urethra

To check your answers, see Appendix G.

the**Point** *For more NCLEX-style questions, log on to http://thepoint.lww.com to access more than 1000 questions.*

Drugs That Affect the Immune System

The immune system is not located in any single portion of the body. Rather, it flows through the entire body as a set of cells and fluid designed to recognize and respond to invasion. The chapters in this unit describe the drugs used to support the immune system in either recognizing invasion of an outside pathogen or identifying the body's own cells growing out of control.

The lymphatic system plays a major role in the immune system. Cells called *T lymphocytes* (T cells) circulate in the bloodstream and lymphatics, prepared to protect the body. The various kinds of T cells include the following:

- Helper T1 cells—increase B-lymphocyte antibody production
- Helper T2 cells—increase activity of cytotoxic (killer) T cells, which attack cells directly by altering the cell membrane and causing cell lysis (destruction)
- Helper T4 cells—function in the bloodstream to identify and destroy antigens
- Suppressor T cells—suppress the immune response
- Memory T lymphocytes—recognize previous contact with antigens and activate an immune response

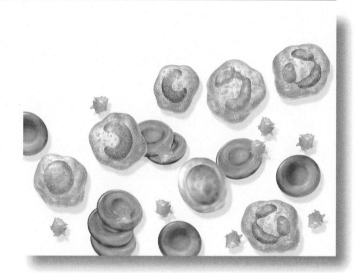

Immunizations, covered in Chapter 49, are individual drugs or a series of drugs given to help the body identify a pathogenic invader. In the past, communicable diseases and injuries were the primary illnesses health care providers treated. Today, some communicable diseases, such as smallpox and polio, have been almost eradicated because of the ability to immunize large populations of people at or near birth. All nurses play an important role in the continued immunization and protection of the population from easily preventable diseases.

Cancer is still a dreaded disease in our culture. At one time, a diagnosis of cancer was akin to a death sentence. With the advent of numerous drugs, known as *chemotherapy*, cancer is now viewed as a chronic illness in which people may be diagnosed and treated, then monitored for the remainder of their lives and treated again should cancer cells re-emerge. The information provided in Chapter 50 about antineoplastic drugs is meant to inform you about these medications—not to prepare you to administer them. Most hospitals and clinics require that nurses receive specialized training and standardized educational preparation before they are permitted to administer antineoplastic drugs. The Oncology Nursing Society has developed guidelines and educational tools for credentialing nurses for certification in administering chemotherapy.

The information in Chapter 50 is based on the need of all nurses to be able to assess and treat patients undergoing chemotherapy, whether they present with adverse reactions in the primary health care provider's outpatient office or hospital emergency department, or are being treated in the acute care setting for other illnesses or injuries.

Many of the treatments today are limited only by the destruction to the good cells in the body. Replacement of these cells from other people is limited by the antibodies we produce. Drugs that help to stimulate the body to make its own platelets and red and white blood cells are described in Chapter 51. With the growing ability to stimulate the body to produce its own blood cell components, many more people may live longer, improved-quality lives.

Immunologic Agents

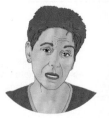

49

KEY TERMS

active immunity • type of immunity that occurs when the person is exposed to a disease and develops the disease, and the body makes antibodies to provide future protection against the disease

antibody • molecule with the ability to bind to a specific antigen

antigen • substance that is capable of inducing a specific immune response

antigen–antibody response • antibodies formed in response to exposure to a specific antigen

attenuate • to weaken

booster • immunogen injected after a specified interval; often after the primary immunization to stimulate and sustain the immune response

cell-mediated immunity • immune reaction caused by white blood cells

globulins • plasma proteins that are insoluble in water

humoral immunity • antibody-mediated immune response of the body

immune globulins • solution obtained from human or animal blood containing antibodies that have been formed by the body to specific antigens; administered to provide passive immunity to one or more infectious diseases

immunity • resistance to infection

immunization • the process in which a person is made immune or resistant to an infectious disease

passive immunity • type of immunity occurring from the administration of ready-made antibodies from another individual or animal

toxin • poisonous substance

toxoid • attenuated toxin that is capable of stimulating the formation of antitoxins

vaccine • substance containing either weakened or killed antigens developed for the purpose of creating resistance to disease

DRUG CLASSES

Active immunity agents	Passive immunity agents
• Vaccines, bacterial and viral	• Immune globulins
• Toxoids	• Antivenins

PHARMACOLOGY IN PRACTICE

Betty Peterson's niece has been staying with Betty since the niece was laid off from her job. She received health insurance from her previous employer; now without it, she has to make choices about when to go to the clinic. She cannot always find the money to pay for the visit. Jimmy is Betty's 4-month-old grandnephew; determine where he is in the immunization schedules assuming he is up-to-date with these.

Immunity refers to the ability of the body to identify and resist microorganisms that are potentially harmful. This ability enables the body to fight or prevent infectious disease and inhibit tissue and organ damage. The immune system is not confined to any one part of the body. Immune stem cells, formed in the bone marrow, may remain in the bone marrow until maturation, or they may migrate to different body sites for maturation. After maturation, most immune cells circulate in the body and exert specific effects. The immune system has two distinct, but overlapping, mechanisms with which to fight invading organisms:

• Cell-mediated defenses (cell-mediated immunity)
• **Antibody**-mediated defenses (humoral immunity)

Cell-Mediated Immunity (T Cells)

Cell-mediated immunity (CMI) results from the activity of many leukocyte actions, reactions, and interactions that range from simple to complex. This type of immunity depends on the actions of the T lymphocytes, which are responsible for a delayed type of immune response. The T lymphocytes defend against viral infections, fungal infections, and some bacterial infections as follows.

• The T lymphocyte becomes sensitized by its first contact with a specific **antigen**.
• Subsequent exposure to an antigen stimulates multiple reactions aimed at destroying or inactivating the offending antigen.
• T lymphocytes and macrophages (large cells that surround, engulf, and digest microorganisms and cellular debris) work together in CMI to destroy the antigen.
• T lymphocytes attack the antigens directly, rather than produce antibodies (as is done in humoral immunity). Cellular reactions may also occur without macrophages.

If CMI is reduced, as in the case of acquired immunodeficiency syndrome (AIDS), the body is unable to protect itself against many viral, bacterial, and fungal infections.

Humoral Immunity (B Cells)

Humoral immunity protects the body against bacterial and viral infections. Special lymphocytes (white blood cells), called *B lymphocytes,* produce circulating antibodies to act against a foreign substance. This type of immunity is based on the **antigen–antibody response**. An *antigen* is a substance, usually a protein, that stimulates the body to produce antibodies. An *antibody* is a globulin (protein) produced by the B lymphocytes as a defense against an antigen.

Specific antibodies are formed for specific antigens—for example, chickenpox antibodies are formed when the person is exposed to the chickenpox virus (the antigen). Once manufactured, antibodies circulate in the bloodstream, sometimes only for a short time, but in other cases for the lifetime of the person. When an antigen enters the body, specific antibodies neutralize the invading antigen; this condition is called *immunity.* Thus, the individual with specific circulating antibodies is immune (or has immunity) to a specific antigen. Immunity is the resistance that an individual has against disease.

Cell-mediated and humoral immunity are interdependent; CMI influences the function of the B lymphocytes, and humoral immunity influences the function of the T lymphocytes.

Active and Passive Immunity

Active and passive immunity involve the use of agents that stimulate antibody formation (**active immunity**) or the injection of ready-made antibodies found in the serum of immune individuals or animals (**passive immunity**). See Figure 49.1.

Active Immunity

When a person is exposed to certain infectious microorganisms (the source of antigens), the body actively builds an immunity (forms antibodies) to the invading microorganism. This is called *active immunity.* There are two types of active immunity: (1) naturally acquired active immunity and (2) artificially acquired active immunity. The Summary Drug

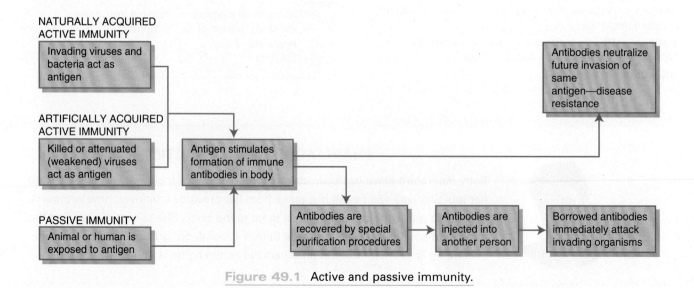

Figure 49.1 Active and passive immunity.

Display 49.1 Example of Naturally Acquired Active Immunity

Naturally acquired active immunity is exemplified by an individual who is exposed to chickenpox for the first time and who has no immunity to the disease. The body immediately begins to manufacture antibodies against the chickenpox virus. However, the production of a sufficient quantity of antibodies takes time, and the individual gets the disease. At the time of exposure and while the individual still has chickenpox, the body continues to manufacture antibodies. These antibodies circulate in the individual's bloodstream for life. In the future, any exposure to the chickenpox virus results in the antibodies mobilizing to destroy the invading antigen.

Display 49.2 Example of Artificially Acquired Active Immunity

Although chickenpox may seem like a minor illness, it can cause herpes zoster (shingles) later in life, which is a painful condition. An example of the use of an attenuated virus is the administration of the varicella virus vaccine to an individual who has not had chickenpox. The varicella (chickenpox) vaccine contains the live, attenuated varicella virus. The individual receiving the vaccine develops a mild or modified chickenpox infection, which then produces immunity against the varicella virus. The varicella vaccine protects the recipient for several years or, for some individuals, for life. An example of a killed virus used for immunization is the yearly influenza vaccine. These vaccines protect those who receive the vaccine for about 3 to 6 months. This is why they are given yearly.

Table: Immunization Agents identifies agents that produce active immunity.

Naturally Acquired Active Immunity

Naturally acquired active immunity occurs when the person is exposed to and experiences a disease, and the body manufactures antibodies to provide future immunity to the disease. This is called *active immunity* because the antibodies are produced by the person who had the disease (see Fig. 49.1). Thus, having the disease produces immunity. Display 49.1 describes an example of naturally acquired active immunity.

Artificially Acquired Active Immunity

Artificially acquired active immunity occurs when an individual is given a killed or weakened antigen, which stimulates the formation of antibodies against the antigen. The antigen does not cause the disease, but the individual still manufactures specific antibodies against the disease. When a **vaccine** containing an **attenuated** (weakened) antigen is given, the individual may experience a few minor symptoms of the disease or even a mild form of the disease, but the symptoms are almost always milder than the disease itself and usually last for a short time.

The decision to use an attenuated rather than a killed virus as a vaccine to provide immunity is based on research in the laboratory to see what form is effective on the virus. Many antigens, when killed, produce a poor antibody response, whereas when the antigen is merely weakened, a good antibody response occurs. Immunization against a specific disease provides artificially acquired active immunity. Display 49.2 gives an example of artificially acquired active immunity.

Artificially acquired immunity against some diseases may require periodic **booster** injections to keep an adequate antibody level (or antibody titer) circulating in the blood. A booster injection is the administration of an additional dose of the vaccine to boost the production of antibodies to a level that will maintain the desired immunity. The booster is given months or years after the initial vaccine and may be needed because the life of some antibodies is short.

Immunization is a form of artificial active immunity and an important method of controlling some of the infectious diseases that are capable of causing serious and sometimes fatal

consequences. The immunization schedule for children and adults is provided in Appendix C. Changes can be made frequently to these schedules. It is best to check the most current immunization schedules for this and other age groups and late start schedules, all of which can be obtained at the Centers for Disease Control and Prevention (CDC) website at http://www.cdc.gov/vaccines/. Currently, many infectious diseases may be prevented by vaccine (artificial active immunity). Examples of some of these diseases can be found in Display 49.3.

Display 49.3 Examples of Diseases Preventable by Vaccination

Diseases Prevented by Routine Vaccination

- *Haemophilus influenzae* type B
- Hepatitis A
- Hepatitis B
- Human papillomavirus
- Influenza
- Mumps
- Measles
- Pertussis
- Pneumococcal disease
- Poliomyelitis
- Rubella
- Tetanus
- Varicella

Diseases Preventable by Vaccination Before Travel to Endemic Areas

- Cholera
- Diphtheria
- Japanese encephalitis
- Lyme disease
- Smallpox
- Typhoid
- Yellow fever

> *Display 49.4* **Example of Passive Immunity**
>
> An example of passive immunity is the administration of immune globulins to prevent organ rejection in patients after organ transplantation surgery.

Passive Immunity

Passive immunity occurs when **immune globulins** or antivenins are administered. This type of immunity provides the individual with ready-made antibodies from another human or an animal (see Fig. 49.1). Passive immunity provides immediate immunity to the invading antigen, but lasts for only a short time. Display 49.4 provides an example of passive immunity.

IMMUNOLOGIC AGENTS

Some immunologic agents capitalize on the body's natural defenses by stimulating the immune response, thereby creating protection against a specific disease within the body. Other immunologic agents supply ready-made antibodies to provide passive immunity. Examples of immunologic agents include vaccines, toxoids, and immune globulins.

Actions and Uses

Vaccines and Toxoids

Antibody-producing tissues cannot distinguish between an antigen that is capable of causing disease (a live antigen), an attenuated antigen, or a killed antigen. Because of this phenomenon, vaccines, which contain either an attenuated or a killed antigen, have been developed to create immunity to certain diseases. The live antigens are either killed or weakened during the manufacturing process. The weakened or killed antigens contained in the vaccine do not have sufficient strength to cause disease. Although it is a rare occurrence, vaccination with any vaccine may not result in a protective antibody response in all individuals given the vaccine.

A **toxin** is a poisonous substance produced by a bacterium (such as *Clostridium tetani,* the bacterium that causes tetanus). A toxin is capable of stimulating the body to produce antitoxins, which are substances that act in the same manner as antibodies. Toxins are powerful substances and, like other antigens, they can be attenuated. A toxin that is attenuated (or weakened) but still capable of stimulating the formation of antitoxins is called a **toxoid**.

Both vaccines and toxoids are administered to stimulate the body's immune response to specific antigens or toxins. These agents must be administered before exposure to the disease-causing organism. The initiation of the immune response, in turn, produces resistance to a specific infectious disease. The immunity produced in this manner is active immunity.

Vaccines and toxoids are used for the following:

• Routine immunization of infants and children
• Immunization of adults against tetanus
• Immunization of adults at high risk for certain diseases (e.g., pneumococcal and influenza vaccines)
• Immunization of children or adults at risk for exposure to a particular disease (e.g., hepatitis A for those going to endemic areas)
• Immunization of prepubertal girls or nonpregnant women of childbearing age against rubella

Immune Globulins and Antivenins

Globulins are proteins present in blood serum or plasma that contain antibodies. *Immune globulins* are solutions obtained from human or animal blood containing antibodies that have been formed by the body to specific antigens. Because they contain ready-made antibodies, they are given for passive immunity against disease. The immune globulins are administered to provide passive immunization to one or more infectious diseases. Those receiving immune globulins receive antibodies only to the diseases to which the donor blood is immune. The onset of protection is rapid but of short duration (1 to 3 months).

Antivenins are used for passive, transient protection from the toxic effects of bites by spiders (black widow and similar spiders) and snakes (rattlesnakes, copperhead and cottonmouth, and coral). The most effective response is obtained when the drug is administered within 4 hours after exposure.

Adverse Reactions

Vaccines and Toxoids

Adverse reactions from the administration of vaccines or toxoids are usually mild. Chills, fever, muscular aches and pains, rash, and lethargy may be present. Pain and tenderness at the injection site may also occur. Although rare, a hypersensitivity reaction may occur. The Summary Drug Table: Immunization Agents provides a listing of the typical adverse reactions.

Immune Globulins and Antivenins

Adverse reactions to immune globulins are rare. However, local tenderness and pain at the injection site may occur. The most common adverse reactions include urticaria, angioedema, erythema, malaise, nausea, diarrhea, headache, chills, and fever. Adverse reactions, if they occur, may last for several hours. Systemic reactions are extremely rare, with the exception of immune globulins given to prevent posttransplantation rejection. These immune globulins are made from equine (horse) or rabbit serum and can produce anaphylactic reactions. They should be administered only under the direction of a physician specializing in transplantation medicine.

The antivenins may cause various reactions, with hypersensitivity being the most severe. Some antivenins are prepared from equine serum, and if a patient is sensitive to equine serum, serious reactions or death may result. The immediate reactions usually occur within 30 minutes after administration of the antivenin. Symptoms include apprehension; flushing; itching; urticaria; edema of the face, tongue, and throat; cough; dyspnea; vomiting; cyanosis; and collapse. Other adverse reactions are included in the Summary Drug Table: Immunization Agents.

Contraindications and Precautions

Vaccines and Toxoids

Immunologic agents are contraindicated in patients with known hypersensitivity to the agent or any component of it. Allergy to eggs is a concern with some vaccines. It is recommended to see a primary health care provider familiar with egg allergies for vaccination if an allergy is suspected. Some people with "hive-only" reactions are able to tolerate vaccines without problem (ACIP, 2012). The measles, mumps, rubella, and varicella vaccines are contraindicated in patients who have had an allergic reaction to gelatin, neomycin, or a previous dose of one of the vaccines. The measles, mumps, rubella, and varicella vaccines are contraindicated during pregnancy, especially during the first trimester, because of the danger of birth defects. Women are instructed to avoid becoming pregnant at least 3 months after receiving these vaccines. Vaccines and toxoids are contraindicated during acute febrile illnesses, leukemia, lymphoma, immunosuppressive illness or drug therapy, and nonlocalized cancer. Always ask about allergy history before preparing a vaccine for administration. See Display 49.5 for additional information on the contraindications to immunologic agents.

Immunologic agents are used with extreme caution in individuals with a history of allergies. Sensitivity testing may be performed in individuals with a history of allergies. Because of potential harm to a fetus no adequate studies have been conducted in pregnant women, and it is also not known whether these agents are excreted in breast milk. Thus, the immunologic agents (pregnancy category C) are used with caution in pregnant women and during lactation.

Immune Globulins and Antivenins

The immune globulins are contraindicated in patients with a history of allergic reactions after administration of human immunoglobulin preparations and in individuals with isolated immunoglobulin A (IgA) deficiency (individuals could have an anaphylactic reaction to subsequent administration of blood products that contain IgA).

 CHRONIC CARE CONSIDERATIONS
Human immune globulin intravenous (IGIV) products have been associated with renal impairment, acute renal failure, osmotic nephrosis, and death. Individuals with a predisposition to acute renal failure (e.g., those with pre-existing renal disease), those with diabetes mellitus, individuals older than 65 years of age, or patients receiving nephrotoxic drugs should not be given human IGIV products.

The antivenins are contraindicated in patients with hypersensitivity to equine serum or any other component of the

---

> ### *Display 49.5* Contraindications to Immunization
>
> - Moderate or severe illness, with or without fever
> - Anaphylactoid reactions (e.g., hives, swelling of the mouth and throat, difficulty breathing [dyspnea], hypotension, and shock)
> - Known allergy to vaccine or vaccine constituents, particularly gelatin, eggs, or neomycin
> - Individuals with an immunologic deficiency should not receive a vaccine (virus is transmissible to the immunocompromised individual).
> - Immunizations are postponed during the administration of steroids, radiation therapy, and antineoplastic (anticancer) drug therapy.
> - Virus vaccines against measles, rubella, and mumps should not be given to pregnant women.
> - Patients who experience severe systemic or neurologic reactions after a previous dose of the vaccine should not be given any additional doses.

serum. The immune globulins and antivenins are administered cautiously during pregnancy and lactation (pregnancy category C) and in children.

Interactions

Vaccines and Toxoids

Vaccinations containing live organisms are not administered within 3 months of immune globulin administration, because antibodies in the globulin preparation may interfere with the immune response to the vaccination. Corticosteroids, antineoplastic drugs, and radiation therapy depress the immune system to such a degree that insufficient numbers of antibodies are produced to prevent the disease. When the salicylates are administered with the varicella vaccination, there is an increased risk of Reye's syndrome developing.

Immune Globulins and Antivenins

Antibodies in the immune globulin preparations may interfere with the immune response to live virus vaccines, particularly measles, but including others such as mumps and rubella. It is recommended that the live virus vaccines be administered 14 to 30 days before or 6 to 12 weeks after administration of immune globulins. No known interactions have been reported with antivenins.

NURSING PROCESS

PATIENT RECEIVING AN IMMUNOLOGIC AGENT

ASSESSMENT

Preadministration Assessment
Before the administration of any vaccine, obtain an allergy history. If the individual is known or thought to have allergies

of any kind, inform the primary health care provider before the vaccine is given. Some vaccines contain antibodies obtained from animals, whereas other vaccines may contain proteins or preservatives to which the individual may be allergic. A highly allergic person may have an allergic reaction that could be serious and even fatal. If the patient has an allergy history, the primary health care provider may decide to perform skin tests for allergy to one or more of the components or proteins in the vaccine. You should also scan the record or ask the patient about any conditions that contraindicate the administration of the agent (e.g., cancer, leukemia, lymphoma, immunosuppressive drug therapy).

Ongoing Assessment

The patient is usually not hospitalized after administration of an immunologic agent (with the exception of transplant recipients). However, the patient may be asked to stay in the clinic or office for observation for about 30 minutes after the injection to observe for any signs of hypersensitivity (e.g., laryngeal edema, hives, pruritus, angioneurotic edema, and severe dyspnea [see Chapter 1 for additional information]). Emergency resuscitation equipment is kept available to be used in the event of a severe hypersensitivity reaction.

NURSING DIAGNOSES

Drug-specific nursing diagnoses include the following:

- **Acute Pain** related to adverse reactions (pain and discomfort at the injection site, muscular aches and pain)
- **Individual Effective Self-Health Management** related to timing of immunization schedule

Nursing diagnoses related to drug administration are discussed in Chapter 4.

PLANNING

The expected outcomes of the patient may include an optimal response to the immunologic agent, support of patient needs related to the management of common adverse drug effects, and confidence in an understanding of and adherence with the prescribed immunization schedule.

IMPLEMENTATION

Promoting an Optimal Response to Therapy

> **! NURSING ALERT**
>
> Most vaccine preparations require refrigeration. Always have a backup plan for storage of the vaccine should the health care facility lose power. Temperature fluctuations can harm the vaccines.

If a vaccine is not in liquid form and must be reconstituted, read the directions enclosed with the vaccine for reconstitution. It is important to follow the enclosed directions carefully to ensure proper action of the vaccine. Package inserts also contain information regarding dosage, adverse reactions, method of administration, administration sites (when appropriate), and, when needed, recommended booster schedules.

 LIFESPAN CONSIDERATIONS
Pediatric

The American Academy of Family Physicians states that children 12 to 15 months of age may receive up to seven injections during a single office visit. Many manufacturers are preparing combination products to reduce the number of injections during the vaccination process. Examples include the measle, mumps, and rubella (MMR) vaccine and the diphtheria, tetanus, pertussis (DTaP), and *Haemophilus* B (TriHIBit) vaccine.

On occasion, it may be necessary to postpone the regular immunization schedule, particularly for children. This is of special concern to parents. The decision to delay immunization because of illness or for other reasons must be discussed with the primary health care provider. However, the decision to administer or delay vaccination because of febrile illness (illness causing an elevated temperature) depends on the severity of the symptoms and the specific disorder. In general, all vaccines can be administered to those with minor illness, such as a cold, and to those with a low-grade fever. However, moderate or severe illness is a temporary contraindication. In instances of moderate or severe illness, vaccination is done as soon as the acute phase of the illness is over. Display 49.5 lists general contraindications to immunizations. Specific contraindications and precautions may be found in the package insert that comes with the drug or at the website of the Immunization Action Coalition (www.immunize.org).

State agencies, drug companies, and immunization organizations all provide standardized forms for parents or caregivers that document immunization history. In addition to your facility documentation, provide or record on the document presented by the parent or caregiver the following information:

- Date of vaccination
- Route and site, vaccine type, manufacturer
- Lot number and expiration date
- Name, address, and title of individual administering vaccine

Monitoring and Managing Patient Needs

Minor adverse reactions, such as fever, rashes, and aching joints, are possible with the administration of a vaccine. In most cases, these reactions subside within 48 hours.

ACUTE PAIN. General interventions, such as increasing the fluids in the diet, allowing for adequate rest, and keeping the atmosphere quiet and nonstimulating, may be beneficial. The primary health care provider may prescribe acetaminophen, every 4 hours, to control these reactions. Using the dominant arm helps aid in absorption of the injection. Also, during the injection aspiration of the syringe contents is not indicated for vaccines. If local irritation at the injection site occurs, it can be treated with warm or cool compresses, depending on the patient's preference. A lump may be palpated at the injection site after a DTaP vaccination or other immunization. This is not abnormal and resolves itself within several days to weeks.

INDIVIDUAL EFFECTIVE SELF-HEALTH MANAGEMENT. Because of the effectiveness of various types of vaccines in the prevention of disease, you should advocate and educate the public about the advantages of immunization. Parents are encouraged to have infants and young children immunized as suggested by the Advisory Committee on Immunization Practices. These schedules are updated and published yearly; an example is provided in Appendix C. If the parents do not bring in a form or booklet to record the immunization, you should provide the parents with a copy of the record of immunizations. This is especially helpful if multiple providers will be involved in the immunization schedule. Because evidence of immunization is required by schools (even at the college level), the record provided to parents by the provider is even more important. Records can be downloaded regarding both information about immunizations and copies of blank record-keeping sheets from the CDC website or the Immunization Action Coalition. This helps to

Immunologic Agents

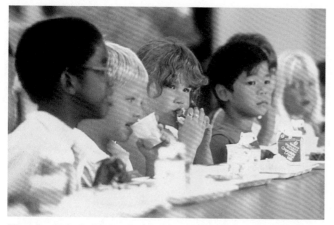

Figure 49.2 By maintaining adherence to immunization schedules children enjoy healthy lives free of debilitating communicable diseases. (Photo courtesy of U.S. Department of Agriculture.)

empower the parent(s) caring for the child, making adherence to the routine immunization schedule likely (Fig. 49.2).

❗ NURSING ALERT

In most cases, the risk of serious adverse reactions from an immunization is much smaller than the risk of contracting the disease for which the immunizing agent is given.

Parents are sometimes concerned about serious adverse reactions that can harm a child following an immunization. Much of this fear stems from a study published in 1998 by Andrew Wakefield, a physician, making a correlation between autism and the MMR vaccine. This study was found to be fraudulent and Wakefield lost his license to practice medicine. Yet, individuals remain fearful of the adverse reactions of immunizations. Although the number of these incidents is small, a risk factor still remains when some vaccines are given.

It is also important for the parents to understand that a risk is also associated with not receiving immunization against infectious diseases. That risk may be higher than and just as serious as the risk associated with the use of vaccines. Keep in mind that when a large segment of the population is immunized, the few not immunized are less likely to be exposed to and be infected with the disease-producing microorganism—they benefit from what is termed *herd immunity*. However, when large numbers of the population are not immunized, there is a great increase in the chances of exposure to the infectious disease and a significant increase in the probability that the individual will experience the disease.

Educating the Patient and Family

When an adult or child is receiving a vaccine for immunization, explain to the patient or a family member the possible reactions that may occur, such as soreness at the injection site or fever.

Advise those traveling to a foreign country to consult their primary health care provider or the CDC website well in advance of their departure date for information about the immunizations that will be needed. Some clinics specialize in overseas travel as immunizations should be given well in advance of departure, because it may take several weeks to produce adequate immunity.

Display 49.6 Vaccine Adverse Event Reporting System

VAERS is a national vaccine safety surveillance program cosponsored by the CDC and the U.S. Food and Drug Administration (FDA). VAERS collects and analyzes information from reports of adverse reactions after immunization. Anyone can report to VAERS. Reports are sent in by vaccine manufacturers, health care providers, and vaccine recipients and their parents or guardians. Any clinically significant adverse event that occurs after the administration of any vaccine should be reported. Individuals are encouraged to provide the information on the form even if the individual is uncertain whether the event was related to the immunization. A copy of the form can be obtained by calling 1-800-822-7967 or by submitting the information through the Internet at http://www.vaers.hhs.gov/.

Encourage the parents or guardians to become educated and advocate for their child's safety. Refer to the Immunization Action Coalition for information both for and against immunization and learn the adverse reactions or serious adverse events that may occur after administration of a vaccine. Build trust and confidence in the parent or caregiver to discuss concerns that may make it necessary to report the event to the Vaccine Adverse Event Reporting System (VAERS) (Display 49.6).

The following list summarizes the information to be included when educating the parents of a child receiving a vaccination:

- Discuss briefly the risks of contracting vaccine preventable diseases and the benefits of immunization.
- Instruct the parents to bring immunization records to all visits.
- Provide the date for return for the next vaccination with reminder mail or telephone messages.
- Discuss common adverse reactions (e.g., fever, soreness at the injection site) and methods to reduce these reactions (e.g., acetaminophen, warm compresses).
- Instruct the parents to report any unusual or severe adverse reactions after the administration of a vaccination.

EVALUATION

- Therapeutic effect is achieved, and the disease for which immunization is given does not present itself.
- Adverse reactions are identified, reported to the primary health care provider, and managed successfully with appropriate nursing interventions:
  - Acute injection pain is managed successfully.
  - Patient or parents/guardians adhere to the immunization schedule.
- Patient and family express confidence and demonstrate an understanding of the drug regimen.

PHARMACOLOGY IN PRACTICE
THINK CRITICALLY

Jimmy Peterson, aged 4 months, has a slight cold with a runny nose when he comes for his regular well-baby check-up. His mother tells you that, because Jimmy is sick, she does not think he needs his immunization at this time. She says that she will bring him in next month for the shot. Looking over his records, you see that the family has no insurance at this time and has to pay out of pocket for all visits and vaccinations. Analyze the situation to determine the best response to Jimmy's mother. Discuss any assessments that you think would be important to make before giving your response.

KEY POINTS

- Immunity is the body's ability to identify and resist potentially harmful microorganisms. There are two types of immunity: cell mediated and antibody mediated.

- Cell-mediated immunity involves the T lymphocytes. When exposed to an antigen, the T cells become sensitized and subsequent exposures stimulate a reaction to destroy the offending antigen.

- Antibody-mediated immunity involves the B lymphocytes and is referred to as humoral immunity. When exposed to an antigen, the B cells produce antibodies as a defense against the offending antigen.

- The active and passive immunity of vaccinations focus on the antibody-mediated immunity. Since the advent of immunizations many childhood diseases have become almost nonexistent (such as polio) and adults can be protected from conditions that can make them severely ill (such as the flu or shingles).

- Adverse reactions typically are minor, yet sensational stories have made some parents or caregivers fearful of the dangers of immunization in comparison with the affliction itself.

Summary Drug Table IMMUNIZATION AGENTS

Generic Drug	Trade Name	Uses	Adverse Reactions	Dosage Ranges
Agents for Active Immunity				
Vaccines, Bacterial (Routine Immunizations)				
Haemophilus influenzae type B conjugate *hee'-mah-fill-uss in-floo-en'-zah kon'-joo-get*	ActHIB, HibTITER, PedvaxHIB	Routine immunization of children	Rare; minor local reactions such as local tenderness, pain at injection site, anorexia, fever, myalgia	0.5 mL IM, see immunization schedule
meningococcal *men-in-joe-kok'-kal*	Menomune, Menactra	Routine immunization of adolescents	Same as *H. influenzae* vaccine	0.5 mL subcut only
pneumococcal (PCV or PPV) *new-moe-kok'-kal*	Pneumovax 23	Routine immunization of children, PPV is recommended for certain high-risk groups who cannot take PCV	Same as *H. influenzae* vaccine	0.5 mL subcut or IM, see immunization schedule

Summary Drug Table IMMUNIZATION AGENTS (continued)

Generic Name	Trade Name	Uses	Adverse Reactions	Dosage Ranges
Vaccines, Bacterial (Special Populations)				
BCG		Prevention of pulmonary tuberculosis (TB) in negative, high-risk populations (health care workers, infants and children in high-TB areas)	Same as *H. influenzae* vaccine	0.2–0.3 mL percutaneous, repeat in 2–3 mo
pneumococcal 7-valent conjugate	Prevnar	Active immunization against *Streptococcus pneumoniae* for infants and toddlers, prevention of otitis media	Rare; minor local reactions such as local tenderness, pain at injection site, decreased appetite, irritability, drowsiness, fever	0.5 mL IM
typhoid *tye'-foyd*	Typhim Vi, Vivotif Berna	Immunization against typhoid	Same as *H. influenzae* vaccine	Oral: total of 4 capsules 1 wk before exposure Parenteral: adults and children 2 yr and older, 1 dose of 0.5 mL IM
Vaccines, Viral (Routine Immunizations)				
measles (rubeola), mumps, rubella, and varicella *mee'-zuls, roo-bee'-oh-lah, roo-bell'-ah*	MMR II (live) ProQuad (attenuated)	Routine immunization of children	Mild fever, rash, cough, rhinitis	0.5 mL subcut
hepatitis A, inactivated *hep-ah-tye'-tuss A*	Havrix, Vaqta	Routine immunization of children	Same as measles vaccine	Administered IM; dosage varies with product; see package insert for specific dosages
hepatitis B, recombinant	Engerix-B, Recombivax HB	Routine immunization of children	Minor local reactions such as local tenderness, pain at injection site, anorexia, fever, myalgia	3–4 doses of 0.5–2 mL IM
poliovirus, inactivated (IPV) *poe'-lee-oh-vye'-russ*	IPOL	Routine immunization of children	Rare; malaise, nausea, diarrhea, fever	0.5 mL IM or subcut; see immunization schedule
varicella *var-ih-sell'-ah*	Varivax	Routine immunization of children	Minor local reactions, such as local tenderness, pain at injection site, rash, fever, cough, irritability	0.5 mL subcut; see immunization schedule
Vaccines, Viral (Special Populations)				
human papillomavirus (HPV)	Cervarix (female), Gardasil (male/female)	Prevention of diseases caused by HPV, genital warts, and certain cancers	Minor local reactions, such as local tenderness, pain at injection site	3 doses of 0.5 mL IM; initial, 2 mo, 6 mo
measles, live, attenuated*	Attenuvax	Selective active immunization against measles	Mild fever, rash, cough, rhinitis	0.5 mL subcut
mumps, live*	Mumpsvax	Selective active immunization against mumps	Same as measles vaccine	0.5 mL subcut
rubella, live*	Meruvax II	Selective active immunization against rubella	Same as measles vaccine	0.5 mL subcut

(table continues on page 548)

Summary Drug Table IMMUNIZATION AGENTS (continued)

Generic Name	Trade Name	Uses	Adverse Reactions	Dosage Ranges
rubella and mumps, live*	Biavax-II	Selective active immunization against rubella and mumps	Same as measles vaccine	0.5 mL subcut
influenza A and B *in-floo-en'-zah*	Afluria, FluMist, Fluarix, FluLaval, Fluvirin, Fluzone	Active immunization against the specific influenza virus strains contained in the formulation	Same as measles vaccine	1 dose 0.5 mL IM Nasal: 1–2 doses (FluMist only)
avian influenza *ay'-vee-an in-floo-en'-zah*	H5N1	Active immunization against avian influenza in adults (18–64 years)	Headache, malaise, nausea	Two 1-mL IM doses given 1 mo apart
rotavirus *roe'-tah-vye'-russ*	RotaTeq	Prevention of gastroenteritis caused by rotavirus serotypes contained in the vaccines	Fever, decreased appetite, abdominal cramping, irritability, decreased activity	Three 2.5-mL doses given orally
rabies vaccine *ray'-beez*	Imovax, RabAvert	Prevention of rabies in people with greater risk (e.g., veterinarians, animal handlers, forest rangers); postexposure prophylaxis: bite by an animal suspected of carrying rabies	Transient pain, erythema, swelling or itching at the injection site, headache, nausea, abdominal pain, muscle aches, dizziness	Pre-exposure prophylaxis: 1 mL IM, see package insert for dosing Postexposure: give vaccine IM after initial immune globulin injection
zoster, live	Zostavax	Prevention of shingles in people older than 60 yr of age	Transient pain, erythema, swelling or itching at the injection site	Single dose subcut
Toxoids (Routine Immunizations)				
diphtheria and tetanus toxoids and acellular pertussis (DtaP) *dif-thair'-ee-ah, tet-ah-nuss tok'-soyds, ay-sell'-yoo-lar per-tuss'-uss*	Daptacel, Infanrix, Tripedia	Active immunization against diphtheria, tetanus, and pertussis	Headache, dizziness, rash, itching, nausea, fever	0.5 mL IM; see immunization schedule
Toxoids (Special Populations)				
diphtheria and tetanus toxoids, combined (DTTd)		Booster immunization against diphtheria and tetanus	Headache, dizziness, rash, itching, nausea, fever	0.5 mL IM, caution with site rotation; see package insert and immunization schedule
Combination Products (Viral/Bacterial Vaccine or Toxoid Together)				
hepatitis A and B combination	Twinrix	Twinrix for those older than 18 yr traveling to endemic areas	See individual vaccines	See package insert for specific dosing
diphtheria, tetanus toxoids, acellular pertussis, and *H. influenzae* type B	TriHIBit	See individual vaccines	See individual vaccines	See package insert for specific dosing
diphtheria, tetanus toxoids and acellular pertussis, hepatitis B (recombinant), and inactivated poliovirus	Pediarix	See individual vaccines	See individual vaccines	See package insert for specific dosing
Haemophilus influenzae type B and hepatitis B	Comvax	See individual vaccines	See individual vaccines	See package insert for specific dosing

Summary Drug Table IMMUNIZATION AGENTS (continued)

Generic Name	Trade Name	Uses	Adverse Reactions	Dosage Ranges
Agents for Passive Immunity				
Immune Globulins				
botulism immune globulin (BIG-IV) *bot'-choo-lih-zum ih-mewn' glob'-yoo-lin*	BabyBIG	Treatment of infant botulism	Headache, chills, fever	IV administration only; see dosing schedule
cytomegalovirus immune globulin (CMV-IGIV) *sye'-toe-meg'-ah-loe-vye-russ*	CytoGam	Prevention of CMV post–organ transplantation	Injection site: tenderness, pain, muscle stiffness Systemic: headache, chills, fever	See dosing schedule, varies weeks out from transplantation
hepatitis B immune globulin (HBIG) *hep-ah-tih'-tuss*	HepaGam B, Nabi-HB	Prevention of hepatitis B after exposure to the disease (use if not previously immunized)	Same as CMV-IGIV	0.06 mL/kg (3–5 mL) IM
immune globulin (gamma globulin; IgG)	GamaSTAN	Prevention of disease after exposure (use if not previously immunized); hepatitis A, measles (rubeola), varicella, rubella, immunoglobulin deficiency	Same as CMV-IGIV	See dosing schedule, varies for disease
immune globulin intravenous (IGIV)	Octagam, Gammagard, Polygam S/D	Immunodeficiency syndrome, idiopathic thrombocytopenia purpura (ITP), chronic lymphocytic leukemia, bone marrow transplantation, pediatric human immunodeficiency virus infection	Headache, chills, fever	IV administration only; see dosing schedule, varies for disease
lymphocyte immune globulin[†] *lim'-foe-syte*	Atgam	Treatment of rejection post–organ transplantation, aplastic anemia	Chills, fever, arthralgia	After skin test dose, IV administration only; see dosing schedule, varies for disease
antithymocyte globulin[†]	Thymoglobulin	Treatment of acute rejection post–kidney transplantation, aplastic anemia	Chills, fever, arthralgia	IV administration only; see dosing schedule
rabies immune globulin (RIG) *ray'-beez*	HyperRAB, Imogam	Prevention of rabies after exposure to the disease (use if not previously immunized)	Same as CMV-IGIV	See dosing schedule
Rh immune globulin (IGIM)	BayRho-D, RhoGAM	Prevention of Rh hemolytic disease after birth	Same as CMV-IGIV	300 mcg (1 vial) IM within 72 hr of delivery
Rh immune globulin (IGIV)	WinRho SDF	Suppression of Rh isoimmunization after termination of pregnancy; ITP	Headache, chills, fever	IV administration only; see dosing schedule

(table continues on page 550)

Summary Drug Table IMMUNIZATION AGENTS (continued)

Generic Name	Trade Name	Uses	Adverse Reactions	Dosage Ranges
Rh immune globulin microdose (IG-microdose)	BayRho-D Mini Dose, MICRho GAM	Suppression of Rh isoimmunization after termination of pregnancy before 12 wk gestation	Same as CMV-IGIV	50 mcg (1 vial) IM
respiratory syncytial virus immune globulin (RSV-IGIV) *sin-sish'-al vye'-russ*	RespiGam	Respiratory syncytial virus	Headache, chills, fever	IV administration only; see dosing schedule
tetanus immune globulin (TIG) *tet'-ah-nuss*	BayTet	Tetanus prophylaxis after injury in patients whose immunization is incomplete or uncertain	Same as CMV-IGIV	250 units IM
varicella-zoster immune globulin (VZIG) *var-ih-sell'-ah zoss'-ter*		Prevention of varicella in compromised patients after exposure to the disease (use if not previously immunized)	Same as CMV-IGIV	IM administration only; see dosing schedule
Antivenins				
Crotalidae polyvalent immune Fab *kroe-tal'-ih-day pol-ee-vay'-lent*	CroFab	For treatment of mild to moderate North American rattlesnake bites	Urticaria, rash	See package insert for mixing and administration
antivenin *(Micrurus fulvius)* *an-tee-venn'-in*		Passive transient protection for toxic effects of venoms of coral snake in United States	Urticaria, rash	See package insert for mixing and administration

*The trivalent MMR vaccine is the preferred immunizing agent for most children and adults.

†Must be prescribed and administered by specialized physicians.

● Chapter Review

Know Your Drugs

Clients sometimes know a medication by the brand (or trade) name and not the generic name. To help you recognize both names, match the brand name with the generic name of the same medication.

Generic Name	Brand Name
1. chickenpox (varicella vaccine)	A. Gardasil
2. HPV vaccine	B. RhoGAM
3. Rh+ (immune globulin)	C. Varivax
4. shingles (varicella-zoster vaccine)	D. Zostavax

Calculate Medication Dosages

1. FluLaval (influenza vaccine) is supplied in 5-mL vials. If each injection is 0.5 mL, how many vials will need to be ordered to inoculate 60 people?

● Prepare for the NCLEX®

Build Your Knowledge

1. Humoral immunity involves which type of white blood cells?

   1. macrophages
   2. basophils
   3. B lymphocytes
   4. T lymphocytes

2. What type of immunity involves injecting ready-made antibodies?

   1. artificially acquired active immunity
   2. naturally acquired active immunity
   3. passive immunity
   4. cell-mediated immunity

3. When discussing the possibility of adverse reactions after receiving a vaccine, the nurse tells the parents of a young child that _____.

   1. adverse reactions may be severe, and the child should be monitored closely for 24 hours
   2. adverse reactions are usually mild
   3. the child will likely experience a hypersensitivity reaction
   4. the most common adverse reaction is a severe headache

4. Which of the following statements made by the client would alert the nurse to a possibility of an allergy to the measles vaccine? "My daughter is allergic to _____."

   1. gelatin
   2. peanut butter
   3. sugar
   4. corn

5. What type of immunity does an antivenin produce?

   1. artificially acquired active immunity
   2. naturally acquired active immunity
   3. passive immunity
   4. cell-mediated immunity

6. What type of immunity is produced by the hepatitis B vaccine recombinant?

   1. artificially acquired active immunity
   2. naturally acquired active immunity
   3. passive immunity
   4. cell-mediated immunity

Apply Your Knowledge

7. The nurse is monitoring a client receiving an intravenous (IV) infusion of RSV-IGIV globulin. Which of the following symptoms may indicate an early allergic reaction?

   1. chills
   2. itching
   3. soreness at infusion site
   4. diarrhea

Alternate-Format Questions

8. Which of the following diseases does the MMR vaccine provide protection against? **Select all that apply**.

   1. HPV infection
   2. measles
   3. chickenpox
   4. mumps
   5. rubella

9. Which of the following provides protection against pertussis? **Select all that apply**.

   1. DTaP
   2. DTTd
   3. TriHiBit
   4. Pediarix
   5. Comvax

To check your answers, see Appendix G.

the**Point** *For more NCLEX-style questions, log on to http://thepoint.lww.com to access more than 1000 questions.*

50

Antineoplastic Drugs

On completion of this chapter, the student will:

1. List the types of drugs used in the treatment of neoplastic diseases.
2. Discuss the uses, general drug actions, general adverse reactions, contraindications, precautions, and interactions of the antineoplastic drugs.
3. Discuss important preadministration and ongoing assessment activities the nurse should perform with the patient taking antineoplastic drugs.
4. List nursing diagnoses particular to a patient taking antineoplastic drugs.
5. Discuss ways to promote an optimal response to therapy, how to manage common adverse reactions, and important points to keep in mind when educating patients about the use of an antineoplastic drug.

KEY TERMS

alopecia • abnormal loss of hair; baldness

anemia • decrease in the number of red blood cells and hemoglobin value below normal

anorexia • loss of appetite

antineoplastic • drug used to treat neoplasia (cancer)

bone marrow suppression • decreased production of all blood cells; also called *myelosuppression*

cell cycle nonspecific • pertaining to a drug used in cancer treatment, effective in any phase of cell division

cell cycle specific • pertaining to a drug used in cancer treatment, affecting a specific phase of cell division

chemotherapy • drug therapy with a chemical, often used when referring to treatment with an antineoplastic drug

extravasation • escape of fluid from a blood vessel into surrounding tissue

leukopenia • decrease in the number of leukocytes (white blood cells)

metastasis • spread of cancer outside the original organ or tissue

myelosuppression • see bone marrow suppression

neoplasm • a group of cells that undergo an abnormal growth pattern

neutropenia • abnormally small number of neutrophils (infection fighting type of white blood cell)

oral mucositis • inflammation of the oral mucous membranes

palliation • therapy designed to treat symptoms, not to produce a cure

stomatitis • inflammation of a cavity opening, such as the oral cavity

thrombocytopenia • decreased number of platelets in the blood

vesicant • caustic drug substance

DRUG CLASSES

Cell cycle–specific agents	Cell cycle–nonspecific agents
• Plant alkaloids	• Alkylates
• Taxanes	• Ethyleneimines
• Podophyllotoxins	• Alkyl sulfonates
• Camptothecin analogs	• Hydrazines
• Antimetabolites	• Nitrosoureas
	• Platinum based
	• Antibiotics

PHARMACOLOGY IN PRACTICE

Patients and families undergoing treatment for a malignant disease need special consideration, understanding, and emotional support. On occasion, these needs are unrecognized by members of the health care profession. Mr. Phillip comes to the clinic for a routine blood pressure check. As he sits at your desk he becomes tearful, telling you his wife fought breast cancer only to die in a car accident. As you read about the drugs used, think about your reaction to his grief situation.

Antineoplastic drugs are one of the tools used in the treatment of malignant diseases (i.e., cancer). The term **chemotherapy** is often used to refer to therapy with antineoplastic drugs. Although these drugs may not always lead to a complete cure of the cancer, they often slow the rate of tumor growth and delay **metastasis** (spreading of the cancer to other sites). These drugs can be used for cure, control, or **palliation** (comfort care, the relief of symptoms at the end of life).

The Cell Cycle

All cells grow in a specific pattern of growth called the *cell cycle* (Fig. 50.1). During the cell cycle, different components of a cell are synthesized, and the cell divides into two new cells.

The five phases of cell growth are:

1. G_1—RNA (ribonucleic acid) and proteins are built
2. S—DNA (deoxyribonucleic acid) is made from the components of the G_1 phase
3. G_2—RNA and protein synthesis preparing for cell division
4. M—mitotic cell division (the cell has doubled its contents and splits into two separate cells)
5. G_0—the dormant or resting phase

When the cell goes into a resting phase, the cell starts performing its usual function in the body (e.g., a white blood cell might "Go" to work, fighting infection) or it prepares to start the cycle of cell division again. Some cells, such as blood cells, rapidly reproduce in a matter of hours. Other cells, such as nerve cells, complete their cell division and then go into the resting phase for years. Some cells tend to stay in the resting phase but quickly divide if the tissue is injured. Liver cells are a good example of this behavior; they do not replicate unless there is damage to the liver.

Antineoplastic drugs are designed to attack a cell during one or many of the phases of cell division. Drugs are categorized as **cell cycle specific** (meaning they target the cell in one of the phases of cell division) or as **cell cycle nonspecific** (they can target the cell at any phase of the cycle). Many subcategories of antineoplastic drugs are available to treat malignancies. The antineoplastic drugs covered in this chapter include the cell cycle–nonspecific and cell cycle–specific drugs. Other drugs, such as biologic and chemoprotective agents, are listed in various tables. Many hormones and antihormones are used in treating cancers associated with the sex organs (see Chapter 47), and new agents that stimulate our bodies to fight cancer are increasingly becoming available (Display 50.1).

The strategy of antineoplastic drug therapy is to affect cells that rapidly divide and reproduce. Malignant **neoplasms** or cancerous tumors usually consist of rapidly growing (abnormal) cells. Cancer cells have no biologic feedback controls to stop their growth or proliferation. Cancer cells are more sensitive to antineoplastic drugs when the cells are in the process of growing and dividing. Chemotherapy is administered at the time the cell population is dividing as part of a strategy to optimize cell death.

Because the drugs are given systemically (i.e., they circulate through the entire body), other rapidly growing cells are usually affected by these drugs. The normal cells that line the oral cavity and gastrointestinal (GI) tract, and cells of the gonads, bone marrow, hair follicles, and lymph tissue are also rapidly dividing cells. Thus, antineoplastic drugs may affect normal as well as malignant cells, causing unpleasant adverse reactions.

Chemotherapy is administered in a series of cycles to allow for recovery of normal cells and to destroy more malignant cells (Fig. 50.2). This timing of drug administration is based on the cell kill theory principle. For example, a group of drugs are selected and this drug regimen is intended to kill about 90% of the cancer cells during the first course of treatment. This means 10% of the cancer cells still remain in the body and continue to grow. Then the second course of chemotherapy, according to this theory, targets the remaining cancer cells and reduces those cells by another 90%. Each cycle of treatment with the antineoplastic drugs kills some, but by no means all, of the cancer cells. Theoretically, when only a few cells remain, the body's own immune system will be triggered and destroy what is left. By understanding the cell kill theory and the cell cycle, one can appreciate the rationale for using repeated doses of chemotherapy with different antineoplastic drugs. Various drugs that target cancer cells at various phases of the cell cycle are administered to kill as many cells as possible. Repeated courses of chemotherapy are used to kill an even greater proportion of the malignant cells until, theoretically, no cells are left.

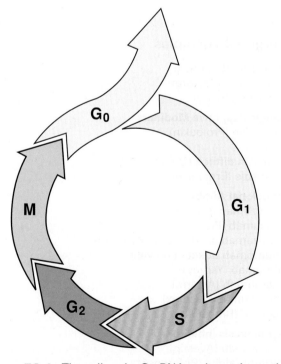

Figure 50.1 The cell cycle: G_1: RNA and protein synthesis; **S**: DNA synthesis; G_2: RNA and protein synthesis; **M**: mitotic cell division; G_0: cell resting phase, during which the cell either differentiates to perform its function or dies.

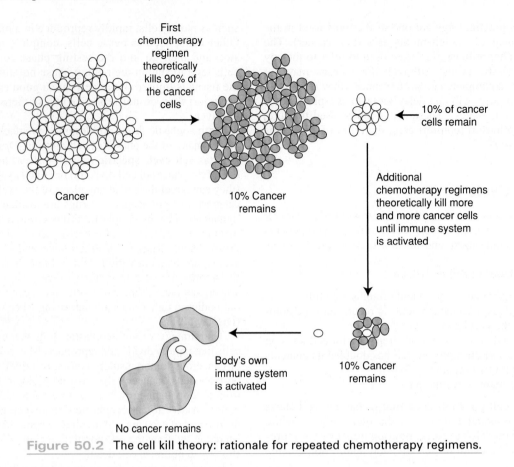

Figure 50.2 The cell kill theory: rationale for repeated chemotherapy regimens.

Display 50.1 New Frontiers in Cancer Treatment: Targeted Therapies

Used in conjunction with conventional antineoplastic drugs, targeted therapies, as the term implies, are agents used to target specific malignant cell components without hurting normal cells. Specific targeting agents include:

bexarotene (Targretin)
bortezomib (Velcade)
cetuximab (Erbitux)
crizotinib (Xalkori)
dasatinib (Sprycel)
erlotinib (Tarceva)
everolimus (Afinitor)
gefitinib (Iressa)
imatinib (Gleevec)
lapatinib (Tykerb)
nilotinib (Tasigna)
pazopanib (Votrient)
pertuzumab (Perjeta)
ruxolitinib (Jakafi)
sorafenib (Nexavar)
sunitinib (Sutent)
temsirolimus (Torisel)
tositumomab (Bexxar)
trastuzumab (Herceptin)

vandetanib (Caprelsa)
vemurafenib (Zelboraf)
vorinostat (Zolina)

Biologic Response Modifiers
aldesleukin (Proleukin)
BCG
denileukin diftitox (Ontak)
levamisole (Ergamisol)

Monoclonal Antibodies
alemtuzumab (Campath)
denosumab (Prolia)
gemtuzumab ozogamicin (Mylotarg)
ibritumomab tiuxetan (Zevalin)
ipilimumab (Yervoy)
ofatumumab (Arzerra)
panitumumab (Vectibix)
rituximab (Rituxan)

Angiogenesis Inhibitors
bevacizumab (Avastin)
interferon-alpha (Roferon-A)
lenalidomide (Revlimid)
romidepsin (Istodax)
thalidomide (Thalomid)

HERBAL CONSIDERATIONS

Green tea and black teas come from the same plant. The difference is in the processing. Green tea is simply dried tea leaves, whereas black tea is fermented, giving it the dark color, stronger flavor, and the lowest amount of tannins and polyphenols. The beneficial effects of green tea lie in the polyphenols, or flavonoids, which have antioxidant properties. Antioxidants are thought to play a major role in preventing disease (e.g., colon cancer) and reducing the effects of aging. Green tea polyphenols are powerful antioxidants. The polyphenols are thought to act by inhibiting the reactions of free radicals in the body that are believed to play a role in aging. The benefits of green tea include an overall sense of well-being, cancer prevention, dental health, and maintenance of heart and liver health. Green tea taken as directed is safe and well tolerated. Because green tea contains caffeine, nervousness, restlessness, insomnia, and GI upset may occur. Green tea should be avoided during pregnancy because of its caffeine content. Patients with hypertension, cardiac conditions, anxiety, insomnia, diabetes, and ulcers should use green tea with caution (DerMarderosian, 2003).

CELL CYCLE–SPECIFIC DRUGS

Actions and Uses

Cell cycle–specific drugs act on the cell in one specific phase of the process of cell division, affecting both malignant and normal cells. A combination of these drugs, all acting at different phases of cell division, is typically used to treat leukemias, lymphomas, and a variety of solid tumors. The site of action of each drug depends on the drug subcategory. See the Summary Drug Table: Antineoplastic Drugs for more information.

Plant Alkaloids

Drugs that are derived from plant alkaloids include vinca alkaloids, taxanes, podophyllotoxins, and camptothecin analog drugs. The vinca alkaloids interfere with amino acid production in the S phase and formation of microtubules in the M phase. Taxanes also interfere in the M phase with microtubules. Cells are stopped during the S and G_2 phases by the podophyllotoxins and thus are unable to divide. DNA synthesis during the S phase is inhibited by camptothecin analog drugs such as topotecan (Hycamtin).

Antimetabolites

Antimetabolite drugs are substances that incorporate themselves into the cellular components during the S phase of cell division. This interferes with the synthesis of RNA and DNA, making it impossible for the cancerous cell to divide into two daughter cells. These drugs are used for many of the leukemias, lymphomas, and solid tumors as well as autoimmune diseases. Methotrexate is an example of the antimetabolite drugs.

CELL CYCLE–NONSPECIFIC DRUGS

Actions and Uses

Cell cycle–nonspecific drugs interfere with the process of cell division of malignant and normal cells. Because they do not exert action specifically on one portion of the cell cycle, they are called *nonspecific* drugs. These drugs are used to cure, control, or provide palliation in the treatment of leukemias, lymphomas, and many different solid tumors, and are also used in the treatment of certain autoimmune diseases.

Alkylating Agents

Alkylating agents make the cell a more alkaline environment, which in turn damages the cell. Malignant cells appear to be more susceptible to the effects of alkylating drugs than normal cells. A number of subcategories are included in this group of cell cycle–nonspecific drugs. Nitrogen mustard derivatives, ethyleneimines, and platinum-based drugs all break or interfere with the crosslinks in the DNA structure. The alkyl sulfonate drug busulfan interferes with DNA of granulocytes and is used primarily for leukemias. The hydrazine group interferes with multiple phases in the synthesis of RNA, DNA, and protein. Nitrosoureas are unique in that they can cross the blood–brain barrier, and therefore are used in treating brain tumors.

Antineoplastic Antibiotics

Antineoplastic antibiotics, unlike their anti-infective antibiotic relatives, do not fight infection. Rather, their action is similar to alkylating drugs. Antineoplastic antibiotics appear to interfere with DNA and RNA synthesis, thereby delaying or inhibiting cell division and blocking the reproductive ability of malignant cells. An example of an antineoplastic antibiotic is doxorubicin, which is used in the treatment of many solid tumors.

Miscellaneous Antineoplastic Drugs

A number of drugs are used for their antineoplastic actions, but they do not belong to any one category. The mechanism of action of many of the drugs in this unrelated group is not entirely clear. Examples of miscellaneous antineoplastics are provided in the Summary Drug Table: Antineoplastic Drugs.

Adverse Reactions

Adverse reactions to antineoplastic drugs can be viewed in three different time frames: immediate (during the actual administration), during therapy cycles, and long term (many years later, during survivorship).

Immediate adverse reactions occur as a result of administration. These include nausea and vomiting from highly emetic drugs or the potential of intravenous (IV) **extravasation** (leakage into the surrounding tissues) of irritating solutions. Antineoplastic drugs are potentially toxic, and their administration is often associated with serious adverse reactions. At times, some of these adverse effects are allowed, because the only alternative is to stop treatment of the cancer. A treatment plan is developed that will prevent, lessen, or treat most or all

---

Display 50.2 Emetic Potential of Antineoplastic Drugs

The following drugs have a 60% or greater chance of causing nausea and vomiting when administered to patients.

Alkylating Agents
carboplatin
carmustine
cisplatin
cyclophosphamide
dacarbazine
ifosfamide
lomustine
mechlorethamine
melphalan
procarbazine
streptozocin

Antibiotics
dactinomycin
daunorubicin
doxorubicin
mitoxantrone

Antimetabolites
cytarabine
methotrexate

Plant Alkaloid
irinotecan

Antineoplastic Drugs. Appropriate references should be consulted when administering these drugs, because there are a variety of uses and dose ranges and, in some instances, many adverse reactions.

Contraindications and Precautions

The information discussed in this section is general, and the contraindications, precautions, and interactions for each antineoplastic drug vary. The chemotherapy nurse should consult appropriate sources before administering any antineoplastic drug.

Antineoplastic drugs are contraindicated in patients with leukopenia, thrombocytopenia, anemia, serious infections, serious renal disease, or known hypersensitivity to the drug, and during pregnancy (see Display 50.3 for pregnancy classifications of selected antineoplastic drugs) or lactation.

Antineoplastic drugs are used cautiously in patients with renal or hepatic impairment, active infection, or other

---

of the symptoms of a specific adverse reaction. An example of prevention is giving an antiemetic before administering an antineoplastic drug known to cause severe nausea and vomiting. Display 50.2 provides a list of those drugs most likely to cause nausea and vomiting.

An example of a treatment for an adverse reaction is the administration of an antiemetic and IV fluids with electrolytes when severe vomiting is anticipated. When the drugs listed in Display 50.2 are given, antiemetic protocols should always be followed to reduce adverse reactions. Some drugs, such as platinum-based agents, may damage certain organs during administration. Again, prechemotherapy protocols for IV fluid administration are initiated to prevent adverse reactions.

Some of these reactions are dose dependent; that is, their occurrence is more common or their intensity is more severe when multiple doses (or cycles) are used. Because the antineoplastic drugs affect cancer cells and rapidly proliferating normal cells (i.e., cells in the bone marrow, GI tract, reproductive tract, and hair follicles), adverse reactions occur as the result of action on these cells.

Adverse reactions common to many of the antineoplastic drugs include **bone marrow suppression (anemia, leukopenia, thrombocytopenia)**, **stomatitis**, diarrhea, and hair loss. The most common reactions are leukopenia and thrombocytopenia, which may cause cycles of chemotherapy to be delayed until blood cell counts can be raised. Some drugs, especially the alkaloids, affect the nervous system. These adverse reactions can range from a peripheral tingling sensation to *hand and foot syndrome* (tiny capillary leaks in extremities, causing symptoms from skin color changes to numbness).

Because the drugs used to treat cancer are effective, many people are living with the disease either cured or in remission. Some of the adverse reactions to antineoplastic drugs can have long-lasting effects. These include damage to the gonads, causing fertility problems, and to other specific organ systems, leading to cardiac, pulmonary, or neurologic problems. In addition, secondary cancers like leukemia can be caused by the original cancer treatment. These problems are listed in the Summary Drug Table:

Display 50.3 Pregnancy Classification for Selected Antineoplastic Drugs

Pregnancy Category C

asparaginase	mitotane	streptozocin
dacarbazine	pegaspargase	

Pregnancy Category D

altretamine	docetaxel	mitoxantrone
azacitidine	doxorubicin	nelarabine
bleomycin	epirubicin	oxaliplatin
busulfan	eribulin	paclitaxel
cabazitaxel	etoposide	pemetrexed
capecitabine	fludarabine	pentostatin
carboplatin	fluorouracil	procarbazine
carmustine	gemcitabine	temozolomide
chlorambucil	hydroxyurea	thioguanine
cisplatin	idarubicin	thiotepa
cladribine	ifosfamide	topotecan
clofarabine	irinotecan	vinblastine
cyclophospha-mide	ixabepilone	vincristine
cytarabine	lomustine	vinorelbine
dactinomycin	mechlo-rethamine	
daunorubicin	melphalan	
decitabine	mercaptopurine	

Pregnancy Category X

methotrexate		

debilitating illnesses, or in those who have recently completed treatment with other antineoplastic drugs or radiation therapy.

Interactions

A number of antineoplastic drugs are harmful to normal cells as well as cancer cells. Cytoprotective agents are drugs used with the antineoplastic drug to protect the normal cells or organs of the body. In this way, enough of the chemotherapeutic drug can be given to eradicate the cancer without irreversible harm to the patient. Cytoprotective agents used with antineoplastic drugs are listed in Display 50.4.

The following table lists selected interactions of the plant alkaloids, antimetabolites, alkylating drugs, antibiotics, and miscellaneous antineoplastic drugs. Typically, additive bone marrow depressive effects occur when any category of antineoplastic drug is administered with another chemotherapy drug or radiation therapy. Appropriate sources should be consulted by the chemotherapy nurse for a more complete listing of interactions before any antineoplastic drug is administered.

Display 50.4 Cytoprotective Agents

The following drugs function to protect cells or counteract adverse reactions resulting from therapeutic doses of the antineoplastic drugs.

- allopurinol, rasburicase (Elitek): Counteract the increase in uric acid and subsequent hyperuricemia resulting from the metabolic waste buildup from rapid tumor lysis (cell destruction)
- amifostine (Ethyol): Binds with metabolites of cisplatin to protect the kidneys from nephrotoxic effects, reduces xerostomia
- dexrazoxane (Zinecard): Cardioprotective agent used with doxorubicin
- leucovorin (Wellcovorin), glucarpidase (Voraxaze): Provide folic acid to cells after methotrexate administration
- mesna (Mesnex): Binds with metabolites of ifosfamide to protect the bladder from hemorrhagic cystitis
- palifermin (Kepivance): Helps epithelial cells in the oral cavity recover after severe mucositis

---

Interacting Drug	Common Use	Effect of Interaction
Plant Alkaloids		
digoxin	Cardiac problems	Decrease serum level of digoxin
phenytoin	Seizure disorders	Increased risk of seizures
oral anticoagulants	Blood thinners	Prolonged bleeding
Antimetabolites		
digoxin	Cardiac problems	Decrease serum level of digoxin
phenytoin	Seizure disorders	Decreased need for antiseizure medication
nonsteroidal anti-inflammatory drugs (NSAIDs)	Pain relief	Methotrexate toxicity
Alkylating Drugs		
aminoglycosides	Anti-infective agents	Increased risk of nephrotoxicity and ototoxicity
loop diuretics	Heart problems and edema	Increased risk of ototoxicity
phenytoin	Seizure disorder	Increased risk of seizure
Antineoplastic Antibiotics		
digoxin	Cardiac problems	Decrease serum level of digoxin

Interacting Drug	Common Use	Effect of Interaction
Miscellaneous Antineoplastic Drugs		
insulin and oral antidiabetic	Diabetes management	Increased risk of hyperglycemia
oral anticoagulants	Blood thinners	Prolonged bleeding
antidepressants, antihistamines, opiates, or sedatives	Depression, allergy, pain relief, or sedation, respectively	Increased risk of central nervous system depression

 HERBAL CONSIDERATIONS

The shiitake mushroom, an edible variety of mushroom, is associated with general health maintenance but not with any severe adverse reactions. Mild side effects, such as skin rashes and GI upset, have been reported. Lentinan, a derivative of the shiitake mushroom, is proving to be valuable in boosting the body's immune system and may prolong the survival time of patients with cancer by supporting immunity. In Japan, lentinan is commonly used to treat cancer. Additional possible benefits of this herb include lowering cholesterol levels by increasing the rate at which cholesterol is excreted from the body. Under no circumstances should shiitake or lentinan be used for cancer or any serious illness without consulting a primary health care provider (DerMarderosian, 2003).

NURSING PROCESS

PATIENT RECEIVING AN ANTINEOPLASTIC DRUG

ASSESSMENT

Preadministration Assessment

The extent of the preadministration assessment depends on the type of cancer and the patient's general physical condition. The initial assessment of the patient scheduled for chemotherapy may include the following:

- Type and location of the neoplastic lesion
- Stage of the disease, for example, early, metastatic, or terminal
- Patient's general physical condition
- Patient's emotional response to the disease
- Anxiety or fears the patient may have regarding chemotherapy treatments
- Previous or concurrent treatments (if any), such as surgery, radiation therapy, other antineoplastic drugs
- Other current nonmalignant disease or disorder, such as congestive heart failure or peptic ulcer, that may or may not be related to the malignant disease
- Patient's knowledge or understanding of the proposed chemotherapy regimen
- Other factors, such as the patient's age, financial problems that may be associated with a long-term illness, family cooperation and interest in patient care, and the adequacy of health insurance coverage (which may be of great concern to the patient)

Immediately before administering the first dose of an antineoplastic drug, take the patient's vital signs and obtain a current weight, because the dose of some antineoplastic drugs is based on the patient's weight in kilograms or pounds. The dosages of some antineoplastic drugs also may be based on body surface measurements and are stated as a specific amount of drug per square meter (m²) of body surface. When an antineoplastic drug has a depressing effect on the bone marrow, laboratory tests, such as a complete blood count, are ordered to determine the effect of the previous drug dosage. Before the first dose of the drug is administered, pretreatment laboratory tests provide baseline data for future reference. The administration route of chemotherapy is routinely monitored; examples include assessment of vessel integrity for IV access or patency of venous access devices.

Some antineoplastic drugs require treatment measures before administration. An example of preadministration treatment is hydration of the patient with 1 to 2 L of IV fluid infused before administration of cisplatin or administration of an antiemetic before the administration of irinotecan (Camptosar). These measures are ordered by the oncology health care provider and, in some instances, may vary slightly from the manufacturer's recommendations.

Ongoing Assessment

The patient who is acutely ill with many physical problems requires different ongoing assessment activities than does one who is ambulating and able to participate in the activities of daily living. Once the patient's general condition is assessed and needs identified, develop a care plan to meet those needs. Patients receiving chemotherapy can be at different stages of their disease; therefore, you should individualize the nursing care of each patient based on the patient's needs, and not just on the type of drug administered.

In general, after the administration of an antineoplastic drug, base your ongoing assessment on the following factors:

- Patient's general condition
- Patient's individual response to the drug
- Adverse reactions that may occur
- Guidelines established by the oncology health care provider or clinic
- Results of periodic laboratory tests and radiographic scans

Different types of laboratory tests may be used to monitor the patient's response to therapy. Some of these tests, such as a complete blood count, may be used to determine the response of the bone marrow to an antineoplastic drug. Other tests, such as kidney function tests, may be used to detect nephrotoxicity, an adverse reaction that sometimes occurs with the administration of some of these drugs. Abnormal laboratory test results may also require a change in the nursing care plan. For example, a significant drop in the neutrophil count may require a delay in treatment, administration of colony-stimulating factors (see Chapter 51), and patient teaching about ways to recognize and prevent infection and sepsis.

Review the results of all laboratory tests at the time they are reported. The oncology health care provider is notified of the results before the administration of successive doses of an antineoplastic drug. If these tests indicate a severe depressant effect on the bone marrow or other test abnormalities, the oncology health care provider may reduce the next drug dose or temporarily stop chemotherapy to allow the affected body systems to recover.

NURSING DIAGNOSES

The nursing diagnoses for the patient with cancer are usually extensive and are based on many factors, such as the patient's physical and emotional condition, the adverse reactions resulting from antineoplastic drug therapy, and the stage of the disease. Drug-specific nursing diagnoses include the following:

- **Imbalanced Nutrition: Less Than Body Requirements** related to anorexia, nausea, vomiting, and stomatitis
- **Fatigue** related to anemia and myelosuppression
- **Risk for Injury** related to thrombocytopenia and myelosuppression
- **Risk for Infection** related to neutropenia, leukopenia, and myelosuppression
- **Disturbed Body Image** related to adverse reactions of antineoplastic drugs (e.g., alopecia, weight loss)
- **Anxiety** related to diagnosis, necessary treatment measures, the occurrence of adverse reactions, other factors
- **Impaired Tissue Integrity** related to adverse reactions of the antineoplastic drugs (radiation recall and extravasation)

Nursing diagnoses related to drug administration are discussed in Chapter 4.

PLANNING

The expected outcomes of the patient may include an optimal response to therapy, support of patient needs related to the management of adverse reactions, and confidence in an understanding of the prescribed treatment modalities.

IMPLEMENTATION

Promoting an Optimal Response to Therapy

Care of the patient receiving an antineoplastic drug depends on factors such as the drug or combination of drugs given, the dosage of the drugs, the route of administration, the patient's physical response to therapy, the response of the tumor to chemotherapy, and the type and severity of adverse reactions. Some drugs may be administered by various routes, depending on the cancer being treated. For example, thiotepa may be administered by the IV route for breast cancer, intravesicular route for superficial bladder cancer, intrapleural route for malignant pleural effusions, and intraperitoneal route for ovarian cancer. As the methods of administration have changed, so has the location for administration. Once given as long IV infusions over days or a week in the hospital, many of the antineoplastic drugs are still given IV but as push or small-volume infusions, and they are delivered in an outpatient setting by highly skilled nurses.

GUIDELINES ESTABLISHED BY THE SETTING FOR CARE. In these settings (hospital, outpatient chemotherapy clinics, or office), policies are established to provide nursing personnel with specific guidelines for the assessment and care of patients receiving a single or combination chemotherapeutic drug regimen. During chemotherapy, the oncology health care provider may write orders for certain nursing procedures, such as measuring fluid intake and output, monitoring the vital signs at specific intervals, and increasing the fluid intake to a certain amount. Even when orders are written, you should increase the frequency of certain assessments, such as monitoring vital signs, if the patient's condition changes. Some settings have written guidelines for nursing management when the patient is receiving a specific antineoplastic drug. Incorporate these guidelines into the nursing care plan with nursing observations and assessments geared to the individual. At any time you may add further assessments to the nursing care plan when the patient's condition changes.

If treatment is given in a setting where guidelines are not provided, it is important for you to review the drugs being given before their administration. These drugs should not be prescribed by a generalist health care provider; rather, antineoplastics should be prescribed only by a provider trained specifically in the care of oncology patients. The clinical pharmacist consults appropriate references to obtain information regarding the preparation and administration of a particular drug, the average dose ranges, all the known adverse reactions, and the warnings and precautions given by the manufacturer.

PROTECTION OF THE PROVIDER. Those involved in the administration of antineoplastic drugs are at risk for many adverse reactions from accidental absorption of the drugs. Because so many of the drugs are given in the outpatient setting,

personnel in clinics and offices are at high risk for exposure. It is important to follow the directions of the manufacturer regarding the type of solution to be used for preparation, dilution, or administration. The Occupational Safety and Health Administration (OSHA) guidelines state that antineoplastic drug preparation is to be performed in a biologic safety cabinet in a designated area. This is to prevent accidental inhalation and exposure to the person preparing the drugs. In addition, nurses need to be protected during administration and cleanup from accidental ingestion, inhalation, or absorption of the drugs. Table 50.1 outlines the protective items that should be available to staff working with antineoplastic drugs.

ORAL ADMINISTRATION. A number of antineoplastic drugs are administered orally. The oral route is convenient and noninvasive. Most oral drugs are well absorbed when the GI tract is functioning normally. Antineoplastic drugs such as capecitabine (Xeloda) or temozolomide (Temodar) are given orally. Most oral drugs are administered by the patient in a home setting. The section on Educating the Patient and Family provides information to include in a teaching plan.

PARENTERAL ADMINISTRATION. Although some of these drugs are given orally, others are given by the parenteral route. Antineoplastic drugs may be administered subcutaneously (subcut), intramuscularly (IM), and IV. When giving these drugs IM, inject into the large muscles using the Z-track method (see Chapter 2), because administration can cause stinging or burning. When the subcutaneous method of administration is used, the injection should contain no more than 1 mL, and injections are given in the usual subcutaneous injection sites (see Chapter 2). If the injections are given

---

Table 50.1 Personal Protective Equipment for Safe Handling of Antineoplastic Drugs

Route of Potential Exposure	Safety Equipment
Skin	Gowns—single-use, disposable gowns with closed front and cuffs and made of impermeable or minimally permeable fabric (to the agents in use)
	Gloves—powder-free; made of latex, nitrile, or neoprene; labeled and tested for use with chemotherapeutic drugs
Ingestion	Safety goggles with face shield—to protect face and eyes from possible splashes
Inhalation	National Institute for Occupational Safety and Health (NIOSH)–approved respirator—when a spill must be cleaned up

Adapted from Polovich, M. (2004). Safe handling of hazardous drugs. Retrieved April 28, 2009, from http://www.guideline.gov/summary/summary. aspx?ss=15&doc_id=4152&nbr=3180/

frequently, the sites should be rotated and charted appropriately.

Intravenous administration may be accomplished using a vascular access device, an Angiocath, or a butterfly needle. These devices have become common methods of drug delivery and, depending on the patient's individual treatment regimen, may be inserted before therapy. Selection of the device depends on the type of therapy the patient is to receive, the condition of the veins, and how long the treatment regimen is to be continued. Special directions for administration, stated by either the oncology health care provider or manufacturer, are also important. For example, cisplatin cannot be prepared or administered with needles or IV administration sets containing aluminum, because aluminum reacts with cisplatin, causing formation of a precipitate and loss of potency.

Nurses who are certified in chemotherapy drug administration administer these drugs, but any nurse may be involved in monitoring patients receiving antineoplastic drugs. Antineoplastic drugs are potentially toxic drugs that can cause a variety of effects during and after their administration. Display 50.5 summarizes important points to keep in mind when administering an antineoplastic drug.

Monitoring and Managing Patient Needs
Not all patients have the same response to a specific antineoplastic drug. For example, an antineoplastic drug may cause vomiting, but the amount of fluid and electrolytes lost through vomiting may vary from patient to patient. One patient may require additional sips of water once nausea and vomiting have subsided, whereas another may require IV fluid and electrolyte replacement. Nursing management is focused not only on what may or what did happen but also on the effects produced by a particular adverse reaction.

IMBALANCED NUTRITION: LESS THAN BODY REQUIREMENTS. Patients may not eat because they are tired or not hungry. Anorexia (loss of appetite resulting in the inability to eat) is a common occurrence with the antineoplastic drugs. This may be due to nausea, taste alterations, or sores in the GI system. Nausea and vomiting are common adverse reactions to some of the highly emetic antineoplastic drugs. To minimize this adverse reaction, the oncology health care provider may order an antiemetic, such as ondansetron (Zofran), to be given before treatment and continued for a few days after administration of the chemotherapy. Because this is an expensive drug, other protocols may include different (and less expensive) antiemetics. Some of these have adverse effects, such as a sedative action, which might add to the patient's lack of desire to eat. In the example of the patient who is vomiting, it is important to track accurately all fluid intake. To prevent handling of contaminated waste, use the patient's weight instead of measuring urine or emesis to assess for fluid loss and observe the patient for signs of dehydration and electrolyte imbalances. These measurements and observations aid the oncology health care provider in determining if fluid replacement is necessary.

Assess the nutritional status of the patient before and during treatment. To stimulate appetite, provide small, frequent meals to coincide with the patient's tolerance for food. Greasy or fatty foods and unpleasant sights, smells, and tastes are avoided. Cold foods, dry foods, and salty foods may be better tolerated. It is a good idea to provide diversional activities, such as music, television, and books. Relaxation, visualization, guided imagery, hypnosis, and other nonpharmacologic measures have been helpful to some patients.

It is not uncommon for the patient to report alterations in the sense of taste during the course of chemotherapy. Some drugs give protein foods such as beef a bitter, metallic taste. Small, frequent meals (five to six meals daily) are usually better tolerated than are three large meals. Breakfast is often the best-tolerated meal of the day. Stress the importance of eating meals high in nutritive value, particularly protein (e.g., eggs, milk products, tuna, beans, peas, and lentils). Some patients prefer to have available high-protein finger foods such as cheese or peanut butter and crackers. Nutritional supplements may also be prescribed. Monitor the patient's body weight weekly (or more often if necessary) and report any weight loss. If the patient continues to lose weight, a feeding tube or total parenteral nutrition (TPN) may be used to supplement nutritional needs. Although this is not ideal, the patient who is malnourished and weak may benefit from this intervention.

Because the cells in the mouth grow rapidly, they are particularly sensitive to the effects of the antineoplastic drugs. Stomatitis (inflammation of the mouth) or oral mucositis (inflammation of the oral mucous membranes) may appear 5 to 7 days after chemotherapy is started and continue up to 10 days after therapy. This adverse reaction is particularly

---

Display 50.5 Points to Keep in Mind About Antineoplastic Drug Administration

Great care and accuracy are important in preparing and administering these drugs. Important points to keep in mind during drug administration follow:

- Wear personal protective equipment when preparing any of these drugs for parenteral administration.
- Administer any prophylactic medications or fluids in a timely manner to prevent reactions.
- Observe the patient closely before, during, and after the administration of an antineoplastic drug.
- Observe the IV site closely to detect any signs of extravasation (leakage into the surrounding tissues). Tissue necrosis can be a serious complication. Discontinue the infusion and notify the oncology health care provider if discomfort, redness along the pathway of the vein, or infiltration occurs.
- Continually update nursing assessments, nursing diagnoses, and nursing care plans to meet the changing needs of the patient.
- Notify the oncology health care provider of all changes in the patient's general condition, the appearance of adverse reactions, and changes in laboratory test results.
- Provide the patient and family with both physical and emotional support during treatment.

uncomfortable, because irritation of the oral mucous membranes affects the nutritional aspects of care. The patient must avoid any foods or products that are irritating to the mouth, such as alcoholic beverages, spices, alcohol-based mouthwash, or toothpaste. Instruct caregivers to provide soft or liquid food high in nutritive value. The oral cavity is inspected for increased irritation. Teach the patient to report any white patches on the tongue (possible *candidiasis* fungal infection), throat, or gums; any burning sensation; and bleeding from the mouth or gums. Mouth care is encouraged, and should be performed every 4 hours, including a rinse with normal saline solution. Lemon/glycerin swabs are avoided because they tend to irritate the oral mucosa and complicate stomatitis. The oncology health care provider may order a topical viscous anesthetic, such as lidocaine viscous, to decrease discomfort.

Fatigue, Risk for Injury, and Risk for Infection. Many antineoplastic drugs interfere with the bone marrow's ability to make new cells. This interference is called *bone marrow suppression* or myelosuppression and is a potentially dangerous adverse reaction. Bone marrow suppression is manifested by abnormal laboratory test results and clinical evidence of leukopenia, thrombocytopenia, or anemia. For example, there is a decrease in the white blood cells or leukocytes (*leukopenia*), a decrease in the thrombocytes (*thrombocytopenia*), and a decrease in the red blood cells, resulting in anemia.

Anemia occurs as the result of a decreased production of red blood cells in the bone marrow and is characterized by fatigue, dizziness, shortness of breath, and palpitations. Teach the patient to prioritize activities to conserve energy. Permission may need to be given to the active patient to slow down and even take daytime naps. In some cases, the administration of blood transfusions may be necessary to correct the anemia.

Patients with neutropenia (reduction in the neutrophil type of white blood cells) have a decreased resistance to infection and must be monitored closely for any signs of infection. Combined therapy, such as chemotherapy and radiation together, can have an additive effect on the reduction of blood cells.

NURSING ALERT

Because of the severity of leukopenia when taking temozolomide (Temodar) in conjunction with radiation to the brain, patients should be started on prophylactic therapy to prevent *Pneumocystis* pneumonia (PCP).

Patients are instructed to stay away from crowds or ill individuals while receiving myelosuppressive drugs. Sepsis, without the typical signs of infection, can affect patients because they lack neutrophils. The oncology health care provider may prescribe colony-stimulating factor injections to promote the production of blood cells between the chemotherapy cycles. Low blood counts are one of the primary reasons a chemotherapy treatment may be delayed.

NURSING ALERT

Report immediately any of the following signs of infection to the health care provider: temperature of 100.4°F (38°C) or higher, cough, sore throat, chills, frequent urination, or a white blood cell count of less than 2500/mm³.

Thrombocytopenia is characterized by a decrease in the platelet count (less than 100,000/mm³). Teach patients to monitor for bleeding tendencies and take precautions to prevent bleeding. Injections and multiple blood draws are avoided but, if necessary, then apply pressure to the injection site for 3 to 5 minutes to prevent bleeding into the tissue and the formation of a hematoma. Instruct the patient to avoid the use of disposable razors, nail trimmers, dental floss, firm toothbrushes, or any sharp objects. The patient is taught to refrain from contact and highly physical activities at this time. The patient is monitored closely for easy bruising, skin lesions, and bleeding from any orifice (opening) of the body.

NURSING ALERT

Teach the patient to report to you or to the health care provider immediately any of the following: bleeding gums, easy bruising, petechiae (pinpoint hemorrhages), increased menstrual bleeding, tarry stools, bloody urine, or coffee-ground emesis.

Disturbed Body Image. Adverse reactions seen with the administration of these drugs may range from very mild to life-threatening. Some of these reactions, such as the loss of hair (alopecia), may have little effect on the physical status of the patient but certainly may have a serious effect on the patient's mental health. Because the practice of nursing is concerned with the whole patient, such physically altering reactions that can have a profound effect on the patient must be considered when planning nursing management.

Some drugs cause severe hair loss, whereas others cause gradual thinning. Examples of drugs commonly associated with severe hair loss are doxorubicin and vinblastine. If hair loss is associated with the antineoplastic drug being given, inform the patient that hair loss may occur. This problem may occur 10 to 21 days after the first treatment cycle. Hair loss is usually temporary, and hair will grow again when the drug therapy is completed. Forewarn the patient that hair loss may occur suddenly and in large amounts. Hair will be lost not only from the head but also from the entire body. Although it is not life-threatening, alopecia can have an impact on both self-esteem and body image, serving as a reminder that the individual is undergoing treatment for cancer.

Depending on the patient, you may need to assist in making plans for the purchase of a wig or cap to disguise the hair loss until the hair grows back. Be aware that this might be as great a problem to a male patient as it is to a female patient. The patient is reminded about the importance of a head covering because of the amount of body heat that can be lost with the hair gone.

Anxiety. The word *cancer* still evokes dread in people. Patients and family members are usually devastated by the diagnosis of cancer. Patients have to absorb much information and make quick, critical decisions about treatment. This can be especially demanding on both family and providers if English is not their first language. Obtaining information in the preferred language and interpreter services for provider interactions is both time consuming and exhausting for the patient and family members. The emphasis on the safety requirements of chemotherapy administration adds to the demands and fears placed on patients. The emotional impact of the disease may be forgotten or put aside by members of the health care team as they plan and institute therapy to control the disease. Because cancer treatment happens over time, you have the opportunity to offer consistent and empathetic emotional support to the patient and family members. This support can help reduce some of the fear and anxiety experienced by the patient and family during treatment.

IMPAIRED TISSUE INTEGRITY. Erythema consists of a red, warm, and sometimes painful area on the skin. Because the skin cells are rapidly growing cells, the integument is at risk for breakdown during antineoplastic drug therapy. Care should be taken by patients to avoid the sun; to wear loose, protective clothing; and to watch areas of skinfolds for breakdown. Some antineoplastic drugs have the ability to sensitize skin that has previously been irradiated. Be sure to instruct the patient about this adverse reaction, because it can be both surprising and painful.

> **! NURSING ALERT**
>
> Radiation recall is a skin reaction in which an area that was previously irradiated becomes reddened when a patient is administered certain specific chemotherapy drugs. This is well differentiated from a reaction exclusive to the drugs, because of the defined outline of the previous radiation treatment field on the body.

Some antineoplastic drugs are vesicants (i.e., they cause tissue necrosis if they infiltrate or extravasate out of the blood vessel and into the soft tissue). If extravasation occurs, underlying tissue is damaged. The damage can be severe, causing physical deformity or loss of vascularity or tendon function. If the damage is severe, skin grafting may be necessary to preserve function. Examples of vesicant drugs are daunorubicin, doxorubicin, and vinblastine.

> **! NURSING ALERT**
>
> Patients at risk for extravasation are those unable to communicate to the nurse about the pain of extravasation, older adults, debilitated patients, or confused patients, and any patient with fragile veins.

When the patient is receiving a vesicant, ensure that extravasation protocol orders are signed and that an extravasation kit is on the unit before vesicant drugs are administered. The IV site is continuously monitored and checks for blood return are made frequently during IV push procedures (every 1 to 2 mL). If a vesicant is prescribed as an infusion, it is given only through a central line and checked every 1 to 2 hours. Keep the extravasation kit containing all materials necessary to manage an extravasation available, along with the extravasation policy and procedure guidelines (see Appendix E for a sample kit).

Extravasation may occur without warning, or minor signs may be detected by an alert nurse. The earlier the extravasation is detected, the less likely soft tissue damage will occur. Signs of extravasation include:

- Swelling (most common)
- Stinging, burning, or pain at the injection site (not always present)
- Redness

- Lack of blood return (if this is the only symptom, the IV line should be re-evaluated; a lack of blood return alone is not always indicative of extravasation, and extravasation can occur even if a blood return is present)

If extravasation is suspected, the infusion is stopped immediately, antidotal procedures initiated, and the extravasation reported to the oncology health care provider.

Educating the Patient and Family

The oncology health care provider usually discusses the proposed treatment and possible adverse drug reactions with the patient and family members. As the nurse, you will briefly review these explanations immediately before administration of any antineoplastic drug.

Some antineoplastic drugs are taken orally at home. The areas included in a patient and family teaching plan for this type of treatment regimen are based on the drug prescribed, the oncology health care provider's explanation of the chemotherapy regimen and instructions for taking the drug, and the needs of the individual. To prevent unintended absorption, some pills or tablets should not be handled by others when administering the drugs. Family members are taught how to take out the medication from its container without touching the drug. Because the drugs are eliminated in body wastes, teach the patient to double flush toilets and if able use a bathroom secluded from other family members. Hospitals, clinics, or primary health care providers give printed instructions in the preferred language to the patient. After the patient has read them you will want to spend time with the patient or family members to allow them to ask questions.

In some instances, a drug to prevent nausea may be prescribed to be taken at home before administration of the antineoplastic drugs in the outpatient setting. To obtain the best possible effects, stress to the patient that the drug must be taken at the time specified by the oncology health care provider. It is important for the patient to comply with the treatment regimen to maximize therapeutic effect. Most patients adhere to antineoplastic therapy; however, some of the drugs have modified schedules, such as when given in conjunction with radiation therapy with certain weeks on therapy and others off therapy, and these administration schedules can become confusing. Stress the importance of maintaining the dosing schedule exactly as prescribed. A calendar or automated medication box indicating the doses to take and dates the drug is to be taken is often helpful for the patient. The patient is instructed to bring the treatment calendar to each appointment, and he or she is questioned about any omitted or delayed doses. Nurses in the clinic, home health nurses, or caregivers are taught to fill the medication boxes. In general, one course of therapy is prescribed at a time to avoid inadvertent overdosing that could be life-threatening.

Include the following points in a patient and family teaching plan when oral therapy is prescribed:

- Take the drug only as directed on the prescription container. Unless otherwise indicated, take the drug on an empty stomach with water to enhance absorption. However, the patient should follow specific directions, such as "take on an empty stomach" or "take at the same time each day"; they are extremely important.

- Familiarize yourself with the brand or trade name and the generic name to avoid confusion. If you live with another person at home, ask that person to help you verify the correct drug and dose of the drug before you take it.

- Never increase, decrease, or omit a dose unless advised to do so by the oncology health care provider.

- If any problems (adverse reactions) occur, no matter how minor, contact the oncology health care provider immediately.

- All recommendations given by the oncology health care provider, such as increasing the fluid intake or eating or avoiding certain foods, are important.

- Some drugs leave the body relatively unchanged; therefore, to prevent contamination men should avoid using urinals and sit to urinate for at least 48 hours following the last dose of the drug. Toilets should be double flushed with the lid down to prevent spray in the bathroom.

- The effectiveness or action of the drug could be altered if these directions are ignored. Other recommendations, such as checking the mouth for sores, rinsing the mouth thoroughly after eating or drinking, or drinking extra fluids, are given to identify or minimize some of the effects these drugs have on the body. It is important to follow these recommendations.

- Keep all appointments for chemotherapy. These drugs must be given at certain intervals to be effective.

- Do not take any nonprescription drug unless the use of a specific drug has been approved by the oncology health care provider.

- ♥ Avoid drinking alcoholic beverages unless the oncology health care provider has approved their use.

- Always inform other physicians, dentists, and medical personnel of therapy with this drug.

- Keep all appointments for the laboratory tests ordered by the oncology health care provider. If you are unable to keep a laboratory appointment, notify the oncology health care provider immediately.

EVALUATION

- Therapeutic effect is achieved.

- Adverse reactions are identified, reported to the primary health care provider, and managed successfully using nursing interventions.
  - Patient maintains an adequate nutritional status.
  - Patient reports fatigue is managed appropriately.
  - No evidence of injury is seen.
  - No evidence of infection is seen.
  - Perceptions of body changes are managed successfully.
  - Anxiety is managed successfully.
  - Skin remains intact.

- Patient and family express confidence and demonstrate an understanding of the drug regimen.

PHARMACOLOGY IN PRACTICE
THINK CRITICALLY

 Some people do not think about survivorship when discussing cancer. Mr. Phillip's wife survived breast cancer, yet he still feels grief after losing her. Review Chapters 21 and 22 regarding the medications used to help him deal with his feelings. What other strategies would you now consider?

KEY POINTS

- A neoplasm is a group of cells that do not maturate, but grow out of control. Antineoplastic drugs are used to retard this process by targeting specific portions of the cell cycle or disturbing the process.

- Although chemotherapy literally means drug therapy, it is typically associated with anticancer drugs used in the cure, control, or palliation of the disease.

- Because antineoplastic drugs enter the body systemically, the same mechanism of action used to kill or retard cancerous cells can also harm other fast-growing cells in the body such as GI, blood component, skin, and other lining cells. Caution should be taken during administration with many of the drugs due to their ability to irritate tissues.

- Adverse reactions to the platelets and red and white blood cells result in fatigue, bleeding, and infection. Nausea, vomiting, and diarrhea result from destruction of GI lining cells. Peripheral nerve damage can result in numbness, tingling, or lack of sensation.

Summary Drug Table ANTINEOPLASTIC DRUGS

Generic Name	Trade Name	Uses	Adverse Reactions
Cell Cycle–Specific Agents			
Plant Alkaloids			
Vinca Alkaloids			
vinblastine *vin-blas'-teen*		Leukemia/lymphomas: Hodgkin's disease, other lymphomas Solid tumors: testicular, breast, Kaposi's sarcoma (KS) Nonmalignant: mycosis fungoides	Immediate: extravasation potential During therapy cycles: alopecia, anemia, leukopenia, paresthesias, nausea, vomiting, constipation Long term: fertility problems
vincristine *vin-kris'-teen*		Leukemia/lymphomas: acute leukemia, other lymphomas Solid tumors: rhabdomyosarcoma, bladder, breast, KS Nonmalignant: idiopathic thrombocytopenic purpura	Immediate: extravasation potential During therapy cycles: alopecia, anemia, leukopenia, paresthesias, nausea, vomiting, stomatitis, constipation Long term: renal, adrenal, fertility problems
vinorelbine *vin-noe'-rell-been*	Navelbine	Solid tumors: non–small cell lung cancer (NSCLC) Unlabeled use: other solid tumors, KS	Immediate: extravasation potential During therapy cycles: leukopenia, paresthesias, nausea, constipation, alopecia, radiation recall
Taxanes			
cabazitaxel *kab-az-tax'-ell*	Jevtana	Solid tumors: prostate	Immediate: hypersensitivity reaction During therapy cycles: nausea, fever, anemia, leukopenia, vomiting, diarrhea, constipation, stomatitis, hematuria
docetaxel *doe-seh-tax'-ell*	Taxotere	Solid tumors: breast, NSCLC, prostate Unlabeled use: other solid tumors	Immediate: extravasation potential During therapy cycles: nausea, peripheral neuropathy, alopecia, cutaneous changes, fever, anemia, leukopenia, vomiting, diarrhea, stomatitis, fluid retention Long term: fertility problems
paclitaxel *pak-leh-tax'-ell*	Abraxane	Solid tumors: ovary, breast, NSCLC, KS Unlabeled use: other solid tumors	Immediate: cardiac changes, hypotension, extravasation potential During therapy cycles: nausea, vomiting, peripheral neuropathy, alopecia, fever, anemia, leukopenia, diarrhea, stomatitis Long term: fertility problems
Podophyllotoxins			
etoposide *eh-toe'-poe-syde*		Solid tumors: testicular, small cell lung cancer (SCLC) Unlabeled use: other solid tumors, leukemias and lymphomas	During therapy cycles: anemia, leukopenia, thrombocytopenia, alopecia, nausea, vomiting
teniposide (VM-26) *teh-nip'-oh-syde*	Vumon	Leukemia/lymphomas: acute lymphocytic leukemia (ALL)	Immediate: extravasation potential During therapy cycles: anemia, leukopenia, thrombocytopenia, alopecia, nausea, vomiting
Camptothecin Analogs			
irinotecan *eye-rin-oh-tee'-kan*	Camptosar	Solid tumors: metastatic colon or rectal	Immediate: nausea, vomiting, diarrhea, inflammation potential (IV site) During therapy cycles: diarrhea, anemia, leukopenia, thrombocytopenia, asthenia, alopecia
topotecan *toe-poh-tee'-kan*	Hycamtin	Solid tumors: metastatic ovarian, SCLC	During therapy cycles: anemia, leukopenia, thrombocytopenia, alopecia, nausea, vomiting, diarrhea, constipation

Summary Drug Table ANTINEOPLASTIC DRUGS (continued)

Generic Name	Trade Name	Uses	Adverse Reactions
Antimetabolites			
azacitidine *ay-za-site'-i-deen*	Vidaza	Myelodysplastic syndrome Unlabeled use: other leukemias and lymphomas	During therapy cycles: anemia, leukopenia, thrombocytopenia, nausea, vomiting
capecitabine *kap-eh-see'-tah-been*	Xeloda	Solid tumors: breast, colon	During therapy cycles: anemia, leukopenia, thrombocytopenia, diarrhea, hand and foot syndrome
cladribine *kla'-drih-been*	Leustatin	Leukemia/lymphomas: hairy cell leukemia Unlabeled use: other leukemias and lymphomas	During therapy cycles: anemia, leukopenia, thrombocytopenia, fever, nausea, rash
clofarabine *kloe-far'-ah-been*	Clolar	Leukemia/lymphomas: ALL	During therapy cycles: anemia, leukopenia, thrombocytopenia, hyperuricemia
cytarabine (ara-C) *sye-tare'-ah-been*	Cytosar-U, DepoCyt	Leukemia/lymphomas: ALL, acute myelocytic leukemia (AML)	Immediate: nausea, vomiting During therapy cycles: anemia, leukopenia, thrombocytopenia
decitabine *dee-sye'-ta-been*	Dacogen	Myelodysplastic syndrome Unlabeled use: other leukemias and lymphomas	During therapy cycles: anemia, leukopenia, thrombocytopenia, nausea, vomiting
fludarabine *floo-dar'-ah-been*		Leukemia/lymphomas: chronic lymphocytic leukemia Unlabeled use: other leukemias and lymphomas	During therapy cycles: anemia, leukopenia, thrombocytopenia
fluorouracil (5-FU) *floo-roh-yoor'-ah-sill*		Palliative treatment for solid tumors: breast, stomach, pancreas, colon, rectum	During therapy cycles: anemia, leukopenia, thrombocytopenia, nausea, vomiting, stomatitis, diarrhea, alopecia
gemcitabine *jem-sye'-tah-been*	Gemzar	Solid tumors: pancreatic, NSCLC	During therapy cycles: anemia, leukopenia, thrombocytopenia, fever, rash, nausea, vomiting, diarrhea, proteinuria
mercaptopurine (6-MP) *mer-kap-toe-pyoor'-een*	Purinethol	Leukemia/lymphomas: ALL, AML Unlabeled use: inflammatory bowel disease	During therapy cycles: anemia, leukopenia, thrombocytopenia, hyperuricemia
methotrexate *meth-oh-trex'-ate*	Trexall	Leukemia/lymphomas; ALL, non-Hodgkin's lymphoma Solid tumors: breast, head/neck, choriocarcinomas, osteosarcomas Nonmalignant: mycosis fungoides, severe psoriasis, rheumatoid arthritis Unlabeled use: multiple sclerosis, inflammatory bowel disease	Immediate: nausea, vomiting (high dose) During therapy cycles: anemia, leukopenia, thrombocytopenia, stomatitis, diarrhea, renal damage Long term: hepatotoxicity
nelarabine *nel-lah-rah'-been*	Arranon	Leukemia/lymphomas: T-cell acute lymphoblastic leukemia and T-cell lymphoblastic lymphoma	During therapy cycles: fatigue, neurologic toxicity
pemetrexed *pem-ah-trex'-ed*	Alimta	Solid tumors: NSCLC, malignant pleural mesothelioma	During therapy cycles: anemia, leukopenia, thrombocytopenia, skin rashes
pentostatin *pen'-toe-stat-in*	Nipent	Leukemia/lymphomas: hairy cell leukemia Unlabeled use: other leukemias and lymphomas	During therapy cycles: anemia, leukopenia, thrombocytopenia, rash, itching, nausea, vomiting, diarrhea
thioguanine *thye-oh-gwah'-neen*		Acute leukemias Unlabeled use: severe psoriasis, inflammatory bowel disease	During therapy cycles: anemia, leukopenia, thrombocytopenia, hyperuricemia

(table continues on page 566)

Antineoplastic Drugs

Summary Drug Table ANTINEOPLASTIC DRUGS (continued)

Generic Name	Trade Name	Uses	Adverse Reactions
Miscellaneous Agents			
eribulin *er'-i-bue-in*	Halaven	Solid tumors: advanced breast	During therapy cycles: fatigue, peripheral neuropathy, neutropenia, alopecia, nausea, diarrhea
ixabepilone *ix'-ah-bep'-ih-loan*	Ixempra	Solid tumors: advanced breast	During therapy cycles: fatigue, peripheral neuropathy, neutropenia, alopecia, nausea, diarrhea
Cell Cycle–Nonspecific Agents			
Alkylating Drugs			
Nitrogen Mustard Derivatives			
chlorambucil *klor-am'-byoo-sill*	Leukeran	Leukemia/lymphomas: chronic lymphocytic leukemia (CLL), lymphomas, Hodgkin's disease	During therapy cycles: anemia, leukopenia, thrombocytopenia Long term: fertility problems
cyclophospha-mide *sye-kloe-foss'-fah-myde*	Cytoxan, Neosar	Leukemia/lymphomas: ALL, AML, CLL, advanced lymphomas, Hodgkin's disease Solid tumors: breast, ovary, neuroblastoma, retinoblastoma Nonmalignant: mycosis fungoides, nephrotic syndrome (children), rheumatoid arthritis, systemic lupus erythematosus, multiple sclerosis	Immediate: nausea, vomiting During therapy cycles: leukopenia, hemorrhagic cystitis, thrombocytopenia Long term: fertility problems, secondary cancers
ifosfamide *eye-foss'-fah-myde*	Ifex	Leukemia/lymphomas: unlabeled use (except AML) Solid tumors: testicular Unlabeled use: lung, breast, ovary, gastric, pancreatic	Immediate: nausea, vomiting During therapy cycles: leukopenia, thrombocytopenia, hemorrhagic cystitis, alopecia, somnolence, confusion
mechlorethamine *meh-klor-eth'-ah-meen*	Mustargen	Palliative treatment for CLL, chronic myelocytic leukemia (CML), advanced lymphomas, Hodgkin's disease Solid tumors: lung, metastatic disease, mycosis fungoides	Immediate: nausea, vomiting, extravasation potential, lymphocytopenia During therapy cycles: anemia, leukopenia, thrombocytopenia, hyperuremia, diarrhea Long term: fertility problems, secondary cancers
melphalan *mel'-fah-lan*	Alkeran	Palliative treatment for multiple myeloma Solid tumors: ovary Unlabeled use: testicular, breast, bone marrow transplantation	Immediate: nausea, vomiting During therapy cycles: leukopenia, thrombocytopenia, diarrhea, alopecia Long term: fertility problems, secondary cancers
Ethyleneimines			
altretamine (hexamethyl melamine) *al-tret'-ah-meen*	Hexalen	Palliative treatment for solid tumors: ovary	During therapy cycles: anemia, leukopenia, thrombocytopenia, nausea, vomiting, peripheral neuropathy, dizziness
bendamustine *ben'-da-mus-teen*	Treanda	Leukemia/lymphomas: CLL, non-Hodgkin's lymphoma	During therapy cycles: anemia, leukopenia, thrombocytopenia, nausea, vomiting, diarrhea
thiotepa *thye-oh-tep'-ah*	Thioplex	Solid tumors: breast, ovary, bladder	During therapy cycles: anemia, leukopenia, thrombocytopenia, alopecia Long term: fertility problems
Alkyl Sulfonate			
busulfan *byoo-sul'-fan*	Busulfex, Myleran	Palliative treatment for CML	Immediate: induce seizures During therapy cycles: anemia, leukopenia, thrombocytopenia, hyperuremia, graft-versus-host disease Long term: fertility problems

Summary Drug Table ANTINEOPLASTIC DRUGS (continued)

Generic Name	Trade Name	Uses	Adverse Reactions
Hydrazines			
dacarbazine *dah-kar'-bah-zeen*	DTIC	Leukemia/lymphomas: Hodgkin's disease Solid tumors: melanoma Unlabeled use: pheochromocytoma, KS	Immediate: nausea, vomiting During therapy cycles: anemia, leukopenia, thrombocytopenia
procarbazine *proe-kar'-bah-zeen*	Matulane	Leukemia/lymphomas: Hodgkin's disease Unlabeled use: other lymphomas, brain, small cell lung cancer, melanoma	Immediate: nausea, vomiting During therapy cycles: anemia, leukopenia, thrombocytopenia, peripheral neuropathy, alopecia
temozolomide *tem-oh-zoll'-oh-myde*	Temodar	Solid tumors: glioblastoma, astrocytoma Unlabeled use: melanoma	During therapy cycles: leukopenia, thrombocytopenia, headache, nausea, vomiting, alopecia
Nitrosoureas			
carmustine (BCNU) *car-muss'-teen*	BiCNU, Gliadel	Palliative treatment for Hodgkin's disease, multiple myeloma, various brain tumors Unlabeled use: T-cell lymphoma, melanoma	Immediate: nausea, vomiting During therapy cycles: leukopenia, thrombocytopenia Long term: pulmonary fibrosis
lomustine (CCNU) *loe-muss'-teen*	CeeNU	Leukemia/lymphomas: secondary treatment for Hodgkin's disease Solid tumors: brain	Immediate: nausea, vomiting During therapy cycles: leukopenia, thrombocytopenia, alopecia, stomatitis Long term: pulmonary fibrosis, fertility problems
streptozocin *strep'-toe-zoh-sin*	Zanosar	Solid tumors: pancreatic	Immediate: nausea, vomiting During therapy cycles: azotemia, proteinuria, stomatitis
Platinum-Based Drugs			
cisplatin *sis-plah'-tin*		Solid tumors: ovarian, testicular, bladder	Immediate: nausea, vomiting, renal damage During therapy cycles: anemia, leukopenia, thrombocytopenia tinnitus, hyperuricemia
oxaliplatin *ox-al'-ih-plah-tin*	Eloxatin	Solid tumors: colon, rectal	During therapy cycles: leukopenia, thrombocytopenia, peripheral neuropathy
carboplatin *kar'-boe-plah-tin*	Paraplatin	Solid tumors: ovarian Unlabeled use: lung, head and neck, testicular	During therapy cycles: anemia, leukopenia, thrombocytopenia
Antibiotics			
bleomycin *blee-oh-mye'-sin*		Palliative treatment for lymphomas, pleural effusion Solid tumors: testicular, various types Unlabeled use: mycosis fungoides, KS	During therapy cycles: anemia, leukopenia, thrombocytopenia, vomiting, alopecia, skin erythema, cutaneous changes Long term: pneumonitis, pulmonary fibrosis
dactinomycin *dak-tih-noe-mye'-sin*	Cosmegen	Solid tumors: various sarcomas, Wilms' tumor, gestational neoplasia, testicular	Immediate: nausea, vomiting, extravasation potential During therapy cycles: anemia, leukopenia, thrombocytopenia, alopecia, skin erythema Long term: fertility problems
daunorubicin *daw-noe-roo'-bih-sin*	DaunoXome	Leukemia/lymphomas: ALL, AML Solid tumors: KS	Immediate: nausea, vomiting, extravasation potential During therapy cycles: anemia, leukopenia, thrombocytopenia, alopecia, stomatitis, hyperuricemia, urine discoloration Long term: cardiotoxicity

(table continues on page 568)

Antineoplastic Drugs

Summary Drug Table ANTINEOPLASTIC DRUGS (continued)

Generic Name	Trade Name	Uses	Adverse Reactions
doxorubicin *dox-oh-roo'-bih-sin*	Doxil	Leukemia/lymphomas; ALL, AML, and various lymphomas Solid tumors: Wilms' tumor, neuroblastoma, KS, various sarcomas, breast, lung, ovary, bladder, thyroid, gastric	Immediate: nausea, vomiting, extravasation potential During therapy cycles: anemia, leukopenia, thrombocytopenia, alopecia, cutaneous changes, stomatitis, hyperuricemia, urine discoloration, radiation recall, hand and foot syndrome Long term: cardiotoxicity
epirubicin *ep-pee-roo'-bih-sin*	Ellence	Solid tumors: breast Unlabeled use: advanced esophageal	Immediate: extravasation potential During therapy cycles: anemia, leukopenia, thrombocytopenia, nausea, vomiting, alopecia, stomatitis, diarrhea, urine discoloration, radiation recall Long term: cardiotoxicity, fertility problems
idarubicin *eye-dah-roo'-bih-sin*		Leukemia/lymphomas: AML	Immediate: extravasation potential During therapy cycles: anemia, leukopenia, thrombocytopenia, alopecia, nausea, vomiting, stomatitis, diarrhea, hyperuricemia, urine discoloration Long term: cardiotoxicity
mitomycin *mye-toe-mye'-sin*		Solid tumors: stomach, pancreas	Immediate: extravasation potential During therapy cycles: anemia, leukopenia, thrombocytopenia, hyperuricemia
mitoxantrone *mye-toe-zan'-trone*		Leukemia/lymphomas: acute nonlymphocytic leukemia Solid tumors: advanced prostate Nonmalignant: multiple sclerosis	Immediate: nausea, vomiting, extravasation potential During therapy cycles: leukopenia, nausea, alopecia Long term: cardiotoxicity, AML
Miscellaneous Agents			
DNA Inhibitor			
hydroxyurea *hye-drox-ee-yoor-ee'-ah*	Hydrea,	Solid tumors: melanoma Unlabeled use: thrombocythemia, human immunodeficiency virus infection, psoriasis	During therapy cycles: anemia, leukopenia, thrombocytopenia, radiation recall
Adrenocortical Inhibitor			
mitotane *mye'-toe-tane*	Lysodren	Solid tumors: adrenal cortex Unlabeled use: Cushing's disease	During therapy cycles: nausea, vomiting, diarrhea
Enzymes			
asparaginase *ah-spare'-ah-gih-nayce*	Elspar	Leukemia/lymphomas: ALL	During therapy cycles: anemia, leukopenia, thrombocytopenia, hyperuricemia, rash, urticaria, acute anaphylaxis
pegaspargase *peg-ah-spar'-gayce*	Oncaspar	Same as asparaginase	Same as asparaginase
Antimicrotubule Agents			
estramustine (estradiol/ nitrogen mustard) *ess-tra-muss'-teen*	Emcyt	Palliative treatment for solid tumors (e.g., prostate)	Immediate: nausea, diarrhea During therapy cycles: breast tenderness, thrombophlebitis, fluid retention Long term: gynecomastia, impotence
Retinoids			
tretinoin *tret'-ih-noyn*		Leukemia/lymphomas: acute promyelocytic leukemia	During therapy cycles: headache, fever, weakness, fatigue, edema, retinoic acid–acute promyelocytic leukemia (RA-APL) syndrome (acute anaphylactic reaction)
bexarotene *bex-air'-oh-teen*	Targretin	Leukemia/lymphomas: cutaneous T-cell lymphoma	During therapy cycles: elevated blood lipids, rash, leukopenia, dry skin

Chapter Review

Know Your Drugs

Clients sometimes know a medication by the brand (or trade) name and not the generic name. To help you recognize both names, match the brand name with the generic name of the same medication.

Generic Name	Brand Name
1. cyclophosphamide	A. Arranon
2. ifosfamide	B. Cytoxan
3. nelarabine	C. Ifex
4. temozolomide	D. Temodar

Calculate Medication Dosages

1. Chlorambucil dosage is calculated based on the patient's body weight. Mrs. Garcia weighs 64 kg. The prescribed dosage of chlorambucil is 0.2 mg/kg of body weight per day. What is the correct daily dosage for Mrs. Garcia?

2. A patient weighing 54 kg is to receive bleomycin 0.25 units/kg of body weight. What is the correct dosage of bleomycin?

Prepare for the NCLEX®

Build Your Knowledge

1. Cancerous cells grow when _____.
   1. the pH is too acid
   2. G_0 phase of the cell cycle is skipped
   3. too much wear and tear on the cells happens
   4. neutrophils are too low

2. During which phase of the cell cycle does a cell split into two daughter cells?
   1. G_1
   2. S
   3. G_2
   4. M

3. Which of the following findings would be most indicative to the nurse that the client has thrombocytopenia?
   1. nausea
   2. blurred vision
   3. headaches
   4. easy bruising

4. Which of the following adverse reactions to the antineoplastic drugs is most likely to affect the client's body image?
   1. hematuria
   2. alopecia
   3. nausea
   4. diarrhea

5. When assessing the client for leukopenia, the nurse _____.
   1. checks the client every 8 hours for hematuria
   2. monitors the client for fever, sore throat, and chills
   3. checks female clients for increased menstrual bleeding
   4. reports a white blood cell count of 5000/mm^3

6. Which of the following interventions would be most helpful for a client with stomatitis?
   1. Mouth care should be provided at least once daily
   2. Swab the mouth with lemon glycerin swabs every 4 hours
   3. Provide frequent mouth care with normal saline
   4. Use a hard-bristle toothbrush to cleanse the mouth and teeth of debris

7. Which of the drugs listed is most likely to cause nausea or vomiting?
   1. temozolomide
   2. cetuximab
   3. cisplatin
   4. vincristine

Apply Your Knowledge

8. Which of the following is the most common symptom of extravasation?
   1. swelling around the injection site
   2. redness along the vein and around the injection site
   3. pain at the injection site
   4. tenderness along the path of the vein

9. A family member calls the nurse to report that the client is losing handfuls of hair. The nurse instructs the family member to:
   1. take the client to the emergency department
   2. have the client scrub the head hard to get it all off
   3. reassure the family member this is normal, and to support the client
   4. rush to the store and purchase a wig or turban

Alternate-Format Questions

10. In what way might the nurse accidentally be exposed to chemotherapy? **Select all that apply**.
    1. direct skin contact
    2. ingestion
    3. inhalation
    4. needle stick

To check your answers, see Appendix G.

thePoint *For more NCLEX-style questions, log on to http://thepoint.lww.com to access more than 1000 questions.*

51

Immunostimulant Drugs

LEARNING OBJECTIVES

On completion of this chapter, the student will:

1. Describe the function of the different types of blood cells.
2. List the drugs used in the treatment of anemia and bleeding and prevention of infection.
3. Discuss the actions, uses, general adverse reactions, contraindications, precautions, and interactions of the agents used in the treatment anemia and bleeding and prevention of infection.
4. Discuss important preadministration and ongoing assessment activities the nurse should perform on a patient receiving an agent used in the treatment of anemia and bleeding and prevention of infection.
5. Identify nursing diagnoses particular to a patient receiving an agent used in the treatment of anemia and bleeding and prevention of infection.
6. Discuss ways to promote an optimal response to therapy and important points to keep in mind when educating patients about the use of an agent used in the treatment of anemia and bleeding and prevention of infection.

KEY TERMS

erythrocytes • red blood cells (RBCs); one of several formed elements in the blood

erythropoiesis • process of making RBCs

folinic acid rescue • *in chemotherapy,* the technique of administering leucovorin after a large dose of methotrexate, thereby allowing normal cells to survive; also called *leucovorin rescue*

hematopoiesis • undifferentiated stem cells are stimulated to become specific blood cells

intrinsic factor • substance produced by the cells in the stomach and necessary for the absorption of vitamin B_{12}

iron deficiency anemia • condition resulting when the body does not have enough iron to meet its need for iron

leukocytes • white blood cells

macrocytic anemia • anemia resulting from abnormal formation (enlargement) of erythrocytes

megakaryocytes • precursor cell to the platelets

megaloblastic anemia • anemia characterized by large, abnormal, immature erythrocytes circulating in the blood; results from folic acid deficiency

thrombopoiesis • formation of platelets (thrombocytes)

DRUG CLASSES

Hematopoietic factors for bleeding and infection
Hematopoietic factors for anemia

An immunostimulant is an agent that stimulates the immune system. In Chapter 49, vaccines (that stimulate us to make specific antibodies) were presented. Two other classes used to boost the immune system are the interferons and the interleukins. Interferons modulate the response of the immune system to viruses, bacteria, cancer, and other foreign substances that invade the body. Interferons do not kill viral or cancer cells; they boost the immune system response and reduce the growth by controlling cellular proteins controlling growth. There are basically three types of interferons: (1) interferon-alpha (α) is used for treating cancers and viral infections, (2) interferon-beta (β) is used

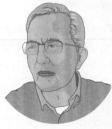

PHARMACOLOGY IN PRACTICE

Mr. Phillip, age 72 years, has chronic kidney disease. He had a friend who was on dialysis about 5 years ago and complained of being tired all the time. They gave him "shots" to perk him up but instead he had a heart attack. Mr. Phillip is concerned about his kidney disease progressing and having to start dialysis, and wonders if the same thing could happen to him.

for treating multiple sclerosis, and (3) interferon-gamma (γ) is used for treating hereditary immune system disorders. Interleukins are a group of chemicals called cytokines. The white blood cells normally make interleukins. Different interleukins help the body's immune system respond to inflammation.

This chapter focuses on the colony-stimulating factors (CSFs), a group of immunostimulants used in cancer treatment and chronic renal failure to support the hematopoietic system. The hematopoietic system is composed of fluids and particles that are known as *blood*. Blood is a complex fluid that circulates continuously through the heart and blood vessels and to the outermost cells of our body tissues. Three distinct cells circulate in the blood:

- Red blood cells (RBCs, **erythrocytes**) that supply our cells with oxygen from the lungs to the tissues
- White blood cells (WBCs, **leukocytes**) that protect our bodies from dangerous microorganisms
- Platelets (**megakaryocytes**) that control the bleeding from microscopic to major tears in our tissues

Chronic diseases such as chronic kidney disease or medical treatments such as chemotherapy can cause a hematologic failure. When this happens, inadequate numbers of cells are produced. As a result, the body can no longer meet the demands for oxygen transportation, blood coagulation, or prevention of invasion of microorganisms. Anemia, bleeding, and infection can result.

The goal for treating these hematologic problems is to stimulate the body to make more of the specific blood cells. This process is called **hematopoiesis**. During this process, undifferentiated stem cells in the bone marrow are signaled to multiply and differentiate into erythrocytes, leukocytes, or megakaryocytes (Fig. 51.1). Hematopoietic drugs help to enhance this process and are used to treat anemia, bleeding, and infection.

HEMATOPOIETIC DRUGS USED IN TREATING POTENTIAL BLEEDING OR INFECTION

There are a number of different WBCs that protect the body from microbial invasion and infection. The WBC known as the neutrophil is one of the major cells in the line of defense from infection. *Neutropenia* is the term for the condition that results when the neutrophil level in the blood is low. Infection is likely to occur when a patient is neutropenic. Neutrophils have an extremely short lifespan (6 to 8 hours), meaning that they rapidly grow and divide. Because of their rapid growth cycle, the neutrophil is a target of the cancer chemotherapy drugs, as well as the cancer cells themselves. Chemotherapy-induced neutropenia is a major reason that cancer treatments may be delayed or cancelled. When this happens, the patient is at a greater risk for continued growth of the cancer or illness from the treatment. CSFs are drugs used to stimulate the growth and production of WBCs to help fight off infection.

Platelets are important to normal blood clotting. They are formed from megakaryocytes in the blood. The megakaryocyte is a large blood cell that can divide into many platelets.

A low platelet count is a condition called *thrombocytopenia*. Decreased platelet production can also be caused by anemia. The interleukin drug oprelvekin is used when sufficient platelets are not made to meet the body's needs. Sometimes the body does not make enough platelets due to unknown causes; this is termed idiopathic (or immune) thrombocytopenic purpura or ITP. Drugs to treat this disorder are appearing in the drug market.

COLONY-STIMULATING FACTORS

Actions and Uses

CSFs are glycoproteins that act on the hematopoietic cells to stimulate proliferation, differentiation, and maturation of WBCs. CSFs are used to treat or prevent infection (by minimizing neutropenia) associated with the following:

- Chemotherapy-induced neutropenia during solid tumor cancer treatment
- Neutropenia during bone marrow transplantation (BMT)
- Production of stem cells for harvest before bone marrow transplant
- Neutropenia in those susceptible to symptomatic chronic infection

Injections of the CSF filgrastim are started at least 24 hours after the completion of a cycle of chemotherapy. The absolute neutrophil count (ANC) is monitored and therapy is continued until an ANC count of at least 10,000/mm^3 is achieved. It is not recommended to use the drug for longer than 2 weeks, and treatment is discontinued at least 1 day before the next chemotherapy cycle is to begin. Special instruction is needed in cases of bone marrow transplant or stem cell harvest.

Pegfilgrastim is similar to filgrastim but is given as a single dose between chemotherapy cycles. Sargramostim is used following BMT, following induction chemotherapy used with leukemia, and to stimulate stem cells for harvest.

Adverse Reactions

General System Reactions

- Bone pain
- Hypertension
- Nausea and vomiting
- Alopecia
- Hypersensitivity or allergic reactions

See the Summary Drug Table: Immunostimulant Drugs for more information on these drugs.

Contraindications, Precautions, and Interactions

CSFs are contraindicated in patients with known hypersensitivity to the drug or any component of the drug. Filgrastim is used cautiously in patients with hypothyroid disease. The CSFs are pregnancy category C drugs, and caution is used when the patient is breastfeeding. Pegfilgrastim can cause a sickle cell crisis in those with the disease. CSFs can cause

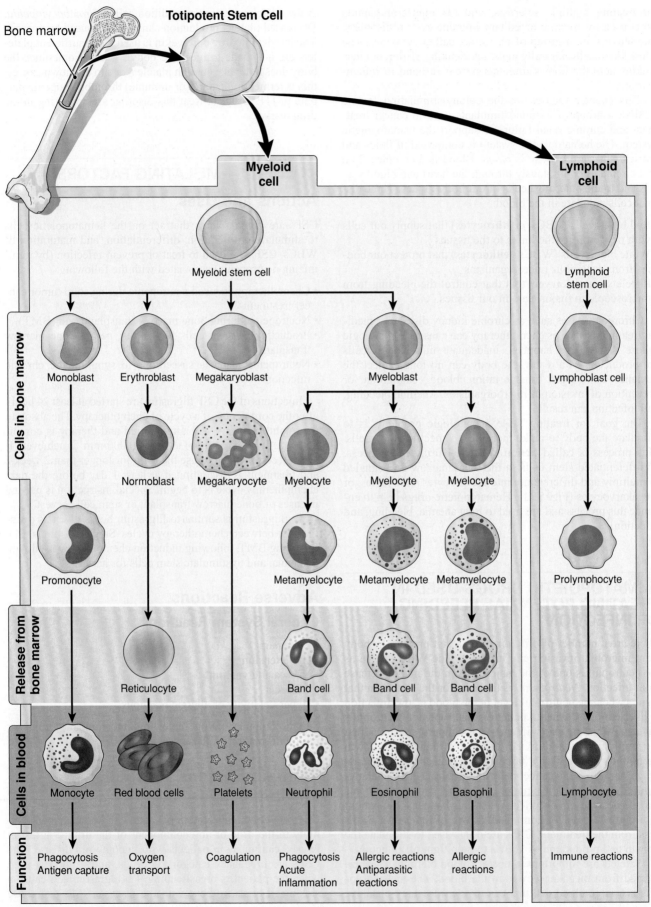

Figure 51.1 Hematopoiesis. (From McConnell, T. H. [2007]. The nature of disease pathology for the health professions. Philadelphia: Lippincott Williams & Wilkins.)

hypersensitive reactions and should be treated with anti-histamines, steroids, and bronchodilators to maintain their use. These drugs can stimulate cancer cell growth in cancer types that are stimulated by growth factors. An even higher increase in neutrophil count can occur when these drugs are taken with lithium, a drug used for the manic phase of mood disorders. The CSFs are currently in study phases to assess safety in children.

DRUGS USED TO TREAT THROMBOCYTOPENIA

Actions and Uses

Oprelvekin is a drug that stimulates **thrombopoiesis**. Thrombopoiesis is the process of making platelets. The drug is used to prevent severe thrombocytopenia and reduces the need for multiple platelet transfusions. Oprelvekin is used to treat or prevent thrombocytopenia associated with chemotherapy for solid tumor cancer treatment.

Injections are started at least 6 hours after the completion of a chemotherapy cycle. Platelet counts are monitored and therapy is continued until a count of at least 50,000/mcL is achieved. It is not recommended for use for more than 21 days; treatment is discontinued at least 2 days before the next chemotherapy cycle is to begin.

ITP can be an acute or chronic bleeding disorder. Sometimes it is associated with other diseases. It is typically diagnosed by signs of bleeding (purple areas on the skin) or fatigue. If it does not resolve on its own, then a course of corticosteroids (see Chapter 43) or removal of the spleen may help. Two products are now available should these treatments prove unsuccessful: eltrombopag and romiplostim. Both of these drugs are used only for ITP and are not to be used to increase platelet count associated with immunosuppression during chemotherapy.

Adverse Reactions

General System Reactions

- Fluid retention
- Peripheral edema
- Dyspnea
- Syncope
- Fever
- Allergic reactions

Cardiovascular System Reactions

- Tachycardia
- Palpitations
- Atrial fibrillation
- Arrhythmias resulting in stroke and pulmonary edema
- Capillary leak syndrome

Eltrombopag can be toxic to the liver. Liver function studies are done prior to starting the drug and every 2 weeks while on drug therapy. See the Summary Drug Table: Immunostimulant Drugs for more information on these drugs.

Contraindications, Precautions, and Interactions

Thrombopoietin drugs are contraindicated in patients with known hypersensitivity to the drug or any component of the drug. Oprelvekin should not be used in patients receiving chemotherapy that is extremely myelosuppressive. These drugs are used cautiously in patients with renal failure, heart failure, or atrial arrhythmias. Severe hypokalemia (low potassium levels) can occur if the patient is receiving the cancer chemotherapy agent ifosfamide. It is a pregnancy category C drug and lactating patients should stop breastfeeding when oprelvekin is prescribed. Safety in children has not been established.

Oprelvekin can cause anaphylactic-type reactions and should be permanently discontinued if these occur. Discontinuing either eltrombopag or romiplostim may result in platelet counts lower than the original diagnosed counts.

HEMATOPOIETIC DRUGS USED IN TREATING ANEMIA

Anemia is a condition caused by an insufficient amount of hemoglobin delivering oxygen to the tissues. Causes of anemia include a decrease in the number of RBCs, a decrease in the amount of hemoglobin in RBCs, or both. There are various types and causes of anemia. For example, anemia can result from blood loss, excessive destruction of RBCs, inadequate production of RBCs, and deficits in various nutrients, as in **iron deficiency anemia**. Once the type and cause have been identified, the primary health care provider selects a method of treatment.

The anemias discussed in this chapter include anemia in patients with chronic illness such as renal disease or caused by treatment, iron deficiency anemia, pernicious anemia, and anemia resulting from a folic acid deficiency. Table 51.1 defines these anemias.

Table 51.1 Anemias	
Type of Anemia	**Description**
Iron deficiency	Anemia characterized by an inadequate amount of iron in the body to produce hemoglobin
Anemia in chronic kidney disease	Anemia resulting from a reduced production of erythropoietin, a hormone secreted by the kidney that stimulates the production of RBCs
Pernicious anemia	Anemia resulting from lack of secretion by the gastric mucosa of the intrinsic factor essential to the formation of RBCs and the absorption of vitamin B_{12}
Folic acid deficiency	Anemia occurring because of a dietary lack of folic acid, a component necessary in the formation of RBCs

DRUGS USED IN TREATING ANEMIA ASSOCIATED WITH CHRONIC ILLNESS

Anemia may occur in patients with chronic illness as a result of disease treatment. Cancer and chronic kidney disease are two diseases that produce disease- or treatment-related anemia. Erythropoiesis-stimulating agents (ESAs) are glycoproteins that stimulate and regulate the production of erythrocytes. Chronic kidney disease reduces the kidney's ability to produce erythropoietin, which stimulates the production of RBCs. Cancer treatment reduces the bone marrow's ability to produce RBCs. Two examples of drugs used to treat anemia associated with chronic illness are epoetin alfa (Epogen) and darbepoetin alfa (Aranesp).

Actions and Uses

ESAs are drugs that, like natural erythropoietin, stimulate **erythropoiesis**, the process of making RBCs. ESAs are used to treat anemia associated with the following:

- Chronic kidney disease
- Chemotherapy for cancer treatment
- Zidovudine (AZT) therapy for human immunodeficiency virus (HIV) infection
- Postsurgical blood replacement in place of allogeneic transfusions

Darbepoetin alfa and methoxy polyethylene–epoetin β are erythropoiesis-stimulating proteins used to treat anemia associated with chronic kidney disease in patients receiving dialysis, as well as in patients who are not receiving dialysis. These drugs elevate or maintain RBC levels and decrease the need for transfusions.

Adverse Reactions

Epoetin alfa (erythropoietin; EPO), darbepoetin alfa, and methoxy polyethylene are usually well tolerated when used to maintain a hemoglobin no higher than 12g/dL. The most common adverse reactions include:

- Hypertension
- Headache
- Nausea, vomiting, diarrhea
- Rashes
- Fatigue
- Arthralgia, and skin reaction at the injection site

See the Summary Drug Table: Immunostimulant Drugs for more information on these drugs.

Contraindications and Precautions

Epoetin alfa is contraindicated in patients with uncontrolled hypertension, those needing an emergency transfusion, and those with a hypersensitivity to human albumin. Darbepoetin alfa (Aranesp) is contraindicated in patients with uncontrolled hypertension or in those allergic to the drug. Polycythemia (an overload of RBCs in the circulation) can occur if the hemoglobin is not carefully monitored and the dosage is too high. This can result in increased mortality, serious cardio or thromboembolic events in any patient, and possible tumor progression in cancer patients.

Epoetin alfa and darbepoetin alfa are used with caution in patients with hypertension, heart disease, congestive heart failure, or a history of seizures. Both of these drugs are pregnancy category C drugs and are used cautiously during pregnancy and lactation.

DRUGS USED IN TREATING IRON DEFICIENCY ANEMIA

When the body does not have enough iron to supply its own needs, the resulting condition is called *iron deficiency anemia*. Iron is the component in hemoglobin that picks up oxygen from the lungs and carries it to the body tissues. Iron deficiency anemia is a very common type of anemia. Approximately 50% of pregnant women and 20% of all women experience anemia. Decreased iron stores result from a decrease in RBCs; causes include heavy menstrual bleeding and poor absorption or lack of iron in the diet.

Actions and Uses

Iron preparations act by elevating the serum iron concentration, which replenishes hemoglobin and depleted iron stores. Oral iron supplements are typically used. Iron is best absorbed on an empty stomach. Supplemental iron is needed during pregnancy and lactation, because normal dietary intake rarely supplies the required amount.

Parenteral iron is used when the patient cannot take oral drugs or when the patient experiences gastrointestinal (GI) intolerance to oral iron administration. Other iron preparations, both oral and parenteral, used in treating iron deficiency anemia can be found in the Summary Drug Table: Immunostimulant Drugs.

Adverse Reactions

Gastrointestinal Reactions

- GI irritation
- Nausea, vomiting
- Constipation, diarrhea
- Darker (black) stools

Generalized System Reactions

- Headache
- Backache
- Allergic reactions

When given parenterally, additional adverse reactions include soreness, inflammation, and sterile abscesses at the intramuscular (IM) injection site. When iron is administered by the IM route, a brownish discoloration of the skin may occur. Intravenous (IV) administration may result in phlebitis at the injection site.

Contraindications and Precautions

Iron supplements are contraindicated in patients with known hypersensitivity to the drug or any component of the drug.

Iron compounds are contraindicated in patients with hemochromatosis or hemolytic anemia. Iron compounds are used cautiously in patients with hypersensitivity to aspirin, because these patients may have a hypersensitivity to the tartrazine or sulfite content of some iron compounds.

The parenteral form of iron can cause anaphylactic-type reactions and should be used only when oral supplement is contraindicated.

Interactions

The following interactions may occur when an iron preparation is administered with another agent:

Interacting Drug	Common Use	Effect of Interaction
antibiotics	Fight infection	Decreased GI absorption of the antibiotic
levothyroxine	Treatment of hypothyroidism	Decreased absorption of levothyroxine
levodopa, methyldopa	Treatment of Parkinson's disease	Decreased effect of antiparkinsonism medication
ascorbic acid (vitamin C)	Vitamin supplement	Increased absorption of iron

DRUGS USED IN TREATING FOLIC ACID DEFICIENCY ANEMIA

Folic acid (folate) is required for the manufacture of RBCs in the bone marrow. Folic acid is found in leafy green vegetables, fish, meat, poultry, and whole grains. A deficiency of folic acid results in **megaloblastic anemia**. Megaloblastic anemia is characterized by the presence of large, abnormal, immature erythrocytes circulating in the blood.

Actions and Uses

Folic acid is used in treating megaloblastic anemias that are caused by a deficiency of folic acid. Although neural tube defects are not related to anemia, studies indicate there is a decreased risk for embryonic neural tube defects if folic acid is taken before conception and during early pregnancy. Neural tube defects occur during early pregnancy, when the embryonic folds forming the spinal cord and brain join together. Defects of this type include anencephaly (congenital absence of brain and spinal cord), spina bifida (defect of the spinal cord), and meningocele (a sac-like protrusion of the meninges in the spinal cord or skull). The U.S. Public Health Service recommends the use of folic acid for all women of childbearing age to decrease the incidence of neural tube defects. Dosages during pregnancy and lactation are as great as 0.8 mg/day.

Oral supplements are the first choice for megaloblastic anemia and folic acid deficiency treatment. If a patient is unable to take oral medications, leucovorin may be used. This drug is a derivative (an active reduced form) of folic acid. Leucovorin is more commonly used to diminish the hematologic effects of methotrexate, a drug used in treating certain types of cancer (see Chapter 50). Leucovorin "rescues" normal cells from the destruction caused by methotrexate and

allows them to survive. This technique of administering leucovorin after a large dose of methotrexate is called **folinic acid rescue** or *leucovorin rescue.*

Adverse Reactions

Few adverse reactions are associated with the administration of folic acid. Rarely, parenteral administration may result in allergic hypersensitivity.

Contraindications and Precautions

Folic acid and leucovorin are contraindicated for treating pernicious anemia or for other anemias in which vitamin B_{12} is deficient. Folic acid is a pregnancy category A drug and is generally considered safe for use during pregnancy. Pregnant women are more likely to experience folate deficiency, because folic acid requirements increase during pregnancy. Pregnant women with a folate deficiency are at increased risk for complications of pregnancy and fetal abnormalities. The recommended dietary allowance (RDA) of folate during pregnancy is 0.4 mg/day and, during lactation, 0.26 to 0.28 mg/day. Although the potential for fetal harm appears remote, the drug should be used cautiously and only within the RDA guidelines.

Interactions

Signs of folate deficiency may occur when sulfasalazine is administered concurrently. An increase in seizure activity may occur when folic acid is administered with the hydantoins (antiseizure drugs).

DRUGS USED IN TREATING VITAMIN B_{12} DEFICIENCY ANEMIA

Vitamin B_{12} is essential to growth, cell reproduction, the manufacture of myelin (which surrounds some nerve fibers), and blood cell manufacture. The **intrinsic factor**, which is produced by cells in the stomach, is necessary for the absorption of vitamin B_{12} in the intestine. A deficiency of the intrinsic factor results in abnormal formation of erythrocytes because of the body's failure to absorb vitamin B_{12}, a necessary component for blood cell formation. The resulting anemia is called **macrocytic anemia**.

Actions and Uses

Vitamin B_{12} (cyanocobalamin) is used to treat patients with a vitamin B_{12} deficiency; this condition is seen in those who have:

- A strict vegetarian (vegan) lifestyle
- Total gastrectomy or subtotal gastric resection (in which the cells producing the intrinsic factor are totally or partially removed)
- Intestinal diseases, such as ulcerative colitis or sprue
- Gastric carcinoma
- Congenital decrease in the number of gastric cells that secrete intrinsic factor

Vitamin B_{12} is also used to perform the Schilling test, which is used to diagnose pernicious anemia.

Pernicious anemia must be diagnosed and treated as soon as possible, because vitamin B_{12} deficiency that is allowed to progress for more than 3 months may result in degenerative lesions of the spinal cord.

A deficiency of vitamin B_{12} caused by a low dietary intake is rare, because the vitamin is found in meats, milk, eggs, and cheese. The body is also able to store this vitamin. A deficiency, for any reason, will not occur for 5 to 6 years from birth. Patients should be assessed for a history of vegan diet or gastric bypass surgery.

Adverse Reactions

Mild diarrhea and itching have been reported with the administration of vitamin B_{12}. Other adverse reactions that may be seen include a marked increase in RBC production, acne, peripheral vascular thrombosis, congestive heart failure, and pulmonary edema.

Contraindications, Precautions, and Interactions

Vitamin B_{12} is contraindicated in patients who are allergic to cyanocobalamin. Vitamin B_{12} is a pregnancy category A drug if administered orally and a pregnancy category C drug if given parenterally. Vitamin B_{12} is administered cautiously during pregnancy and in patients with pulmonary disease and anemia. Alcohol, neomycin, and colchicine may decrease the absorption of oral vitamin B_{12}.

NURSING PROCESS

PATIENT RECEIVING A DRUG USED IN THE TREATMENT OF ANEMIA, BLEEDING, OR INFECTION

ASSESSMENT

Preadministration Assessment

When obtaining a general health history, ask about the symptoms of the anemia, bleeding, or infection. A patient may not readily report fatigue, oozing from the gums, or an ongoing cough. The primary health care provider may order laboratory tests to determine the type, severity, and possible cause of the anemia, bleeding, or infection. When the patient is undergoing treatment such as for cancer, the blood counts will be used to titrate the drug doses.

Take the vital signs to provide a baseline during therapy. Other physical assessments may include the patient's general appearance and, in the severely ill patient, an evaluation of the patient's ability to carry out the activities of daily living. General symptoms may include fatigue, shortness of breath, sore tongue, headache, and pallor.

If iron dextran is to be given, an allergy history is necessary, because this drug is given with caution to those with significant allergies or asthma. The patient's weight and hemoglobin level are required for calculating the dosage.

Ongoing Assessment

During the ongoing assessment, if the vital signs such as heart or respiration rate increase, this can indicate low RBCs; these should be frequently monitored especially if the patient is moderately to acutely ill. Additionally, ask the patient about adverse reactions and report any occurrence of adverse reactions to the primary health care provider before the next dose is due. Immediately report severe adverse reactions.

Monitor the patient for relief of the symptoms (fatigue, shortness of breath, sore tongue, headache, pallor). Some patients may note a relief of symptoms after a few days of therapy. Periodic laboratory tests are necessary to monitor the results of therapy. Check for signs of bleeding and infection during the first few days of therapy with the CSF since an increase in blood cells may take a few days once therapy is started.

When the patient is receiving oral iron supplements, inform the patient that the color of the stool will become darker or black. If diarrhea or constipation occurs, contact the primary health care provider.

If parenteral iron dextran is administered, inform the patient that soreness at the injection site may occur. Teach the patient to check injection sites daily for signs of inflammation, swelling, or abscess formation.

NURSING DIAGNOSES

Drug-specific nursing diagnoses include the following:

- **Fatigue** related to dilutional anemia caused by fluid retention
- **Imbalanced Nutrition: Less Than Body Requirements** related to lack of iron, folic acid, other (specify) in the diet
- **Constipation** related to adverse reaction to iron therapy

Nursing diagnoses related to drug administration are discussed in Chapter 4.

PLANNING

The expected outcomes for the patient may include an optimal response to therapy, supporting the patient needs related to the management of adverse reactions, and confidence in an understanding of and compliance with the prescribed treatment regimen.

IMPLEMENTATION

Promoting an Optimal Response to Therapy

EPOETIN ALFA. When epoetin alfa is administered to a patient with hypertension, monitor the blood pressure closely. Report any rise of 20 mm Hg or more in the systolic or diastolic pressure to the primary health care provider. The hematocrit is usually measured before each dose during therapy with epoetin alfa.

The drug is given three times weekly IV or subcutaneously (subcut); if the patient is receiving dialysis, the drug is administered into the venous access line. The drug is mixed gently during preparation for administration. Shaking may denature the glycoprotein. The vial is used for only one dose; any remaining or unused portion is discarded.

NURSING ALERT

The target hemoglobin is no more than 11 g/dL. Myocardial infarction and stroke are more likely to occur when the hemoglobin rises higher. Additionally, report any increase in the hematocrit of 4 points within any 2-week period, because an exacerbation of hypertension is associated with an excessive rise of hematocrit. Withholding the drug lowers the blood levels.

IRON. Iron supplements are preferably given between meals with water, but many people cannot tolerate this and may need to take them with food. Milk and antacids may interfere with absorption of iron and should not be taken at the same time as iron supplements. If the patient is receiving other drugs, check with the clinical pharmacist regarding the simultaneous administration of iron salts with other drugs.

Iron dextran is given by the IM or IV route. Before iron dextran is administered, a test dose (0.5 mL iron dextran) may be administered IV at a gradual rate over a period of 30 seconds or more. A test dose is also given before administering the first dose of iron dextran IM by injecting 0.5 mL into the upper outer quadrant of the buttocks. Then monitor the patient for an allergic response for at least 1 hour after the test dose and before administering the remaining dose. Epinephrine is kept on standby in the event of severe anaphylactic reaction.

NURSING ALERT

Parenteral administration of iron has resulted in fatal anaphylactic-type reactions. Report immediately any of the following adverse reactions: dyspnea, urticaria, rashes, itching, and fever.

After the test dose, the prescribed dose of iron is administered IM. The drug is given into the muscle mass of the buttocks' upper outer quadrant (never into an arm or other area) using the Z-track method (see Chapter 2) to prevent leakage into the subcutaneous tissue. A large-bore needle is required. If the patient is standing, have the patient place weight on the leg not receiving the injection.

VITAMIN B_{12}. Patients with vitamin B_{12} anemia are treated with vitamin B_{12} IM administered weekly. The parenteral route is used because the vitamin is ineffective orally, owing to the absence of the intrinsic factor in the stomach, which is necessary for utilization of vitamin B_{12}. After stabilization, maintenance (usually monthly) injections may be necessary for life. Vitamin B_{12} is available in an intranasal form for those who are on maintenance therapy.

Monitoring and Managing Patient Needs

FATIGUE. During administration of the CSF drugs, the patient may experience fluid retention. With the increase in fluid volume, this makes the ratio of cells to fluid in the blood less, which results in a dilutional anemia. The patient may experience fatigue due to this anemia. The patient may need an explanation of this situation and to be given permission to feel tired. Teach the patient and family energy-saving skills to help maintain the same level of activities of daily living.

IMBALANCED NUTRITION: LESS THAN BODY REQUIREMENTS. A balanced diet is recommended with an emphasis on foods that are high in iron (e.g., lean red meats, cereals, dried beans, and leafy green vegetables), folic acid (e.g., green leafy vegetables, liver, and yeast), or vitamin B_{12} (e.g., beef, pork, eggs, milk, and milk products). If the patient is a vegetarian, a dietitian may need to be consulted to provide menus with appropriate iron-rich foods.

If appetite is poor or eating is inadequate to maintain normal nutrition, consultation with the dietitian may be necessary. Small portions of food may be more appealing than large or moderate portions. Provide a pleasant atmosphere and allow ample time for eating. If the patient is unable to eat well, note this on the patient's chart and bring the problem to the attention of the primary health care provider.

CONSTIPATION. Constipation may be a problem when a patient is taking oral iron preparations. Instruct the patient to increase fluid intake to 10 to 12 glasses of water daily (if the condition permits), eat a diet high in fiber, and increase activity. An active lifestyle and regular exercise (if condition permits) help to decrease the constipating effects of iron. If constipation persists, the primary health care provider may prescribe a stool softener.

Educating the Patient and Family

Explain the medical regimen thoroughly to the patient and family and emphasize the importance of following the prescribed treatment regimen. Include the following points in a patient and family teaching plan:

HEMATOPOIETIC FACTORS

- Keep all appointments with the primary health care provider. The drug is administered up to three times per week (by the subcutaneous or IV route or through a dialysis access line). Periodic blood tests are performed to determine the effects of the drug and to determine dosage.

- Strict compliance with the antihypertensive drug regimen is important in patients with known hypertension during epoetin alfa therapy.

- The following adverse reactions may occur: dizziness, headache, fatigue, joint pain, nausea, vomiting, or diarrhea. Report any of these reactions.

- Patients might have heard about problems with the drug Leukine. The product was withdrawn temporarily, because of reports of adverse reactions including syncope (fainting). This was correlated with a change in the formulation of the drug, which included edetate disodium (EDTA). That formula has been taken off the market and Leukine is now considered safe.

- If the patient or caregiver is administering the injections at home, use puncture-resistant containers for disposal and return full containers to the proper agency for disposal.

IRON

- Take this drug with water on an empty stomach. If GI upset occurs, take the drug with food or meals.

- Do not take antacids, tetracyclines, penicillamine, or fluoroquinolones at the same time or 2 hours before or after taking iron without first checking with the primary health care provider.

- This drug may cause a darkening of the stools, constipation, or diarrhea. If constipation or diarrhea becomes severe, contact the primary health care provider.

- Mix the liquid iron preparation with water or juice and drink through a straw to prevent staining the teeth.
- Avoid the indiscriminate use of advertised iron products. If a true iron deficiency occurs, the cause must be determined and therapy should be under the care of a health care provider.
- Have periodic blood tests during therapy to determine the therapeutic response.

Folic Acid

- Avoid the use of multivitamin preparations unless it has been approved by the primary health care provider.
- Follow the diet recommended by the primary health care provider, because diet and drug are necessary to correct anemia associated with folic acid deficiency.

Leucovorin

- Megaloblastic anemia—Adhere to the diet prescribed by the primary health care provider. If the purchase of foods high in protein (which can be expensive) becomes a problem, discuss this with the primary health care provider.

Vitamin B_{12}

- Nutritional deficiency of vitamin B_{12}—Eat a balanced diet that includes seafood, eggs, meats, and dairy products.
- Pernicious anemia—Lifetime therapy is necessary. Eat a balanced diet that includes seafood, eggs, meats, and dairy products. Avoid contact with infections, and report any signs of infection to the primary health care provider immediately, because an increase in dosage may be necessary.

- Adhere to the treatment regimen and keep all appointments with the clinic or primary health care provider. The drug is given at periodic intervals (usually monthly for life). In some instances, parenteral or intranasal self-administration or parenteral administration by a family member is allowed (instruction in administration is necessary).

EVALUATION

- Therapeutic effect of the drug is achieved.
- Adverse reactions are identified, reported to the primary health care provider, and managed successfully with appropriate nursing interventions:
  - Patient reports fatigue is manageable.
  - Patient maintains an adequate nutritional status.
  - Patient reports adequate bowel movements.
- Patient and family express confidence and demonstrate an understanding of the drug regimen.

PHARMACOLOGY IN PRACTICE
THINK CRITICALLY

You learn that Mr. Phillip's wife was given colony-stimulating factors during her breast cancer treatment. How could you explain the differences and similarities between these medications?

KEY POINTS

- The hematopoietic system is composed of fluid and three types of cells. RBCs supply the body with oxygen, WBCs protect the body from microorganisms, and platelets control bleeding.

- Chronic diseases such as kidney failure or treatments such as chemotherapy can reduce the number of cells in the circulation, causing fatigue, bleeding, or infection. Colony-stimulating factors are one type of immunostimulant that can boost the number of cells.

- These drugs are fragile and must be mixed before administration. They are given subcutaneously or intravenously. Adverse reactions include flu-like symptoms. Dramatic reduction in cell lines stimulated occurs when the injections are stopped.

- Anemia is a condition caused by reduced amounts of hemoglobin causing less oxygen to be delivered to the tissues. Anemia occurs due to chronic illnesses or specific deficiencies such as iron.

Summary Drug Table IMMUNOSTIMULANT DRUGS

Generic Name	Trade Name	Uses	Adverse Reactions	Dosage Ranges
Hematopoietic Factors for Infection				
filgrastim *fill-grah'-stim*	Neupogen	Treat or prevent severe neutropenia	Bone pain, nausea, vomiting, diarrhea, alopecia	5–10 mcg/kg subcut or IV daily
pegfilgrastim *peg-fill-grah'-stim*	Neulasta	Treat or prevent severe neutropenia	Bone pain, nausea, vomiting, diarrhea, alopecia	Single 6-mg subcut injection per cycle
sargramostim *sar-gram'-oh-stim*	Leukine	Treat or prevent severe neutropenia following BMT, induction chemotherapy	Headache, bone pain, nausea, vomiting, diarrhea, alopecia, skin rash	250 mcg/m² IV daily
Hematopoietic Factors for Bleeding				
eltrombopag *el-trom'-boe-pag*	Promacta	Treatment of severe chronic thrombocytopenia (ITP)	Nausea, excessive menstrual bleeding	Max. dose 75 mg/day orally
oprelvekin *oh-prel'-veh-kin*	Neumega	Treat or prevent severe thrombocytopenia associated with cancer chemotherapy	Edema, dyspnea, tachycardia, palpitations, syncope, atrial fibrillation, fever	50 mcg/kg subcut daily
romiplostim *roe-mi-ploe'-stim*	Nplate	Treatment of severe chronic thrombocytopenia (ITP)	Muscle pain, dizziness, insomnia	1 mcg/kg subcut weekly
Hematopoietic Factors for Anemia				
darbepoetin alfa *dar-beh-poe-eh'-tin*	Aranesp	Anemia associated with chronic kidney disease (CKD) and nonmyeloid cancers	Hypertension, hypotension, headache, diarrhea, vomiting, nausea, myalgia, arthralgia, cardiac arrhythmias, cardiac arrest	Titrated to hemoglobin level
epoetin alfa (erythropoietin; EPO) *eh-poe-eh'-tin*	Epogen, Procrit	Anemias associated with CKD, zidovudine therapy in HIV-infected patients, patients with cancer receiving chemotherapy, patients undergoing elective nonvascular surgery	Hypertension, headache, nausea, vomiting, fatigue, skin reaction at injection site	Titrated to hemoglobin level
methoxy polyethylene (epoetin β)	Mircera	Anemia associated with CKD	Hypertension, hypotension, headache, diarrhea, vomiting, nausea	Titrated to hemoglobin level
peginesatide *peg'-in-es-a-tide*	Omontys	Anemia associated with CKD	Hypertension, hypotension, headache, diarrhea, vomiting, nausea, dyspnea, atrioventricular shunt problems	Titrated to hemoglobin level
ferrous *fair'-us*	Feostat, Fergon, Feosol, Fer-In-Sol	Prevention and treatment of iron deficiency anemia	GI irritation, nausea, vomiting, constipation, diarrhea, allergic reactions	Daily requirements: males, 10 mg/day orally; females, 18 mg/day orally; during pregnancy and lactation: 30–60 mg/day orally Replacement in deficiency states: 90–300 mg/day (6 mg/kg/day) orally for 6–10 mo
folic acid *foe'-lik*	Folvite	Megaloblastic anemia due to deficiency of folic acid	Allergic sensitization	Up to 1 mg/day orally, IM, IV, subcut
iron dextran	Dexferrum, INFeD	Iron deficiency anemia (only when oral form is contraindicated)	Anaphylactoid reactions, soreness and inflammation at injection site, chest pain, arthralgia, backache, convulsions, pruritus, abdominal pain, nausea, vomiting, dyspnea	Dosage (IV, IM) based on body weight and grams percent (g/dL) of hemoglobin

(table continues on page 580)

Summary Drug Table IMMUNOSTIMULANT DRUGS (continued)

Generic Name	Trade Name	Uses	Adverse Reactions	Dosage Ranges
iron sucrose	Venofer	Iron deficiency anemia in kidney disease, via dialysis machine	Hypotension, cramps, leg cramps, nausea, headache, vomiting, diarrhea, dizziness	100 mg elemental iron by slow IV infusion or during dialysis session
leucovorin *loo-koe-vor'-in*	Wellcovorin	Treatment of megaloblastic anemia; leucovorin rescue after high-dose methotrexate therapy	Allergic sensitization, urticaria, anaphylaxis	See cancer therapy
sodium ferric gluconate complex	Ferrlecit	Iron deficiency	Flushing, hypotension, syncope, tachycardia, dizziness, pruritus, dyspnea, conjunctivitis, hyperkalemia	125 mg of elemental iron IV over at least 10 min
vitamin B12 (cyanocobalamin) *sye-an-oh-koe-bal'-ah-min*		Vitamin B_{12} deficiencies, GI pathology; Schilling's test	Mild diarrhea, itching, edema, anaphylaxis	Schilling's test: 100–1000 mcg/day for 2 wk, then 100–1000 mcg IM every month
Immunomodulators Used for Multiple Sclerosis and Other Autoimmune Conditions				
fingolimod *fin-gol'-i-mod*	Gilenya	Multiple sclerosis	Back pain, diarrhea, headache	0.5 mg daily
natalizumab *nat-ta-liz'-yoo-mab*	Tysabri	Multiple sclerosis, Crohn's disease	Headache, fatigue, GI distress, depression, diarrhea, urinary tract infection, vaginitis, upper respiratory infection symptoms	300 mg IV every 4 wk

● Chapter Review

Know Your Drugs

Clients sometimes know a medication by the brand (or trade) name and not the generic name. To help you recognize both names, match the brand name with the generic name of the same medication.

Generic Name	Brand Name
1. epoetin alfa	A. Neulasta
2. filgrastim	B. Neumega
3. pegfilgrastim	C. Neupogen
4. oprelvekin	D. Procrit

Calculate Medication Dosages

1. The primary health care provider prescribes 25 mg iron dextran IM. The drug is available in a vial with 50 mg/mL. The nurse administers _____.

2. Folvite (folic acid) 1 mg subcut is prescribed. The drug is available in a vial with 5 mg/mL. The nurse administers _____.

● Prepare for the NCLEX®

Build Your Knowledge

1. An erythrocyte is commonly know as a _____.
   1. white blood cell
   2. basophil
   3. red blood cell
   4. platelet

2. Which of the following drugs is approved to treat ITP?
   1. folic acid
   2. filgrastim
   3. leucovorin
   4. romiplostim

3. Which is the most common type of anemia?
   1. iron deficiency anemia
   2. folic acid anemia
   3. pernicious anemia
   4. megaloblastic anemia

4. Which of the following substances would decrease the absorption of oral iron?
   1. antacids
   2. levothyroxine
   3. ascorbic acid
   4. vitamin B_{12}

5. Filgrastim is contraindicated in which of the following conditions?
   1. hypothyroidism
   2. hyperthyroidism
   3. pernicious anemia
   4. pregnancy

Apply Your Knowledge

6. When monitoring a client taking epoetin alfa, which of the following laboratory results would be most important for the nurse to report immediately?
   1. any increase in hematocrit of 4 points within a 2-week period
   2. any increase in hematocrit of 2 points within a 2-week period
   3. a daily change in the hematocrit of 1 point or more
   4. a stabilization in the hematocrit in any 2-day period

7. When teaching a client about the use of vitamin B_{12}, the nurse would include which of the following statements?
   1. Take the oral form of vitamin B_{12} daily at bedtime on an empty stomach.
   2. Take the oral form of vitamin B_{12} when you begin to feel weak or experience a headache.
   3. You will require vitamin B_{12} injections monthly for life.
   4. You will require vitamin B_{12} injections every 2 weeks until remission occurs.

8. A vegan client has been diagnosed with iron deficiency. Which of the following foods would be recommended?
   1. lean red meats
   2. dried beans
   3. egg yolks
   4. pork

Alternate-Format Questions

9. A client with limited health literacy is prescribed oral iron tablets for anemia following blood loss during a surgical procedure. The iron is available in 10-mg tablets. The primary health care provider has ordered 30 mg on the first day, followed by 10 mg on days 2 to 5. The nurse shows the client how many tablets to be taken on the first day? _____ And on the last day of therapy? _____

10. Match the colony-stimulating factor with the sign or symptom it is used to treat:

1. filgrastim	A. Fatigue
2. oprelvekin	B. Bleeding
3. darbepoetin	C. Infection

To check your answers, see Appendix G.

Drugs That Affect Other Body Systems

This unit covers a variety of drugs affecting body systems not covered earlier in this book, including topical drugs used to treat skin disorders, otic (ear) and ophthalmic (eye) preparations, and fluids and electrolytes. Chapter 52 discusses topical drugs used in the treatment of skin disorders. The skin forms a barrier between the outside environment and the structures located beneath the skin. The *epidermis* is the outermost layer of the skin. Immediately below the epidermis is the *dermis,* which contains small capillaries that supply nourishment to the dermis and epidermis, sebaceous (oil-secreting) glands, sweat glands, nerve fibers, and hair follicles. Because of the skin's proximity to the outside environment, it is subject to various types of injury and trauma, as well as to changes in the skin itself. Topical drugs discussed include anti-infectives, corticosteroids, antipsoriatics, enzymes, keratolytics, and anesthetics.

Chapter 53 discusses drugs used to treat disorders of the eye and ear. Otic drugs may be used to treat infection and inflammation of the ear or to soften and remove cerumen (wax). Ophthalmic drugs are used for diagnostic and therapeutic purposes. As a diagnostic tool, ophthalmic drugs are used to anesthetize the eye, dilate the pupil, and stain the cornea to identify anomalies. Therapeutic purposes include the treatment of infection, allergy, and eye disorders such as glaucoma. Ophthalmic drugs discussed include an alpha (α)$_2$-adrenergic agonist, sympathomimetics, α-adrenergic blocking drugs, beta (β)-adrenergic blocking drugs, miotics (direct acting and cholinesterase inhibitors), carbonic anhydrase inhibitors, prostaglandin agonists, mast cell stabilizers, nonsteroidal anti-inflammatory drugs, corticosteroids, cycloplegics, mydriatics, artificial tears, and various anti-infectives.

The composition of body fluids remains relatively constant despite the many demands placed on the body each day. On occasion, these demands cannot be met, and

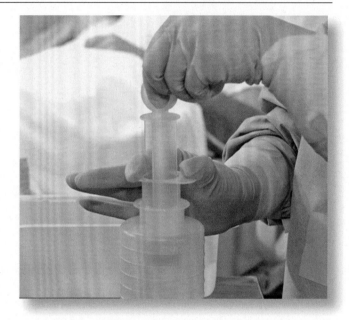

electrolytes and fluids must be given intravenously (IV) in an attempt to restore equilibrium. In the many facilities where nurses work, the role you will play in IV therapy differs. No matter where you practice nursing it is important to understand the basic concepts of fluid and electrolyte balance. The solutions used in managing body fluids discussed in Chapter 54 include intravenous fluid and electrolyte replacement, blood products, and total parenteral nutrition. Electrolytes are charged particles (ions) that are essential for normal cell function and are involved in various metabolic activities. The major electrolytes discussed include potassium, calcium, magnesium, sodium, and bicarbonate. Chapter 54 discusses the use of electrolytes to replace one or more electrolytes that may be lost by the body.

52

Skin Disorder Topical Drugs

LEARNING OBJECTIVES

On completion of this chapter, the student will:

1. List the types of drugs used in the treatment of skin disorders.
2. Discuss the general drug actions, uses, and reactions to and any contraindications, precautions, and interactions associated with drugs used in treating skin disorders.
3. Discuss important preadministration and ongoing assessment activities the nurse should perform on patients receiving a drug used to treat skin disorders.
4. List nursing diagnoses particular to a patient using a drug to treat a skin disorder.
5. Discuss ways to promote an optimal response to therapy and important points to keep in mind when educating the patient about a skin disorder.

KEY TERMS

antipsoriatic • drug used to treat psoriasis

antiseptic • agent that stops, slows, or prevents the growth of microorganisms

bactericidal • drug or agent that destroys or kills bacteria

bacteriostatic • drug or agent that slows or retards the multiplication of bacteria

germicide • agent that kills bacteria

keratolytic • agent that removes excessive growth of the epidermis (top layer of skin)

necrotic • pertaining to death of tissue

onychomycosis • finger or toenail fungal infection

proteolysis • enzymatic action that helps remove dead soft tissues by reducing proteins to simpler substances

purulent exudate • fluid discharge of pus and white cells

superinfection • overgrowth of bacterial or fungal microorganisms not affected by the antibiotic being administered

tinea corporis • superficial fungal infection, commonly called *ringworm*

tinea cruris • superficial fungal infection of the groin region, commonly called *jock itch*

tinea pedis • superficial fungal infection of the foot, commonly called *athlete's foot*

tinea versicolor • fungal infection that concentrates on the trunk of the body occurring in adolescents and young adults

DRUG CLASSES

Antibiotic topicals	Corticosteroids
Antifungal topicals	Antipsoriatic topicals
Antiviral topicals	Enzymes and
Antiseptics and	Keratolytics
germicides	Local anesthetics

This chapter discusses the following types of topical drugs: anti-infectives, corticosteroids, antipsoriatics, enzymes, keratolytics, and anesthetics. Each of the following sections discusses only select topical drugs. See the Summary Drug Table: Topical Drugs for a more complete listing of the drugs and additional information.

PHARMACOLOGY IN PRACTICE

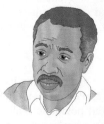

The medication nurse in the long-term care facility caring for Mr. Park asks you about his shingles outbreak. Her cousin has cold sores and uses an acyclovir ointment when they first appear. She questions why Mr. Park was not prescribed a topical drug to ease the pain and irritation from the shingles lesions. Would not the same help Mr. Park? As you read about topical preparations, consider her question.

TOPICAL ANTI-INFECTIVES

Localized skin infections may require the use of a topical anti-infective. The topical anti-infectives include antibiotic, antifungal, and antiviral drugs.

Actions and Uses

Topical Antibiotic Drugs

Topical antibiotics exert a direct local effect on specific microorganisms and may be **bactericidal** (i.e., lethal to bacteria) or **bacteriostatic** (i.e., inhibit bacterial growth). Bacitracin inhibits cell wall synthesis and is an example of a topical antibiotic.

These drugs are used to:

• Treat primary and secondary skin infections
• Prevent infection in minor cuts, wounds, scrapes, and minor burns
• Treat acne vulgaris

Topical Antifungal Drugs

Superficial mycotic infections occur on the surface of, or just below, the skin or nails. Superficial infections include athlete's foot (**tinea pedis**), jock itch (**tinea cruris**), ringworm (**tinea corporis**), and nail fungus (**onychomycosis**). In hot and humid climates a generalized fungal infection (**tinea versicolor**) is bothersome. Antifungal drugs exert a local effect by inhibiting growth of fungi. Antifungal drugs are used for treating:

• Athlete's foot, jock itch, ringworm
• Cutaneous candidiasis
• Other superficial fungal infections of the skin

Topical Antiviral Drugs

Acyclovir and penciclovir are topical forms of antiviral drugs used to treat oral herpes simplex virus (HSV). These drugs are used to inhibit viral activity:

• During initial episodes of HSV (prodrome phase)
• Directly on lesions to speed up recovery

Docosanol is a cream sold over the counter (OTC) and speeds healing as well.

Adverse Reactions

Adverse reactions to topical anti-infectives are usually mild. Occasionally, the patient may experience a rash, itching, urticaria (hives), dermatitis, irritation, or redness, which may indicate a hypersensitivity (allergic) reaction to the drug. Prolonged use of topical antibiotic preparations may result in a superficial **superinfection** (an overgrowth of bacterial or fungal microorganisms not affected by the antibiotic being administered).

Contraindications, Precautions, and Interactions

These drugs are contraindicated in patients with known hypersensitivity to the drugs or any components of the drug.

The topical antibiotics are pregnancy category C drugs and are used cautiously during pregnancy and lactation. Acyclovir and penciclovir are pregnancy category B drugs and are used cautiously during pregnancy and lactation. The pregnancy categories of the antifungals are unknown except for econazole, which is in pregnancy category C, and ciclopirox, which is in pregnancy category B; both are used with caution during pregnancy and lactation. There are no significant interactions for the topical anti-infectives.

HERBAL CONSIDERATIONS

Aloe vera is used to prevent infection and promote healing of minor burns (e.g., sunburn) and wounds. When used externally, aloe helps to repair skin tissue and reduce inflammation. Aloe gel is naturally thick when taken from the leaf but quickly becomes watery because of the action of enzymes in the plant. Commercially available preparations have additive thickeners to make the aloe appear like the fresh gel. The agent can be applied directly from the fresh leaf by cutting the leaf in half lengthwise and gently rubbing the inner gel directly onto the skin. Commercially prepared products are applied externally as needed. Rare reports of allergy have been reported with the external use of aloe (DerMarderosian, 2003).

TOPICAL ANTISEPTICS AND GERMICIDES

An **antiseptic** is a drug that stops, slows, or prevents the growth of microorganisms. A **germicide** is a drug that kills bacteria.

Actions

The exact mechanism of action of topical antiseptics and germicides is not well understood. These drugs affect a variety of microorganisms. Some of these drugs have a short duration of action, whereas others have a long duration of action. The action of these drugs may depend on the strength used and the time the drug is in contact with the skin or mucous membrane.

Chlorhexidine

Chlorhexidine affects a wide range of microorganisms, including gram-positive and gram-negative bacteria.

Hexachlorophene

Hexachlorophene (pHisoHex) is a bacteriostatic drug that acts against staphylococci and other gram-positive bacteria. Cumulative antibacterial action develops with repeated use.

Iodine

Iodine has anti-infective action against many bacteria, fungi, viruses, yeasts, and protozoa. Povidone–iodine (Betadine) is a combination of iodine and povidone that liberates free iodine. Povidone–iodine is often preferred over iodine solution or tincture, because it is less irritating to the skin and treated areas may be bandaged or taped.

Uses

Topical antiseptics and germicides are used for the following:

- To reduce the number of bacteria on skin surfaces
- As a surgical scrub and preoperative skin cleanser
- For performing hand hygiene before and after caring for patients
- In the home to cleanse the skin
- On minor cuts and abrasions to prevent infection

Adverse Reactions

Topical antiseptics and germicides provoke few adverse reactions. Occasionally, an individual may be allergic to the drug, and a skin rash or itching may occur. If an allergic reaction is noted, use of the topical drug is discontinued.

Contraindications, Precautions, and Interactions

These drugs are contraindicated in patients with known hypersensitivity to the individual drug or any component of the preparation. There are no significant precautions or interactions when the drugs are used as directed.

TOPICAL CORTICOSTEROIDS

Topical corticosteroids vary in potency, depending on the concentration (percentage) of the drug, the vehicle (lotion, cream, aerosol spray) in which the drug is suspended, and the area (open or denuded skin, unbroken skin, thickness of the skin over the treated area) to which the drug is applied.

Actions and Uses

Topical corticosteroids exert localized anti-inflammatory activity. When applied to inflamed skin, they reduce itching, redness, and swelling. These drugs are used in treating skin disorders such as:

- Psoriasis
- Dermatitis
- Rashes
- Eczema
- Insect bites
- First- and second-degree burns, including sunburn

Adverse Reactions

Localized reactions may include burning, itching, irritation, redness, dryness of the skin, allergic contact dermatitis, and secondary infection. These reactions are more likely to occur if occlusive dressings are used. Systemic reactions may also occur with hypothalamic-pituitary-adrenal axis suppression, Cushing's syndrome, hyperglycemia, and glycosuria.

Contraindications, Precautions, and Interactions

Topical corticosteroids are contraindicated in patients with known hypersensitivity to the drug or any component of the drug; as monotherapy for bacterial skin infections; for use on the face, groin, or axilla (only the high-potency corticosteroids); and for ophthalmic use (may cause steroid-induced glaucoma or cataracts). The topical corticosteroids are not used as sole therapy in widespread plaque psoriasis. The topical corticosteroids are pregnancy category C drugs and are used cautiously during pregnancy and lactation. There are no significant interactions when these drugs are administered as directed.

TOPICAL ANTIPSORIATICS
Action and Uses

Topical **antipsoriatic** drugs are drugs used to treat psoriasis (a chronic skin disease manifested by bright red patches covered with silvery scales or plaques) by helping to remove the plaques associated with the disorder.

Adverse Reactions

These drugs may cause burning, itching, and skin irritation. Anthralin may cause skin irritation, as well as temporary discoloration of the hair and fingernails.

Contraindications, Precautions, and Interactions

Topical antipsoriatics are contraindicated in patients with known hypersensitivity to the drugs. Anthralin and calcipotriene, pregnancy category C drugs, are used cautiously during pregnancy and lactation.

TOPICAL ENZYMES
Actions and Uses

A topical enzyme is used to help remove **necrotic** (dead) tissue from:

- Chronic dermal ulcers
- Severely burned areas

These enzymes aid in the removal of dead soft tissues by hastening the reduction of proteins into simpler substances. The process is called **proteolysis** or a proteolytic action. The components of certain types of wounds, namely, necrotic tissues and **purulent exudates** (pus-containing fluid), prevent proper wound healing. Removal of this type of debris by application of a topical enzyme aids in healing. Examples of conditions that may respond to application of a topical enzyme include second- and third-degree burns, pressure ulcers, and ulcers caused by peripheral vascular disease. An example of a topical enzyme is collagenase.

Adverse Reactions

The application of collagenase may cause mild, transient pain and possibly numbness and dermatitis. There is a low incidence of adverse reactions to collagenase.

Contraindications, Precautions, and Interactions

Topical enzyme preparations are contraindicated in patients with known hypersensitivity to the drugs, in wounds in contact with major body cavities or where nerves are exposed, and in fungating neoplastic ulcers. These drugs are pregnancy category B drugs and are used cautiously during pregnancy and lactation. Enzymatic activity may be impaired by certain detergents and heavy metal ions, such as mercury and silver, which are used in some antiseptics. The optimal pH for collagenase is 6 to 8. Higher or lower pH conditions decrease the enzyme's activity.

KERATOLYTICS

Actions and Uses

A **keratolytic** is a drug that removes excess growth of the epidermis (top layer of skin) in disorders such as warts. These drugs are used to remove:

- Warts
- Calluses
- Corns
- Seborrheic keratoses (benign, variously colored skin growths arising from oil glands of the skin)

Examples of keratolytics include salicylic acid and masoprocol. Some strengths of salicylic acid are available as nonprescription products for the removal of warts on the hands and feet.

Adverse Reactions

These drugs are usually well tolerated. Occasionally a transient burning sensation, rash, dry skin, scaling, or flu-like syndrome may occur.

Contraindications, Precautions, and Interactions

Keratolytics are contraindicated in patients with known hypersensitivity to the drugs and for use on moles, birthmarks, or warts with hair growing from them, on genital or facial warts, on warts on mucous membranes, or on infected skin. Prolonged use of the keratolytics in infants and in patients with diabetes or impaired circulation is contraindicated. Salicylic acid may cause salicylate toxicity with prolonged use. These drugs are pregnancy category C drugs and are used cautiously during pregnancy and lactation.

TOPICAL LOCAL ANESTHETICS

A topical anesthetic may be applied to the skin or mucous membranes.

Actions and Uses

Topical anesthetics temporarily inhibit the conduction of impulses from sensory nerve fibers. These drugs may be used to relieve itching and pain due to skin conditions, such as minor burns, fungal infections, insect bites, rashes, sunburn, and plant poisoning (e.g., poison ivy). Some are applied to mucous membranes as local anesthetics.

Adverse Reactions

Occasionally, local irritation, dermatitis, rash, burning, stinging, and tenderness may be noted.

Contraindications, Precautions, and Interactions

These drugs are contraindicated in those with a known hypersensitivity to any component of the preparation. Topical anesthetics are used cautiously in patients receiving class I antiarrhythmic drugs such as tocainide and mexiletine, because the toxic effects are additive and potentially synergistic.

NURSING PROCESS
PATIENT RECEIVING A TOPICAL DRUG FOR A SKIN DISORDER

ASSESSMENT

Preadministration Assessment
The preadministration assessment involves a visual inspection and palpation of the involved area(s). Carefully measure and document the areas of involvement, including the size, color, and appearance. The appearance of the skin lesions, such as rough, itchy patches; cracks between the toes; and sore and reddened areas, is noted so treatment can begin with an accurate database. A specific description is important so that changes indicating worsening or improvement of the lesions can be readily identified. Figure 52.1 illustrates common types of lesions found on the skin. Note any subjective reports, such as pain, burning, or any complaint of itching. Some agencies may provide a figure on which the lesions can be drawn, indicating the shape and distribution of the involved areas. Other agencies may document the appearance of the lesions using photography.

Ongoing Assessment
At the time of each application, inspect the affected area for changes (e.g., signs of improvement or worsening of the

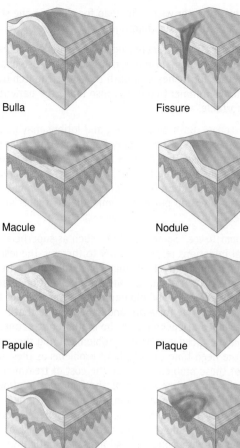

Bulla

Fissure

Macule

Nodule

Papule

Plaque

Pustule

Ulcer

Vesicle

Wheal

Figure 52.1 Types of skin lesions. (From Cohen, B. J. [2003]. *Medical terminology* [4th ed.]. Philadelphia: Lippincott Williams & Wilkins.)

infection) and for adverse reactions, such as redness or rash. Contact the primary health care provider, and do not apply the drug if these or other changes are noted or if the patient reports new problems, such as itching, pain, or soreness at the site. You may be responsible for checking the treatment sites 1 day or more after application and should inform the primary health care provider of any signs of extreme redness or infection at the application site.

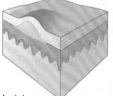

LIFESPAN CONSIDERATIONS
Pediatric

Because infants and children have a high ratio of skin surface area to body mass, they are at greater risk than adults for systemic adverse effects when treated with topical medication.

NURSING DIAGNOSES

Drug-specific nursing diagnoses include the following:

- **Impaired Skin Integrity** related to the inflammatory process (increased sensitivity to the drug)
- **Acute Pain** related to skin condition or increased sensitivity to drug therapy
- **Risk for Infection** related to entry of pathogens into affected areas
- **Disturbed Body Image** related to changes in skin and mucous membranes

Nursing diagnoses related to drug administration are discussed in Chapter 4.

PLANNING

The expected outcomes of the patient may include an optimal response to drug therapy, support of patient needs related to management of adverse drug reactions, and confidence in an understanding of the application or the reason for use of a topical drug.

IMPLEMENTATION

Promoting an Optimal Response to Therapy

Patients with wound healing issues using these drugs may be institutionalized in acute rehab care or long-term care facilities. Oftentimes devices to promote wound healing will be utilized and the application of the drug and device is carried out by a nurse in these facilities. When the patient is at home, frequently the nurse's involvement will be instructing the patient or caregiver in the methods used to apply topical drugs.

TOPICAL ANTI-INFECTIVES. Before each application, the area is cleansed with soap and warm water unless the primary health care provider orders a different method. The anti-infective is applied as prescribed (e.g., thin layer or applied liberally) and the area is either covered or left exposed as prescribed.

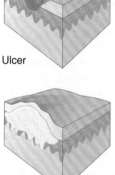

NURSING ALERT

Care must be exercised when applying anti-infectives or any topical drug near or around the eyes.

TOPICAL ANTIFUNGAL INFECTION PREPARATIONS. When these drugs are applied topically to the skin, the area is inspected at the time of each application for localized skin reactions. When these drugs are administered vaginally, ask the patient about any discomfort or other sensations experienced after insertion of the antifungal preparation. Note improvement or deterioration of lesions of the skin, mucous membranes, or vaginal secretions in the patient record (see Chapter 12 for nursing care of vaginal yeast infections). It is important to evaluate and chart the patient's response to therapy, too.

TOPICAL ANTISEPTICS AND GERMICIDES. Antiseptics and germicides are instilled or applied as directed by the primary health care provider or by the label on the product. Topical antiseptics and germicides are not a substitute for clean or aseptic techniques. Occlusive dressings are not to be used after application of these products unless a dressing is specifically ordered by the primary health care provider. Iodine permanently stains clothing and temporarily stains the skin. Care should be taken to remove or protect the patient's personal clothing when applying iodine solution or tincture.

Antiseptic and germicidal drugs kept at the patient's bedside must be clearly labeled with the name of the product, the strength, and, when applicable, the date of preparation of the solution. Be sure to replace hard-to-read or soiled, stained labels as needed. These solutions are not kept at the bedside of any patient who is confused or disoriented, because the solution may be mistaken for water or another beverage.

TOPICAL CORTICOSTEROIDS. Before drug application, the area is washed with soap and warm water unless the primary health care provider directs otherwise. Topical corticosteroids are usually ordered to be applied sparingly. The primary health care provider also may order the area of application to be covered or left exposed to the air. Some corticosteroids are applied with an occlusive dressing. The drug is applied while the skin is still moist after washing with soap and water and a dressing is applied if ordered by the primary health care provider.

LIFESPAN CONSIDERATIONS
Pediatric
Do not use tight-fitting diapers or pants on a child treated in the diaper area. These types of clothing may work like an occlusive dressing and cause more of the drug to be absorbed into the child's body, resulting in a greater risk for adverse reactions.

TOPICAL ENZYMES. Certain types of wounds may require special preparations before applying the topical enzyme. The area is cleansed or prepared and the topical enzyme is applied as directed by the primary health care provider. Often a wound suction device may be applied to promote healing.

TOPICAL ANTIPSORIATICS. Care is exercised so that the product is applied only to the psoriatic lesions and not to surrounding skin. Instruct the patient or caregiver to bring signs of excessive irritation to the attention of the primary health care provider.

LIFESPAN CONSIDERATIONS
Gerontology
Adults older than 65 years have more skin-related adverse reactions to calcipotriene (antipsoriatic). Use calcipotriene cautiously in older adults.

TOPICAL ANESTHETICS. The anesthetic is applied as directed by the primary health care provider. Before the first application, cleanse and dry the area. For subsequent applications, all previous residue of the anesthetic should be removed.

When a topical gel, such as lidocaine viscous, is used for oral anesthesia, instruct the patient not to eat food for 1 hour after use, because local anesthesia of the mouth or throat may impair swallowing and increase the possibility of aspiration.

Monitoring and Managing Patient Needs
Most topical drugs cause few adverse reactions and, if they occur, discontinuing use of the drug may be all that is necessary to relieve the symptoms.

IMPAIRED SKIN INTEGRITY. Dry skin increases the risk of skin breakdown from scratching. Advise the patient to keep nails

short, use warm water with mild soap for cleaning the skin, and rinse and dry the skin thoroughly.

ACUTE PAIN. Occasionally, increased skin sensitivity occurs, causing greater redness, discomfort, and itching. Use cool, wet compresses for rashes or a bath to relieve the itching. Keeping the environment cool may also make the patient more comfortable.

RISK FOR INFECTION. Bath oils, creams, and lotions may be used, if necessary, as long as the primary health care provider is consulted before use. Dry, flaky skin is subject to breakdown and infection. Instruct the patient or caregiver to observe the skin for signs of infection (e.g., redness, heat, pus, and elevated temperature and pulse) and immediately report any sign of infection.

DISTURBED BODY IMAGE. Some infections such as superficial and deep fungal infections respond slowly to therapy. The lesions caused by the fungal infections may cause the patient to feel negatively about the body or a body part. In addition, many patients experience anxiety and depression over the fact that therapy must continue for a prolonged period and that results are slow to appear. Depending on the method of treatment, patients may be faced with many problems during therapy and therefore need time to talk about problems as they arise. Examples of these problems may be the cost of treatment, institutionalization (when required), the failure of treatment adequately to control the infection, and loss of income. It is important to develop a therapeutic nurse–patient relationship that conveys an attitude of caring and fosters a sense of trust. Listen to the patient's concerns and assist the patient in accepting the situation as temporary. Encourage the patient to verbalize any feelings or anxiety about the effect of the disorder on body image. Explain the disorder and the treatment regimen in terms the patient can understand and discuss the need at times for long-term treatment to eradicate the infection. Help the patient and the family to understand that therapy must be continued until the infection is under control. In some cases, therapy may take weeks or months.

Educating the Patient and Family
If the primary health care provider has prescribed or recommended the use of a topical drug, note that most of the adverse effects that occur with topical drugs are a result of applying the drug improperly. Typically, if applied correctly, the drug usually is not systemically absorbed. However, sometimes patients think that if a little is good, then "more is better." Applying more than the amount necessary increases the patient's risk for systemic absorption (see Patient Teaching for Improved Patient Outcomes: Application of Topical Drugs).

GENERAL TEACHING POINTS

- Wash the hands thoroughly before and after applying the product.
- If the enclosed directions state that the product will stain clothing, be sure clothing is moved away from the treated area. If the product stains the skin, wear disposable gloves when applying the drug.
- Follow the directions on the label or use as directed by the primary health care provider. Read any enclosed directions for use of the product carefully.

Patient Teaching for Improved Patient Outcomes

Application of Topical Drugs

Often patients are required to apply topical drugs in the home setting. To ensure that the patient applies the topical drug properly, *when you teach, make sure your patient understands the following:*

✔ Gather all necessary supplies and wash hands before starting.
✔ Wash the area first to remove any debris and old drug.
✔ Pat the area dry with a clean cloth.
✔ Open the container (or tube) and place the lid or cap upside down on the counter or surface.
✔ Use a tongue blade, gloved finger (either with a nonsterile gloved hand or finger cot), cotton swab, or gauze pad to remove the drug, and then apply it to the skin.
✔ Wipe the drug onto the affected area using long smooth strokes in the direction of hair growth.
✔ Apply a thin layer of drug to the area (more is not better).
✔ Use a new tongue blade, applicator, or clean gloved finger to remove additional drug from the container (if necessary).
✔ Apply a clean, dry dressing (if appropriate) over the area.
✔ Wrap items for disposal and perform hand hygiene before engaging in other activities.

- Prepare the area to be treated as recommended by the primary health care provider or as described in the directions supplied with the product.
- Do not apply to areas other than those specified by the primary health care provider. Apply the drug as directed (e.g., thin layer or apply liberally).
- Follow the directions of the primary health care provider regarding covering the treated area or leaving it exposed to air. The effectiveness of certain drugs depends on keeping the area covered or leaving it open.
- Keep the product away from the eyes (unless use in or around the eye has been recommended or prescribed). Do not rub or put the fingers near the eyes unless the hands have been thoroughly washed and all remnants of the drug removed from the fingers. If the product is accidentally spilled, sprayed, or splashed in the eye, wash the eye immediately with copious amounts of running water. Contact the primary health care provider immediately if burning, pain, redness, discomfort, or blurred vision persists for more than a few minutes.
- The drug may cause momentary stinging or burning when applied.
- Discontinue use of the drug and contact the primary health care provider if rash, burning, itching, redness, pain, or other skin problems occur.

ANTI-INFECTIVES

- Gentamicin may cause photosensitivity. Take measures to protect the skin from ultraviolet rays (e.g., wear protective clothing and use a sunscreen when out in the sun).
- Topical clindamycin can be absorbed in sufficient amounts to cause systemic effects. If severe diarrhea, stomach cramps, or bloody stools occur, contact the primary health care provider immediately.

ANTIFUNGALS

- Clean the involved area and apply the ointment or cream to the skin as directed by the primary health care provider.
- Do not increase or decrease the amount used or the number of times the ointment or cream should be applied unless directed to do so by the primary health care provider.
- During treatment for a ringworm infection, keep towels and facecloths for bathing separate from those of other family members to avoid the spread of the infection. It is important to keep the affected area clean and dry.

ANTIVIRALS

- When applying ointment, use a finger cot (a medical supply used to cover one or more fingers when a full glove is unnecessary) or glove to prevent autoinoculation of other body sites.
- This product will not prevent transmission of infection to others.
- Transient burning, itching, and rash may occur.

TOPICAL CORTICOSTEROIDS

- Apply ointments, creams, or gels sparingly in a light film; rub in gently.
- Use only as directed. Do not use bandages, dressings, cosmetics, or other skin products over the treated area unless so directed by the primary health care provider.

ENZYME PREPARATIONS

- If, for any reason, it becomes necessary to inactivate collagenase, this can be accomplished by washing the area with povidone–iodine.

EVALUATION

- Therapeutic drug response is achieved.
- Adverse reactions are identified, reported to the primary health care provider, and managed successfully with appropriate nursing interventions:
  - Skin remains intact.
  - Patient is free of pain.
  - No evidence of infection is seen.
  - Perceptions of body changes are managed successfully.
- Patient or family member expresses confidence and demonstrates an understanding of the use and application of the prescribed or recommended drug.

PHARMACOLOGY IN PRACTICE
THINK CRITICALLY

 You point out to the medication nurse that Mr. Park is taking acyclovir orally. How would you explain the use of this medication in a systemic form rather than a topical form like the cousin's use for HSV?

KEY POINTS

- A variety of topical drugs exist for many purposes. Anti-infectives treat bacterial, fungal, and viral infections of the skin. Antiseptic or germicidal solutions help to clean or kill bacteria on the skin or in wounds. Topical corticosteroids when used reduce the itching, redness, and swelling associated with inflammation.

- When used as directed, adverse reactions are minor, consisting of mild irritation or discomfort. Some products

make the skin more sensitive to sunlight, and the patient will need to wear protective clothing or use sunscreen when these products are used.

- Agents used to treat plaques or wounds can be used alone or in conjunction with wound healing systems.

- Important nursing measures include thorough documentation of the site to be treated and instruction of appropriate use of drugs for the skin.

Summary Drug Table TOPICAL DRUGS

Generic Name	Trade Name	Uses	Adverse Reactions	Dosage Ranges
Antibiotic Drugs				
azelaic acid *ah-zeh'-lay-ik*	Azelex, Finacea	Acne vulgaris, rosacea	Mild and transient pruritus, burning, stinging, erythema	Apply BID
bacitracin *bah-sih-tray'-sin*	Various brand names	Relief of skin infections, to help prevent infections in minor cuts and burns	Rare; occasionally redness, burning, pruritus, stinging	Apply daily to TID
benzoyl peroxide *ben'-zoil per-ox'-syde*	Various brand names	Mild to moderate acne vulgaris and oily skin	Excessive drying, stinging, peeling, erythema, possible edema, allergic dermatitis	Apply daily or BID
clindamycin *clin-dah-mye'-sin*	Cleocin T, ClindaMax, Clindets, Clindagel	Acne vulgaris	Dryness, erythema, burning, itching, peeling, oily skin, diarrhea, bloody diarrhea, abdominal pain, colitis	Apply a thin film daily (Clindagel) or BID to affected area
erythromycin *ee-rith-roe-mye'-sin*	Akne-Mycin, Emgel, Erygel	Acne vulgaris	Skin irritation, tenderness, pruritus, erythema, peeling, oiliness, burning sensation	Apply to affected area BID
gentamicin *jen-tah-mye'-sin*	Various brand names	Relief of primary and secondary skin infections	Mild and transient pruritus, burning, stinging, erythema, photosensitivity	Apply TID or QID to affected area
metronidazole *meh-troe-nye'-dah-zoll*	Metro-Gel, MetroLotion, Noritate	Rosacea	Watery (tearing) eyes, redness, mild dryness, burning, skin irritation, nausea, tingling/numbness of extremities	Apply a thin film daily or BID to affected areas

Summary Drug Table TOPICAL DRUGS (continued)

Generic Name	Trade Name	Uses	Adverse Reactions	Dosage Ranges
mupirocin *mew-peer'-oh-sin*	Bactroban, Bactroban Nasal	Impetigo infections caused by *Staphylococcus aureus* and *Streptococcus pyogenes* Nasal: eradication of methicillin-resistant *S. aureus* (MRSA) as part of an infection control program to reduce the risk of institutional outbreaks of MRSA	Ointment: burning, stinging, pain, itching, rash, nausea, erythema, dry skin Cream: headache, rash, nausea, abdominal pain, burning at application site, dermatitis Nasal: headache, rhinitis, respiratory disorders (e.g., pharyngitis), taste perversion, burning, stinging, cough	Ointment: apply TID for 3–5 days Cream: apply TID for 10 days Nasal: divide the single-use tube between nostrils and apply BID for 5 days
retapamulin *reh'-tah-pam'-yoo-lin*	Altabax	Impetigo due to *Staphylococcus* or *Streptococcus*	Headache, pruritus	Apply a thin film daily or BID to affected areas
Antifungal Drugs				
butenafine *byoo-ten'-ah-feen*	Mentax, Lotrimin Ultra	Dermatologic infections, tinea versicolor, tinea corporis (ringworm), tinea cruris (jock itch)	Burning, stinging, itching, worsening of the condition, contact dermatis, erythema, irritation	Apply daily or BID for 2–4 wk
ciclopirox *sik-loe-peer'-ox*	Loprox, Penlac Nail Lacquer	Loprox, cream and suspension: tinea pedis (athlete's foot), tinea cruris, tinea corporis, cutaneous candidiasis Gel: interdigital tinea pedis and tinea corporis, seborrheic dermatitis of the scalp Penlac: mild to moderate onychomycosis of fingernails and toenails	Cream: pruritus at the application site, worsening of clinical signs and symptoms, burning Loprox Gel: burning sensation on application, contact dermatitis, pruritus, dry skin, acne, rash, alopecia, eye pain, facial edema Loprox shampoo: increased itching, burning, erythema, rash, headache Penlac: periungual erythema, nail disorders, irritation, ingrown toenail, burning of the skin	Apply to affected areas daily or BID Shampoo: see directions Penlac: Apply daily preferably at bedtime or 8 hr before washing
clotrimazole *kloe-trim'-ah-zoll*	Cruex, Lotrimin AF, Desenex	Tinea pedis, tinea cruris, and other skin infections caused by ringworm	Burning, itching, erythema, peeling, edema, general skin irritation	Apply thin layer to affected areas BID for 2–4 wk
econazole *ee-kon'-ah-zoll*	Spectazole	Tinea pedis, tinea cruris, tinea corporis, tinea versicolor, cutaneous candidiasis	Local burning, itching, stinging, erythema, pruritic rash	Apply to affected areas daily or BID
gentian violet *jen'-shun*		External treatment of abrasions, minor cuts, surface injuries, superficial fungal infections of the skin	Local irritation or sensitivity reactions	Apply locally BID Do not bandage

(table continues on page 594)

Summary Drug Table TOPICAL DRUGS (continued)

Generic Name	Trade Name	Uses	Adverse Reactions	Dosage Ranges
ketoconazole *kee-toe-koe'-nah-zoll*	Nizoral	Cream: tinea cruris, tinea corporis, tinea versicolor Shampoo: reduction of scaling due to dandruff	Cream: Severe itching, pruritus, stinging Shampoo: increase in hair loss, abnormal hair texture, scalp pustules, mild dryness of the skin, itching, oiliness/dryness of the hair	Cream: apply daily to affected areas for 2–6 wk Shampoo: twice a week for 4 wk with at least 3 days between each shampoo
miconazole *mi-kon'-ah-zoll*	Tetterine, Micatin, Monistat-Derm, Micatin, Fungoid Tincture	Tinea pedis, tinea cruris, tinea corporis, cutaneous candidiasis	Local irritation, burning, maceration, allergic contact dermatitis	Cover affected areas BID
naftifine *naf'-tih-feen*	Naftin	Topical treatment of tinea pedis, tinea cruris, tinea corporis	Burning, stinging, erythema, itching, local irritation, rash, tenderness	Apply BID for 4 wk
nystatin *nye-stat'-in*	Mycostatin, Nystex	Mycotic infections caused by *Candida albicans* and other *Candida* species	Virtually nontoxic and nonsensitizing; well tolerated by all age groups, even with prolonged administration; if irritation occurs, discontinue use	Apply BID or TID until healing is complete
oxiconazole *ox-ee-kon'-ah-zoll*	Oxistat	Tinea pedis, tinea cruris, tinea corporis	Pruritus, burning, stinging, irritation, contact dermatitis, scaling, tingling	Apply daily or BID for 1 mo
sertaconazole *ser-ta-kon'-ah-zoll*	Ertaczo	Tinea pedis	Pruritus, burning, stinging, irritation, contact dermatitis, scaling, tingling	Apply daily or BID for 1 mo
sulconazole *soo-kon'-ah-zoll*	Exelderm	Same as oxiconazole	Pruritus, burning, stinging, irritation	Apply daily or BID for 3–6 wk
terbinafine *ter-bin'-ah-feen*	Lamisil	Same as oxiconazole	Same as oxiconazole	Apply BID until infection clears (1–4 wk)
tolnaftate *toll-naf'-tate*	Aftate, Genaspor, Tinactin, Ting	Same as oxiconazole	Same as oxiconazole	Apply BID for 2–3 wk (4–6 wk may be needed)

Topical Antivirals

acyclovir *ay-sye'-kloe-veer*	Zovirax	HSV infections, varicella-zoster	Ointment: Mild pain with transient burning/stinging Cream: pruritus, rash, vulvitis, edema or pain at application site	Ointment: apply to all lesions q 3 hr 6 times daily for 7 days Cream: apply 5 times daily for 4 days
docosanol *doe-koe-nah'-zoll*	Abreva	HSV-1 and -2	Headache, skin irritation	Apply to lesions 5 times daily
imiquimod *im-ee'-kwee-mod*	Aldara	External genitalia and perianal warts	Local skin irritation, itching, excoriation, flaking	Apply externally 3 times weekly
penciclovir *pen-sye'-kloe-veer*	Denavir	HSV-1 and -2	Headache, taste perversion	Apply q 2 hr for 4 days during waking hours
vidarabine *vye-dare'-ah-been*	Ara-A, Vira-A	Keratitis, keratoconjunctivitis caused by HSV-1 and -2	Burning, itching, irritation, tearing, sensitivity to light	Ophthalmic ointment: 0.5 inch into lower conjunctival sac 2–5 times daily

Antiseptics and Germicides

chlorhexidine *klor-hex'-eh-deen*	Bacto Shield 2, Betasept, Exidine-2 Scrub, Hibiclens	Surgical scrub, skin cleanser, preoperative skin preparation, skin wound cleanser, preoperative showering and bathing	Irritation, dermatitis, photosensitivity (rare), deafness, mild sensitivity reactions	Varies, depending on administration

Summary Drug Table TOPICAL DRUGS (continued)

Generic Name	Trade Name	Uses	Adverse Reactions	Dosage Ranges
hexachlorophene *hex-ah-klor'-oh-feen*	pHisoHex, Septisol	Surgical scrub and bacteriostatic skin cleanser, control of an outbreak of gram-positive infection when other procedures are unsuccessful	Dermatitis, photosensitivity, sensitivity to hexachlorophene, redness or mild scaling or dryness	Surgical wash or scrub: as indicated Bacteriostatic cleansing: wet hand with water and squeeze approx. 5 mL into palm, add water and work up lather, apply to area to be cleansed, rinse thoroughly
povidone–iodine *poe'-vih-doan*	Acu-Dyne, Aerodine, Betadine	Microbicidal against bacteria, fungi, viruses, spores, protozoa, yeasts	Dermatitis, irritation, burning, sensitivity reactions	Varies, depending on administration
sodium hypochlorite	Dakin's Solution	Antiseptic against bacteria, fungi, viruses, spores, protozoa, yeasts; deodorizing properties	Chemical reaction or burn	Varies, depending on administration
triclosan *trye'-kloe-san*	Clearasil Daily Face Wash	Skin cleanser and de-germer	None significant	Apply 5 mL on hands or face and rub thoroughly for 30 sec, rinse thoroughly, pat dry
Corticosteroids, Topical				
alclometasone *al-kloe-met'-ah-soan*	Aclovate	Treatment of various allergic/immunologic skin problems	Allergic contact dermatitis, burning, dryness, edema, irritation	Apply 1–6 times daily according to directions
amcinonide *am-sin'-oh-nyde*	Cyclocort	Same as alclometasone	Same as alclometasone	Apply 1–6 times daily according to directions
betamethasone *bay-tah-meth'-ah-soan*	Alphatrex, Betatrex, Diprolene, Diprosone, Maxivate	Same as alclometasone	Same as alclometasone	Apply 1–4 times daily according to directions
desoximetasone *dess-ox-ih-met'-ah-soan*	Topicort	Same as alclometasone	Same as alclometasone	Apply 1–4 times daily according to directions
dexamethasone *dex-ah-meth'-ah-soan*	Decadron Phosphate	Same as alclometasone	Same as alclometasone	Apply 1–4 times daily according to directions
diflorasone *dye-flor'-ah-soan*	Florone, Maxiflor	Same as alclometasone	Same as alclometasone	Apply 1–4 times daily according to directions
fluocinolone *floo-oh-sin'-oh-loan*	Fluonid, Flurosyn, Synalar	Same as alclometasone	Same as alclometasone	Apply 1–4 times daily according to directions
fluocinonide *floo-oh-sin'-oh-nyde*	Lidex	Same as alclometasone	Same as alclometasone	Apply 1–4 times daily according to directions
flurandrenolide *flor-an-dren'-oh-lyde*	Cordran	Same as alclometasone	Same as alclometasone	Apply 1–4 times daily according to directions
hydrocortisone *hye-droe-kore'-tih-soan*	Bactine, Cort-Dome, Hytone, Locoid, Pandel	Same as alclometasone	Same as alclometasone	Apply 1–4 times daily according to directions
triamcinolone *trye-am-sin'-oh-loan*	Aristocort, Flutex, Kenalog, Triacet	Same as alclometasone	Same as alclometasone	Apply 1–4 times daily according to directions
Antipsoriatic Drugs				
anthralin *an-thra'-lin*	Anthra-Derm Drithocreme, Miconal	Psoriasis	Few; transient irritation of normal skin or uninvolved skin	Apply daily

(table continues on page 596)

Summary Drug Table TOPICAL DRUGS (continued)

Generic Name	Trade Name	Uses	Adverse Reactions	Dosage Ranges
calcipotriene *cal-sip-oh-trye'-een*	Dovonex	Psoriasis	Burning, itching, skin irritation, erythema, dry skin, peeling, rash, worsening of psoriasis, dermatitis, hyperpigmentation	Apply BID
selenium sulfide *seh-leh'-nee-um*	Exsel, Head and Shoulders Intensive Treatment Dandruff Shampoo, Selsun Blue	Treatment of dandruff, seborrheic dermatitis of the scalp, and tinea versicolor	Skin irritation, greater than normal hair loss, hair discoloration, oiliness or dryness of hair	Massage 5–10 mL into wet scalp and allow to remain on scalp for 2–3 min, rinse
Enzyme Preparations				
collagenase *koll-ah'-geh-nace*	Santyl	For débriding chronic dermal ulcers and severely burned areas	Well tolerated and nonirritating; transient burning sensation may occur	Apply daily according to directions
enzyme combinations	Accuzyme, Granul-Derm Granulex, Panafil	Débridement of necrotic tissue and liquefaction of slough in acute and chronic lesions such as pressure ulcers, varicose and diabetic ulcers, burns, wounds, pilonidal cyst wounds, and miscellaneous traumatic or infected wounds	Well tolerated and nonirritating; transient burning sensation may occur	Aerosol: apply BID or TID according to directions Ointment: apply daily or BID according to directions
Keratolytic Drugs				
masoprocol *mah-soe'-proe-koll*	Actinex	Actinic keratoses	Erythema, flaking, dryness, itching, edema, burning, soreness, bleeding, crusting, skin roughness	Apply BID
salicylic acid *sal-ih-sill'-ik*	Duofilm, Wart Remover, Fostex, Fung-O, Mosco, Panscol	Aids in the removal of excessive keratin in hyperkeratotic skin disorders, including warts, psoriasis, calluses, and corns	Local irritation	Apply as directed in individual product labeling
Local Anesthetics				
benzocaine *ben'-zoh-kane*	Lanacane	Topical anesthesia in local skin disorders	Rare; hypersensitivity, local burning, stinging, tenderness, sloughing	Apply to affected area
dibucaine *dih'-byoo-kane*	Nupercainal	Topical anesthesia in local skin disorders, local anesthesia of accessible mucous membranes	Same as benzocaine	Topical: apply to affected area as needed Mucous membranes: dosage varies and depends on the area to be anesthetized
lidocaine *lye'-doe-kane*	DentiPatch, ELA-Max, Lidocaine Viscous, Xylocaine	Same as dibucaine	Same as benzocaine	Topical: apply to affected area as needed Mucous membranes: dosage varies and depends on the area to be anesthetized
butamben picrate *byoo'-tam-ben*		Topical anesthesia	Rare; local burning, stinging, tenderness	Apply to affected area

● Chapter Review

Know Your Drugs

Clients sometimes know a medication by the brand (or trade) name and not the generic name. To help you recognize both names, match the brand name with the generic name of the same medication.

Generic Name	Brand Name
1. acyclovir	A. Desenex
2. chlorhexidine	B. Hibiclens
3. clotrimazole	C. pHisoHex
4. hexachlorophene	D. Zovirax

● Prepare for the NCLEX®

Build Your Knowledge

1. Which is the outermost layer of skin tissue?
   1. dermis
   2. epidermis
   3. subcutaneous
   4. tendon

2. What reaction could occur with prolonged use of the topical antibiotics?
   1. water intoxication
   2. superficial superinfection
   3. outbreak of eczema
   4. cellulitis

3. Which of the following drugs has a proteolytic action?
   1. amcinonide
   2. collagenase
   3. bacitracin
   4. ciclopirox

4. A keratolytic agent would be safe to use on which of the following skin conditions?
   1. moles
   2. birthmarks
   3. facial warts
   4. calluses

5. What type of action do the corticosteroids have when used topically?
   1. bactericidal activity
   2. anti-inflammatory activity
   3. antifungal activity
   4. antiviral activity

6. What reaction could happen when a topical drug is covered with a heating pad?
   1. increased drug absorption
   2. slower wound healing
   3. decreased drug absorption
   4. bruising of surrounding area

Apply Your Knowledge

7. The nurse is about to débride and cleanse an ulcerated wound. How should the nurse determine if pain medication is needed before starting the procedure?
   1. wait for the client to ask for medication
   2. check facial grimace when removing dressing
   3. use the 0 to 10 scale for pain assessment
   4. review medication administration record for past medication

8. The nurse is gathering supplies to change the dressing of a client's central line (IV). Which of the following drugs is best suited to be used as a topical antiseptic?
   1. amphotericin B
   2. benzocaine
   3. iodine
   4. povidone–iodine

Alternate-Format Questions

9. Name the type of skin lesion illustrated below.

   _____

10. Dakin's solution is ordered for home irrigation of a wound. The primary health care provider orders a 3:1 solution (water:Dakin's) to be mixed with distilled water. How much water should be added to 10 mL of the Dakin's solution?

To check your answers, see Appendix G.

the**Point** *For more NCLEX-style questions, log on to http://thepoint.lww.com to access more than 1000 questions.*

53

Otic and Ophthalmic Preparations

LEARNING OBJECTIVES

On completion of this chapter, the student will:

1. Discuss the general actions, uses, adverse reactions, contraindications, precautions, and interactions of otic and ophthalmic preparations.
2. Discuss important preadministration and ongoing assessment activities the nurse should perform on a patient receiving otic and ophthalmic preparations.
3. List nursing diagnoses particular to a patient taking an otic or ophthalmic preparation.
4. Discuss ways to promote an optimal response to therapy, how to administer the preparations, and important points to keep in mind when educating patients about the use of otic or ophthalmic preparations.

KEY TERMS

cerumen • ear wax

cycloplegia • paralysis of the ciliary muscle, resulting in an inability to focus the eye

intraocular pressure • pressure within the eye

miosis • constriction of the pupil of the eye

mydriasis • dilation of the pupil

ophthalmic • pertaining to the eye

otic • pertaining to the ear, means *auditory* in Latin

otitis media • infection of the middle ear

superinfection • overgrowth of bacterial or fungal microorganisms not affected by the antibiotic being administered

DRUG CLASSES

Otic preparations
Ophthalmic
Preparations

This chapter provides information on drugs that are topically applied to the eyes and ears. Because the eyes and ears help us to interpret our environment, any disease or injury that has the potential for partial or total loss of function of these organs should be treated.

OTIC PREPARATIONS

The term "**otic**" means *auditory* in Latin. It is important to remember the connection between the words "otic" and "ear," because harm can be done when these preparations are swallowed or administered into the eye.

Disorders of the ear are categorized according to the part of the ear affected: the outer, the middle, or the inner ear (Fig. 53.1). The disorders of the outer and middle ear are discussed in this chapter. **Otitis media**, by far the most common disorder of the middle ear, is fluid in the middle ear accompanied by symptoms of intense local or systemic infection. Symptoms include pain in the ear, drainage of fluid from the ear canal, and hearing loss. Other symptoms that may be present if the disorder becomes systemic include fever, irritability, headache, and anorexia. The most common causes are viruses and bacteria.

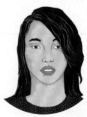

PHARMACOLOGY IN PRACTICE

Janna Wong, a 16-year-old high school student, recently switched from eyeglasses to contact lenses. She is experiencing minor eye irritation. In this chapter learn how to teach Janna the correct way to use her eye drops.

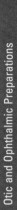

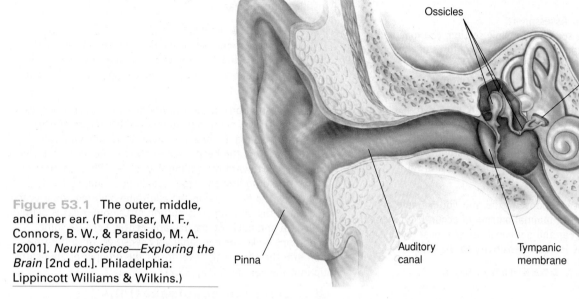

Figure 53.1 The outer, middle, and inner ear. (From Bear, M. F., Connors, B. W., & Parasido, M. A. [2001]. *Neuroscience—Exploring the Brain* [2nd ed.]. Philadelphia: Lippincott Williams & Wilkins.)

Actions

Otic preparations can be divided into three categories: (1) antibiotics, (2) antibiotic/steroid combinations, and (3) miscellaneous preparations. The miscellaneous preparations usually contain one or more of the following ingredients:

- Benzocaine—a local anesthetic used to temporally relieve pain
- Phenylephrine—a vasoconstrictor decongestant
- Hydrocortisone—corticosteroid for anti-inflammatory and antipruritic effects
- Glycerin—an emollient and a solvent
- Antipyrine—an analgesic
- Acetic acid, boric acid, benzalkonium, aluminum, benzethonium—provide antifungal or antibacterial action
- Carbamide peroxide—aids in removing **cerumen** (yellowish or brownish ear wax) by softening and breaking up the wax

Examples of otic preparations are given in the Summary Drug Table: Selected Otic Preparations.

Uses

Otic preparations are instilled in the external auditory canal and may be used to:

- Relieve pain
- Treat infection and inflammation
- Aid in the removal of cerumen

When the patient has an inner ear infection, systemic antibiotic therapy is indicated.

Adverse Reactions

When otic drugs are applied topically, the amount of drug that enters the systemic circulation usually is not sufficient to produce adverse reactions. Local adverse reactions that may occur include:

- Ear irritation
- Itching
- Burning

Prolonged use of otic preparations containing an antibiotic, such as ofloxacin, may result in a **superinfection** (an overgrowth of bacterial or fungal microorganisms not affected by the antibiotic being administered).

Contraindications, Precautions, and Interactions

These drugs are contraindicated in patients with a known hypersensitivity to the drugs. The otic drugs are used with caution during pregnancy and lactation. The pregnancy category of most of these drugs is unknown when they are used as otic drugs. Drugs to remove cerumen are not used if ear drainage, discharge, pain, or irritation is present; if the eardrum is perforated; or after ear surgery. Otic drugs may be available in dropper bottles and can be dangerous if ingested. Therefore, these drugs are stored safely out of the reach of children and pets.

If an allergy is suspected, the drug is not administered. Ofloxacin is a pregnancy category C drug and should be administered in pregnancy only if the potential benefit justifies the risk to the fetus. No significant interactions have been reported with use of the otic preparations.

NURSING PROCESS
PATIENT RECEIVING AN OTIC PREPARATION

ASSESSMENT

Preadministration Assessment
When a patient is seen in the clinic setting, you may be responsible for examining the outer structures of the ear (i.e., the earlobe and the skin around the ear) as part of the intake procedure. Be sure to document a description of any drainage or visible wax. Before prescribing an otic preparation, the primary health care provider examines the ear's external and internal structures. Perforated eardrums may be a contraindication to some of the otic preparations. Check with the primary health care provider before administering an otic preparation to a patient with a perforated eardrum.

Ongoing Assessment
Assess the patient's response to therapy. For example, a decrease in pain or inflammation should occur. Examine and palpate the outer ear and ear canal for any local redness or irritation that may indicate sensitivity to the drug.

>
> **LIFESPAN CONSIDERATIONS**
> **Pediatric**
> When assessing the infant, look for pulling, grabbing, or tugging at his or her ears. Because infants cannot tell you about pain, this may be a sign that the child's ear hurts. Since infants do pull their ears for all kinds of reasons or for no reason at all, validate this behavior with the parent or caregiver. Additional signs include a change in behavior, crying, fussiness or irritability, or a fever.

NURSING DIAGNOSES
Drug-specific nursing diagnoses include the following:

- **Risk for Infection** (superinfection) related to prolonged use of the anti-infective otic drug
- **Anxiety** related to ear pain or discomfort, changes in hearing, diagnosis, or other factors

Nursing diagnoses related to drug administration are discussed in Chapter 4.

PLANNING
The expected outcomes of the patient depend on the reason for administering the drug and may include an optimal response to the drug, support of patient needs related to the management of adverse reactions, a reduction in anxiety, and confidence in an understanding of the application and use of an otic preparation.

IMPLEMENTATION

Promoting an Optimal Response to Therapy
Ear disorders may result in symptoms such as pain, a feeling of fullness in the ear, tinnitus, dizziness, or a change in hearing. Some of these same sensations may be felt by the patient from the solutions used for treatment. Before instilling an otic solution, tell the patient that a feeling of fullness may be felt in the ear and that hearing in the treated ear may be impaired while the solution remains in the ear canal.

Before instillation of otic preparations, hold the container in your hand for a few minutes to warm it to body temperature. Cold and too warm (above body temperature) preparations may cause dizziness or other sensations after being instilled into the ear.

> **! NURSING ALERT**
> Only preparations labeled as "otic" are instilled in the ear. Check the label of the preparation carefully for the name of the drug and a statement indicating that the preparation is for *otic* use.

To keep solutions in the ear when instilling ear drops, have the patient lie on his or her side with the affected ear up toward the ceiling. If the patient wishes to remain in an upright position, the head is tilted toward the untreated side with the ear toward the ceiling (Fig. 53.2). When administering an otic drug, the ear canal should be straightened. To straighten the ear canal in the adult and children age 3 years and older, the cartilaginous portion of the outer ear is gently pulled up and back. Be particularly gentle, because some conditions make the ear canal very sensitive. Drop the solution into the ear canal; never insert the dropper or applicator tip into the ear canal (Fig. 53.2).

>
> **LIFESPAN CONSIDERATIONS**
> **Pediatric**
> In children younger than 3 years of age, the ear canal is straighter and needs less manipulation. Gently pull the outer ear down (instead of up) and back.

The patient is kept lying on the untreated side after the medication is instilled for approximately 5 minutes to facilitate the penetration of the drops into the ear canal. If medication is needed in the other ear, it is best to wait at least 5 minutes after instillation of the first ear drops before

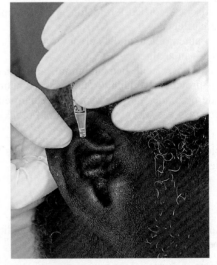

Figure 53.2 Instilling ear drops. With the head turned toward the unaffected side, pull the cartilaginous portion of the outer ear (pinna) up and back in the adult and instill the prescribed number of drops on the side of the auditory canal.

administering drops to the other ear. Once the patient is upright, the solution running out of the ear may be gently removed with gauze. A piece of cotton can be loosely inserted into the ear canal to prevent the medication from flowing out. The cotton is not inserted too deeply, because it may cause increased pressure within the ear canal.

Cerumen is a natural product of the ear and is produced by modified sweat glands in the auditory canal. Sometimes too much cerumen is produced, particularly in older adults. Drugs that loosen cerumen, such as Cerumenex, work by softening the dried ear wax inside the ear canal. Cerumenex is available by prescription and is not allowed to stay in the ear canal more than 30 minutes before irrigation. When Cerumenex is administered, the ear canal is filled with the solution and a cotton plug is inserted. The drug is allowed to remain in the ear for 15 to 30 minutes, and then the ear is flushed with warm water using a soft rubber bulb ear syringe.

LIFESPAN CONSIDERATIONS
Gerontology
Cerumen is thicker in the older adult, making the accumulation of excess wax more likely. When hearing loss is suspected in the older adult, mentally impaired, or debilitated patient, the ear should be checked for excess cerumen.

Monitoring and Managing Patient Needs
RISK FOR INFECTION. When using the otic antibiotics there is a danger of a superinfection, or another infection on top of the original one, from prolonged use of the drug (see Chapter 9 for a discussion of superinfection). If after administering the drops as directed for 1 week the infection does not improve, the primary health care provider should be notified.

ANXIETY. Patients with an ear disorder or injury usually have great concern over the effect the problem will have on their hearing. Reassure the patient that every effort is being made to treat the disorder and relieve the symptoms.

Educating the Patient and Family
Provide the patient or a family member written instructions or a demonstration of the instillation technique of an otic preparation.

LIFESPAN CONSIDERATIONS
Pediatric
Because some children are prone to recurrent attacks of acute otitis media, parents should be taught to identify early signs and symptoms of otitis media and seek medical attention when their child exhibits these symptoms.

The following information may be given to the patient when an ear ointment or solution is prescribed:

- Wash the hands thoroughly before cleansing the area around the ear (when necessary) and instilling ear drops or ointment.

- If the solution is cool or cold, warm to room temperature by holding solution in the hand for 1 to 2 minutes before administering.

- Instill the prescribed number of drops in the ear. Do not put the applicator or dropper tip in the ear or allow the tip to become contaminated from the fingers or other sources.

- Immediately after use, replace the cap or dropper and refrigerate the solution if so stated on the label.

- If the drops are in a suspension form, shake the container well for 10 seconds before using.

- Keep the head tilted or lie on the untreated side for approximately 5 minutes to allow the solution to remain in contact with the ear. Excess solution and solution running out of the ear can be wiped off with a tissue.

- Do not insert anything into the ear canal before or after applying the prescribed drug unless advised to do so by the primary health care provider. At times a soft cotton plug may be inserted into the affected ear.

- Complete a full course of treatment with the prescribed drug to achieve satisfactory results.

- Do not use nonprescription ear products during or after treatment unless such use has been approved by the primary health care provider.

- Remember that temporary changes in hearing or a feeling of fullness in the ear may occur for a short time after the drug has been instilled.

- Notify the primary health care provider if symptoms do not improve or become worse.

DRUGS USED TO REMOVE CERUMEN

- Do not put anything in the ear canal such as a Q-tip.

- Do not use a drug to remove cerumen if ear drainage, discharge, pain, or irritation occurs.

- Do not use for more than 4 days. If excessive cerumen remains, consult the primary health care provider.

- Any wax remaining after the treatment may be removed by gently flushing the ear with warm water using a soft rubber bulb ear syringe.

- If dizziness occurs, consult the primary health care provider.

EVALUATION

- Therapeutic effect is achieved.

- Adverse reactions are identified, reported to the primary health care provider, and managed successfully with appropriate nursing interventions:
  - No evidence of infection is seen.
  - Anxiety is managed successfully.

- Patient and family express confidence and demonstrate an understanding of the drug regimen.

OPHTHALMIC PREPARATIONS

Various types of preparations are used for treating **ophthalmic** (eye) disorders, such as glaucoma, to lower the **intraocular pressure** (IOP; the pressure within the eye); and to treat bacterial or viral infections of the eye, inflammatory conditions, and symptoms of allergy related to the eye.

Glaucoma

Glaucoma is a condition of the eye in which there is an increase in the IOP, causing progressive atrophy of the optic nerve with deterioration of vision and, if untreated, blindness. The eye's lens, iris, and cornea are continuously bathed and nourished by a fluid called *aqueous humor*. As aqueous humor is produced, excess fluid normally flows out through a complex network of tissue called the *canal of Schlemm*. An angle is formed where the canal of Schlemm and iris meet. This forms a filtration angle that maintains the normal pressure within the eye by allowing excess aqueous humor to leave the anterior chamber of the eye (Fig. 53.3).

There are two types of glaucoma: angle-closure glaucoma and open-angle, or chronic, glaucoma (Fig. 53.4). The limitation of outflow in both types of glaucoma causes an accumulation of intraocular fluid, followed by increased IOP. As a result, the higher the IOP, the greater the risk of optic nerve damage, visual loss, and blindness. Some individuals have an anatomic defect that causes the angle to be more narrow than normal but do not have any symptoms and do not develop glaucoma under normal circumstances. However, certain situations, such as medication that causes dilation of the eye, fear, or pain, may precipitate an attack. The aim of treatment in glaucoma is to lower the IOP. The Summary Drug Table: Selected Ophthalmic Preparations provides examples of the drugs used to treat both glaucoma and other ophthalmic problems.

Actions and Uses

The drugs used to treat ophthalmic conditions are from the same classes of drugs used in other body systems and conditions. Systemic effects are rare because only small amounts of these preparations may be absorbed systemically.

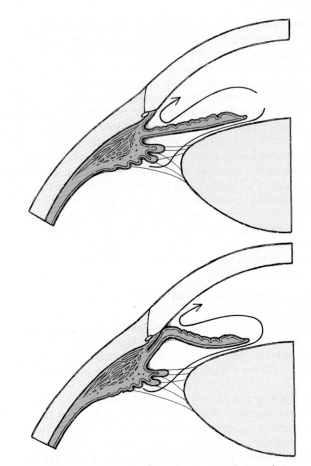

Figure 53.4 In open-angle glaucoma, the angle where aqueous humor drains is normal but does not function properly and excess fluid cannot leave the anterior chamber as shown in the top picture. In angle-closure glaucoma, the iris blocks the canal and limits the flow of aqueous humor from the anterior chamber of the eye as shown in the bottom picture.

Alpha (α)₂-Adrenergic Drugs

Brimonidine is an α_2-adrenergic receptor agonist used to lower IOP in patients with open-angle glaucoma or ocular hypertension. This drug acts to reduce production of aqueous humor and increase the outflow of aqueous humor.

Sympathomimetic Drugs

Sympathomimetics have α- and beta (β)-adrenergic activity (see Chapter 24 for a detailed discussion of adrenergic drugs). These drugs lower the IOP by increasing the outflow of aqueous humor in the eye and are used to treat glaucoma. Apraclonidine is used to control or prevent postoperative elevations in IOP.

α-Adrenergic Blocking Drugs

Dapiprazole acts by blocking the α-adrenergic receptor in smooth muscle and produces **miosis** (constriction of the pupil) through an effect on the dilator muscle of the iris.

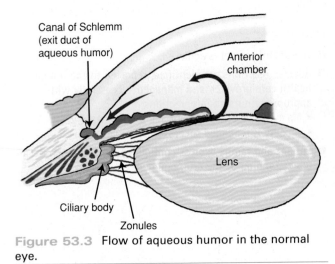

Figure 53.3 Flow of aqueous humor in the normal eye.

Canal of Schlemm (exit duct of aqueous humor)

Anterior chamber

Lens

Ciliary body

Zonules

The drug is used primarily after ophthalmic examinations to reverse the diagnostic **mydriasis** (dilation of the pupil).

β-Adrenergic Blocking Drugs

The β-adrenergic blocking drugs decrease the rate of production of aqueous humor and thereby lower the IOP. These drugs are used to treat glaucoma.

Miotics, Direct Acting, and Cholinesterase Inhibitors

Miotics contract the pupil of the eye (miosis), resulting in an increase in the space through which the aqueous humor flows, decreasing IOP. The miotics were, for a number of years, the drug of choice for glaucoma. These drugs have lost that first-choice treatment status to the β-adrenergic blocking drugs.

Carbonic Anhydrase Inhibitors

Carbonic anhydrase is an enzyme found in many tissues of the body, including the eye. Inhibition of carbonic anhydrase in the eye decreases aqueous humor secretion, resulting in a decrease of IOP. These drugs are used in the treatment of elevated IOP seen in open-angle glaucoma. Except for dorzolamide and brinzolamide, carbonic anhydrase inhibitors are administered systemically.

Prostaglandin Agonists

Prostaglandin agonists are used to lower IOP in patients with open-angle glaucoma and ocular hypertension who do not tolerate other IOP-lowering medications or have an insufficient response to these medications. These drugs act to lower IOP by increasing the outflow of aqueous humor through the trabecular meshwork.

Mast Cell Stabilizers

Mast cell stabilizers currently approved for ophthalmic use are nedocromil and pemirolast. These drugs are used to prevent itching of the eyes caused by allergic conjunctivitis. Mast cell stabilizers inhibit the antigen-induced release of inflammatory mediators (e.g., histamine) from human mast cells.

Nonsteroidal Anti-Inflammatory Drugs

Nonsteroidal anti-inflammatory drugs (NSAIDs) inhibit prostaglandin synthesis (see Chapter 14 for a discussion of the NSAIDs), thereby exerting anti-inflammatory action. These drugs are used to treat postoperative pain and inflammation after cataract surgery, for the relief of itching of the eyes caused by seasonal allergies, and during eye surgery to prevent miosis.

Corticosteroids

These drugs possess anti-inflammatory activity and are used for inflammatory conditions, such as allergic conjunctivitis, keratitis, herpes zoster keratitis, and inflammation of the iris. Corticosteroids also may be used after injury to the cornea or after corneal transplantation to prevent rejection.

Antibiotics and Sulfonamides

Antibiotics possess antibacterial activity and are used in the treatment of eye infections. Sulfonamides possess a bacteriostatic effect against a wide range of gram-positive and gram-negative microorganisms. They are used in treating conjunctivitis, corneal ulcer, and other superficial infections of the eye. See Chapter 6 for additional information on the sulfonamides.

Silver

Silver possesses antibacterial activity against gram-positive and gram-negative microorganisms. Silver proteinate is occasionally used in the treatment of eye infections. Silver nitrate is occasionally used to prevent gonorrheal ophthalmia neonatorum (gonorrheal infection of the newborn's eyes). Ophthalmic tetracycline and erythromycin have largely replaced the use of silver nitrate in newborns.

Antiviral Drugs

Antiviral drugs interfere with viral reproduction by altering DNA synthesis. These drugs are used in the treatment of herpes simplex infections of the eye, in the treatment of immunocompromised patients with cytomegalovirus (CMV) retinitis, and for the prevention of CMV retinitis in patients undergoing transplantation.

Antifungal Drugs

Natamycin is the only ophthalmic antifungal in use. This drug possesses antifungal activity against a variety of yeast and other fungi.

Vasoconstrictors/Mydriatics

Mydriatics are drugs that dilate the pupil (mydriasis), constrict superficial blood vessels of the sclera, and decrease the formation of aqueous humor. Depending on the specific drug and strength, these drugs may be used before eye surgery in the treatment of glaucoma, for relief of minor eye irritation, and to dilate the pupil for examination of the eye.

Cycloplegic Mydriatics

Cycloplegic mydriatics cause mydriasis and **cycloplegia** (paralysis of the ciliary muscle, resulting in an inability to focus the eye). These drugs are used in the treatment of inflammatory conditions of the iris and uveal tract of the eye and for examination of the eye.

Artificial Tear Solutions

These products lubricate the eyes and are used for conditions such as dry eyes and eye irritation caused by inadequate tear production. Inactive ingredients may be found in some preparations. Examples of these inactive ingredients include preservatives and antioxidants, which prevent deterioration of the product, and drugs that slow drainage of the drug from the eye into the tear duct.

Adverse Reactions

Although adverse reactions are rare, these drugs can cause visual impairment such as blurring of vision and local irritation and burning. These reactions are most often self-limiting and resolve if the patient waits a few minutes. Visual impairment that does not clear within 30 minutes after therapy should be reported to the primary health care provider.

Drugs to Treat Glaucoma

Drugs used to treat glaucoma may cause transient local reactions and systemic reactions. Although side effects are usually mild they may include:

- Locally in or near the eye—burning and stinging, headache, visual blurring, tearing, foreign body sensation, ocular allergic reactions, and ocular itching
- Systemic effects—fatigue and drowsiness, palpations, nausea

Corticosteroids

Local adverse reactions associated with administration of the corticosteroid ophthalmic preparations include elevated IOP with optic nerve damage, loss of visual acuity, cataract formation, delayed wound healing, secondary ocular infection, exacerbation of corneal infections, dry eyes, ptosis, blurred vision, discharge, ocular pain, foreign body sensation, and pruritus.

Antibiotics, Sulfonamides, and Silver

The antibiotic and sulfonamide ophthalmics are usually well tolerated, and few adverse reactions are seen. Local adverse reactions include occasional transient irritation, burning, itching, stinging, inflammation, and blurred vision. With prolonged or repeated use, a superinfection may occur.

Antiviral Drugs

Administration of the antiviral ophthalmics may cause local reactions such as irritation, pain, pruritus, inflammation, edema of the eyes or eyelids, foreign body sensation, and corneal clouding. Systemic reactions include photophobia and allergic reactions.

Antifungal Drugs

Adverse reactions are rare. Occasional local irritation to the eye may occur.

Artificial Tear Solutions

Adverse reactions are rare, but on occasion redness or irritation may occur.

Contraindications, Precautions, and Interactions

Drugs Used to Treat Glaucoma

These drugs are contraindicated in patients with hypersensitivity to the drug or any component of the drug. Adrenergic-based drugs are contraindicated in patients taking monoamine oxidase inhibitors (MAOIs). Epinephrine is contraindicated in patients with narrow-angle glaucoma, or patients with a narrow angle but no glaucoma, and aphakia (absence of the crystalline lens of the eye). Patients wearing soft contact lenses should be cautioned, because the preservative in the drug may be absorbed by soft contact lenses and discoloration of the lenses may occur. The drug is used cautiously during pregnancy (epinephrine, pregnancy category B; and apraclonidine, pregnancy category C) and lactation and in patients with cardiovascular disease, depression, cerebral or coronary insufficiency, hypertension, diabetes, hyperthyroidism, or Raynaud's phenomenon. When brimonidine is used with central nervous system (CNS) depressants, such as alcohol, barbiturates, opiates, sedatives, or anesthetics, there is a risk for an additive CNS depressant effect. Use the drugs cautiously in combination with antihypertensive drugs and cardiac glycosides, because a synergistic effect may occur.

Adrenergic blocking drugs are contraindicated in patients with bronchial asthma, obstructive pulmonary disease, sinus bradycardia, heart block, cardiac failure, or cardiogenic shock, and in patients with hypersensitivity to the drug or any components of the drug. These drugs should not be used in conditions in which pupil constriction is not desirable, such as in acute iritis (inflammation of the iris), and in the treatment of IOP in open-angle glaucoma.

These drugs are in pregnancy category C (dapiprazole is pregnancy category B) and are used cautiously during pregnancy and lactation and in patients with cardiovascular disease, diabetes (may mask the symptoms of hypoglycemia), and hyperthyroidism (may mask symptoms of hyperthyroidism). The patient taking β-adrenergic blocking drugs for ophthalmic reasons may experience increased or additive effects when the drugs are administered with the oral β-adrenergic blockers. Coadministration of timolol and calcium antagonists may cause hypotension, left ventricular failure, and condition disturbances within the heart. There is a potential additive hypotensive effect when the β-adrenergic blocking ophthalmic drugs are administered with the phenothiazines.

Miotic drugs are contraindicated in patients with hypersensitivity to the drug or any component of the drug and in conditions where constriction is undesirable (e.g., iritis, uveitis, and acute inflammatory disease of the anterior chamber). The drugs are used cautiously in patients with corneal abrasion, pregnancy (pregnancy category C), lactation, cardiac failure, bronchial asthma, peptic ulcer, hyperthyroidism, gastrointestinal spasm, urinary tract infection, Parkinson's disease, renal or hepatic impairment, recent myocardial infarction, hypotension, or hypertension. These drugs are also used cautiously in patients with angle-closure glaucoma, because miotics occasionally can precipitate angle-closure glaucoma by increasing the resistance to aqueous flow from posterior to anterior chamber.

Cholinesterase inhibitors are used cautiously in patients with myasthenia gravis (may cause additive adverse effects), before and after surgery, and in patients with chronic angle-closure (narrow-angle) glaucoma or those with anatomically narrow angles (may cause papillary block and increase the angle blockage). When cholinesterase inhibitors are administered with systemic anticholinesterase drugs, there is a risk for additive effects. Individuals such as farmers, warehouse workers, or gardeners working with carbamate–organophosphate insecticides or pesticides are at risk for systemic effects of cholinesterase inhibitors from absorption of the pesticide or insecticide through the respiratory tract or the skin. Individuals working with pesticides or insecticides containing carbamate–organophosphate and taking a cholinesterase inhibitor should be advised to wear respiratory masks, change clothes frequently, and wash exposed clothes thoroughly.

Drugs Used to Treat Inflammation

These drugs are contraindicated in patients with hypersensitivity to the drug or any component of the drug. The mast cell stabilizers are used cautiously in patients who wear contact lenses (preservative may be absorbed by the soft contact lenses). NSAIDs are used cautiously in patients with bleeding tendencies. When used topically, there is less risk of interactions with drugs or other substances. There is a possibility of a cross-sensitivity reaction when NSAIDs are administered to patients allergic to salicylates. Corticosteroids and antibiotics are used cautiously in patients with sulfite sensitivity, because an allergic-type reaction may result. The corticosteroid ophthalmic preparations are used cautiously in patients with infectious conditions of the eye. Prolonged use of corticosteroids may result in elevated IOP and optic nerve damage. The antibiotic and sulfonamide ophthalmics are contraindicated

in patients with epithelial herpes simplex keratitis, varicella, mycobacterial infection of the eye, and fungal diseases of the eye. These drugs are pregnancy category B or C drugs and are used cautiously during pregnancy and lactation.

Artificial tears are contraindicated in patients who are allergic to any component of the solution. No precautions or interactions have been reported.

⚕ HERBAL CONSIDERATIONS

Bilberry, also known as whortleberry, blueberry, and huckleberry, is a shrub with bluish flowers that appear in early spring and ripen in July and August. A beneficial use appears to be in promoting healthy eyes. Other benefits reportedly include improved visual acuity, improved night vision, prevention of free radical damage, and promotion of capillary blood flow in the eyes, hands, and feet. Bilberry extract has been used in treating nonspecific, mild diarrhea and as a mouthwash or gargle for inflammation of the mouth and throat. Bilberry fruit is a safe substance with no known adverse reactions or toxicity. There are no known contraindications to its use as directed unless the individual has an allergy to bilberry. The dosage of standard extract is 80 to 160 mg per day (DerMarderosian, 2003).

NURSING PROCESS
PATIENT RECEIVING AN OPHTHALMIC PREPARATION

ASSESSMENT

Preadministration Assessment
The primary health care provider examines the eye and external structures surrounding the eye and prescribes the drug indicated to treat the disorder. During the intake procedure you may perform a baseline assessment by examining the eye for irritation, redness, and the presence of any exudate, being careful to document the findings in the patient's record. A purulent discharge is often found with infection of the eye. Pruritus (itching) is often present with allergic conditions of the eye. Review the primary health care provider's diagnosis and comments, take a general patient health history, and evaluate the patient's ability to carry out the activities of daily living, especially if the patient is older or has limited vision. Assess the patient for any hypersensitivity to the specific medication being administered and note any cautions to the drug as well.

Ongoing Assessment
During the ongoing assessment observe for a therapeutic drug response and report any increase in symptoms and the presence of any redness, irritation, or pain in the eye. Patients admitted for treatment of acute glaucoma should be assessed every 2 hours for relief of pain. Pain in the eye may indicate increased IOP.

NURSING DIAGNOSES
Drug-specific nursing diagnoses include the following:

- **Risk for Injury** related to adverse reactions to drug therapy (blurring of the vision)
- **Acute Pain** related to eye disorder or adverse reaction to medication

- **Anxiety** related to eye pain or discomfort, diagnosis, other factors

Nursing diagnoses related to drug administration are discussed in Chapter 4.

PLANNING
The expected outcomes of the patient depend on the reason for administration but may include an optimal response to therapy, support of patient needs related to the management of adverse reactions, minimized anxiety, and confidence in an understanding of the application and use of an ophthalmic preparation (see the Patient Teaching for Improved Patient Outcomes: Instilling an Ophthalmic Preparation).

IMPLEMENTATION

Promoting an Optimal Response to Therapy
Many patients will self-administer ophthalmic preparations. In some instances when hospitalized, the patient may have been using an ophthalmic preparation for a long time and the primary health care provider may allow the patient to instill his or her own eye drops. When this is stated on the patient's orders, consult with the pharmacy about leaving the drug at the patient's bedside. Even though the drug is self-administered, check the patient at intervals to be sure that the drug is instilled at the prescribed time using the correct technique for ophthalmic instillation. Always review basic administration steps with the patient no matter whether the medication is given by you or the patient. Steps to be reviewed include:

- The drug label must indicate that the preparation is for ophthalmic use.
- Check the medication to make sure the solution is clear and not discolored.

Patient Teaching for Improved Patient Outcomes

Instilling an Ophthalmic Preparation

Many eye surgeries are performed in ambulatory clinics, requiring the patient to instill eye drops or ointment at home. If the patient is unable to do so, a family member or friend may have to instill the preparation. Teaching the steps of preparation and administration are important for good outcomes. Discuss, demonstrate, and watch a "teach-back" from the patient on the procedure before this becomes a self-administered task.

Be sure the patient understands the following:

✔ Wash hands thoroughly before beginning.
✔ Look at the solution each time; if discolored or unclear, don't use it!
✔ Hold bottle (drops) or tube (ointment) in hand for a few minutes before using to warm the solution.
✔ Cleanse the area around the eye of any secretions.
✔ Squeeze the eye dropper bulb to release and then refill the dropper, squeeze the bottle to fill the drop chamber, or squeeze ointment to tip of the tube.
✔ Tilt head slightly backward and toward the eye to be treated.
✔ Pull affected lower lid down.
✔ Position dropper, bottle, or tube over lower conjunctival sac.
✔ Steady hand by resting fingers against cheek or by resting base of hand on cheek.
✔ Look up at ceiling and squeeze dropper, bottle, or tube.
✔ Drop ordered number of drops into the middle of lower conjunctival sac; instill prescribed amount of ointment to eyelid or lower conjunctival sac.
✔ Close eye briefly and gently and release lower lid (do not squeeze eyes shut after instilling the drug).
✔ Place finger on inner canthus to avoid absorption through the tear duct (when instilling drops and only if ordered).
✔ Repeat procedure with other eye (if ordered).
✔ If more than one type of ophthalmic preparation is being instilled, wait the recommended time before instilling the second drug (usually 5 minutes for drops and 10–15 minutes for ointment).
✔ Replace the cap of the eye preparation immediately after instilling the eye drops or ointment. Do not touch the tip of the dropper, bottle, or tube.

- Ophthalmic ointments are applied to the eyelids or dropped into the lower conjunctival sac; ophthalmic solutions are dropped into the middle of the lower conjunctival sac, not directly on the eyeball (Fig. 53.5).
- Avoid touching the eye with the tip of the dropper or container to prevent contamination of the product.
- When eye solutions are instilled, apply gentle pressure on the inner canthus to delay drainage of the drug down the tear duct. This prevents the drug from being absorbed systemically.

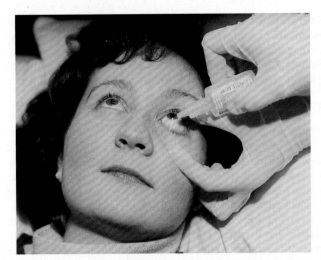

Figure 53.5 Instilling eye medication. While the patient looks upward, gently pull the lower lid down and instill the correct number of drops into the lower conjunctival sac.

Consult the primary health care provider regarding use of this technique before the first dose is instilled, because this technique can be potentially dangerous in some eye conditions, for example, after recent eye surgery. When two eye drops are prescribed for use at the same time, wait at least 5 minutes before instilling the second drug. This helps prevent dilution of the drug and loss of some therapeutic effect from tearing.

When a patient is scheduled for eye surgery, it is most important that the eye drops ordered by the primary health care provider are instilled at the correct time. This is especially important when the purpose of the drug is to change the size of the pupil (dilate the pupil).

> **! NURSING ALERT**
> Only preparations labeled as "*ophthalmic*" are instilled in the eye. Check the label of the preparation carefully for the name of the drug, the percentage of the preparation, and a statement indicating that the preparation is for ophthalmic use.

Monitoring and Managing Patient Needs

RISK FOR INJURY. When the ophthalmic drugs produce blurring of vision, this can result in falls and other injuries. Keeping the patient's room dimly lit at night is helpful, because night vision may be decreased. Obstacles that may hinder ambulation or result in falls, such as slippers, chairs, and tables, are placed out of the way, especially during the night. Warn patients to exercise care when getting out of bed when the vision is impaired by these drugs. If needed, provide assistance with ambulation to prevent injury from falls.

ACUTE PAIN. Pain can occur with eye conditions such as glaucoma and eye infections. Patients with acute glaucoma are assessed for relief of pain. Pain in the eye may indicate increased IOP and should be reported to the primary health care provider. Pain associated with infection should decrease with administration of medication. Any increase in pain or no decrease in the symptoms after 1 to 2 days of treatment should be reported to the primary health care provider. Headache and brow ache are associated with adverse reactions of some of the ophthalmic agents and are usually self-limiting.

ANXIETY. Eye injuries and some eye infections are very painful. Other eye conditions may result in discomfort or a loss of or change in vision. The patient with an eye disorder or injury usually has great concern about the effect the problem will have on his or her vision. Reassure the patient that every effort is being made to treat the disorder.

Educating the Patient and Family
The patient or a family member will require instruction in the technique of instilling an ophthalmic preparation (see Patient Teaching for Improved Patient Outcomes: Instilling an Ophthalmic Preparation). In addition, give the following information to the patient and family member when an eye ointment or solution is prescribed:

- Eye preparations may cause a momentary stinging or burning sensation; this is normal.
- Temporary blurring of vision may occur. Avoid activities requiring visual acuity until vision returns to normal.
- If more than one topical ophthalmic drug is being used, administer the drugs at least 5 to 10 minutes apart or as directed by the physician.
- Complete a full course of treatment with the prescribed drug to achieve satisfactory results.
- Do not rub the eyes, and keep hands away from the eyes.
- Do not use nonprescription eye products during or after treatment unless such use has been approved by the primary health care provider.
- Some of these preparations cause sensitivity (photophobia) to light; to minimize this, wear sunglasses.
- Notify the primary health care provider if symptoms do not improve or if they worsen.

DRUGS TO TREAT GLAUCOMA

- The eye preparation may sting on instillation, especially the first few doses.
- Do not use if solution is brown or contains a precipitate.
- Do not use while wearing soft contact lenses.
- Headache or brow ache may occur.

- Report any decrease in visual acuity. Use caution when driving at night or performing activities in poor illumination.
- If using the ocular therapeutic system, check the system before retiring at night and on arising. Follow instructions in the package insert.
- If more than one ophthalmic drug is being used, administer the drugs 5 minutes apart.
- Changes may occur to the lashes—length, thickness, pigmentation, and number—in the eye being treated.
- The color of the iris may change because of an increase in the brown pigment. This may be more noticeable in patients with blue, green, gray-brown, or other light-colored eyes. This discoloration may be permanent.

DRUGS TO TREAT INFLAMMATION

- If improvement in the condition being treated does not occur within 2 days, or pain, redness, itching, or swelling of the eye occurs, notify the primary health care provider.

EVALUATION

- Therapeutic effect is achieved.
- Adverse reactions are identified, reported to the primary health care provider, and managed successfully with appropriate nursing interventions:
  - No evidence of injury is seen.
  - Patient has minimal to no pain.
  - Anxiety is reduced.
- Patient and family express confidence and demonstrate an understanding of the drug regimen.

PHARMACOLOGY IN PRACTICE
THINK CRITICALLY

 The primary health care provider has prescribed eye drops. Janna is fidgety and tells you she just can't put those drops in her eyes. Design an age-appropriate teaching plan for this individual.

KEY POINTS

- Otitis media is one of the most common middle ear conditions consisting of fluid buildup that may or may not be infected. Otic preparations are topical solutions used to treat the outer and middle ear conditions. The categories of otics include antibiotics, antibiotic/steroid combinations, and different miscellaneous solutions.
- Minimal drug enters the systemic circulation when administered properly; therefore, local adverse reactions predominate—irritation, itching, or a burning sensation. It is important never to touch the ear canal with an implement, even when administering ear medicines.

- Glaucoma is one of the common ophthalmic conditions requiring medications. Ophthalmic solutions may also treat infections, inflammation, or allergies in the eye.
- The drugs used to treat ophthalmic conditions are from the same classes of drugs used in other body systems and conditions. Systemic effects are rare because only small amounts of these preparations may be absorbed systemically. Local adverse reactions consist of irritation, a burning sensation, and temporary blurriness.
- Take time to check solutions: *otic* preparations are for ears, whereas *ophthalmic* preparations are for eyes.

Summary Drug Table SELECTED OTIC PREPARATIONS

Generic Combinations	Trade Name	Uses	Adverse Reactions	Dosage Ranges
Corticosteroid and Antibiotic Combinations, Solutions				
1% hydrocortisone, 5 mg neomycin, 10,000 units polymyxin B	Antibiotic Ear Solution, AntibiOtic, Cortisporin Otic, Drotic, Ear-Eze, Otic-Care, Oticair Otic, Otocort, Otosporin	Bacterial infections of the external auditory canal	Few; can cause ear irritation, burning, or itching; when used for prolonged periods there is a danger of a superinfection	4 gtt instilled TID or QID
0.5% hydrocortisone, 10,000 units polymyxin B	Otobiotic Otic	Same as 1% hydrocortisone solution	Same as 1% hydrocortisone solution	4 gtt instilled TID or QID
Corticosteroid and Antibiotic Combinations, Suspensions				
1% hydrocortisone, 5 mg neomycin, 10,000 units polymyxin B	AK-Spore, AntibiOtic, Antibiotic Ear Suspension, Otocort, UAD Otic, Pediotic	Same as 1% hydrocortisone solution	Same as 1% hydrocortisone solution	4 gtt instilled TID or QID
1% hydrocortisone, 4.71 mg neomycin	Coly-Mycin S Otic	Same as 1% hydrocortisone solution	Same as 1% hydrocortisone solution	4 gtt instilled TID or QID
1% hydrocortisone, 3.3 mg neomycin	Cortisporin-TC Otic	Same as 1% hydrocortisone solution	Same as 1% hydrocortisone solution	4 gtt instilled TID or QID
2 mg ciprofloxacin, 10 mg hydrocortisone/mL	Cipro HC Otic	Same as 1% hydrocortisone solution	Same as 1% hydrocortisone solution	4 gtt instilled TID or QID
Otic Antibiotic				
ofloxacin (otic)	Floxin Otic	Otitis externa, chronic suppurative otitis media, acute otitis media	Local irritation, itching, burning, earache	Ages 1–12 yr: 5 gtt BID into affected ear for 10 days. Ages 12 yr and older: 10 gtt BID into affected ear for 10–14 days
Select Miscellaneous Preparations				
1% hydrocortisone, 2% acetic acid, 3% propylene glycol, 0.015% sodium, 0.02% benzethonium chloride	Acetasol HC, VoSoL HC Otic	Relieve pain, inflammation, and irritation in the external auditory canal	Local irritation, itching, burning	Insert saturated wick into ear; leave for 24 hr, keeping moist with 3–5 gtt q 4–6 hr. Keep moist for 24 hr; remove wick and instill 5 gtt TID or QID
1% hydrocortisone, 1% pramoxine, 0.1% chloroxylenol, 3% propylene glycol and benzalkonium chloride	Cortic	Same as 1% hydrocortisone solution	Same as 1% hydrocortisone solution	Insert saturated wick into ear; leave in for 24 hr, keeping moist with 3–5 gtt q 4–6 hr; remove wick and instill 5 gtt TID or QID
1% hydrocortisone, 2% acetic acid glacial, 3% propylene glycol, 0.02% benzethonium chloride, 0.015% sodium, 0.2% citric acid	AA-HC Otic	Same as 1% hydrocortisone solution	Same as 1% hydrocortisone solution	Insert saturated wick into the ear; leave in for 24 hr, keeping moist with 3–5 gtt q 4–6 hr; remove wick and instill 5 gtt TID or QID

Summary Drug Table SELECTED OTIC PREPARATIONS (continued)

Generic Combinations	Trade Name	Uses	Adverse Reactions	Dosage Ranges
1.4% benzocaine, 5.4% antipyrine glycerin	Allergen Ear Drops, Auralgan Otic, Auroto Otic Ear Drops, Otocalm Ear	Relieve ear pain	Local irritation, itching, burning	Fill ear canal with 2–4 gtt; insert saturated cotton pledget; repeat TID or QID or q 1–2 hr
20% benzocaine, 0.1% benzethonium chloride, 1% glycerin, PEG 300	Americaine Otic, Otocain	Relieve ear pain temporarily	Local irritation, itching, burning	Instill 4–5 gtt; insert cotton pledget; repeat q 1–2 hr
10% triethanolamine polypeptide oleate condensate, 0.5% chlorobutanol, propylene glycol	Cerumenex Drops	Aid in the removal of ear wax	Local irritation, itching, burning	Fill ear canal, insert cotton plug, allow to remain 15–30 min, flush ear
1 mg chloroxylenol, 10 mg hydrocortisone, 10 mg/mL pramoxine	Otomar-HC	Relieve pain and irritation in the external auditory canal	Local irritation, itching, burning	Instill 5 gtt into affected ear TID or QID
2% acetic acid in aluminum acetate solution	Burow's Otic, Otic Domeboro	Relieve pain and irritation in the external auditory canal	Local irritation, itching, burning	Insert saturated wick; keep moist for 24 hr; instill 4–6 gtt q 2–3 hr

Summary Drug Table SELECTED OPHTHALMIC PREPARATIONS

Generic Name	Trade Name	Uses	Dosage Ranges
α₂-Adrenergic Agonist			
brimonidine *brih-moe'-nih-deen*	Alphagan-P	Lowers IOP in patients with open-angle (chronic) glaucoma	1 gtt in affected eye(s) TID
Sympathomimetics			
apraclonidine *app-rah-kloe'-nih-deen*	Iopidine	1% Solution: control or prevention of postoperative elevations in IOP 5% Solution: short-term therapy in patients receiving maximal medical therapy who require additional IOP reduction	1% Solution: 1 gtt in operative eye 1 hr before surgery and 1 gtt immediately after surgery 5% Solution: 1–2 gtt in the affected eye(s) TID
dipivefrin *dye-pih'-veh-frin*	Propine, AKPro	Open-angle glaucoma	1 gtt into affected eye(s) q 12 hr
epinephrine *epp-ih-neff'-rin*	Epifrin, Glaucon Solution	Open-angle (chronic) glaucoma; may be used in combination with miotics, β blockers, or carbonic anhydrase inhibitors	1–2 gtt into affected eye(s) daily or BID
α-Adrenergic Blocking Drugs			
dapiprazole *dap-ih-pray'-zoll*	Rev-Eyes	Reverse diagnostic mydriasis after ophthalmic examination	2 gtt into the conjunctiva of each eye, followed 5 min later by an additional 2 gtt

(table continues on page 610)

Summary Drug Table SELECTED OPHTHALMIC PREPARATIONS (continued)

Generic Name	Trade Name	Uses	Dosage Ranges
β-Adrenergic Blocking Drugs			
betaxolol *beh-tax'-oh-lahl*	Betoptic, Betoptic S	Chronic open-angle glaucoma, ocular hypertension	1–2 gtt in the affected eye(s) BID
carteolol *car'-tee-oh-lahl*	Ocupress	Same as betaxolol	1 gtt in affected eye(s) TID
levobetaxolol *lee'-voe-beh-tax'-oh-lahl*	Betaxon	Same as betaxolol	1 gtt in affected eye(s) BID
levobunolol *lee'-voe-byoo'-noe-lahl*	AKBeta, Betagan Liquifilm	Same as betaxolol	0.5% Solution: 1–2 gtt in affected eye(s) daily 0.25% Solution: 1–2 gtt in affected eye(s) BID
metipranolol *meh-tih-pran'-oh-lahl*	OptiPranolol	Treatment of elevated IOP in patients with ocular hypertension or open-angle glaucoma	1 gtt in affected eye(s) BID
timolol *tih'-moe-lahl*	Betimol, Timoptic, Timoptic-XE	Reduces IOP in ocular hypertension or open-angle glaucoma	1 gtt in affected eye(s) daily or BID Gel: invert the closed container and shake once before each use; administer 1 gtt/day
Miotics, Direct Acting and Cholinesterase Inhibitor			
carbachol *car'-bah-koll*	Carboptic, Isopto Carbachol	Glaucoma	1–2 gtt up to TID
pilocarpine *pye-loe-car'-peen*	Isopto Carpine, Pilopine HS	Glaucoma, preoperative and postoperative intraocular hypertension	Solution: 1–2 gtt in affected eye(s) Gel: apply a 0.5-in ribbon in the lower conjunctival sac of affected eye(s) daily at bedtime
echothiophate iodide *eck-oh-thye'-oh-fate* *eyé-oh-dyde*	Phospholine Iodide	Chronic open-angle glaucoma, accommodative esotropia Esotropia: 1 gtt daily	Glaucoma: 2 doses/day in the morning and at bedtime or 1 dose every other day
Carbonic Anhydrase Inhibitors			
brinzolamide *brin-zoll'-ah-myde*	Azopt	Open-angle glaucoma, ocular hypertension	1 gtt in affected eye(s) TID
dorzolamide *dore-zoll'-ah-myde*	Trusopt	Open-angle glaucoma, ocular hypertension	1 gtt in affected eye(s) TID
Prostaglandin Agonists			
latanoprost *lah-tan'-oh-prahst*	Xalatan	First-line treatment of open-angle glaucoma, ocular hypertension	1 gtt in affected eye(s) daily in the evening
travoprost *trav'-oh-prahst*	Travatan	Reduction of increased IOP in patients with glaucoma who do not respond to or cannot take other drugs to lower IOP	1 gtt in affected eye(s) daily in the evening
bimatoprost *bih-mat'-oh-prahst*	Lumigan	Same as travoprost	1 gtt in affected eye(s) daily in the evening
unoprostone isopropyl *yoo-noh-pross'-toan*	Rescula	Same as travoprost	1 gtt in affected eye(s) BID
Combinations Used to Treat Glaucoma			
brimonidine/timolol	Combigan	Glaucoma	1 gtt in the affected eye(s) 2 times daily
dorzolamide/timolol *dore-zoll'-ah-myde*	Cosopt	Open-angle glaucoma and ocular hypertension	1 gtt into the affected eye(s) BID

Summary Drug Table SELECTED OPHTHALMIC PREPARATIONS (continued)

Generic Name	Trade Name	Uses	Dosage Ranges
Mast Cell Stabilizers			
nedocromil *neh-doe'-roe-mill*	Alocril	Allergic conjunctivitis	1–2 gtt in each eye BID
pemirolast *peh-meer'-oh-last*	Alamast	Allergic conjunctivitis	1–2 gtt in each eye QID
Nonsteroidal Anti-Inflammatory Drugs			
bromfenac *brom'-fen-ak*	Xibrom	Postoperative pain and inflammation after cataract surgery	1 gtt BID
diclofenac *dye-kloe'-fen-ak*	Voltaren	Postoperative inflammation after cataract surgery	1 gtt QID
flurbiprofen *floor-bye'-proe-fen*	Ocufen	Inhibition of intraoperative miosis	1 gtt q 30 min beginning 2 hr before surgery (total of 4 gtt)
ketorolac *keh-tor'-oh-lak*	Acular	Relief of ocular itching due to seasonal allergies, pain after corneal refractive surgery	Allergies: 1 drop QID Postoperative pain: 1 gtt in operated eye
nepafenac *neh-pah'-fen-ak*	Nevanac	Postoperative pain and inflammation after cataract surgery	1 gtt TID
Corticosteroids			
dexamethasone *dex-ah-meth'-ah-soan*	AK-Dex, Maxidex	Treatment of inflammatory conditions of the conjunctiva, eyelid, cornea, anterior segment of the eye	Solution: 1–2 gtt q hr during the day and q 2 hr at night, reduced to 1 gtt q 4 hr when response noted, then 1 gtt TID or QID Ointment: thin coating in lower conjunctival sac TID or QID
fluorometholone *floo-roh-meth'-oh-loan*	Flarex, Fluor-Op	Treatment of inflammatory conditions of the conjunctiva, lid, cornea, anterior segment of the eye	Suspension: 1–2 gtt BID–QID, may increase to 2 gtt q 2 hr Ointment: thin coating in lower conjunctival sac 1–3 times daily (up to 1 application q 4 hr)
loteprednol *loe-teh-pred'-noll*	Alrex, Lotemax	Allergic conjunctivitis	1–2 gtt QID
prednisolone *pred-niss'-oh-loan*	AK-Pred, Pred Forte, Pred Mild	Treatment of inflammatory conditions of the conjunctiva, lid, cornea, anterior segment of the eye	1–2 gtt/hr during the day and q 2 hr at night, reduced to 1 gtt q 4 hr, then 1 gtt TID or QID Suspensions: 1–2 gtt BID–QID
Antibiotics			
azithromycin *ah-zith-roe-mye'-sin*	AzaSite	Treatment of eye infections	See package insert
bacitracin *bass-ih-tray'-sin*	AK-Tracin	Same as azithromycin	See package insert
ciprofloxacin *sih-proe-flox'-ah-sin*	Ciloxan	Same as azithromycin	See package insert
erythromycin *eh-rith-roe-mye'-sin*		Same as azithromycin	See package insert
gatifloxacin *gah-tah-flox'-ah-sin*	Zymar	Same as azithromycin	Days 1 and 2: instill 1 gtt in affected eye(s) q 2 hr while awake, up to 8 times daily Days 3–7: instill 1 gtt in affected eye up to QID while awake

(table continues on page 612)

Summary Drug Table **SELECTED OPHTHALMIC PREPARATIONS** (continued)

Generic Name	Trade Name	Uses	Dosage Ranges
gentamicin *jen-tah-mye'-sin*	Gentak	Same as azithromycin	See package insert
levofloxacin *lee-voe-flox'-ah-sin*	Quixin	Same as azithromycin	Days 1 and 2: instill 1–2 gtt in affected eye(s) q 2 hr while awake, up to 8 times daily Days 3–7: instill 1–2 gtt in affected eye up to QID while awake
moxifloxacin *mox-ah-flox'-ah-sin*	Vigamox	Same as azithromycin	Adults and children at least 1 year of age: 1 drop in affected eye TID for 7 days
norfloxacin *nor-flox'-ah-sin*	Chibroxin	Same as azithromycin	Adults and children age 1 year and older: 1 or 2 gtt applied topically in the affected eye(s) QID for up to 7 days; dosage may be 1 or 2 gtt q 2 hr during waking hours the first day of treatment if the infection is severe
ofloxacin *oh-flox'-ah-sin*	Ocuflox	Same as azithromycin, corneal ulcers	Bacterial conjunctivitis: days 1 and 2: 1–2 gtt q 2–4 hr in the affected eye(s); days 3–7: 1–2 gtt QID Bacterial corneal ulcer: days 1 and 2: 1–2 gtt into the affected eye q 30 min while awake; awaken approximately q 4–6 hr and instill 1–2 gtt; days 3 through 7–9: instill 1–2 drops QID
polymyxin B *pah-lee-mix'-in*		Same as azithromycin	See package insert
tobramycin *toe-brah-mye'-sin*	Tobrex, Defy	Same as azithromycin	See package insert
sulfacetamide *sul-fah-see'-tah-myde*	Sulster, AK-Sulf, Bleph-10, Ocusulf-10	Ocular infections, trachoma	Ocular infections: 1–2 gtt q 1–4 hr Trachoma: 2 gtt q 2 hr Ointments: 0.5 in. into lower conjunctival sac TID or QID
sulfisoxazole *sul-fah-sox'-ah-zoll*		Ocular infections, trachoma	Ocular infections: 1–2 gtt q 1–4 hr Trachoma: 2 gtt q 2 hr
Silver Compound			
silver nitrate *nye'-trate*		Prevention of ophthalmia neonatorum	2 gtt of 1% solution in each eye
Antiviral Drugs			
ganciclovir *gan-sih'-kloe-veer*	Vitrasert	CMV retinitis	Implant used for 5–8 mo
idoxuridine *eye-dox-yoor'-ih-deen*	Herplex	Herpes simplex keratitis	1 gtt q hr during the day and q 2 hr at night

Summary Drug Table SELECTED OPHTHALMIC PREPARATIONS (continued)

Generic Name	Trade Name	Uses	Dosage Ranges
trifluridine *tri-floor'-ih-deen*	Viroptic	Keratoconjunctivitis keratitis, epithelial keratitis	Adults and children older than 6 yr: 1 gtt onto the corners of affected eye(s) while awake Maximum daily dose: 9 gtt until corneal ulcer has completely re-epithelialized, treat for an additional 7 days with 1 gtt q 4 hr for a maximum of 5 gtt/day
vidarabine *vye-dare'-ah-been*		Treatment of herpes simplex keratitis and conjunctivitis	0.5 in. of ointment into lower conjunctival sac 5 times daily at 3-hr intervals
Antifungal Drug			
natamycin *nah-tah-mye'-sin*	Natacyn	Fungal infections of the eye	1 gtt q 1–2 hr
Vasoconstrictors/Mydriatics			
oxymetazoline *ox-ih-met-az'-oh-leen*	OcuClear, Visine LR	Relief of redness of eye due to minor irritation	1–2 gtt q 6 hr
phenylephrine *fen-ill-eff'-rin*	AK-Dilate 2.5%, Neo-Synephrine 10%, AK-Nephrin	0.12% for relief of redness of eye due to minor irritation; 2.5% and 10% for treatment of uveitis and glaucoma, refraction procedures, before eye surgery	0.12%: 1–2 gtt up to QID 2.5% and 10%: 1–2 gtt in the eye up to QID (may have up to 8 gtt/day)
tetrahydrozoline *tet-trah-hye-drah'-zoh-leen*	Murine Plus Eye Drops, Visine	Relief of eye redness due to minor irritation	1–2 gtt up to QID
Cycloplegics/Mydriatics			
atropine *at'-troe-peen*	Isopto-Atropine	Mydriasis/cycloplegia	1–2 gtt up to TID
homatropine hydrobromide *hoe-mah'-troe-peen*	Isopto Homatropine	Mydriasis/cycloplegia	1–2 gtt q 3–4 hr
Ocular Lubricants			
benzalkonium chloride *benz-al-koe'-nee-um*	Artificial Tears	Treatment of dry eyes	1–2 gtt TID or QID
0.25% glycerin, EDTA sodium chloride, benzalkonium chloride	Eye-Lube-A	Treatment of dry eyes	1–2 gtt TID or QID

Chapter Review

Know Your Drugs

Clients sometimes know a medication by the brand (or trade) name and not the generic name. To help you recognize both names, match the brand name with the generic name of the same medication.

Generic Name	Brand Name
1. ofloxacin otic	A. Ocuflox
2. diclofenac	B. Alamast
3. ofloxacin ophthalmic	C. Floxin
4. pemirolast	D. Voltaren

Calculate Medication Dosages

1. The primary health care provider orders 0.5 mL of Burow's solution for ear pain. If the dropper used delivers 0.1 mL/drop, how many drops should be instilled into the ear?

2. If the ophthalmic drug Latisse comes in a 3-mL container and each drop is 0.05 mL, how many doses are there in the container?

Prepare for the NCLEX®

Build Your Knowledge

1. The cochlea and ossicles are in which segment of the ear?

   1. inner ear
   2. middle ear
   3. outer ear

2. In glaucoma intraocular pressure builds because _____.

   1. the client has a headache
   2. the drainage of the anterior eye chamber is blocked
   3. hypertension causes increased pressure
   4. the sinus cavities drain into the eye

3. When administering an otic solution, the drug is instilled into the _____.

   1. inner canthus
   2. auditory canal
   3. canal of Schlemm
   4. upper canthus

4. Which of the following adverse reactions would the nurse suspect in a client receiving prolonged treatment with an antibiotic otic drug?

   1. congestive heart failure
   2. superinfection
   3. anemia
   4. hypersensitivity reactions

5. When administering an ophthalmic solution, the drug is instilled into the _____.

   1. inner canthus
   2. upper conjunctival sac
   3. lower conjunctival sac
   4. upper canthus

6. Which of the following instructions would be included in a teaching plan for the client prescribed an ophthalmic solution?

   1. Squeeze the eyes tightly after the solution is instilled.
   2. Immediately wipe the eye using pressure to squeeze out excess medication.
   3. After the drug is instilled, remain upright with the head bent slightly forward for about 2 minutes.
   4. A temporary stinging or burning may be felt at the time the drug is instilled.

Apply Your Knowledge

7. What is the rationale for warming an otic solution that has been refrigerated before instilling the drops into the client's ear?

   1. The drug becomes thick when refrigerated, and warming liquefies the solution.
   2. It helps to prevent dizziness on instillation.
   3. A cold solution could significantly increase the client's blood pressure.
   4. A cold solution could damage the tympanic membrane.

8. The client has vision problems yet has been instilling his own eye solutions for years. He brings his own medication to the hospital, and the nurse notes that the half-used bottle is yellow and cloudy. What is the *first* intervention the nurse should perform?

   1. contact the primary health care provider immediately
   2. set the solution out for the client to use
   3. ask the client when he last used this specific container
   4. throw it away and get a new bottle of solution

Alternate-Format Questions

9. Which sections of the ear are typically treated with topical preparations? **Select all that apply**.

   1. inner ear
   2. middle ear
   3. outer ear
   4. the eye

To check your answers, see Appendix G.

thePoint *For more NCLEX-style questions, log on to http://thepoint.lww.com to access more than 1000 questions.*

Fluids, Electrolytes, and Parenteral Therapy

On completion of this chapter, the student will:

1. List the types and uses of solutions used in the parenteral management of body fluids.
2. List the steps involved in the intravenous (IV) administration of a solution or electrolyte used in the management of body fluids.
3. Describe the calculations used to establish IV flow rates.
4. List the types and uses of electrolytes used in the management of electrolyte imbalances.
5. Discuss the more common signs and symptoms of electrolyte imbalance.
6. Discuss preadministration and ongoing assessment activities the nurse should perform with the patient administered an electrolyte or an IV solution to manage body fluids.
7. List nursing diagnoses particular to a patient receiving an electrolyte or a solution to manage body fluids.
8. Discuss ways to promote an optimal response to therapy and important points to keep in mind when educating patients about the use of an electrolyte or a solution to manage body fluids.

KEY TERMS

electrolyte • electrically charged substance essential to the normal functioning of all cells

extravasation • escape of fluid from a blood vessel into surrounding tissue

fluid overload • condition in which the body's fluid requirements are met and the administration of fluid occurs at a rate that is greater than the rate at which the body can use or eliminate the fluid; also called *circulatory overload*

heparin (or saline) lock • equipment consisting of an adapter and tubing introduced into a vein to maintain access to circulation

infiltration • collection of fluid into tissue

normal saline • solution of 0.9% sodium chloride and water, which is the proportion of salt and water normally circulating in body fluid

parenteral • administration of a substance, such as a drug, by any route other than through the gastrointestinal (GI) system (e.g., oral or rectal route)

total parenteral nutrition • complex admixture of nutrients combined in a single container and administered to the body by an IV route

DRUG CLASSES

Electrolytes	• Potassium
• Calcium	• Sodium
• Magnesium	Alkaline/acidifying agents

PHARMACOLOGY IN PRACTICE

Alfredo Garcia is a 55-year-old man being seen in the clinic for an upper respiratory infection. During the intake assessment, you find that his blood pressure is high and he continues to complain of "heartburn." Mr. Garcia attempted to use home remedies (e.g., drinking cream) to decrease acid production. You have taught him about ulcer treatment, yet his heartburn persists. He continues to rely on home remedies, which are causing other problems. Mr. Garcia's weight is up, and looking at his legs, you note +2 pitting edema bilaterally. While reading the chapter, you will learn about some of the problems that can happen with electrolyte imbalances.

Over 50% of our body is made up of fluid. It gives our cells shape, acts as a cushion by filling the void between cells, and travels throughout our bodies with elements to help cells work or eliminate waste. The electrolytes also play important roles in our daily function. This chapter offers information about our fluids and electrolytes as well as basics on parenteral (IV) therapy. The clinical setting where nurses work determines the role you will play in IV therapy. Who starts the IV, monitors it, and accesses the line for medication administration is different in each setting. No matter where you practice nursing, it is important to understand the basic concepts of fluid and electrolyte balance.

Fluid makes up a major portion of our body tissues. When individuals become ill, they may lose excess amounts of fluid or not feel well enough to maintain the daily intake of fluid needed for basic survival. Without fluids, the body's ability to transport oxygen and nutrients to the various tissues is compromised. Individual cells or organs are not able to function and the person becomes even more ill. Various solutions are used in the management of body fluids. These solutions are used when the body cannot sustain the fluid or **electrolyte** balance needed for normal functioning.

Parenteral Management of Body Fluids

Parenteral administration includes the injecting of drugs or solutions directly into a vein. In the acute care or urgent care setting, solutions used to manage body fluids are usually administered IV. Intravenous replacement solutions are used for the following:

- As a parenteral source of electrolytes, calories, or water for hydration
- To facilitate nutrition and maintain electrolyte balance when the patient cannot eat
- As a method to deliver drugs when a less invasive method is not suitable due to drug pharmacokinetics or patient status

Establishing Intravenous Access

All facilities have specific policies and procedures for cleaning, access, and stabilization of IV sites. Basic steps are outlined in this section. When selecting a vein for IV access, the nondominant arm is typically selected and inspected, and a site is often picked at the most distal point. Larger, more proximal veins may be selected, depending on the need for the IV therapy. You should ask the patient about previous IV therapy. The patient can frequently tell you if a specific site gives providers trouble when access is attempted. This can save time and reduce the pain of an unsuccessful attempt when the patient's knowledge of previous care is considered.

When a site has been selected for venipuncture, place a tourniquet above the selected vein. It is important to tighten the tourniquet so that venous blood flow is blocked but arterial blood flow is not. Cleanse the site according to facility policy. The vein fills (distends) and then the skin is pulled taut (to anchor the vein and the skin) and the needle is inserted into the vein bevel up, and at a low angle to the skin. Blood should immediately flow into the syringe if the needle is properly inserted into the vein. If the IV is being placed for a period of time, a device with a cannula is used. With this device, the needle is then removed, and a flexible cannula remains in the vein. The cannula is secured in place, and the device is ready for administration of drugs or fluids.

Performing a venipuncture requires practice. A suitable vein for venipuncture may be hard to find, and some veins are difficult to enter. Never repeatedly and unsuccessfully attempt a venipuncture. Depending on clinical judgment, two unsuccessful attempts on the same patient warrant having a more skilled individual attempt the procedure.

Maintaining Intravenous Access

Intermittent Intravenous Access

Fluids, electrolytes, and drugs are given by direct IV push, intermittent infusion, or continuous infusion. When the direct IV method or intermittent infusion is used, the cannula that stays in the vein, an adapter, and small tubing are called a **heparin (or saline) lock**, and it is secured to the arm (Fig. 54.1). The device allows for a dose to be given directly into a vein or via intermittent IV administration without having to maintain an infusion. A lock also gives the patient the ability to move about more freely without cumbersome IV lines or machines to impede activities such as ambulation.

To maintain the patency of the lock, a solution of saline or dilute heparin may be ordered for injection into the heparin lock before and after the administration of a drug administered via the IV route. This is called a *lock flush*. The flush solution aids in preventing small clots from obstructing the cannula of the IV administration set. Patients may hear providers refer to the device as both a saline and a heparin lock. The primary health care provider or institutional policy dictates the use and strength of heparin lock flush solution. It is important to know the policies of your institution to be sure that you access the device with the appropriate solution. Should the policy of your institution be the use of heparin, be sure to prevent incompatibility of heparin with other drugs, and flush with sterile **normal saline** solution before and after any drug is given through the IV line.

> **! NURSING ALERT**
>
> Do not mix multiple IV medications in a syringe (e.g., benzodiazepines and furosemide) without consulting the clinical pharmacist about compatibility. When injecting multiple drugs sequentially, always flush thoroughly and monitor the IV site for phlebitis and/or thrombosis.

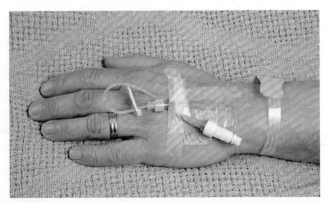

Figure 54.1 IV access (saline/heparin lock) for intermittent infusions or direct administration of drugs.

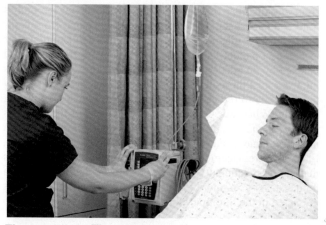

Figure 54.2 The nurse sets the electronic IV device to deliver a specific amount of IV fluid.

Continuous Infusion Access

Continuous infusion involves a continual flow of fluid into a vein for replacement purposes and continuous or frequent drug administration. Electronic infusion devices monitor the rate and flow of intravenous fluids (Fig. 54.2). The purpose of the device is to monitor the flow of the intravenous solution. An alarm is set to sound if the rate of infusion is more or less than the preset rate. These machines are classified as either infusion controllers or infusion pumps. The primary difference between the two is that an infusion pump adds pressure to the infusion, whereas an infusion controller does not.

When any problem is detected by the device, an alarm is activated to alert the nurse. Controllers and pumps have detectors and alarms that sound when various problems occur, such as air in the line, an occlusion, low battery, completion of an infusion, or an inability to deliver the preset rate.

> **NURSING ALERT**
> Use of an infusion pump or controller still requires nursing supervision and frequent monitoring of the IV infusion.

It is important to monitor frequently for signs of **infiltration** (the collection of fluid into tissues), such as edema or redness at the site. Infiltration can progress rapidly, because with the increased pressure the infusion will not slow until considerable edema has occurred. Careful monitoring of the pump or controller is also necessary to make sure the flow rate is correct.

When the patient needs fluid replacement and drugs are to be administered, a secondary line is established using the IV route. Intermittent IV infusion is given using "Y" tubing while another solution is being given on a continuous basis. When this method is used, depending on the machine you may have to clamp off the IV fluid given on a continuous basis while the drug is allowed to infuse or the two solutions may infuse at the same time.

Calculating Intravenous Flow Rates

When fluid replacement is indicated, the amount (or volume) of fluid to be administered is ordered over a specified time period, such as 125 mL/hr or 1000 mL over 8 hours. Many infusion machines work by setting the volume of fluid to be infused over a specific time period. If the IV is not infused

through a machine or if the machine monitors the drip rate, then the IV flow rate must be calculated.

The IV flow rate is obtained by counting the number of drops in the drip chamber and using the amount of fluid in each drop to calculate the volume. Drip chambers on the various types of IV fluid administration sets vary. Some deliver 15 drops/mL and others deliver more or less than this number. This is called the *drop factor.* The drop factor (number of drops/mL) is given on the package containing the drip chamber and IV tubing. Three methods for determining the IV infusion rate follow. Methods 1 and 2 can be used when the known factors are the total amount of solution, the drop factor, and the number of hours over which the solution is to be infused.

Method 1
Step 1. Total amount of solution ÷ number of hours = number of mL/hr
Step 2. mL/hr ÷ 60 min/hr = number of mL/min
Step 3. mL/min × drop factor = number of drops/min

Example
1000 mL of an IV solution is to infuse over a period of 8 hours. The drop factor is 15.

Step 1. 1000 mL ÷ 8 hours = 125 mL/hr
Step 2. 125 mL ÷ 60 minutes = 2.08 mL/min
Step 3. 2.08 × 15 = 31.2 or (31 to 32) drops/min

Method 2
Step 1. Total amount of solution ÷ number of hours = number of mL/hr
Step 2. mL/hr × drop factor ÷ 60 = number of drops/min

Example
1000 mL of an IV solution is to infuse over a period of 6 hours. The drop factor is 10.

Step 1. 1000 mL ÷ 6 hours = 166.6 mL/hr
Step 2. 166.6 × 10 ÷ 60 = 26.66 or (26 to 27) drops/min

Method 3
This method may be used when the desired amount of solution to be infused in 1 hour is known or written as a physician's order.

$$\frac{\text{drops/mL of given set (drop factor)}}{60 \times \text{(minutes in an hour)}} \times \text{total hourly volume} = \text{drops/min}$$

Example
If a set delivers 15 drops/min and 240 mL is to be infused in 1 hour:

$$\frac{15}{60} \times 240 = \frac{1}{4} \times 240 = 60 \text{ drops/min}$$

Fluid Overload

One problem commonly associated with all solutions administered by the parenteral route is fluid overload, that is, the administration of more fluid than the body is able to handle.

The term **fluid overload** (also *circulatory overload*) describes a condition when the body's fluid requirements are met and the administration of fluid occurs at a rate that is

---

Display 54.1 Signs and Symptoms of Fluid Overload

- Headache
- Weakness
- Blurred vision
- Behavioral changes (confusion, disorientation, delirium, drowsiness)
- Weight gain
- Isolated muscle twitching
- Hyponatremia
- Rapid breathing
- Wheezing
- Coughing
- Rise in blood pressure
- Distended neck veins
- Elevated central venous pressure
- Convulsions

---

greater than the rate at which the body can use or eliminate the fluid. Thus, the amount of fluid and the rate of administration of fluid that will cause fluid overload depend on several factors, such as the patient's cardiac status and adequacy of renal function. The signs and symptoms of fluid overload are listed in Display 54.1.

Solutions Used in the Management of Body Fluids

The next section gives a brief overview of the following IV replacement solutions: electrolytes, blood products and expanders, and **total parenteral nutrition** (TPN). One of the primary purposes of administering an IV solution is to provide proper electrolyte balance in the body.

ELECTROLYTES

An *electrolyte* is an electrically charged particle essential to the normal functioning of all cells. Intracellular and extracellular fluids have specific chemical compositions of electrolytes. Major electrolytes in intracellular fluid include:

- Potassium
- Magnesium

Major electrolytes in extracellular fluid include:

- Sodium
- Calcium

Electrolytes circulate in the blood at specific levels, where they are available for use when needed by the cells. An electrolyte imbalance occurs when the concentration of an electrolyte in the blood is either too high or too low. In some instances, an electrolyte imbalance may be present without an appreciable disturbance in fluid balance. An electrolyte imbalance can profoundly affect a patient's physiologic functioning, the body's water distribution, neuromuscular activity, and acid-base balance. An electrolyte imbalance can occur

from any disorder that alters electrolyte levels in the body's fluid compartments. An imbalance can also occur from vomiting, surgery, diagnostic tests, or drug administration. For example, a patient taking a diuretic is able to maintain fluid balance by an adequate oral intake of water, which replaces the water lost through diuresis. However, the patient is likely to be unable to replace the potassium that is also lost during diuresis. When the potassium concentration in the blood is too low, as may occur with the administration of a diuretic, an imbalance may occur that requires the addition of potassium. Electrolyte replacement drugs are inorganic or organic salts that increase deficient electrolyte levels that help to maintain homeostasis. Commonly used electrolyte replacement drugs are listed in the Summary Drug Table: Electrolytes.

INTRACELLULAR ELECTROLYTES

Action and Uses

Potassium (K$^+$)

Potassium is the major electrolyte in intracellular fluid and must be consumed daily because it cannot be stored. It is necessary for the transmission of impulses; the contraction of smooth, cardiac, and skeletal muscles; and other important physiologic processes. Potassium may be given to correct hypokalemia (low blood potassium) resulting from increased potassium excretion or depletion. Examples of causes of hypokalemia are a marked loss of GI fluids (severe vomiting, diarrhea, nasogastric suction, draining intestinal fistulas), diabetic acidosis, marked diuresis, severe malnutrition, use of a potassium-depleting diuretic, excess antidiuretic hormone, and excessive urination. Potassium as a drug is available as potassium chloride (KCl) and potassium gluconate, and is measured in milliequivalents (mEq)—for example, 40 mEq in 20 mL or 8-mEq controlled-release tablet.

Magnesium (Mg^{++})

Magnesium plays an important role in the transmission of nerve impulses. It is also important in the activity of many enzyme reactions, such as carbohydrate metabolism. Magnesium sulfate (MgSO$_4$) is used as replacement therapy in hypomagnesemia. Magnesium is also used in the prevention and control of seizures in obstetric patients with pregnancy-induced hypertension (PIH; also referred to as *eclampsia* and *preeclampsia*). It may also be added to TPN mixtures.

Adverse Reactions, Contraindications, Precautions, and Interactions

Potassium (K$^+$)

Nausea, vomiting, diarrhea, abdominal pain, and phlebitis have been seen with oral and IV administration of potassium. Adverse reactions related to hypokalemia or hyperkalemia are listed in Display 54.2.

Potassium is contraindicated in patients who are at risk for hyperkalemia, such as those with renal failure, oliguria, azotemia (the presence of nitrogen-containing compounds in the blood), anuria, severe hemolytic reactions, untreated

---

Display 54.2 Signs and Symptoms of Electrolyte Imbalances

Calcium
Normal laboratory values: 4.5–5.3 mEq/L or
9–11 mg/dL*

Hypocalcemia
Hyperactive reflexes, carpopedal spasm, perioral
paresthesias, positive Trousseau's sign, positive
Chvostek's sign, muscle twitching, muscle cramps,
tetany (numbness, tingling, and muscular twitching
usually of the extremities), laryngospasm, cardiac
arrhythmias, nausea, vomiting, anxiety, confusion,
emotional lability, convulsions

Hypercalcemia
Anorexia, nausea, vomiting, lethargy, bone tenderness or pain, polyuria, polydipsia, constipation, dehydration, muscle weakness and atrophy, stupor, coma,
cardiac arrest

Magnesium
Normal laboratory values: 1.5–2.5 mEq/L or
1.8–3 mg/dL*

Hypomagnesemia
Leg and foot cramps, hypertension, tachycardia,
neuromuscular irritability, tremor, hyperactive deep
tendon reflexes, confusion, disorientation, visual or
auditory hallucinations, painful paresthesias, positive
Trousseau's sign, positive Chvostek's sign, convulsions

Hypermagnesemia
Lethargy, drowsiness, impaired respiration, flushing,
sweating, hypotension, weak to absent deep tendon
reflexes

Potassium
Normal laboratory values: 3.5–5 mEq/L*

Hypokalemia
Anorexia, nausea, vomiting, mental depression,
confusion, delayed or impaired thought processes,
drowsiness, abdominal distention, decreased bowel
sounds, paralytic ileus, muscle weakness or fatigue,
flaccid paralysis, absent or diminished deep tendon
reflexes, weak and irregular pulse, paresthesias, leg
cramps, electrocardiographic changes

Hyperkalemia
Irritability, anxiety, listlessness, mental confusion,
nausea, diarrhea, abdominal distress, GI hyperactivity, paresthesias, weakness and heaviness of the legs,
flaccid paralysis, hypotension, cardiac arrhythmias,
electrocardiographic changes

Sodium
Normal laboratory values: 132–145 mEq/L*

Hyponatremia
Cold and clammy skin, decreased skin turgor, apprehension, confusion, irritability, anxiety, hypotension,
postural hypotension, tachycardia, headache, tremors,
convulsions, abdominal cramps, nausea, vomiting,
diarrhea

Hypernatremia
Fever; hot, dry skin; dry, sticky mucous membranes;
rough, dry tongue; edema; weight gain; intense thirst;
excitement; restlessness; agitation; oliguria or anuria

*These laboratory values may not concur with the normal range of values in all hospitals and
laboratories. The hospital policy manual or laboratory values sheet should be consulted for the
normal ranges of all laboratory tests.

Addison's disease, acute dehydration, heat cramps, and any form of hyperkalemia. Potassium is used cautiously in patients with renal impairment or adrenal insufficiency, heart disease, metabolic acidosis, or prolonged or severe diarrhea.

Concurrent use of potassium with angiotensin-converting enzyme (ACE) inhibitors may result in an elevated serum potassium level. Potassium-sparing diuretics and salt substitutes used with potassium can produce severe hyperkalemia. The use of digitalis with potassium increases the risk of digoxin toxicity.

Magnesium (Mg⁺⁺)

Adverse reactions from magnesium administration are most likely related to overdose and may include flushing, sweating, hypotension, depressed reflexes, muscle weakness, respiratory failure, and circulatory collapse (see Display 54.2). Magnesium is contraindicated in patients with heart block or myocardial damage and in women with PIH during the 2 hours before delivery. Magnesium is a pregnancy category A drug, and there is no increased risk of fetal abnormalities

if the agent is used during pregnancy. Nevertheless, caution is used when administering magnesium during pregnancy.

Magnesium is used with caution in patients with renal function impairment. When magnesium is used with alcohol, antidepressants, antipsychotics, barbiturates, hypnotics, general anesthetics, and opioids, an increase in central nervous system depression may occur. Prolonged respiratory depression and apnea may occur when magnesium is administered with the neuromuscular blocking agents. When magnesium is used with digoxin, heart block may occur.

EXTRACELLULAR ELECTROLYTES

Action and Uses

Sodium (Na⁺)

Sodium is a major electrolyte in extracellular fluid and is important in maintaining acid-base balance and normal heart action, and in the regulation of osmotic pressure in body cells (water balance). Sodium is administered for hyponatremia (low blood sodium). Examples of causes of hyponatremia are excessive diaphoresis, severe vomiting or diarrhea, excessive diuresis, diuretic use, wound drainage, and draining intestinal fistulas.

Sodium, as sodium chloride (NaCl), may be given IV. A solution containing 0.9% NaCl is called *normal saline,* and a solution containing 0.45% NaCl is called half-normal saline. Sodium also is available combined with dextrose, such as dextrose 5% and sodium chloride 0.9% (D5NS).

Calcium (Ca⁺⁺)

Calcium is necessary for the functioning of nerves and muscles, the clotting of blood, the building of bones and teeth, and other physiologic processes. Examples of calcium salts are calcium gluconate and calcium carbonate. Calcium may be given for the treatment of hypocalcemia (low blood calcium), which may be seen in those with parathyroid disease or after accidental removal of the parathyroid glands during surgery of the thyroid gland. Calcium may also be given during cardiopulmonary resuscitation, particularly after open heart surgery, when epinephrine fails to improve weak or ineffective myocardial contractions. Calcium may be used as adjunct therapy of insect bites or stings to reduce muscle cramping, such as occurs with black widow spider bites. Calcium may also be recommended for those eating a diet low in calcium or as a dietary supplement when there is an increased need for calcium, such as during pregnancy.

Combined Electrolyte Solutions

Combined electrolyte solutions are available for oral and IV administration. The IV solutions contain various electrolytes and dextrose. The amount of electrolytes, given as milliequivalents per liter (mEq/L), also varies. The IV solutions are used to replace fluid and electrolytes that have been lost and to provide calories through their carbohydrate content. Examples of IV electrolyte solutions are dextrose 5% with 0.9% NaCl, lactated Ringer's, and Plasma-Lyte. The primary health care provider selects the type of combined electrolyte solution that will meet the patient's needs.

Oral electrolyte solutions contain a carbohydrate and various electrolytes. Examples of combined oral electrolyte solutions are Pedialyte and Rehydralyte. Oral electrolyte solutions are most often used to replace lost electrolytes and fluids in conditions such as severe vomiting or diarrhea.

Adverse Reactions, Contraindications, Precautions, and Interactions

Sodium (Na⁺)

Sodium as the salt (e.g., NaCl) has no adverse reactions except those related to overdose (see Display 54.2). In some instances, excessive oral use may produce nausea and vomiting.

Sodium is contraindicated in patients with hypernatremia or fluid retention, and when the administration of sodium or chloride could be detrimental. Sodium is used cautiously in surgical patients and those with circulatory insufficiency, hypoproteinemia, urinary tract obstruction, heart failure (HF), edema, or renal impairment. Sodium is a pregnancy category C drug and is used cautiously during pregnancy.

Calcium (Ca⁺⁺)

Irritation of the vein used for administration, tingling, a metallic or chalky taste, and "heat waves" may occur when calcium is given IV. Rapid IV administration (calcium gluconate) may result in bradycardia, vasodilation, decreased blood pressure, cardiac arrhythmias, and cardiac arrest. Oral administration may result in GI disturbances. Administration of calcium chloride may cause peripheral vasodilation, a temporary fall in blood pressure, and a local burning. Display 54.2 lists adverse reactions associated with hypercalcemia and hypocalcemia.

BLOOD PRODUCTS AND EXPANDERS

Actions and Uses

Blood Plasma

Blood plasma is the liquid part of blood, containing water, sugar, electrolytes, fats, gases, proteins, bile pigment, and clotting factors. Human plasma, also called human pooled plasma, is obtained from donated blood. Although whole blood must be typed and crossmatched because it contains red blood cells carrying blood type and Rh factors, human plasma does not require this procedure. Because of this, plasma can be given in acute emergencies.

Plasma administered IV is used to increase blood volume when severe hemorrhage has occurred and it is necessary partially to restore blood volume while waiting for whole blood to be typed and crossmatched or when plasma alone has been lost, as may be seen in severe burns.

Plasma Protein Fractions

Plasma protein fractions include human plasma protein fraction 5% and normal serum albumin 5% (Albuminar-5, Buminate 5%) and 25% (Albuminar-25, Buminate 25%). Plasma protein fraction 5% is an IV solution containing 5% human plasma proteins. Serum albumin is obtained from donated whole blood and is a protein found in plasma. The albumin fraction of human blood acts to maintain plasma colloid osmotic pressure and as a carrier of intermediate metabolites in the transport and exchange of tissue products. It is critical in regulating the volume of circulating blood. When blood is lost from shock, such as in hemorrhage, there is a reduced plasma volume. When blood volume is reduced, albumin quickly restores the volume in most situations.

Plasma protein fractions are used to treat hypovolemic (low blood volume) shock that occurs as the result of burns, trauma, surgery, and infections, or in conditions where shock is not currently present but likely to occur. As with human pooled plasma, blood type and crossmatch are not needed when plasma protein fractions are given. Adverse reactions are rare when plasma protein fractions are administered, but nausea, chills, fever, urticaria, and hypotensive episodes may occasionally be seen. Plasma proteins are contraindicated in those with a history of allergic reactions to albumin, severe anemia, or cardiac failure; in the presence of normal or increased intravascular volume; and in patients on cardiopulmonary bypass. Plasma protein fractions are used cautiously in patients who are in shock or dehydrated and in those with heart failure or hepatic or renal failure.

Most of these solutions should not be combined with any other solutions or drugs but should be administered alone. Consult the drug insert or other appropriate sources before combining any drug with any plasma protein fraction. Solutions used in the management of body fluids are contraindicated in patients with hypersensitivity to any component of the solution. All solutions used to manage body fluids discussed in this chapter are pregnancy category C drugs and are used cautiously during pregnancy and lactation. No interactions have been reported.

Plasma Expanders

The IV solutions of plasma expanders include hetastarch (Hespan), low–molecular-weight dextran (Dextran 40), and high–molecular-weight dextran (Dextran 70, Dextran 75).

Plasma expanders are used to expand plasma volume when shock is caused by burns, hemorrhage, surgery, and other trauma or for prophylaxis of venous thrombosis and thromboembolism. When used in the treatment of shock, plasma expanders are not a substitute for whole blood or plasma, but they are of value as emergency measures until the latter substances can be used.

Administration of hetastarch, a plasma expander, may be accompanied by vomiting, a mild temperature elevation, itching, and allergic reactions. Allergic reactions are evidenced by wheezing, swelling around the eyes (periorbital edema), and urticaria. Other plasma expanders may result in mild cutaneous eruptions, generalized urticaria, hypotension, nausea, vomiting, headache, dyspnea, fever, tightness of the chest, bronchospasm, wheezing, and, rarely, anaphylactic shock.

Plasma expanders are contraindicated in patients with hypersensitivity to any component of the solution and those with severe bleeding disorders, severe cardiac failure, renal failure with oliguria, or anuria. Plasma expanders are used cautiously in patients with renal disease, HF, pulmonary edema, and severe bleeding disorders. Plasma expanders are pregnancy category C drugs and are used cautiously during pregnancy and lactation. Consult the drug insert or other appropriate sources before combining a plasma expander with another drug for IV administration.

TOTAL PARENTERAL NUTRITION

When normal enteral feeding is not possible or is inadequate to meet an individual's nutritional needs, IV nutritional therapy or TPN is required. TPN is a method of administering nutrients to the body by an IV route. TPN uses a complex admixture of chemicals combined in a single container. The components of the TPN mixture may include proteins (amino acids), fats, glucose, electrolytes, vitamins, minerals, and sterile water. Products used to meet the IV nutritional requirements of the patient include protein substrates (amino acids), energy substrates (dextrose and fat emulsions), fluids, electrolytes, and trace minerals.

Total parenteral nutrition is used to prevent nitrogen and weight loss or to treat negative nitrogen balance (a situation in which more nitrogen is used by the body than is taken in) in the following situations:

- Oral, gastrostomy, or jejunostomy route cannot or should not be used.
- GI absorption of protein is impaired by obstruction.
- Inflammatory disease or antineoplastic therapy prevents normal GI functioning.
- Bowel rest is needed (e.g., after bowel surgery).
- Metabolic requirements for protein are significantly increased (e.g., in hypermetabolic states such as serious burns, infections, or trauma).
- Morbidity and mortality may be reduced by replacing amino acids lost from tissue breakdown (e.g., renal failure).
- Tube feeding alone cannot provide adequate nutrition.

If a patient's intake of protein nutrients is significantly less than is required by the body to meet energy expenditures, a state of negative nitrogen balance occurs. The body begins to convert protein from the muscle into carbohydrate for energy to be used by the body. This results in weight loss and muscle wasting. In these situations, traditional IV fluids do not provide sufficient calories or nitrogen to meet the body's daily requirements. TPN may be administered through a peripheral vein or a central venous catheter in a highly concentrated form to improve nutritional status, establish a positive nitrogen balance, and enhance the healing process. Peripheral TPN is used for relatively short periods (no more than 5 to 7 days) and when the central venous route is not possible or necessary. An example of a solution used in TPN is amino acids with electrolytes. These solutions may be used alone or combined with dextrose (5% or 10%) solutions.

Total parenteral nutrition through a central vein is indicated to promote protein synthesis in patients who are severely hypercatabolic or severely depleted of nutrients, or who require long-term parenteral nutrition. For example, amino acids combined with hypertonic dextrose and IV fat emulsions are infused through a central venous catheter to promote protein synthesis. Vitamins, trace minerals, and electrolytes may be added to the TPN mixture to meet the patient's individual needs. The daily dose depends on the patient's daily protein requirement and his or her metabolic state and clinical responses.

TPN is delivered with an infusion pump. The pump infuses a small amount (0.1 to 10 mL/hr) continuously to keep the vein open. Feeding schedules vary; one example is administration of the feeding continuously over a few hours, leveling off the rate for several hours, and then increasing the rate of administration for several hours to simulate a normal set of meal times.

! NURSING ALERT

Hyperglycemia is a common metabolic complication. If an infusion of TPN is given too rapidly it may result in hyperglycemia, glycosuria, mental confusion, and loss of consciousness. Assess blood glucose levels every 4 to 6 hours to monitor for hyperglycemia and guide the dosage of dextrose and insulin (if required). To minimize these complications, the primary health care provider may decrease the rate of administration, reduce the dextrose concentration, or administer insulin.

To prevent a rebound hypoglycemic reaction from the sudden withdrawal of TPN containing a concentrated dose of dextrose, the rate of administration is slowly reduced or the concentration of dextrose gradually decreased. If TPN must be abruptly withdrawn, a solution of 5% or 10% dextrose is begun to reduce gradually the amount of dextrose administered. The primary health care provider is notified if the patient exhibits symptoms of hypoglycemia, including weakness, tremors, diaphoresis, headache, hunger, and apprehension. Other complications of TPN include bacterial infection, sepsis, embolism, metabolic problems, and hemothorax or pneumothorax.

An IV fat emulsion contains soybean or safflower oil and a mixture of natural triglycerides, predominantly unsaturated fatty acids. It is used in the prevention and treatment of essential fatty acid deficiency. It also provides nonprotein calories for those receiving TPN when calorie requirements cannot be met by glucose. Examples of IV fat emulsion include Intralipid 10% and 20%, Liposyn II 10% and 20%, and Liposyn III 10% and 20%. Fat emulsion is used as a source of calories and essential fatty acids for patients requiring parenteral nutrition for extended periods (usually more than 5 days). No more than 60% of the patient's total caloric intake should come from fat emulsion, with carbohydrates and amino acids making up the remaining 40% or more of caloric intake.

The most common adverse reaction associated with the administration of fat emulsion is sepsis caused by administration equipment and thrombophlebitis caused by venous irritation from concurrently administering hypertonic solutions. Less frequent adverse reactions include dyspnea, cyanosis, hyperlipidemia, hypercoagulability, nausea, vomiting, headache, flushing, increased body temperature, sweating, sleepiness, chest and back pain, slight pressure over the eyes, and dizziness. Intravenous fat emulsions are contraindicated in conditions that interfere with normal fat metabolism (e.g., acute pancreatitis) and in patients allergic to eggs. IV fat emulsions are used with caution in those with severe liver impairment, pulmonary disease, anemia, and blood coagulation disorders. These solutions are pregnancy category C drugs and are used cautiously during pregnancy and lactation.

In general, fat emulsions should not be combined with any other solutions or drugs except when combined in TPN. Consult appropriate sources before combining any drug with a fat emulsion.

ALKALINIZING AND ACIDIFYING DRUGS

Alkalinizing and acidifying drugs are used to correct an acid-base imbalance in the blood. The acid-base imbalances are:

- Metabolic acidosis—decrease in the blood pH caused by an excess of hydrogen ions in the extracellular fluid (treated with alkalinizing drugs)
- Metabolic alkalosis—increase in the blood pH caused by an excess of bicarbonate in the extracellular fluid (treated with acidifying drugs)

ALKALINIZING DRUG: BICARBONATE (HCO_3^-)

Action and Uses

A low blood pH means the body is in an acidic condition, and a high blood pH indicates an alkaline condition. To raise the pH, an alkalinizing drug must be administered. Sodium bicarbonate, an alkalinizing drug, separates in the blood and

the bicarbonate functions as a buffer to decrease the hydrogen ion concentration and raise the blood pH.

Bicarbonate (HCO_3^-) plays a vital role in the acid-base balance of the body. Alkalinizing drugs are used to treat metabolic acidosis and to increase blood pH. Bicarbonate may be given IV as sodium bicarbonate ($NaHCO_3$) in the treatment of metabolic acidosis, a state of imbalance that may be seen in diseases or conditions such as severe shock, diabetic acidosis, severe diarrhea, extracorporeal circulation of blood, severe renal disease, and cardiac arrest. Oral sodium bicarbonate is used as a gastric and urinary alkalinizer. It may be used as a single drug or may be found as one of the ingredients in some antacid preparations. It is also useful in treating severe diarrhea accompanied by bicarbonate loss.

Adverse Reactions, Contraindications, Precautions, and Interactions

In some instances, excessive oral use of bicarbonate may produce nausea and vomiting. Some individuals may use sodium bicarbonate (baking soda) for the relief of GI disturbances such as pain, discomfort, symptoms of indigestion, and gas. Prolonged use of oral sodium bicarbonate or excessive doses of IV sodium bicarbonate may result in systemic alkalosis.

Bicarbonate is contraindicated in patients losing chloride by continuous GI suction or through vomiting; in patients with metabolic or respiratory alkalosis, hypocalcemia, renal failure, or severe abdominal pain of unknown cause; and in those on sodium-restricted diets.

Bicarbonate is used cautiously in patients with HF or renal impairment and those receiving glucocorticoid therapy. Bicarbonate is a pregnancy category C drug and is used cautiously during pregnancy.

Oral administration of bicarbonate may decrease the absorption of ketoconazole. Increased blood levels of quinidine, flecainide, or sympathomimetics may occur when these agents are administered with bicarbonate. There is an increased risk of crystalluria when bicarbonate is administered with the fluoroquinolones. Possible decreased effects of lithium, methotrexate, chlorpropamide, salicylates, and tetracyclines may occur when these drugs are administered with sodium bicarbonate. Sodium bicarbonate is not administered within 2 hours of enteric-coated drugs, because the protective enteric coating may disintegrate before the drug reaches the intestine.

ACIDIFYING DRUG: AMMONIUM CHLORIDE

Actions and Uses

Ammonium chloride lowers the blood pH by being metabolized first into urea, then to hydrochloric acid, which is further metabolized to hydrogen ions to acidify the blood.

Adverse Reactions and Interactions

Adverse reactions to ammonium chloride include metabolic acidosis and loss of electrolytes, especially potassium. Use of ammonium chloride and spironolactone may increase systemic acidosis.

NURSING PROCESS

PATIENT RECEIVING A SOLUTION FOR MANAGEMENT OF BODY FLUIDS

ASSESSMENT

Preadministration Assessment

Before administering an IV solution, assess the patient's general status, review recent laboratory test results (when appropriate), weigh the patient (when appropriate), and take vital signs. Blood pressure, pulse, and respiratory rate provide a baseline, which is especially important when the patient is receiving fluids for shock or other serious disorders. Ask the patient how he or she feels to help assess for signs of an electrolyte imbalance (see Display 54.2). Review all recent laboratory and diagnostic tests appropriate to the imbalance.

Ongoing Assessment

During the ongoing assessment of an IV line, check the needle site every 15 to 30 minutes or more frequently if the patient is restless or confused. The needle site is inspected for signs of extravasation (escape of fluid from a blood vessel into surrounding tissues) or infiltration (the collection of fluid into tissues). If signs of extravasation or infiltration are apparent, restart the infusion in another vein.

When the patient is in a critical condition, a central venous pressure line may be inserted to monitor the patient's response to therapy. Central venous pressure readings are taken as ordered. During administration of fluids and electrolytes in the critical setting, the blood pressure, pulse, and respiratory rate are continuously monitored. For example, a patient in shock and receiving a plasma expander is monitored continuously, whereas the patient with a saline lock 3 days after surgery may require monitoring only once or twice a shift.

During therapy, serum electrolyte or bicarbonate studies are drawn to monitor therapy.

POTASSIUM. Patients receiving oral potassium should have their blood pressure and pulse monitored every 4 hours, especially during early therapy. Observe the patient for signs of hyperkalemia (see Display 54.2), which would indicate that the dose of potassium is too high. Signs of hypokalemia may also occur during therapy and may indicate that the dose of potassium is too low and must be increased. If signs of hypokalemia or hyperkalemia are apparent or suspected, contact the primary health care provider. In some instances, frequent laboratory monitoring of the serum potassium may be ordered.

When infusing potassium, inspect the IV needle site every 30 minutes for signs of extravasation. Potassium is irritating to the tissues. If extravasation occurs, discontinue the IV immediately and notify the primary health care provider. Many facilities have protocols for treatment of the tissues to delay further tissue damage.

The acutely ill patient and the patient with severe hypokalemia require monitoring of the blood pressure and pulse rate every 15 to 30 minutes during the IV infusion. Measure and record the intake and output every 8 hours. The infusion rate is slowed to keep the vein open, and the primary health care provider is notified if an irregular pulse is noted.

CALCIUM. Before, during, and after the administration of IV calcium, monitor the blood pressure, pulse, and respiratory rate every 30 minutes until the patient's condition has stabilized. After administration of calcium, observe the patient for signs of hypercalcemia (see Display 54.2).

> **! NURSING ALERT**
>
> Systemic overloading of calcium ions in the systemic circulation results in acute hypercalcemic syndrome. Symptoms of hypercalcemic syndrome include elevated plasma calcium, weakness, lethargy, severe nausea and vomiting, coma, and, if left untreated, death. Report signs of hypercalcemic syndrome immediately to the primary health care provider.

To combat hypercalcemic syndrome, the primary health care provider may prescribe IV sodium chloride and a potent diuretic such as furosemide. When used together, these two drugs markedly increase calcium renal clearance and reduce hypercalcemia.

SODIUM. When NaCl is administered by IV infusion, observe the patient during and after administration for signs of hypernatremia (see Display 54.2). Check the rate of IV infusion as ordered by the primary health care provider, usually every 15 to 30 minutes. More frequent monitoring of the infusion rate may be necessary when the patient is restless or confused. To minimize venous irritation during administration of sodium or any electrolyte solution, use a small-bore needle placed well within the lumen of a large vein.

Patients receiving a 3% or 5% NaCl solution by IV infusion are observed closely for signs of pulmonary edema (i.e., dyspnea, cough, restlessness, bradycardia). If any one or more of these symptoms occurs, the IV infusion is slowed to keep the vein open and the primary health care provider is contacted immediately. Patients receiving NaCl by the IV route have their intake and output measured every 8 hours. Observe the patient for signs of hypernatremia every 3 to 4 hours and contact the primary health care provider if this condition is suspected.

MAGNESIUM. When magnesium is ordered to treat convulsions or severe hypomagnesemia, the patient requires constant observation. Obtain the patient's blood pressure, pulse, and respiratory rate immediately before the drug is administered, as well as every 5 to 10 minutes during the time of IV infusion, or place the patient on a device for continuous monitoring. Continue monitoring these vital signs at frequent intervals until the patient's condition has stabilized. Because magnesium is eliminated by the kidneys, it is used with caution in patients with renal impairment. Monitor the urine output to verify an output of at least 100 mL every 4 hours. Voiding less than 100 mL of urine every 4 hours is reported to the primary health care provider.

BICARBONATE. When given in the treatment of metabolic acidosis, the drug may be added to the IV fluid or given as a prepared IV sodium bicarbonate solution. Frequent laboratory monitoring of the blood pH and blood gases is usually ordered, because dosage and length of therapy depend on test results. Observe frequently for signs of clinical improvement and monitor the blood pressure, pulse, and respiratory rate every 15 to 30 minutes or as ordered by the primary health care provider. Extravasation of the drug requires selection of another needle site, because the drug is irritating to the tissues.

Fᴀᴛ Eᴍᴜʟsɪᴏɴs. When a fat emulsion is administered, monitor the patient's ability to eliminate the infused fat from the circulation, because the lipidemia must clear between daily infusions. Additionally, monitor for lipidemia by assessing the results of the following laboratory examinations: hemogram, blood coagulation, liver function tests, plasma lipid profile, and platelet count. Report an increase in the results of any of these laboratory examinations as abnormal.

NURSING DIAGNOSES
Drug-specific nursing diagnoses include the following:

■ **Excess Fluid Volume** related to adverse effects resulting from too rapid intravenous infusion
■ **Deficient Fluid Volume** related to inability to take oral fluids, abnormal fluid loss, other factors (specify cause of deficient fluid volume)
■ **Imbalanced Nutrition: Less Than Body Requirements** related to anorexia caused by opioids
■ **Risk for Injury** related to adverse drug effects (muscular weakness)
■ **Acute Confusion** related to adverse drug effects
■ **Risk for Decreased Cardiac Output** related to adverse drug effects (cardiac arrhythmias)

Nursing diagnoses related to drug administration are discussed in Chapter 4.

PLANNING
The expected outcomes of the patient depend on the specific drug, dose, route of administration, and reason for administration of an electrolyte or fluid but may include an optimal response to therapy, supporting the patient needs related to the management of adverse reactions, and confidence in an understanding of the treatment regimen.

IMPLEMENTATION
Promoting an Optimal Response to Therapy
The extremity used for administration should be made comfortable and supported as needed by a small pillow or other device. An IV infusion pump may be ordered for the administration of these solutions. Set the alarm of the infusion pump and check the functioning of the unit at frequent intervals.

> **❗ NURSING ALERT**
> Administer all IV solutions with great care. At no time should any IV solution be infused at a rapid rate, unless there is a specific written order to do so.

Unless otherwise directed, the IV solution should be administered at room temperature. If the solution is refrigerated, allow the solution to warm by exposing it to room temperature 30 to 45 minutes before use. The average length of time for infusion of 1000 mL of an IV solution is 4 to 8 hours. One exception is when there is a written or verbal order by the primary health care provider to give the solution at a rapid rate because of an emergency. In this instance, the order must specifically state the rate of administration as drops per minute, milliliters per minute, or the period of time over which a specific amount of fluid is to be infused (e.g., 125 mL/hr or 1000 mL in 8 hours).

In some situations, electrolytes are administered when an electrolyte imbalance may potentially occur. For example, the patient with nasogastric suction is prescribed one or more electrolytes added to an IV solution, such as 5% dextrose or a combined electrolyte solution, to be given IV to make up for the electrolytes that are lost through nasogastric suction. In other instances, electrolytes are given to replace those already lost, such as the patient admitted to the hospital with severe vomiting and diarrhea of several days' duration.

When electrolytes are administered parenterally, the dosage is expressed in milliequivalents (mEq)—for example, calcium gluconate 7 mEq IV. When administered orally, sodium bicarbonate, calcium, and magnesium dosages are expressed in milligrams (mg). Potassium liquids and effervescent tablet dosages are expressed in milliequivalents; capsule or tablet dosages may be expressed as milliequivalents or milligrams.

Electrolyte disturbances can cause varying degrees of confusion, muscular weakness, nausea, vomiting, and cardiac irregularities (see Display 54.2 for specific symptoms). Serum electrolyte blood levels have a very narrow therapeutic range. Careful monitoring is needed to determine if blood levels fall above or below normal. Normal values may vary with the laboratory, but a general range of normal values for each electrolyte is found in Display 54.2. Adverse reactions are usually controlled by maintaining blood levels of the various electrolytes within the normal range.

Aᴅᴍɪɴɪsᴛᴇʀɪɴɢ Pᴏᴛᴀssɪᴜᴍ. When given orally, potassium may cause GI distress. Therefore, it is given immediately after meals or with food and a full glass of water. Oral potassium must not be crushed or chewed. If the patient has difficulty swallowing, consult the primary health care provider regarding the use of a solution or an effervescent tablet, which fizzes and dissolves on contact with water. Potassium in the form of effervescent tablets, powder, or liquid must be thoroughly mixed with 4 to 8 ounces of cold water, juice, or other beverage. Effervescent tablets must stop fizzing before the solution is sipped slowly during a period of 5 to 15 minutes. Oral liquids and soluble powders that have been mixed and dissolved in cold water or juice are also sipped slowly over a period of 5 to 15 minutes. Advise patients that liquid potassium solutions have a salty taste. Some of these products are flavored to make the solution more palatable.

> **❗ NURSING ALERT**
> Concentrated potassium solutions are for IV mixtures only and should never be used undiluted. Direct IV injection of potassium could result in sudden death. When potassium is given IV, it is always diluted in 500 to 1000 mL of an IV solution. The maximum recommended concentration of potassium is 80 mEq in 1000 mL of IV solution (although in acute emergency situations a higher concentration of potassium may be required).

Aᴅᴍɪɴɪsᴛᴇʀɪɴɢ Mᴀɢɴᴇsɪᴜᴍ. Magnesium may be ordered intramuscularly (IM), IV, or by IV infusion diluted in a specified type and amount of IV solution. When ordered to be given IM, this drug is given undiluted as a 50% solution for adults and a 20% solution for children. Magnesium is given deep IM in a large muscle mass, such as the gluteus muscle.

LIFESPAN CONSIDERATIONS
Gerontology
Older adults may need a reduced dosage of magnesium because of decreased renal function. Closely monitor serum magnesium levels when magnesium is administered to older adults.

Monitor the patient for early signs of hypermagnesemia (see Display 54.2) and contact the primary health care provider immediately if this imbalance is suspected. Frequent plasma magnesium levels are usually ordered. Contact the primary health care provider if the magnesium level is higher or lower than the normal range.

❗ NURSING ALERT
As plasma magnesium levels rise above 4 mEq/L, the deep tendon reflexes are first decreased and then disappear as the plasma levels reach 10 mEq/L. The knee-jerk reflex is tested before each dose of magnesium. If the reflex is absent or a slow response is obtained, the nurse withholds the dosage and notifies the primary health care provider. IV calcium is kept available to reverse the respiratory depression and heart block that may occur with magnesium overdose.

TOTAL PARENTERAL NUTRITION. A microscopic filter is attached to the IV line when TPN solutions are administered. The filter prevents microscopic aggregates (particles that may form in the IV bag) from entering the bloodstream, where they could cause massive emboli.

LIPID SOLUTIONS. Fat solutions (emulsions) should be handled with care to decrease the risk of separation or "breaking out of the oil." Separation can be identified by yellowish streaking or the accumulation of yellowish droplets in the emulsion. Fat solutions are administered to adults at a rate no greater than 1 to 2 mL/min.

❗ NURSING ALERT
During the first 30 minutes of infusion of a fat solution, carefully observe the patient for difficulty in breathing, headache, flushing, nausea, vomiting, or signs of a hypersensitivity reaction. If any of these reactions occur, discontinue the infusion, keep the IV line open with fluid running, and immediately notify the primary health care provider.

ADMINISTERING BICARBONATE. Give oral sodium bicarbonate tablets with a full glass of water; the powdered form is dissolved in a full glass of water. If oral sodium bicarbonate is used to alkalinize the urine, check the urine pH two or three times a day or as ordered by the primary health care provider. If the urine remains acidic, contact the primary health care provider, because an increase in the dose of the drug may be necessary. IV sodium bicarbonate is given in emergency situations, such as metabolic acidosis or certain types of drug overdose, when alkalinization of the urine is necessary to hasten drug elimination.

Monitoring and Managing Patient Needs
When electrolyte solutions are administered, adverse reactions are most often related to overdose. Correcting the

imbalance by decreasing the dosage or discontinuing the solution usually works, and the adverse reactions subside quickly. Frequent serum electrolyte levels are used to monitor blood levels.

EXCESS FLUID VOLUME. Monitor patients receiving IV solutions at frequent intervals for signs of fluid overload. If signs of fluid overload (see Display 54.1) are observed, slow the IV infusion rate and immediately contact the primary health care provider.

LIFESPAN CONSIDERATIONS
Gerontology
Older adults are at increased risk for fluid overload because of the increased incidence of cardiac disease and decreased renal function that may accompany old age. Careful monitoring for signs and symptoms of fluid overload is extremely important when administering fluids to older adults.

DEFICIENT FLUID VOLUME AND IMBALANCED NUTRITION: LESS THAN BODY REQUIREMENTS. Often, the solutions used in the management of body fluids are given to correct a fluid volume deficit and to supply carbohydrates (nutrition). Review the patient's record for a full understanding of the rationale for administration of the specific solution.

When appropriate, nursing measures that may be instituted to correct a fluid volume and carbohydrate deficit may be included in a plan of care. Examples of these measures include offering oral fluids at frequent intervals and encouraging the patient to take small amounts of nourishment between meals and to eat as much as possible at mealtime.

Electrolyte imbalances may cause nausea, vomiting, and other GI disturbances. If GI disturbances occur from oral administration, taking the drug with meals may decrease the nausea. Offering smaller, more frequent meals may help to stabilize nutritional status. Correcting the electrolyte imbalance usually solves the problem of nausea and vomiting.

RISK FOR INJURY. The patient is at increased risk of falling because of weakness or muscular cramping. Frequent observation and quickly answering the call light help to maintain the patient's safety. If weakness or muscular cramping occurs, assist the patient when ambulating to prevent falls or other injury.

ACUTE CONFUSION. The patient with an electrolyte imbalance may be confused or disoriented. Approach the patient in a calm and nurturing manner. Gently reorient or redirect the individual and explain any procedures carefully before performing any procedures with the patient. Reassure the patient that these symptoms are part of the imbalance but can recede as the imbalance improves (if applicable).

RISK FOR DECREASED CARDIAC OUTPUT. Some electrolytes may cause cardiac irregularities. Check the pulse rate at regular intervals, usually every 4 hours or more often if an irregularity in the heart rate is observed. Depending on the patient's condition, cardiac monitoring may be indicated when administering the electrolytes (particularly when administering potassium or calcium). For example, if potassium is administered to a patient with cardiac disease, a cardiac monitor is needed to monitor the heart rate and rhythm continuously during therapy.

Mild (5.5 to 6.5 mEq/L) to moderate (6.5 to 8 mEq/L) potassium blood level increases may be asymptomatic and manifested only by increased serum potassium concentrations and characteristic electrocardiographic changes, such as disappearance of P waves or spreading (widening) of the QRS complex.

Educating the Patient and Family

When IV therapy is started, give the patient or family a brief explanation of the reason for and the method of administration of an IV solution. Sometimes, when alarms go off patients and families may feel the staff is too busy to respond and tamper with or adjust the rate of flow of IV administration sets. Emphasize the importance of calling for your help if there appears to be a problem with the IV site or the IV administration set or the equipment.

To ensure accurate adherence to the prescribed drug regimen, carefully explain the dose and time intervals to the patient or a family member. Because overdose (which can be serious) may occur if the patient does not adhere to the prescribed dosage and schedule, it is most important that the patient completely understands how much and when to take the drug. Stress the importance of adhering to the prescribed dosage schedule during patient teaching.

The primary health care provider may order periodic laboratory and diagnostic tests for some patients receiving oral electrolytes. Encourage the patient to keep all appointments for these tests, as well as primary health care provider or clinic visits. Persons with a history of using sodium bicarbonate (baking soda) as an antacid are warned that overuse can result in alkalosis and could disguise a more serious problem.

EVALUATION

■ Therapeutic response is achieved; fluid and electrolyte imbalances are corrected.

■ Adverse reactions are identified, reported to the primary health care provider, and managed successfully with appropriate nursing interventions:
  • Patient maintains an adequate fluid volume.
  • Patient maintains an adequate nutritional status.
  • No evidence of injury is seen.
  • Orientation and mentation remain intact.
  • Cardiac output is maintained.

■ Patient and family express confidence and demonstrate an understanding of the drug regimen.

PHARMACOLOGY IN PRACTICE
THINK CRITICALLY

Mr. Garcia tells you that he has not deviated from the sodium-restricted diet that he was given. He cannot figure out why he has gained weight. He states that, with his heartburn, he knows he has been eating less. He also mentions that the soda bicarbonate he uses does little to relieve the heartburn. Describe how you would teach him about the side effects he is experiencing from the sodium bicarbonate.

KEY POINTS

• Fluids and electrolytes make up a major component of our bodies. Without fluids the body's ability to transport oxygen and nutrients to the various tissues is compromised.

• Solutions used to manage body fluids are frequently delivered parenterally. Electrolytes, calories, or water is supplemented IV. IV access policies are written by each institution and include who may start lines, access them for administration, and monitor them. Venous access is typically initiated on a distal limb. Any provider should attempt venous access no more than two times before requesting assistance. IV sites should be routinely monitored no matter whether used for intermittent or continuous fluid.

• Solutions frequently infused include electrolytes, blood products, blood expanders, and total parenteral nutrition. Electrolytes circulate in the blood at specific levels, where they are available for use when needed by the cells. An electrolyte imbalance occurs when the concentration of an electrolyte in the blood is either too high or too low. An imbalance can also occur from vomiting, surgery, diagnostic tests, or drug administration. Blood products are used to increase blood volume from conditions such as hemorrhage or shock. TPN is used when the body cannot take in nutrients via the GI system.

• Conditions of acid-base imbalance can be corrected using drugs such as sodium bicarbonate.

Summary Drug Table ELECTROLYTES

Generic Name	Trade Name	Uses	Adverse Reactions	Dosage Ranges
calcium	PhosLo	Control of hyperphosphatemia in end-stage renal failure	See Display 54.2	3–4 tablets orally with each meal
calcium carbonate	Calcium-600, Apo-Cal, Caltrate, Oyster Shell Calcium Tums, Rolaids, Calcium Rich, Tums E-X	Dietary supplement for prevention or treatment of calcium deficiency for conditions such as pregnancy and lactation, chronic diarrhea, osteoporosis, osteomalacia, rickets, and latent tetany, and to reduce the symptoms of premenstrual syndrome	Rare; see Display 54.2 for signs of hypercalcemia	500–2000 mg/day orally
calcium citrate	Citracal, Citracal Liquitab	Same as calcium carbonate	Same as calcium carbonate	500–2000 mg/day orally
calcium gluconate		Hypocalcemic tetany, hyperkalemia with secondary cardiac toxicity, magnesium intoxication, exchange transfusion	Same as calcium carbonate	Adults: dosage range 1.35–70 mEq/day IV Children: 2.3 mEq/kg/day well diluted; give slowly in divided doses
calcium lactate	Cal-Lac	Same as calcium carbonate	Same as calcium carbonate	500–2000 mg/day orally
magnesium	Magonate, Mag-Ox 400, Magtrate, Mag-200, Slow-Mag	Dietary supplement, hypomagnesemia	Rare; see Display 54.2 for signs of hypermagnesemia	54–483 mg/day orally
magnesium sulfate		Mild to severe hypomagnesemia, seizures	Toxicity, weak or absent deep tendon reflexes, flaccid paralysis, drowsiness, stupor, weak pulse, arrhythmias, hypotension, circulatory collapse, respiratory paralysis	Hypomagnesemia: 2–5 g IV in 1 L of solution; 4–5 g over 3 hr Seizures: 4–5 g magnesium sulfate in 250 mL D_5W; simultaneously give 4–5 g magnesium sulfate (undiluted) IM to each buttock for initial dose of 10–14 g; followed by 1–2 g/hr IV infusion until seizure controlled
oral electrolyte mixtures	Infalyte Oral Solution, Naturalyte, Pedialyte, Pedialyte Electrolyte, Pedialyte Freezer Pops, Rehydralyte, Resol Solution	Maintenance of water and electrolytes after corrective parenteral therapy of severe diarrhea; maintenance to replace mild to moderate fluid losses when food and liquid intake are discontinued, to restore fluid and minerals lost in diarrhea and vomiting in infants and children	Rare	Individualize dosage following the guidelines on the product labeling

(table continues on page 628)

Summary Drug Table ELECTROLYTES (continued)

Generic Name	Trade Name	Uses	Adverse Reactions	Dosage Ranges
potassium replacements	Effer-K, K Norm, Kaon Cl, K-Dur, Klor-Con, K-Lyte, K-Tab, Micro-K, Slow-K	Hypokalemia	See Display 54.2; most common: nausea, vomiting, diarrhea, flatulence, abdominal discomfort, skin rash	40–100 mEq/day orally
sodium chloride	Slo-Salt	Prevention or treatment of extracellular volume depletion, dehydration, sodium depletion, aid in the prevention of heat prostration	Nausea, vomiting, diarrhea, abdominal cramps, edema, irritability, restlessness, weakness, hypertension, tachycardia, fluid accumulation, pulmonary edema, respiratory arrest (see Display 54.2)	Individualize dosage
Alkalinizing Drugs				
bicarbonate		Metabolic acidosis, cardiac arrest, systemic and urinary alkalinization	Tetany, edema, gastric distention, flatulence, belching, hypokalemia, metabolic alkalosis	Metabolic acidosis and cardiac arrest: dosage varies depending on laboratory results and patient's condition Urinary alkalinization: 4 g orally initially, followed by 1–2 g orally q 6 hr
tromethamine	Tham	Metabolic acidosis during cardiac bypass surgery or cardiac arrest	Fever, hypoglycemia, hyperkalemia, respiratory depression, hemorrhagic hepatic necrosis, venospasm, vein necrosis	9 mL/kg (not to exceed total single dose of 500 mL)
Acidifying Drug				
ammonium chloride		Metabolic alkalosis	Loss of electrolytes, especially potassium, metabolic acidosis	Varies depending on patient's tolerance and condition

● Chapter Review

Know Your Drugs

Clients sometimes know a medication by the brand (or trade) name and not the generic name. To help you recognize both names, match the brand name with the generic name of the same medication.

Generic Name	Brand Name
1. calcium carbonate	A. Citracal
2. calcium citrate	B. Micro-K
3. magnesium	C. Slow-Mag
4. potassium	D. Tums

Calculate Medication Dosages

1. The client is to receive 1000 mL of 5% dextrose in water during a period of 10 hours. Calculate how many milliliters should be infused each hour.

2. The client is prescribed potassium 40 mEq orally. The drug is available from the pharmacy in a solution of 20 mEq/15 mL. The nurse administers _____.

● Prepare for the NCLEX®

Build Your Knowledge

1. Fluid and electrolytes make up what percentage of the body?

   1. 10%
   2. 33%
   3. 50%
   4. 99%

2. Parenteral therapy is initiated _____.

   1. because client is too tired to eat
   2. for provider ease
   3. because of inability to handle GI nutrition
   4. because of better outcomes

3. Which of the following is a symptom of fluid overload?

   1. tinnitus
   2. hypotension
   3. decreased body temperature
   4. behavioral changes

4. Which of the following symptoms would indicate hypocalcemia?

   1. tetany
   2. constipation
   3. muscle weakness
   4. hypertension

5. Which of the following potassium plasma concentration laboratory results would the nurse report immediately to the primary health care provider?

   1. 3.5 mEq/L
   2. 4.0 mEq/L
   3. 4.5 mEq/L
   4. 5.5 mEq/mL

6. Which of the following symptoms would most likely indicate hypernatremia?

   1. fever, increased thirst
   2. cold, clammy skin
   3. decreased skin turgor
   4. hypotension

7. Which of the following is a common metabolic complication of TPN?

   1. hypomagnesemia
   2. hypermagnesemia
   3. hypoglycemia
   4. hyperglycemia

Apply Your Knowledge

8. When monitoring a client with an IV line, the nurse observes that the area around the needle insertion site is swollen and red. The first action of the nurse is to _____.

   1. check the client's blood pressure and pulse
   2. check further for possible extravasation
   3. ask the client if the IV site has been accidentally injured
   4. immediately notify the primary health care provider

9. Which of the following IV solutions must be typed and crossmatched for administration?

   1. lipid solutions
   2. platelets
   3. whole blood
   4. normal saline

Alternate-Format Questions

10. Order the steps used to start an IV access in a client.

    1. Apply tourniquet about intended puncture site
    2. Inspect the limb
    3. Cleanse the site for puncture
    4. Ask the client about previous IV sites
    5. Pull the skin taut for access

To check your answers, see Appendix G.

the**Point** *For more NCLEX-style questions, log on to http://thepoint.lww.com to access more than 1000 questions.*

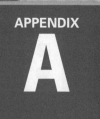

Drug Categories: Controlled Substances and FDA Pregnancy Risk

Schedules of Controlled Substances

Schedule I (C-I)
- High abuse potential
- Lack of accepted safety, not approved for medical use in the United States
- Examples: heroin, marijuana,* ecstasy (MDMA), peyote

Schedule II (C-II)
- Potential for high abuse with severe physical or psychological dependence
- Approved for medical use in the United States (and all categories below)
- Examples: opioids such as fentanyl, meperidine, methadone, morphine, oxycodone, amphetamines, and cocaine

Schedule III (C-III)
- Less abuse potential than schedule II drugs
- Potential for moderate or low physical or psychological dependence
- Examples: anabolic steroids, ketamine, hydrocodone/codeine compounded with a nonsteroidal anti-inflammatory drug

Schedule IV (C-IV)
- Less abuse potential than schedule III drugs
- Limited dependence potential
- Examples: some sedatives and anxiety agents, nonopioid analgesics, "diet drugs"

Schedule V (C-V)**
- Limited abuse potential
- Examples: small amounts of opioid (codeine) used as antitussives or antidiarrheals, pregabalin (Lyrica)

*Eighteen states and the District of Columbia allow marijuana for medicinal purposes. State-specific requirements determine how a person applies for permission to purchase and use the product.
**Under federal law, limited quantities of certain schedule V drugs may be purchased without a prescription directly from a pharmacist if allowed under state law. The purchaser must be at least 18 years of age and must furnish identification. All such transactions must be recorded by the dispensing pharmacist.

FDA Pregnancy (Fetal) Risk Categories

Pregnancy Category A
- Adequate, well-controlled studies in pregnant women have not shown an increased risk of fetal abnormalities to the fetus in any trimester of pregnancy.

Pregnancy Category B
- Animal studies have revealed no evidence of harm to the fetus; however, there are no adequate and well-controlled studies in pregnant women.
OR
- Animal studies have shown an adverse effect, but adequate and well-controlled studies in pregnant women have failed to demonstrate a risk to the fetus in any trimester.

Pregnancy Category C
- Animal studies have shown an adverse effect and there are no adequate and well-controlled studies in pregnant women.
OR
- No animal studies have been conducted and there are no adequate and well-controlled studies in pregnant women.

Pregnancy Category D
- Adequate well-controlled or observational studies in pregnant women have demonstrated a risk to the fetus.
- However, potential benefits may outweigh the risk to the fetus. If needed in a life-threatening situation or a serious disease, the drug may be acceptable if safer drugs cannot be used or are ineffective.

Pregnancy Category X
- Adequate well-controlled or observational studies in animals or pregnant women have demonstrated positive evidence of fetal abnormalities or risks.
- The use of the product is contraindicated in women who are or may become pregnant.

Pregnancy Category N
- The drug is not classified by the FDA.

Regardless of the pregnancy category or the presumed safety of the drug, no drug should be administered during pregnancy unless it is clearly needed and the potential benefits outweigh the potential harm to the fetus.

ISMP Institute for Safe Medication Practices

FDA and ISMP Lists of
Look-Alike Drug Names with Recommended Tall Man Letters

The look-alike drug names in the Tables that follow have been modified using tall man (mixed case) letters to help draw attention to the dissimilarities in their names. Several studies have shown that highlighting sections of drug names using tall man letters can help distinguish similar drug names,[1] making them less prone to mix-ups.[2-3] ISMP, FDA, The Joint Commission, and other safety-conscious organizations have promoted the use of tall man letters as one means of reducing confusion between similar drug names.

Table 1 provides an alphabetized list of FDA-approved established drug names with recommended tall man letters, which were first identified during the FDA Name Differentiation Project (www.fda.gov/Drugs/DrugSafety/MedicationErrors/ucm164587.htm).

Table 2 provides an alphabetized list of additional drug names with recommendations from ISMP regarding the use and placement of tall man letters. This is not an official list approved by FDA. It is intended for voluntary use by healthcare practitioners and drug information vendors. Any product label changes by manufacturers require FDA approval.

One of the difficulties with the use of tall man letters includes inconsistent application in health settings and lack of standardization regarding which letters to present in uppercase. A new study by Gerrett[4] describes several ways to determine which of the dissimilar letters in each drug name should be highlighted. To promote standardi-

zation, ISMP followed one of these tested methodologies whenever possible. Called the CD3 rule, the methodology suggests working from the left of the word first by capitalizing all the characters to the right once two or more dissimilar letters are encountered, and then, working from the right of the word back, returning two or more letters common to both words to lowercase letters. When the rule cannot be applied because there are no common letters on the right side of the word, the methodology suggests capitalizing the central part of the word only. ISMP suggests that the tall man lettering scheme provided in Tables 1 and 2 be followed when presenting these drug names to healthcare providers to promote consistency. At this time, scientific studies do not support the use of tall man letters when presenting drug names to patients.

References: 1) Filik R, Purdy K, Gale A, Gerrett D. Drug name confusion: evaluating the effectiveness of capital ("Tall Man") letters using eye movement data. *Social Science & Medicine* 2004;59(12):2597-2601. **2)** Filik R, Purdy K, Gale A, Gerrett D. Labeling of medicines and patient safety: evaluating methods of reducing drug name confusion. *Human Factors* 2006;48(1):39-47. **3)** Grasha A. Cognitive systems perspective on human performance in the pharmacy: implications for accuracy, effectiveness, and job satisfaction. Alexandria (VA): NACDS; 2000 Report No. 062100. **4)** Gerrett D, Gale AG, Darker IT, Filik R, Purdy KJ. Tall man lettering. Final report of the use of tall man lettering to minimize selection errors of medicine names in computer prescribing and dispensing systems. Loughborough University Enterprises Ltd.; 2009 (www.connectingforhealth.nhs.uk/systemsandservices/eprescribing/refdocs/tallman.pdf).

Table 1. FDA-Approved List of Generic Drug Names with Tall Man Letters

Drug Name with Tall Man Letters	Confused with
aceta**ZOLAMIDE**	aceto**HEXAMIDE**
aceto**HEXAMIDE**	aceta**ZOLAMIDE**
bu**PROP**ion	bus**PIR**one
bus**PIR**one	bu**PROP**ion
chlorpro**MAZINE**	chlorpro**PAMIDE**
chlorpro**PAMIDE**	chlorpro**MAZINE**
clomi**PHENE**	clomi**PRAMINE**
clomi**PRAMINE**	clomi**PHENE**
cyclo**SERINE**	cyclo**SPORINE**
cyclo**SPORINE**	cyclo**SERINE**
DAUNOrubicin	**DOXO**rubicin
dimenhy**DRINATE**	diphenhydr**AMINE**
diphenhydr**AMINE**	dimenhy**DRINATE**
DOBUTamine	**DOP**amine
DOPamine	**DOBUT**amine

continued on next page

www.ismp.org

ISMP Institute for Safe Medication Practices

FDA and ISMP Lists of
Look-Alike Drug Names with Recommended Tall Man Letters (continued)

Table 1. FDA-Approved List of Generic Drug Names with Tall Man Letters (continued)

Drug Name with Tall Man Letters	Confused with
DOXOrubicin	DAUNOrubicin
glipiZIDE	glyBURIDE
glyBURIDE	glipiZIDE
hydrALAZINE	hydrOXYzine
hydrOXYzine	hydrALAZINE
medroxyPROGESTERone	methylPREDNISolone – methylTESTOSTERone
methylPREDNISolone	medroxyPROGESTERone – methylTESTOSTERone
methylTESTOSTERone	medroxyPROGESTERone – methylPREDNISolone
niCARdipine	NIFEdipine
NIFEdipine	niCARdipine
prednisoLONE	predniSONE
predniSONE	prednisoLONE
sulfADIAZINE	sulfiSOXAZOLE
sulfiSOXAZOLE	sulfADIAZINE
TOLAZamide	TOLBUTamide
TOLBUTamide	TOLAZamide
vinBLAStine	vinCRIStine
vinCRIStine	vinBLAStine

Table 2. ISMP List of Additional Drug Names with Tall Man Letters

Drug Name with Tall Man Letters	Confused with
ALPRAZolam	LORazepam
aMILoride	amLODIPine
amLODIPine	aMILoride
ARIPiprazole	RABEprazole
AVINza*	INVanz*
azaCITIDine	azaTHIOprine
azaTHIOprine	azaCITIDine
carBAMazepine	OXcarbazepine
CARBOplatin	CISplatin
ceFAZolin	cefoTEtan – cefOXitin – cefTAZidime – cefTRIAXone
cefoTEtan	ceFAZolin – cefOXitin – cefTAZidime – cefTRIAXone
cefOXitin	ceFAZolin – cefoTEtan – cefTAZidime – cefTRIAXone
cefTAZidime	ceFAZolin – cefoTEtan – cefOXitin – cefTRIAXone
cefTRIAXone	ceFAZolin – cefoTEtan – cefOXitin – cefTAZidime
CeleBREX*	CeleXA*
CeleXA*	CeleBREX*
chlordiazePOXIDE	chlorproMAZINE
chlorproMAZINE	chlordiazePOXIDE
CISplatin	CARBOplatin
clonazePAM	cloNIDine – cloZAPine – LORazepam

* Brand names always start with an uppercase letter. Some brand names incorporate tall man letters in initial characters and may not be readily recognized as brand names. An asterisk follows all brand names in Table 2.

continued on next page

ISMP
INSTITUTE FOR SAFE MEDICATION PRACTICES
www.ismp.org

ISMP Institute for Safe Medication Practices

FDA and **ISMP** Lists of
Look-Alike Drug Names with Recommended Tall Man Letters **(continued)**

Table 2. ISMP List of Additional Drug Names with Tall Man Letters (continued)	
Drug Name with Tall Man Letters	**Confused with**
cloNIDine	clonazePAM – cloZAPine - KlonoPIN*
cloZAPine	clonazePAM – cloNIDine
DACTINomycin	DAPTOmycin
DAPTOmycin	DACTINomycin
DOCEtaxel	PACLitaxel
DOXOrubicin	IDArubicin
DULoxetine	FLUoxetine – PARoxetine
ePHEDrine	EPINEPHrine
EPINEPHrine	ePHEDrine
fentaNYL	SUFentanil
flavoxATE	fluvoxaMINE
FLUoxetine	DULoxetine – PARoxetine
fluPHENAZine	fluvoxaMINE
fluvoxaMINE	fluPHENAZine - flavoxATE
guaiFENesin	guanFACINE
guanFACINE	guaiFENesin
HumaLOG*	HumuLIN*
HumuLIN*	HumaLOG*
HYDROcodone	oxyCODONE
HYDROmorphone	morphine
IDArubicin	DOXOrubicin
inFLIXimab	riTUXimab
INVanz*	AVINza*
ISOtretinoin	tretinoin
KlonoPIN*	cloNIDine
LaMICtal*	LamISIL*
LamISIL*	LaMICtal*
lamiVUDine	lamoTRIgine
lamoTRIgine	lamiVUDine
levETIRAcetam	levOCARNitine
levOCARNitine	levETIRAcetam
LORazepam	ALPRAZolam – clonazePAM
metFORMIN	metroNIDAZOLE
metroNIDAZOLE	metFORMIN
mitoMYcin	mitoXANtrone
mitoXANtrone	mitoMYcin
NexAVAR*	NexIUM*
NexIUM*	NexAVAR*
niCARdipine	niMODipine – NIFEdipine
NIFEdipine	niMODipine – niCARdipine
niMODipine	NIFEdipine – niCARdipine
NovoLIN*	NovoLOG*

* Brand names always start with an uppercase letter. Some brand names incorporate tall man letters in initial characters and may not be readily recognized as brand names. An asterisk follows all brand names in Table 2.

continued on next page

ISMP
INSTITUTE FOR SAFE MEDICATION PRACTICES
www.ismp.org

ISMP Institute for Safe Medication Practices

FDA and ISMP Lists of
Look-Alike Drug Names with Recommended *Tall Man Letters* (continued)

Table 2. ISMP List of Additional Drug Names with Tall Man Letters (continued)	
Drug Name with Tall Man Letters	**Confused with**
NovoLOG*	NovoLIN*
OLANZapine	QUEtiapine
OXcarbazepine	carBAMazepine
oxyCODONE	HYDROcodone – OxyCONTIN*
OxyCONTIN*	oxyCODONE
PACLitaxel	DOCEtaxel
PARoxetine	FLUoxetine – DULoxetine
PEMEtrexed	PRALAtrexate
PENTobarbital	PHENobarbital
PHENobarbital	PENTobarbital
PRALAtrexate	PEMEtrexed
PriLOSEC*	PROzac*
PROzac*	PriLOSEC*
QUEtiapine	OLANZapine
quiNIDine	quiNINE
quiNINE	quiNIDine
RABEprazole	ARIPiprazole
RisperDAL*	rOPINIRole
risperiDONE	rOPINIRole
riTUXimab	inFLIXimab
romiDEPsin	romiPLOStim
romiPLOStim	romiDEPsin
rOPINIRole	RisperDAL*– risperiDONE
SandIMMUNE*	SandoSTATIN*
SandoSTATIN*	SandIMMUNE*
SEROquel*	SINEquan*
SINEquan*	SEROquel*
sitaGLIPtin	SUMAtriptan
Solu-CORTEF*	Solu-MEDROL*
Solu-MEDROL*	Solu-CORTEF*
SORAfenib	SUNItinib
SUFentanil	fentaNYL
sulfADIAZINE	sulfaSALAzine
sulfaSALAzine	sulfADIAZINE
SUMAtriptan	sitaGLIPtin – ZOLMitriptan
SUNItinib	SORAfenib
TEGretol*	TRENtal*
tiaGABine	tiZANidine
tiZANidine	tiaGABine
traMADol	traZODone
traZODone	traMADol

* Brand names always start with an uppercase letter. Some brand names incorporate tall man letters in initial characters and may not be readily recognized as brand names. An asterisk follows all brand names in Table 2.

continued on next page

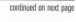

ISMP
INSTITUTE FOR SAFE MEDICATION PRACTICES
www.ismp.org

FDA and ISMP Lists of *Look-Alike Drug Names with Recommended Tall Man Letters*

ISMP Institute for Safe Medication Practices

FDA and ISMP Lists of
Look-Alike Drug Names with Recommended Tall Man Letters **(continued)**

Table 2. ISMP List of Additional Drug Names with Tall Man Letters (continued)

Drug Name with Tall Man Letters	Confused with
TRENtal*	TEGretol*
valACYclovir	valGANciclovir
valGANciclovir	valACYclovir
ZOLMitriptan	SUMAtriptan
ZyPREXA*	ZyrTEC*
ZyrTEC*	ZyPREXA*

* Brand names always start with an uppercase letter. Some brand names incorporate tall man letters in initial characters and may not be readily recognized as brand names. An asterisk follows all brand names in Table 2.

www.ismp.org

Typical Immunization Schedules

Part 1: Immunization Schedule for Children 0–18 Years

Figure 1. Recommended immunization schedule for persons aged 0 through 18 years – 2013.
(FOR THOSE WHO FALL BEHIND OR START LATE, SEE THE CATCH-UP SCHEDULE [FIGURE 2]).

These recommendations must be read with the footnotes that follow. For those who fall behind or start late, provide catch-up vaccination at the earliest opportunity as indicated by the green bars in Figure 1. To determine minimum intervals between doses, see the catch-up schedule (Figure 2). School entry and adolescent vaccine age groups are in bold.

Vaccines	Birth	1 mo	2 mos	4 mos	6 mos	9 mos	12 mos	15 mos	18 mos	19–23 mos	2-3 yrs	4-6 yrs	7-10 yrs	11-12 yrs	13–15 yrs	16–18 yrs
Hepatitis B¹ (HepB)	1ˢᵗ dose	←---- 2ⁿᵈ dose ----→			←------------------ 3ʳᵈ dose ------------------→											
Rotavirus² (RV) RV-1 (2-dose series); RV-5 (3-dose series)			1ˢᵗ dose	2ⁿᵈ dose	See footnote 2											
Diphtheria, tetanus, & acellular pertussis³ (DTaP: <7 yrs)			1ˢᵗ dose	2ⁿᵈ dose	3ʳᵈ dose		←------ 4ᵗʰ dose ------→					5ᵗʰ dose				
Tetanus, diphtheria, & acellular pertussis⁴ (Tdap: ≥7 yrs)														(Tdap)		
Haemophilus influenzae type b³ (Hib)			1ˢᵗ dose	2ⁿᵈ dose	See footnote 5		3ʳᵈ or 4ᵗʰ dose, see footnote 5									
Pneumococcal conjugate⁶ᵇᶜ (PCV13)			1ˢᵗ dose	2ⁿᵈ dose	3ʳᵈ dose		←-- 4ᵗʰ dose --→									
Pneumococcal polysaccharide⁶ᵇᶜ (PPSV23)																
Inactivated Poliovirus⁷ (IPV) (<18years)			1ˢᵗ dose	2ⁿᵈ dose	←------------------ 3ʳᵈ dose ------------------→							4ᵗʰ dose				
Influenza⁸ (IIV; LAIV) 2 doses for some : see footnote 8					Annual vaccination (IIV only)								Annual vaccination (IIV or LAIV)			
Measles, mumps, rubella⁹ (MMR)							←---- 1ˢᵗ dose ----→					2ⁿᵈ dose				
Varicella¹⁰ (VAR)							←---- 1ˢᵗ dose ----→					2ⁿᵈ dose				
Hepatitis A¹¹ (HepA)							←----- 2 dose series, see footnote 11 -----→									
Human papillomavirus¹² (HPV2: females only; HPV4: males and females)														(3-dose series)		
Meningococcal¹³ (Hib-MenCY ≥ 6 weeks; MCV4-D≥9 mos; MCV4-CRM ≥ 2 yrs.)				see footnote 13										1ˢᵗ dose		booster

Range of recommended ages for all children	Range of recommended ages for catch-up immunization	Range of recommended ages for certain high-risk groups	Range of recommended ages during which catch-up is encouraged and for certain high-risk groups	Not routinely recommended

This schedule includes recommendations in effect as of January 1, 2013. Any dose not administered at the recommended age should be administered at a subsequent visit, when indicated and feasible. The use of a combination vaccine generally is preferred over separate injections of its equivalent component vaccines. Vaccination providers should consult the relevant Advisory Committee on Immunization Practices (ACIP) statement for detailed recommendations, available online at http://www.cdc.gov/vaccines/pubs/acip-list.htm. Clinically significant adverse events that follow vaccination should be reported to the Vaccine Adverse Event Reporting System (VAERS) online (http://www.vaers.hhs.gov) or by telephone (800-822-7967). Suspected cases of vaccine-preventable diseases should be reported to the state or local health department. Additional information, including precautions and contraindications for vaccination, is available from CDC online (http://www.cdc.gov/vaccines) or by telephone (800-CDC-INFO [800-232-4636]).

This schedule is approved by the Advisory Committee on Immunization Practices (http://www.cdc.gov/vaccines/acip/index.html), the American Academy of Pediatrics (http://www.aap.org), the American Academy of Family Physicians (http://www.aafp.org), and the American College of Obstetricians and Gynecologists (http://www.acog.org).

NOTE: The above recommendations must be read along with the footnotes of this schedule.

Footnotes — Recommended immunization schedule for persons aged 0 through 18 years—United States, 2013

For further guidance on the use of the vaccines mentioned below, see: http://www.cdc.gov/vaccines/pubs/acip-list.htm.

1. **Hepatitis B (HepB) vaccine. (Minimum age: birth)**
   Routine vaccination:
   At birth
   - Administer monovalent HepB vaccine to all newborns before hospital discharge.
   - For infants born to hepatitis B surface antigen (HBsAg)–positive mothers, administer HepB vaccine and 0.5 mL of hepatitis B immune globulin (HBIG) within 12 hours of birth. These infants should be tested for HBsAg and antibody to HBsAg (anti-HBs) 1 to 2 months after completion of the HepB series, at age 9 through 18 months (preferably at the next well-child visit).
   - If mother's HBsAg status is unknown, within 12 hours of birth administer HepB vaccine to all infants regardless of birth weight. For infants weighing <2,000 grams, administer HBIG in addition to HepB within 12 hours of birth. Determine mother's HBsAg status as soon as possible and, if she is HBsAg-positive, also administer HBIG for infants weighing ≥2,000 grams (no later than age 1 week).
   Doses following the birth dose
   - The second dose should be administered at age 1 or 2 months. Monovalent HepB vaccine should be used for doses administered before age 6 weeks.
   - Infants who did not receive a birth dose should receive 3 doses of a HepB-containing vaccine on a schedule of 0, 1 to 2 months, and 6 months starting as soon as feasible. See Figure 2.
   - The minimum interval between dose 1 and dose 2 is 4 weeks and between dose 2 and 3 is 8 weeks. The final (third or fourth) dose in the HepB vaccine series should be administered no earlier than age 24 weeks, and at least 16 weeks after the first dose.
   - Administration of a total of 4 doses of HepB vaccine is recommended when a combination vaccine containing HepB is administered after the birth dose.
   Catch-up vaccination:
   - Unvaccinated persons should complete a 3-dose series.
   - A 2-dose series (doses separated by at least 4 months) of adult formulation Recombivax HB is licensed for use in children aged 11 through 15 years.
   - For other catch-up issues, see Figure 2.
2. **Rotavirus (RV) vaccines. (Minimum age: 6 weeks for both RV-1 [Rotarix] and RV-5 [RotaTeq]).**
   Routine vaccination:
   - Administer a series of RV vaccine to all infants as follows:
     1. If RV-1 is used, administer a 2-dose series at 2 and 4 months of age.
     2. If RV-5 is used, administer a 3-dose series at ages 2, 4, and 6 months.
     3. If any dose in series was RV-5 or vaccine product is unknown for any dose in the series, a total of 3 doses of RV vaccine should be administered.
   Catch-up vaccination:
   - The maximum age for the first dose in the series is 14 weeks, 6 days.
   - Vaccination should not be initiated for infants aged 15 weeks 0 days or older.
   - The maximum age for the final dose in the series is 8 months, 0 days.
   - If RV-1(Rotarix) is administered for the first and second doses, a third dose is not indicated.
   - For other catch-up issues, see Figure 2.
3. **Diphtheria and tetanus toxoids and acellular pertussis (DTaP) vaccine. (Minimum age: 6 weeks)**
   Routine vaccination:

- Administer a 5-dose series of DTaP vaccine at ages 2, 4, 6, 15–18 months, and 4 through 6 years. The fourth dose may be administered as early as age 12 months, provided at least 6 months have elapsed since the third dose.
   Catch-up vaccination:
   - The fifth (booster) dose of DTaP vaccine is not necessary if the fourth dose was administered at age 4 years or older.
   - For other catch-up issues, see Figure 2.
4. **Tetanus and diphtheria toxoids and acellular pertussis (Tdap) vaccine. (Minimum age: 10 years for Boostrix, 11 years for Adacel).**
   Routine vaccination:
   - Administer 1 dose of Tdap vaccine to all adolescents aged 11 through 12 years.
   - Tdap can be administered regardless of the interval since the last tetanus and diphtheria toxoid-containing vaccine.
   - Administer one dose of Tdap vaccine to pregnant adolescents during each pregnancy (preferred during 27 through 36 weeks gestation) regardless of number of years from prior Td or Tdap vaccination.
   Catch-up vaccination:
   - Persons aged 7 through 10 years who are not fully immunized with the childhood DTaP vaccine series, should receive Tdap vaccine as the first dose in the catch-up series; if additional doses are needed, use Td vaccine. For these children, an adolescent Tdap vaccine should not be given.
   - Persons aged 11 through 18 years who have not received Tdap vaccine should receive a dose followed by tetanus and diphtheria toxoids (Td) booster dose every 10 years thereafter.
   - An inadvertent dose of DTaP vaccine administered to children aged 7 through 10 years can count as part of the catch-up series. This dose can count as the adolescent Tdap dose, or the child can later receive a Tdap booster dose at age 11–12 years.
   - For other catch-up issues, see Figure 2.
5. **Haemophilus influenzae type b (Hib) conjugate vaccine. (Minimum age: 6 weeks)**
   Routine vaccination:
   - Administer a Hib vaccine primary series and a booster dose to all infants. The primary series doses should be administered at 2, 4, and 6 months of age; however, if PRP-OMP (PedvaxHib or Comvax) is administered at 2 and 4 months of age, a dose at age 6 months is not indicated. One booster dose should be administered at age 12 through 15 months.
   - Hiberix (PRP-T) should only be used for the booster (final) dose in children aged 12 months through 4 years, who have received at least 1 dose of Hib.
   Catch-up vaccination:
   - If dose 1 was administered at ages 12-14 months, administer booster (as final dose) at least 8 weeks after dose 1.
   - If the first 2 doses were PRP-OMP (PedvaxHIB or Comvax), and were administered at age 11 months or younger, the third (and final) dose should be administered at age 12 through 15 months and at least 8 weeks after the second dose.
   - If the first dose was administered at age 7 through 11 months, administer the second dose at least 4 weeks later and a final dose at age 12 through 15 months, regardless of Hib vaccine (PRP-T or PRP-OMP) used for first dose.
   - For unvaccinated children aged 15 months or older, administer only 1 dose.

For further guidance on the use of the vaccines mentioned below, see: http://www.cdc.gov/vaccines/pubs/acip-list.htm.

- For other catch-up issues, see Figure 2.

Vaccination of persons with high-risk conditions:
- Hib vaccine is not routinely recommended for patients older than 5 years of age. However one dose of Hib vaccine should be administered to unvaccinated or partially vaccinated persons aged 5 years or older who have leukemia, malignant neoplasms, anatomic or functional asplenia (including sickle cell disease), human immunodeficiency virus (HIV) infection, or other immunocompromising conditions.

6a. Pneumococcal conjugate vaccine (PCV). (Minimum age: 6 weeks)

Routine vaccination:
- Administer a series of PCV13 vaccine at ages 2, 4, 6 months with a booster at age 12 through 15 months.
- For children aged 14 through 59 months who have received an age-appropriate series of 7-valent PCV (PCV7), administer a single supplemental dose of 13-valent PCV (PCV13).

Catch-up vaccination:
- Administer 1 dose of PCV13 to all healthy children aged 24 through 59 months who are not completely vaccinated for their age.
- For other catch-up issues, see Figure 2.

Vaccination of persons with high-risk conditions:
- For children aged 24 through 71 months with certain underlying medical conditions (see footnote 6c), administer 1 dose of PCV13 if 3 doses of PCV were received previously, or administer 2 doses of PCV13 at least 8 weeks apart if fewer than 3 doses of PCV were received previously.
- A single dose of PCV13 may be administered to previously unvaccinated children aged 6 through 18 years who have anatomic or functional asplenia (including sickle cell disease), HIV infection or an immunocompromising condition, cochlear implant or cerebrospinal fluid leak. See MMWR 2010;59 (No. RR-11), available at http://www.cdc.gov/mmwr/pdf/rr/rr5911.pdf.
- Administer PPSV23 at least 8 weeks after the last dose of PCV to children aged 2 years or older with certain underlying medical conditions (see footnotes 6b and 6c).

6b. Pneumococcal polysaccharide vaccine (PPSV23). (Minimum age: 2 years)

Vaccination of persons with high-risk conditions:
- Administer PPSV23 at least 8 weeks after the last dose of PCV to children aged 2 years or older with certain underlying medical conditions (see footnote 6c). A single revaccination with PPSV should be administered after 5 years to children with anatomic or functional asplenia (including sickle cell disease) or an immunocompromising condition.

6c. Medical conditions for which PPSV23 is indicated in children aged 2 years and older and for which use of PCV13 is indicated in children aged 24 through 71 months:
- Immunocompetent children with chronic heart disease (particularly cyanotic congenital heart disease and cardiac failure); chronic lung disease (including asthma if treated with high-dose oral corticosteroid therapy), diabetes mellitus; cerebrospinal fluid leaks; or cochlear implant.
- Children with anatomic or functional asplenia (including sickle cell disease and other hemoglobinopathies, congenital or acquired asplenia, or splenic dysfunction).
- Children with immunocompromising conditions: HIV infection, chronic renal failure and nephrotic syndrome, diseases associated with treatment with immunosuppressive drugs or radiation therapy, including malignant neoplasms, leukemias, lymphomas and Hodgkin disease; or solid organ transplantation, congenital immunodeficiency.

7. Inactivated poliovirus vaccine (IPV). (Minimum age: 6 weeks)

Routine vaccination:
- Administer a series of IPV at ages 2, 4, 6–18 months, with a booster at age 4–6 years. The final dose in the series should be administered on or after the fourth birthday and at least 6 months after the previous dose.

Catch-up vaccination:
- In the first 6 months of life, minimum age and minimum intervals are only recommended if the person is at risk for imminent exposure to circulating poliovirus (i.e., travel to a polio-endemic region or during an outbreak).
- If 4 or more doses are administered before age 4 years, an additional dose should be administered at age 4 through 6 years.
- A fourth dose is not necessary if the third dose was administered at age 4 years or older and at least 6 months after the previous dose.
- If both OPV and IPV were administered as part of a series, a total of 4 doses should be administered, regardless of the child's current age.
- IPV is not routinely recommended for U.S. residents aged 18 years or older.
- For other catch-up issues, see Figure 2.

8. Influenza vaccines. (Minimum age: 6 months for inactivated influenza vaccine [IIV]; 2 years for live, attenuated influenza vaccine [LAIV])

Routine vaccination:
- Administer influenza vaccine annually to all children beginning at age 6 months. For most healthy, nonpregnant persons aged 2 through 49 years, either LAIV or IIV may be used. However, LAIV should NOT be administered to some persons, including 1) those with asthma, 2) children 2 through 4 years who had wheezing in the past 12 months, or 3) those who have any other underlying medical conditions that predispose them to influenza complications. For all other contraindications to use of LAIV see MMWR 2010; 59 (No. RR-8), available at http://www.cdc.gov/mmwr/pdf/rr/rr5908.pdf.
- Administer 1 dose to persons aged 9 years and older.

For children aged 6 months through 8 years:
- For the 2012–13 season, administer 2 doses (separated by at least 4 weeks) to children who are receiving influenza vaccine for the first time. For additional guidance, follow dosing guidelines in the 2012 ACIP influenza vaccine recommendations, MMWR 2012;61:613–618, available at http://www.cdc.gov/mmwr/pdf/wk/mm6132.pdf.
- For the 2013–14 season, follow dosing guidelines in the 2013 ACIP influenza vaccine recommendations.

9. Measles, mumps, and rubella (MMR) vaccine. (Minimum age: 12 months for routine vaccination)

Routine vaccination:
- Administer the first dose of MMR vaccine at age 12 through 15 months, and the second dose at age 4 through 6 years. The second dose may be administered before age 4 years, provided at least 4 weeks have elapsed since the first dose.
- Administer 1 dose of MMR vaccine to infants aged 6 through 11 months before departure from the United States for international travel. These children should be revaccinated with 2 doses of MMR vaccine, the first at age 12 through 15 months (12 months if the child remains in an area where disease risk is high), and the second dose at least 4 weeks later.
- Administer 2 doses of MMR vaccine to children aged 12 months and older, before departure from the United States for international travel. The first dose should be administered on or after age 12 months and the second dose at least 4 weeks later.

Catch-up vaccination:
- Ensure that all school-aged children and adolescents have had 2 doses of MMR vaccine; the minimum interval between the 2 doses is 4 weeks.

10. Varicella (VAR) vaccine. (Minimum age: 12 months)

Routine vaccination:
- Administer the first dose of VAR vaccine at age 12 through 15 months, and the second dose at age 4 through 6 years. The second dose may be administered before age 4 years, provided at least 3 months have elapsed since the first dose. If the second dose was administered at least 4 weeks after the first dose, it can be accepted as valid.

Catch-up vaccination:
- Ensure that all persons aged 7 through 18 years without evidence of immunity (see MMWR 2007;56 [No. RR-4], available at http://www.cdc.gov/mmwr/pdf/rr/rr5604.pdf) have 2 doses of varicella vaccine. For children aged 7 through 12 years the recommended minimum interval between doses is 3 months (if the second dose was administered at least 4 weeks after the first dose, it can be accepted as valid); for persons aged 13 years and older, the minimum interval between doses is 4 weeks.

11. Hepatitis A vaccine (HepA). (Minimum age: 12 months)

Routine vaccination:
- Initiate the 2-dose HepA vaccine series for children aged 12 through 23 months; separate the 2 doses by 6 to 18 months.
- Children who have received 1 dose of HepA vaccine before age 24 months, should receive a second dose 6 to 18 months after the first dose.
- For any person aged 2 years and older who has not already received the HepA vaccine series, 2 doses of HepA vaccine separated by 6 to 18 months may be administered if immunity against hepatitis A virus infection is desired.

Catch-up vaccination:
- The minimum interval between the two doses is 6 months.

Special populations:
- Administer 2 doses of Hep A vaccine at least 6 months apart to previously unvaccinated persons who live in areas where vaccination programs target older children, or who are at increased risk for infection.

12. Human papillomavirus (HPV) vaccines. (HPV4 [Gardasil] and HPV2 [Cervarix]). (Minimum age: 9 years)

Routine vaccination:
- Administer a 3-dose series of HPV vaccine on a schedule of 0, 1-2, and 6 months to all adolescents aged 11-12 years. Either HPV4 or HPV2 may be used for females, and only HPV4 may be used for males.
- The vaccine series can be started beginning at age 9 years.
- Administer the second dose 1 to 2 months after the **first** dose and the third dose 6 months after the **first** dose (at least 24 weeks after the first dose).

Catch-up vaccination:
- Administer the vaccine series to females (either HPV2 or HPV4) and males (HPV4) at age 13 through 18 years if not previously vaccinated.
- Use recommended routine dosing intervals (see above) for vaccine series catch-up.

13. Meningococcal conjugate vaccines (MCV). (Minimum age: 6 weeks for Hib-MenCY, 9 months for Menactra [MCV4-D], 2 years for Menveo [MCV4-CRM]).

Routine vaccination:
- Administer MCV4 vaccine at age 11–12 years, with a booster dose at age 16 years.
- Adolescents aged 11 through 18 years with human immunodeficiency virus (HIV) infection should receive a 2-dose primary series of MCV4, with at least 8 weeks between doses. See MMWR 2011; 60:1018–1019 available at: http://www.cdc.gov/mmwr/pdf/wk/mm6030.pdf.
- For children aged 2 months through 10 years with high-risk conditions, see below.

Catch-up vaccination:
- Administer MCV4 vaccine at age 13 through 18 years if not previously vaccinated.
- If the first dose is administered at age 13 through 15 years, a booster dose should be administered at age 16 through 18 years with a minimum interval of at least 8 weeks between doses.
- If the first dose is administered at age 16 years or older, a booster dose is not needed.
- For other catch-up issues, see Figure 2.

Vaccination of persons with high-risk conditions:
- For children younger than 19 months of age with anatomic or functional asplenia (including sickle cell disease), administer an infant series of Hib-MenCY at 2, 4, 6, and 12-15 months.
- For children aged 2 through 18 months with persistent complement component deficiency, administer either an infant series of Hib-MenCY at 2, 4, 6, and 12 through 15 months or a 2-dose primary series of MCV4-D starting at 9 months, with at least 8 weeks between doses. For children aged 19 through 23 months with persistent complement component deficiency who have not received a complete series of Hib-MenCY or MCV4-D, administer 2 primary doses of MCV4-D at least 8 weeks apart.
- For children aged 24 months and older with persistent complement component deficiency or anatomic or functional asplenia (including sickle cell disease), who have not received a complete series of Hib-MenCY or MCV4-D, administer 2 primary doses of either MCV4-D or MCV4-CRM. If MCV4-D (Menactra) is administered to a child with asplenia (including sickle cell disease), do not administer MCV4-D until 2 years of age and at least 4 weeks after the completion of all PCV13 doses. See MMWR 2011;60:1391–2, available at http://www.cdc.gov/mmwr/pdf/wk/mm6040.pdf.
- For children aged 9 months and older who are residents of or travelers to countries in the African meningitis belt or to the Hajj, administer an age appropriate formulation and series of MCV4 for protection against serogroups A and W-135. Prior receipt of Hib-MenCY is not sufficient for children traveling to the meningitis belt or the Hajj. See MMWR 2011;60:1391–2, available at http://www.cdc.gov/mmwr/pdf/wk/mm6040.pdf.
- For children who are present during outbreaks caused by a vaccine serogroup, administer or complete an age and formulation-appropriate series of Hib-MenCY or MCV4.
- For booster doses among persons with high-risk conditions refer to http://www.cdc.gov/vaccines/pubs/acip-list.htm#mening.

Additional information
- For contraindications and precautions to use of a vaccine and for additional information regarding that vaccine, vaccination providers should consult the relevant ACIP statement available online at http://www.cdc.gov/vaccines/pubs/acip-list.htm.
- For the purposes of calculating intervals between doses, 4 weeks = 28 days. Intervals of 4 months or greater are determined by calendar months.
- Information on travel vaccine requirements and recommendations is available at http://wwwnc.cdc.gov/travel/page/vaccinations.htm.
- For vaccination of persons with primary and secondary immunodeficiencies, see Table 13, "Vaccination of persons with primary and secondary immunodeficiencies," in General Recommendations on Immunization (ACIP), available at http://www.cdc.gov/mmwr/preview/mmwrhtml/rr6002a1.htm; and American Academy of Pediatrics. Immunization in Special Clinical Circumstances. In: Pickering LK, Baker CJ, Kimberlin DW, Long SS eds. Red book: 2012 report of the Committee on Infectious Diseases. 29th ed. Elk Grove Village, IL: American Academy of Pediatrics.

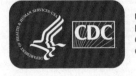

U.S. Department of Health and Human Services
Centers for Disease
Control and Prevention

Part 2: Immunization Schedule for Adults

Recommended Adult Immunization Schedule—United States - 2013

Note: These recommendations must be read with the footnotes that follow containing number of doses, intervals between doses, and other important information.

VACCINE ▼ AGE GROUP ▶	19-21 years	22-26 years	27-49 years	50-59 years	60-64 years	≥ 65 years
Influenza [2,*]	1 dose annually					
Tetanus, diphtheria, pertussis (Td/Tdap) [3,*]	Substitute 1-time dose of Tdap for Td booster; then boost with Td every 10 yrs					
Varicella [4,*]	2 doses					
Human papillomavirus (HPV) Female [5,*]	3 doses					
Human papillomavirus (HPV) Male [5,*]	3 doses					
Zoster [6]					1 dose	
Measles, mumps, rubella (MMR) [7,*]	1 or 2 doses					
Pneumococcal polysaccharide (PPSV23) [8,9]	1 or 2 doses					1 dose
Pneumococcal 13-valent conjugate (PCV13) [10]	1 dose					
Meningococcal [11,*]	1 or more doses					
Hepatitis A [12,*]	2 doses					
Hepatitis B [13,*]	3 doses					

*Covered by the Vaccine Injury Compensation Program

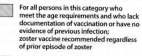

For all persons in this category who meet the age requirements and who lack documentation of vaccination or have no evidence of previous infection; zoster vaccine recommended regardless of prior episode of zoster

Recommended if some other risk factor is present (e.g., on the basis of medical, occupational, lifestyle, or other indication)

No recommendation

Report all clinically significant postvaccination reactions to the Vaccine Adverse Event Reporting System (VAERS). Reporting forms and instructions on filing a VAERS report are available at www.vaers.hhs.gov or by telephone, 800-822-7967.

Information on how to file a Vaccine Injury Compensation Program claim is available at www.hrsa.gov/vaccinecompensation or by telephone, 800-338-2382. To file a claim for vaccine injury, contact the U.S. Court of Federal Claims, 717 Madison Place, N.W., Washington, D.C. 20005; telephone, 202-357-6400.

Additional information about the vaccines in this schedule, extent of available data, and contraindications for vaccination is also available at www.cdc.gov/vaccines or from the CDC-INFO Contact Center at 800-CDC-INFO (800-232-4636) in English and Spanish, 8:00 a.m. - 8:00 p.m. Eastern Time, Monday - Friday, excluding holidays.

Use of trade names and commercial sources is for identification only and does not imply endorsement by the U.S. Department of Health and Human Services.

The recommendations in this schedule were approved by the Centers for Disease Control and Prevention's (CDC) Advisory Committee on Immunization Practices (ACIP), the American Academy of Family Physicians (AAFP), the American College of Physicians (ACP), American College of Obstetricians and Gynecologists (ACOG) and American College of Nurse-Midwives (ACNM).

VACCINE ▼ INDICATION ▶	Pregnancy	Immuno-compromising conditions (excluding human immunodeficiency virus [HIV]) [4,6,7,10,13]	HIV infection CD4+ T lymphocyte count [4,6,7,10,14,15] < 200 cells/µL	HIV infection CD4+ T lymphocyte count ≥ 200 cells/µL	Men who have sex with men (MSM)	Heart disease, chronic lung disease, chronic alcoholism	Asplenia (including elective splenectomy and persistent complement component deficiencies) [10,14]	Chronic liver disease	Kidney failure, end-stage renal disease, receipt of hemodialysis	Diabetes	Healthcare personnel
Influenza [2,*]	1 dose IIV annually				1 dose IIV or LAIV annually	1 dose IIV annually					1 dose IIV or LAIV annually
Tetanus, diphtheria, pertussis (Td/Tdap) [3,*]	1 dose Tdap each pregnancy	Substitute 1-time dose of Tdap for Td booster; then boost with Td every 10 yrs									
Varicella [4,*]	Contraindicated				2 doses						
Human papillomavirus (HPV) Female [5,*]	3 doses through age 26 yrs				3 doses through age 26 yrs						
Human papillomavirus (HPV) Male [5,*]	3 doses through age 26 yrs				3 doses through age 21 yrs						
Zoster [6]	Contraindicated				1 dose						
Measles, mumps, rubella (MMR) [7,*]	Contraindicated				1 or 2 doses						
Pneumococcal polysaccharide (PPSV23) [8,9]	1 or 2 doses										
Pneumococcal 13-valent conjugate (PCV13) [10]	1 dose										
Meningococcal [11,*]	1 or more doses										
Hepatitis A [12,*]	2 doses										
Hepatitis B [13,*]	3 doses										

*Covered by the Vaccine Injury Compensation Program

For all persons in this category who meet the age requirements and who lack documentation of vaccination or have no evidence of previous infection; zoster vaccine recommended regardless of prior episode of zoster

Recommended if some other risk factor is present (e.g., on the basis of medical, occupational, lifestyle, or other indications)

No recommendation

These schedules indicate the recommended age groups and medical indications for which administration of currently licensed vaccines is commonly indicated for adults ages 19 years and older, as of January 1, 2013. For all vaccines being recommended on the Adult Immunization Schedule: a vaccine series does not need to be restarted, regardless of the time that has elapsed between doses. Licensed combination vaccines may be used whenever any components of the combination are indicated and when the vaccine's other components are not contraindicated. For detailed recommendations on all vaccines, including those used primarily for travelers or that are issued during the year, consult the manufacturers' package inserts and the complete statements from the Advisory Committee on Immunization Practices (www.cdc.gov/vaccines/pubs/acip-list.htm). Use of trade names and commercial sources is for identification only and does not imply endorsement by the U.S. Department of Health and Human Services.

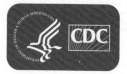

U.S. Department of Health and Human Services
Centers for Disease Control and Prevention

Footnotes — Recommended Immunization Schedule for Adults Aged 19 Years and Older—United States, 2013

1. **Additional information**
   - Additional guidance for the use of the vaccines described in this supplement is available at http://www.cdc.gov/vaccines/pubs/acip-list.htm.
   - Information on vaccination recommendations when vaccination status is unknown and other general immunization information can be found in the General Recommendations on Immunization at http://www.cdc.gov/mmwr/preview/mmwrhtml/rr6002a1.htm.
   - Information on travel vaccine requirements and recommendations (e.g., for hepatitis A and B, meningococcal, and other vaccines) are available at http://wwwnc.cdc.gov/travel/page/vaccinations.htm.

2. **Influenza vaccination**
   - Annual vaccination against influenza is recommended for all persons aged 6 months and older.
   - Persons aged 6 months and older, including pregnant women, can receive the inactivated influenza vaccine (IIV).
   - Healthy, nonpregnant persons aged 2–49 years without high-risk medical conditions can receive either intranasally administered live, attenuated influenza vaccine (LAIV) (FluMist), or IIV. Health-care personnel who care for severely immunocompromised persons (i.e., those who require care in a protected environment) should receive IIV rather than LAIV.
   - The intramuscularly or intradermally administered IIV are options for adults aged 18–64 years.
   - Adults aged 65 years and older can receive the standard dose IIV or the high-dose IIV (Fluzone High-Dose).

3. **Tetanus, diphtheria, and acellular pertussis (Td/Tdap) vaccination**
   - Administer one dose of Tdap vaccine to pregnant women during each pregnancy (preferred during 27–36 weeks' gestation), regardless of number of years since prior Td or Tdap vaccination.
   - Administer Tdap to all other adults who have not previously received Tdap or for whom vaccine status is unknown. Tdap can be administered regardless of interval since the most recent tetanus or diphtheria-toxoid containing vaccine.
   - Adults with an unknown or incomplete history of completing a 3-dose primary vaccination series with Td-containing vaccines should begin or complete a primary vaccination series including a Tdap dose.
   - For unvaccinated adults, administer the first 2 doses at least 4 weeks apart and the third dose 6–12 months after the second.
   - For incompletely vaccinated (i.e., less than 3 doses) adults, administer remaining doses.
   - Refer to the Advisory Committee on Immunization Practices (ACIP) statement for recommendations for administering Td/Tdap as prophylaxis in wound management (see footnote #1).

4. **Varicella vaccination**
   - All adults without evidence of immunity to varicella (as defined below) should receive 2 doses of single-antigen varicella vaccine or a second dose if they have received only 1 dose.
   - Special consideration for vaccination should be given to those who have close contact with persons at high risk for severe disease (e.g., health-care personnel and family contacts of persons with immunocompromising conditions) or are at high risk for exposure or transmission (e.g., teachers; child care employees; residents and staff members of institutional settings, including correctional institutions; college students; military personnel; adolescents and adults living in households with children; nonpregnant women of childbearing age; and international travelers).
   - Pregnant women should be assessed for evidence of varicella immunity. Women who do not have evidence of immunity should receive the first dose of varicella vaccine upon completion or termination of pregnancy and before discharge from the health-care facility. The second dose should be administered 4–8 weeks after the first dose.
   - Evidence of immunity to varicella in adults includes any of the following:
     — documentation of 2 doses of varicella vaccine at least 4 weeks apart;
     — U.S.-born before 1980 except health-care personnel and pregnant women;
     — history of varicella based on diagnosis or verification of varicella disease by a health-care provider;
     — history of herpes zoster based on diagnosis or verification of herpes zoster disease by a health-care provider; or
     — laboratory evidence of immunity or laboratory confirmation of disease.

5. **Human papillomavirus (HPV) vaccination**
   - Two vaccines are licensed for use in females, bivalent HPV vaccine (HPV2) and quadrivalent HPV vaccine (HPV4), and one HPV vaccine for use in males (HPV4).
   - For females, either HPV4 or HPV2 is recommended in a 3-dose series for routine vaccination at age 11 or 12 years, and for those aged 13 through 26 years, if not previously vaccinated.
   - For males, HPV4 is recommended in a 3-dose series for routine vaccination at age 11 or 12 years, and for those aged 13 through 21 years, if not previously vaccinated. Males aged 22 through 26 years may be vaccinated.
   - HPV4 is recommended for men who have sex with men (MSM) through age 26 years for those who did not get any or all doses when they were younger.
   - Vaccination is recommended for immunocompromised persons (including those with HIV infection) through age 26 years for those who did not get any or all doses when they were younger.
   - A complete series for either HPV4 or HPV2 consists of 3 doses. The second dose should be administered 1–2 months after the first dose; the third dose should be administered 6 months after the first dose (at least 24 weeks after the first dose).
   - HPV vaccines are not recommended for use in pregnant women. However, pregnancy testing is not needed before vaccination. If a woman is found to be pregnant after initiating the vaccination series, no intervention is needed; the remainder of the 3-dose series should be delayed until completion of pregnancy.
   - Although HPV vaccination is not specifically recommended for health-care personnel (HCP) based on their occupation, HCP should receive the HPV vaccine as recommended (see above).

6. **Zoster vaccination**
   - A single dose of zoster vaccine is recommended for adults aged 60 years and older regardless of whether they report a prior episode of herpes zoster. Although the vaccine is licensed by the Food and Drug Administration (FDA) for use among and can be administered to persons aged 50 years and older, ACIP recommends that vaccination begins at age 60 years.
   - Persons aged 60 years and older with chronic medical conditions may be vaccinated unless their condition constitutes a contraindication, such as pregnancy or severe immunodeficiency.
   - Although zoster vaccination is not specifically recommended for HCP, they should receive the vaccine if they are in the recommended age group.

7. **Measles, mumps, rubella (MMR) vaccination**
   - Adults born before 1957 generally are considered immune to measles and mumps. All adults born in 1957 or later should have documentation of 1 or more doses of MMR vaccine unless they have a medical contraindication to the vaccine, or laboratory evidence of immunity to each of the three diseases. Documentation of provider-diagnosed disease is not considered acceptable evidence of immunity for measles, mumps, or rubella.

   Measles component:
   - A routine second dose of MMR vaccine, administered a minimum of 28 days after the first dose, is recommended for adults who
     — are students in postsecondary educational institutions;
     — work in a health-care facility; or
     — plan to travel internationally.
   - Persons who received inactivated (killed) measles vaccine or measles vaccine of unknown type during 1963–1967 should be revaccinated with 2 doses of MMR vaccine.

   Mumps component:
   - A routine second dose of MMR vaccine, administered a minimum of 28 days after the first dose, is recommended for adults who
     — are students in a postsecondary educational institution;
     — work in a health-care facility; or
     — plan to travel internationally.
   - Persons vaccinated before 1979 with either killed mumps vaccine or mumps vaccine of unknown type who are at high risk for mumps infection (e.g., persons who are working in a health-care facility) should be considered for revaccination with 2 doses of MMR vaccine.

   Rubella component:
   - For women of childbearing age, regardless of birth year, rubella immunity should be determined. If there is no evidence of immunity, women who are not pregnant should be vaccinated. Pregnant women who do not have evidence of immunity should receive MMR vaccine upon completion or termination of pregnancy and before discharge from the health-care facility.

   HCP born before 1957:
   - For unvaccinated health-care personnel born before 1957 who lack laboratory evidence of measles, mumps, and/or rubella immunity or laboratory confirmation of disease, health-care facilities should consider vaccinating personnel with 2 doses of MMR vaccine at the appropriate interval for measles and mumps or 1 dose of MMR vaccine for rubella.

8. **Pneumococcal polysaccharide (PPSV23) vaccination**
   - Vaccinate all persons with the following indications:
     — all adults aged 65 years and older;

   — adults younger than age 65 years with chronic lung disease (including chronic obstructive pulmonary disease, emphysema, and asthma); chronic cardiovascular diseases; diabetes mellitus; chronic renal failure; nephrotic syndrome; chronic liver disease (including cirrhosis); alcoholism; cochlear implants; cerebrospinal fluid leaks; immunocompromising conditions; and functional or anatomic asplenia (e.g., sickle cell disease and other hemoglobinopathies, congenital or acquired asplenia, splenic dysfunction, or splenectomy [if elective splenectomy is planned, vaccinate at least 2 weeks before surgery]);
     — residents of nursing homes or long-term care facilities; and
     — adults who smoke cigarettes.
   - Persons with immunocompromising conditions and other selected conditions are recommended to receive PCV13 and PPSV23 vaccines. See footnote #10 for information on timing of PCV13 and PPSV23 vaccinations.
   - Persons with asymptomatic or symptomatic HIV infection should be vaccinated as soon as possible after their diagnosis.
   - When cancer chemotherapy or other immunosuppressive therapy is being considered, the interval between vaccination and initiation of immunosuppressive therapy should be at least 2 weeks. Vaccination during chemotherapy or radiation therapy should be avoided.
   - Routine use of PPSV23 is not recommended for American Indians/Alaska Natives or other persons younger than age 65 years unless they have underlying medical conditions that are PPSV23 indications. However, public health authorities may consider recommending PPSV23 for American Indians/Alaska Natives who are living in areas where the risk for invasive pneumococcal disease is increased.
   - When indicated, PPSV23 should be administered to patients who are uncertain of their vaccination status and there is no record of previous vaccination. When PCV13 is also indicated, a dose of PCV13 should be given first (see footnote #10).

9. **Revaccination with PPSV23**
   - One-time revaccination 5 years after the first dose is recommended for persons aged 19 through 64 years with chronic renal failure or nephrotic syndrome; functional or anatomic asplenia (e.g., sickle cell disease or splenectomy); and for persons with immunocompromising conditions.
   - Persons who received 1 or 2 doses of PPSV23 before age 65 years for any indication should receive another dose of the vaccine at age 65 years or later if at least 5 years have passed since their previous dose.
   - No further doses are needed for persons vaccinated with PPSV23 at or after age 65 years.

10. **Pneumococcal conjugate 13-valent vaccination (PCV13)**
    - Adults aged 19 years or older with immunocompromising conditions (including chronic renal failure and nephrotic syndrome), functional or anatomic asplenia, CSF leaks or cochlear implants, and who have not previously received PCV13 or PPSV23 should receive a single dose of PCV13 followed by a dose of PPSV23 at least 8 weeks later.
    - Adults aged 19 years or older with the aforementioned conditions who have previously received one or more doses of PPSV23 should receive a dose of PCV13 one or more years after the last PPSV23 dose was received. For those that require additional doses of PPSV23, the first such dose should be given no sooner than 8 weeks after PCV13 and at least 5 years since the most recent dose of PPSV23.
    - When indicated, PCV13 should be administered to patients who are uncertain of their vaccination status history and there is no record of previous vaccination.
    - Although PCV13 is licensed by the Food and Drug Administration (FDA) for use among and can be administered to persons aged 50 years and older, ACIP recommends PCV13 for adults aged 19 years and older with the specific medical conditions noted above.

11. **Meningococcal vaccination**
    - Administer 2 doses of meningococcal conjugate vaccine quadrivalent (MCV4) at least 2 months apart to adults with functional asplenia or persistent complement component deficiencies.
    - HIV-infected persons who are vaccinated also should receive 2 doses.
    - Administer a single dose of meningococcal vaccine to microbiologists routinely exposed to isolates of Neisseria meningitidis, military recruits, and persons who travel to or live in countries in which meningococcal disease is hyperendemic or epidemic.
    - First-year college students up through age 21 years who are living in residence halls should be vaccinated if they have not received a dose on or after their 16th birthday.
    - MCV4 is preferred for adults with any of the preceding indications who are aged 55 years and younger; meningococcal polysaccharide vaccine (MPSV4) is preferred for adults aged 56 years and older.
    - Revaccination with MCV4 every 5 years is recommended for adults previously vaccinated with MCV4 or MPSV4 who remain at increased risk for infection (e.g., adults with anatomic or functional asplenia or persistent complement component deficiencies).

12. **Hepatitis A vaccination**
    - Vaccinate any person seeking protection from hepatitis A virus (HAV) infection and persons with any of the following indications:
      — men who have sex with men and persons who use injection or noninjection illicit drugs;
      — persons working with HAV-infected primates or with HAV in a research laboratory setting;
      — persons with chronic liver disease and persons who receive clotting factor concentrates;
      — persons traveling to or working in countries that have high or intermediate endemicity of hepatitis A; and
      — unvaccinated persons who anticipate close personal contact (e.g., household or regular babysitting) with an international adoptee during the first 60 days after arrival in the United States from a country with high or intermediate endemicity. (See footnote #1 for more information on travel recommendations.) The first dose of the 2-dose hepatitis A vaccine series should be administered as soon as adoption is planned, ideally 2 or more weeks before the arrival of the adoptee.
    - Single-antigen vaccine formulations should be administered in a 2-dose schedule at either 0 and 6–12 months (Havrix), or 0 and 6–18 months (Vaqta). If the combined hepatitis A and hepatitis B vaccine (Twinrix) is used, administer 3 doses at 0, 1, and 6 months; alternatively, a 4-dose schedule may be used, administered on days 0, 7, and 21–30, followed by a booster dose at month 12.

13. **Hepatitis B vaccination**
    - Vaccinate persons with any of the following indications and any person seeking protection from hepatitis B virus (HBV) infection:
      — sexually active persons who are not in a long-term, mutually monogamous relationship (e.g., persons with more than one sex partner during the previous 6 months); persons seeking evaluation or treatment for a sexually transmitted disease (STD); current or recent injection-drug users; and men who have sex with men;
      — health-care personnel and public-safety workers who are potentially exposed to blood or other infectious body fluids;
      — persons with diabetes younger than age 60 years as soon as feasible after diagnosis; persons with diabetes who are age 60 years or older at the discretion of the treating clinician based on increased need for assisted blood glucose monitoring in long-term care facilities, likelihood of acquiring hepatitis B infection, its complications or chronic sequelae, and likelihood of immune response to vaccination;
      — persons with end-stage renal disease, including patients receiving hemodialysis; persons with HIV infection; and persons with chronic liver disease;
      — household contacts and sex partners of hepatitis B surface antigen-positive persons; clients and staff members of institutions for persons with developmental disabilities; and international travelers to countries with high or intermediate prevalence of chronic HBV infection; and
      — all adults in the following settings: STD treatment facilities; HIV testing and treatment facilities; facilities providing drug-abuse treatment and prevention services; health-care settings targeting services to injection-drug users or men who have sex with men; correctional facilities; end-stage renal disease programs and facilities for chronic hemodialysis patients; and institutions and nonresidential daycare facilities for persons with developmental disabilities.
    - Administer missing doses to complete a 3-dose series of hepatitis B vaccine to those persons not vaccinated or not completely vaccinated. The second dose should be administered 1 month after the first dose; the third dose should be given at least 2 months after the second dose (and at least 4 months after the first dose). If the combined hepatitis A and hepatitis B vaccine (Twinrix) is used, give 3 doses at 0, 1, and 6 months; alternatively, a 4-dose Twinrix schedule, administered on days 0, 7, and 21–30 followed by a booster dose at month 12 may be used.
    - Adult patients receiving hemodialysis or with other immunocompromising conditions should receive 1 dose of 40 µg/mL (Recombivax HB) administered on a 3-dose schedule at 0, 1, and 6 months or 2 doses of 20 µg/mL (Engerix-B) administered simultaneously on a 4-dose schedule at 0, 1, 2, and 6 months.

14. **Selected conditions for which Haemophilus influenzae type b (Hib) vaccine may be used**
    - 1 dose of Hib vaccine should be considered for persons who have sickle cell disease, leukemia, or HIV infection, or who have anatomic or functional asplenia if they have not previously received Hib vaccine.

15. **Immunocompromising conditions**
    - Inactivated vaccines generally are acceptable (e.g., pneumococcal, meningococcal, and influenza [inactivated influenza vaccine]), and live vaccines generally are avoided in persons with immune deficiencies or immunocompromising conditions. Information on specific conditions is available at http://www.cdc.gov/vaccines/pubs/acip-list.htm.

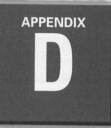

Select Herbs and Natural Products Used for Medicinal Purposes

Common Name(s)	Scientific Name	Uses	Adverse Reactions	Significant Considerations
Aloe vera	*Aloe vera*	To inhibit infection and promote healing of minor burns and wounds; as a laxative	None significant if used as directed; may cause burning sensation in wound	Rare reports of delayed healing when used in the gel form on a wound. If taken internally as a laxative, do not take longer than 1–3 wk without consulting primary health care provider. Decrease dosage if cramping occurs.
Bilberry	*Vaccinium myrtillus*	For vision enhancement and eye health, microcirculation, spider veins and varicose veins, capillary strengthening before surgery	No adverse effects reported in clinical studies	None.
Black cohosh (black snakeroot, squawroot)	*Cimicifuga racemosa*	For management of some symptoms of menopause and as an alternative to hormone replacement therapy; may be beneficial for hypercholesterolemia or peripheral vascular disease	Overdose causes nausea, dizziness, nervous system and visual disturbances, decreased pulse rate and increased perspiration	Should not be used during pregnancy. Possible interactions with hormone therapy.
Capsicum (hot peppers)	*Capsicum frutescens*	For neuralgic pain relief, bladder pain and hyperreflexia; as an antipruritic for psoriasis	Burning sensation upon application	Creams should be applied with gloves and hands washed thoroughly before touching face or eyes.
Chamomile	*Matricaria chamomilla*	Drunk as an infusion for gastrointestinal (GI) disturbances (e.g., diarrhea, flatulence, stomatitis); as a sedative and as an anti-inflammatory agent	Possible contact dermatitis and, in rare instances, anaphylaxis	Chamomile is a member of the ragweed family and those allergic to ragweed should not take the herb. Avoid use during pregnancy. May enhance anticoagulant effect when administered with anticoagulants. Do not administer to a child without checking with primary health care provider.
Chondroitin	Chondroitin sulfate, chondroitin sulfuric acid, chonsurid	For arthritis—particularly osteoarthritis	None significant if used as directed	Because chondroitin is concentrated in cartilage, theoretically it produces no toxic or teratogenic effects.

(table continues on page 642)

Common Name(s)	Scientific Name	Uses	Adverse Reactions	Significant Considerations
Cranberry	*Vaccinium macrocarpon*	To prevent urinary tract infection (UTI) by acidifying the urine; lower pH also reduces the ammonia odor of urinary incontinence.	Large doses can produce GI symptoms (e.g., diarrhea)	None. Safe for use during pregnancy and while breastfeeding. Inform patient that sugar-free cranberry juice or supplements are available if the patient has diabetes mellitus. Antibiotic is usually needed to treat active UTI.
Eucalyptus oil	*E. globules Labillardiere*	As a decongestant, expectorant for respiratory conditions; topically for antimicrobial effect	Pain, nausea, vomiting; individuals with acute intermittent porphyria should not take	Used in mouthwashes for antimicrobial properties. Adverse reactions of slowing the central nervous system (CNS), drowsiness, seizures, and coma when taken orally. Blood sugar levels may decrease with use.
Feverfew	*Tanacetum parthenium*	As an antipyretic; for migraine headaches, asthma, arthritis, relief of menstrual cramps	Most are mild; rash or contact dermatitis may indicate allergy and herb should be withdrawn	Possible interaction with anticoagulants. Patient should be observed for abnormal bleeding. Do not use during pregnancy or lactation.
Garlic	*Allium sativum*	To lower blood glucose, cholesterol, and lipid levels; as topical antifungal	May cause abnormal blood glucose levels	Increased risk of bleeding in patients taking the warfarin, salicylates, or antiplatelet drugs.
Ginger (ginger root, black ginger)	*Zingiber officinale*	As antiemetic, cardiotonic, antithrombotic, antibacterial, antioxidant, antitussive, anti-inflammatory, prophylaxis for nausea and vomiting; for GI disturbances, colic; to lower cholesterol	Excessive doses may cause CNS depression and interfere with cardiac functioning or anticoagulant activity	Theoretically, ginger could enhance the effects of the antiplatelet drugs, such as coumarin. Observe for excessive bleeding (e.g., nose bleeding, easy bruising). Consult primary health care provider for use during pregnancy.
Ginkgo (maiden hair tree, kew tree)	*Ginkgo biloba*	For cerebral insufficiency dementias, circulatory problems, headaches, macular degeneration, diabetic retinopathy, premenstrual syndrome	Rare if used as directed; possible effects include headache, dizziness, heart palpitations, GI effects, rash, allergic dermatitis	Do not take with antidepressant drugs, such as the monoamine oxidase inhibitors (MAOIs), or antiplatelet drugs, such as coumarin, unless advised to do so by the primary health care provider. Discontinue use at least 2 wk before surgery.
Goldenseal	*Hydrastis canadensis*	As antiseptic for skin (topical), astringent for mucous membranes (mouthwash), wash for inflamed eyes, anti-diarrheal	Large doses may cause dry or irritated mucous membranes and injury to the GI system	Should not be taken for more than 3–7 days. Contraindicated in pregnancy and hypertension.
Glucosamine (chitosamine)	*2-Amino-2-deoxy-glucose*	As antiarthritic in osteoarthritis	Usually well tolerated; mild adverse reactions such as heartburn, diarrhea, nausea, and itching have been reported	No direct toxic effects have been reported. Cautious use is recommended in diabetes because there is a potential for altering blood glucose levels.
Green tea	*Camellia sinensis*	To reduce cancer risk, lower lipid levels, help prevent dental caries; for antimicrobial and antioxidative effects	Well tolerated; contains caffeine (may cause mild stimulant effects such as anxiety, nervousness, heart irregularities, restlessness, insomnia, and digestive irritation)	No direct toxic effects have been reported. Contains caffeine and should be avoided during pregnancy and by individuals with hypertension, anxiety, eating disorders, insomnia, diabetes, and ulcers. Inform patient to avoid taking green tea with iron supplements because green tea interferes with iron absorption.

(table continues on page 643)

Common Name(s)	Scientific Name	Uses	Adverse Reactions	Significant Considerations
Hawthorne	*Crataegus oxyacantha*	For regulation of blood pressure and heart rhythm; to treat athero-sclerosis and angina pectoris; as a sedative	Hypotension and sedation (in high doses)	May interfere with serum digoxin effects. Notify primary health care provider and pharmacist if taking the herb.
Kava (kawa, kava-kava, awa yangona)	*Piper methys-ticum*	For mild to moderate anxiety; as a sedative	Scaly skin rash; disturbances in visual accommodation, habituation	Limit use to no more than 3 mo.
Melatonin	*Melatonin*	For insomnia; topically to protect against ultraviolet light	Headache, depression, possi-ble additive effects when taken with alcohol	Avoid hazardous activities until the CNS effects of this supplement are known. Do not take for prolonged periods, because effects of pro-longed use are not known. May interfere with conception.
Passionflower (passion fruit, granadilla, water lemon, apricot vine)	*Passiflora incarnata*	To promote sleep; as a treatment for pain and nervous exhaustion	None if used as directed; excessively large doses may cause CNS depression	May interact with anticoagulants and MAOIs.
Red yeast	*Monascus purpureus*	To reduce cholesterol lev-els in healthy people, gas-tric and circulation health	Same reactions as statin drugs; headache, dizziness, nausea, constipation	Should not be taken with other antihyperlipidemia drugs.
Saw palmetto (cabbage palm, fan palm, scrub palm)	*Serenoa repens*	For symptoms of benign prostatic hypertrophy	Generally well tolerated; occa-sional GI effects	May interact with hormones such as oral contraceptive drugs and hormone replacement therapy.
St. John's wort (Klamath weed, goatweed, rosin rose)	*Hypericum perforatum*	As an antidepressant or antiviral	Usually mild; may cause dry mouth, dizziness, constipa-tion, other GI symptoms, pho-tosensitivity	May decrease efficacy of protease inhibitors, theophylline, warfarin, and digoxin; use with other antide-pressant prescriptions is not recommended.
Tea tree oil	*Melaleuca alternifolia*	As topical antimicrobial, antifungal	Contact dermatitis	For topical use only; do not take orally.
Valerian	*Valeriana officinalis*	For restlessness, sleep disorders	Rare if used as directed	May interact with the barbiturates (e.g., phenobarbital), the benzodi-azepines (e.g., diazepam), and the opioids, (e.g., morphine).
Willow bark (weidenrinde, white willow, purple osier willow, crack willow)	*Salix alba, S. purpurea, S. fragilis*	As an analgesic	Adverse reactions are those associated with the salicylates	Do not use with aspirin or other nonsteroidal anti-inflammatory drugs. Do not use in patients with peptic ulcers and other medical conditions in which the salicylates are contraindicated.

Select Herbs and Natural Products Used for Medicinal Purposes

Improving Patient Outcomes Using Standardized Drug Protocols

Nurses work in many different practice settings. Part of your job is to provide up-to-date, innovative care strategies to improve patient outcomes. By sharing what works in your institution with others, we can achieve good outcomes. Here are some examples of standardized drug protocols if your agency has not adopted a protocol for similar situations that are not frequented by all patient populations.

Before you implement any of these protocols, bring together providers from different agency resources and be sure to have experts such as a clinical pharmacist review the information from that area of expertise. Then test it out and see if it works for your institution.

Hospice Comfort Kit

This is a set of medications prescribed and kept at the patient's home when service begins, to be used in the event of a comfort emergency. This kit includes different medications to relieve distress caused by the disease or treatment process and can support symptom management without the delay of having to wait for providers, orders, and medication pick-up. Typical medications in a comfort kit include:

- morphine or oxycodone (or another pain medication), to treat pain and shortness of breath
- lorazepam, to treat anxiety, agitation, nausea, or insomnia
- atropine (or another anticholinergic), to reduce excessive secretions
- prochlorperazine or promethazine, to treat nausea and vomiting
- laxative of choice, to treat constipation

(Used with permission from Franciscan Hospice and Palliative Care, Tacoma, Washington)

Intravenous Extravasation of Vesicant Drugs

Although few incidences of extravasation are reported, when it happens the skin is at risk for injury. Supplies and protocols for treatment of extravasations should be readily available when vesicant intravenous (IV) medication is prescribed. All members of the health care team should diligently monitor the patient. Supplies include:

- Warm pack
- Cold pack
- hyaluronidase (150 units/mL) solution
- phentolamine for dilution in 0.9% sodium chloride (for use with vasopressor vesicant)

(Hadaway, 2007)

Sexual Assault (Prophylaxis) Medication

One out of six women in the United States reports experiencing sexual assault in her lifetime. When reported, adherence to follow-up visits is poor. Therefore, protocols for one-time-only prophylactic treatment can be administered following an assault to help prevent sexually transmitted infections following exposure. These include:

- ceftriaxone 250 mg intramuscular (IM) in a single dose OR cefixime 400 mg orally in a single dose
- metronidazole 2 g orally in a single dose
- azithromycin 1 g orally in a single dose OR doxycycline 100 mg orally twice a day for 7 days
- Hepatitis B vaccine series

(Centers for Disease Control and Prevention, 2010)

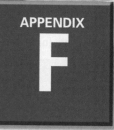

Less Frequently Used Calculations, Measurements, and Basic Mathematical Review

Body Surface Area Nomograms

Nomogram for Estimating Body Surface Area of Infants and Young Children

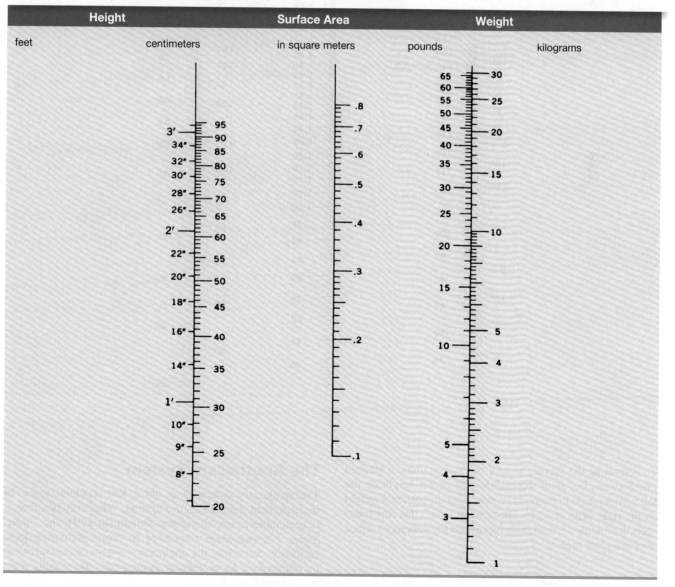

Nomogram for Estimating Body Surface Area of Older Children and Adults

Height	Surface Area	Weight
feet centimeters	in square meters	pounds kilograms

To determine the surface area of the patient, draw a straight line between the point representing his or her height on the left vertical scale to the point representing the patient's weight on the right vertical scale. The point at which this line intersects the middle vertical scale represents the patient's surface area in square meters.

The Apothecary System

The apothecary system is an older, less accurate system of measurement than the metric system. Whenever possible, it is preferable to use the metric system. In 1994, the *United States Pharmacopeia* responded to errors stemming from confusion caused by the apothecary system of measurement by eliminating an apothecary system conversion table from its national formulary.

Approximate Equivalents of Systems of Measurement

Metric	Apothecary	Household
Weight		
0.1 mg	gr 1/600	
0.15 mg	gr 1/400	
0.2 mg	gr 1/300	
0.3 mg	gr 1/200	
0.4 mg	gr 1/150	
0.6 mg	gr 1/100	
1 mg	gr 1/60	
2 mg	gr 1/30	
4 mg	gr 1/15	
6 mg	gr 1/10	
8 mg	gr 1/8	
10 mg	gr 1/6	
15 mg	gr 1/4	
20 mg	gr 1/3	
30 mg	gr ss (1/2)	
60 mg	gr 1	
100 mg	gr i ss (1 1/2)	
120 mg	gr ii	
1 g (1000 mg)	gr xv	
Volume		
0.06 mL	min i	
1 mL	min xv or xvi	
4 mL	fluid dram i	1 teaspoon
15 mL	fluid drams iv	1/2 ounce
30 mL	fluid ounce i	1 ounce
500 mL	1 pint	1 pint
1000 mL (1 liter)	1 quart	1 quart

In 2002, the Joint Commission adopted recommendations from the Institute for Safe Medication Practices' list of error-prone medication abbreviations, symbols, and dose designations for use in its National Patient Safety Goals. It has proven very difficult to convince practitioners of all types to relinquish use of the apothecary system. In keeping with current health care standards, this information is provided for situations in which conversion is necessary.

Mathematical Review

This section of Appendix F provides a review of basic math concepts. Should the drug dosage calculations in Chapter 3 cause confusion or if they are hard to understand, look here to find out how to perform the basic math before adding drug names or amounts.

Fractions

The two parts of a fraction are the numerator and the denominator.

$$\frac{2}{3} \begin{array}{l} \leftarrow \text{numerator} \\ \leftarrow \text{denominator} \end{array}$$

A proper fraction may be defined as a part of a whole or any number less than a whole number. An improper fraction is a fraction having a numerator the same as or larger than the denominator. For example,

$$\text{proper fraction } \frac{1}{2}$$

$$\text{improper fraction } \frac{7}{3}$$

The numerator and the denominator must be of *like entities or terms,* that is:

Correct (like terms)	Incorrect (unlike terms)
$\dfrac{2\,\text{acres}}{3\,\text{acres}}$	$\dfrac{2\,\text{acres}}{3\,\text{miles}}$
$\dfrac{2\,\text{grams}}{3\,\text{grams}}$	$\dfrac{2\,\text{grams}}{5\,\text{milliliters}}$

Mixed Numbers and Improper Fractions

A mixed number is a whole number and a proper fraction. A whole number is a number that stands alone; 3, 25, and 117 are examples of whole numbers. A proper fraction is a fraction whose numerator is *smaller than* the denominator; 1/8, 2/5, and 3/7 are examples of proper fractions.

These are mixed numbers:

2 2/3   2 is the whole number and 2/3 is the proper fraction
3 1/4   3 is the whole number and 1/4 is the proper fraction

When doing certain calculations, it is sometimes necessary to change a mixed number to an improper fraction or change an improper fraction to a mixed number. An improper fraction is a fraction whose numerator is *larger than* the denominator; 5/2, 16/3, and 12 3/2 are examples of improper fractions.

To change a *mixed number* to an *improper fraction,* multiply the denominator of the fraction by the whole number, add the numerator, and place the sum over the denominator.

EXAMPLE: Mixed number 3 3/5

1. Multiply the denominator of the fraction (5) by the whole number (3), or $5 \times 3 = 15$:

$$3 \times \frac{3}{5}$$

2. Add the result of multiplying the denominator of the fraction (15) to the numerator (3), or $15 + 3 = 18$:

$$\frac{15}{5} + \frac{3}{5}$$

3. Then place the sum (18) over the denominator of the fraction:

$$\frac{18}{5}$$

To change an *improper fraction to a mixed number,* divide the denominator into the numerator. The quotient (the result of the division of these two numbers) is the whole

number. Then place the remainder over the denominator of the improper fraction.

EXAMPLE: Improper fraction 15/4

$$\frac{15 \leftarrow \text{numerator}}{4 \leftarrow \text{denominator}}$$

1. Divide the denominator (4) into the numerator (15), or 15 divided by 4 (15 ÷ 4):

$$\begin{array}{r} 3 \leftarrow \text{quotient} \\ 4\overline{)15} \\ \underline{12} \\ 3 \leftarrow \text{remainder} \end{array}$$

2. The quotient (3) becomes the whole number:

$$3\frac{3}{4}$$

3. The remainder (3) now becomes the numerator of the fraction of the mixed number:

$$3\frac{3}{-}$$

4. And the denominator of the improper fraction (4) now becomes the denominator of the fraction of the mixed number:

$$3\frac{3}{4}$$

Adding Fractions With Like Denominators

When the denominators are the *same,* fractions can be added by adding the numerators and placing the sum of the numerators over the denominator.

EXAMPLES

$2/7 + 3/7 = 5/7$

$1/10 + 3/10 = 4/10$

$2/9 + 1/9 + 4/9 = 7/9$

$1/12 + 5/12 + 3/12 = 9/12$

$2/13 + 1/13 + 3/13 + 5/13 = 11/13$

When giving a final answer, fractions are *always* reduced to the lowest possible terms. In the examples above, the answers of 5/7, 7/9, and 11/13 cannot be reduced. The answers of 4/10 and 9/12 can be reduced to 2/5 and 3/4.

To reduce a fraction to the lowest possible terms, determine if any number, which always must be the same, can be divided into both the numerator and the denominator.

4/10: the numerator *and* the denominator can be divided by 2.
9/12: the numerator *and* the denominator can be divided by 3.

For example:

$$\frac{4 \div 2 = 2}{10 \div 2 = 5}$$

If when adding fractions the answer is an improper fraction, it may then be changed to a mixed number.

2/5 + 4/5 = 6/5 (improper fraction)

6/5 changed to a mixed number is 1 1/5.

Adding Fractions With Unlike Denominators

Fractions with *unlike denominators* cannot be added until the denominators are changed to like numbers or numbers that are the same. The first step is to find the *lowest common denominator*, which is the lowest number divisible by (or that can be divided by) all the denominators.

EXAMPLE: Add 2/3 and 1/4

$\frac{2}{3}$
$\frac{1}{4}$

The lowest number that can be divided by these two denominators is 12; therefore, 12 is the lowest common denominator.

1. Divide the lowest common denominator (which in this example is 12) by each of the denominators in the fractions (in this example 3 and 4):

$$\frac{2}{3} = \frac{}{12} \quad (12 \div 3 = 4)$$

$$\frac{1}{4} = \frac{}{12} \quad (12 \div 4 = 3)$$

2. Multiply the results of the divisions by the numerator of the fractions (12 ÷ 3 = 4 × the numerator 2 = 8 and 12 ÷ 4 = 3 × the numerator 1 = 3) and place the results in the numerator:

$$\frac{2}{3} = \frac{}{12} \qquad \frac{8}{12}$$

$$\frac{1}{4} = \frac{}{12} \qquad \frac{3}{12}$$

3. Add the numerators (8 + 3) and place the result over the denominator (12):

$$\frac{8}{12}$$

$$\frac{3}{12}$$

$$\frac{11}{12}$$

Adding Mixed Numbers or Fractions With Mixed Numbers

When adding two or more mixed numbers or adding fractions and mixed numbers, the mixed number is first changed to an improper fraction.

EXAMPLE: Add 3 3/4 and 3 3/4

$3\frac{3}{4}$ changed to an improper fraction → $\frac{15}{4}$

$3\frac{3}{4}$ changed to an improper fraction → $\frac{15}{4}$

The numerators are added → $\frac{30}{4} = 7\ 2/4 = 7\ 1/2$

The improper fraction (30/4) is changed to a mixed number (7 2/4) and the fraction of the mixed number (2/4) changed to the lowest possible terms (1/2).

EXAMPLE: Add 2 1/2 and 3 1/4

$2\frac{1}{2}$ changed to an improper fraction $\frac{5}{2}$

$3\frac{1}{4}$ changed to an improper fraction $\frac{13}{4}$

In the example above, 5/2 and 13/4 cannot be added because the denominators are not the same. It will be necessary to find the lowest common denominator first. For these two fractions the lowest common denominator is 4.

$\frac{5}{2}$ $\qquad$ $\frac{13}{4}$ becomes $\frac{10}{4}$ $\qquad$ $\frac{13}{4}$

The numerators are added $\frac{23}{4}$ changed to a mixed number $= 5\frac{3}{4}$

Comparing Fractions

When fractions with *like* denominators are compared, the fraction with the *largest numerator* is the *largest* fraction.

EXAMPLES

Compare: 5/8 and 3/8   Answer: 5/8 is larger than 3/8.

Compare: 1/4 and 3/4   Answer: 3/4 is larger than 1/4

When the denominators are *not* the same, for example, comparing 2/3 and 1/10, the lowest common denominator must first be determined. The same procedure is followed when adding fractions with unlike denominators (see above).

EXAMPLE: Compare 2/3 and 1/10 (fractions with unlike denominators)

$$\frac{2}{3} = \frac{20}{30}$$

$$\frac{1}{10} = \frac{3}{30} \quad \text{lowest common denominator}$$

The largest numerator in these two fractions is 20; therefore, 2/3 is larger than 1/10.

Multiplying Fractions

When fractions are multiplied, the numerators are multiplied *and* the denominators are multiplied.

EXAMPLES

$$\frac{1}{8} \times \frac{1}{4} = \frac{1}{32} \qquad \frac{1}{2} \times \frac{2}{3} = \frac{2}{6} = \frac{1}{3}$$

In the above examples, it was necessary to reduce one of the answers to its lowest possible terms.

Multiplying Whole Numbers and Fractions

When whole numbers are multiplied with fractions, the numerator is multiplied by the whole number and the product is placed over the denominator. When necessary, the fraction is reduced to its lowest possible terms. If the answer is an improper fraction, it may be changed to a mixed number.

EXAMPLES

$$2 \times \frac{1}{2} = \frac{2}{2} = 1 \text{ (answer reduced to lowest possible terms)}$$

$$2 \times \frac{3}{8} = \frac{6}{8} = \frac{3}{4} \text{ (answer reduced to lowest possible terms)}$$

$$4 \times \frac{2}{3} = \frac{8}{3} = 2\frac{2}{3} \text{ (improper fraction changed to a mixed number)}$$

Multiplying Mixed Numbers

To multiply mixed numbers, the mixed numbers are changed to *improper fractions* and then multiplied.

EXAMPLES

$$2\frac{1}{2} \times 3\frac{1}{4} = \frac{5}{2} \times \frac{13}{4} = \frac{65}{8} = 8\frac{1}{8}$$

$$3\frac{1}{3} \times 4\frac{1}{2} = \frac{10}{3} \times \frac{9}{2} = \frac{90}{6} = 15$$

Multiplying a Whole Number and a Mixed Number

To multiply a whole number and a mixed number, *both* numbers must be changed to improper fractions.

EXAMPLES

$$3 \times 2\frac{1}{2} = \frac{3}{1} \times \frac{5}{2} = \frac{15}{2} = 7\frac{1}{2}$$

$$2 \times 4\frac{1}{2} = \frac{2}{1} \times \frac{9}{2} = \frac{18}{2} = 9$$

A whole number is converted to an improper fraction by placing the whole number over 1. In the above examples, 3 becomes 3/1 and 2 becomes 2/1.

Dividing Fractions

When fractions are divided, the *second* fraction (the divisor) is inverted (turned upside down) and then the fractions are multiplied.

EXAMPLES

$$\frac{1}{3} \div \frac{3}{7} = \frac{1}{3} \times \frac{7}{3} = \frac{7}{9}$$

$$\frac{1}{8} \div \frac{1}{4} = \frac{1}{8} \times \frac{4}{1} = \frac{4}{8} = \frac{1}{2}$$

$$\frac{3}{4} \div \frac{1}{2} = \frac{3}{4} \times \frac{2}{1} = \frac{6}{4} = 1\frac{1}{2}$$

In the above examples, the second answer was reduced to its lowest possible terms and the third answer, which was an improper fraction, was changed to a mixed number.

Dividing Fractions and Mixed Numbers

Some problems of division may be expressed as (1) fractions and mixed numbers, (2) two mixed numbers, (3) whole numbers and fractions, or (4) whole numbers and mixed numbers.

Mixed Numbers and Fractions

When a mixed number is divided by a fraction, the whole number is first changed to a fraction.

EXAMPLES

$$2\frac{1}{3} \div \frac{1}{4} = \frac{7}{3} \div \frac{1}{4} = \frac{7}{3} \times \frac{4}{1} = \frac{28}{3} = 9\frac{1}{3}$$

$$2\frac{1}{2} \div \frac{1}{2} = \frac{5}{2} \div \frac{1}{2} = \frac{5}{2} \times \frac{2}{1} = \frac{10}{2} = 5$$

Mixed Numbers

When two mixed numbers are divided, they are both changed to improper fractions.

EXAMPLE

$$3\frac{3}{4} \div 1\frac{1}{2} = \frac{15}{4} \div \frac{3}{2} = \frac{15}{4} \times \frac{2}{3} = \frac{30}{12}$$

$$= 2\frac{6}{12} = 2\frac{1}{2}$$

Whole Numbers and Fractions

When a whole number is divided by a fraction, the whole number is changed to an improper fraction by placing the whole number over 1.

EXAMPLE

$$2 \div \frac{2}{3} = \frac{2}{1} \div \frac{2}{3} = \frac{2}{1} \times \frac{3}{2} = \frac{6}{2} = 3$$

Whole Numbers and Mixed Numbers

When whole numbers and mixed numbers are divided, the whole number is changed to an improper fraction and the mixed number is changed to an improper fraction.

EXAMPLE

$$4 \div 2\frac{2}{3} = \frac{4}{1} \div \frac{8}{3} = \frac{4}{1} \times \frac{3}{8} = \frac{12}{8} = 1\frac{4}{8} = 1\frac{1}{2}$$

Ratios

A ratio is a way of expressing *a part of a whole* or *the relation of one number to another*. For example, a ratio written as 1:10 means 1 in 10 parts, or 1 to 10. A ratio may also be written as a fraction; thus, 1:10 can also be expressed as 1/10.

EXAMPLES

1:1000 is 1 part in 1000 parts, or 1 to 1000, or 1/1000.

1:250 is 1 part in 250 parts, or 1 to 250, or 1/250.

Some drug solutions are expressed in ratios; for example, 1:100 or 1:500. These ratios mean that there is 1 part of a drug in 100 parts of solution or 1 part of the drug in 500 parts of solution.

Percentages

The term *percentage* or *percent* (%) means *parts per hundred*.

EXAMPLES

25% is 25 parts per hundred.
50% is 50 parts per hundred.

A percentage may also be expressed as a fraction.

EXAMPLES

25% is 25 parts per hundred or 25/100.
50% is 50 parts per hundred or 50/100.
30% is 30 parts per hundred or 30/100.

The above fractions may also be reduced to their lowest possible terms:

$$25/100 = 1/4, \ 50/100 = 1/2, \ 30/100 = 3/10.$$

Changing a Fraction to a Percentage

To change a fraction to a percentage, divide the denominator by the numerator and multiply the results (quotient) by 100 and then add a percent sign (%).

EXAMPLES

Change 4/5 to a percentage.

$$4 \div 5 = 0.8$$
$$0.8 \times 100 = 80\%$$

Change 2/3 to a percentage.

$$2 \div 3 = 0.666$$
$$0.666 \times 100 = 66.6\%$$

Changing a Ratio to a Percentage

To change a ratio to a percentage, the ratio is first expressed as a fraction with the first number or term of the ratio becoming the numerator and the second number or term becoming the denominator. For example, the ratio 1:500 when changed to a fraction becomes 1/500. This fraction is then changed to a percentage by the same method shown in the preceding section.

EXAMPLES

Change 1:125 to a percentage.
1:125 written as a fraction is 1/125.

$$1 \div 125 = 0.008$$
$$0.008 \times 100 = 0.8$$

add the percent sign = 0.8%

Changing a Percentage to a Ratio

To change a percentage to a ratio, the percentage becomes the numerator and is placed over a denominator of 100.

EXAMPLES

Changing 5% and 10% to ratios

$$5\% \text{ is } \frac{5}{100} = \frac{1}{20} \text{ or } 1:20$$

$$10\% \text{ is } \frac{10}{100} = \frac{1}{10} \text{ or } 1:10$$

Proportions

A proportion is a method of expressing equality between two ratios. An example of two ratios expressed as a proportion is as follows: 3 is to 4 as 9 is to 12. This may also be written as:

$$3:4 \text{ as } 9:12$$

or

$$3:4::9:12$$

or

$$\frac{3}{4} = \frac{9}{12}$$

Proportions may be used to find an unknown quantity. The unknown quantity is assigned a letter, usually X. An example of a proportion with an unknown quantity is 5:10::15:X.

The first and last terms of the proportion are called the *extremes*. In the above expression 5 and X are the extremes. The second and third terms of the proportion are called the *means*. In the above proportion, 10 and 15 are the means:

$$\text{means} \quad 5:10::15:X \quad \text{extremes}$$

$$\text{extreme} \frac{5}{10} = \frac{15}{X} \text{mean} \quad \text{extreme}$$

To solve for X:

1. Multiply the extremes and place the product (result) to the *left* of the equal sign.

$$\mathbf{5}:10::15:\mathbf{X}$$
$$5X =$$

2. Multiply the means and place the product to the *right* of the equal sign.

$$5:\mathbf{10}::\mathbf{15}X$$
$$5X = 150$$

3. Solve for X by dividing the number to the right of the equal sign by the number to the left of the equal sign (150 ÷ 5).

$$5X = 150$$
$$X = 30$$

4. To prove the answer is correct, substitute the answer (30) for X in the equation.

$$5:10::15:X$$
$$5:10::15:30$$

Then multiply the means and place the product to the left of the equal sign. Then multiply the extremes and place the product to the right of the equal sign.

$$5:10::15:30$$
$$150 = 150$$

If the numbers are the same on both sides of the equal sign, the equation has been solved correctly.

If the proportion has been set up as a fraction, cross-multiply and solve for X.

$$\frac{5}{10} = \frac{15}{X}$$

5 times X = 5X and 10 times 15 = 150

$$5X = 150$$
$$X = 30$$

To set up a proportion, remember that a sequence *must* be followed. If a sequence is not followed, the proportion will be stated incorrectly.

EXAMPLES

If a man can walk 6 *miles* in 2 *hours,* how many *miles* can he walk in 3 *hours?*

miles is to *hours* and *miles* is to *hours*
or
miles:hours::miles:hours
or

$$\frac{miles}{hours} = \frac{miles}{hours}$$

The unknown fact is the number of miles walked in 3 hours:

6 miles:2 hours::X miles:3 hours

$$2X = 18$$

X = 9 miles (he can walk 9 miles in 3 hours)

If there are 15 *grains* in 1 *gram,* 30 *grains* equals how many *grams?*

15 grains:1 gram::30 grains:X grams

$$15X = 30$$

X = 2 grams (30 grains equals 2 grams)

Decimals

Decimals are used in the metric system. A decimal is a fraction in which the denominator is 10 or some power of 10. For example, 2/10 (read as two tenths) is a fraction with a denominator of 10; 1/100 (read as one one hundredth) is an example of a fraction with a denominator that is a power of 10 (i.e., 100).

A power (or multiple) of 10 is the *number 1 followed by one or more zeros.* Therefore, 100, 1000, 10,000, and so on are powers of 10 because the number 1 is followed by two, three,

and four zeros, respectively. Fractions whose denominators are 10 or a power of 10 are often expressed in decimal form.

Parts of a Decimal
There are three parts to a decimal:

	1.25	
number(s) to the left of the decimal	**d e c i m a l**	number(s) to the right of the decimal

Types of Decimals
A decimal may consist only of numbers to the right of the decimal point. This is called a decimal fraction. Examples of decimal fractions are 0.05, 0.6, and 0.002.

A decimal may also have numbers to the left *and* right of the decimal point. This is called a mixed decimal fraction. Examples of mixed decimal fractions are 1.25, 2.5, and 7.5.

Reading Decimals
To read a decimal, the position of the number to the left or right of the decimal point indicates how the decimal is to be expressed.

0 hundred thousands
0 ten thousands
0 thousands
0 hundreds
0 tens
0 units

Decimal Point
0 tenths
0 hundredths
0 thousandths
0 ten thousandths
0 hundred thousandths

Adding Decimals
When adding decimals, place the numbers in a column so that the whole numbers are aligned to the left of the decimal and the decimal fractions are aligned to the right of the decimal.

EXAMPLE

20.45 + 2.56	2 + 0.25
is written as:	is written as:
20.45 + 2.56	2.00 + 0.25
23.01	2.25

Subtracting Decimals

When subtracting decimals, the numbers are aligned to the left and right of the decimal in the same manner as for the addition of decimals.

EXAMPLE

$20.45 - 2.56$ $9.74 - 0.45$

is written as: is written as:

$$\begin{array}{r} 20.45 \\ -\ 2.56 \\ \hline 17.89 \end{array} \qquad \begin{array}{r} 9.74 \\ -\ 0.45 \\ \hline 9.29 \end{array}$$

Multiplying a Whole Number by a Decimal

To multiply a whole number by a decimal, move the decimal point of the product (answer) as many places to the left as there are places to the right of the decimal point.

EXAMPLES

$$\begin{array}{r} 500 \\ \times\ .05 \leftarrow \\ \hline 2500. \end{array}$$ there are two places to the right of the decimal

the decimal point is moved two places to the left

After moving the decimal point, the answer reads 25.

$$\begin{array}{r} 250 \\ \times\ .3 \leftarrow \\ \hline 750. \end{array}$$ there is one place to the right of the decimal

the decimal point is moved one place to the left

After moving the decimal point, the answer reads 75.

Multiplying a Decimal by a Decimal

To multiply a decimal by a decimal, move the decimal point of the product (answer) as many places to the left as there are places to the right in *both* decimals.

EXAMPLE

$$\begin{array}{r} \\ 2.75 \leftarrow \\ \times\ .05 \leftarrow \\ \hline 1375. \end{array}$$ there are two places to the right of the decimal

plus two places to the right of the decimal, move

the decimal point *four* places to the left

After moving the decimal point, the answer reads 0.1375.

Dividing Decimals

The divisor is a number that is divided into the dividend.

EXAMPLE

$$0.69 \div 0.3 \qquad 0.3\overline{)0.69}$$

$$\uparrow \qquad \uparrow \qquad\qquad \uparrow \quad \uparrow$$

dividend divisor   divisor dividend

This may be written or spoken as 0.69 divided by 0.3. To divide decimals:

1. The *divisor* is changed to a whole number. In this example, the decimal point is moved one place to the right so that 0.3 now becomes 3, which is a whole number.

$$0.3\overline{)0.69}$$

2. The decimal point in the *dividend* is now moved the *same number of places* to the right. In this example, the decimal point is moved one place to the right, the same number of places the decimal point in the divisor was moved.

$$0.3\overline{)0.69}$$

3. The numbers are now divided.

$$3\overline{)6.9}^{\,2.3}$$

When only the dividend is a decimal, the decimal point is carried to the quotient (answer) in the same position.

EXAMPLES

$$2\overline{)0.750}^{\,.375} \qquad 2\overline{)3.472}^{\,1.736}$$

To divide when only the divisor is a decimal, for example,

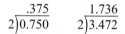

$$.3\overline{)66}$$

1. The divisor is changed to a whole number. In this example, the decimal point is moved one place to the right.

$$3\overline{)66}$$

2. The decimal point in the dividend must also be moved one place to the right.

$$3\overline{)66.0}$$

3. The numbers are now divided.

$$3\overline{)660}^{\,220}$$

Whenever the decimal point is moved in the dividend it must *also* be moved in the divisor, and whenever the decimal point in the divisor is moved it must *also* be moved in the dividend.

Changing a Fraction to a Decimal

To change a fraction to a decimal, divide the numerator by the denominator.

EXAMPLES

$$\frac{1}{5} = 5\overline{)1.0}^{\,.2} \qquad \frac{3}{4} = 4\overline{)3.00}^{\,.75} \qquad \frac{1}{6} = 6\overline{)1.000}^{\,.166}$$

Changing a Decimal to a Fraction

To change a decimal to a fraction:

1. Remove the decimal point and make the resulting whole number the numerator: 0.2 = 2.
2. The denominator is stated as 10 or a power of 10. In this example, 0.2 is read as two tenths, and therefore the denominator is 10.

$0.2 = \dfrac{2}{10}$ reduced to the lowest possible number is $\dfrac{1}{5}$

ADDITIONAL EXAMPLES

$$0.75 = \dfrac{75}{100} = \dfrac{3}{4} \qquad 0.025 = \dfrac{25}{1000} = \dfrac{1}{40}$$

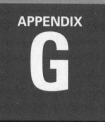

Answers to Review Questions and Medication Dosage Problems

Unit I Nursing Foundation of Clinical Pharmacology

Chapter 1 General Principles of Pharmacology

Review Questions: Prepare for the NCLEX

1. 3
2. 3
3. 2
4. 2
5. 4
6. 1
7. 1
8. 4
9. 1, 2, 4, 3
10. 1, 3, 4

Chapter 2 Administration of Drugs

Review Questions: Prepare for the NCLEX

1. 3
2. 4
3. 3
4. 2
5. 4
6. 2
7. 3
8. 2
9. 2, 3, 4
10. 2, 3

Chapter 3 Making Drug Dosing Safer

Questions

1. Tagamet is the brand name; cimetidine is the generic name.
2. The form of the drug is a Tiltab tablet and 400 milligrams is in each tablet of Tagamet.
3. Zyprexa and olanzapine are the names; it comes in tablet form and the dose strength is 5 milligrams.
4. Lanoxin and digoxin are the names; it comes in tablet form and the dose strength is 250 micrograms or 0.25 milligrams.
5. Augmentin and amoxicillin/clavulanate are the names; it comes in liquid form and the dose strength is 250 milligrams in 5 milliliters.

Calculations

1. 1 tablet after breakfast
2. 2 tablets after every meal
3. 2 tablets daily
4. 2 tablets daily
5. 5 milliliters in each dose
6. Patient's weight in kilograms: $142 \div 2.2 = 64.5$ kg; child's weight in kilograms: $43 \div 2.2 = 19.5$ kg

Review Questions: Prepare for the NCLEX

1. 2
2. 4
3. 4
4. 4
5. 3
6. 1
7. 3
8. 3
9. 2
10. 2

Chapter 4 The Nursing Process

Review Questions: Prepare for the NCLEX

1. 3
2. 4
3. 4
4. 3
5. 3
6. 1
7. 4
8. 4
9. 2, 1, 5, 4, 3
10. 1, 4

Chapter 5 Patient and Family Teaching

Hints for Pharmacology in Practice: Think Critically
Reviewing the patients presented, look at Display 5.1. Are any of them potential high-risk patients? What should you refrain from asking when you question the patients to assess if they have limited health literacy? Make a list of questions you could use with any patients that you interact with in your daily practice.

Review Questions: Prepare for the NCLEX

1. 4
2. 4
3. 3
4. 1
5. 2
6. 2
7. 3
8. 2
9. 3, 2, 1, 4
10. 1, 3, 4

Unit II Drugs Used to Fight Infections

Chapter 6 Antibacterial Drugs—Sulfonamides

Hints for Pharmacology in Practice: Think Critically
What is the relationship between urinary tract infections, memory, and cognitive processes in older adults? What do you know about limited health literacy? Would Mrs. Moore be at high risk for problems? Check Chapter 5 for hints to help her remember to take the medication. When should you reassess her mental status?

Review Questions: Know Your Drugs

1. C
2. A
3. B

Calculate Medication Dosages

1. 10 mL
2. 2 tablets

Prepare for the NCLEX

1. 2
2. 4
3. 1
4. 3
5. 3
6. 2
7. 2
8. 3
9. 4, 2, 3, 1
10. 2, 3, 4

Chapter 7 Antibacterial Drugs That Disrupt the Cell Wall

Hints for Pharmacology in Practice: Think Critically
Review Chapter 5 for methods to assess health literacy and limited English proficiency. When you teach should you be using Mrs. Garcia for interpretation? Because Mr. Garcia is taking a cephalosporin, what do you need to tell him specifically about alcohol, and why?

Review Questions: Know Your Drugs

1. C
2. D
3. A
4. B

Calculate Medication Dosages

1. 1 teaspoon (t) = 5 mL, then 1 teaspoon = 250 mg of amoxicillin. The nurse will teach the caregiver to administer 2 teaspoons (t) or 10 mL of amoxicillin.
2. 1 gram cefoxitin = 4 mL of solution; this would require 2 IM injections.

Prepare for the NCLEX

1. 1
2. 4
3. 2
4. 2
5. 1
6. 2
7. 4
8. 2
9. 4
10. 1, 2, 4

Chapter 8 Antibacterial Drugs That Interfere With Protein Synthesis

Hints for Pharmacology in Practice: Think Critically
Review the drug–drug interactions in this chapter. What may happen with the medication combinations that Mrs. Moore is taking? Look for teaching hints in Chapter 5.

Review Questions: Know Your Drugs

1. D
2. C
3. B
4. A

Calculate Medication Dosages

1. 2 mL
2. 20 mL

Prepare for the NCLEX

1. 3
2. 2
3. 4
4. 1
5. 2
6. 1
7. 2
8. 4
9. 1, 3, 4
10. Day 1 = 2 tablets, days 2 through 5 = 1 tablet daily

Chapter 9 Antibacterial Drugs That Interfere With DNA/RNA Synthesis

Hints for Pharmacology in Practice: Think Critically
Think about what diarrhea means when someone is taking an anti-infective. Look at the information in this chapter's Patient Teaching for Improved Patient Outcomes. What factors could be contributing to this condition? What assessment should be carried out?

Review Questions: Know Your Drugs

1. B
2. A
3. C

Calculate Medication Dosages

1. 1 tablet every 12 hours
2. 3 tablets each dose

Prepare for the NCLEX

1. 4
2. 3
3. 1
4. 1
5. 3
6. 1
7. 2
8. 4
9. 30 mL of solution
10. 2, 3, 4

Chapter 10 Antitubercular Drugs

Hints for Pharmacology in Practice: Think Critically
Think about the risk factors for TB and what Betty Peterson's perceptions of her living situation are in relation to those factors.

Review Questions: Know Your Drugs

1. A
2. B
3. C
4. D

Calculate Medication Dosages

1. 6 mL
2. 4 tablets

Prepare for the NCLEX

1. 4
2. 3
3. 2
4. 4
5. 1
6. 2
7. 1
8. 4
9. 1, 2, 4, 5
10. 2

Chapter 11 Antiviral Drugs

Hints for Pharmacology in Practice: Think Critically
Think about the mode of transmission of the herpes zoster (shingles) virus. What childhood disease would alert you to which staff or residents would be at risk to get the infection? Review information about the drug, and then think about drug interactions and the medications that Mr. Park is currently taking.

Review Questions: Know Your Drugs

1. D
2. A
3. B
4. C

Calculate Medication Dosages

1. 2 tablets
2. 10 mL

Prepare for the NCLEX

1. 2
2. 2
3. 1
4. 1
5. 1
6. 2
7. 3
8. 1
9. 2 dose inhalations total in 24 hours, which is 10 mg of zanamivir in 24 hours
10. 1 = C, 2 = E, 3 = A, 4 = B, 5 = D

Chapter 12 Antifungal and Antiparasitic Drugs

Hints for Pharmacology in Practice: Think Critically
Review information about collecting pinworm samples. Do you need face-to-face instruction or could you relay this information accurately over the telephone? Review patient education for information to include about treating both the patient and the entire household when infection is suspected.

Review Questions: Know Your Drugs

1. C
2. A
3. D
4. B

Calculate Medication Dosages

1. 2 tablets
2. 2 capsules

Prepare for the NCLEX

1. 2
2. 2
3. 3
4. 2
5. 4
6. 1
7. 1
8. 2
9. 1, 2, 3
10. 95.4 mg (140 lb = 63.6 kg) 1.5 mg/63.6 kg/day = 95.4 mg or 95 mg if rounding to the nearest whole number

Unit III Drugs Used to Manage Pain

Chapter 13 Nonopioid Analgesics: Salicylates and Nonsalicylates

Hints for Pharmacology in Practice: Think Critically
Review information on GI distress and the nonopioid analgesics. What problems could the aspirin product be causing? If Betty does switch to an acetaminophen product, what other drugs or foods should Betty avoid that might contain salicylates?

Review Questions: Know Your Drugs
1. A, D
2. B, C, E

Calculate Medication Dosages
1. 1.5 or 1½ mL
2. 2 tablets

Prepare for the NCLEX
1. 4
2. 3
3. 1
4. 3
5. 3
6. 2
7. 3
8. 4
9. 1, 4, 5
10. 12 tablets in 1 day (3900 mg); each tablet is 325 mg, maximum dose is 4000 mg (4 grams) per day

Chapter 14 Nonopioid Analgesics: Nonsteroidal Anti-Inflammatory Drugs (NSAIDs) and Migraine Headache Medications

Hints for Pharmacology in Practice: Think Critically
As you assess drug use, what are some of the adverse reactions to salicylate therapy? With regard to GI-related adverse reactions when using a COX-2 inhibitor, would you see a difference? Think about the daughter's concerns; what could be causing the hearing difficulty, and would that change with a change of medications?

Review Questions: Know Your Drugs
1. C
2. A
3. B
4. D

Calculate Medication Dosages
1. 10 mL
2. 2 tablets

Prepare for the NCLEX
1. 2
2. 4
3. 1
4. 1

5. 4
6. 2
7. 4
8. 3
9. 2, 3, 4
10. 1, 3, 4

Chapter 15 Opioid Analgesics

Hints for Pharmacology in Practice: Think Critically
How would you measure adequate pain relief with regard to heart-related problems? How would you modify your assessment strategies for someone 85 years old?

Review Questions: Know Your Drugs
1. C
2. B
3. A
4. D

Calculate Medication Dosages
1. 1.2 mL
2. 2 capsules

Prepare for the NCLEX
1. 4
2. 3
3. 3
4. 1
5. 4
6. 3
7. 2
8. 3, 4
9. Vicodin contains 500 mg acetaminophen in each tablet (Table 15.2), 6 tablets = 3000 mg
10. 1 mL

Chapter 16 Opioid Antagonists

Hints for Pharmacology in Practice: Think Critically
Think about all components of a pain assessment; which ones were neglected in the patient interview? Who is the opioid-naive patient, and what steps should you take to facilitate breathing before administering an opioid antagonist?

Review Questions: Calculate Medication Dosages
1. 0.8 mL

Prepare for the NCLEX
1. 2
2. 3
3. 3
4. 4 injections; 0.4 mg + 0.2 mg + 0.2 mg + 0.2 mg = 1 mg
5. 2, 3

Chapter 17 Anesthetic Drugs

Hints for Pharmacology in Practice: Think Critically
Think about what you learned about the additive epinephrine in this chapter. When should it be used and when should it not be used?

Review Questions: Know Your Drugs
1. D
2. A
3. B
4. C

Calculate Medication Dosages
1. 1 mL

Prepare for the NCLEX
1. 3
2. 2
3. 3
4. 1
5. 2
6. 4
7. 4
8. 1 = C, 2 = A, 3 = D, 4 = B
9. 3, 2, 4, 1
10. 0.3 mg

Unit IV Drugs That Affect the Central Nervous System

Chapter 18 Central Nervous System Stimulants

Hints for Pharmacology in Practice: Think Critically
Key assessment items would include inattention, hyperactivity, and impulsiveness. What is the importance of maintaining a specific weight to a gymnast? Could the mother be looking for an anorexiant to maintain Janna's weight?

Review Questions: Know Your Drugs
1. B
2. D
3. A
4. C

Calculate Medication Dosages
1. 2 capsules
2. 2 tablets

Prepare for the NCLEX
1. 3
2. 3
3. 1
4. 4
5. 4
6. 1
7. 2
8. 1
9. 1, 2, 4
10. 24 mg; yes it is appropriate.

Chapter 19 Cholinesterase Inhibitors

Hints for Pharmacology in Practice: Think Critically
What are the primary adverse reactions of the cholinesterase inhibitors? Why would Mrs. Moore have on multiple patches?

Review Questions: Know Your Drugs
1. A
2. D
3. C
4. B

Calculate Medication Dosages
1. 3 mL
2. 2 tablets

Prepare for the NCLEX
1. 1
2. 2
3. 3
4. 1
5. 4
6. 3
7. 3
8. 2
9. 1, 2, 3, 5
10. 2, 3

Chapter 20 Antianxiety Drugs

Hints for Pharmacology in Practice: Think Critically
Do Mr. Garcia's vital signs indicate anxiety? What are the cultural implications to consider with this patient if he is displaying anxiety? How will you interact when an interpreter is involved in patient teaching?

Review Questions: Know Your Drugs
1. D
2. B
3. C
4. A

Calculate Medication Dosages
1. 1 mL
2. 2 tablets

Prepare for the NCLEX
1. 2
2. 1
3. 4
4. 2
5. 3
6. 2
7. 2
8. 4
9. 1, 2, 3, 4, 5
10. 2 mL

Chapter 21 Sedatives and Hypnotics

Hints for Pharmacology in Practice: Think Critically
How long and for what reasons should hypnotics be used? Is this an appropriate use of the drug? What other nonpharmacologic interventions would be helpful?

Review Questions: Know Your Drugs

1. C
2. D
3. A, B

Calculate Medication Dosages

1. 1 tablet
2. 2 tablets

Prepare for the NCLEX

1. 4
2. 2
3. 3
4. 1
5. 4
6. 3
7. 1
8. 2
9. 1, 3, 4
10. 1, 2, 3

Chapter 22 Antidepressant Drugs

Hints for Pharmacology in Practice: Think Critically
How long does it take for antidepressant medications to take effect? In Chapter 21, we learned that Mr. Phillip was prescribed a hypnotic for sleep. What are the drug interactions when using these medications together?

Review Questions: Know Your Drugs

1. C, D
2. A
3. B

Calculate Medication Dosages

1. 3 tablets
2. 25 mL

Prepare for the NCLEX

1. 4
2. 3
3. 2
4. 2
5. 3
6. 3
7. 3
8. 4
9. 1, 2, 3
10. 2, 3, 4

Chapter 23 Antipsychotic Drugs

Hints for Pharmacology in Practice: Think Critically
What type of symptoms does she have, positive or negative? Mrs. Moore had a UTI earlier; what is the relationship between UTI and cognition? Does she have a condition that contradicts the use of the medication? How would you present this information to the daughter?

Review Questions: Know Your Drugs

1. A
2. C
3. D
4. B

Calculate Medication Dosages

1. 2 tablets
2. 0.6 mL will be 3 mg of haloperidol

Prepare for the NCLEX

1. 2
2. 3
3. 3
4. 2
5. 4
6. 3
7. 3
8. 2
9. 1, 2, 3
10. 1 = B, 2 = A, C, D, E

Unit V Drugs That Affect the Peripheral Nervous System

Chapter 24 Adrenergic Drugs

Hints for Pharmacology in Practice: Think Critically
Review the patient teaching for improved outcomes; how could you use this information to decrease Mrs. Wong's concerns? Check Chapter 5 for suggestions.

Review Questions: Know Your Drugs

1. C
2. B
3. A

Calculate Medication Dosages

1. 2 mL
2. 0.5 mL

Prepare for the NCLEX

1. 2
2. 3
3. 2
4. 1
5. 4
6. 4
7. 2
8. 4
9. 1, 3
10. 0.6 mg

Chapter 25 Adrenergic Blocking Drugs

Hints for Pharmacology in Practice: Think Critically
When are the blood levels of a drug taken daily the highest and the lowest? What items should Mr. Garcia be taught each time he changes position?

Review Questions: Know Your Drugs

1. C
2. B
3. A
4. D

Calculate Medication Dosages

1. 2 tablets
2. 1 capsule

Prepare for the NCLEX

1. 2
2. 4
3. 4
4. 1
5. 2
6. 2
7. 3
8. 2 (12 mL of propranolol oral solution + 30 mL of flush solution = 42 mL total)
9. 2, 3
10. 4 tablets

Chapter 26 Cholinergic Drugs

Hints for Pharmacology in Practice: Think Critically
In addition to considering the drugs to help stimulate the bladder to contract and produce urine, review Chapter 24 and apply the information learned to the situation with Mr. Park's bladder when the sympathetic system was activated by the stressful state of the initial hip fracture.

Review Questions: Know Your Drugs

1. A, C
2. B

Calculate Medication Dosages

1. 0.5 mL

Prepare for the NCLEX

1. 4
2. 4
3. 2
4. 3
5. 1, 2, 4
6. 10 tablets

Chapter 27 Cholinergic Blocking Drugs

Hints for Pharmacology in Practice: Think Critically
Review the side effects that can occur with the different cholinergic blocking drugs. What is the impact specifically on the bowels and mobility?

Review Questions: Know Your Drugs

1. A
2. D
3. B
4. C

Calculate Medication Dosages

1. 0.5 mL
2. 10 mL

Prepare for the NCLEX

1. 1
2. 2
3. 2
4. 4
5. 2
6. 3
7. 4
8. 3
9. 2, 4
10. 1, 3, 4, 5

Unit VI Drugs That Affect the Neuromuscular System

Chapter 28 Antiparkinsonism Drugs

Hints for Pharmacology in Practice: Think Critically
What is the cluster of symptoms described in the case study? What are some of the adverse reactions to medications that Betty is currently using?

Review Questions: Know Your Drugs

1. D
2. B
3. C
4. A

Calculate Medication Dosages

1. One 500-mg tablet and one 250-mg tablet = 750 mg or 0.75 grams
2. 3 tablets

Prepare for the NCLEX

1. 2
2. 1
3. 2
4. 3
5. 2
6. 4
7. 4
8. 2
9. 1, 3
10. 2, 4, 3, 1

Chapter 29 Anticonvulsants

Hints for Pharmacology in Practice: Think Critically
What type of seizures do you think Ms. Chase had following her accident? What questions would you ask before you discuss your findings with the primary health care provider regarding Ms. Chase's intermittent use of the medications?

Review Questions: Know Your Drugs

1. C
2. D

3. A
4. B

Calculate Medication Dosages

1. 2 tablets
2. 10 mL

Prepare for the NCLEX

1. 3
2. 3
3. 1
4. 3
5. 1
6. 3
7. 2
8. 2
9. 2 mL
10. Dilantin

Chapter 30 Skeletal Muscle, Bone, and Joint Disorder Drugs

Hints for Pharmacology in Practice: Think Critically
Review the drug administration requirements and the fact that Mrs. Moore suffers from periodic confusion.

Review Questions: Know Your Drugs

1. C
2. D
3. A
4. B

Calculate Medication Dosages

1. 3 tablets
2. 3 tablets

Prepare for the NCLEX

1. 2
2. 1
3. 3
4. 4
5. 4
6. 1
7. 4
8. 4
9. 1, 2, 4, 5
10. 252 mg

Unit VII Drugs That Affect the Respiratory System

Chapter 31 Upper Respiratory System Drugs

Hints for Pharmacology in Practice: Think Critically
Janna Wong competes on her school's gymnastic team. How might her abilities be altered by the influence of either the antihistamine or nasal decongestant? Check earlier pain relief chapters; what do you need to discuss with teens independently taking medications?

Review Questions: Know Your Drugs

1. A
2. D
3. C
4. B

Calculate Medication Dosages

1. 5 mL
2. 2 tablets

Prepare for the NCLEX

1. 2
2. 1
3. 1
4. 2
5. 3
6. 4
7. 1
8. 1
9. 1
10. 2, 3, 4

Chapter 32 Lower Respiratory System Drugs

Hints for Pharmacology in Practice: Think Critically
Check the chapter for the medication taken. What medication did Mrs. Chase's mother use in the inhalation device, and how are Mrs. Chase's medications different?

Review Questions: Know Your Drugs

1. B
2. A
3. C
4. D

Calculate Medication Dosages

1. 0.25 mL
2. 2 tablets, 40 mg each day

Prepare for the NCLEX

1. 2
2. 3
3. 4
4. 1
5. 1
6. 4
7. 2
8. 3
9. 1, 3
10. 1, 3

Unit VIII Drugs That Affect the Cardiovascular System

Chapter 33 Diuretics

Hints for Pharmacology in Practice: Think Critically
What are some recommendations you can make to facilitate correct use of the medication? Review Mrs. Moore's status in

Chapters 6 and 23; what could be contributing to her urinary tract infections? Think about fluids.

Review Questions: Know Your Drugs

1. B
2. C
3. D
4. A

Calculate Medication Dosages

1. 2 tablets
2. 2.5 mL

Prepare for the NCLEX

1. 4
2. 4
3. 4
4. 3
5. 4
6. 4
7. 2
8. 2
9. 1, 2, 3
10. 1 = C; 2 = B, E; 3 = D; 4 = A

Chapter 34 Antihyperlipidemic Drugs

Hints for Pharmacology in Practice: Think Critically
Review Chapter 5 and principles of adult learning. What information from the two sets of lab values and vital signs can be used to motivate adherence to Lillian's lifestyle changes? What information about her medications can help reduce constipation symptoms?

Review Questions: Know Your Drugs

1. B
2. C
3. A
4. D

Calculate Medication Dosages

1. 2 tablets
2. Dose requirement = four 20-mg tablets or two 40-mg tablets; the 40-mg tablet size is less in number

Prepare for the NCLEX

1. 3
2. 2
3. 3
4. 1
5. 2
6. 1
7. 3
8. 4
9. 1, 4, 5
10. Yes, 200 mg is an appropriate dosage. However, if the client requires 200 mg, it is preferable to give a 200-mg

capsule rather than three 67-mg capsules. The nurse should notify the primary health care provider that only 67-mg capsules are available.

Chapter 35 Antihypertensive Drugs

Hints for Pharmacology in Practice: Think Critically
Where can you access information for clients with limited English proficiency (LEP)? What are some diet resources? What questions do you need to ask Mr. Garcia about flavor preferences?

Review Questions: Know Your Drugs

1. C
2. D
3. A
4. B

Calculate Medication Dosages

1. 2 tablets
2. 3 capsules

Prepare for the NCLEX

1. 2
2. 3
3. 3
4. 3
5. 4
6. 2
7. 4
8. 3
9. 1, 3
10. 90-mg tablets and give 2 tablets

Chapter 36 Antianginal and Vasodilating Drugs

Hints for Pharmacology in Practice: Think Critically
A likely choice may be the transdermal system; check Chapter 19. Is this a good solution for Mrs. Moore? Is she able to remember when to replace patches, and what would happen if she forgot to remove an old one?

Review Questions: Know Your Drugs

1. B
2. A
3. C
4. D

Calculate Medication Dosages

1. 3 tablets
2. 2 tablets

Prepare for the NCLEX

1. 2
2. 1
3. 2
4. 2
5. 3

6. 2
7. 4
8. 4
9. 1, 2, 3
10. In 1 minute, and then again in 5 more minutes

Chapter 37 Anticoagulant and Thrombolytic Drugs

Hints for Pharmacology in Practice: Think Critically
What could be the effect of taking a different strength of Coumadin for each dose?

Review Questions: Know Your Drugs
1. D
2. C
3. A
4. B

Calculate Medication Dosages
1. 2 mL
2. 2 tablets

Prepare for the NCLEX
1. 3
2. 4
3. 4
4. 2
5. 1
6. 4
7. 2
8. 1
9. 1, 4, 5
10. 1 = C, 2 = A, 3 = B

Chapter 38 Cardiotonics and Inotropic Drugs

Hints for Pharmacology in Practice: Think Critically
Compare the cardiotonics with the ACE inhibitors. Can you ease the daughter's concerns with the medication order change?

Review Questions: Calculate Medication Dosages
1. 2 mL

Prepare for the NCLEX
1. 2
2. 4
3. 1
4. 3
5. One 0.5-mg tablet and one 0.25-mg tablet

Chapter 39 Antiarrhythmic Drugs

Hints for Pharmacology in Practice: Think Critically
Mr. Phillip has multiple medications and schedules. Review patient teaching and medication administration. How can you help him safely self-administer the medications?

Review Questions: Know Your Drugs
1. D
2. C
3. A
4. B

Calculate Medication Dosages
1. 2 tablets
2. 2 tablets

Prepare for the NCLEX
1. 1
2. 2
3. 1
4. 4
5. 1
6. 4
7. 3
8. 1
9. 2 tablets daily
10. 1 = D, 2 = C, 3 = A, 4 = B

Unit IX Drugs That Affect the Gastrointestinal System

Chapter 40 Upper Gastrointestinal System Drugs

Hints for Pharmacology in Practice: Think Critically
Where can you access information for patients with LEP? Review in Chapter 5 how to handle what may be a long-standing cultural practice. Do antacids actually coat the stomach lining? What do they actually do? By examining the different elements, determine what a person should reduce in his or her diet when dealing with hypertensive disease. Which elements promote constipation?

Review Questions: Know Your Drugs
1. C
2. A
3. B
4. D

Calculate Medication Dosages
1. 2 capsules
2. 20 mL

Prepare for the NCLEX
1. 3
2. 4
3. 2
4. 3
5. 2
6. 2
7. 2
8. 1 = B, C; 2 = A, D
9. 2 tablets
10. 1 tablet

Chapter 41 Lower Gastrointestinal System Drugs

Hints for Pharmacology in Practice: Think Critically
What do the medications listed do to the bowel? There are different preparations to add bulk, soften stool, and so forth. Which does Betty need based on the drugs she is currently taking?

Review Questions: Know Your Drugs
1. B
2. A
3. D
4. C

Calculate Medication Dosages
1. 3 capsules
2. 5 milligrams

Prepare for the NCLEX
1. 3
2. 3
3. 3
4. 1
5. 4
6. 4
7. 2
8. 3
9. 1, 3, 4
10. 3 hours (2.7, question asks in hours so round to within 3 hours)

Unit X Drugs That Affect the Endocrine System

Chapter 42 Antidiabetic Drugs

Hints for Pharmacology in Practice: Think Critically
Review strategies to promote patient adherence to medication regimens. What skills can you sequence to provide a positive learning experience for Mr. Phillip?

Review Questions: Know Your Drugs
1. A
2. B
3. D
4. C

Calculate Medication Dosages
1. 4 tablets
2. 45 units

Prepare for the NCLEX
1. 2
2. 1
3. 3
4. 4
5. 3
6. 2
7. 3
8. C, B, D, A

9. 45 units; inject air into NPH vial, inject air into regular vial, draw out 5 units, then draw out 40 units NPH
10. 2 tablets per dose; total daily dose = 2000 mg

Chapter 43 Pituitary and Adrenocortical Hormones

Hints for Pharmacology in Practice: Think Critically
Desmopressin replaces which hormone made by the pituitary gland? What is the function of this hormone, and why would you want more in the system at night than in the daytime when you are more active?

Review Questions: Know Your Drugs
1. D
2. C
3. B
4. A

Calculate Medication Dosages
1. 2 tablets
2. 2 tablets

Prepare for the NCLEX
1. 3
2. 4
3. 2
4. 1
5. 3
6. 3
7. 2
8. 2
9. 1
10. 1 = A, B, D; 2 = C

Chapter 44 Thyroid and Antithyroid Drugs

Hints for Pharmacology in Practice: Think Critically
Be sure to assess why Betty believes there is danger before you work to educate her about the radioactive iodine. This will make it easier to clarify unrealistic beliefs.

Review Questions: Know Your Drugs
1. C
2. D
3. B
4. A

Calculate Medication Dosages
1. 4 tablets
2. 2 tablets

Prepare for the NCLEX
1. 3
2. 1
3. 2
4. 2
5. 3
6. 1
7. 3
8. 2

9. 1, 2
10. 1, 2, 4

Chapter 45 Male and Female Hormones

Hints for Pharmacology in Practice: Think Critically
Is Janna sexually active, or does she want to begin birth control for another reason? What is the best method for her to use? Are there any indications from previous chapters that would negate the use of any specific methods?

Review Questions: Know Your Drugs

1. B
2. C
3. D
4. A

Calculate Medication Dosages

1. 1.6 mL
2. 1 mL

Prepare for the NCLEX

1. 4
2. 3
3. 4
4. 3
5. 2
6. 1
7. 1
8. 3
9. 1, 2
10. 1, 2, 3, 4

Chapter 46 Uterine Drugs

Hints for Pharmacology in Practice: Think Critically
Be sure to assess Betty's health literacy regarding the birth process. How can you explain what oxytocin does to induce labor in terminology that is easy for her to understand?

Review Questions: Know Your Drugs

1. C
2. A
3. D
4. B

Calculate Medication Dosages

1. ½ tablet
2. 1 mL

Prepare for the NCLEX

1. 4
2. 2
3. 4
4. 2
5. 1
6. 4
7. 4

8. 2
9. 5 mL/min
10. 1 = indomethacin, NSAID; 2 = nifedipine, calcium channel blocker; 3 = terbutaline, bronchodilator

Unit XI Drugs That Affect the Urinary System

Chapter 47 Menopause and Andropause Drugs

Hints for Pharmacology in Practice: Think Critically
What happens to urinary structures when fluids are reduced, since that is contrary to recommended practices for treating urinary symptoms?

Review Questions: Know Your Drugs

1. D
2. C
3. A
4. B

Calculate Medication Dosages

1. 2 tablets
2. 2 tablets

Prepare for the NCLEX

1. 3
2. 4
3. 3
4. 2
5. 1
6. 2
7. 2
8. 2
9. 1, 3, 5
10. 2, 3, 4

Chapter 48 Urinary Tract Anti-Infectives and Other Urinary Drugs

Hints for Pharmacology in Practice: Think Critically
Review the Patient Teaching for Improved Patient Outcomes. What behaviors do you need to address?

Review Questions: Know Your Drugs

1. B
2. D
3. C
4. A

Calculate Medication Dosages

1. 2 tablets
2. 10 mL

Prepare for the NCLEX

1. 1
2. 4
3. 3
4. 4
5. 1 = A, 2 = C, 3 = B, 4 = D

Unit XII Drugs That Affect the Immune System

Chapter 49 Immunologic Agents

Hints for Pharmacology in Practice: Think Critically
Think about the consequences to the child should he acquire the illness in the timeframe of the delay in immunization.

Review Questions: Know Your Drugs
1. C
2. A
3. B
4. D

Calculate Medication Dosages
1. 6 vials of the FluLaval vaccine

Prepare for the NCLEX
1. 3
2. 3
3. 2
4. 1
5. 3
6. 1
7. 2
8. 2, 4, 5
9. 1, 3, 4

Chapter 50 Antineoplastic Drugs

Hints for Pharmacology in Practice: Think Critically
Mr. Phillip is now ready to discuss his losses. What in addition to the medications prescribed should be recommended?

Review Questions: Know Your Drugs
1. B
2. C
3. A
4. D

Calculate Medication Dosages
1. 12.8 mg/day
2. 13.5 units

Prepare for the NCLEX
1. 2
2. 4
3. 4
4. 2
5. 2
6. 3
7. 3
8. 1
9. 3
10. 1, 2, 3, 4

Chapter 51 Immunostimulant Drugs

Hints for Pharmacology in Practice: Think Critically
What are the stipulations for use of erythropoiesis-stimulating agents (ESAs) in dialysis?

Review Questions: Know Your Drugs
1. D
2. C
3. A
4. B

Calculate Medication Dosages
1. 0.5 mL
2. 0.2 mL

Prepare for the NCLEX
1. 3
2. 4
3. 1
4. 1
5. 1
6. 1
7. 3
8. 2
9. 3 tablets day 1, 1 tablet day 5
10. 1 = C, 2 = B, 3 = A

Unit XIII Drugs That Affect Other Body Systems

Chapter 52 Skin Disorder Topical Drugs

Hints for Pharmacology in Practice: Think Critically
What are the differences in the treatment of herpes simplex virus (HSV) oral lesions and the varicella-zoster virus that presents on the skin?

Review Questions: Know Your Drugs
1. D
2. B
3. A
4. C

Prepare for the NCLEX
1. 2
2. 2
3. 2
4. 4
5. 2
6. 1
7. 3
8. 4
9. Fissure
10. 30 mL

Chapter 53 Otic and Ophthalmic Preparations

Hints for Pharmacology in Practice: Think Critically
Appealing to principles of personal growth and development and using the concepts you learned about health literacy, what would be the best way to interact with and teach Janna?

Review Questions: Know Your Drugs

1. C
2. D
3. A
4. B

Calculate Medication Dosages

1. 5 (gtt) drops
2. 60 doses

Prepare for the NCLEX

1. 1
2. 2
3. 2
4. 2
5. 3
6. 4
7. 2
8. 3
9. 2, 3

Chapter 54 Fluids, Electrolytes, and Parenteral Therapy

Hints for Pharmacology in Practice: Think Critically
Describe what electrolyte imbalance is occurring as a result of taking sodium bicarbonate for stomach ailments.

Review Questions: Know Your Drugs

1. D
2. A
3. C
4. B

Calculate Medication Dosages

1. 100 mL/hour
2. 30 mL

Prepare for the NCLEX

1. 3
2. 3
3. 4
4. 1
5. 4
6. 1
7. 4
8. 2
9. 3
10. 4, 2, 1, 3, 5

NCLEX-PN Prep

See the following pages for a pictorial diagram of how a sampling of 'Prepare for the NCLEX' review questions in each chapter are correlated with the most recent NCLEX—PN Test plan.

At the end of each chapter in the section Prepare for the NCLEX, you are provided approximately 10 questions to test your knowledge. The first section, Build Your Knowledge, provides questions about information and content retention. In the section Apply Your Knowledge, analysis and application questions are provided that are designed using the 2011 NCLEX-PN Detailed Test Plan. An Alternate-Format Questions section gives you exposure to the different ways in

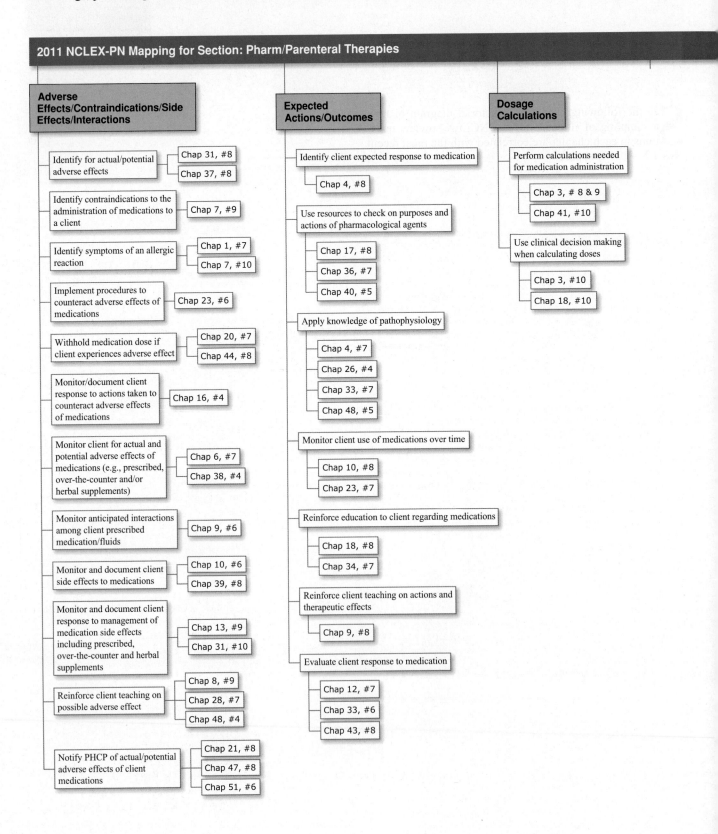

2011 NCLEX-PN Mapping for Section: Pharm/Parenteral Therapies

Adverse Effects/Contraindications/Side Effects/Interactions

- Identify for actual/potential adverse effects
  - Chap 31, #8
  - Chap 37, #8
- Identify contraindications to the administration of medications to a client
  - Chap 7, #9
- Identify symptoms of an allergic reaction
  - Chap 1, #7
  - Chap 7, #10
- Implement procedures to counteract adverse effects of medications
  - Chap 23, #6
- Withhold medication dose if client experiences adverse effect
  - Chap 20, #7
  - Chap 44, #8
- Monitor/document client response to actions taken to counteract adverse effects of medications
  - Chap 16, #4
- Monitor client for actual and potential adverse effects of medications (e.g., prescribed, over-the-counter and/or herbal supplements)
  - Chap 6, #7
  - Chap 38, #4
- Monitor anticipated interactions among client prescribed medication/fluids
  - Chap 9, #6
- Monitor and document client side effects to medications
  - Chap 10, #6
  - Chap 39, #8
- Monitor and document client response to management of medication side effects including prescribed, over-the-counter and herbal supplements
  - Chap 13, #9
  - Chap 31, #10
- Reinforce client teaching on possible adverse effect
  - Chap 8, #9
  - Chap 28, #7
  - Chap 48, #4
- Notify PHCP of actual/potential adverse effects of client medications
  - Chap 21, #8
  - Chap 47, #8
  - Chap 51, #6

Expected Actions/Outcomes

- Identify client expected response to medication
  - Chap 4, #8
- Use resources to check on purposes and actions of pharmacological agents
  - Chap 17, #8
  - Chap 36, #7
  - Chap 40, #5
- Apply knowledge of pathophysiology
  - Chap 4, #7
  - Chap 26, #4
  - Chap 33, #7
  - Chap 48, #5
- Monitor client use of medications over time
  - Chap 10, #8
  - Chap 23, #7
- Reinforce education to client regarding medications
  - Chap 18, #8
  - Chap 34, #7
- Reinforce client teaching on actions and therapeutic effects
  - Chap 9, #8
- Evaluate client response to medication
  - Chap 12, #7
  - Chap 33, #6
  - Chap 43, #8

Dosage Calculations

- Perform calculations needed for medication administration
  - Chap 3, # 8 & 9
  - Chap 41, #10
- Use clinical decision making when calculating doses
  - Chap 3, #10
  - Chap 18, #10

which questions are presented in the examination. Here we provide you a diagram to help you understand and connect your learning to the items of the NCLEX-PN test plan. Below, you will find how specific questions from each chapter correspond directly to the items of the Detailed Test Plan, Pharmacological and Parenteral Therapies section. In this way you can prepare for the NCLEX-PN exam by practicing with sample questions that are of the type used in the exam.

Pharmacological Pain Management

Identify client need for pain medication
- Chap 21, #7
- Chap 52, #7

Monitor client non-verbal signs of pain/discomfort (e.g., grimacing, restlessness)
- Chap 14, #10

Monitor and document client response to pharmacological interventions (e.g., pain rating scale, verbal reports)
- Chap 15, #9

Medication Administration

Identify client need for PRN medication — Chap 40, #6

Mix client medication from two vials as necessary — Chap 42, # 8 & 9

Follow the rights of medication administration — Chap 2, #8

Maintain medication safety practices (e.g., storage, checking for expiration dates or compatibility)
- Chap 2, #7
- Chap 5, #8
- Chap 11, #7
- Chap 50, #10

Reconcile and maintain medication list or medication administration record — Chap 11, #8

Review pertinent data prior to medication administration — Chap 7, #8

Assist in preparing client for insertion of central line — Chap 52, #8

Administer a medication by the oral route — Chap 5, #7

Administer IVPB medications — Chap 29, #9

Administer medication by gastrointestinal tube
- Chap 25, #8
- Chap 35, #8

Administer a subcutaneous medication — Chap 27, #8

Administer a medication by the topical route — Chap 6, #8 & 9

Dispose of client unused medication according to proper policy — Chap 19, #7

Count controlled substances — Chap 1, #8

Regulate client IV rate — Chap 46, #9

Monitor transfusion of blood product — Chap 54, #9

Monitor client IV site and flow rate
- Chap 49, #7
- Chap 50, #7
- Chap 54, #8

Reinforce client teaching on client self administration of medications (e.g., insulin, subcutaneous insulin pump)
- Chap 14, #7
- Chap 24, #7
- Chap 45, #7

Bibliography

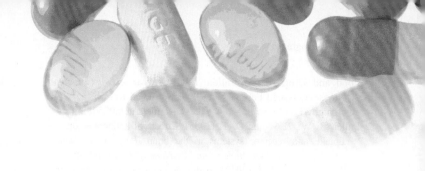

Unit I

Carpenito-Moyet, L. (2006). *Nursing diagnosis: Application to clinical practice* (11th ed., pp. 473–480). Philadelphia: Lippincott Williams & Wilkins.

Eisenhauer, L., Nichols, L., Spencer, R., & Bergan, F. (1998). *Clinical pharmacology and nursing management* (5th ed., p. 189). Philadelphia: Lippincott-Raven.

Fontaine, K. L. (2000). *Healing practices: Alternative therapies for nursing* (pp. 126–127). Upper Saddle River, NJ: Prentice Hall.

Herbal products and supplements: What you should know. Retrieved from the American Academy of Family Physicians FamilyDoctor.org website: http://familydoctor.org/familydoctor/en/drugs-procedures-devices/over-the-counter/herbal-products-and-supplements.html

Health Resources and Services Administration (HRSA) training course: Effective Communication Tools for Healthcare Professionals 101, June 26, 2012.

Hughes, R. G., & Blegen, M. A. (2008). Medication administration safety. In R. G. Hughes (Ed.), *Patient safety and quality: An evidence-based handbook for nurses.* Rockville, MD: Agency for Healthcare Research and Quality. Available from: http://www.ncbi.nlm.nih.gov/books/NBK2656/

Institute of Medicine. (1999). *To err is human: Building a safer health system.* Washington, DC: National Academy Press.

Just culture and its critical link to patient safety. (2012, July 12). *ISMP Medication Safety Alert – Acute Care* (pp. 1–2). Horsham, PA: Institute for Safe Medication Practice (ISMP).

Lorig, K., Halstead, H., Sobel, D., Laurent, D., Gonzalez, V., & Minor, M. (2012). *Living a healthy life with chronic conditions* (4th ed., pp. 31–33). Boulder, CO: Bull Publishing.

Pape, T. M., Guerra, D. M., Muzquiz, M., Bryant, J. B., Ingram, M., Schranner, B., ... Welker, J. (2005). Innovative approaches to reducing nurses' distractions during medication administration. *Journal of Continuing Education in Nursing, 36*(3), 108–116.

Side tracks on the safety express, interruptions lead to errors and unfinished...wait what was I doing? (2012, November 29). *ISMP Medication Safety Alert – Acute Care* (pp. 1–3). Horsham, PA: Institute for Safe Medication Practice (ISMP).

Websites for Information

Institute for Safe Medication Practices: http://www.ismp.org/
Joint Commission: http://www.jointcommission.org
LactMed: http://toxnet.nlm.nih.gov/cgi-bin/sis/htmlgen?LACT
MedWatch program: http://www.fda.gov/medwatch/index.html
Texas Tech University (Dr. Hale Breastfeeding Scale): http://www.infantrisk.com/

Unit II

Brown, T. (2012). Protection against urinary tract infections seen with cranberry products. *Archives of Internal Medicine,* 172, 988–996.

Centers for Disease Control and Prevention. (2010). *STD treatment guidelines, 2010.* Retrieved from http://www.cdc.gov/std/treatment/2010/sexual-assault.htm

DerMarderosian, A., & Beutler, J. (Eds.). (2003). *Guide to popular natural products* (3rd ed.). St. Louis, MO: Lippincott Williams & Wilkins.

Healthcare-associated methicillin resistant Staphylococcus aureus (HA-MRSA). (2008). Retrieved from http:www.cdc.gov/hai/organisms/organisms.html#m

Munsiff, S., Kambili, C., & Ahuja, S. (2006). Rifapentine for the treatment of pulmonary tuberculosis. *Clinical Infectious Diseases,* 43(11), 1468–1475.

Reports

World Health Organization: *Global tuberculosis report 2012:* http://www.who.int/tb/publications/global_report/en/

Unit III

DerMarderosian, A., & Beutler, J. (Eds.). (2003). *Guide to popular natural products* (3rd ed.). St. Louis, MO: Lippincott Williams & Wilkins.

International Association for the Study of Pain. (1979). Subcommittee on Taxonomy: Pain terms: A list with definitions and notes on usage. *Pain,* 6, 249.

World Health Organization. *WHO's pain ladder for adults.* Retrieved from http://www.who.int/cancer/palliative/painladder/en/index.html

Reports

A scientific review paper and recommendation statement from CDER's Acetaminophen Hepatotoxicity Working Group. Finalized February 26, 2008. Retrieved from http://www.fda.gov/downloads/AdvisoryCommittees/CommitteesMeetingMaterials/Drugs/DrugSafetyandRiskManagementAdvisoryCommittee/UCM164897.pdf

Unit IV

Alzheimer's Association. (2012). *Alzheimer's disease facts and figures.* Retrieved from http://www.alz.org/downloads/facts_figures_2012.pdf

Billioti de Gage, S., et al. (2012). Benzodiazepine use and risk of dementia: Prospective population based study. *British Medicine Journal,* 345, 6231.

DerMarderosian, A., & Beutler, J. (Eds.). 2003. *Guide to popular natural products* (3rd ed.). St. Louis, MO: Lippincott Williams & Wilkins.

Diagnostic criteria and guidelines for Alzheimer's disease. Retrieved from https://www.alz.org/research/diagnostic_criteria/

Food and Drug Administration. (2009). *Kava—FDA Consumer Advisory*. Issued February 7, 2009. Retrieved from http://www.fda.gov/Food/ResourcesForYou/Consumers/ucm085482.htm

Fuller, R. W., & Wong, D. T. (1985). Effects of antidepressants on uptake and receptor systems in the brain. *Progress in Neuropsychopharmacology, Biology, and Psychiatry*, 9(5–6), 485–490.

Gallagher, P. J., et al. (2012). Antidepressant response in patients with major depression exposed to NSAIDs: A pharmacovigilance study. *American Journal of Psychiatry*, 169(10), 1065–1072.

Jack, Jr., C. R., Albert, M. S., Knopman, D. S., McKhann, G. M., Sperling, R. A., Carrillo, M. C., ... Phelps, C. H. (2011). Introduction to the recommendations from the National Institute on Aging – Alzheimer's Association workgroups on diagnostic guidelines for Alzheimer's disease. *Alzheimer's & Dementia: The Journal of the Alzheimer's Association*, 7(3), 257–262.

Llorente, M., & Urrutia, V. (2006). Diabetes, psychiatric disorders, and the metabolic effects of antipsychotic medications. *Clinical Diabetes*, 24(1), 18–24.

Manos, M. J., Tom-Revzon, C., Bukstein, O. G., & Crismon, M. L. (2007). Changes and Challenges: managing ADHD in a fast-paced world. *Journal of Managed Care Pharmacy*, 13(9), 2–13.

Snitz, B. E., et al. (2009). Ginkgo Evaluation of Memory (GEM) Study Investigators. Ginkgo biloba for preventing cognitive decline in older adults: a randomized trial. *Journal of the American Medical Association*, 302(24), 2663–2670.

University of Maryland Medical Center. (2011). *Facts on ginkgo biloba*. University of Maryland Center for Integrative Medicine. Retrieved from http://www.umm.edu/altmed/articles/ginkgo-biloba-000247.htm#ixzz2By34P8T2

Websites for Information

National Sleep Foundation: http://www.sleepfoundation.org/

Unit V

Chaudhry, R., Portnoy, J., & Purser, J. (2012). *Patients forget how to use EpiPens after 3 months*. Abstract 59. Presented at the American College of Allergy, Asthma & Immunology (ACAAI) 2012 Annual Scientific Meeting, November 12, 2012.

DerMarderosian, A., & Beutler, J. (Eds.). 2003. *Guide to popular natural products* (3rd ed.). St. Louis, MO: Lippincott Williams & Wilkins.

Ferdinand, K., & Armani, A. (2007). The management of hypertension in African Americans. *Critical Pathways in Cardiology*, 6(2), 67–71.

Huang, H., & Fox, K. (2012). The impact of beta-blockers on mortality in stable angina: A meta-analysis. *Scottish Medical Journal*, 57, 69–75.

Magee, L., et al. (2000). Risks and benefits of beta-receptor blockers for pregnancy hypertension: Overview of the randomized trials. *European Journal of Obstetrics, Gynecology, and Reproductive Biology*, 88(1), 15–26.

Unit VI

DerMarderosian, A., & Beutler, J. (Eds.). 2003. *Guide to popular natural products* (3rd ed.). St. Louis, MO: Lippincott Williams & Wilkins.

Li, F., et al. (2012). Tai Chi and postural stability in patients with Parkinson's disease. *New England Journal of Medicine*, 366, 511–519.

Unit VII

DerMarderosian, A., & Beutler, J. (Eds.). 2003. *Guide to popular natural products* (3rd ed.). St. Louis, MO: Lippincott Williams & Wilkins.

Institute for Safe Medication Practices. (2007, January 11). Seasonal mix-ups. *ISMP Medication Safety Alert – Acute Care* (p. 1). Horsham, PA: Institute for Safe Medication Practice (ISMP).

Reports

U.S. Department of Health and Human Services, National Institutes of Health, National Heart, Lung, and Blood Institute. (2007). *The Expert Panel Report 3 (EPR–3) full report 2007: Guidelines for the Diagnosis and Management of Asthma*. Developed by an expert panel commissioned by the National Asthma Education and Prevention Program (NAEPP) Coordinating Committee (CC), coordinated by the National Heart, Lung, and Blood Institute (NHLBI) of the National Institutes of Health.

Unit VIII

Butt, D., et al. (2012). The risk of hip fracture after initiating antihypertensive drugs in the elderly. *Archives of Internal Medicine*, 172(22), 1739–1744.

Couris, R., et al. (2006). Dietary vitamin K variability affects international normalized ration (INR) coagulation indices. *International Journal of Vitamin and Nutrition Research*, 76(2), 65–74.

DerMarderosian, A., & Beutler, J. (Eds.). 2003. *Guide to popular natural products* (3rd ed.). St. Louis, MO: Lippincott Williams & Wilkins.

Reports

National Heart, Lung, and Blood Institute. (2003). *The Seventh Report of the Joint National Committee on Prevention, Detection, Evaluation, and Treatment of High Blood Pressure*. Bethesda, MD: National Institutes of Health. Retrieved from http://www.nhlbi.nih.gov/guidelines/hypertension/

Websites for Information

Health-Alicious.com (National Center for Complementary and Alternative Medicine): http://healthaliciousness.com/

Red Yeast Rice: http://nccam.nih.gov/health/redyeastrice

Unit IX

DerMarderosian, A., & Beutler, J. (Eds.). 2003. *Guide to popular natural products* (3rd ed.). St. Louis, MO: Lippincott Williams & Wilkins.

Manoguerra, A. S., & Cobaugh, D. J. (2005). Guideline on the use of ipecac syrup in the out-of-hospital management of ingested poisons. *Clinical Toxicology*, 43(1), 1–10.

Moukarbel, G. V., et al. (2012). Antiplatelet therapy and proton pump inhibition. *Circulation*, 125, 375–380.

Websites for Information

Crohn's and Colitis Foundation of America: http://www.ccfa.org/
State Medical Marijuana Laws (National Conference of State
Legislatures): http://www.ncsl.org/issues-research/health/state-
medical-marijuana-laws.aspx

Unit X

Barusiban, A. (2006). An effective long-term treatment of oxyto-
cin-induced preterm labor in nonhuman primates. *Biological*
Reproduction, 75(5), 809–814; published ahead of print August
16, 2006, doi:10.1095/biolreprod.106.053637

Cowley, K. (2005). Psychogenic and pharmacologic induction of
the let-down reflex can facilitate breastfeeding by tetraplegic
women: A report of 3 cases. *Archives of Physical and Medical*
Rehabilitation, 86(6), 1261–1264.

Craft, S., et al. (2012). Intranasal insulin therapy for Alzheimer disease and amnestic mild cognitive impairment: A pilot clinical
trial. *Archives of Neurology,* 69(1), 29–38.

DerMarderosian, A., & Beutler, J. (Eds.). 2003. *Guide to popular*
natural products (3rd ed.). St. Louis, MO: Lippincott Williams
& Wilkins.

Fewtrell, M., et al. (2006). Randomised, double blind trial of oxytocin nasal spray in mothers expressing breast milk for preterm
infants. *Archives of Disease in Childhood: Fetal and Neonatal*
Edition, 91, F169–F174.

Franklyn, J., & Boelaert, K. (2012). Thyrotoxicosis. *Lancet,*
379(9821), 1155–1166.

Lower, A. (2003). Sliding scale insulin regimens demonstrate no
added benefit for patients with type 2 diabetes mellitus. *Annals*
of Family Medicine, May. Retrieved from http://www.aafp.org/
online/annals/home/tips/05-29-03.html

Valdés, E, et al. (2012). Nifedipine versus fenoterol in the management of preterm labor: A randomized, multicenter clinical study.
Gynecologic and Obstetric Investigation, 74(2), 109–115.

Unit XI

Bent, S., et al. (2006). Saw palmetto for benign prostate hyperplasia.
New England Journal of Medicine, 354(6), 557–566.

Brown, T. (2012). Protection against urinary tract infections seen with
cranberry products. *Archives of Internal Medicine,* 172, 988–996.

Dhingra, N., & Bhagwat, D. (2011). Benign prostate hyperplasia: An
overview of existing treatment. *Indian Journal of Pharmacology,*
43(1), 6–12.

Unit XII

Advisory Committee of Immunization Practices. (2012). Prevention
and control of influenza with vaccines: Recommendations of the
Advisory Committee of Immunization Practices (ACIP) – United
States, 2012–13 influenza season, August 17. 61(32), 613–618.

DerMarderosian, A., & Beutler, J. (Eds.). 2003. *Guide to popular*
natural products (3rd ed.). St. Louis, MO: Lippincott Williams
& Wilkins.

Polovich, M. (2004). *Safe handling of hazardous drugs.* Retrieved
April 28, 2009, from http://www.guideline.gov/summary/
summary.aspx?ss=15&doc_id=4152&nbr=3180/

Reports

IOM Childhood Immunization Schedule and Safety (2013): http://
books.nap.edu/openbook.php?record_id=13563

Unit XIII

Bertolino, G., et al. (2012). Intermittent flushing with heparin versus
saline for maintenance of peripheral intravenous catheters in a
medical department: A pragmatic cluster-randomized controlled
study. *Worldviews in Evidence-Based Nursing,* 9(4), 221–226.
published ahead of print March 5, 2012. doi:10.1111/j.1741–
6787.2012.00244.x

DerMarderosian, A., & Beutler, J. (Eds.). 2003. *Guide to popular*
natural products (3rd ed.). St. Louis, MO: Lippincott Williams
& Wilkins.

Goode, C., et al. (1993). Improving practice through research: The
case of heparin vs. saline for peripheral intermittent infusion
devices. *Medsurg Nursing,* 2(1), 23–27.

Hadaway, L. (2007). Infiltration and extravasation, preventing
a complication of IV catheterization. *American Journal of*
Nursing, 107(8), 64–72.

Schallom, M., et al. (2012). Heparin or 0.9% sodium chloride
to maintain central venous catheter patency: A randomized
trial. *Critical Care Medicine,* 40(6), 1820–1826. doi:10.1097/
CCM.0b013e31824e11b4

Index

Note: Page numbers followed by f, t, and d, indicate figures, tables, and display material respectively.